D1159687

PEDIATRIC CLINICAL ADVISOR

Instant Diagnosis and Treatment

PEDIATRIC CLINICAL ADVISOR

Instant Diagnosis and Treatment

SECOND EDITION

Editors

Lynn C. Garfunkel, MD
Associate Professor of Pediatrics
University of Rochester School of Medicine & Dentistry
Rochester, New York

Jeffrey M. Kaczorowski, MD
Associate Professor of Pediatrics
University of Rochester School of Medicine & Dentistry
Rochester, New York

Cynthia Christy, MD
Associate Professor of Pediatrics
University of Rochester School of Medicine & Dentistry
Rochester, New York

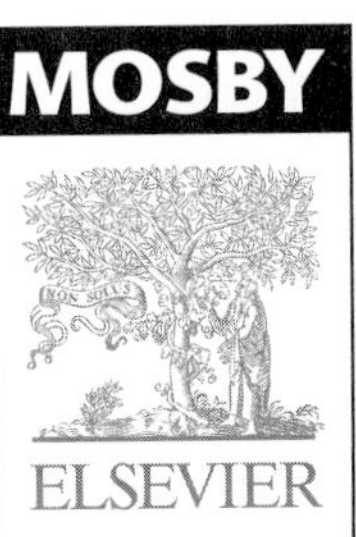

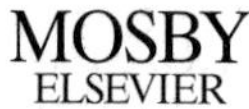

1600 John F. Kennedy Blvd.
Ste 1800
Philadelphia, PA 19103-2899

PEDIATRIC CLINICAL ADVISOR

ISBN-13: 978-0-323-03506-4
ISBN-10: 0-323-03506-X

Notice

Knowledge and best practice in this field are constantly changing. As new research and experience broaden our knowledge, changes in practice, treatment and drug therapy may become necessary or appropriate. Readers are advised to check the most current information provided (i) on procedures featured or (ii) by the manufacturer of each product to be administered, to verify the recommended dose or formula, the method and duration of administration, and contraindications. It is the responsibility of the practitioner, relying on their own experience and knowledge of the patient, to make diagnoses, to determine dosages and the best treatment for each individual patient, and to take all appropriate safety precautions. To the fullest extent of the law, neither the Publisher nor the Editors assume any liability for any injury and/or damage to persons or property arising out or related to any use of the material contained in this book.

The Publisher

Library of Congress Cataloging-in-Publication Data

Pediatric clinical advisor : instant diagnosis and treatment / [edited by] Lynn C. Garfunkel, Jeffrey M. Kaczorowski, Cynthia Christy. – 2nd ed.
p.; cm.
Rev. ed. of: Mosby's pediatric clinical advisor. c2002.
Includes bibliographical references and index.
ISBN 0-323-03506-X
1. Pediatrics–Handbooks, manuals, etc. 2. Children–Diseases–Handbooks, manuals, etc. 3. Diagnosis, Differential–Handbooks, manuals, etc. I. Garfunkel, Lynn C. II. Kaczorowski, Jeffrey. III. Christy, Cynthia. IV. Mosby's pediatric clinical advisor.
[DNLM: 1. Pediatrics–Handbooks. 2. Diagnosis, Differential–Handbooks. 3. Therapeutics–Handbooks. WS 39 P3703 2007]
RJ48.M627 2007
618.92–dc22 2006048103

Acquisitions Editor: Judith Fletcher
Developmental Editor: Joanie Milnes
Project Manager: Mary Stermel
Design Direction: Steve Stave
Marketing Manager: Matt Latuchie

Printed in the United States

Last digit is the print number: 9 8 7 6 5 4 3 2 1

To our spouses
Craig Orlowski,
Laura Jean Shipley, and
Ralph Manchester

To our children
Zachary and Rachel Orlowski,
Daniel Shipley, Emma and Jack Kaczorowski,
Eric, Alison, and Ian Manchester

And to our
Parents, mentors, colleagues, students, and friends,
who have encouraged and inspired us

Thank you all,
LCG, JK, CC

Contributors

BARBARA L. ASSELIN, MD
Associate Professor of Pediatrics and Oncology
Department of Pediatrics
University of Rochester School of Medicine & Dentistry
James P. Wilmot Cancer Center
Rochester, New York

GEORGIANNE ARNOLD, MD
Associate Professor of Pediatrics and Genetics
University of Rochester School of Medicine & Dentistry
Rochester, New York

SHERRY L. BAYLIFF, MD, MPH
Assistant Professor of Pediatrics
Division of Pediatric Hematology-Oncology
University of Kentucky, Markey Cancer Center
Lexington, Kentucky

CHRISTOPHER E. BELCHER, MD, FAAP
Pediatric Infectious Diseases
Infectious Disease of Indiana
Indianapolis, Indiana

DEENA BERKOWITZ, MD, MPH
Clinical Fellow, Division of Emergency Medicine
Children's National Medical Center
Washington, D.C.

JEFFREY BLAKE, MD
Fellow, Division of Emergency Medicine
Children's National Medical Center
Department of Pediatrics
The George Washington University School of Medicine and Health Sciences
Washington, D.C.

CHRISTOPHER F. BOLLING, MD
Voluntary Associate Professor
Department of Pediatrics
University of Cincinnati College of Medicine
Cincinnati, Ohio
Pediatrician
Pediatric Associates, PSC
Crestview Hills, Kentucky

DEBORAH BORCHERS, MD
Eastgate Pediatric Center
Cincinnati, Ohio

BRITTANNY LIAM BOULANGER, MD
Practitioner
Department of Pediatrics
Harvard Vanguard Medical Associates
West Roxbury, Massachusetts

PETER N. BOWERS, MD
Assistant Professor
Section of Pediatric Cardiology
Department of Pediatrics
Yale University School of Medicine
New Haven, Connecticut

PAULA K. BRAVERMAN, MD
Professor of Pediatrics
Cinncinati Children's Medical Center
Cinnciati, Ohio

CARMELITA V. BRITTON, MD, FAAP
Guthrie Clinic Pediatrics
Fort Drum, New York

ROBERT A. BROUGHTON, MD
Professor of Pediatrics
Division of Critical Care
Chief
Division of Infectious Diseases
University of Kentucky Medical Center
Lexington, Kentucky

ANN BUCHANAN, MD
Cary, North Carolina

GALE R. BURSTEIN, MD, MPH
Medical Officer
Division of STD Prevention
Centers for Disease Control and Prevention
Atlanta, Georgia

JAMES R. CAMPBELL, MD, MPH
Associate Professor
Department of Pediatrics
University of Rochester School of Medicine & Dentistry
Rochester, New York

KATHLEEN M. CAMPBELL, MD
Assistant Professor of Pediatrics
Division of Gastroenterology, Hepatology and Nutrition
Cincinnati Children's Hospital Medical Center
Cincinnati, Ohio

LYNN R. CAMPBELL, MD
Associate Professor of Pediatrics
Director, Pediatric Residency Training Program
University of Kentucky Medical Center
Lexington, Kentucky

MARGARET-ANN CARNO, PhD, RN
Assistant Clinical Professor of Nursing and Pediatrics
School of Nursing
University of Rochester School of Medicine & Dentistry
Rochester, New York

PATRICK L. CAROLAN, MD
Medical Director
Minnesota Sudden Infant Death Center
Children's Hospitals and Clinics of Minnesota
Minneapolis, Minnesota
Adjunct Associate Professor of Pediatrics
Family Medicine and Community Health
University of Minnesota Medical School
Minneapolis, Minnesota

MARY T. CASERTA, MD
Associate Professor of Pediatrics
Department of Pediatrics
University of Rochester School of Medicine & Dentistry
Rochester, New York

HEIDI A. CASTILLO, MD
Fellow, Division of Developmental and Behavioral Pediatrics
Cincinnati Children's Hospital Medical Center
Cincinnati, Ohio

KATHRYN CASTLE, PhD
Assistant Professor
Psychiatry and Pediatrics
University of Rochester School of Medicine & Dentistry
Rochester, New York

PETER CHANG, MD
Fellow, Pediatric Cardiology
University of Rochester School of Medicine & Dentistry
Rochester, New York

SHARON F. CHEN, MD
Instructor, Pediatric Infectious Diseases
Department of Pediatrics
University of Minnesota School of Medicine
Minneapolis, Minnesota

EULALIA R. Y. CHENG, MD
Assistant Clinical Professor
Division of Pediatric Pulmonology
University of Rochester School of Medicine & Dentistry
Rochester, New York

ELIZABETH K. CHEROT, MD
Assistant Professor
Department of Obstetrics and Gynecology
Robert Wood Johnson Medical School
University of Medicine and Dentistry
New Brunswick, New Jersey

PATRICIA R. CHESS, MD
Associate Professor of Pediatrics and Biomedical Engineering
Division of Neonatology
University of Rochester School of Medicine & Dentistry
Rochester, New York

OLIVIA CHIANG, PsyD
Dept of Psychiatry (Psychology)
University of Rochester School of Medicine & Dentistry
Rochester General Hospital
Rochester, New York

BARBARA A. CHINI, MD
Associate Professor of Pediatrics
Division of Pediatric Pulmonology
Division of Pulmonary Medicine
Department of Pediatrics
Cincinnati Children's Hospital Medical Center
Cincinnati, Ohio

JILL M. CHOLETTE, MD
Pediatric Critical Care Fellow
Department of Pediatrics
University of Rochester School of Medicine & Dentistry
Rochester, New York

CYNTHIA CHRISTY, MD
Associate Professor of Pediatrics
University of Rochester School of Medicine & Dentistry
Rochester, New York

EMMA CIAFALONI, MD
Assistant Professor of Neurology
Department of Neurology
University of Rochester School of Medicine & Dentistry
Rochester, New York

CAROLYN CLEARY, MD
Elmwood Pediatric Group
Clinical Faculty
University of Rochester School of Medicine & Dentistry
Rochester, New York

LISA LOEB COLTON, MD
Partner, Panorama Pediatric Group, RLLP
Courtesy Attending
Golisano Children's Hospital, Highland Hospital
Associate Attending
Rochester General Hospital
Rochester, New York

GREGORY P. CONNERS, MD, MPH, MBA, FAAP
Associate Professor of Emergency Medicine and Pediatrics
Departments. of Emergency Medicine & Pediatrics
University of Rochester School of Medicine & Dentistry
Rochester, New York

HEIDI V. CONNOLLY, MD
Director, Pediatric Sleep Services
Strong Sleep Disorders Center
Assistant Professor of Pediatrics
University of Rochester School of Medicine & Dentistry
Rochester, New York

STEPHEN COOK, MD
Senior Instructor, Pediatrics
Golisano Children's Hospital at Strong
University of Rochester School of Medicine & Dentistry
Research Associate
Center for Child Health Research
American Academy of Pediatrics
Rochester, New York

CHRISTOPHER COPENHAVEN, MD
Allentown Asthma & Allergy
Lehigh Valley Hospital
Department of Pediatrics
Allentown, Pennsylvania

ELLIOTT L. CROW, MD, FPCC
Private Practice
Albuquerque, New Mexico

THERESE CVETKOVICH, MD, FPCC
Medical Officer
Division of Vaccines and Related Products Applications
Office of Vaccines Research and Review
Center for Biologics Evaluation and Research, US Food and Drug Administration
Rockville, Maryland

DAVID CYWINSKI, MD
Fingerlakes Bone and Joint Center
Geneva, New York

KRISTEN SMITH DANIELSON, MD
General Pediatrics
Fallon Medical Clinic
Worcester, Massachussetts

DOROTHY M. DELISLE, MD
Pediatrician
Co-Chair, Department of Pediatrics
Medical Associates Health Centers
Waukesha, Wisconsin

LARRY DENK, MD
Clinical Assistant Professor of Pediatrics
University of Rochester School of Medicine & Dentistry
Rochester, New York

LEE A. DENSON, MD
Assistant Professor of Pediatrics
Division of Gastroenterology, Hepatology and Nutrition
Cincinnati Children's Hospital Medical Center
Cincinnati, Ohio

GEORGE T. DRUGAS, MD
Associate Professor, Pediatric Surgery
University of Rochester School of Medicine & Dentistry
Rochester, New York

CAROLYN PIVER DUKARM, MD
Director
Center for Eating Disorders
Department of Pediatrics
Specialty Center for Women
Sisters of Charity Hospital
Buffalo, New York

JASON G. EMMICK, MD, FAAP
Director of Pediatrics for Elliot Hospital
Section Chief of Pediatrics for Elliot Hospital
Internal Medicine and Pediatrics
Manchester, New Hampshire

GUS GIBBONS EMMICK, MD
Departments of Internal Medicine and Pediatrics
Elliot Hospital and Elliot Physician Network
Manchester, New Hampshire

OSCAR ESCOBAR, MD
Assistant Professor of Pediatrics
Division of Endocrinology
University of Pittsburgh School of Medicine
Children's Hospital of Pittsburgh
Pittsburgh, Pennsylvania

ANNA F. FAKADEJ, MD, FAAO, FACS
Chairman, Division of Ophthalmology
First Health Moore Regional Hospital
Caroline Eye Associates
Southern Pines, North Carolina

RICHARD A. FALCONE, JR., MD
Assistant Professor of Surgery
Division of Pediatric and Thoracic Surgery
Cincinnati Children's Hospital Medical Center
Department of Surgery
University of Cincinnati
Cincinnati, Ohio

S. NICHOLE FEENEY, MD
Internal Medicine and Pediatrics Physician
Memphis, Tennessee

THOMAS J. FISCHER, MD
Professor of Clinical Pediatrics
University of Cincinnati College of Medicine
Division of Allergy and Clinical Immunology
Cincinnati Children's Hospital Medical Center
Cincinnati, Ohio

DONNA J. FISHER, MD
Assistant Professor of Pediatrics
Baystate Medical Center Children's Hospital
Tufts University School of Medicine
Springfield, Massachusetts

AMY FIX, MD
Instructor of Clinical Medicine and Pediatrics
Department of Internal Medicine and Department of Pediatrics
University of Rochester School of Medicine & Dentistry
Rochester, New York

CHIN-TO FONG, MD
Associate Professor of Pediatrics
Department of Pediatrics & Genetics
University of Rochester School of Medicine & Dentistry
Rochester, New York

CYNTHIA L. FOX, MD
Private Practice
Fairhaven, Massachusetts

D. STEVEN FOX, MD, MSc
Consulting Specialist
Olive View, UCLA Medical Center
Department of Primary Care
Sylmar, California

ROBERT J. FREISHTAT, MD, MPH
Assistant Professor of Pediatrics and Emergency Medicine
Division of Emergency Medicine
Children's National Medical Center
George Washington University School of Medicine and Health Sciences
Washington, D.C.

MADELYN GARCIA, MD
Fellow, Pediatric Emergency Medicine
Dept. of Emergency Medicine
University of Rochester
Rochester, New York

LYNN C. GARFUNKEL, MD
Associate Professor of Pediatrics
University of Rochester School of Medicine & Dentistry
Rochester, New York

MATTHEW D. GEARINGER, MD
Assistant Professor
Ophthalmology and Pediatrics
University of Rochester School of Medicine & Dentistry
Rochester, New York

MARY ELLEN GELLERSTEDT, MD
Director, Development and Behavioral Pediatrics
Eastern Maine Medical Center
Bangor, Maine

JOHN GIROTTO, MD
Assistant Professor
Plastic Surgery
University of Rochester School of Medicine & Dentistry
Rochester, New York

MICHELLE A. GRENIER, MD
Assistant Professor Pediatric Cardiology
Baylor College of Medicine
Houston, Texas

ALKA GOYAL, MD
Assistant Professor of Pediatrics
Division of Gastroenterology
Children's Hospital of Pittsburgh
University of Pittsburgh
Pittsburgh, Pennsylvania

MARYELLEN E. GUSIC, MD
Associate Dean for Clinical Education
Associate Professor of Pediatrics
Department of Pediatrics
Penn State College of Medicine
Hershey, Pennsylvania

CAROLINE B. HALL, MD
Professor of Pediatrics and Medicine
University of Rochester School of Medicine & Dentistry
Rochester, New York

JILL S. HALTERMAN, MD, MPH
Assistant Professor of Pediatrics
University of Rochester School of Medicine & Dentistry
Rochester, New York

DAVID W. HANNON, MD
Professor
Department of Pediatrics
East Carolina University Brody School of Medicine
Greenville, North Carolina

WILLIAM G. HARMON, MD
Assistant Professor of Pediatrics
Divisions of Pediatric Cardiology and Critical Care Medicine
University of Rochester School of Medicine & Dentistry
Rochester, New York

J. PETER HARRIS, MD
Professor of Pediatrics and Associate Chair for Education
University of Rochester School of Medicine & Dentistry
Rochester, New York

AMY HENEGHAN, MD
Associate Professor of Pediatrics
Case Western Reserve University School of Medicine
Cleveland, Ohio

NEIL E. HERENDEEN, MD
Associate Professor of Pediatrics
University of Rochester School of Medicine & Dentistry
Rochester, New York

JOELI HETTLER, MD
Attending Physician,
Division of Emergency Medicine,
Childrens National Medical Center
Washington, D.C.

JOHN L. HICK, MD
Hennepin County Medical Center
Department of Emergency Medicine
Assistant Professor of Emergency Medicine
University of Minnesota
Minneapolis, Minnesota

ANDREA S. HINKLE, MD
Associate Professor
Division of Pediatric Hematology/Oncology
University of Rochester School of Medicine & Dentistry
Rochester, New York

ALEJANDRO HOBERMAN, MD
Chief, Division of General Academic Pediatrics
Children's Hospital of Pittsburgh
Pittsburgh, Pennsylvania

CHRISTOPHER H. HODGMAN, MD
Clinical Professor of Pediatrics and Professor Emeritus of Psychiatry
University of Rochester School of Medicine & Dentistry
Rochester, New York

ALLISON L. HOLM, MD
Dermatology Partners of WNY, LLP
Rochester, New York

MARK A. HOSTETLER, MD, MPH
Assistant Professor
Department of Pediatrics
The University of Chicago
Pritzker School of Medicine
Medical Director, Pediatric Emergency Department
The University of Chicago Children's Hospital
Chicago, Illinois

CYNTHIA R. HOWARD, MD, MPH, FAAP
Associate Professor of Pediatrics
Division of General Pediatrics
University of Rochester School of Medicine & Dentistry
Pediatric Director Mother Baby Unit
Rochester General Hospital
Rochester, New York

STEPHANIE SANSONI HSU, MD
Private Practice
Reisterstown, Maryland

WILLIAM C. HULBERT, MD
Associate Professor of Urology and Pediatrics
University of Rochester School of Medicine & Dentistry
Rochester, New York

ROBERT HUMPHREYS, MD
Fellow, Nephrology
University of Rochester School of Medicine & Dentistry
Rochester, New York

JON HUTCHINSON, MD
Fellow, Pediatric Cardiology
University of Rochester School of Medicine & Dentistry
Rochester, New York

SUSAN L. HYMAN, MD
Strong Center for Developmental Disabilities
University of Rochester School of Medicine & Dentistry
Rochester, New York

CAROLYN JACOBS PARKS, MD
Department of Pediatrics
Rochester General Hospital
Rochester, New York

ANDREE JACOBS-PERKINS, MD
Clinical Instructor
University of Rochester School of Medicine & Dentistry
Pediatrician
Genesee Health Service
Rochester, New York

SANDRA H. JEE, MD, MPH
Assistant Professor of Pediatrics
University of Rochester School of Medicine & Dentistry
Rochester, New York

NICHOLAS JOSPE, MD
Associate Professor
Chief, Division of Pediatric Endocrinology
Department of Pediatrics
University of Rochester School of Medicine & Dentistry
Rochester, New York

STEVEN JOYCE, MD
Clinical Assistant Professor of Pediatrics
University of Iowa
Associate Director
Family Practice
Siouxland Medical Education Foundation
University of Iowa
Sioux City, Iowa

JEFFREY M. KACZOROWSKI, MD
Associate Professor of Pediatrics
University of Rochester School of Medicine & Dentistry
Rochester, New York

INDRA KANCITIS, MD
Assistant Professor
Division of General Pediatrics and Emergency Medicine
Department of Pediatrics
Virginia Commonwealth University
Richmond, Virginia

JAMES W. KENDIG, MD
Professor of Pediatrics
Penn State Children's Hospital
Hershey, Pennsylvania

JOHN KNIGHT, MD
Associate Professor of Pediatrics
Harvard Medical School
Director, Center for Adolescent Substance Abuse Research
Children's Hospital Boston
Boston, Massachusetts

DAVID N. KORONES, MD
Associate Professor of Pediatrics, Oncology, and Neurology
Department of Pediatrics
University of Rochester School of Medicine & Dentistry
Rochester, New York

PETER A. KOUIDES, MD
Research Director
Mary M. Gooley Hemophilia Center
Associate Professor of Medicine
University of Rochester School of Medicine & Dentistry
Rochester, New York

RICHARD KREIPE, MD
Professor of Pediatrics
Adolescent Medicine
University of Rochester School of Medicine & Dentistry
Rochester, New York

DIANA BARNETT KUDES, MD
Panorama Pediatric Group
Rochester, New York

JENNIFER M. KWON, MD
Assistant Professor
Pediatrics and Neurology
University of Rochester School of Medicine & Dentistry
Rochester, New York

MARC S. LAMPELL, MD, FAAP, FACEP
Clinical Assistant Professor of Emergency Medicine
Clinical Assistant Professor of Pediatrics
University of Rochester School of Medicine & Dentistry
Rochester, New York

MEREDITH LANDORF, MD
Private Practice
Edgewood, Kentucky

NANCY E. LANPHEAR, MD
Associate Professor of Pediatrics
Division of Developmental and Behavioral Pediatrics
Cincinnati Children's Hospital Medical Center
Cincinnati, Ohio

JEFFREY H. LEE, MD
Instructor in Pediatrics and Internal Medicine
University of Massachusetts Medical School
Worcester, Massachusetts

LUCIA H. LEE, MD
Medical Officer
Food and Drug Administration
Rockville, Maryland

THOMAS J. A. LEHMAN, MD
Chief
Division of Pediatric Rheumatology
Hospital for Special Surgery
Professor of Clinical Pediatrics
Weill Medical College
Cornell University
New York, New York

PAUL LEHOULLIER, MD
Attending Physician
Department of Pediatrics
Rochester General Hospital
Rochester, New York

NORMA B. LERNER, MD
Associate Professor of Pediatrics
Division of Pediatric Hematology/Oncology
University of Rochester School of Medicine & Dentistry
Rochester, New York

GREGORY S. LIPTAK, MD, MPH
Professor of Pediatrics
University of Rochester School of Medicine & Dentistry
Rochester, New York

ANN M. LOEFFLER, MD
Pediatric Infectious Diseases Attending
Legacy Emanuel Children's Hospital
Portland, Oregon
Pediatric Consultant
Francis J. Curry National TB Center
San Francisco, California

KATHI MAKOROFF, MD
Assistant Professor of Pediatrics
Cincinnati Children's Hospital Medical Center
Cincinnati, Ohio

ELIZABETH MANNICK, MD
Associate Professor of Pediatrics
Tulane University Hospital and Clinic
New Orleans, Louisiana

CHRISTINA M. MCCANN, PhD
Private Practice
Rochester, New York

CAROL A. MCCARTHY, MD
Associate Professor of Pediatrics
University of Vermont College of Medicine
Burlington, Vermont
Director
Pediatric Infectious Disease
Maine Medical Center
Portland, Maine

MICHAEL E. MCCONNELL, MD
Associate Clinical Professor
Department of Pediatrics
Emory University School of Medicine
Atlanta, Georgia

ALAN M. MENDELSOHN, MD, FACC
Director
Clinical Immunology Research
Centocor
Malvern, Pennsylvania

RAM K. MENON, MD
Professor of Pediatrics
Professor of Molecular and Integrative Physiology
Director, Division of Endocrinology
Department of Pediatrics
University of Michigan Medical School
Ann Arbor, Michigan

ROBERT A. MEVORACH, MD
Associate Professor of Urology and Pediatrics
University of Rochester School of Medicine & Dentistry
Rochester, New York

AYESA N. MIAN, MD
Assistant Professor of Pediatrics and Nephrology
University of Maryland School of Medicine
Baltimore, Maryland

HEATHER MICHALAK, MD
English Road Pediatrics and Adolescent Medicine
Rochester, New York

DANIEL E. MIGA, MD
Associate Professor of Pediatrics
Director of Interventional Pediatric Cardiology
University of Rochester Medical Center
Rochester, New York

NICOLE L. MIHALOPOULOS, MD, MPH
Department of Pediatrics
Division of Adolescent Medicine
Department of Community and Preventive Medicine
University of Rochester School of Medicine & Dentistry
Rochester, New York

JONATHAN W. MINK, MD, PhD
Associate Professor of Neurology
Neurobiology & Anatomy, and Pediatrics
Chief, Child Neurology
University of Rochester School of Medicine & Dentistry
Rochester, New York

M. SUSAN MOYER, MD
Professor
Department of Pediatrics
University of Cincinnati College of Medicine
Attending, Division of Gastroenterology, Hepatology and Nutrition
Cincinnati Children's Hospital Medical Center
Cincinnati, Ohio

SUZANNE FREDRICKSON MULLIN, MD
Associate Medical Director of Rochester General Pediatric Associates
Department of Pediatrics
Rochester General Hospital
Rochester, New York

CHARLES M. MYER, III, MD
Professor of Pediatric Otolaryngology
Department of Otolaryngology
Head and Neck Surgery
Cincinnati Children's Hospital Medical Center
Cincinnati, Ohio

RAN NAMGUNG, MD, PhD
Professor
Department of Pediatrics
Yonsei University College of Medicine
Seoul, Korea

JONATHAN F. NASSER, MD
Department of Internal Medicine and Pediatrics
Crystal Run Health Care
Middletown, New York

ROBERT NEEDLMAN, MD
Associate Professor of Pediatrics
Case School of Medicine
Cleveland, Ohio

JOSEPH A. NICHOLAS, MD
Fellow in Preventive Medicine
State University of New York at Albany
School of Public Health
Albany, New York

MAUREEN NOVAK, MD
Vice Chair
Reed Bell Chair of Pediatrics
Department of Pediatrics
University of Florida
Gainesville, Florida

SAMUEL NURKO, MD, MPH
Director Motility Program
Pediatric Gastroenterology
Children's Hospital Boston
Boston, Massachusetts

CRAIG ORLOWSKI, MD
Associate Professor
Pediatric Endocrinology
University of Rochester School of Medicine & Dentistry
Rochester, New York

PONRAT PAKPREO, MD
Adolescent Medicine Fellow
Department of Pediatrics, Division of Adolescent Medicine
University of Rochester School of Medicine & Dentistry
Rochester, New York

JAMES PALIS, MD
Associate Professor
Department of Pediatrics, Cancer Center, and Biomedical Genetics
University of Rochester Medical Center
Rochester, New York

MURRAY H. PASSO, MD
Clinical Director
Division of Rheumatology
Department of Pediatrics
University of Cincinnati
Cincinnati Children's Hospital Medical Center
Cincinnati, Ohio

JOANNE PEDRO-CARROLL, PhD
Associate Professor of Psychology
Clinical Associate Professor of Psychiatry
Director of Program Development
University of Rochester School of Medicine & Dentistry
Rochester, New York

WALTER PEGOLI, JR., MD
Division Chief, Pediatric Surgery
University of Rochester School of Medicine & Dentistry
Rochester, New York

KAREN S. POWERS, MD
Associate Professor of Pediatrics
University of Rochester School of Medicine & Dentistry
Rochester, New York

SUSAN HALLER PSAILA, MD
Clinical Instructor
Dermatology and Pediatrics
University of Rochester School of Medicine & Dentistry
Rochester, New York.

RONALD RABINOWITZ, MD
Professor of Urology and Pediatrics
University of Rochester School of Medicine & Dentistry
Rochester, New York

MARC A. RASLICH, MD
Assistant Professor, Internal Medicine and Pediatrics
Program Director, Combined Med-Peds Residency Program
Wright State University School of Medicine
Dayton, Ohio

KAREN L. RESCH, MD
Clinical Assistant Professor of Emergency Medicine
University of Minnesota
Children's Healthcare
Minneapolis, Minnesota

MEREDITH E. REYNOLDS, MD
Assistant Professor
Department of Pediatrics
University of New Mexico, Health Sciences Center
University of New Mexico Children's Hospital
Albuquerque, New Mexico

MATTHEW RICHARDSON, MD
Assistant Professor of Pediatrics
Department of Pediatrics
Section Pediatric Hematology/Oncology
Baystate Medical Center Children's Hospital
Springfield, Massachusetts

BRETT ROBBINS, MD
Assistant Professor
Internal Medicine and Pediatrics
University of Rochester School of Medicine & Dentistry

MARK RODDY, MD
Adjunct Professor of Pediatrics and Emergency Medicine
Pediatric Emergency Medicine Fellow
Division of Emergency Medicine
Children's National Medical Center
George Washington University School of Medicine and Health Sciences
Washington, D.C.

DENNIS ROY, MD
Orthopaedic Attending
Shriners Hospital for Children
Portland, Oregon

LETICIA MANNING RYAN, MD
Clinical Fellow
Division of Emergency Medicine
Children's National Medical Center
Washington, DC

SHERYL A. RYAN, MD
Chief, Section of Adolescent Medicine
Department of Pediatrics
Yale University School of Medicine
New Haven, Connecticut

STANLEY J. SCHAFFER, MD, MS
Professor
Department of Pediatrics
University of Rochester School of Medicine & Dentistry
Rochester, New York

LORA L. SCHAUER, MD, FAAP
Department of Pediatrics
Cox Health Systems
Springfield, Missouri

CHARLES SCHUBERT, MD
Associate Professor of Clinical Pediatrics
Cincinnati Children's Hospital Medical Center
Cincinnati, Ohio

GEORGE J. SCHWARTZ, MD
Professor of Pediatrics and Medicine
Chief, Pediatric Nephrology
University of Rochester School of Medicine & Dentistry
Rochester, New York

STEVEN SCOFIELD, MD
Assistant Professor
Departments of Internal Medicine and Pediatrics
University of Rochester School of Medicine & Dentistry
Rochester, New York

GEORGE B. SEGEL, MD
Professor of Pediatrics and Medicine
Vice Chair, Department of Pediatrics
University of Rochester School of Medicine & Dentistry
Rochester, New York

EDGARD A. SEGURA, MD
Internist and Pediatrician
Loudoun Medical Office
Mid-Atlantic Permanente Medical Group
Lansdowne, Virginia

LORNA M. SEYBOLT, MD, MPH
Fellow
Department of Medicine, Infectious Diseases
Department of Pediatrics
Maine Medical Center
Portland, Maine

NADER SHAIKH, MD, MPH
Assistant Professor of Pediatrics
General Academic Pediatrics
Children's Hospital of Pittsburgh
Pittsburgh, Pennsylvania

RONALD L. SHAM, MD
Department of Medicine
Rochester General Hospital
Rochester, New York

LAURA JEAN SHIPLEY, MD
Clinical Associate Professor
Department of Pediatrics
University of Rochester
Rochester, New York

BENJAMIN L. SHNEIDER, MD
Professor of Pediatrics
Chief, Division of Pediatric Hepatology
Mount Sinai School of Medicine
New York, New York

DAVID M. SIEGEL, MD, MPH
Professor of Pediatrics and Medicine
Edward H. Townsend Chief of Pediatrics
Rochester General Hospital
Chief, Division of Pediatric Rheumatology/Immunology, Department of Pediatrics
University of Rochester School of Medicine & Dentistry
Rochester, New York

MARK SCOTT SMITH, MD
Professor of Pediatrics
Chief, Adolescent Medicine Section
Division of General Pediatrics
University of Washington School of Medicine
Seattle, Washington

R. DENNIS STEED, MD
Associate Professor of Pediatrics
Section of Pediatric Cardiology
The Brody School of Medicine
Greenville, North Carolina

MOIRA A. SZILAGYI, MD, PhD
Associate Professor of Pediatrics
Medical Director, Foster Care Pediatrics
University of Rochester
Rochester, New York

SUSANNE E. TANSKI, MD
Assistant Professor of Pediatrics
Dartmouth Medical School
Dartmouth Hitchcock Medical Center
Lebanon, New Hampshire

DANIELLE THOMAS-TAYLOR, MD
Department of Pediatrics
University of Rochester School of Medicine & Dentistry
Rochester General Hospital
Rochester, New York

SVETLANA TISMA-DUPANOVIC, MD
Fellow, Department of Pediatrics
University of Rochester School of Medicine & Dentistry
Rochester, New York

JOHN J. TREANOR, MD
Professor
Division of Infectious Diseases
University of Rochester School of Medicine & Dentistry
Rochester, New York

C. ELIZABETH TREFTS, MD
General Pediatrics
Penobscot Pediatrics
Bangor, Maine
Assistant Clinical Professor of Pediatrics
Tufts University School of Medicine
Boston, Massachusetts

WILLIAM T. TSAI, MD
Clinical Fellow
Division of General Pediatrics
University of Washington School of Medicine
Seattle, Washington

REGINALD TSANG, MBBS
Professor
Department of Pediatrics
University Cincinnati College of Medicine
Cincinnati, Ohio

ELISE W. VAN DER JAGT, MD, MPH
Professor of Pediatrics and Critical Care
Department of Pediatrics/Critical Care
University of Rochester School of Medicine & Dentistry
Rochester, New York

JON A. VANDERHOOF, MD
Chief, Pediatric Gastroenterology and Nutrition
University of Nebraska Medical Center
Omaha, Nebraska

WILLIAM S. VARADE, MD
Associate Professor of Pediatrics
Department of Pediatrics (Pediatric Nephrology)
University of Rochester School of Medicine & Dentistry
Rochester, New York

KATHLEEN M. VENTRE, MD
Division of Critical Care Medicine
Primary Children's Medical Center
Salt Lake City, Utah

MICHAEL K. VISICK, MD
Attending Physician
Department of Pediatrics
Department of Internal Medicine
Logan Regional Hospital
IHC Budge Clinic
Logan, Utah

BRAD W. WARNER, MD
Professor
Department of Surgery
University of Cincinnati College of Medicine
Attending Surgeon
Division of Pediatric and Thoracic Surgery
Cincinnati Children's Hospital Medical Center
Cincinnati, Ohio

GEOFFREY A. WEINBERG, MD
Professor of Pediatrics
Department of Pediatrics
Division of Infectious Diseases
Director, Pediatric HIV Program
University of Rochester School of Medicine & Dentistry
Rochester, New York

MELANIE WELLINGTON, MD
Assistant Professor
Department of Pediatrics
University of Rochester School of Medicine & Dentistry
Rochester, New York

DAVID R. WHITE, MD
Fellow, Pediatric Otolaryngology
Department of Otolaryngology, Head and Neck Surgery
Cincinnati Children's Hospital Medical Center
Cincinnati, Ohio

SUSAN WILEY, MD
Assistant Professor of Pediatrics
Division of Developmental and Behavioral Pediatrics
Cincinnati Children's Hospital Medical Center
Cincinnati, Ohio

ROBERT R. WITTLER, MD
Professor
Department of Pediatrics
Kansas University School of Medicine—Wichita
Wichita, Kansas

BRYAN J. WOHLWEND, MD
Chief Resident, Pediatrics
University of Missouri
Kansas City School of Medicine
Kansas City, Missouri

JONATHAN P. WOOD, MD
Medical Director
Pediatric Intensive Care Unit
Eastern Maine Medical Center
Bangor, Maine

KIMBERLY A. WORKOWSKI, MD, FACP
Associate Professor of Medicine
Division of Infectious Diseases
Emory University
Division of STD Prevention
Centers for Disease Control and Prevention
Atlanta, Georgia

DANIEL YAWMAN, MD
Attending Physician
Rochester General Hospital
Department of Pediatrics
Rochester, New York

ROGER A. YEAGER, PhD
Psychologist and Director
Behavioral Pediatrics Program
Department of Pediatrics
Rochester General Hospital
Rochester, New York

ROSEMARY J. YOUNG, RN, MS
Pediatric Gastroenterology Clinical Nurse Specialist
University of Nebraska Medical Center
Omaha, Nebraska

Preface to the Second Edition

In this second edition of the *Pediatric Clinical Advisor,* the ready reference for busy pediatric clinicians, we reordered the major sections at the urging of our publishers. We have also added many new chapters at the advice and suggestions of our residents, students, and colleagues who realized that there were important missing topics in the first edition.

This "five-books-in-one" format includes updated or new information in each section. **Section I, Diseases and Disorders** covers nearly 400 clinical topics in easy to read bulleted format; **Section II, Differential Diagnosis** encompasses some 50 common differentials in table format; **Section III, Clinical Algorithms** leads the busy practitioner through diagnoses of more than 40 common signs and symptoms; **Section IV, Charts, Formulas, Tables, and Tests,** provides readers with those frequently used, difficult to locate when needed, tables, graphs, equations and charts. This section is organized by broad topic area to include: dermatology, development, emergency medicine (burns and concussion), equations and nomograms, growth charts, neurology, sports medicine and orthopedics (maneuvers, diagrams and conditions for participation), as well as selected vital sign charts and laboratory tests and interpretations. The new **Section V, Prevention** would seem to be amiss in a "rapid diagnosis" textbook; however, for most pediatricians and pediatric practitioners, primary and secondary prevention is part of every patient encounter. Whether it be an office visit for a child with asthma or otitis media with a parent who smokes; a well child check with an internationally adopted 2 year old, an 8 year old in foster care, or a sexually active teen; or an infant hospitalized with dehydration whose mother is depressed—prevention plays a key role in treatment. We have not only included routine immunization schedules and websites, but immunization and infectious disease prevention for travel and chronic diseases; nutrition guidelines and formula content; adolescent screening and birth control; smoking cessation assistance; risks and screening needs of internationally adopted children, children of incarcerated parents, and children in foster care; and screening and referral information for parental depression, divorce, and domestic violence.

We would like to take this opportunity to thank our many contributors and in particular would like to acknowledge Jean Brockmann for her steadfast dedication to the completion of this project.

Preface to the First Edition

You are between patients; the waiting room is full; and you are falling further behind. You need to review a clinical topic, broaden your differential diagnosis, initiate a diagnostic workup, or remember the latest treatment of a less common disease—this is what we had in mind when we created *Mosby's Pediatric Clinical Advisor.*

This textbook is meant to be a user-friendly, ready reference for the primary care physician, nurse practitioner, physician assistant, resident, or student. It is organized to lead you from signs and symptoms to comprehensive information about specific diseases and clinical problems, with supporting diagrams, tables, and formulas.

Part I presents differential diagnoses of more than 40 common signs and symptoms paired with diagnostic algorithms. **Part II** covers more than 350 clinical topics in a bulleted format including ICD-9CM codes, etiology, epidemiology and demographics, differential diagnosis, diagnostic workup, and therapeutic plans; it also contains pertinent websites and references. **Part III** includes those frequently sought graphs, equations, and charts that you can never seem to get your hands on, such as endocarditis prophylaxis, developmental screening tools, and the body mass index calculation with normative tables.

We wish to express our deepest appreciation to Jean Brockmann, our coordinator, who has worked kindly and tirelessly to facilitate and organize the production of this book. Thanks, Jean.

LCG, JK, CC

Contents

Detailed Contents

SECTION I Diseases and Disorders

SECTION II Differential Diagnosis

SECTION III Clinical Algorithms

SECTION IV Charts, Formulas, Tables and Tests

SECTION V **Prevention**

Section I

Diseases and Disorders

BASIC INFORMATION

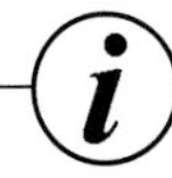

DEFINITION

Acetaminophen (*N*-acetyl-*p*-aminophenol) is widely available as a single agent for relief of fever and pain. It is also widely available in combination cold and pain preparations. Acute and chronic types of over-ingestion are associated with gastrointestinal disturbance and potentially with fatal hepatotoxicity.

SYNONYMS

Acephen
APAP
Aspirin-free Anacin
Cetafen
Feverall
Genapap
Genebs
Infantaire
Liquiprin
Mapap
Medpap
Panadol
Paracetamol
Redutemp
Silapap
Tempra
Tylenol
Valorin

ICD-9-CM CODE
965.4 Acetaminophen poisoning

EPIDEMIOLOGY & DEMOGRAPHICS

- Acetaminophen is the most common potentially toxic ingestion in children younger than 6 years.
- In 2003, there were almost 40,000 acetaminophen exposures in children 0 to 6 years old.
  - Less than 2% of fatalities from acetaminophen toxicity occur in this age group; the reasons for this are not known.
  - Children younger than 6 years may have increased glutathione synthesis and turnover.
- Overall, acetaminophen-related fulminant hepatic failure and mortality are rare and tend to be associated with delays in initiating therapy.

CLINICAL PRESENTATION

History

- It is often possible to obtain history of ingestion. As with all potentially toxic exposures, the clinician should inquire specifically about the following:
  - Time of ingestion
  - Liquid, tablet, or sustained-release preparation
  - Exact preparation ingested (so that effects of a coingestant may be anticipated)
  - Quantity ingested
  - Where the ingestant was stored
  - Degree of supervision at the time of ingestion
  - History of prior ingestions
  - Nature of ingestion (intentional versus accidental)
- Risks of unintended, inappropriate dosing include using an adult preparation, using an incorrect measuring device, using a sustained-release preparation, use in combination with cold or pain medications that also contain acetaminophen, administration by another child, or rectal administration.
- Risks that may contribute to toxicity at appropriate doses include genetic polymorphisms involving the cytochrome P450 enzyme system, decreased oral intake, protein-calorie malnutrition, poorly controlled diabetes, chronic liver disease (by prolongation of elimination half-life), and exposure to cytochrome P450-inducing drugs (e.g., carbamazepine, phenobarbital, rifampin, isoniazid [INH]).
- If an acute over-ingestion history cannot be obtained, inquire about recent routine Tylenol dosing, because chronic over-ingestion of acetaminophen can result in clinical toxicity.
- Generally, acute ingestion of more than 120 to 150 mg/kg in pediatric patients or more than 6 g in adult-sized patients is considered potentially toxic. In chronic over-ingestion, 150 to 175 mg/kg, taken over 2 to 4 days, can result in toxicity.
  - Acetaminophen toxicity should be considered in the differential diagnosis when evaluating any patient with anorexia, nausea, and vomiting.
  - Acetaminophen toxicity should be considered with serum transaminase elevation or other liver function abnormalities (as occurs later in the course).
- Many experts advocate routinely obtaining serum acetaminophen levels on all patients presenting with potentially significant ingestion of any kind because acetaminophen is a common coingestant.

Physical Examination

- Initially, patients may be asymptomatic.
- The first symptoms are anorexia, nausea, and vomiting. At 24 to 72 hours, patients may develop right upper quadrant pain.
- Serum transaminase levels often start to increase.
- Prolongation of the prothrombin time (PT) and elevation of the total bilirubin level may be seen.
- Oliguria may develop during this period.
- Further clinical evidence of hepatic dysfunction typically peaks at 72 to 96 hours.
  - Jaundice
  - Excessive bleeding
  - Encephalopathy
- Acute renal failure may also develop during this period.
- After 96 hours, the severely toxic patient may develop irreversible hepatic failure.
  - The ultimate outcome is usually known by 2 weeks after ingestion.
  - Complete recovery of hepatic function is expected in most appropriately treated patients.
- The clinical picture may be dominated early on by the effects of the coingestant (e.g., anticholinergic effects from combination cold preparations, respiratory depression from combination pain medications).

ETIOLOGY

- Hepatotoxic effects result from cytochrome P450 metabolism of acetaminophen to a toxic metabolite, *N*-acetyl-*p*-benzoquinoneimine (NAPQI).
  - It binds irreversibly to liver proteins to cause centrilobular hepatic necrosis unless it is conjugated with endogenous glutathione.
- Other pathways available for APAP metabolism include the following:
  - Sulfation (predominant in neonates)
  - Glucuronidation (a well-developed pathway by 3 years of age)
- Factors important in the development of acetaminophen-related hepatotoxicity include the following:
  - Over-ingestion of acetaminophen
  - Decreased capacity for metabolism by means of glucuronidation or sulfation
  - Increased activity of the cytochrome P450 system
  - Glutathione depletion

DIAGNOSIS

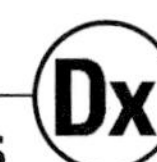

DIFFERENTIAL DIAGNOSIS

- Acute gastroenteritis
- Viral hepatitis
- Other toxic or chemical hepatitis
- Reye's syndrome
- Inborn error of metabolism
- Wilson disease
- α_1-Antitrypsin deficiency

LABORATORY TESTS

- The serum acetaminophen level should be determined at 4 hours after ingestion.
  - An 8-hour level may also be helpful, especially in cases of exposure to sustained-release acetaminophen preparations.
  - The relationship of initial and subsequent serum levels to time of ingestion should be interpreted according to the Rumack-Matthew nomogram.
  - Four-hour serum levels between 150 and 200 μg/mL are potentially toxic, and 4-hour levels in excess of 200 μg/mL are probably toxic.
- Obtain serum chemistries, including blood glucose, blood urea nitrogen (BUN), the creatinine level, and baseline serum transaminases, ammonia level, PT, and partial thromboplastin time (PTT).
- Consider obtaining serum levels of other common coingestants, such as a salicylate (aspirin).

- Broad-spectrum urine or serum toxicology screens are of uncertain value in acute management.
- Evidence of a significant coingestion is usually clinically apparent.

• In cases of potentially toxic ingestion, hepatic function status should be monitored by obtaining levels of serum transaminases and the PT and PTT (the PT is primarily affected) at 24 hours after ingestion and periodically thereafter if a laboratory abnormality has developed.
   - Special attention should be given to monitoring hepatic function in patients who are at high risk for development of hepatotoxicity.
   - Clinical or laboratory evidence of hepatic dysfunction is usually evident by 48 to 72 hours after ingestion.

• Clinical and laboratory markers of renal function should also be followed because renal failure may develop in the presence or absence of hepatic failure.

TREATMENT

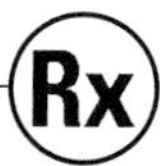

NONPHARMACOLOGIC THERAPY

Maintain the airway, assist ventilation if necessary, and support intravascular volume.

ACUTE GENERAL Rx

• For initial gastrointestinal decontamination, a single dose (1g/kg body weight) of activated charcoal should be administered within 6 to 8 hours after the ingestion.
   - Activated charcoal adsorbs acetaminophen effectively in the gastrointestinal tract.
   - Many experts believe that it can be given concurrently with the first dose of oral *N*-acetylcysteine (NAC) with no appreciable loss of NAC activity.

• While awaiting the initial serum level, if significant ingestion is suspected or if the 4-hour level is 150 µg/mL or more (or if the initial level relative to time of ingestion falls above the lower line in the Rumack-Matthew nomogram), specific antidotal therapy with 20% oral NAC (Mucomyst) or 20% intravenous acetylcysteine (Acetadote, Cumberland Pharmaceuticals) is indicated.
   - NAC decreases the potential for ongoing hepatotoxicity by acting as a glutathione substitute, by enhancing glutathione stores, and by enhancing metabolism by the alternative sulfation pathway.
   - When given orally, the initial dose is 140 mg/kg, and complete treatment consists of 17 subsequent enteral doses of 70 mg/kg. Doses are given at 4-hour intervals.

• Ondansetron and high-dose metoclopramide have been used with some success to control vomiting.
   - Because of its noxious odor and taste, oral NAC often potentiates ongoing nausea and vomiting.
   - Vomiting caused by the acute ingestion should be controlled as much as possible, because ongoing emesis interferes with administration of appropriate oral treatment.

• In January 2004, the U.S. Food and Drug Administration (FDA) approved an intravenous formulation of NAC (Acetadote, Cumberland Pharmaceuticals) for the treatment of suspected acetaminophen toxicity in adults and children.
   - This preparation is especially useful for patients who cannot tolerate enteral dosing.
   - Patients presenting within 8 to 10 hours of the ingestion should receive a loading dose, followed immediately by a maintenance infusion.
      - Loading dose: 150 mg/kg given intravenously over 15 minutes
      - Maintenance dose: 50 mg/kg given intravenously over 4 hours
      - Continued maintenance dose: 100 mg/kg given intravenously over 16 hours
   - A variable incidence of anaphylactoid reactions has been reported with the use of intravenous NAC.
      - It may be dose related.
      - Most reported cases have been easily managed with symptomatic therapies.
      - Lowering the infusion rate may be considered in these cases.
      - Individuals with a history of bronchospasm may be at increased risk for serious anaphylactic reactions to intravenous NAC.
      - Asthmatics were more likely to develop systemic side effects, but these events were not more severe.
   - Maximal benefit is derived from NAC if it is administered before the toxic metabolite of acetaminophen accumulates or within 8 to 10 hours of acute ingestion.
      - Although it may be of diminishing value in protecting against hepatotoxicity if initiated later, NAC should still be initiated, even if presentation is delayed beyond 24 hours after ingestion.
      - Some experts believe that oral NAC is more effective than intravenous NAC when presentation is longer than 16 hours after ingestion.

CHRONIC Rx

• Hepatic transplantation may be necessary in rare cases.

• Patients who develop severe acidosis, coagulopathy, or encephalopathy may be candidates for transport to a transplant facility.

DISPOSITION

• All patients with intentional ingestions should receive a psychiatric evaluation and treatment after they are medically stable.

• In cases of accidental ingestion, a consultation with a social worker is often helpful to assess the degree of supervision in the home.

REFERRAL

• In general, all patients suspected of having a potentially toxic exposure should be stabilized immediately and then referred to the nearest tertiary care facility with experience in managing critically ill children.

• The nearest regional poison center should be consulted in all cases of intentional or accidental toxic ingestion.

PEARLS & CONSIDERATIONS

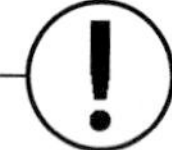

COMMENTS

• Oral NAC may be better tolerated if given by nasogastric tube or if diluted to at least 5% by mixing 1 part of the 20% stock formulation with 3 parts cola or juice. The addition of ice may improve compliance with the regimen.

• Serum levels of acetaminophen may be falsely elevated if the patient also ingested salicylate compounds, cephalosporins, or sulfonamides.

PREVENTION

• The danger of accidental poisoning in the home should be discussed routinely at pediatric health supervision visits, beginning at the 6-month visit.

• Parents should be instructed to childproof the home, including locking all medications and other toxic products out of the reach of children.

• Parents should be provided with the phone number of the regional poison center.

• Parents should be instructed to call the poison center immediately when they suspect that an inappropriate ingestion has occurred.

• Parents should be cautioned that many over-the-counter cold preparations contain acetaminophen and that these should not be given concurrently with acetaminophen.

• Rectal acetaminophen should be avoided because peak drug levels vary and the appropriate dosing interval may be longer than 4 to 6 hours. Parents should also avoid dividing suppositories because the medication is often not evenly distributed within them.

PATIENT/FAMILY EDUCATION

• Parents should be educated about the potential toxicity of acetaminophen (and preparations containing acetaminophen) in the home. These and other medications should be kept in a locked cabinet and out of reach of children, even if they are packaged with childproof caps.

- Families should be provided with the phone number (1-800-222-1222) of the nearest regional poison center.

SUGGESTED READINGS

AAP Committee on Drugs: Acetaminophen toxicity in children. *Pediatrics* 108:1020, 2001.

Alander SW et al: Pediatric acetaminophen overdose. Risk factors associated with hepatocellular injury. *Arch Pediatr Adolesc Med* 154:346, 2000.

Appelboam AV et al: Fatal anaphylactoid reaction to *N*-acetylcysteine: caution in patients with asthma. *Emerg Med J* 19:594, 2002.

Bromer MQ et al: Acetaminophen hepatotoxicity. *Clin Liver Dis* 7:351, 2003.

Burns MJ et al: Pathophysiology and diagnosis of acetaminophen (paracetamol) intoxication. UpToDate Online 12.3. Available at http://www.utdol.com/Accessed November 5, 2004.

Clark RF et al: The use of ondansetron in the treatment of nausea and vomiting associated with acetaminophen poisoning. *J Toxicol Clin Toxicol* 34:163, 1996.

Dargan PI et al: Management of paracetamol poisoning. *Trends Pharmacol Sci* 24:154, 2003.

Mack RB: Introduction: if I can stop one heart from breaking, I shall not live in vain. *Pediatr Ann* 25:12, 1996.

Nolan RJ: Poisoning. *In* Hoekelman RA et al (eds): *Primary Pediatric Care,* 3rd ed. St Louis, Mosby, 1997.

Olson K (ed): *Poisoning and Drug Overdose.* Englewood Cliffs, NJ, Appleton & Lange, 1994.

Perry HE et al: Efficacy of oral versus intravenous *N*-acetylcysteine in acetaminophen overdose: results of an open-label, clinical trial. *J Pediatr* 132:149, 1998.

Schmidt LE et al: Risk factors in the development of adverse reactions to *N*-acetylcysteine in patients with paracetamol poisoning. *Br J Clin Pharmacol* 51:87, 2001.

Smilkstein MJ et al: Efficacy of oral *N*-acetylcysteine in the treatment of acetaminophen overdose: analysis of the National Multicenter Study (1976–1985). *N Engl J Med* 319:1557, 1988.

Spooner JB et al: Paracetamol overdose: facts, not misconceptions. *Pharmaceutical J* 251:706, 1993.

Watson WA et al: 2003 Annual report of the American association of poison control centers toxic exposure surveillance system. *Am J Emerg Med* 22:335, 2004.

Wright RO et al: Effect of metoclopramide dose on preventing emesis after oral administration of *N*-acetylcysteine for acetaminophen overdose. *J Toxicol Clin Toxicol* 37:35, 1999.

AUTHORS: **MEREDITH E. REYNOLDS, MD** and **KATHLEEN M. VENTRE, MD**

Acne Vulgaris

BASIC INFORMATION

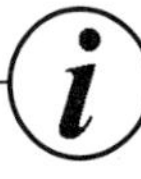

DEFINITION

Acne vulgaris is a disorder of the hair follicle and sebaceous gland affecting most people during adolescence or young adulthood.

SYNONYM

Comedonal acne

ICD-9-CM CODE

706.1 Acne vulgaris

EPIDEMIOLOGY & DEMOGRAPHICS

- Most common skin disease, affecting nearly 80% of people at some time between the ages of 11 and 30 years
- Most prevalent during adolescence, with greater severity in males

CLINICAL PRESENTATION

- Located in areas of highest sebaceous gland concentration; therefore the face, chest, and back are common sites of involvement.
- Ninety-eight percent of patients with acne have facial involvement; a smaller percentage have involvement on back and chest.
- Classic lesions are open and closed comedones (blackheads and whiteheads), formed by sebum-plugged pilosebaceous follicles.
- Inflammatory papules, pustules, and cysts develop after proliferation of *Propionibacterium acnes* in noninflammatory comedones, with rupture of contents into surrounding dermis.
- Cystic acne manifests by fluctuant and painful nodules and cysts that heal with postinflammatory pigment changes and scar formation.

ETIOLOGY

- There is a multifactorial etiology.
- Androgen production causes increasing sebum levels.
- Obstruction of pilosebaceous follicles is caused by excessive sebum combined with desquamated epithelial cells from follicle.
- *P. acnes* proliferates in an environment of excessive sebum and follicular cells.
- Inflammation is caused by mediators and chemotactic factors produced by bacteria.

DIAGNOSIS

DIFFERENTIAL DIAGNOSIS

- Papular scars
- Eosinophilic folliculitis
- Syringomas
- Adenoma sebaceum
- Drug eruption (lithium, corticosteroids)

WORKUP

Diagnosis is usually made on the basis of a characteristic clinical picture.

TREATMENT

NONPHARMACOLOGIC THERAPY

- Wash with mild soap (Dove, Purpose, Neutrogena, Basis) one to two times a day.
- Apply mild moisturizer (Cetaphil, Purpose, Moisturel) as needed.
- Avoid rubbing and scrubbing, which may worsen the condition.

ACUTE GENERAL Rx

All treatments are for several months.

CHRONIC Rx

- No single agent addresses all etiologic factors.
- Combination regimens are the mainstay of treatment.
- Benzoyl peroxide is antibacterial and comedolytic.
  - Available in 1% to 10% gels, creams, pads, and cleansers.
  - Also available in combination with erythromycin (Benzamycin) or clindamycin (BenzaClin, Duac).
  - Use one to two times a day.
  - Side effects include burning, erythema, dryness or peeling, and staining of clothes.
- Topical antibiotics are antibacterial and anti-inflammatory.
  - Erythromycin is available as a solution, gel, ointment, and pad.
  - Clindamycin is available as a solution, gel, lotion, foam, and pad.
  - Use one to two times per day.
  - Side effects include erythema, peeling, and drying.
- Topical retinoids increase cell turnover in the follicle wall and thereby allow expulsion of keratin plugs from microcomedones.
  - Available in many concentrations and forms (cream, gel, microsponge).
  - Begin with lowest concentration and slowly increase if needed.
  - Apply small amount (pea-size for full face) every night.
  - Side effects include transient worsening of acne, irritation, and photosensitivity.
- Systemic antibiotics have an antibacterial and anti-inflammatory mechanism of action.
  - The goal is 2 to 3 months of therapy and then tapering as topical agents are continued.
  - Tetracycline is administered as 500 mg twice a day (take on empty stomach).
  - Erythromycin is administered as 500 mg twice a day (can cause stomach upset).
  - Minocycline is administered as 50 to 100 mg twice a day (can cause hyperpigmentation, autoimmune hepatitis, lupus-like syndrome).
  - Doxycycline is administered as 50 to 100 mg twice a day (can cause sun sensitivity).
- Hormonal therapy (oral contraceptive pills) may be used.
  - A low-dose oral contraceptive containing nonandrogenic progestin, such as norgestimate or desogestrel, may be effective (Ortho-Tri-Cyclen or Yasmin).
  - Treatment for 2 to 4 months is required before any improvement occurs.
- Isotretinoin (systemic retinoids) may be used specifically with consultation of dermatologist.
  - It is indicated for severe nodulocystic acne.
  - It decreases sebum production.
  - It decreases "stickiness" of follicular cells.
  - Side effects include severe teratogen, increased triglycerides, dry skin and mucous membranes, decreased night vision, hyperostosis, and pseudotumor cerebri.
  - Usual course is 20 to 24 weeks.

PEARLS & CONSIDERATIONS

COMMENTS

- The dark color of a blackhead results from oxidized lipids, melanin, and densely packed keratinocytes, not dirt.
- Stress may aggravate acne, but it is not a major primary factor.
- There is no proven link between acne and diet.
- Strains of *P. acnes* that are less sensitive to antibiotics have become more prevalent.

SUGGESTED READINGS

American Academy of Dermatology: AcneNet. Available at www.derm-infonet.com/acnenet/

James WD: Clinical practice. Acne. *N Engl J Med* 352(14):1463, 2005.

Purdy S: Acne vulgaris. *Clin Evid* 13:2038, 2005.

Simonart T, Dramaix M: Treatment of acne with topical antibiotics: lessons from clinical studies. *Br J Dermatol* 153(2):395, 2005.

Society for Pediatric Dermatology. Available at www.spdnet.org

Tanghetti EA: Combination therapy is the standard of care. *Cutis* 76(2):8, 2005.

AUTHOR: **SUSAN HALLER PSAILA, MD**

the duration of illness (hydrocortisone, approximately 50 mg/m^2/day).

 - Illness with vomiting: Parenteral (intravenous or intramuscular) administration of stress-dose glucocorticoids is indicated.

REFERRAL

- All patients with adrenal insufficiency should be referred to an endocrinologist for complete evaluation and initial management.
- Treatment of suspected adrenal insufficiency should not be delayed until consultation because fatal adrenal crisis may occur in the interim.

PEARLS & CONSIDERATIONS

COMMENTS

- Addisonian crisis with hypotension can occur with only glucocorticoid deficiency and therefore with a relatively normal profile of electrolytes. Addisonian crisis and the need for stress-dose glucocorticoids cannot be ruled out by a finding of normal electrolyte levels.
- All patients should have medical alert bracelet or equivalent to alert medical emergency personal of their condition. Failure to treat with stress doses promptly during significant trauma or illness is potentially fatal.

PREVENTION

Patients known to have ALD or PGA should be tested for adrenal insufficiency.

PATIENT/FAMILY EDUCATION

- Education regarding stress-dose glucocorticoids is imperative.
- All patients should have injectable glucocorticoids at home for emergency dosing if they are unable to take a stress dose orally because of vomiting.

SUGGESTED READINGS

Agwu JC et al: Tests of adrenal insufficiency. *Arch Dis Child* 80:330, 1999.

Miller W: The adrenal cortex. *In* Sperling MA (ed): *Pediatric Endocrinology.* Philadelphia, WB Saunders, 2002, pp 385–438.

Perry R et al: Primary adrenal insufficiency in children: twenty years' experience at the Sainte-Justine Hospital, Montreal. *J Clin Endocrinol Metab* 90:3243, 2005.

AUTHOR: **CRAIG ORLOWSKI, MD**

BASIC INFORMATION

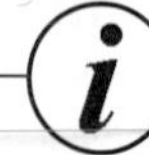

DEFINITION

Infection caused by human immunodeficiency virus type 1 (HIV-1), leading to a spectrum of illness from an early asymptomatic latent period to progressive immunologic deterioration and associated opportunistic infections and malignancies. The final stage is acquired immunodeficiency syndrome (AIDS). A similar illness is caused by HIV-2 in some areas of the world.

ICD-9-CM CODES

042 HIV-1 infection or AIDS
079.53 HIV-2 infection
795.71 Infant born to HIV-infected mother, not yet diagnosed with certainty by HIV polymerase chain reaction (PCR) or culture assays
V65.44 Code to be used for pre- and post-test counseling

EPIDEMIOLOGY & DEMOGRAPHICS

- HIV infection is a pandemic disease affecting mostly young adults. However, the HIV pandemic has a significant impact upon children and adolescents—directly by pediatric and maternal infection, and indirectly by HIV effects on the dissolution of families, death of parents and siblings, and depression of the economy of many developing nations.
- Modes of transmission include the following:
  - Vertical transmission (mother-to-child transmission, MTCT): the current mode of transmission for more than 95% of U.S. children, and still the major mode of pediatric HIV infection globally
  - Heterosexual or homosexual contact: increasingly common mode of transmission among adolescents, predominant mode of spread in young adults
  - Injection drug use: mode of transmission in some adolescents and young adults
  - Transfusion of contaminated blood or clotting factor concentrates: now rare in the United States and wherever adequate screening of donors and manufacture of concentrates takes place
  - Breastfeeding: a significant mode of transmission globally; should not occur in the United States, or in areas with availability of clean water and infant formula (where breastfeeding is contraindicated)
  - Remarkably few well-documented cases of HIV transmission have occurred after bites, or routine care in hospitals, clinics, or child-care settings—only a handful of cases reported in the entire history of the global pandemic!
- Incidence and prevalence of HIV infection among children less than 15 years of age (year 2004 data)

Global:
  - Prevalence: approximately 2.2 million (6% of the world caseload among all ages)
  - Annual incidence: 640,000 new cases per year (13% of the new cases per year worldwide among all ages)
  - Annual death rate: 510,000 deaths per year (16% of deaths from HIV among all ages)

United States:
  - Prevalence: estimated at about 4500 (<1% of total U.S. caseload among all ages)
  - Annual incidence: fewer than 300 new cases among infants from MTCT per year (<1% of the new infections among all ages in United States). However, among adolescents and young adults 15 to 24 years of age, HIV infection rates increase dramatically, with 5- to 10-fold greater numbers in this age group compared to children less than 15 years of age. As many as 10% of new cases of HIV infection per year occur in young adults 15 to 24 years of age.
  - Annual death rate: estimated at less than 100 deaths per year (compared to total U.S. HIV/AIDS death rate of about 18,000 per year)
- Risk factors and affected groups:
  - Infants born to HIV-infected mother
  - Risk of MTCT is 13% to 39% if no antiretroviral therapy is delivered to mother/infant; with appropriate therapy of pregnant woman and newborn, the risk may be lowered to less than 2%.
  - Risk factors for MTCT include maternal viral load and degree of immunodeficiency; prolonged rupture of membranes; lack of maternal antiretroviral therapy; and mode of delivery (cesarean versus vaginal), especially for those women with higher viral loads.
  - In developing countries, HIV transmission by breastfeeding occurs at incidence rates of 6000 per 100,000 breastfed children per year (i.e., 6% per year). As much as one third to one half of the entire MTCT rates in some areas would be preventable if clean water and infant formula were available for women, without social stigmatization.
  - Adolescents engaging in unprotected sexual contact, or injecting drugs with shared/contaminated equipment

CLINICAL PRESENTATION

History and Physical Examination

- Risk factors discussed above (e.g., infant born to HIV-infected mother; adolescents with high-risk behaviors; children or adolescents with history of opportunistic infections including recurrent bacteremia)
- Failure to thrive; generalized lymphadenopathy; organomegaly; oral thrush; lymphoid interstitial pneumonitis; developmental delay or chronic encephalopathy; scars from recurrent herpes simplex virus (HSV) or herpes zoster infections; chronic infiltrative parotitis
- Predominant clinical syndromes (variable, may include all organ systems; antiretroviral therapy may delay onset/modify syndromes):
  - HIV-infected infants: generally asymptomatic for first few months of life; median age of onset of symptoms is 3 years, but some remain asymptomatic for more than 5 years
    - Two patterns of symptoms are recognized: rapid progressors, approximately 10% to 15% of infected infants, who likely acquired true in utero infection; they exhibit a rapid progression to symptoms by 6 to 12 months, and death by 2 to 4 years. Nonrapid progressors represent 85% to 90% of infected infants who acquired HIV immediately pre- or intrapartum; they exhibit a slower progression, with survival beyond 5 years.
    - Common manifestations in infancy: failure to thrive, hepatosplenomegaly, oral candidiasis, *Pneumocystis carinii* pneumonia between 3 and 6 months of age
  - HIV-infected children:
    - Common manifestations include generalized lymphadenopathy, hepatosplenomegaly, failure to thrive, oral candidiasis, recurrent diarrhea, chronic parotitis, developmental delay (either static or progressive), recurrent bacterial infections, lymphocytic interstitial pneumonitis, opportunistic infections, nephropathy, malignancy, hepatitis, cardiomyopathy.
    - Opportunistic infections: *P. carinii* pneumonia most common; also *Candida* esophagitis, chronic or disseminated cytomegalovirus (CMV), HSV, or varicella zoster virus (VZV) infections. Rarely, tuberculosis, atypical *Mycobacterium* infections, toxoplasmosis, cryptococcosis.
    - Malignancies: Uncommon compared to adults with HIV infection, but leiomyosarcomas, lymphomas (especially primary central nervous system lymphoma, or non-Hodgkin's B-cell Burkitt type lymphoma) can occur. Kaposi's sarcoma is very rare in children.
  - Acute retroviral syndrome
    - An estimated 40% to 90% of adolescents or adults acutely infected with HIV will experience symptomatic acute retroviral syndrome; however, the illness is often not recognized as HIV infection by clinicians because of its nonspecific nature. (This syndrome is *not* to be expected in perinatally infected children!)

- The signs and symptoms (expected frequency) include fever (96%); lymphadenopathy (74%); pharyngitis (70%); erythematous maculopapular rash on face, trunk, and sometimes palms and soles, often with mucocutaneous ulceration of mouth, genitals (70%); myalgia or arthralgia (54%); and diarrhea, nausea and vomiting, or headache (each about 30%). Infrequently neurologic symptoms (10%) are seen, including peripheral neuropathy, aseptic meningitis or meningoencephalitis, and Guillain-Barré syndrome.

ETIOLOGY

- HIV-1 (often abbreviated simply as HIV), a human retrovirus, is the major etiologic agent worldwide.
  - A related retrovirus, HIV-2, causes a similar illness predominantly in West Africa.
- HIV has a very high mutation rate during replication, resulting in significant variation in antigenic reactivity and antiviral resistance of virus isolates recovered from different individuals and even from within the same individual.

DIAGNOSIS

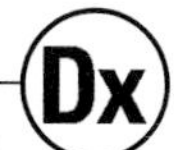

DIFFERENTIAL DIAGNOSIS

- Perinatally acquired HIV:
  - Congenital primary immunodeficiency syndromes
  - Congenital or early infancy infections (CMV, syphilis, EBV [Epstein-Barr virus], toxoplasmosis)
- Acute retroviral syndrome:
  - Infectious mononucleosis syndrome (EBV, CMV)
  - Influenza, influenza-like viral infections
  - Erythema multiforme

WORKUP

- Laboratory indicators of possible HIV infection:
  - Anemia, neutropenia, or thrombocytopenia
  - Progressive loss of total lymphocytes, especially with CD4 lymphopenia and inversion of normal CD4:CD8 subset ratio
  - Progressive humoral immune dysfunction, often with elevations in serum total IgG, IgM, IgA (much more characteristic than hypogammaglobulinemia)

LABORATORY TESTS

- Children older than 18 months: HIV infection diagnosed by positive HIV antibody test (reactive enzyme immunoassay [EIA] confirmed by Western blot)
- Children younger than 18 months: Antibody tests are confounded by transplacental maternal antibody. Diagnosis at this age requires virologic tests such as HIV PCR or culture. HIV DNA PCR testing has become the assay of choice in most laboratories because of its increased ease and safety compared with HIV culture. (Note: The DNA PCR is not the same test as the HIV RNA PCR or "viral load" assay used for prognosis and following the efficacy of therapy.)
  - HIV DNA PCR should be performed at 1 month *and* 4 to 6 months of age at minimum; some experts perform additional PCR tests at less than 1 month of age.
  - Positive results constitute presumptive evidence of HIV infection and should be immediately confirmed by repeat testing.
  - Two negative DNA PCR tests, both of which are performed at greater than 1 month and one of which is performed at greater than 4 months of age exclude HIV infection with reasonable certainty (>95%); such children are followed until antibody tests revert to negative (generally at 15 to 18 months of age) to absolutely exclude infection.
- Pregnant women and newborns:
  - Some states mandate routine HIV antibody screening of pregnant women and newborns to increase the opportunity for successful interruption of vertical transmission by antenatal therapy.
- Local laws requiring oral or written consent should be followed as applicable. As of 2003, five states required HIV testing of pregnant women (with right of refusal); ten states required the offering of voluntary testing; and two states (New York and Connecticut) required mandatory testing of newborns for HIV in addition to requiring or offering maternal testing with right of refusal.
  - Newly available rapid tests for HIV antibody are derivatives of the EIA tests that provide results within minutes to hours. These tests can be performed as point-of-care tests on oral secretions, whole blood, or serum; they may be useful in labor and delivery suites to test women of unknown serostatus in order to allow counseling and commencement of therapy to prevent MTCT, if needed. However, rapid assays require confirmatory Western blot testing for final diagnostic accuracy.
- Acute retroviral syndrome:
  - Acute HIV infection symptoms may occur before the development of HIV antibody. In adolescents with compatible clinical syndromes and recent high-risk behavior, both serum HIV antibody *and* plasma HIV RNA PCR ("viral load") tests should be obtained.

IMAGING STUDIES

Children with HIV encephalopathy may show cerebral cortical atrophy and symmetric calcifications of the basal ganglia.

TREATMENT

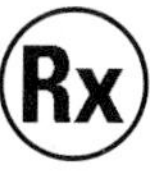

NONPHARMACOLOGIC THERAPY

- None

ACUTE GENERAL Rx

- Whether therapy of acute antiretroviral syndrome results in improved long-term virologic, immunologic, or clinical benefit is unknown; prompt consultation with an expert in pediatric or adult HIV infection should be obtained.

CHRONIC Rx

- The overall goal of pediatric HIV infection therapy is to maintain or achieve a normal CD4 T-lymphocyte count and percentage, by maximally suppressing the plasma HIV RNA viral load with highly active antiretroviral therapy (HAART). Nearly two dozen antiretroviral drugs are available in the United States, including multidrug combinations. Newer drugs, immunomodulators, and vaccines are under evaluation.
  - Primary care physicians are encouraged to participate actively in the care of HIV-infected children in consultation with specialists who have expertise in the treatment of pediatric HIV infection.
  - Expert opinions and knowledge about diagnostic and therapeutic approaches are changing rapidly, making frequent consultation crucial.
  - It is becoming more common for perinatally infected children to survive into adulthood, making further research to maximize long-term efficacy, while at the same time minimizing adverse effects, critical. Where possible, enrollment of the HIV-infected child into available clinical trials should be encouraged.
- The decisions of how and when to initiate antiretroviral therapy in children depend upon multiple factors including age, clinical presentation, CD4 T-lymphocyte percentages, HIV RNA viral loads, risk of disease progression, and readiness of the child and caregivers to adhere to a possibly complex medical regimen. Treatment is generally suggested for:
  - Infected infants less than 12 months of age
  - Symptomatic (clinically or immunologically) children more than 12 months of age
  - Asymptomatic children more than 12 months of age with high viral loads
  - Most commonly, HAART consists of a "backbone" of 2 nucleoside analogue reverse transcriptase inhibitors (NRTIs: zidovudine, didanosine, stavudine, lamivudine, abacavir, zalcitabine, or the NRTI-related drug tenofovir), given in combination with either a non-nucleoside reverse transcriptase inhibitor (NNRTI:

nevirapine, delavirdine, efavirenz) or a protease inhibitor (PI: saquinavir, ritonavir, indinavir, nelfinavir, amprenavir, fosamprenavir, lopinavir, or atazanavir).
  - Regimens are adjusted based upon virologic suppression, tolerance of adverse effects and drug interactions, and palatability of medications.
  - In general, monotherapy or two-drug therapy is avoided in favor of three or more drug HAART.
- Prophylaxis against opportunistic infections is an important adjunct to antiretroviral therapy.
  - Trimethoprim-sulfamethoxazole (TMP-SMX) should be given to all infants born to HIV-infected mothers beginning at 4 to 6 weeks of age through such time that HIV infection is excluded by serial negative PCR tests, in order to prevent *P. carinii* disease. It is also given throughout the first year of life to children whose infection status remains undetermined (e.g., for those in whom PCR results are not available) and to those children of all ages who are HIV-infected and who have advanced immunosuppression (CD4 lymphocyte percentage <15%).
  - Prophylaxis against other organisms such as atypical mycobacteria, CMV, and *Candida* are occasionally used for some children with advanced AIDS.
- Appropriate immunization is the third component of pediatric HIV therapy. Consultation with an expert in pediatric HIV infection is recommended, as certain vaccines are used differently than in noninfected children.
  - In general, live vaccines (e.g., OPV, BCG) are contraindicated.
  - Exceptions include *MMR vaccine*, which is indicated for asymptomatic and symptomatic HIV-infected children except those with severe immunocompromise, and *varicella vaccine*, which has been shown recently to be safe in asymptomatic and early stage HIV-infected children.
  - Killed (inactivated) vaccines such as HBV, DTaP, and Hib and pneumococcal conjugate vaccines are routinely indicated for all HIV-infected children, as are annual inactivated influenza vaccinations.

DISPOSITION

- In New York State, must be reported to local/state health departments
- See Laboratory Test and Chronic Rx sections
- Routine monitoring of children and adolescents with HIV infection includes:
  - CBC, CD4 lymphocyte subset and quantitative HIV RNA viral load determinations every 3 months
  - Serum electrolytes, blood urea nitrogen (BUN), creatinine, liver function tests, amylase, lipase, cholesterol, and triglycerides every 3 to 6 months
  - For sexually active adolescents, Pap smears, pregnancy test, and test for sexually transmitted disease (STDs) including serum rapid plasma reagent (RPR) test for syphilis every 6 to 12 months

REFERRAL

- Infectious diseases specialist with expertise in pediatric HIV
- Referral to the nearest AIDS center at least for initial consultation; continue contact with AIDS center or expert in pediatric/adolescent HIV infection

PEARLS & CONSIDERATIONS

COMMENTS

- Clinical manifestations seen more often in pediatric HIV than in adult HIV include:
  - Rapid progression
  - Recurrent invasive bacterial infection
  - Occurrence of lymphocytic interstitial pneumonitis
  - Progressive encephalopathy
- Clinical manifestations seen *much less often* in pediatric HIV than in adult HIV include:
  - Cerebral toxoplasmosis
  - Cryptococcal meningitis
  - CMV retinitis
  - Kaposi's sarcoma
  - TMP-SMX hypersensitivity

PREVENTION

- Antiretroviral therapy of HIV-infected women during pregnancy, labor, and to the infant for 6 weeks is very effective at interrupting vertical transmission, and should be routinely employed.
- HIV-infected women must be counseled *not to breastfeed* their infants (nor should they donate breast milk to milk banks) in order to prevent MTCT (recommendations in developing countries, where clean water and formula are not available, may differ).
- Safer sex practices, including appropriate use of condoms as well as avoidance of shared/unclean injectable drug equipment, are effective in preventing HIV infection among adolescents and adults, and should be promoted.
- Blood or bloody fluids in hospitals, schools, child-care settings, or on athletic fields should be disinfected with freshly diluted household bleach (1:10 to 1:100).

PATIENT/FAMILY EDUCATION

- www.aidsinfo.nih.gov—HIV/AIDS Information Service (AIDSInfo), a federal government site sponsored by the Department of Health and Human Services, Centers for Disease Control and Prevention (CDC), and National Institutes of Health; continually updated source of approved treatment guidelines for adult and pediatric HIV/AIDS, summaries of available clinical trials, fact sheets, help lines.
- www.cdc.gov/hiv/hivinfo.htm—CDC HIV/AIDS information site, containing a number of multimedia tools and information resources, including a fax information service and information in Spanish.
- www.hivguidelines.org—HIV/AIDS information site maintained by the New York State AIDS Institute; continually updated source of approved treatment guidelines and information on adult and pediatric HIV/AIDS.
- www.womenchildrenhiv.org—Site maintained by University of California at San Francisco and the National Pediatric and Family HIV Resource Center at the University of Medicine and Dentistry at New Jersey; contains treatment guidelines, patient educational materials, newsletters, other information.

SUGGESTED READINGS

American Academy of Pediatrics: Human immunodeficiency virus infection. *In* Pickering LK (ed): *2003 Red Book: Report of the Committee on Infectious Diseases,* 26th ed. Elk Grove Village, IL, American Academy of Pediatrics, 2003.

Hanson IC, Shearer WT: Lentiviruses (human immunodeficiency virus type 1 acquired immunodeficiency syndrome). *In* Feigin RD et al (eds): *Textbook of Pediatric Infectious Diseases,* 5th ed. Philadelphia, WB Saunders, 2004.

Weinberg GA, Burchett SK: Human immunodeficiency virus (HIV) infection in children. *In* Mandell GL et al (eds): *Mandell, Douglas, Bennett's Principles and Practice of Infectious Diseases,* 6th ed. Philadelphia, Elsevier, 2005.

AUTHOR: **GEOFFREY A. WEINBERG, MD**

BASIC INFORMATION

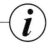

DEFINITION

Acute intoxication is caused by the excessive oral intake of ethyl alcohol.

SYNONYMS

Inebriation, drunkenness (acute alcohol intoxication)
Alcohol abuse (recurrent heavy drinking with associated risks or problems)
Binge-drinking (five or more drinks in a row for males, four or more for females)
Alcoholism, alcohol dependence (a chronic disorder characterized by compulsive use of alcohol, loss of control over drinking, and continued drinking despite serious adverse consequences)
Alcohol poisoning (acute pathologic intoxication)

ICD-9-CM CODES
291.4 Pathologic intoxication
303.0 With alcoholism
303.9 Alcoholism
305.0 Acute intoxication
980.9 Acute alcohol poisoning, specify ethyl alcohol

EPIDEMIOLOGY & DEMOGRAPHICS

- Ethyl alcohol is widely available in adult beverages; therefore large numbers of children and adolescents are exposed.
- Approximately 80% of ninth- to twelfth-grade students have drunk alcohol at least once, 50% are current drinkers, and 33% are current binge-drinkers (five or more drinks in a row).
- Males are more likely to engage in heavy drinking than females, and whites and Hispanic Americans are more likely to engage in heavy drinking than are African American students.
- Almost 17% of high school students report drinking and driving.
- More than 36% ride in cars with an intoxicated driver.
- Alcohol-related motor vehicle crashes are a leading cause of death among young people.

CLINICAL PRESENTATION

History

- Accidental injury or trauma
- Concurrent use of illicit drugs or prescription medications
- Associated health-risk behaviors (e.g., drinking and driving, unprotected sex)
- Prior alcohol use or abuse
- Friends who drink or use drugs
- Parent or family history of alcohol abuse or alcoholism

Physical Examination

- Classic physical findings include odor of alcohol on breath, nystagmus, conjunctival injection, hyporeflexia, ataxia, and orthostatic hypotension.
- Signs and symptoms vary with blood alcohol concentration (BAC, in mg/dL):
  - BAC lower than 100: incoordination, decreased reflexes, and emotional lability
  - BAC 100 to 250: slurred speech, ataxia, confusion, nausea, and vomiting
  - BAC 250 to 400: stupor, unresponsiveness, incontinence, and respiratory depression
  - BAC higher than 400: hypothermia and death (may occur at lower BAC in children)
- Check carefully for signs of trauma, aspiration, or other drug use.

ETIOLOGY

- Accidental ingestion of alcoholic beverages (younger children)
- Accidental over-ingestion by inexperienced older children and adolescents
- Purposeful intoxication (adolescent binge-drinking, alcohol abuse, alcoholism)

DIAGNOSIS

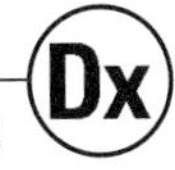

DIFFERENTIAL DIAGNOSIS

- Head trauma
- Other drug intoxication
- Hypoglycemia
- Sepsis, shock
- Central nervous system infection
- Hepatic encephalopathy
- Any other condition that can cause alteration in mental status

LABORATORY TEST(S)

- BAC (see previous listing for interpretation)
- Blood and urine toxicology
- Serum glucose, blood urea nitrogen (BUN), and electrolytes

IMAGING STUDIES

- Head computed tomography (CT) scan or magnetic resonance imaging (MRI) scan should be considered in the following cases:
  - Trauma is known or suspected.
  - Mental status fails to improve during a brief period of observation.

TREATMENT

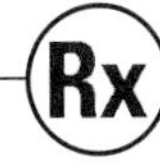

NONPHARMACOLOGIC THERAPY

- Mild alcohol intoxication usually requires observation only.

ACUTE GENERAL Rx

- Intravenous hydration (10% glucose to prevent hypoglycemia)
- If unresponsive:
  - Assess integrity of the gag reflex.
  - Secure the airway if necessary.
  - Support ventilation.
  - Perform gastric lavage after airway is secure.
- Consider hemodialysis if hepatic damage is present or BAC is higher than 300 in a comatose patient. If ingestion occurred within 2 to 3 hours, administer activated charcoal (30 to 60 g for young children; 60 to 100 g for adolescents) and magnesium sulfate 250 mg/kg.
- Administer naloxone if concurrent drug use is suspected.

CHRONIC Rx

- If alcohol dependence is suspected:
  - Administer multivitamins, thiamine, and folate.
  - Admit for observation and possible treatment of alcohol withdrawal.

DISPOSITION

- Rapid clearing of sensorium is to be expected. If steady improvement is not seen over the first few hours, patient must be reassessed for other possible causes of altered mental status (e.g., head trauma, drug intoxication).
- Assessment and therapy for substance abuse disorders (see "Patient/Family Education")
- Assessment and therapy for co-occurring mental health problems

REFERRAL

Physicians should be familiar with substance abuse treatment resources in their own community. For most adolescents, outpatient counseling is the appropriate initial treatment.

PEARLS & CONSIDERATIONS

COMMENTS

BAC may be estimated by calculating serum osmolal gap (serum osmolality [2 × Na + BUN/2.8 + glucose/18]); then estimating BAC of 100 mg/dL for every 22 to 25 osmolal gap increment.

PREVENTION

- According to the American Medical Association's Guidelines for Adolescent Preventive Services, every adolescent should be screened for alcohol and drug use as part of routine care.
- The CRAFFT test (following) is a valid and reliable screening test for adolescents (Box 1-1).

PATIENT/FAMILY EDUCATION

- For an isolated occurrence of intoxication in an adolescent, the physician should emphasize risk reduction.
  - Provide information and advice about drinking and driving or riding in a car with an intoxicated driver.
  - Negotiate or "contract" for specific changes in behavior and arrange follow-up.
- For youth with recurrent episodes of intoxication or other alcohol-related problems, physicians should make a referral to a developmentally appropriate substance abuse treatment program.

BOX 1-1 CRAFFT Screening Test

C Have you ever ridden in a CAR driven by someone (including yourself) who was "high" or had been using alcohol or drugs?
R Do you ever use alcohol or drugs to RELAX, feel better about yourself, or fit in?
A Do you ever use alcohol or drugs while you are ALONE?
F Do you ever FORGET things you did while using alcohol or drugs?
F Do your family or FRIENDS ever tell you that you should cut down on your drinking or drug use?
T Have you ever gotten into TROUBLE while you were using alcohol or drugs?
Two or more "yes" answers suggest a significant problem and need for additional assessment.

SUGGESTED READINGS

American Academy of Pediatrics, Committee on Substance Abuse: Tobacco, alcohol, and other drugs: the role of the pediatrician in prevention and management of substance abuse. *Pediatrics* 101:125, 1998.

Knight JR, et al: Validity of the CRAFFT substance abuse screening test among general adolescent clinic patients. *Arch Pediatr Adolesc Med* 156:607, 2002.

Kleinschmidt K, Delaney K: Ethanol. *In* Haddad L, et al (eds): *Clinical Management of Poisoning and Drug Overdose.* Philadelphia, WB Saunders, 1997.

Knight J: Substance use, abuse, and dependency. *In* Levine M, et al (eds): *Developmental-Behavioral Pediatrics.* Philadelphia, WB Saunders, 1999.

National Center for Alcohol and Drug Information (NCADI): Available at: http://www.health.org/index.htm

Schydlower M: *Substance Abuse: A Guide for Health Professionals.* Elk Grove Village, IL, American Academy of Pediatrics, 2002.

AUTHOR: **JOHN KNIGHT, MD**

BASIC INFORMATION

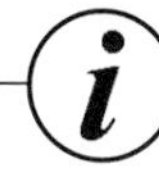

DEFINITION

Allergic bronchopulmonary aspergillosis (ABPA) is a hypersensitivity pulmonary disease occurring in individuals with asthma or cystic fibrosis. In these patients, it is characterized by transient pulmonary infiltrates, reversible airway obstruction, eosinophilia, and evidence of hypersensitivity to the fungus: *Aspergillus fumigatus*.

SYNONYMS

Allergic aspergillosis
Bronchopulmonary aspergillosis

ICD-9-CM CODE
518.6 ABPA

EPIDEMIOLOGY & DEMOGRAPHICS

- Present in 8% to 11% of patients with cystic fibrosis (CF)
- Occurs in 6% to 20% of adults with asthma; rare in pediatric patients with asthma
- Reported from most countries of the world

CLINICAL PRESENTATION

History

- Medical history of asthma, atopy, or CF
- Episodic wheezing of increasing frequency or severity
- Productive cough, occasionally of brown plugs
- Possibly fever, weight loss, anorexia, dyspnea, malaise, chest pain, fatigue, or hemoptysis

Physical Examination

- Generalized airway obstruction with wheezes and rhonchi
- Signs of hyperaeration (e.g., barrel chest, prolonged expiratory phase)
- Localized crackles may be heard
- Digital clubbing is present in those with more severe disease
- Five stages:
  - Stage I (acute): symptoms; chest radiograph and laboratory findings
  - Stage II (remission): clearing of infiltrates; decline in IgE for 6 months after steroids
  - Stage III (exacerbation): new infiltrates and more than twofold rise in IgE
  - Stage IV: corticosteroid-dependent asthma
  - Stage V (fibrotic end stage): irreversible obstructive and restrictive defects

ETIOLOGY

- Ubiquitous *A. fumigatus* spores are inhaled and trapped in obstructed airways with impaired clearance.
- Colonization is helped by small spore size and temperatures at which *A. fumigatus* grows.
- High colonization rate of *A. fumigatus* is seen in patients with asthma or CF.
- Continuous source of antigenic stimulation leads to both type I IgE-mediated and type III immune complex-mediated hypersensitivity reactions.

DIAGNOSIS

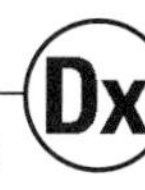

DIFFERENTIAL DIAGNOSIS

- Other lung diseases caused by *A. fumigatus*: invasive aspergillosis, aspergilloma, IgE-mediated asthma from *A. fumigatus* sensitivity, hypersensitivity pneumonitis
- Bacterial, fungal, viral, tuberculous, or eosinophilic pneumonia
- Inadequately controlled asthma
- Cystic fibrosis

WORKUP

- Full diagnostic criteria
  - Episodic bronchial obstruction; deterioration not due to another etiology
  - Serum total IgE concentration greater than 1000 IU/mL in patients not receiving systemic steroids
  - Immediate cutaneous reactivity to *A. fumigatus* antigen, or in vitro presence of *A. fumigatus*-specific IgE antibodies
  - Precipitating antibodies to *A. fumigatus* antigen or serum *A. fumigatus*-specific IgG antibodies by an in vitro test
  - New or recent abnormalities on chest radiograph or chest computed tomography (CT) that have not cleared with antibiotics and standard physiotherapy
- Minimal diagnostic criteria
  - Criteria 1 and 3 above, total serum IgE greater than 500 IU/mL and *either* criteria 4 or 5 above
- Other criteria
  - Peripheral blood eosinophilia
  - Fumigatus in sputum
  - Expectoration of brown plugs or flecks
  - Arthus (late) skin reactivity to *Aspergillus* antigen

LABORATORY TEST(S)

- Blood work: total IgE; blood eosinophil count; precipitating antibodies to *A. fumigatus* antigen by RAST (radioallergosorbent) testing; specific IgE and IgG antibodies to *A. fumigatus* by enzyme-linked immunosorbent assay (ELISA)
- Skin test reaction to *A. fumigatus* antigen
- Sputum smear and culture for fungus
- Pulmonary function testing: airway obstruction, flow limitation, air trapping

IMAGING STUDIES

- Chest radiograph: transient or migratory opacities; upper lobe predominance; atelectasis of a segment, lobe, or entire lung; central bronchiectasis; hyperinflation; bronchial mucoid impaction; tram-line shadows; gloved-finger shadows; fibrosis
- Chest CT scan: all of the above; better for detection of bronchiectasis

TREATMENT

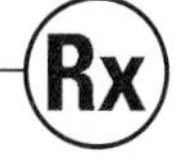

NONPHARMACOLOGIC THERAPY

- Airway clearance with chest physiotherapy and postural drainage

ACUTE GENERAL Rx

- Systemic corticosteroids are the treatment of choice for acute disease and exacerbations.
- Prednisone 0.5 mg/kg/day is given for 2 weeks, then an alternate-day regimen for 3 to 6 months.
- Possible adjunctive therapies include itraconazole, inhaled steroids, cromolyn sodium.
- Immunotherapy has no role.

CHRONIC Rx

- Serial total serum IgE should be monitored monthly for the first year.
- Serial chest radiographs are recommended every 3 to 4 months for 2 years, then every 6 to 12 months.
- ABPA exacerbation is suggested by a significant increase in total IgE level, or recurrence of infiltrates, and is an indication for resumption of prednisone therapy as above.

DISPOSITION

- The prognosis is good if diagnosed early, before severe lung destruction.
- Death occurs from end-stage fibrotic lung disease in the presence of cor pulmonale.

REFERRAL

- Since diagnosis can be difficult, refer to pediatric pulmonology or allergist.

PEARLS & CONSIDERATIONS

COMMENTS

- This condition may be the initial presentation of CF.
- Early diagnosis and treatment are essential to prevent pulmonary fibrosis and insufficiency.
- Overlap of symptoms and radiographic findings in ABPA and CF can make the diagnosis difficult.
- A clue to ABPA in CF: infiltrates progress despite antibiotics and resolve with steroid therapy.

PREVENTION

- Avoidance of farm buildings and compost heaps.

SUGGESTED READINGS

Gibson RL et al: State of the art: pathophysiology and management of pulmonary infections in cystic fibrosis. *Am J Respir Crit Care Med* 168:918, 2003.

Stevens DA et al: Allergic bronchopulmonary aspergillosis in cystic fibrosis—state of the art; Cystic Fibrosis Foundation Consensus Conference. *Clin Infect Dis* 37(Suppl 3):S225, 2003.

AUTHOR: **BARBARA A. CHINI, MD**

BASIC INFORMATION

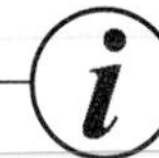

DEFINITION

Allergic rhinitis is a symptom complex of nasal congestion, rhinorrhea, sneezing, and nasal itching resulting from an IgE-mediated allergic reaction and inflammation of the mucosal lining of the nose and contiguous mucosal membranes, usually occurring in temporal relationship to an airborne allergen exposure.

SYNONYMS

Hay fever
Rose fever

ICD-9-CM CODES
477 Allergic rhinitis (seasonal and nonseasonal)
477.0 Allergic rhinitis caused by pollen
477.8 Allergic rhinitis caused by other allergies
477.9 Allergic rhinitis—cause unspecified
493.0 Allergic rhinitis with asthma

EPIDEMIOLOGY & DEMOGRAPHICS

- Allergic rhinitis is a disease predominantly occurring in childhood (mean onset, 10.6 years).
- Prevalence rates of 10% are reported in those younger than 12 years and 20% to 30% are reported among adolescents.
- The incidence is slightly higher in males.
- Allergic rhinitis has a strong association with wheezing symptoms and asthma.
- Although racial differences have been reported, migration studies suggest that environmental factors play a more important role.
  - A 17% prevalence of allergic rhinitis among children born to parents without allergic rhinitis
  - A 26% prevalence in children with one parent with allergic rhinitis
  - A 52% prevalence rate in children with both parents with allergic rhinitis

CLINICAL PRESENTATION

History

- Typical symptoms are sneezing, nasal itching, nasal congestion, clear rhinorrhea, and palatal itching.
- These symptoms can coexist with ocular symptoms of itching, tearing, and redness.
- Pattern and chronicity is seasonal, perennial, or episodic.
- This can be associated with specific triggers:
  - Indoor: dust mites, animal dander, molds
  - Outdoor: molds, pollens
  - Nonallergic triggers: cigarette smoke
- Significant risk factors are a personal and family history of allergic disorders.

Physical Examination

- External examination: allergic facies
  - Allergic shiners: infraorbital dark skin discoloration
  - Allergic crease: a transverse nasal crease caused by rubbing and pushing the tip of the nose upward to relieve obstruction and itching
  - Puffy eyelids
- Examination of the interior of the nose:
  - Clear, watery discharge
  - Pale, edematous mucosa
    - Nasal turbinates may completely occlude the nasal passages.
    - Examination after placement of topical nasal decongestant drops is needed to exclude nasal polyps and other abnormalities.
- Conjunctival injection
- Examination of the lungs: may show wheezing (asthma is a comorbid condition)
- Examination of skin: may show eczema

ETIOLOGY

- Airborne allergens (e.g., pollens, cat dander, dust mites) contact the respiratory mucosa in a susceptible patient who has had IgE sensitization to the antigen or antigens.
- Immediate phase:
  - This results from allergen contact with IgE on mucosal mast cells or basophils.
  - This leads to cell degranulation and release of mediators.
    - Preformed mediators (e.g., histamine)
    - Preformed but slowly eluted mediators (e.g., heparin, trypsin)
    - Newly synthesized mediators (e.g., leukotrienes, prostaglandins)
    - These mediators increase vascular permeability, tissue edema, and begin cellular recruitment.
- Late phase:
  - This phase occurs 4 to 24 hours after mast cell activation.
  - Cellular infiltration plays a more significant role and produces nasal obstruction that is less responsive to antihistamines and decongestants.

DIAGNOSIS

DIFFERENTIAL DIAGNOSIS

- Vasomotor rhinitis (physical or irritant rhinitis, including gustatory and cold-induced)
- Nonallergic rhinitis with eosinophilia (NARES syndrome)
- Acute infectious rhinitis
- Acute or chronic sinusitis, or both
- Drug-induced (rhinitis medicamentosa)
- Anatomic abnormalities
  - Septal deviation
  - Hypertrophic turbinates
  - Nasal polyps
  - Adenoidal adenopathy
  - Foreign bodies
  - Choanal atresia or stenosis
  - Nasal tumors (benign and malignant)
  - Cerebrospinal rhinorrhea
- Hormonal (e.g., hypothyroidism, pregnancy)

WORKUP

Diagnosis is based on history and physical examination, along with response to therapy.

LABORATORY TEST(S)

- The presence of antigen-specific IgE antibodies can be demonstrated by allergy skin testing or in vitro tests (e.g., radioallergosorbent assay or modifications of it such as the Immuno Cap System).
  - The presence of positive results can help differentiate the symptoms from nonallergic causes to better direct therapy.
- Total serum IgE may be elevated but is generally not helpful in making diagnosis.
- Nasal smears often show eosinophils.

TREATMENT

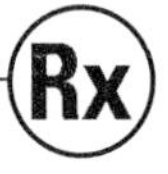

NONPHARMACOLOGIC THERAPY

Environmental control is key.

- Pollens
  - Keep windows closed and air conditioners on automatic.
- Molds
  - Dehumidification
  - Avoidance of outdoor sources such as mowing the lawn or raking leaves
- House dust mites
  - Enclose mattresses and pillowcases in allergen-proof materials.
  - Wash bed linens in hot water (above 130°F).
    - Exercise caution with water temperatures in homes with young children because of scalding risks.
  - Avoid bedroom carpeting.
- Animals
  - Remove pets shedding dander and hair from home or isolate (less optimal) from patient.
  - Eliminate cockroach, mice, or rat infestations.
- Irritants
  - Eliminate exposure to cigarette smoke, perfumes, chalk dust, and other irritating materials.

ACUTE GENERAL Rx

- Oral antihistamines effectively reduce rhinorrhea, sneezing, itching, and ocular symptoms.
  - They have little effect on nasal congestion.
  - Nonsedating antihistamines, although more costly, are preferred over sedating antihistamines because they pose little risk of performance impairment.
- Decongestants, alone or in combination with antihistamines, can help reduce congestion.
  - Side effects of oral decongestants include nervousness, insomnia, and appetite loss.
  - Topical decongestants are effective, but prolonged use (more than 3 days) can lead to rebound congestion.
- Intranasal corticosteroids are the most effective agents to control sneezing, rhinorrhea, nasal itching, and congestion. The onset of action may be several days.
  - Concerns have arisen over the potential to affect childhood growth.

- Medication should be used at the lowest possible dosage for the shortest duration possible.
- Heights should be monitored if use extended.

- Intranasal cromolyn spray is less effective than intranasal corticosteroids but is associated with few side effects.
  - Recommended frequent dosing (three to four times a day) adversely affects adherence.
- Other therapies include the following:
  - Nasal saline washes
  - Intranasal antihistamines
    - Azelastine hydrochloride nasal spray (Astelin): For children 12 years and older use 2 sprays to each nostril twice daily; for children 5 to 11 years use 1 spray to each nostril twice daily.
    - Has bitter taste and can cause drowsiness.
  - Intranasal anticholinergic agents
    - Ipratropium bromide nasal spray (Atrovent) 0.03%: For children 6 years and older use 2 sprays to each nostril two to three times a day.
    - Helpful for the rhinorrhea component of allergic rhinitis.
- For severe cases of allergic rhinitis, a one-time short course of oral corticosteroids (e.g., prednisone 1 mg/kg/day for 3 days) may provide more immediate relief and improve effectiveness of other therapies.

CHRONIC Rx

- Continuation of acute pharmacologic therapy as indicated.
- Immunotherapy (e.g., hyposensitization, allergy shots) can modify disease.
  - An effective treatment option for selected patients with moderate to severe symptoms lasting several months of the year or for those who are unresponsive to other treatment options, including both environmental control and pharmacotherapy.
  - Vaccine composition is based on a careful patient history and results of allergy testing.
  - Allergy injections should be given only in an appropriately equipped office with a physician immediately available to treat anaphylactic reactions.
  - Patients should stay in the office 30 minutes after the injection or injections.
    - Patients should be instructed to immediately report any adverse reactions.
    - Report changes in chronic medication use—the use of β-blocking agents can intensify anaphylactic reactions.

DISPOSITION

- Ongoing follow-up is needed; allergic rhinitis resolves in only 10% to 20% of children within 10 years.
- Asthmatic children with rhinitis have higher risks of hospitalizations and their asthma can benefit from treatment of their rhinitis.

REFERRAL

- Consider referral to an allergist for patients with prolonged manifestations or allergic rhinitis that impairs functioning or quality of life, contributes to comorbid conditions like sinusitis, or requires prolonged use of medications or unsatisfactory response to them.
- Elucidation of allergic rhinitis triggers and more extensive patient education can be helpful.

PEARLS & CONSIDERATIONS

COMMENTS

- Adequate examination of the nasal airway in active allergic rhinitis may require placement of topical decongestants a few moments before examination.
- For nasal inhaler use, providing instructions to the patient with a sample inhaler may improve the patient's technique and adherence to the regimen. Some patients prefer "unscented" inhalers over "scented" ones and vice versa.

PREVENTION

- Lifelong responsiveness to aeroallergens appears to ultimately be determined early in life.
- Proposed strategies of prevention include the following:
  - Identification of high-risk infants before or after birth
  - Avoidance of infant exposure to more allergenic food allergens (e.g., peanuts, nuts)
    - Breastfeeding for the first year of life
    - Maternal lactation with no eggs, cows' milk, peanuts, tree nuts, and fish
    - Supplementation or weaning with a hypoallergenic formula
    - Delay of solid foods for 6 months and then adding least allergenic food first
    - For high-risk foods such as eggs, peanuts, tree nuts, and fish, waiting until 2 to 3 years of age before introducing
  - Early avoidance of aeroallergens by environmental control measures (as noted previously)

PATIENT/FAMILY EDUCATION

- Education of parents and patients about symptoms and triggers of allergic rhinitis
- Environmental control of allergens and irritants
- Appropriate use of medications
  - In particular, patients (or parents) should be shown and be able to demonstrate correct use of prescribed nasal inhalers.
- Expected results and precautions for allergy immunotherapy

SUGGESTED READINGS

American Academy of Allergy, Asthma, and Immunology: Available at:www.aaaai.org

American College of Allergy, Asthma, and Immunology: Available at:www.acaai.org

Dykewicz MS, et al: Diagnosis and management of rhinitis: complete guidelines of the Joint Task Force on Practice Parameters in Allergy, Asthma, and Immunology. *Ann Allergy Asthma Immunol* 81:478, 1998.

Howarth PH: Allergic non allergic rhinitis. *In* Adkinson NF Jr, et al: *Middleton's Allergy: Principles and Practice.* St. Louis, Mosby, 2003, pp 1391–1410.

Li JT, Bernstein IL, et al: Allergy immunotherapy: a practice parameter. *Ann Allergy, Asthma, Immunol* 90:1, 2003.

Mutius E, Martinez FD: Natural history, development, prevention of allergic disease in childhood. *In* Adkinson NF Jr, et al: *Middleton's Allergy: Principles and Practice.* St. Louis, Mosby, 2003, pp 1169–1174.

Wright AL, et al: Epidemiology of physician-diagnosed allergic rhinitis in childhood. *Pediatrics* 94:895, 1994.

AUTHOR: **THOMAS J. FISCHER, MD**

BASIC INFORMATION

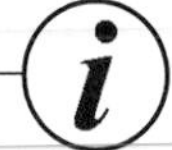

DEFINITION

Alpha-1-antitrypsin (A1AT) deficiency is an inherited autosomal recessive disease caused by homozygosity for the mutant type "Z" A1AT protein. A1AT deficiency is the most common genetic cause of liver disease in children and panacinar emphysema in adults.

ICD-9-CM CODE
277.6 Alpha-1-antitrypsin deficiency

EPIDEMIOLOGY & DEMOGRAPHICS

- The incidence of A1AT deficiency (PiZZ) in most populations is 1 in 1600 to 1 in 2000 live births.
- The prevalence of A1AT deficiency (PiZZ) in the United States is 1 in 4800; an additional 1 in 600 individuals is heterozygous for the Z allele.
- From 10% to 15% of all PiZZ homozygotes develop clinically significant liver disease during the first 30 years of life.
- Liver disease most commonly presents in infancy (as neonatal cholestasis), but may also present as chronic liver disease in childhood or adulthood.
- Neonatal cholestasis may be more common in males.
- Clinically significant pulmonary dysfunction is not apparent until the third decade of life.
- A1AT deficiency occurs worldwide and affects all major racial subgroups.
- Heterozygote carriers of A1AT deficiency (PiMZ) may be at increased risk for a number of other liver or lung diseases.

CLINICAL PRESENTATION

- Persistent jaundice in infancy
- Late hemorrhagic disease in infancy
- Feeding difficulties
- Poor growth
- Pruritis
- Melena/hematemesis (from esophageal varices)
- Asymptomatic elevated transaminases
- Hepatomegaly or splenomegaly, or both
- Ascites (with advanced liver disease)
- Chronic cough, exercise intolerance, wheezing (not apparent until late in second decade of life)
- Increased anteroposterior diameter of chest, prolonged expiratory phase, clubbing, hyperresonant lung fields, poor air exchange (not apparent until late in second decade)
- Membranoproliferative glomerulonephritis, relapsing panniculitis, and systemic vasculitis associated with A1AT deficiency in adults

ETIOLOGY

- A1AT is a protease inhibitor that is produced primarily in the liver.
- A1AT deficiency results in synthesis of a defective A1AT protein that cannot be excreted from the hepatocytes.
- Liver disease is caused by accumulation of abnormal protein polymers in the hepatocytes; in some patients this may be aggravated by an additional defect in the ability to break down the abnormal protein.
- Lung disease (pulmonary emphysema) is caused by a lack of active A1AT in the lung, leading to uninhibited proteolytic destruction of the connective tissue backbone.
- The onset of lung disease is hastened and the severity of disease worsened by exposure to tobacco smoke.

DIAGNOSIS

DIFFERENTIAL DIAGNOSIS

- Other causes of neonatal cholestasis (see Jaundice/Hyperbilirubinemia in Differential Diagnosis [Section II])
- Chronic hepatitis (viral, autoimmune, drug-induced, Wilson disease)
- Asthma (in adults)
- Chronic obstructive pulmonary disease (COPD)

WORKUP

- Liver biopsy
  - May show a variety of findings depending on the clinical presentation, including hepatocellular necrosis, inflammatory cell infiltrate, periportal fibrosis, biliary epithelial cell injury, cholestasis, and even cirrhosis.
  - Will show characteristic periodic acid-Schiff (PAS)–positive, diastase-resistant globules in liver cells (this characteristic finding may be absent in children less than 3 months of age).
- Pulmonary function tests (PFTs)
  - PFT abnormalities precede clinically significant symptoms.
  - By 18 years of age a decrease in forced expiratory volume in 1 second (FEV_1)/vital capacity may be seen.
  - Abnormalities of diffusion capacity (DL_{CO}) are seen as alveolar surface area is lost.

LABORATORY TEST(S)

- Liver function tests often show a modest elevation of transaminases and an elevated γ-glutamate transferase; the conjugated bilirubin may or may not be elevated.
- Prolonged prothrombin time (PT) and decreased serum albumin may be seen with more advanced liver disease.
- Diagnosis depends on demonstration of an A1AT phenotype (Pi) of ZZ by altered migration of the A1AT protein in a polyacrylamide isoelectric-focusing gel.

IMAGING STUDIES

- Abdominal ultrasound with Doppler flow studies to assess the degree of portal hypertension and splenomegaly, and rule out a mass or anatomic cause for liver dysfunction

TREATMENT

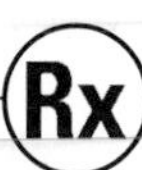

NONPHARMACOLOGIC THERAPY

- Provide adequate nutritional support.
- Avoid additional insults to the liver (avoid alcohol and hepatotoxic medications, immunize for hepatitis A and hepatitis B).
- Avoid additional insults to the lungs, particularly tobacco smoke.
- Liver transplantation is curative in patients with end-stage liver disease from A1AT deficiency.
- Shunt procedures may be an alternative to liver transplantation in patients with complications of portal hypertension but adequate hepatic synthetic function.
- Lung transplantation is an option for treatment of end-stage emphysema.

CHRONIC Rx

- Supportive therapy for cholestasis includes choleretics, fat-soluble vitamin supplementation, antipruritics.
- Supportive therapy for complications of portal hypertension includes diuretics for ascites, β-blockers for esophageal varices.
- Replacement of the defective A1AT protein with intravenous preparations of purified human A1AT (Prolastin, Zemaira, Aralast) may be effective at slowing lung disease in adult patients with emphysema.
- Delivery of A1AT by inhalation, and vector-associated delivery of the normal A1AT gene, are promising future therapies for A1AT pulmonary disease.
- Highly experimental gene therapy directed at inhibiting the production of abnormal A1AT protein, and increasing the production of normal A1AT protein, may one day correct both liver and lung manifestations of A1AT deficiency.

DISPOSITION

- Children with A1AT deficiency should be examined closely at every doctor's visit for hepatosplenomegaly; with ultrasound confirmation when suspected.
- Significant pulmonary dysfunction is unlikely during childhood.

REFERRAL

- All children with A1AT deficiency should be referred to a pediatric gastroenterologist at diagnosis for initial assessment and ongoing surveillance.
- All children with A1AT deficiency should be referred to a pulmonologist in adolescence for initial evaluation and discussion of therapeutic options.

PEARLS & CONSIDERATIONS

COMMENTS

- A1AT is an acute phase reactant and may be elevated to a normal range in patients with A1AT deficiency and liver inflammation; therefore, a phenotype should always be determined.

- A1AT phenotype should be included in the evaluation of every patient with unexplained liver disease.
- In infants with A1AT deficiency, classic PAS-positive, diastase-resistant globules may not be identified on liver biopsy.

PREVENTION

- Avoidance of tobacco smoke will markedly slow the development and progression of lung disease.

PATIENT/FAMILY EDUCATION

- Any exposure to tobacco smoke (active or passive) should be strictly avoided, as this will hasten the progression of lung disease.
- Signs and symptoms of progressive liver disease (i.e., poor growth, gastrointestinal bleeding, increasing jaundice, and abdominal distension) should be promptly reviewed with the child's physician.
- Even in the absence of overt symptoms, children may experience progression of liver disease and eventually require liver transplantation.
- Relatives with unexplained liver or lung disease should be tested for A1AT deficiency.
- Support groups: Alpha-1 Foundation (www.alphaone.org), Alpha-1 Association (www.alpha1.org), American Liver Foundation (www.liverfoundation.org), American Lung Association (www.lungusa.org), AlphaNet (www.alphanet.org).

SUGGESTED READINGS

De Serres FJ, et al: Genetic epidemiology of alpha–1 antitrypsin deficiency in North America and Australia/New Zealand: Australia, Canada, New Zealand and the United States of America. *Clin Genet* 64:382, 2003.

Perlmutter DH: Alpha-1-antitryspin deficiency: Diagnosis and treatment. *Clin Liver Dis* 8:839, 2004.

Perlmutter DH: α_1-Antitrypsin deficiency. *In* Suchy FJ, et al (eds): *Liver Disease in Children.* Philadelphia, 2001, Lippincott Williams & Wilkins, pp 523–547.

Piitulainen E, et al: Effect of environmental and clinical factors on lung function and respiratory symptoms in adolescents with alpha$_1$-antitrypsin deficiency. *Acta Paediatr* 87:1120, 1998.

Primhak RA, et al: Alpha-1 antitrypsin deficiency. *Arch Dis Child* 85:2, 2001.

Sveger T, et al: The liver in adolescents with alpha$_1$-antitrypsin deficiency. *Hepatology* 22:514, 1995.

AUTHORS: **KATHLEEN M. CAMPBELL, MD** and **LEE A. DENSON, MD**

BASIC INFORMATION

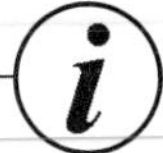

DEFINITION

In the setting of a recent gain in altitude, headache plus at least one of the following symptoms: fatigue and/or weakness, nausea and/or vomiting and/or anorexia, dizziness and/or light-headedness, or difficulty sleeping.

SYNONYMS

Acute mountain sickness (AMS)
Altitude mountain sickness
High-altitude sickness
Mountain illness

ICD-9-CM CODE

993.2 Other and unspecified effects of high altitude

EPIDEMIOLOGY & DEMOGRAPHICS

- Approximately 20% of people who rapidly reach 2400 meters (8000 feet) from sea level develop AMS.
- The development or degree of AMS is not predicted by physical condition or previous experiences at altitude.
- AMS is more likely the higher the altitude and the faster the altitude is achieved.
- Patients with blunted hypoxic ventilatory response (HVR) are more likely to develop AMS than those with brisk HVR.

CLINICAL PRESENTATION

History

- Rapid ascent from sea level to high altitude, usually more than 2400 meters (8000 feet)
- Symptoms occurring 12 to 24 hours after altitude reached
    - Subside in 2 to 7 days
- Symptoms include the following: headache, weakness, fatigue, gastrointestinal symptoms (nausea, vomiting, anorexia), dizziness, light-headedness, difficulty sleeping.

Physical Examination

- Tired-appearing: dyspnea with exertion but none at rest, lungs clear, normal neurologic examination.
- High-altitude pulmonary edema (HAPE), a life-threatening condition: pronounced tachypnea, dyspnea at rest, rales, wheezes, severe cough, cyanosis.
- High-altitude cerebral edema (HACE), life-threatening: ataxia, confusion, severe headache.

ETIOLOGY

- Rapid exposure to hypobaric, hypoxic conditions
- Made worse by a poor hypoxic ventilatory response
- Hyperventilation occurs to maintain adequate arterial oxygen saturation

DIAGNOSIS

DIFFERENTIAL DIAGNOSIS

- Carbon monoxide poisoning
- Post-alcohol intoxication headache (hang-over)
- Early HAPE or HACE
- Influenza
- Vertigo
- Other causes of headache, respiratory distress, and fatigue

WORKUP

- Based primarily on history and physical examination

LABORATORY TEST(S)

- Consider arterial blood gas if respiratory distress present

IMAGING STUDIES

- Chest X-ray if significant pulmonary symptoms present
- Computed tomography (CT) of head if neurologic symptoms present

TREATMENT

NONPHARMACOLOGIC THERAPY

- Stop ascent.
- If symptoms are mild or tolerable, remain at present altitude until symptoms stop.
- If symptoms are severe or intolerable, descend until symptoms stop.

ACUTE GENERAL Rx

- Nonsteroidal anti-inflammatory drugs (NSAIDs) are given for headache.
- Acetazolamide 125 to 250 mg twice a day lessens symptoms in adults.
    - Effectiveness in children is unknown.
- If symptoms of HAPE:
    - Supplemental oxygen
    - Nifedipine (effectiveness in children unknown)
    - Hyperbaric chamber if available
    - Descend at least 610 meters (2000 feet) and continue descent until symptoms stop
- If symptoms of HACE:
    - Supplemental oxygen
    - Dexamethasone (dose for pediatric HACE unknown)
    - Hyperbaric chamber if available
    - Descend at least 610 meters (2000 feet) and continue descent until symptoms stop

COMPLEMENTARY & ALTERNATIVE MEDICINE

- Gingko biloba
    - Decreased incidence of AMS and milder symptoms
    - Dosing: 120 mg orally twice a day beginning 5 days before ascent and continuing at altitude
    - Not studied in children

DISPOSITION

- Watch for symptoms of HAPE or HACE over 1 to 3 days after presentation of AMS

REFERRAL

- Anyone with evidence of HAPE or HACE should be referred to a tertiary center for support.

PEARLS & CONSIDERATIONS

COMMENTS

- Physical condition does not predict development of AMS.
- Oxygen desaturations during sleep increase the likelihood of developing AMS.
    - Try to sleep at lower altitudes.
    - Follow the old mountaineering adage: "climb high, sleep low."
- In general, once above 2400 meters (8000 feet), climb about 300 meters (1000 feet) per day.
    - Acclimate for 1 to 2 days for each ascent of 600 meters (2000 feet).
        - Denver is at 1610 meters (5280 feet) above sea level
        - The top of Mt. McKinley is 6200 meters (20,320 feet)
        - The top of Mt. Everest is 8850 meters (29,028 feet)

PREVENTION

- Attain altitude slowly.
- In adults, take acetazolamide 125 to 250 mg twice a day 1 to 2 days before going to altitude and continue for 48 hours after attaining altitude.
    - Decreases incidence of AMS
    - Effectiveness in children unknown

PATIENT/FAMILY EDUCATION

- Stop ascent if symptoms of AMS develop.
- Ascend gradually.
- Watch for cough, wheezes, sputum production, and ataxia.
- If AMS in past, attain altitude slowly.
- General information on AMS from healthanswers.com
- See also High Altitude Medicine Guide at www.high-altitude-medicine.com

SUGGESTED READINGS

Carpenter T, et al: Altitude-related illness in children. *Curr Probl Pediatr* 28:181, 1998.

Hackett PH, Roach RC: High-altitude illness. *New Engl J Med* 345:107, 2001.

Krieger B, de la Hoz RE: Altitude-related pulmonary disorders. *Crit Care Clin* 15:265, 1999.

Maakestad K, et al: Gingko biloba reduces incidence and severity of acute mountain sickness [abstract]. Proceedings of Wilderness Medical Society Summer Conference. Park City, UT, 2000.

AUTHOR: **MATTHEW RICHARDSON, MD**

BASIC INFORMATION

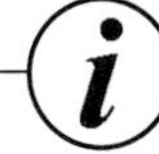

DEFINITION

Ambiguity of the external genitalia occurs either when a female fetus is virilized or when a male fetus is under-virilized during sexual differentiation in the first trimester.

- *Female pseudohermaphroditism* refers to masculinization of the external genitalia in a patient with a female karyotype from exposure to abnormally elevated levels of androgens. If exposure occurs before the 12th fetal week, fusion of the labioscrotal folds and formation of a urogenital sinus occur. In severe cases, the urethra may traverse the phallus. The external genitalia may look like those of a male infant with severe hypospadias and undescended testes. If exposure occurs after the 12th fetal week, only clitoral hypertrophy will occur.
- *Male pseudohermaphroditism* occurs when the genitalia of a male infant are under-virilized.

SYNONYMS

Ambiguous genitalia
Disorders of sex differentiation
Intersex

ICD-9-CM CODES
253.2 Hypopituitarism
255.2 Congenital adrenal hyperplasia (CAH)
257.8 Androgen insensitivity—testicular feminization (syndrome)
752.49 Clitoromegaly
752.51 Cryptorchidism
752.61 Hypospadias
752.65 Hidden penis
752.8 Anorchia/hypoplastic testes
752.9 Unspecified anomaly of female genitalia

EPIDEMIOLOGY & DEMOGRAPHICS

- The incidence of the most common form of CAH, 21-hydroxylase deficiency, is approximately 1 in 10,000 to 15,000.
  - Autosomal recessive inheritance.
  - Three fourths of affected children have severe or salt-wasting CAH.
- Other disorders of adrenal steroidogenesis are exceedingly rare.
- Androgen insensitivity syndrome is X-linked.

CLINICAL PRESENTATION

- Newborn screening is performed in the United States and other countries. Hence, often there is no history because the diagnosis is usually made shortly after birth for affected males and at birth for affected females, based on the physical exam that indicates ambiguity of the external genitalia.
- The patient may have positive family history (previously affected sibling[s]).
- Rule out maternal androgen use.

ETIOLOGY

Multiple etiologies, based on karyotype and sex steroid abnormalities (see "Differential Diagnosis")

DIAGNOSIS

DIFFERENTIAL DIAGNOSIS

- Dependent on genetic sex
- Differential diagnosis of female pseudohermaphroditism—XX genotype
  - Multiple congenital anomalies
  - Midline defects
  - Prune-belly syndrome
  - Bladder exstrophy
  - Increased in utero androgen exposure
    - Excessive fetal androgen—CAH
    - Exogenous androgens—oral progestins (e.g., 17-ethinyl testosterone, danazol)
    - Excessive maternal androgens—ovarian or adrenal tumors
- Differential diagnosis of male pseudohermaphroditism—XY genotype
  - Disorders of testicular differentiation
  - Abnormalities of placental or fetal gonadotropins
  - Defective gonadal (5α-reductase deficiency) and adrenal sex steroid synthesis
  - End-organ resistance (androgen insensitivity) and defective androgen action

WORKUP

- Female pseudohermaphroditism
  - Karyotype: 46,XX
  - 17-OH progesterone and androstenedione levels very elevated in CAH
  - Urogenital sinogram to outline the urogenital sinus
  - Pelvic and abdominal ultrasound to show presence of uterus and to look for hyperplastic adrenal glands
- Male pseudohermaphroditism
  - Palpable gonads
  - Karyotype: 46,XY
  - Adrenal and gonadal steroid levels, testosterone, and dihydrotestosterone
    - Elevated adrenal precursors (pregnenolone, 17-OH pregnenolone, dehydroepiandrosterone [DHEA], or androstenedione) and low gonadal testosterone may be indicative of defective gonadal and adrenal sex steroid synthesis.
    - Elevated testosterone and low dihydrotestosterone are indicative of 5α-reductase deficiency.
    - Normal to elevated levels of testosterone may be consistent with androgen insensitivity.
    - Luteinizing hormone and follicle-stimulating hormone, thyroid-stimulating hormone, growth hormone: low in hypopituitarism

LABORATORY TESTS

- See "Workup" discussed earlier
- 17-OH progesterone and androstenedione, testosterone and dihydrotestosterone.

IMAGING STUDIES

- See "Workup" discussed earlier
- Pelvic and abdominal ultrasound
- Urogenital sinogram to outline the urogenital sinus

TREATMENT

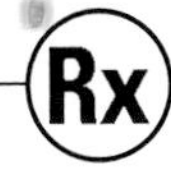

NONPHARMACOLOGIC THERAPY

- One of few pediatric endocrine emergencies. Rapid decision should be made with experienced team (pediatrician, endocrinologist, urologist, geneticist) regarding gender decision.
- Ongoing psychological support for the family to deal with the implications of genital abnormalities.

ACUTE GENERAL Rx

Therapy depends on cause and decision regarding gender rearing.

CHRONIC Rx

- Female pseudohermaphroditism from CAH
  - Oral glucocorticosteroids—cortisol 20 mg/M^2/day divided three times a day
  - Mineralocorticoid—fludrocortisone 0.1 mg/day
- Male pseudohermaphroditism
  - Consider periodic testosterone throughout childhood if needed to increase penile size
    - See "Disposition"

DISPOSITION

- Avoid determining the sex of rearing before an accurate diagnosis is reached.
- The decision to pursue surgical genitoplasty for ambiguity of the external genitalia is becoming increasingly controversial.
- Provide full support (medical and psychologic) for adaptation to and development of chosen sex of rearing.
- Physicians who care for children who have ambiguous genitalia must appreciate the family's cultural, religious, and psychological needs.

REFERRAL

- Care should be coordinated with a pediatric endocrinologist and a pediatric urologist.

PEARLS & CONSIDERATIONS

COMMENTS

- In salt-wasting CAH, electrolyte abnormalities first occur at about 1 week of age, with hyperkalemia.

- Hyponatremia occurs by 2 to 3 weeks of age, and addisonian shock occurs at 4 to 5 weeks of age.
- With vomiting in the 2- to 5-week-old child, be sure to think about salt-wasting CAH. If the electrolytes show hyponatremia and hyperkalemia, CAH is the likely diagnosis.

PREVENTION

- For CAH, prenatal diagnosis and therapy are available but still experimental.
- In several states, newborn screening for detection of CAH is practiced.

PATIENT/FAMILY EDUCATION

- Androgen Insensitivity Syndrome Support Group (AISSG): www.medhelp.org/www/ais/
- CARES (Congenital Adrenal hyperplasia Research, Education and Support) Foundation, Inc: www.caresfoundation.org/
- Intersex Society of North America: www.isna.org
- The Magic Foundation: www.magicfoundation.org/cah.html
- The National Organization of Rare Diseases: www.rarediseases.org/

SUGGESTED READINGS

Anhalt H et al: Ambiguous genitalia. *Pediatr Rev* 17:213, 1996.

Long DN et al: Gender role across development in adult women with congenital adrenal hyperplasia due to 21-hydroxylase deficiency. *J Pediatr Endocrinol* 17(10):1367, 2004.

Speiser PW, White PC: Congenital adrenal hyperplasia. *N Engl J Med* 349(8):776, 2003.

Warne GL, Zajac JD: Disorders of sexual differentiation. *Endocrinol Metab Clin North Am* 27:945, 1998.

Zaontz MR, Packer MG: Abnormalities of the external genitalia. *Pediatr Clin North Am* 44:1267, 1997.

AUTHOR: **NICHOLAS JOSPE, MD**

BASIC INFORMATION

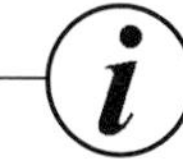

DEFINITION

Amblyopia is the decrease in visual acuity that has resulted from an abnormality in visual stimulation. The word amblyopia comes from the Greek and means "dull sight."

SYNONYM

Lazy eye

ICD-9-CM CODES
368.00 Amblyopia, unspecified
368.01 Strabismic amblyopia
368.02 Deprivation amblyopia
368.03 Refractive amblyopia

EPIDEMIOLOGY & DEMOGRAPHICS

- Amblyopia affects at least 2% of the population.
- It is the leading cause of preventable visual loss in children.
- Any condition causing poor visual input before the age of 9 years can result in amblyopia.

Risk factors include prematurity and a family history of amblyopia.

CLINICAL PRESENTATION

- The most important clinical finding is poor visual acuity.
- The patient may have a normal-appearing eye and may not complain of poor vision.
- Amblyopia often is associated with strabismus.
  - A complete eye examination to screen for strabismus should be a part of every well-child visit (see "Strabismus" in Diseases and Disorders [Section I]).
  - Especially important in the preverbal infant/toddler because of the difficulty in accurately assessing visual acuity in this age range.

Check for red reflex to assess for cataracts, glaucoma, retinoblastoma, or opacity.

ETIOLOGY

There are three major types of amblyopia:

- **Strabismic amblyopia**
  - Misalignment of the eyes results in abnormal binocular interaction.
  - Eventual unconscious suppression of visual stimulation to an affected eye creates amblyopia.
- **Deprivation amblyopia**
  - Eyes fail to receive clearly formed images on the retina
  - Due to a cataract, other opacity, or obstruction (hemangioma of lid)
- **Refractive (anisometropic) amblyopia**
  - Difference in refractive error between the two eyes
  - Clearer image favored
  - Visual loss (amblyopia) in eye with higher refractive error

Difficult to diagnose in the preverbal patient because of a lack of associated strabismus.

DIAGNOSIS

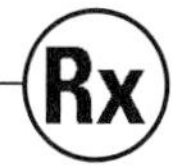

DIFFERENTIAL DIAGNOSIS

- Uncorrected refractive error (need for glasses)
- Ocular or visual pathway lesion accounting for visual loss
  - Pituitary tumor
  - Other brain tumor
  - Optic nerve inflammation
  - Retinoblastoma

WORKUP

- A thorough history and eye examination are the keys to the diagnostic evaluation.
- Laboratory tests and imaging are generally unnecessary in the outpatient setting.

TREATMENT

Rx

NONPHARMACOLOGIC THERAPY

- Identify the cause (i.e., strabismus, deprivation, or refractive error)
- Train the amblyopic eye to fixate
  - Strabismic—with glasses, occlusion of the good eye, or surgery (Occlusion therapy includes patching, cycloplegic drops, or filtering optical devices.)
  - Deprivation—provide a clear visual pathway
  - Refractive-glasses and occlusion therapy
- Older children generally require longer therapy.
- All treatment for amblyopia should be directed by an ophthalmologist.

DISPOSITION

- Determined by the eye care provider; dependent on the child's age, diagnosis, severity of amblyopia, and method of treatment

REFERRAL

- All patients who are suspected to have amblyopia from any etiology should be referred to an ophthalmologist.

PEARLS & CONSIDERATIONS

COMMENTS

- Amblyopia is the leading cause of reduced vision in children.
- Amblyopia is often not detected because children "peek" during the eye examination given by the primary care provider or school.
- Early detection and therapy are essential to maximize visual recovery.

PREVENTION

- Prompt diagnosis of strabismus, obstruction of the visual axis, and refractive errors are the key to preventing amblyopia.

PATIENT/FAMILY EDUCATION

- Most cases of amblyopia are correctable.
- Early detection yields the best prognosis.
- After age 7 to 9 years, amblyopia is usually irreversible.

SUGGESTED READINGS

American Academy of Pediatrics: Policy Statement, Committee on Practice and Ambulatory Medicine and Section of Ophthalmology: Eye Examination in Infants, Children, and Young Adults by Pediatricians. *Pediatrics* 111:902, 2003.

Avallone J: Amblyopia strabismus in toddlers. *In* Hertle R, et al (eds): *Pediatric Eye Disease Color Atlas and Synopsis.* New York, McGraw-Hill, 2002, pp 119–128.

Mittelman D: Amblyopia. *Pediatr Clin North Am* 50:189, 2003.

AUTHOR: **DANIEL YAWMAN, MD**

BASIC INFORMATION

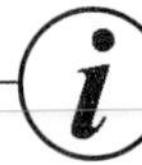

DEFINITION

Amenorrhea is the absence of menses; it is divided into primary and secondary.

- Primary amenorrhea is defined as:
  - Absence of menarche by age 16 years in presence of normal pubertal development *or*
  - Absence of menarche by age 14 years in absence of normal pubertal development *or*
  - Absence of menarche 2 years after completion of sexual maturation
- Secondary amenorrhea is defined by:
  - Absence of menstruation for at least 3 cycles or at least 6 months in females who have already established menstruation

SYNONYMS

Primary amenorrhea
Secondary amenorrhea

ICD-9-CM CODE
626.0 Amenorrhea

EPIDEMIOLOGY & DEMOGRAPHICS

- Median age of menarche in the United States is 12.43 years.
- Approximately 95% to 97% of females reach menarche by 16 years of age.
- Ten percent of all girls in the United States are menstruating by 11.1 years of age and 90% are menstruating by 13.75 years of age.

CLINICAL PRESENTATION

Physical Examination

- Growth parameters, growth pattern, pubertal spurt
- Stigmata of Turner syndrome or anorexia nervosa
- Hair distribution; quality of skin, hair, and nails
  - Hirsutism and acne may indicate androgen excess.
  - Dry skin and pitted nails may indicate hypothyroidism.
  - *Acanthosis nigricans* indicates insulin resistance.
  - Hypertrichosis or excessive vellus hair occurs with anorexia nervosa.
  - Scant pubic and axillary hair may indicate androgen insensitivity.
- Funduscopic examination, gross visual fields, examination of cranial nerves
- Palpation of thyroid
- Breast examination to elicit galactorrhea
- Abdominal examination for masses
- Complete neurologic examination (including sense of smell)
- Pelvic examination with assessment of the following:
  - External genitalia for pubic hair, hymenal opening, clitoral size
  - Vaginal mucosa for assessment of estrogenization
  - Vaginal patency
  - Visualization of cervix
- Bimanual examination with rectovaginal examination for masses

ETIOLOGY

- Amenorrhea is a symptom of any of the following:
  - Central nervous system dysfunction
  - Ovarian dysfunction
  - Genital tract abnormality
  - Pregnancy

DIAGNOSIS

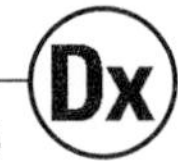

DIFFERENTIAL DIAGNOSIS

- Pregnancy
- Hormonal contraception
- Hypothalamic
  - Chronic or systemic illness
  - Eating disorder
  - Hypothalamic pituitary axis immaturity
  - Infiltration (hemochromatosis)
  - Isolated gonadotropin-releasing hormone deficiency
  - Kallmann's syndrome (associated with defects in olfaction)
  - Obesity
  - Strenuous exercise
  - Stress
  - Substance abuse
  - Tumor (craniopharyngioma)
- Pituitary
  - Hypopituitarism
  - Infiltration (hemochromatosis)
  - Infarction (Sheehan's syndrome, sickle cell disease)
  - Tumor (prolactinoma)
- Adrenal
  - Congenital adrenal hyperplasia (classic, nonclassic)
- Ovarian
  - Agenesis (46,XX)
  - Dysgenesis (Turner syndrome [45,XO] or variant with abnormal X chromosome)
  - Hyperandrogenic chronic anovulation (also known as *polycystic ovary syndrome*)
  - Premature ovarian failure (autoimmune, chemotherapy, radiation)
  - Tumor
- Uterus, cervix, vagina
  - Agenesis (Mayer-Rokitansky-Kuster-Hauser syndrome)
  - Androgen insensitivity syndrome (testicular feminization)
  - Imperforate hymen
  - Synechiae (Asherman's syndrome)
  - Transverse vaginal septum
- Other
  - Endocrinopathies (thyroid disease, Cushing's syndrome)
  - Prader-Willi syndrome
  - Laurence-Moon-Biedl syndrome

LABORATORY TESTS

- A pregnancy test is essential.
- It is helpful to divide the laboratory evaluation into adolescents with the following characteristics:
  - Absent breast development with absent uterus
  - Absent breast development with normal uterus
  - Normal breast development with absent uterus
  - Normal breast development with normal uterus
- For absent breast development with absent uterus:
  - Evaluation includes karyotype, luteinizing hormone (LH), follicle-stimulating hormone (FSH), progesterone, and 17α-hydroxyprogesterone.
  - Differential diagnosis includes vanishing testes syndrome or enzyme block (17,20-desmolase defect).
- For absent breast development with normal uterus:
  - Evaluation should include FSH, LH, and karyotype.
  - Differential diagnosis includes gonadal dysgenesis, hypothalamic/pituitary disorder, or a genetic defect in ovarian steroid production.
  - A low or normal FSH suggests a hypothalamic or pituitary abnormality, and a careful neuroendocrine evaluation is in order.
  - A high FSH and normal blood pressure suggest a genetic disorder or gonadal dysgenesis such as Turner syndrome.
  - A high FSH with hypertension suggests a 17α-hydroxylase deficiency. This is confirmed by elevated progesterone, low 17α-hydroxyprogesterone, and elevated serum deoxycorticosterone.
- For normal breast development with absent uterus:
  - Evaluation includes karyotype and testosterone level.
  - Differential diagnosis includes androgen insensitivity or müllerian agenesis.
    - A patient with androgen insensitivity will have XY karyotype with normal *male* levels of testosterone.
    - A patient with müllerian agenesis will have XX karyotype with normal *female* levels of testosterone.
- For normal breast development with normal uterus:
  - Evaluation includes thyroid-stimulating hormone (TSH), prolactin, and pregnancy test.
    - A normal prolactin level rules out prolactinoma. Elevated levels or symptoms of visual changes *require magnetic resonance imaging* to exclude prolactinoma.
  - Differential diagnosis includes vaginal outlet obstruction or disturbance in hypothalamic/pituitary axis.
  - If physical examination reveals androgen excess, the evaluation should also include serum dehydroepiandrosterone sulfate

(DHEA-S), hydroxyprogesterone (17-OHP), and testosterone levels.
  - If TSH and prolactin are normal and the patient is not pregnant, a progesterone challenge should be performed.
    - Withdrawal bleeding after the challenge indicates chronic anovulation with estrogen production.
    - No response suggests ovarian failure or hypothalamic dysfunction; FSH, LH, and estradiol levels should be performed.
      - A high FSH suggests ovarian failure, and a karyotype and evaluation for autoimmune disease should be performed.
      - A low or normal FSH should demand a search for risk factors of hypothalamic dysfunction, such as chronic disease, eating disorder, or strenuous exercise.

IMAGING STUDIES

- A pelvic ultrasound may be helpful in defining anatomy.
  - May be difficult to do and to interpret
  - Results not always accurate

TREATMENT

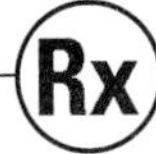

CHRONIC Rx

- Varies depending on cause of amenorrhea
  - Patients with hyperandrogenic chronic anovulation benefit from combined oral contraceptives.
  - Patients who are hypoestrogenic and anovulatory because of hypothalamic suppression (e.g., anorexia, exercise) should be given calcium and oral contraceptives to reduce the long-term risks of osteoporosis.
  - Patients with Turner syndrome or ovarian failure require hormonal replacement therapy beginning with gradually increasing doses of estrogen and a progestational agent.

DISPOSITION

- If ectopic pregnancy is suspected, admit to hospital urgently.
- If pituitary tumor is suspected, check visual fields for defects and measure prolactin urgently to rule out prolactinoma causing mass lesion.

REFERRAL

- Refer patients with menstrual outflow obstruction to a gynecologist for further investigation.
- Refer patients with suspected tumors to the appropriate specialist for further investigation.
- Refer patients with suspected endocrine disorder to a pediatric endocrinologist.
- Karyotyping may miss mosaic cases; specialist assessment is essential if a genetic abnormality is suspected.

PEARLS & CONSIDERATIONS

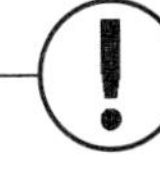

COMMENTS

- Pregnancy is the most common cause of secondary amenorrhea; thus, regardless of sexual history reported, a pregnancy test is essential.
- Turner syndrome (because of associated primary ovarian failure) is the most common cause of primary amenorrhea.

SUGGESTED READINGS

Hoffman B, Bradshaw K: Delayed puberty and amenorrhea. *Semin Reprod Med* 21:353, 2003.

Rosen D et al: Delayed puberty. *Peds Rev* 22:309, 2001.

AUTHOR: **STEPHANIE SANSONI HSU, MD**

BASIC INFORMATION

DEFINITION

- *Anal fissure (fissure-in-ano):* superficial linear disruption of the anal epithelium around the anal verge, often leading to local pain and bleeding
- *Anal fistula (fistula-in-ano):* persistently patent tract originating in the crypt of Morgagni at the anal valves and terminating at the perianal skin; often the secondary consequence of draining a perianal or perirectal abscess
- *Perianal abscess:* abscess formed from an infection within the crypt of Morgagni, presenting on the perianal skin; initial and often persistent communication to the anus results in enteric organism infection
- *Perirectal abscess:* uncommon in children; presents as perirectal collections but do not communicate with a fistula-in-ano
- Imperforate anus—see "Imperforate Anus" in Diseases and Disorders (Section I)

SYNONYMS

Rectal abscess
Rectal fistula

ICD-9-CM CODES
565.0 Anal fissure
565.1 Anal fistula
566 Perianal and perirectal abscess

EPIDEMIOLOGY & DEMOGRAPHICS

- Anal fissures are common in infants and children.
- In infants, boys and girls are affected equally.
- In older children there is a slight male predominance.
- Anal fistulas have a male predominance and are most often observed in infants.

CLINICAL PRESENTATION

Anal Fissure

- Most common cause of minor rectal bleeding in infancy.
- Mild constipation with dehydration is often responsible for the initial event, followed by a cycle of stool withholding, further constipation, and continuing trauma to the anal canal.
- Infants over 1 year of age may present with a fissure during the transition from formula to whole milk.
- Firm stool with blood streaking should suggest the diagnosis.
- Examination of the anal canal by eversion of the anal skin allows visualization of the fissure, most commonly located posteriorly.
- In chronic cases a "sentinel" skin tag indicates the site of the fissure.

Anal Fistula

- Generally proceeded by a small perianal abscess that either drains spontaneously or has been drained.
- Drainage site persists and recurrent spontaneous discharge of a small amount of pus or mucus is observed.
- There is a persistent communication from the skin site and an abnormally deep crypt at the dentate line.
- The involved crypt is inflamed and can be recognized on gentle speculum exam.

Perianal Abscess

- Develops from an infection within a deep crypt at the base of the columns of Morgagni.
- Presents with perianal redness and pain as well as pain with defecation.

Perirectal Abscess

- Rare in children but may be seen especially with inflammatory bowel disease.
- Presents with pain and redness.
- There may be only minimal induration of the buttock but the deep extension may be appreciated on rectal exam or by computed tomography (CT) scan.

ETIOLOGY

- Anal fissure—tearing of mucosal surface with passage of large, hard stool
- Anal fistula:
  - Secondary to infection of the crypt of Morgagni.
- Perianal/perirectal abscess:
  - Bacterial (usually enteric) and inflammatory collection of fluid.

DIAGNOSIS

Dx

DIFFERENTIAL DIAGNOSIS

- Constipation with painful defecation
- Hemorrhoids (uncommon in pediatrics)
- Buttock impetigo, cellulitis, or folliculitis
- Diaper dermatitis, especially perianal with group A β-hemolytic streptococcus
- If recurrent or if multiple tracts seen, should consider inflammatory bowel disease (IBD), chronic granulomatous disease (CGD), and immune dysfunction

WORKUP

- Generally a clinical diagnosis.

LABORATORY TESTS

- In unusual or recurrent cases, neutrophil studies and T- and B-cell studies may be useful.
- Complete blood cell count (CBC), sedimentation rate, ASCA, ANCA may be warranted if IBD is suspected.

IMAGING STUDIES

- When there is a suspicion of IBD a barium enema or colonoscopy may be warranted.
- CT scan of the pelvis may be useful in complex perirectal abscesses.

TREATMENT

Rx

NONPHARMACOLOGIC THERAPY

- Anal fissure—dietary modifications to avoid constipation
- Abscesses and fistulas—sitz baths after surgical therapy
- Anal fistula:
  - Under general anesthesia a probe is inserted through the fistula until the involved crypt is identified.
  - An incision is then made along the entire length of the tract.
  - The base of the tract is then curetted.
- Perianal/perirectal abscess:
  - Superficial abscesses can be surgically drained under local anesthesia.
  - More complex abscesses require drainage under general anesthesia.
  - Packing is generally removed in 24 to 48 hours and sitz baths can begin.

ACUTE GENERAL Rx

- A short (3- to 5-day) course of antibiotics is given when cellulitis or induration is significant.
- No surgical therapy is needed for anal fissures.

DISPOSITION

- Local wound care with sitz baths until healing.
- Bowel regimen as needed to avoid constipation.
- Sphincter involvement is rare; continence is not disturbed.
- Recurrence is uncommon.
- When the abscesses are recurrent, multiple tracts are seen; if healing is not forthcoming after drainage, IBD, CGD, or immune dysfunction should be sought.

REFERRAL

In general, infants and children with possible abscess or fistula should be referred to general pediatric surgeons.

PEARLS & CONSIDERATIONS

!

COMMENTS

- Perirectal abscesses are one of three types of abscesses that require drainage despite lack of fluctuance as they enlarge (others are breast and brain).
- Consider barium enema or other imaging study (MRI or CT) if in doubt.

PATIENT/FAMILY EDUCATION

- Maintain soft, easily passed stool to avoid fissuring and painful defecation.

SUGGESTED READING

Drugas G, Pegoli W: Perirectal abscess fistula. *In* Mattei P (ed): *Surgical Directives: Pediatric Surgery.* Philadelphia, Lippincott, Williams & Wilkins, 2003, pp 425–429.

Touloukian R: Anorectal prolapse, abscess, fissure. *In* Ziegler MM, et al (eds): *Operative Pediatric Surgery.* New York, McGraw-Hill, 2003, pp 735–738.

AUTHOR: **RICHARD A. FALCONE, JR., MD**

BASIC INFORMATION

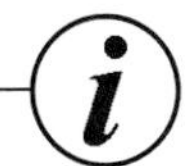

DEFINITION

Erythroid aplastic crisis is characterized by a relative failure of red blood cell production, usually in response to an infectious agent such as parvovirus.

ICD-9-CM CODES
284.8 Aplastic anemia—acquired
284.9 Aplastic anemia

EPIDEMIOLOGY & DEMOGRAPHICS

- Children with the most significant hemolysis (i.e., the shortest red cell life span or highest reticulocyte percentage) are at highest risk for aplastic crisis. Transient aplasia has little effect in persons with no hemolysis and a normal red cell life span.
- Consider in all children with chronic hemolysis (e.g., sickle cell disease, hereditary spherocytosis, pyruvate kinase deficiency) who are evaluated for febrile illnesses.
- The frequency of aplastic crisis varies with the prevalence of erythrotropic viruses. When parvovirus is prevalent, aplastic crisis is a particular risk for those with chronic hemolysis.

CLINICAL PRESENTATION

History
- Acute onset of pallor or fatigue, or both, especially in patients with a hemolytic disease.
- Fever is common, as is history of a recent febrile illness.
- Usually, no history of heightened jaundice is elicited.
- Abrupt onset in patients with hemolysis; can be life-threatening.

Physical Examination
- Tachycardia
- Pallor
- Systolic (high output) cardiac murmur

ETIOLOGY

- Parvovirus B12 is particularly erythrotropic and infects the marrow red cell precursors.
- Severe anemia occurs most commonly in patients with hemolysis who acquire viral infections (particularly parvovirus B19) that cause erythroid marrow suppression.
- In hemolytic anemias, the red cell life span can be fewer than 20 days (normal is 120 days), leading to a precipitous decrease in hemoglobin concentration if red cell production is suppressed even for a few days.
- Transient erythroid marrow failure can occur in any person infected with parvovirus or similar viruses, but with little clinical effect if the red cell life span is normal.
- Aplastic crisis may result from viruses other than parvovirus.

DIAGNOSIS

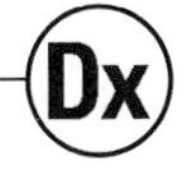

DIFFERENTIAL DIAGNOSIS

- Diamond-Blackfan syndrome
- Transient erythroblastopenia of childhood (TEC)
- Fanconi anemia (pancytopenia)
- Aplastic anemia (pancytopenia)

LABORATORY TEST(S)

- The hallmark of the diagnosis is a decrease in the baseline reticulocyte percentage.
  - Hemoglobin and hematocrit initially may be sustained, particularly if the child is dehydrated.
- Bone marrow evaluation may reveal giant proerythroblasts and a paucity of erythroid precursors compatible with parvovirus infection.
- Bone marrow recovery follows shortly after antiparvovirus antibodies are detectable in the serum.
- Viral DNA may be detectable by polymerase chain reaction (PCR) technique.

TREATMENT

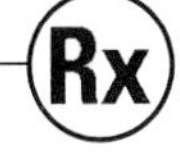

NONPHARMACOLOGIC THERAPY

- If hemodynamically stable, the patient may be observed for signs of deterioration.

ACUTE GENERAL Rx

- Transfusions may be needed for severe anemia in patients with chronic hemolysis until erythropoiesis is restored.

CHRONIC Rx

- No specific long-term therapy for aplastic crisis, which is usually self-limited.

DISPOSITION

- The erythroid aplasia caused by parvovirus is usually transient; recovery typically occurs within 1 to 2 weeks.
- Provide the usual follow-up of a patient with hemolytic disease.

REFERRAL

- Pediatric hematologist

PEARLS & CONSIDERATIONS

COMMENTS

- Note that some patients have hemolysis without anemia (e.g., mild hereditary spherocytosis).
  - The shortened red cell life span, however, makes these patients susceptible to aplastic crises.

PREVENTION

- Avoid exposure to Fifth disease.

PATIENT/FAMILY EDUCATION

- Patient and parents should understand that acute changes in appetite or activity may represent anemia in young children.
- Fever, a concern for patients with sickle cell disease because of the risk of sepsis, is also a concern for aplastic crises in children with other hemolytic anemias.

SUGGESTED READINGS

Krijanovski OI, Sieff CA: Diamond-Blackfan anemia. *Hematol Oncol Clin North Am* 11:1061, 1997.

Nathan DG, Orkin SH (eds): *Nathan and Oski's Hematology of Infancy and Childhood*, 6th ed. Philadelphia, WB Saunders, 2003.

AUTHORS: **JILL S. HALTERMAN, MD, MPH** and **GEORGE B. SEGEL, MD**

Section I DISEASES AND DISORDERS

BASIC INFORMATION

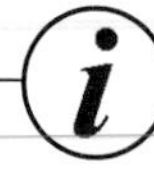

DEFINITION

Vitamin B_{12} megaloblastic anemia is associated with impaired nuclear maturation of the hematopoietic cells in the marrow. The characteristic finding in the marrow is a delay of nuclear maturation compared with cytoplasmic maturation. This may result in a macrocytic anemia, thrombocytopenia, hypersegmentation and reduction of granulocytes.

SYNONYMS

Vitamin B_{12} deficiency
Pernicious anemia

ICD-9-CM CODES
281.0 Pernicious anemia
281.1 Vitamin B_{12} deficiency anemia
281.2 Folate and B_{12} deficiency

EPIDEMIOLOGY & DEMOGRAPHICS

- The most common cause of vitamin B_{12} deficiency in infants is maternal vitamin B_{12} deficiency.
- Children who are on strict vegan diets (no milk, eggs, or animal products) are at risk for Vitamin B_{12} deficiency.
- Pernicious anemia rarely occurs in children (failure of intrinsic factor secretion due to gastric atrophy and autoimmune disease).

CLINICAL PRESENTATION

- Children may present with irritability, anorexia, and listlessness.
- Neurologic manifestations can precede megaloblastic changes and anemia and include:
  - Ataxia
  - Paresthesias
  - Hyporeflexia
  - Clonus
  - Coma
- Neurologic problems can become irreversible if not treated promptly and adequately.
- Newborns may manifest failure to thrive and slowed development even without anemia and macrocytosis.

ETIOLOGY

- Body stores of vitamin B_{12} are relatively large, and daily requirements are low.
  - Vitamin B_{12} is present in many foods, making dietary deficiency very rare.
  - However, dietary deficiency may be seen in vegans (who consume no milk, eggs, or animal products) because vegetables do not contain vitamin B_{12}.
- Newborn infants whose mothers are deficient in vitamin B_{12} may develop severe B_{12} deficiency in the first few weeks of life.
- Inborn errors of vitamin B_{12} metabolism also can cause inadequate B_{12} availability in newborns and infants.
- Vitamin B_{12} combines with intrinsic factor produced by parietal cells in the stomach and is absorbed in the terminal ileum.
- Deficiency in older children and adolescents may stem from the following:
  - Surgery or diseases involving the stomach (diminished amount of intrinsic factor) or terminal ileum (decreased absorption of B_{12})
  - Congenital lack of intrinsic factor
  - Pernicious anemia (Autoimmune antibodies may be directed to parietal cells or to intrinsic factor. Antiparietal cell antibodies are present in 85% of patients but are not specific to pernicious anemia. Anti-intrinsic factor antibodies are present in only 50%, but are specific to the disease.)
  - Human immunodeficiency virus infection (likely caused by B_{12} malabsorption secondary to small intestinal disease and infection)

DIAGNOSIS

DIFFERENTIAL DIAGNOSIS

- Megaloblastic
  - Folate deficiency
  - Thiamine deficiency (rare)
  - Dyserythropoietic anemia
  - Drugs (e.g., phenytoin, primidone, phenobarbital, pyrimethamine, trimethoprim)
  - Transcobalamin II deficiency
  - Inborn errors of metabolism (oroticaciduria, homocystinuria)
  - Myelodysplastic syndromes
- Macrocytosis
  - Hemolytic anemias with increased reticulocytes
  - Liver disease

WORKUP

- History, family history
- Complete neurologic examination to rule out signs of subacute combined degeneration

LABORATORY TESTS

- Complete blood cell count, platelet count, reticulocyte percentage
- Blood film for macro-ovalocytes, Howell-Jolly bodies (nuclear remnants), nucleated red cells, hypogranulated platelets, and hypersegmented granulocytes
- Macrocytic anemia, mean corpuscular volume greater than 100 fL/cell
- Granulocytopenia and thrombocytopenia may occur, particularly with more prolonged vitamin deficiency.
- Serum B_{12} levels are typically less than 100 pg/mL; this finding alone is not specific for vitamin B_{12} deficiency.
- Elevated serum levels of methylmalonic acid and total homocysteine, in conjunction with low serum levels of the vitamin, provide evidence of functional B_{12} deficiency.
- Children with juvenile pernicious anemia may have detectable antibodies to intrinsic factor or parietal cells and a positive Schilling test (correction of vitamin B_{12} malabsorption with administration of oral radiolabeled vitamin B_{12} and intrinsic factor).
- Marrow exam would reveal dissociation between nuclear and cytoplasmic maturation (megaloblasts and giant metamyelocytes).

TREATMENT

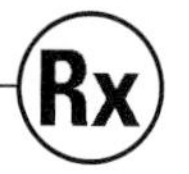

ACUTE GENERAL Rx

- Initial subcutaneous injections of 1000 μg/day of vitamin B_{12} for 7 days and then 100 μg subcutaneously weekly for 1 month are given to replenish body stores.

CHRONIC Rx

- Maintenance therapy is administered with monthly subcutaneous injections of 100 μg of vitamin B_{12}.
- For individuals with rare dietary deficiency, the requirement is 1 to 5 μg/day orally.

DISPOSITION

- Most rapid improvement occurs in the indices of ineffective erythropoiesis. Within days there is a reticulocyte increase and within 1 to 2 months the hemoglobin and hematocrit normalize.
- There is a rapid improvement in the sense of well-being within hours. However, the improvement in neurologic signs and symptoms is variable.

REFERRAL

- Referral to a hematologist and neurologist may be warranted.

PEARLS & CONSIDERATIONS

COMMENTS

- The neurologic manifestations of B_{12} deficiency can present in the absence of hematologic findings.

PREVENTION

- Dietary B_{12} deficiency can be prevented by avoiding strict vegan diets.

SUGGESTED READINGS

Nathan DG, Orkin SH (eds): *Nathan and Oski's Hematology of Infancy and Childhood*, 6th ed. Philadelphia, WB Saunders, 2003.

Rosenblatt DS, Whitehead VM: Cobalamin folate deficiency: acquired and hereditary disorders in children. *Semin Hematol* 36:19, 1999.

AUTHORS: **JILL S. HALTERMAN, MD, MPH** and **GEORGE B. SEGEL, MD**

BASIC INFORMATION

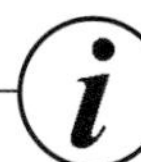

DEFINITION

- Diamond-Blackfan syndrome is a congenital pure red cell aplasia that usually presents at birth or soon thereafter.
- Anemias of erythroid failure result from the failure of the erythroid marrow to produce red cells.

SYNONYMS

Congenital hypoplastic anemia
Erythrogenesis imperfecta
Chronic congenital aregenerative anemia
Josephs-Diamond-Blackfan anemia
Blackfan-Diamond syndrome

ICD-9-CM CODES
284.0 Congenital hypoplastic anemia

EPIDEMIOLOGY & DEMOGRAPHICS

- Some 700 cases have been reported. More than 350 patients are enrolled in the Diamond-Blackfan Anemia (DBA) registry of North America.
- Fifty percent of children are diagnosed by 2 months of age, 75% are diagnosed by 6 months, and 90% by 1 year of age.
- Familial occurrence, with both autosomal dominant and autosomal recessive patterns, is described in approximately 20% of patients, suggesting a genetic basis for the disease in some families.
- There is a predisposition to hematopoietic and other malignancy.

CLINICAL PRESENTATION

History

- Children most commonly present with progressive anemia within the first 2 to 6 months of age.
  - Poor feedings
  - Easy fatigue
  - Pallor
  - Lethargy or fretfulness

Physical Examination

- Increased heart rate
- Systolic murmur
- Pallor
- Congenital abnormalities (in approximately 30% of patients)
  - Dysmorphic facies such as orofacial clefts
  - Defects of the upper extremities
  - Short stature

ETIOLOGY

- Diamond-Blackfan syndrome is a severe aregenerative anemia often associated with other congenital anomalies.
- The genetic basis remains unclear, but approximately 25% of patients have some mutation in the gene DBA1, that codes for RPS 19, a ribosomal protein.
- The disease may be related to haploinsufficiency of the protein product. How this relates to the accelerated erythroid apoptosis and erythroid failure is unclear.

DIAGNOSIS

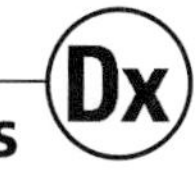

DIFFERENTIAL DIAGNOSIS

- Transient erythroblastopenia of childhood (TEC)
- Aplastic crises in patients with hemolytic anemias
- Fanconi anemia (pancytopenia)
- Aplastic anemia (pancytopenia)

LABORATORY TESTS

- Severely low hemoglobin and hematocrit are noted.
- Blood film reveals macrocytosis, anisocytosis, and teardrop cells.
- Marked reticulocytopenia (less than 0.5%) is observed.
- The red cells have elevated fetal hemoglobin (HbF), increased expression of the "i" antigen, and elevated adenosine deaminase.
- White blood cell and platelet counts usually are normal.
- Marrow evaluation reveals erythroid hypoplasia or total erythroid aplasia.

TREATMENT

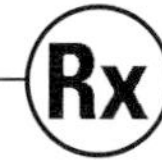

ACUTE GENERAL Rx

- Glucocorticoids are the mainstay of therapy.
  - Initial dosage of prednisone is 2 mg/kg/day. This dose may be titrated up or down to achieve an ongoing therapeutic effect.
- Blood transfusions may be needed for glucocorticoid-resistant patients.
- Other therapies include danazol (attenuated androgen), 6-mercaptopurine, cyclophosphamide, and hematopoietic growth factors, but their value is not established.

CHRONIC Rx

- For many patients, prednisone is needed lifelong. Few remit and do not require future therapy.
- The anemia is progressive and usually requires repeated transfusions if drug therapy is not administered.
- Iron chelation eventually will be necessary if the patient requires chronic transfusions.
- Marrow transplantation may be considered for patients who do not respond to glucocorticoids.

DISPOSITION

- The patients with the best prognosis are those who respond well to glucocorticoid therapy (approximately 50%).
- Approximately one third require chronic transfusions.
- Approximately 15% of patients undergo spontaneous remission.
- An elevated risk of leukemia and other cancers is present.

REFERRAL

- All patients with progressive anemia and severe reticulocytopenia should be referred to a pediatric hematologist.

PEARLS & CONSIDERATIONS

COMMENTS

- The diagnosis of Diamond-Blackfan syndrome is unlikely if the reticulocyte percentage is higher than 0.5%.

PATIENT/FAMILY EDUCATION

- Information for families is available through the Diamond-Blackfan Anemia Foundation.
  www.dbafoundation.org
  info@dbafoundation.org
  DBA Foundation
  PO Box 1092
  West Seneca, NY 14224

SUGGESTED READINGS

Da Costa L, et al: Diamond-Blackfan anemia. *Curr Opin Pediatr* 13:10, 2001.
Nathan DG, Orkin SH (eds): *Nathan and Oski's Hematology of Infancy and Childhood*, 6th ed. Philadelphia, WB Saunders, 2003.
Vlachos A, et al: The Diamond-Blackfan Anemia Registry. *J Pediatr Hematol Oncol.* 23:377, 2001.

AUTHORS: **JILL S. HALTERMAN, MD, MPH** and **GEORGE B. SEGEL, MD**

BASIC INFORMATION

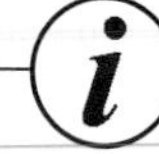

DEFINITION

Folate deficiency megaloblastic anemia is associated with impaired nuclear maturation of the hematopoietic cells in the marrow. The characteristic finding in the marrow is a delay of nuclear maturation compared with cytoplasmic maturation. This may result in a macrocytic anemia, thrombocytopenia, and hypersegmentation and reduction of granulocytes.

ICD-9-CM CODES
281.2 Folate deficiency anemia

EPIDEMIOLOGY & DEMOGRAPHICS

- Body stores of folic acid are small in comparison to daily requirements; therefore deficiency may result relatively quickly from inadequate folate intake or poor folate absorption.
- Folate requirements are greatest per kilogram in newborn infants, young children, and pregnant and lactating women.
- Other groups with increased folate requirements are those with malabsorption syndromes, premature infants, children receiving chronic antiepileptic therapy, and children with chronic hemolysis with or without anemia.
- Human and cow's milk provide adequate amounts of folic acid; goat's milk contains very little folic acid.

In adolescents and adults, chronic alcoholism and inadequate diet may result in folic acid deficiency.

CLINICAL PRESENTATION

History

- Goat's milk ingestion
- Chronic diarrhea (malabsorption)
- Failure to gain weight

ETIOLOGY

- Decreased dietary folate intake: goat's milk, alcoholism
- Malabsorption: celiac disease, inflammatory bowel disease, short gut syndromes

DIAGNOSIS

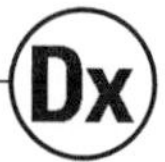

DIFFERENTIAL DIAGNOSIS

- Megaloblastic: vitamin B_{12} deficiency, rarely thiamine deficiency, dyserythropoietic anemia, drugs, transcobalamin II deficiency, inborn errors of metabolism (oroticaciduria, homocystinuria), myelodysplastic syndromes
- Pernicious anemia
- Macrocytosis: hemolytic anemias with increased reticulocytes, liver disease

WORKUP

- Family history
  - Complete neurologic examination to rule out signs of subacute combined degeneration in B_{12} deficiency

LABORATORY TESTS

- Complete blood cell count, platelet count, reticulocyte percentage
  - In more severe deficiency, laboratory evaluation reveals a macrocytic anemia with a mean corpuscular volume greater than 100 fL/cell.
- Review of blood film for macro-ovalocytes, Howell-Jolly bodies (nuclear remnants), nucleated red cells, hypogranulated platelets, and hypersegmented granulocytes
- Granulocytopenia and thrombocytopenia may be present.
- Low serum folate (less than 3 ng/mL; normal, 5 to 20 ng/mL), in addition to low red cell folate
  - Mild folate deficiency can be detected by a decrease in red cell folate.
- Marrow exam would reveal dissociation between nuclear and cytoplasmic maturation (megaloblasts and giant metamyelocytes).
- Total plasma homocysteine level is increased above normal in most patients with folate deficiency.
- Concomitant vitamin B_{12} deficiency must be ruled out because treatment with folic acid may mask the diagnosis of B_{12} deficiency by correcting the hematologic findings. Such children would remain at risk for the neurologic manifestations of vitamin B_{12} deficiency.

TREATMENT

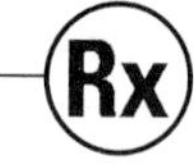

NONPHARMACOLOGIC THERAPY

- Dietary insufficiency should be corrected to provide adequate folate intake.

ACUTE GENERAL Rx

- Treatment is initiated with physiologic quantities of folate (50 to 100 μg/day) and monitoring of the reticulocyte percentage.
- Reticulocytosis should occur after the first week of treatment if folate deficiency was present.
- Therapy consists of 1 mg/day of folic acid.
- Larger amounts of folate (5 mg/day) may be needed for children with malabsorption.

CHRONIC Rx

- Continue folate if malabsorption not effectively resolved
- Treat for other associated problems (alcoholism)

DISPOSITION

- Follow-up based on etiology and ongoing associated medical or psychological problems.

REFERRAL

- For patients with megaloblastic anemia caused by folate deficiency, both hematology and gastroenterology consultations may be reasonable.

PEARLS & CONSIDERATIONS

COMMENTS

- Supplement with folic acid if patient is a known goat's milk drinker.
- All patients with chronic hemolysis should receive supplemental folic acid.
- Alcoholism is a major underlying factor in folate deficiency in adolescents and older patients.

SUGGESTED READINGS

Nathan DG, Orkin SH (eds): *Nathan and Oski's Hematology of Infancy and Childhood*, 6th ed. Philadelphia, WB Saunders, 2003.

Rosenblatt DS, Whitehead VM: Cobalamin and folate deficiency: acquired and hereditary disorders in children. *Semin Hematol* 36:19, 1999.

AUTHORS: **JILL S. HALTERMAN, MD, MPH** and **GEORGE B. SEGEL, MD**

BASIC INFORMATION

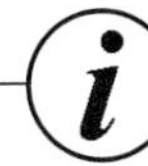

DEFINITION

Iron deficiency anemia is caused by insufficient iron for the normal formation of hemoglobin.

ICD-9-CM CODES

280.9 Iron deficiency anemia, unspecified

EPIDEMIOLOGY & DEMOGRAPHICS

- Iron deficiency is the most prevalent hematologic disorder in childhood.
- Affects 5% to 10% of infants.
- Infants who consume large amounts of cow's milk as well as foods not supplemented with iron may develop dietary iron deficiency.
- Cow's milk contains essentially no iron.
- Excessive intake of cow's milk impairs adequate intake of other foods rich in iron.
- Proteins in the cow's milk may cause bleeding from irritation of the gastrointestinal (GI) tract in infants, compounding iron deficiency.
- The small amount of iron in breast milk is absorbed efficiently but is not sufficient for the growing infant after 6 months.

CLINICAL PRESENTATION

History

- Pallor may be apparent.
- When anemia is severe (hemoglobin < 5 g/dL), of irritability, anorexia, and exertional intolerance, reflect the systemic effects of iron deficiency.
- Pica may include consumption of laundry starch, ice, and soil clay.
- Iron deficiency with or without concomitant anemia impairs growth and intellectual development in children.

Physical Examination

- Tachycardia, pallor, irritability, systolic murmur, growth failure, developmental delay

ETIOLOGY

- Iron deficiency may be caused by insufficient dietary intake, GI or other bleeding, or rarely, chronic intravascular hemolysis and urinary iron loss.
- Iron deficiency is common from 9 to 24 months of age because iron stores are depleted during periods of accelerated growth.
- Adolescent girls also may develop iron deficiency because of poor dietary intake, high iron requirements related to rapid growth, and menstrual blood loss.
- Blood loss must be considered, particularly in the older child who is likely to have adequate dietary intake.
  - The most common location for blood loss is the GI tract.
  - Rarely, iron loss may result from bleeding into the lungs (idiopathic pulmonary hemosiderosis or Goodpasture's syndrome) or urinary tract.
- Rare iron malabsorption syndromes occur.

DIAGNOSIS

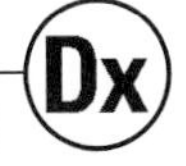

DIFFERENTIAL DIAGNOSIS

- Other causes of hypochromic, microcytic anemias (see Anemia in Section IV).
- β-Thalassemia trait
  - Elevated hemoglobin A_2
  - Mentzer index (mean corpuscular volume/red blood cell count, MCV/RBC) less than 13
- Anemia of chronic inflammatory disease
  - Low iron and iron-binding capacity
  - Normal or increased ferritin
- Lead poisoning
  - Dietary iron deficiency and elevated lead often occur together.

LABORATORY TESTS

- Low serum ferritin (<10 ng/ml).
  - Ferritin may be high in inflammatory states.
- A decrease in serum iron (<30 μg/dL).
- Iron-binding capacity is increased (>350 μg/dL).
- Subsequently, the percentage of iron saturation falls to less than 15%.
- Accumulation of heme precursors results in an elevated free erythrocyte protoporphyrin.
- As iron deficiency progresses, the MCV falls the hemoglobin content decreases, and the RBC becomes deformed.
- Iron deficiency alters the red cell size unevenly, leading to an elevated red cell distribution width (RDW).
- The Mentzer index is high in:
  - Iron deficiency: greater than 13
  - Thalassemia: less than 13
- The reticulocyte percentage is typically normal or slightly elevated.
- Thrombocytosis or thrombocytopenia.

TREATMENT

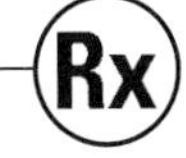

NONPHARMACOLOGIC THERAPY

- Limit cow's milk intake to 16 oz/day in young children.

ACUTE GENERAL Rx

- Ferrous salts should be administered orally until the hemoglobin and hematocrit levels are normal. This can be administered as ferrous sulfate (6 mg/kg elemental iron in three divided doses for infants and children) or as one of the new iron polysaccharide complexes that can be administered once a day.
  - Iron is better absorbed if given between meals.
  - Juices containing ascorbic acid increase iron absorption.
  - Cow's milk and tannins in tea decrease iron absorption.
- Therapy should be continued for an additional 1 to 2 months after the hemoglobin and hematocrit levels are normal to replenish iron stores.
- Parenteral iron is available but is rarely indicated.
  - Administered with careful observation for local and systemic allergic reactions.
  - Newer parenteral iron preparations appear to have fewer side effects.
- Transfusions should be reserved for profoundly anemic children.
  - If needed, give transfusions slowly.
  - Consider diuretics or exchange transfusion to prevent hypervolemia and cardiac compromise.

PEARLS & CONSIDERATIONS

COMMENTS

- A "trial of iron therapy" may be warranted in infants younger than 2 years of age, when dietary iron deficiency is common.
- Test stool for occult blood in all children to ensure that there is no GI blood loss.
- In children older than 2 years, a more extensive evaluation is needed.
- Poor response to oral iron therapy may represent problems with adherence, poor absorption, continuing unrecognized blood loss, or an incorrect diagnosis.
- Black stools are observed soon after the initiation of ferrous sulfate therapy and can serve as an index of adherence.
- Iron deficiency increases the rate of uptake of both iron and lead from the GI tract. Therefore iron deficiency and lead intoxication often occur together.

PREVENTION

- Dietary iron deficiency can be prevented by avoiding excessive cow's milk consumption.
- Adequate iron replacement is recommended in menstruating females.

SUGGESTED READINGS

Booth IW, Aukett MA: Iron deficiency anemia in infancy and early childhood. *Arch Dis Child* 76:549, 1997.

Nathan DG, Orkin SH (eds): *Nathan and Oski's Hematology of Infancy and Childhood*, 6th ed. Philadelphia, WB Saunders, 2003.

Provan D: Mechanisms and management of iron deficiency anemia. *Br J Hematol* 105(Suppl 1):19, 1999.

AUTHORS: **JILL S. HALTERMAN, MD, MPH** and **GEORGE B. SEGEL, MD**

BASIC INFORMATION

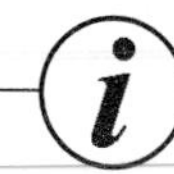

DEFINITION

Transient erythroblastopenia of childhood (TEC) is a severe, slowly developing, transient inability of the erythroid marrow to produce red blood cells (hypoplastic anemia). The other cell lines are not affected.

SYNONYMS

TEC
Anemia of erythroid failure
Aplastic anemia, acquired

ICD-9-CM CODES
284.8 Acquired aplastic anemia

EPIDEMIOLOGY & DEMOGRAPHICS

- This disease mainly affects previously healthy children at 6 months to 5 years of age: the mean age of presentation is 2 years.
  - It has been reported in patients less than age 6 months and as old as 10 years.
  - More than 600 cases have been reported, but without specific gender, ethnic, or known genetic factors.
- A history of a preceding viral illness is often present, but such illnesses are common in children of this age range.
- Patients do not have congenital anomalies as in Diamond-Blackfan syndrome, and there is no evidence for toxic, immune, or specific viral causes.

CLINICAL PRESENTATION

History

- Progressive onset of pallor
- Symptoms related to progressive anemia include:
  - Fatigue, irritability
  - Vague decrease in activity or feeding
  - Potential heart failure with edema and respiratory symptoms

Physical Examination

- Usually normal except for pallor and signs of anemia (e.g., congenital pallor, elevated heart rate, systolic flow murmur).
- Splenomegaly is not present.
- Malformations (e.g., craniofacial, skeletal, and genitourinary anomalies) suggest Diamond-Blackfan anemia.

ETIOLOGY

- An uncommon disease of unknown origin that results in transient acquired erythroid marrow failure.
- Immunologic and viral causes have been suggested but not substantiated.
- Rare familial cases may be related to the DBA RPS19 gene locus.

DIAGNOSIS

DIFFERENTIAL DIAGNOSIS

- Diamond-Blackfan syndrome
- Aplastic anemia (pan bone marrow suppression)
- Fanconi anemia
- Aplastic crisis (seen when underlying hemolytic disorder exists)
- Iron deficiency anemia
- Other forms of anemia (hemolytic, megaloblastic)

LABORATORY TESTS

- Children slowly develop a normochromic, normocytic anemia with marked reticulocytopenia.
  - The mean hemoglobin level is 6 g/dL; the reticulocyte percentage is usually below 0.5%, unless the patient is recovering.
  - The mean corpuscular volume is normal.
  - The white blood cell and platelet counts are normal in most cases.
- 20% have mild neutropenia.
- Marrow contains few red blood cell precursors, unless the patient is recovering.
- No specific diagnostic test is available.
  - In contrast to Diamond-Blackfan anemia, fetal hemoglobin (HbF) levels and adenosine deaminase levels are normal.
- Check Parvovirus and other viral titers if underlying hemolysis is suspected.

TREATMENT

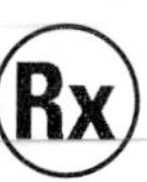

NONPHARMACOLOGIC THERAPY

- Watchful waiting is appropriate if no signs of congestive heart failure, respiratory distress, or growth failure are present.
- Spontaneous remission usually occurs within months.

ACUTE GENERAL Rx

- Red cell transfusions may be required for children with severe anemia in the absence of signs of early recovery.
- Glucocorticoid therapy is not helpful.

DISPOSITION

- Recurrence of the disease is rare.

REFERRAL

- Referral to a hematologist is warranted.

PEARLS & CONSIDERATIONS

COMMENTS

- Although TEC and Diamond-Blackfan syndrome can have similar presentations, patients with TEC are usually older than 1 year of age.
- The level of reticulocyte depression cannot be used to distinguish between TEC and Diamond-Blackfan syndrome.
- In other marrow failure syndromes the reticulocyte percentage may not be as profoundly depressed.

PREVENTION

- No known preventive measures

SUGGESTED READINGS

Nathan DG, Orkin SH (eds): *Nathan and Oski's Hematology of Infancy and Childhood*, 6th ed. Philadelphia, WB Saunders, 2003.

AUTHORS: **JILL S. HALTERMAN, MD, MPH** and **GEORGE B. SEGEL, MD**

BASIC INFORMATION

DEFINITION

Bites may occur from a variety of animals including dogs, cats, and rodents; most are minor and do not require medical attention. An animal bite is medically significant when the injury is severe, if cosmetic appearance or infection of the wound is a concern, or when rabies or tetanus prophylaxis is indicated.

SYNONYMS

Dog bite
Cat bite

ICD-9-CM CODES

879.8 Open wound

EPIDEMIOLOGY & DEMOGRAPHICS

- The true incidence is unknown as most bites are trivial and do not require medical care. An estimated 2 million animal bites occur annually. In 2001, an estimated 368,245 persons were treated in U.S. hospital emergency departments for dog-bite related injuries.
- Children (aged 5 to 9 years) are the most common victims. Younger children are more likely to be male.
- Animal bites tend to occur most often in warm climates or during warm seasons. The majority of dog and cat bites occur with domestic pets. Non-neutered male dogs and aggressive breeds of dogs typically pose a greater risk.

CLINICAL PRESENTATION

- Identify the specific animal involved, including its whereabouts and immunization status, to consider need for antibiotic and rabies prophylaxis.
- Determine the time elapsed since the injury, which is an important factor in infection control and wound closure.
- Describe the location and type of wound.
- Search for underlying structural damage including neurovascular or tendon injury, joint involvement, and fractures. (Dog bites are most commonly associated with significant occult injury.)
- Bites may result in lacerations, puncture wounds, and superficial abrasions as well as underlying structural damage.

ETIOLOGY

- The most common perpetrators of animal bites are dogs, which account for 80% to 90% of animal bites.
- Wound infections are frequently polymicrobial; *Pasteurella multocida* and *Staphylococcus aureus* are commonly implicated organisms.

DIAGNOSIS

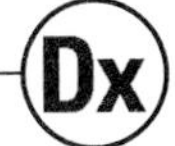

DIFFERENTIAL DIAGNOSIS

- Human bite
- Other penetrating trauma

WORKUP

- The diagnosis of an animal bite is usually made based on information from history and physical examination.

LABORATORY TESTS

- No routine laboratory tests are indicated.
- Cultures of a noninfected bite are not helpful in predicting the likelihood or etiology of subsequent infections.

IMAGING STUDIES

- Consider the need for radiographic imaging to evaluate for underlying fractures, particularly with dog bites of the scalp.

TREATMENT

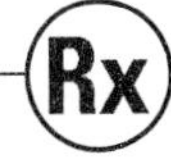

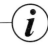

NONPHARMACOLOGIC THERAPY

- Copious irrigation, wound cleansing, and débridement should be performed and may prevent infectious complications.
- Fresh nonpuncture wounds can be sutured. Contaminated wounds and puncture wounds should not be closed.
- Tendon or vascular injury should be identified and repaired as needed.

ACUTE GENERAL Rx

- Antibiotic prophylaxis is controversial. Generally, prophylaxis should be considered for dog bites that are more than 12 hours old, difficult to clean, in the hand or foot, or in an infection-susceptible patient. All cat bites should receive prophylaxis.
- Amoxicillin/clavulanate is considered first-line antibiotic prophylaxis.
- Update the patient's tetanus status if needed.
- Consider the need for rabies prophylaxis.

CHRONIC Rx

- Three to five days of antibiotic prophylaxis may be adequate, if indicated. Wounds should be closely monitored for signs of infection.

DISPOSITION

- Most patients can be treated as outpatients. Patients with extensive injury may require hospitalization and long-term cosmetic follow-up.
- Follow-up in 24 to 48 hours is useful to monitor for infection.

REFERRAL

- Extensive injury, underlying structural damage, or a cosmetically concerning location may require surgical consultation.
- Follow-up may be indicated for the psychological effects of these traumatic injuries.

PEARLS & CONSIDERATIONS

COMMENTS

- Remember to evaluate for occult injury.
- Infection is the most common complication of animal bites; prevention is crucial for a good long-term outcome.
- Bites to the hand and puncture wounds (typically from cats) are the most likely animal bites to become infected.
- Consider cosmetic and psychological issues.

PREVENTION

- Supervise all children around animals.
- Socialize and appropriately train household pets.
- Consult with a professional before choosing a pet.
- Teach children basic safety around animals.

PATIENT/FAMILY EDUCATION

- Advise patients regarding the risk and signs of infection as well as the need to seek immediate medical care if infection occurs.
- Additional information regarding treatment of animal bites is available at the following Mayo Clinic web site: www.mayoclinic.com/health/first_aid_animal_bites
- Additional information regarding dog bite prevention is available at the following Centers for Disease Control web site: www.cdc.gov/ncipc/duip/biteprevention.htm

SUGGESTED READINGS

Centers for Disease Control: Nonfatal dog bite-related injuries treated in hospital emergency departments—United States. *MMWR* 52:605, 2003.

Garcia VF: Animal bites and *Pasteurella* infections. *Pediatr Rev* 18:127, 1997.

Talan DA et al: Bacteriologic analysis of infected dog and cat bites. *N Engl J Med* 340:85, 1999.

AUTHORS: **LETICIA MANNING RYAN, MD** and **ROBERT J. FREISHTAT, MD, MPH**

BASIC INFORMATION

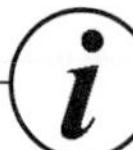

DEFINITION

An ankle sprain is an injury to the ankle caused by a sudden twisting motion that stretches or tears the supporting ligaments.

SYNONYMS

Sprained ankle
Twisted ankle
Wrenched or turned ankle

ICD-9-CM CODE
845.0 Sprain, ankle

EPIDEMIOLOGY & DEMOGRAPHICS

- Thirty million children in the United States participate in organized sports programs.
- The annual cost, including health care and lost time at work, have been estimated to be as high as $1.8 billion.
- More than 2 million people in the United States sustain ankle injuries every year.
- On average, individuals experience two to three ankle injuries in a lifetime.
- Ankle sprains account for 12% of all injuries seen in emergency departments.
- In the athletic population, ankle injuries are the most common injury, accounting for 15% of all musculoskeletal injuries.
  - Basketball has the highest incidence of ankle sprains (40% of all their injuries), followed by football, volleyball, soccer, and cross-country running.
- Sports with the highest ankle sprain injury rates emphasize jumping, cutting, or running on uneven ground.
- Most ankle injuries occur in people 21 to 30 years old.
  - Injuries in younger age groups tend to be more serious.
- Of all ankle injuries, 85% are ankle sprains.
  - Five percent are eversion injuries.
  - Ten percent involve the syndesmosis.

CLINICAL PRESENTATION

History

- Consider the time since the injury.
- Assess the patient's ability to bear weight immediately and later.
  - Able to continue the game?
  - Able to walk off the field?
- Consider the mechanism of injury.
  - A lateral ankle sprain occurs with the foot in plantar-flexion with an inversion force applied. The patient describes "rolling" the foot under.
  - A deltoid sprain occurs with the foot in dorsiflexion with an eversion force applied, such as when a wrestler tries to get a wider stance on the mat.
  - A syndesmosis injury occurs when the foot is forcibly rotated, such as in football when a player falls on top of the ankle of another player who is lying prone.
- Was a "pop" or "snap" heard?
- What was the site of initial pain and swelling?
- Is there a history of previous injury and treatment?

Physical Examination

- It is best to examine the patient as soon as possible after the injury.
  - Pain, swelling, and ecchymosis increase with time, making examination more difficult.
- Inspect for swelling, ecchymosis, and deformity.
- Assess skin integrity.
- Assess neurovascular integrity.
- Range of motion may be limited because of pain; attempt active and passive assessment of the following six cardinal movements:
  - Dorsiflexion
  - Dorsiflexion with inversion and eversion
  - Plantar-flexion
  - Plantar-flexion with inversion and eversion
- Palpate the following areas that are most often injured during ankle trauma:
  - Entire length of the fibula
  - Malleoli
  - Base of the fifth metatarsal
  - Navicular
  - Peroneal tendons behind the lateral malleolus
  - Anterior, medial, and lateral joint lines
  - Achilles tendon
- Point tenderness or crepitation may indicate a fracture.
- Palpate ankle ligaments.
  - The anterior talofibular ligament (ATFL) is palpated two fingerbreadths anteroinferior to the lateral malleolus.
  - The calcaneofibular ligament (CFL) is palpated two fingerbreadths inferior to the lateral malleolus.
  - The posterior talofibular ligament (PTFL) is palpated posteroinferior to the posterior edge of the lateral malleolus.
- The anterior drawer test is performed as follows:
  - Place the patient's ankle in a neutral position with the knee flexed at 90 degrees.
  - Place one hand 3 inches above the ankle joint to stabilize the tibia-fibula.
  - Grip the heel with the other hand to apply anterior force.
  - If there is more than a 5-mm difference from the uninjured side, it indicates an incompetent ATFL ligament.
- The talar tilt test is performed with the patient and examiner in the same position as the anterior drawer test.
  - The hand that cups the heel applies an inversion force in neutral and 20-degree plantar-flexion.
  - If the head of the talus is felt laterally, the ATFL and CFL are incompetent.
- To test the tibiofibular syndesmosis, perform the following actions:
  - Interlace the fingers together behind the distal third of the calf.
  - Use the heels of the hands to squeeze the tibia and fibula together.
  - If there is a tear in the syndesmosis or a fibula fracture, the patient will experience pain with squeeze and release of squeeze.
- Assess the ability to bear weight or walk.
- Perform a modified Romberg's test to evaluate balance and proprioception.
  - Have the patient balance on the injured leg with the eyes closed.

ETIOLOGY

- A traumatic event, such as twisting or rapidly rotating about the talar or subtalar joints
  - Causes the ankle joint to move outside its normal range of movement
  - Causes supporting ligaments to stretch or tear

DIAGNOSIS

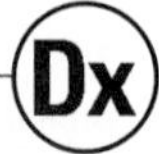

DIFFERENTIAL DIAGNOSIS

- Fractures should be considered; 15% of all ankle injuries have an associated fracture.
- Prepubescent children are at risk for physeal injury because the ligaments are stronger than the physis at this age.
- Be suspicious of prepubescent "ankle sprains."
- Consider peroneal tendon injuries:
  - The patient experiences point tenderness behind the lateral malleolus and pain on dorsiflexion.
  - Achilles tendinitis or rupture consists of local tenderness, crepitus, and pain on passive dorsiflexion and resisted plantar-flexion.
  - The patient may hear a "pop" and notice weakness on plantar-flexion.
  - If the tendon is completely ruptured, the foot will not plantar-flex when the calf is squeezed (i.e., positive Thompson's test).

WORKUP

- Three independent factors are significantly associated with ankle fractures in adults:
  - Inability to walk immediately after the traumatic event
  - Inability to bear weight for four steps in the emergency department
  - Tender deltoid ligament
- If one or more of these factors were present, the sensitivity for predicting ankle fractures was 93%, and the specificity was 27%.
  - The sensitivity for applying the Ottawa rules in children was 83%, and the specificity was 50%; therefore, the Ottawa rules cannot be applied to children with the same sensitivity as in adult cases.
  - Indications for an ankle radiograph (Fig. 22-1) are known as the Ottawa rules.

- Pain in the area of the malleoli *and* one of the following:
  - Inability to bear weight (four steps)
  - Bony tenderness at the posterior edge of the distal tibia or fibula
- A foot radiograph is necessary if there is pain in the area of the midfoot *and* one of the following:
  - Inability to bear weight (four steps)
  - Bony tenderness of the navicular or the base of the fifth metatarsal
- Arthroscopy may be useful to evaluate persistent ankle pain.

IMAGING STUDIES

- For mild to moderate ankle sprains, stress x-ray films are usually unnecessary.
- Stress radiographs to rule out ligamentous rupture may also be needed for prolonged pain and dysfunction after a typical healing period.
  - The anterior drawer test is performed as lateral views are taken. (The test result is considered abnormal if anterior subluxation of the talus is greater than 6 mm.)
  - The talar tilt test is performed as the mortise view is taken. (Any talar tilt of more than 5 degrees is considered abnormal.)
- Computed tomography (CT), and magnetic resonance imaging (MRI) may be useful in the evaluation of persistent chronic ankle pain after an acute sprain.
- MRI may be especially useful if a double ligament tear is suspected and surgery is being considered.

TREATMENT

Rx

NONPHARMACOLOGIC THERAPY

PRICEMMS (**p**rotection, **r**est, **i**ce, **c**ompression, **e**levation, **m**edication, **m**obilization, **s**trengthening) is an extension of the commonly used mnemonic RICE (**r**est, **i**ce, **c**ompression, **e**levation):

- **P** = Protection from further injury
  - Air stirrup is used to allow dorsiflexion and plantar-flexion and to limit inversion and eversion.
  - Stirrups should be used continuously during the initial phases of healing.
- **R** = Relative rest
  - Do nothing that hurts.
  - Use crutches if needed.
- **I** = Ice is effective as long as there is swelling. Cold should be applied for at least 20 minutes, four times each day.
- **C** = Compression dressings (most useful in the first 48 to 72 hours)
  - Do not obstruct distal venous return.
  - Use an elastic wrap bandage, Unna boot, or air stirrup.
- **E** = Elevation (optimally above the level of the heart)
- **M** = Medications (analgesics and anti-inflammatory agents)
- **M** = Mobilization (start after an initial 24- to 72-hour period of rest)
  - Active plantar-flexion and dorsiflexion: ankle pumps
  - Writing the alphabet in the air with the big toe: alphabets
  - Rising up on toes and lowering heel back down: heel raises
- **S** = Strength training of the peroneal and gastrocnemius muscles (start as soon as possible to minimize deconditioning)

ACUTE GENERAL Rx

Analgesia and anti-inflammatory agents as discussed above.

CHRONIC Rx

This is addressed below in "Disposition".

DISPOSITION

- A grading system for ankle ligament injuries is based on the degree of injury of each ligament and helps predict the return to full activities (Table 1-1).
- The goal of rehabilitation is to regain full strength, range of motion, and proprioception while minimizing the loss of cardiovascular fitness.
- Isometric exercises used to strengthen the peroneals involve pushing the lateral aspect of the forefoot against a fixed surface.
- Using a series of rubber bands of graduated strengths provides isotonic exercises for strengthening dorsiflexors and evertors.
- Range of motion incorporates ankle pumps and alphabets.
- A progressive walking program should be initiated after 10 toe raises have been accomplished:
  - Walk on a circular track for 20 minutes per day.
  - Then walk the curved portion and jog the straight portion.
  - Then jog the entire track.
- Proprioceptive retraining is achieved by standing on one foot with and then without support.
  - The next step is balancing with eyes closed with and without support.
  - When balance is maintained for 2 to 3 minutes, proprioception is recovered.
- After the athlete is ready to return to practice, he or she should start with simple drills and progress to a level without restrictions.
- All exercises should be performed with a protective brace because this support improves proprioceptive feedback.
  - The benefit of ankle taping diminishes with exercise. The more exercise, the less taping is effective, because the tape loosens and does not limit range of motion adequately.
  - There is good evidence for the beneficial effect of ankle supports in the form of semirigid orthoses or Aircast braces to prevent ankle sprains during high-risk sporting activities by reducing ankle inversion, and they may be preferred over taping.
  - High-top sneakers significantly increase the passive resistance to inversion and may be advisable for children predisposed to ankle sprains, although the protective effect of these shoes remains to be established.

REFERRAL

- Orthopedic consultation should be considered for all patients with third-degree ankle sprains.
- Consider sports medicine or physical therapy referrals.

PEARLS & CONSIDERATIONS

COMMENTS

- The Ottawa rules offer guidelines for determining when ankle radiographs are necessary.

TABLE 1-1 **Ankle Sprain Grading**

Severity	Pathology	Signs and Symptoms	Disability	Stress Examination
Grade 1	Ligament stretch	Minimal swelling, small area of tenderness, little or no hemorrhage, minimal decreased range of motion	Little or no limp with walking, difficulty hopping, expected 7-10 days with rehabilitation	Normal
Grade 2	Partial ligament tear	Moderate swelling, more generalized tenderness, some hemorrhage, decreased range of motion	Limping with walking, unable to hop/run/toe raise, expected recovery 2-4 weeks with rehabilitation	Anterior drawer and Talar tilt tests may be positive or negative
Grade 3	Complete ligament tear	Diffuse swelling, diffuse tenderness, evident hemorrhage, pronounced decreased range of motion	Unable to bear weight, expected recovery 5-10 weeks with rehabilitation	Anterior drawer and Talar tilt tests positive

- Be very suspicious of prepubescent ankle sprains.
- The essential elements for the management of ankle sprains may be remembered by the use of the mnemonic *PRICEMMS.*

PREVENTION

Excellent strengthening and stretching with appropriate attention to proprioception. Use of ankle support brace (see Disposition above) in children and adolescents may be beneficial in decreasing injury.

SUGGESTED READINGS

Adamson C, Cymet T: Ankle sprains: evaluation, treatment, rehabilitation. *Md Med J* 46:530, 1997.

Adirim TA, Cheng TL: Overview of injuries in the young athlete. *Sports Med* 33:75, 2003.

Allerston J, Justham D: A case-control study of the transit times through an accident and emergency department of ankle injured patients assessed using the Ottawa ankle rules. *Accid Emerg Nurs* 8:148, 2000.

Bennett WF: Lateral ankle sprains. Part I. Anatomy, biomechanics, diagnosis, and natural history. *Orthop Rev* 23:381, 1994.

Bennett WF: Lateral ankle sprains. Part II. Acute and chronic treatment. *Orthop Rev* 23:504, 1994.

Chorley J, Hergenroeder A: Management of ankle sprains. *Pediatr Ann* 26:56, 1997.

Clark KD, Tanner S: Evaluation of the Ottawa ankle rules in children. *Pediatr Emerg Care* 19:73, 2003.

Fallat L et al: Sprained ankle syndrome: prevalence and analysis of 639 acute injuries. *J Foot Ankle Surg* 37:280, 1998.

Handoll HH et al: Interventions for preventing ankle ligament injuries. *Cochrane Database Syst Rev* (3):CD000018, 2001.

Karpas A et al: Utilization of the Ottawa ankle rules by nurses in a pediatric emergency department. *Acad Emerg Med* 9:130, 2002.

Kuwada G: Current concepts in the diagnosis and treatment of ankle sprains. *Clin Podiatr Med Surg* 12:653, 1995.

Lord J, Winell JJ: Overuse injuries in pediatric athletes. *Curr Opin Pediatr* 16:47, 2004.

MDConsult. Available at www.mdconsult.com

MedScope. Available at www.medscope.com

Pigman E et al: Evaluation of the Ottawa clinical decision rules for the use of radiography in acute ankle and midfoot injuries in the emergency department: an independent site assessment. *Ann Emerg Med* 24:41, 1994.

Quinn K et al: Interventions for preventing ankle ligament injuries. *Cochrane Database Syst Rev* (2): CD000018, 2000.

Shapiro M et al: Ankle sprain prophylaxis: an analysis of the stabilizing effects of braces and tape. *Am J Sports Med* 22:78, 1994.

WebMD. Available at www.webmd.com

AUTHOR: **MARC S. LAMPELL, MD, FAAP, FACEP**

BASIC INFORMATION

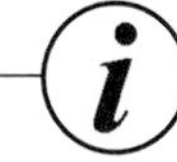

DEFINITION

Juvenile ankylosing spondylitis (JAS) is a chronic arthropathy, which includes chronic inflammation of the sacroiliac joints (SIJs), spine, peripheral joints, and entheses (i.e., tendon, ligament, and fascia insertion to bone). It is the prototype of the spondyloarthropathies. These enthesitis-related arthritides share a common link with inflammation in the ligament, tendon, and fascia insertion sites on the bone, as well as the synovium, uveal tract, and gastrointestinal tract. The class I HLA-B27 gene allele is present in most of these patients.

SYNONYMS

Marie-Strümpell disease
Juvenile spondyloarthropathy (JSPA)
Juvenile ankylosing spondylitis (JAS)

ICD-9-CM CODE
720.00 Juvenile spondylitis

EPIDEMIOLOGY & DEMOGRAPHICS

- Older studies indicate a male-to-female ratio of 4.5:1 to 6:1; later data suggest a 2:1 to 3:1 ratio.
- There is a strong (75% to 90%) genetic link with HLA-B27.
- The prevalence of JAS is approximately 1.6 cases per 100,000 adolescents; the rate for total juvenile spondyloarthropathies is approximately 20 cases per 100,000 adolescents (Cabral DA et al).
  - The prevalence may be higher, but slow progression makes diagnosis difficult during childhood and adolescence.
- The age at onset is 10 years or younger.

CLINICAL PRESENTATION

History

- Usually, JAS occurs in an older boy who presents with pain and stiffness in lower extremity joints, especially the feet (tarsal disease), knees, and hips. Upper extremity involvement is uncommon.
- Inflammation in entheses is common: plantar fascia, Achilles tendon insertion, and tibial tubercle.
- Lumbar or sacroiliac pain and stiffness occur early in disease in 13% to 24% of patients.
- Fever, lymphadenopathy, and uveitis (acute) may occur early in the disease.

Physical Examination

- The examiner may find signs of inflammation with swelling or loss of motion with pain in lower extremity joints, especially the feet, knees, ankles, and subtalar joints. Hips may be involved early in the disease.
- Tenderness and swelling of entheses may be seen. Inspect the Achilles tendon with the insertion site on calcaneus. Palpate over the plantar fascia, tibial tubercles, greater trochanters, and ischial tuberosities.
- Pain may be elicited in the SIJ with provocative compression.
  - Simultaneous, bilateral compression of the hips by the examiner may elicit pain in the SIJ.
  - In the Patrick test, the patient lies supine, and the examiner flexes, abducts, and externally rotates the patient's test leg while placing the foot on the top of the opposite knee. The examiner lowers the test leg toward the examining table while compressing the opposite anterior superior iliac spine. A positive result occurs when the test leg remains above the opposite leg, usually with pain and may indicate hip disease, iliopsoas spasm, or sacroiliac disease.
  - Gaenslen's sign is demonstrated by having the patient in a supine position, with the hip flexed and the knee on the chest; the other thigh is extended over the edge of the table. Pain in the hip that is extended over the edge of the table (contralateral to the flexed hip) may have pathology, especially if pain is elicited in the SIJ.
- Limited lumbar flexion and reduced chest expansion are uncommon early in the disease.
- Examine carefully for evidence of acute iritis, psoriasis, nail changes (i.e., pitting or onycholysis), oral mucosal lesions, perianal fissure or fistula (e.g., Crohn's disease), right lower quadrant mass, and aortic insufficiency.

ETIOLOGY

- The cause is unknown.
- A strong predisposition for JAS is associated with the HLA-B27 marker.
- Suspected antigenic stimulation is suggested by bacterial infections, such as *Salmonella*, *Shigella*, *Yersinia*, and *Campylobacter* species; *Mycobacterium tuberculosis*; and *Chlamydia* species, which trigger reactive arthritis in the HLA-B27 host.
- How the antigen works to invoke or what peptides provoke the inflammatory response and interaction with HLA-B27 are not understood.

DIAGNOSIS

DIFFERENTIAL DIAGNOSIS

- Juvenile rheumatoid arthritis (JRA) versus JAS:
  - Tarsal, enthesis, and lower extremity joint inflammation predict JAS.
  - Presence of sacroiliac involvement strongly suggests JAS.
- Arthritis associated with psoriasis, Reiter's disease, and inflammatory bowel disease (IBD) must be considered.

LABORATORY TESTS

- Test results for antinuclear antibodies and rheumatoid factor are usually negative.
- Up to 95% of patients are HLA-B27 positive.
- Complete blood cell count (CBC) with differential, erythrocyte sedimentation rate, urinalysis, and renal and liver chemistries are necessary to follow the patient for medication toxicities and systemic complications.

IMAGING STUDIES

- Radiographs are *not* usually abnormal early in the disease.
  - Radionuclide scan, computed tomography, magnetic resonance imaging (MRI) of SIJs may be helpful if suspected involvement needs to be confirmed.
  - MRI, particularly if used with gadolinium contrast, is a superb modality to identify disease of synovium and tenosynovium in selected cases.

TREATMENT

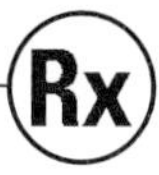

NONPHARMACOLOGIC THERAPY

- Physical therapy is essential and should include range-of-motion, strengthening, flexibility, and postural exercises, along with heat or whirlpool treatments.
- Swimming as an avocational sport is strongly encouraged.
- Orthotics are recommended for foot and enthesis pain relief and support.
- Later, total-joint arthroplasty may be necessary, especially hip replacement.

ACUTE GENERAL Rx

- Initiate anti-inflammatory drugs and physiotherapy, along with general principles of self-management of pain and stiffness (see "Chronic Rx").

PHARMACOLOGIC THERAPY

CHRONIC Rx

- Nonsteroidal anti-inflammatory drugs (NSAIDs)
  - Indomethacin, 1 to 2 mg/kg/day divided into three to four doses; slow release product (75 mg total dose) lasts 12 hours in larger patients
  - Tolmetin sodium, 20 to 30 mg/kg/day divided into three doses
  - Naproxen, 10 to 20 mg/kg/day divided into two doses; maximum 1000 mg/day
- Second-line medications
  - Sulfasalazine (this is not only for IBD), up to 50 mg/kg/day divided every 6 to 12 hours
  - Methotrexate, 5 to 15 mg/m^2/week given orally or subcutaneously; higher doses may be tolerated later if initial low dose is not effective
- Intra-articular corticosteroid injections
  - Triamcinolone hexacetonide, 1 mg/kg per joint (up to 40 mg per joint)

- Avoid tendon insertion injection because of weakening of the tendon and potential rupture.
- Third-line medications
    - Tumor necrosis factor (TNF) blockade can be used; etanercept or infliximab may be beneficial in refractory cases.

DISPOSITION

- Carefully follow range of motion of peripheral joints and lumbar flexion.
- Follow for loss of lumbar flexion; chest expansion; cervical flexion, extension, and rotation; postural alterations; this should be done every 3 to 6 months.
- Radiographic re-evaluation is done as necessary but may not reveal bone or joint space changes for several years.
- Monitor CBC with differential cell count, blood urea nitrogen (BUN), creatinine, alanine aminotransferase (ALT), albumin, and erythrocyte sedimentation rate or C-reactive protein.
- Encourage ongoing physiotherapy; an often neglected component of therapy.
- Complications include cartilage and bone erosion, sacroiliac and spinal ankylosis with severe loss of motion, aortic insufficiency, atlantoaxial subluxation, IgA nephropathy, and cauda equina syndrome.

REFERRAL

- A pediatric rheumatologist can be invaluable in helping to establish a diagnosis and to follow the patient's progress.
- Provide an interdisciplinary team for physical management.

PEARLS & CONSIDERATIONS

COMMENTS

- Watch for psoriasis, IBD, and uveitis.
- Pauciarticular-onset JRA in older boys may evolve into JAS; prospectively follow for axial involvement.
- Enthesitis in an older boy with signs of inflammation may have early JAS, although repetitive activity (overuse) syndromes are more common.

PREVENTION

- Physiotherapy is essential to prevent the loss of axial and peripheral joint motion.

PATIENT/FAMILY EDUCATION

- Educate about slow progression.
- Educate about importance of exercise.
- Advise regarding development of acute, painful red eye (i.e., acute iritis), which needs prompt ophthalmologic evaluation.
- Advise regarding diarrhea, blood in stools, weight loss; clinical IBD develops in some of these patients.
- Advise regarding development of dyspepsia and epigastric pain caused by NSAIDs.
- Educational materials and support groups are provided by the National Ankylosing Spondylitis Foundation, local Arthritis Foundation groups, and American Juvenile Arthritis Organization (AJAO) (www.spondylytis.org, www.kickas.org).

SUGGESTED READINGS

Bukulmez H, Colbert R: Juvenile spondyloarthropathies and related arthritis. *Curr Opin Rheumatol* 14:531, 2002.

Burgos-Vargas R et al: Juvenile-onset spondyloarthropathies. *Rheum Dis Clin North Am* 23:569, 1997.

Burgos-Vargas R et al: The juvenile-onset spondyloarthritides: Rationale for clinical evaluation. *Best Pract Res Clin Rheumatol* 16:551, 2002.

Burgos-Vargas R, Vásquez-Mellado J: The early clinical recognition of juvenile-onset ankylosing spondylitis and its differentiation from juvenile rheumatoid arthritis. *Arthritis Rheum* 38:835, 1995.

Cabral DA et al: Spondyloarthropathies of childhood. *Pediatr Clin North Am* 42:1051, 1995.

Calin A, Elswood J: The natural history of juvenile-onset ankylosing spondylitis: A 24-year retrospective case-control study. *Br J Rheumatol* 27:91, 1998.

AUTHOR: **MURRAY H. PASSO, MD**

BASIC INFORMATION

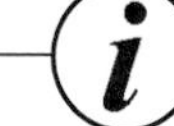

DEFINITION

Anorexia nervosa is characterized by refusal to maintain body weight over a minimum necessary for height and weight loss up to 85% of ideal body weight (IBW) or body mass index (BMI) of 17.5 kg/m^2. In early adolescence, anorexia nervosa can exist without a history of weight loss; instead, there is a failure to achieve expected weight gain during a period of growth, intense fear of weight gain, body image distortion, and amenorrhea (i.e., absence of three consecutive menstrual cycles) in postmenarchal girls. In the first 1 to 2 years after menarche, healthy adolescents may have periods of amenorrhea for longer than 3 months. Subtypes include restricting anorexia nervosa and binge-eating and purging anorexia nervosa.

SYNONYMS

Eating disorder
Eating disorder, not otherwise specified (EDNOS)
Anorexia

ICD-9-CM CODES
307.1 Anorexia nervosa
307.50 Eating disorder, not otherwise specified

EPIDEMIOLOGY & DEMOGRAPHICS

- Incidence: The rates are 19 cases per 100,000 females per year, 2 cases per 100,000 males per year, and 51 cases per 100,000 13- to 19-year-old girls per year.
- Prevalence: The rate is 0.5% among 15- to 19-year-old girls in the United States.
- Gender: More than 90% of patients with anorexia nervosa are female.
- Age: The typical age of onset is between 15 and 19 years of age. There is a bimodal distribution, with peaks at 14.5 and 18 years.
- Genetics: There are increased rates of eating disorders in first-degree relatives of adolescents with eating disorders.
- Risk factors: Patients may have a family history of anorexia nervosa, bulimia nervosa, depression, anxiety, obsessive-compulsive disorder, or obsessive-compulsive personality disorder; may exhibit perfectionism; and may have a negative self-evaluation.

CLINICAL PRESENTATION

History

- Weight loss or failure to gain weight
- Restrictive intake (requires careful review of dietary intake)
- Excessive exercise
- Use of diuretics or appetite suppressants
- Purging, including self-induced vomiting, Ipecac to induce vomiting, laxative abuse, and purging that may exist with or without binge eating in anorexia nervosa
- Amenorrhea
- Physical symptoms, including fatigue, cold intolerance, constipation, headaches, and syncope
- Affective symptoms, including distorted body image, intense fear of weight gain, anxiety, depression, and irritability

Physical Examination

- Weight and height: calculation of appropriateness of weight for height, age, and sex
  - Body mass index (BMI): weight (kg) ÷ height (m)^2
  - Percentage of ideal body weight (% IBW): weight ÷ IBW
- Estimate of IBW for postmenarchal females: 100 pounds at 5 feet, plus 5 pounds per inch over 5 feet
- Vital signs: hypotension, bradycardia, hypothermia, orthostatic pulse changes
- Skin: dry skin, lanugo, alopecia, calluses or abrasions over the knuckles from self-induced vomiting
- Head and neck: parotid gland enlargement, dental enamel erosion caused by vomiting
- Extremities: acrocyanosis, decreased capillary refill, edema, loss of muscle mass

ETIOLOGY

- Multifactorial causes
- Contributing factors include
  - Genetic predisposition (increased rates of eating disorders in first-degree relatives of adolescents with eating disorders)
  - Neurochemical factors (in several studies, altered serotonin activity persisted after weight and nutritional rehabilitation)
  - Psychological factors (developmental transitions, comorbid anxiety, depression)
  - Sociocultural influences (societal emphasis on thinness)
- Biologic effects of starvation
  - Restrictive eating produces a state of semistarvation.
  - Starvation contributes to many of the abnormal cognitive and behavioral symptoms exhibited in anorexia nervosa and perpetuates the disorder.

DIAGNOSIS

Dx

DIFFERENTIAL DIAGNOSIS

- Bulimia nervosa
- Inflammatory bowel disease
- Diabetes mellitus
- Thyroid disease
- Neoplastic disease
- Malnutrition
- Depression
- Anxiety
- Obsessive-compulsive disorder
- Substance abuse

WORKUP

- Diagnosis is primarily based on history from the patient and family and on results of the physical examination.
- Laboratory data vary based on the degree of malnutrition and presence or absence of purging.
- Laboratory tests in anorexia nervosa are often within normal limits.
- There is no confirmatory laboratory test.

LABORATORY TESTS

- Serum electrolytes: hypokalemic, hypochloremic metabolic alkalosis (associated with vomiting) or hyponatremia
- Blood urea nitrogen: elevated levels
- Complete blood cell count and platelets: mild anemia, leukopenia, thrombocytopenia
- Erythrocyte sedimentation rate: low
- Electrocardiogram: prolonged QTc interval, T-wave abnormalities, low voltage, conduction defects

TREATMENT

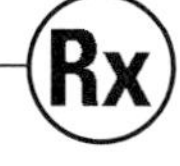

NONPHARMACOLOGIC THERAPY

- Interdisciplinary approach: biologic, nutritional, and psychosocial
- Biologic approach: medical and nutritional stabilization
  - Weight gain to within appropriate range of 90% to 110% of IBW
  - Correction of medical complications caused by malnutrition and purging
  - Physical examination and close monitoring of weight and vital signs
- Nutritional approach: education about nutrition and caloric intake
  - Structured meal planning to establish healthy patterns of eating
  - Identification of events that trigger abnormal eating behaviors
- Psychosocial approach: combinations of individual, group, and family treatment
- Indications for hospitalization
  - Presence of severe malnutrition (weight < 75% IBW)
  - Physiologic instability
  - Vital sign instability: severe bradycardia, hypotension, hypothermia, orthostatic changes
  - Dehydration
  - Significant electrolyte disturbances
  - Cardiac dysrhythmia
  - Syncope
  - Acute food refusal
  - Failure of outpatient treatment
  - Acute psychiatric emergencies

ACUTE GENERAL Rx

- Antidepressant medication (e.g., selective serotonin reuptake inhibitors such as fluoxetine) should be considered for coexisting depression.

- ○ Psychopharmacologic agents have not been effective in reducing the primary symptoms of anorexia nervosa during the acutely malnourished state.
- ○ Fluoxetine may help reduce the risk of relapse in weight-recovered patients with anorexia nervosa.
- There is no evidence of efficacy of hormone replacement therapy in preventing osteopenia in anorexia nervosa.
- Supplementation with calcium (1000 to 1500 mg/day) and a multivitamin, including vitamin D (400 IU/day), should be recommended to all patients.

REFERRAL

- Referral to an interdisciplinary treatment team (i.e., adolescent medicine specialist, mental health provider, and nutritionist) with expertise in managing adolescents with eating disorders is highly recommended.
- Communication among members of the treatment team is essential.

PEARLS & CONSIDERATIONS

COMMENTS

- Ninety percent of the IBW should be established as the initial goal weight, based on probable return of menstrual function.
- Patients with anorexia nervosa who are taking oral contraceptive pills may have a false sense of health because they have monthly menstrual bleeding even at low weights.
- Many patients with anorexia nervosa consider their eating disorder to be a helpful "coping mechanism."
- Patients may be resistant to treatment. Acknowledging this conflict can be beneficial.

PREVENTION

- Early intervention is associated with improved outcome.

PATIENT/FAMILY EDUCATION

- Education should be developmentally appropriate.
- Family involvement is an essential part of treatment for adolescents.
- Confidentiality is essential.

SUGGESTED READINGS

Becker AE, et al: Eating disorders. *N Engl J Med* 340:1092, 1999.

Kreipe RE, Dukarm CP: Eating disorders in adolescents and older children. *Pediatr Rev* 20:410, 1999.

Rome ES, et al: Children and adolescents with eating disorders: the state of the art. *Pediatrics* 111:e98, 2003.

AUTHOR: **CAROLYN PIVER DUKARM, MD**

BASIC INFORMATION

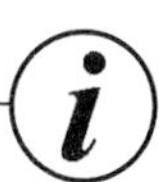

DEFINITIONS

Separation anxiety disorder (i.e., anxiety) is characterized by developmentally inappropriate symptoms that are excessive and caused by separation from home or parents or other loved ones. **Generalized anxiety disorder** (i.e., overanxious disorder) is characterized by excessive and unrealistic worry and behavior about past or future events. **Reactive attachment disorder** is characterized by a disturbance of social attachment; patients may be inhibited, with persistent failure to initiate or respond to attachment figures, or they may have uninhibited diffuse attachments or excessive familiarity with strangers. **Social phobia** refers to excessive anxiety in social or performance situations; in younger children, symptoms include tantrums, freezing, blushing, and timidity. **Simple** or **specific phobias** are irrational or excessive and persistent fears of a specific object or situation, associated with avoidance behavior and functional or social impairment. **Common phobias** involve fear of animals, blood, the dark, fire, germs or dirt, heights, insects, small or closed spaces, snakes, spiders, strangers, or thunder. **Selective mutism** is characterized by a failure to speak in specific social situations (e.g., school) and the ability to speak in other situations (e.g., home). **Panic disorder** refers to recurrent spontaneous episodes of panic that are associated with physiologic and psychological symptoms; less than one half of affected persons also develop agoraphobia.

SYNONYMS

Separation anxiety disorder, including school phobia and school avoidance

Generalized anxiety disorder, including overanxious disorder

Social phobia, including avoidant disorder

ICD-9-CM CODES

309.21 Separation anxiety disorder
300.02 Generalized anxiety disorder
313.89 Reactive attachment disorder
300.12 Social phobia
300.29 Specific phobia
313.23 Selective mutism
300.01 Panic disorder without agoraphobia
300.21 Panic disorder with agoraphobia

EPIDEMIOLOGY & DEMOGRAPHICS

- The prevalence of anxiety disorders is high, but they are often unrecognized and undertreated.
- The 1-year prevalence of anxiety disorder is 15.4% overall for children and all adolescents.
  - Prevalence rate is based on parent and child interviews.
  - Simple phobia, separation anxiety disorder, and overanxious disorder are the most prevalent, with rates of 9.2%, 4.1%, and 4.6%, respectively.
- Separation anxiety disorder more commonly affects children between the ages of 2 to 6 years, those with lower socioeconomic status, and children from single-parent families.
- Reactive attachment disorder is more common with insecure attachment early in life.
- Generalized anxiety disorder and social phobia are more common in several groups: females, whites, middle- and upper-class families, and children older than 8 years to those in their midteens.
- The usual onset for panic disorder is during adolescence or early adulthood.

CLINICAL PRESENTATION

History

- Children who are passive, shy, and fearful and who avoid new situations are more likely to exhibit anxiety.
- Increased tension is felt in the throat.
- Behavioral inhibition to the unfamiliar (i.e., avoidance of new situations) is an enduring, temperamental trait.
- Separation anxiety can manifest in several ways:
  - Bedtime difficulties, including refusal to go to sleep and insistence on sleeping with parents
  - Pattern of abdominal pain associated with separation anxiety disorder and often involving pain on Sunday night, Monday morning, or at the end of a school vacation
  - Excessive worry about harm befalling a loved one
  - Nightmares
  - Anticipatory anxiety with separations
- Generalized anxiety is associated with
  - Extremely self-conscious behavior
  - Need for excessive reassurance
  - Inability to relax
  - Headaches
  - Abdominal pain
  - Muscle tension
  - Sleep problems
  - Symptoms that may worsen with stress
- Reactive attachment disorder is associated with
  - Maternal anxiety or depression
  - Maltreatment or neglect
  - Chaotic environment
- Social phobia is associated with
  - Fear of humiliation or embarrassment
  - Avoidance or inability to function
  - Hypersensitivity to criticism
  - Poor social skills
- With simple or specific phobias, patients often recognize their own irrational fears.

Physical Examination

- Usually normal despite complaints of abdominal pain, throat tightness, or headache
- Increased heart rate
- Pupillary dilation

ETIOLOGY

- Neurotransmitters, including γ-aminobutyric acid (GABA), serotonin, and norepinephrine, are associated with anxiety phenomena in the central nervous system.
- Genetic predispositions are evident.
  - Family history of anxiety disorder, depression, alcoholism, or somatization disorder is a risk factor.
  - Family history is also associated with earlier onset and increased severity.

DIAGNOSIS

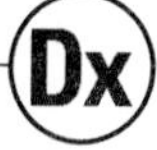

DIFFERENTIAL DIAGNOSIS

- For all anxiety disorders
  - Depression and other mood disorders
  - Substance abuse
  - Attention deficit/hyperactivity disorder
- Separation anxiety disorder
  - This type of anxiety overlaps with depression in one third of cases.
  - Truancy (during adolescence) is not associated with anxiety about leaving loved ones or home.
  - Medical causes for recurrent abdominal pain should be considered.
- Generalized anxiety
  - Overuse of caffeine or other stimulants is common in adolescents.
  - Reactions may occur to medications.
  - Other medical causes may include cardiac arrhythmias, hyperthyroidism, and excessive catecholamine (pleochromocytoma) and hypoglycemic reactions.
- Reactive attachment disorder
  - Normal developmental variations must be considered. Indiscriminate acceptance of strangers is common until about 8 months.
  - Autistic and mentally retarded children may display disturbed social relationships.
  - Failure to thrive may have a medical cause associated with malnutrition and metabolic disturbance compromising mood and social relationships.
- Social phobia
  - In schizophrenia and other psychotic disorders, individuals do not recognize their fears as unreasonable or excessive.
- Simple phobia
  - Developmentally appropriate fears may be seen.
  - Other anxiety disorders may manifest.
- Panic disorder
  - Rule out organic causes such as cardiac problems, pain, or asthma.
  - Catecholamine excess and hyperthyroidism may occur.
  - Real fears may result from trauma (e.g., family stressors, abusive relationship, sibling abuse, unsafe neighborhood or school).

WORKUP

- Developmental, medical, school, social, and family histories, as well as recent stressors, often lead to the appropriate diagnosis.

- Diagnostic interviews are generally used by psychologists.
  - Schizophrenia and Affective Disorders Scale for Children (K-SADS): a semistructured clinical diagnostic interview tool
  - Diagnostic Interview for Children and Adolescents (DICA): a semistructured clinical diagnostic interview tool
  - Diagnostic Interview Scale for Children (DISC): a structured clinical diagnostic interview
  - Anxiety Diagnostic Interview Scale for Children and Parents (ADIS IV-C/P): a semistructured clinical diagnostic interview tool
- The following clinician rating scales are available:
  - Hamilton Anxiety Rating Scale (14 items)
  - Anxiety Rating for Children–Revised (22 items)
- Parent or self-report instruments include the following:
  - State-Trait Anxiety Inventory for Children (two 20-item scales)
  - Children's Manifest Anxiety Scale (37 items)
- If the history or physical examination is suggestive, consider a workup for the following:
  - Hyperthyroidism
  - Caffeine intoxication
  - Medication reactions
  - Substance abuse
  - Cardiac arrhythmias
  - Pheochromocytoma
  - Seizure disorders
  - Migraine
  - Other central nervous system disorders
- As part of the workup, usually screen for misdiagnosed or comorbid psychiatric disorders, including mood disorders, attention deficit/hyperactivity disorder, substance abuse, and eating disorders.

LABORATORY TESTS

- Correlates of behavioral inhibition include the following:
  - Elevated cortisol
  - Elevated catecholamine levels

TREATMENT

NONPHARMACOLOGIC THERAPY

- For infants and preschool children, the clinician should attend to parents whose anxiety, losses, and traumatic experiences may affect attachment relationships.
- Behavioral programs for separation anxiety disorder should include a plan for return to school as soon a possible.
  - Home tutoring is generally contraindicated.
  - Behavioral techniques such as systematic desensitization, relaxation training, extinction, exposure, and response prevention may be helpful.
- For separation anxiety disorder, family interventions and family therapy are critical.
- Treatment for all anxiety disorders includes the following:
  - Cognitive-behavioral therapy integrates behavioral approaches and cognitive techniques.
  - Individual therapy is more effective when combined with pharmacologic intervention.
- For social phobia and selective mutism, group therapy with peers may promote social skills peer involvement, and age-appropriate assertiveness.
- For panic disorder, a panic attack diary, which describes the number, intensity, and type of panic attacks, allows the clinician to evaluate triggers and to plan for effective and focused intervention.

ACUTE GENERAL Rx

- Use of selective serotonin reuptake inhibitors (SSRIs) is controversial because of reports of suicides during treatment initiation, requiring a black box warning.
- When considering the use of antidepressant treatment, weigh the risks and benefits of medications.
- Separation anxiety disorder treatment is based on the following ideas:
  - Studies have not replicated positive results of earlier reports of the effectiveness of imipramine for the treatment of school phobia.
  - Small dose after a finite (short) period of short-acting benzodiazepines may be part of a multimodal treatment plan for anxiety.
  - SSRIs may be effective when used in multimodal treatment.
- Generalized anxiety disorder treatment is based on the following ideas:
  - Little research has been done about the role of pharmacotherapy.
  - Anecdotal reports suggest possible role for SSRIs or buspirone.
- For reactive attachment disorder, no role for pharmacotherapy has been defined.
- Social phobia treatment is based on the following ideas:
  - Pharmacotherapy has not been well studied in children and adolescents.
  - There is some evidence for the usefulness of SSRIs or buspirone in treating social anxiety for children and adolescents.
- Panic disorder treatment is based on the following ideas:
  - Pharmacotherapy has not been well studied in children and adolescents.
  - Some studies show effectiveness of benzodiazepines and SSRIs.
  - SSRIs may cause worsening of panic-anxiety when treatment is initiated. Low initial dosages (5 mg of fluoxetine, 10 mg of paroxetine) may protect against this. Almost 50% of adults show a significant treatment response to placebo, suggesting the need for psychotherapeutic approach and multimodal treatment.
- Benzodiazepines in children and adolescents are controversial.
  - Psychopharmacology consultation should be considered.
  - Problems with benzodiazepine use include dependency, sedation, memory dysfunction, disinhibition, ataxia, and drug interactions.

CHRONIC Rx

- Long-term and intermittent therapies (e.g., cognitive-behavioral therapy) and family counseling are often warranted.

DISPOSITION

- Anxiety disorders are recurrent.
- Medication (if used) should be tapered slowly before discontinuation, and ongoing consultation and therapy can help to identify risks of decompensation.

REFERRAL

- Psychopharmacologic consultations, behavioral treatment, and family therapy are important because there is a high risk for recurrence of anxiety disorders.
- The treatment course is often extended.

PEARLS & CONSIDERATIONS

COMMENTS

- Successful treatment of school phobia requires family therapy interventions.
  - Pharmacotherapy alone is rarely helpful.
  - Home tutoring is generally contraindicated.
- Cognitive-behavioral therapy with a trained practitioner is effective for a range of anxiety disorders.
- Adolescents who receive inadequate treatment for anxiety disorders may resort to self-medication and substance abuse.
- Distinguish clinically significant anxiety disorders from age-related, transient fears and anxieties by the following features:
  - Intensity: The reaction is out of proportion to the actual threat or demands of the situation.
  - Frequency: The fear reaction or anxiety symptoms occur with increased frequency and cannot be explained or reasoned away.
  - Content: The worry or fear is usually focused on a nonthreatening situation or stimulus that is not likely to cause harm.
  - Avoidance: The fear reaction leads to avoidance of or escape from the stimulus.
  - Stage of development: The reaction is not specific to the child's age or stage of development.
  - Nonadaptive and persistent nature: The reaction is persistent and not helpful.

 - Interference: Reactions interfere with the individual or the family's functions.
- Comorbidity with other psychiatric disorders is significant.
 - With depression (22% to 44%)
 - With disruptive behavior disorders, including attention deficit/hyperactivity disorder (8% to 50%)
 - Co-occurrence of more than one anxiety disorder (65% to 95% lifetime prevalence)

PREVENTION

- Address anxiety as early as possible, and maintain ongoing treatment to decrease the likelihood of recurrence.
- Offer anticipatory guidance to families regarding upcoming transitions or stressors as potential triggers for recurrent anxiety.

PATIENT/FAMILY EDUCATION

- Use of medication in combination with behavioral, individual, and family therapy is more effective than any one approach.
- Parents and caregivers should be educated about the signs of recurrence and ways in which to identify stressors.
- Cognitive-behavioral techniques may prevent recurrence.
- Education and consultation for school personnel is valuable.

SUGGESTED READINGS

American Academy of Child and Adolescent Psychiatry: AACAP practice parameters. *J Am Acad Child Adolesc Psychiatry* 36:69S, 1997.
American Academy of Child and Adolescent Psychiatry: www.aacap.org
American Psychiatric Association: *Diagnostic and Statistical Manual of Mental Disorders,* 4th ed, text revision. Washington, DC, American Psychiatric Association, 2000.
Anxiety Disorders Association of America (ADAA) home page: www.adaa.org
March JS, Morris TL: *Anxiety Disorders in Children and Adolescents,* 2nd ed. New York, Guilford Publications, 2004.
NIMH Anxiety Disorders Education Program: www.nimh.nih.gov/anxiety/index.htm
Varley CK, Smith CJ: Anxiety disorders in the child and teen. *Pediatr Clin North Am* 50:5, 2003.
Waslick B: Interventions for pediatric anxiety disorder: a research update. *Child Adolesc Psychiatry Clin North Am* 15:1, 2006.
Werry JS, Aman MG: *Practitioner's Guide to Psychoactive Drugs for Children and Adolescents,* 2nd ed. New York, Plenum Medical Book Company, 1999.

AUTHOR: **OLIVIA CHIANG, PSYD**

BASIC INFORMATION

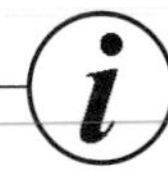

DEFINITION

Left ventricular outflow tract (LVOT) obstruction is an anatomic blockage of left ventricular output. Obstruction can occur at multiple levels, including subvalvar, valvular, supravalvar, and aortic sites. These lesions can occur in isolation or in combination. The most severe form is hypoplastic left ventricle syndrome with aortic valve atresia and aortic hypoplasia.

SYNONYMS

Aortic stenosis (AS)
Coarctation of the aorta
"Coarct"

ICD-9-CM CODE
746.3 Congenital aortic valve stenosis
746.7 Hypoplastic left heart syndrome
746.81 Subaortic stenosis
747.10 Coarctation of the aorta
747.11 Interruption of the aortic arch
747.22 Supravalvar aortic stenosis

EPIDEMIOLOGY & DEMOGRAPHICS

- LVOT obstruction occurs in 10% of cases of congenital heart disease.
- The true incidence of bicuspid aortic valve is unknown.
- Multifactorial inheritance patterns are possible.
- Other anomalies are frequently associated.
  - Ventricular septal defect
  - Mitral valve abnormalities
  - Patent ductus arteriosus

CLINICAL PRESENTATION

History

- Aortic stenosis
  - A murmur is usually heard at birth in patients with significant aortic stenosis.
  - Severe obstruction manifests in the neonate as congestive heart failure.
  - Other features include poor feeding, poor growth, lethargy, and a rapid respiratory rate.
- Cardiovascular collapse
  - Older children are usually asymptomatic.
  - Patients with moderate to severe obstruction may develop exertional chest pain, syncope (ominous sign), or fatigability.
  - Congestive heart failure in older children is rare but may develop in adulthood.
- Coarctation of the aorta in the neonate
  - It may manifest in the neonatal period with sudden cardiovascular collapse at 7 to 10 days of age when the ductus arteriosus closes.
  - Coarctation in later infancy and childhood is possible.
  - It usually is identified by diminished or absent femoral pulses and relative (but not necessarily absolute) upper extremity hypertension.
  - Symptoms are uncommon but may include headaches and exertional leg pain.
- Aortic valve stenosis (usually progressive)
  - A narrow pulse pressure is detected.
  - Systolic ejection murmur is present in the middle left sternal border and radiates into the aortic region.
  - The murmur increases in intensity as obstruction increases in severity.
  - A palpable thrill may be present over the murmur and in the suprasternal notch.
  - An ejection click is heard when the valve is mobile.
  - An associated decrescendo diastolic murmur of aortic valve regurgitation may be present.
- Subaortic stenosis (usually progressive, often rapidly)
  - Murmur is better localized to middle left sternal border or midsternum.
  - No ejection click is heard.
  - The patient may have an associated diastolic murmur of aortic valve insufficiency.
  - Supravalvar aortic stenosis may be part of the Williams syndrome, whose features include elfin facies; mental retardation; "cocktail personality;" and small, pointed, and irregular teeth.
- Peripheral pulmonary artery stenosis
  - It may occur in Williams syndrome.
  - A systolic ejection murmur with or without a thrill is heard at the aortic region with radiation into the carotid arteries.
  - No ejection click is heard.
  - The aortic closure sound may be accentuated.
  - The right arm blood pressure may be higher than the left arm pressure, even without arch obstruction.
- Coarctation of aorta in the neonate
  - Infant may have no pulses if cardiac function is poor or there is only a palpable right arm pulse.
  - Congestive heart failure
  - Pallor or grayness may be evident.
  - No characteristic murmur, but the patient may have a murmur in pulmonic area.
- Coarctation in later infancy and childhood
  - This can occur in a well-developed, well-nourished child.
  - Arm pulses more vigorous than leg pulses; leg pulses are delayed.
  - Arm blood pressure exceeds the leg blood pressure.
  - Normal leg blood pressure should be higher than arm pressure by at least 10 mm Hg.
  - Palpable collateral vessels may be felt in the neck and the parascapular area.
  - No characteristic murmur is present, but there may be a bruit in the back over the area of coarctation.
  - The patient may have murmurs caused by the associated defects of aortic valve stenosis, mitral valve regurgitation, or ventricular septal defect.

ETIOLOGY

- Multifactorial inheritance patterns are associated with strong genetic determinants for LVOT obstruction (i.e., male predominance and associated syndromes such as Turner syndrome, Williams syndrome, DiGeorge syndrome).
- Environmental and developmental factors include abnormal in utero flow patterns and abnormal in utero valve formation.
- Other anomalies, including ventricular septal defect, mitral valve abnormalities, and patent ductus arteriosus, are frequently associated with the stenosis.

DIAGNOSIS

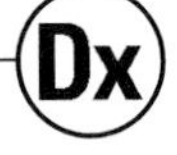

DIFFERENTIAL DIAGNOSIS

- Careful attention to location and characteristics helps differentiate aortic stenosis from other systolic murmurs.
  - Pulmonary stenosis murmur is heard at the upper left sternal border with radiation into the clavicular region and lung fields.
  - Ventricular septal defect murmur is heard at the lower left sternal border and is harsh and holosystolic.
- Presence of an ejection click helps to localize the region of aortic stenosis.
- Differential arm-leg blood pressures and pulses signify arch obstruction.

WORKUP

- Aortic valve stenosis
  - Electrocardiogram: normal to left ventricular hypertrophy with ischemia
  - Chest radiograph: normal to prominent ascending aorta (poststenotic dilation), enlarged left ventricle
  - Echocardiogram: valve structure, including number and equality of leaflets; left ventricular hypertrophy, dilation, and function; valve gradient; diameter of aortic and pulmonic annuli (for surgical correction)
  - Cardiac catheterization and angiography: typically performed only if intervention indicated; direct measurement of valve gradient, left ventricular function, evaluation of associated anomalies
- Subaortic stenosis
  - Electrocardiogram: same as valve stenosis
  - Chest radiograph: same as aortic valve stenosis, except no poststenotic dilation
  - Echocardiogram: defines location of obstruction; defines type (e.g., ridge versus muscular); estimates gradient; evaluates left ventricular hypertrophy, dilation, and function; defines associated defects
- Supravalvar aortic stenosis
  - Electrocardiogram: same as for aortic valve stenosis
  - Chest radiograph: same as for valve stenosis; no poststenotic dilation, although ascending aorta may be prominent

- Echocardiogram: locates obstruction; estimates gradient; evaluates left ventricular hypertrophy, dilation, and function; defines associated defects
- Cardiac catheterization and angiocardiography: anatomic evaluation of aorta; evaluation of coronary arteries, which may be involved in stenosis; evaluation for surgical repair

- Coarctation of aorta in the neonate
  - Electrocardiogram: not diagnostic; usually finds right axis deviation with right ventricular hypertrophy; may indicate increased or decreased left ventricular forces
  - Chest radiograph: detects cardiomegaly with increased pulmonary arterial flow or pulmonary venous congestion
  - Echocardiogram: delineates poor myocardial function, visible coarctation or arch hypoplasia, and associated defects
  - Cardiac catheterization and angiocardiography: not usually indicated
- Coarctation in later infancy and childhood
  - Electrocardiogram: usually normal, although may indicate left ventricular hypertrophy
  - Chest radiograph: usually normal but may show left ventricular hypertrophy; possible rib notching
  - Echocardiography: confirms coarctation and provides localization, estimates gradient across coarctation, evaluates associated defects and left ventricular hypertrophy, dilation, and function
  - Catheterization and angiography: not always indicated; used for delineation of coarctation in older patients; can evaluate associated defects, pulmonary hypertension, and left ventricular function; possible catheter intervention (i.e., angioplasty, stent implantation)

TREATMENT

Rx

NONPHARMACOLOGIC THERAPY

- Aortic valve stenosis
  - Follow clinically if not severe (gradient <60 mm Hg, no symptoms and normal electrocardiogram).
  - Good dental hygiene is important.

ACUTE GENERAL Rx

- Aortic valve stenosis
  - For infants with cardiovascular collapse, administer prostaglandin to improve systemic cardiac output.
  - Add conventional agents for congestive heart failure and decreased cardiac output.
- Aortic stenosis (all forms)
  - Subacute bacterial endocarditis prophylaxis
  - Treatment of congestive heart failure if necessary
- Neonatal coarctation
  - Administer prostaglandin to reopen ductus to improve systemic circulation and renal blood flow.
  - Provide general supportive measures and treatment for congestive heart failure and poor systemic output.

CHRONIC Rx

- Aortic valve stenosis, if severe gradient (>60 mm Hg), electrocardiographic change, congestive heart failure, or left ventricular dysfunction:
  - Relieve obstruction by balloon valvuloplasty.
  - Surgical valvotomy may be needed.
  - Aortic valve replacement may be required.
  - The Ross procedure substitutes pulmonic valve for an abnormal aortic valve, prosthetic valve, or tissue valve (not usually required for first procedure unless associated with aortic insufficiency).
- Subvalvar aortic stenosis
  - Surgical resection must remove all traces of abnormal tissue to prevent recurrence.
  - Obstruction by muscle, mitral valve, and so forth may not be surgically approachable.
- Supravalvar aortic stenosis
  - Surgical repair is technically difficult.
  - Outcome depends on left ventricular function and aortic and coronary anatomy more than on the gradient.
- Neonatal coarctation
  - Surgical resection (or bypass) is possible when the patient is stable.
  - The patient may require repeat relief of obstruction in later childhood by balloon dilation or repeat surgery.
- Coarctation in later infancy or childhood
  - Relief of aortic obstruction may be achieved by balloon angioplasty or surgical resection or bypass.
  - Treatment is usually attempted in the preschool period.

DISPOSITION

- Although surgical approaches are available for most types of LVOT obstruction, they generally are palliative rather than curative, and repeated surgery is often needed.
- All these patients deserve lifelong surveillance and follow-up for recurrence after surgery.
- Appropriate protection against bacterial endocarditis is necessary at times of possible bacteremia.
- Patients with coarctation need long-term follow-up for restenosis, aneurysm formation, systemic hypertension, and development of aortic valve stenosis.

REFERRAL

- All patients with suspected LVOT obstruction should be referred to a cardiologist for diagnosis and management.

PEARLS & CONSIDERATIONS

!

COMMENTS

- The presence of a systolic ejection murmur at birth may signify ventricular outflow tract obstruction.
- An ejection click signifies a thin, mobile valve and signifies valvar stenosis.
- LVOT obstruction may be minor, severe, or lethal.
- Consider aortic stenosis or coarctation of the aorta in an infant with cardiovascular collapse because there may be no suggestive physical findings.
- A normal electrocardiogram does not necessarily correlate with a mild degree of obstruction.
- A family history may include members with any degree of LVOT obstructive disease.
- Isometric exercise increases left ventricular work by increasing systemic vascular resistance and should be avoided.
- Children with LVOT obstruction should be encouraged to develop an interest in nonsustained, noncompetitive sports, such as bowling, swimming, and archery. They should be exposed to music and the arts, allowing them to develop interest in activities that do not depend on hard physical work.
- LVOT obstruction is usually a progressive disease, particularly when the valve or the immediate subvalvar and supravalvar areas are involved.
- Surgical approaches to LVOT obstruction are palliative, not curative, and repeat surgery may be necessary.

PATIENT/FAMILY EDUCATION

- Patients and parents need to understand fully the concept of infective endocarditis prophylaxis.
- Patients and parents need to understand that surgical approaches to LVOT obstruction are palliative, not curative.
- Although small children may not need activity restriction, older children and those with more severe disease may be limited in sports participation.
- Isometric exercise imposes a significant extra workload on the heart, and sports such as weightlifting, wrestling, and rope climbing may not be permitted.

SUGGESTED READINGS

American Heart Association: www.americanheart.org.

Congenital Heart Information Network: www.tchin.org/pdheart.htm

Emedicine: www.emedicine.com

Heart Center Online: www.heartcenteronline.com

Moss, Adams: *Heart Disease in Infants, Children and Adolescents including the Fetus and Young Adult,* 6th ed. Baltimore, Williams & Wilkins, 2001, pp 970–1026.

Park MK: *Pediatric Cardiology for Practitioners,* 4th ed. St. Louis, Mosby, 2002, pp 158–172.

Pedi heart: www.pediheart.org

AUTHOR: **DANIEL E. MIGA, MD**

BASIC INFORMATION

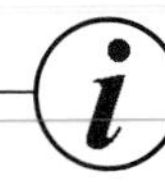

DEFINITION

Aphthous ulcers are benign but painful oral lesions whose precise cause is unknown.

SYNONYMS

Aphthosis
Aphthous stomatitis
Benign aphthous ulcers
Canker sores
Common oral ulcers
Herpetiform RAU
Periadenitis mucosa necrotica recurrens
Recurrent aphthous stomatitis (RAS)
Recurrent aphthous ulcers (RAU)
RAU major
RAU minor
Sutton disease

ICD-9-CM CODE
528.2 Aphthous ulcer

EPIDEMIOLOGY & DEMOGRAPHICS

- RAU accounts for most oral ulcers in North America.
  - Estimated in 20% of the general population in the United States, children and adults
  - Peak age of 10 to 19 years
  - Slightly more common in females than males
  - RAUs in approximately 1% of U.S. children
- Aphthous ulcers are found in all ethnic groups and geographic locations worldwide.
  - There are some reports of increased occurrence in more affluent countries and higher socioeconomic groups.
  - The ulcers are reported in the pediatric and adult age groups.
  - Of childhood RAU, RAU minor is the most common type (80% to 85%).
  - Onset is typically before age 5 years.
  - RAU major (10% to 15% of cases) usually develops after puberty and may endure for 20 years.
  - Herpetiform apthous ulcers account for 10% of all cases.
- A family history of aphthous ulcers is common. Aphthous ulcers are associated with HLA haplotypes B51, Cn7, A2, B12, and Dr5.
- There are many predisposing factors: emotional or physical stress; higher cortisol and anxiety levels; hormonal levels; outbreaks associated with menstruation and ovulation; regression of recurrent ulcers with pregnancy; infection; food sensitivity; flavoring agents, essential oils, and benzoic acid; cinnamon, gluten, cow's milk, coffee, chocolate, cheese, figs, nuts, potatoes, and citrus fruits; trauma; accidental bites, dental injections, toothbrush injury, ingestion of sharp foods; salivary gland dysfunction; toxin exposure; nitrates in drinking water; immune deficiency; familial tendency; poor nutritional status; allergic reaction; sodium lauryl sulfate (i.e., toothpaste detergent); recent chemotherapy or radiation treatment.

CLINICAL PRESENTATION

- Patients may complain of a burning or itching sensation 24 to 48 hours before ulcer development.
- Pain usually lasts 3 to 4 days.
- Exclude constitutional symptoms and other concerning complaints that may indicate the concurrent presence of a systemic disease.
- Investigation of family history may be helpful if clinical suspicion of systemic disease exists. Inquire about (Inflammatory bowel disease, Behçet's disease, systemic lupus erythematosus, celiac disease, and RAU).
- The typical course includes development of clearly defined, round, small, painful oral ulcers that spontaneously heal within 10 to 14 days without scarring. More severe disease occurs when lesions are larger than 5 mm in diameter; such lesions may last 6 weeks.
- Lesions classically occur on the poorly or nonkeratinized and loosely attached areas of oral mucosa. The remainder of the mouth should be normal. Common sites of involvement include the buccal mucosa, floor of the mouth, ventral surface of the tongue, soft palate, and labial mucosa.
- Three distinct categories exist based on clinical presentation:
  - Minor AU lesions are 1 to 10 mm in diameter with a shallow base.
    - Lesions are covered by a yellow-gray pseudomembrane and surrounded by an erythematous halo.
    - Usually, one to five ulcers are present at any time.
    - Spontaneous resolution occurs within 7 to 10 days.
  - Major AU are larger than 10 mm in diameter and more oval than minor ones.
    - They often have an irregular, raised border.
    - One to 10 major aphthae can be present at a time.
    - Healing may take 30 days.
    - They can coalesce and cause distortion of the oral and pharyngeal mucosa.
    - Scarring may result.
  - Herpetiform ulcers are multiple, clustered, 1- to 3-mm lesions that heal within 7 to 10 days.
    - They can coalesce into larger plaques, simulating the appearance of a major aphthous ulcer.
    - Typically, there are only 2 to 10 ulcers, but patients may suffer from as many as 100 lesions at once.
- The remainder of physical examination should be normal.
  - Abnormalities in the skin, joints, eyes, or genital or lymphatic systems should raise concern about systemic disease. Submandibular lymphadenopathy can occur with isolated aphthous ulcers.
  - Dehydration with severe disease or in susceptible age groups may occur.
- Most patients have an isolated outbreak approximately three or four times per year. Continuous outbreaks are reported.

ETIOLOGY

- The cause is considered idiopathic and likely multifactorial.
- The pathogenesis is not well established. Alterations in immune function, familial predisposition, nutritional deficiencies, and bacterial infection have all been implicated.
  - Immune dysfunction: Alterations in local cell-mediated immunity have been proposed. Presumably, immune-mediated destruction of the epithelium is the ultimate result.
  - Genetics: A familial pattern is recognized in some patients. There is a high correlation of RAU in identical twins. A relationship between specific HLA haplotypes and RAU has been proposed.
  - Hematinic deficiency: Some studies report that iron, folic acid, and vitamin B_{12} deficiencies are twice as common in RAU patients as in controls. Up to 20% of patients with RAU are diagnosed with hematinic deficiency.
  - Infection: Controversy exists about the role of microbes in RAU development. Pathogens such as *Helicobacter pylori* and *Streptococcus sanguis* have been implicated.

DIAGNOSIS

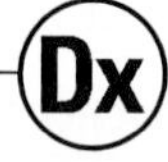

DIFFERENTIAL DIAGNOSIS

- Dermatologic
  - Bullous pemphigoid
  - Cicatricial pemphigoid
  - Epidermolysis bullosa
  - Erythema multiforme
  - Lichen planus
  - Linear IgA disease
  - Pemphigus vulgaris
  - Stevens-Johnson syndrome
- Gastrointestinal
  - Celiac Disease
  - Crohn's disease
  - Ulcerative colitis
- Iatrogenic
  - Antimetabolite use
  - Methotrexate therapy
- Immunodeficiencies, primary and secondary
  - Human immunodeficiency virus (HIV)-related or -associated ulcers
  - Syphilis, cytomegalovirus infection, Kaposi's sarcoma, non-Hodgkin's lymphoma, *Mycobacterium avium*

- Neutropenia: medication-related, cyclic neutropenia, Sweet syndrome
- T-cell disorders
- Infectious
  - Coxsackie virus
  - Herpes simplex virus (HSV)
  - Histoplasmosis
  - HIV
  - Human herpesvirus–6
  - Necrotizing ulcerative gingivostomatitis
  - Syphilis
  - Varicella
  - Varicella-zoster
- Miscellaneous
  - Contact or irritant stomatitis
  - PFAPA syndrome (Periodic fever, aphthosis, pharyngitis, adenitis)
  - Marshall's syndrome
- Nutritional
  - Folic acid deficiency
  - Iron deficiency
  - Thiamine deficiency
  - Vitamin B_1, B_2, B_6, and B_{12} deficiencies
  - Vitamin C deficiency
  - Zinc deficiency
- Oral and genital ulcer disease
  - Behçet's disease
  - MAGIC syndrome (i.e., mouth and genital ulcers with inflamed cartilage syndrome)
  - Tuberculosis enterocolitis
  - Typhoid fever
  - *Yersinia enterocolitica* infection
- Rheumatologic
  - Reiter syndrome
  - Systemic lupus erythematosus (SLE)
- Traumatic
  - Chemical
  - Mechanical
  - Self-injury
  - Thermal

WORKUP

- This is primarily a clinical diagnosis based on the history and physical examination.
- No laboratory tests are available for a definitive diagnosis.

LABORATORY TESTS

- For severe RAU, consider a complete blood cell count, erythrocyte sedimentation rate, chemistry panel, and nutritional evaluation (e.g., iron, ferritin, folate, vitamin B_{12} levels).
- Consider potassium hydroxide examination if concerned about fungal disease.
- Consider viral culture to exclude HSV.
- A pediatric patient with secondary dehydration may benefit from urinalysis and chemistry panel, depending on the clinical scenario.
- When systemic disease is suspected, appropriately tailor the evaluation.

TREATMENT

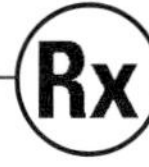

NONPHARMACOLOGIC THERAPY

- Advise consumption of cool, bland beverages.
- Avoid spicy or salty foods.
- Other interventions, although not cost-effective or practical, include laser treatment and low-intensity ultrasound application for severe cases.

ACUTE GENERAL Rx

- Empirical treatment of minor aphthous ulcers or herpetiform ulcers is achieved with local anesthetics.
  - Over-the-counter, topical benzocaine-use sparingly in children, especially in those younger than 2 years old.
  - Lidocaine (2% gel) can be applied to lesions with a cotton-tipped applicator in older children.
  - Local application or swish and spit diphenhydramine may help.
- Major aphthous ulcers may benefit from anti-inflammatory agent use, specifically locally applied corticosteroids.
  - If applied early, high-potency corticosteroids in gel form improve symptoms and shorten course.
  - Corticosteroid sprays can be considered for large areas of ulceration.
  - Liquid preparations can be used for a 2-minute swish and spit routine three or four times per day.
  - Corticosteroid injections may alleviate pain in severe cases.
  - A short course of pulsed oral corticosteroids may be considered in refractory cases.
- Immunomodulatory agents provide an alternative to the use of anti-inflammatory agents.
  - Cyclosporin
  - Retinoids
- Various systemic agents may play a role in the treatment of aphthous ulcers, but experience in children is limited.
  - Colchicine
  - Cimetidine
  - Azathioprine
  - Thalidomide
- Attapulgite (Kaopectate) is a coating agent that may protect and improve the natural mucosal barrier. The swish and spit preparation is recommended.

CHRONIC Rx

Treatment of severe and refractory cases is discussed in the "Acute General Rx" section.

DISPOSITION

- Complications from aphthous ulcers are rare. Most patients recover fully without difficulty.
- The most common problem is dehydration in patients whose oral intake is limited because of pain.
- Patients with major RAU may suffer from local scarring.

REFERRAL

- Consider referral to appropriate specialist if systemic disease is suspected.

PEARLS & CONSIDERATIONS

COMMENTS

- Consider laboratory screening if symptoms are refractory, severe, continuous, or lasting more than 6 months.
- If a nutritional deficiency is suspected, initiate evaluation urgently.

PREVENTION

- Avoid toothpaste or mouthwash containing sodium lauryl sulfate.
- Dietary supplementation for those at risk for vitamin, iron, and zinc deficiencies.
- Patients should maintain healthy oral hygiene. The goal is to limit inflammatory effect and reduce bacteria.
  - Chlorhexidine gluconate
  - Betadine and salt water rinses
  - Dilute hydrogen peroxide rinses

PATIENT/FAMILY EDUCATION

- Reassure patient and family that aphthous ulcers are benign and self-limited.
- Maintain proper oral hygiene, avoid aggravating foods, use nonirritating gargles, and increase oral fluid intake during ulcer outbreak.

SUGGESTED READINGS

Delaney JE et al: Pediatric oral pathology. Soft tissue and periodontal conditions. *Pediatr Clin North Am* 47:1125, 2000.

Field EA et al: Recurrent aphthous ulceration in children—a review. *Int J Paediatr Dent* 2:1, 1992.

McBride DR: Management of aphthous ulcers. *Am Fam Physician* 62:149, 2000.

Natah SS et al: Recurrent aphthous ulcers today: A review of growing knowledge. *Int J Oral Maxillofac Surg* 33:221, 2004.

Scully C: Aphthous ulcers. *eMedicine: Emergency Medicine [serial outline]*, 2004. Available at: http://www.emedicine.com/ent/topic700.htm

AUTHOR: **BRITTANNY LIAM BOULANGER, MD**

BASIC INFORMATION

DEFINITION

An apparent life-threatening event (ALTE) is an episode that is frightening to the observer and that is characterized by some combination of apnea (central or obstructive), change in color (pallor, cyanosis, or suffusion), change in muscle tone (usually diminished), and choking or gagging. In some cases, the observer fears that the infant has died. Previously used terminology (e.g., near-miss SIDS, aborted crib death) should be abandoned because use of these terms implies a possibly misleading close association between this type of spell and sudden infant death syndrome (SIDS) according to the National Institutes of Health (NIH) Consensus Development Conference on Infantile Apnea and Home Monitoring.

SYNONYMS

ALTE
Apnea
Spells

ICD-9-CM CODE
786.09 Apparent life-threatening event

EPIDEMIOLOGY & DEMOGRAPHICS

- The estimated frequency is 1% to 3% among healthy, term infants.
- Risk of subsequent infant death is 1% to 2% among infants experiencing an ALTE.
  - Risk for mortality increases to 4% among infants whose ALTE is associated with respiratory syncytial virus (RSV).
  - Risk for subsequent death increases to 8% to 10% for a small subset of infants who experience ALTEs during sleep or require some form of cardiopulmonary resuscitation (CPR).
- Among victims of SIDS, only 5% have history of an ALTE preceding the death.

CLINICAL PRESENTATION

History

- State of the infant during the event: awake, asleep, location (e.g., crib, car seat, caretaker's arms), position relation to most recent feeding, duration of event
- Appearance of the infant during the event: color (e.g., suffused, pale, cyanotic), respiratory effort (e.g., normal, distressed, apnea), muscle tone (i.e., diminished or increased), abnormal posturing or motor movements, skin temperature and appearance (e.g., cool or warm to touch, mottling, diaphoresis)
- Environmental conditions at the scene: location of event, ambient temperature
- Intervention in response to the event: none, stimulation, rescue breaths, chest compressions, oxygen, assisted ventilations
- Duration of intervention: until resumption of spontaneous respirations
- Medical history
  - Acute (<48 hours): fever, illness symptoms, behavior or feeding change, sleep disruption, immunization
  - Chronic (>48 hours): stridor, snoring, chronic poor feeding or poor weight gain, vomiting or regurgitation, perspiring, excessive or reduced total sleep
  - Birth history: premature birth, oxygen requirement, BPD, apnea, bradycardia, oxygen desaturation, seizures, intraventricular hemorrhage, risk factors for sepsis, congenital anomalies
  - Pregnancy history: maternal history of anemia, diabetes, thyroid disease, seizures, medications, cigarette smoking, drug or alcohol use
- Family history
  - History of SIDS in immediate or remote family, verified by postmortem examination
  - Unexplained death in infancy or childhood without postmortem examination
  - History of sudden death of adolescents or adults (e.g., long QT syndrome)

Physical Examination

- General: persistent change in tone, vigor, mental status, or responsiveness; quality of hydration and perfusion
- Head and neck: characteristics of the fontanelle, pupillary responses, patency of the nasopharyngeal airway, abnormalities of the mandible
- Respiratory: adequacy of oxygenation, pattern of breathing, work of breathing, signs of obstructed airway
- Cardiac: presence of murmur, adequacy and symmetry of pulses, comparison of upper and lower extremity blood pressures
- Abdomen: findings suggesting bowel obstruction, intussusception
- Neurologic: focal or general abnormality in tone, movement, strength, deep tendon reflexes, or sensation

In most cases, the infant appears entirely normal on examination after the initial presentation.

ETIOLOGY

- As many as 50% of ALTEs remain unexplained after a thorough evaluation.
- The principal identifiable causes of ALTE include gastroesophageal reflux, RSV bronchiolitis, pertussis, sepsis or meningitis, seizure, apnea of infancy or apnea associated with premature birth, or breath-holding spells.
- Less common causes include cardiac dysrhythmia (e.g., long QT syndrome); anemia; structural central nervous system (CNS), cardiac, or airway anomalies; or metabolic disturbances manifesting with hypoglycemia.

DIAGNOSIS

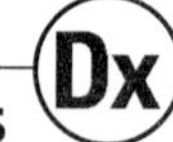

DIFFERENTIAL DIAGNOSIS

- Congenital disorders
  - Craniofacial anomalies producing airway obstruction (e.g., small mandible syndromes, macroglossia, choanal atresia or stenosis)
  - Laryngotracheal anomalies (e.g., laryngotracheomalacia, vascular rings, mucoceles, cysts, hemangiomas)
  - Structural CNS abnormalities associated with apnea
  - Central alveolar hypoventilation syndrome
- Infection
  - Sepsis
  - Meningitis or meningoencephalitis
  - Laryngotracheobronchitis
  - Pneumonia
  - Bronchiolitis
  - Pertussis
  - Enterocolitis with severe dehydration
- Endocrine or metabolic causes
  - Conditions associated with hypoglycemia (e.g., disorders of fatty acid oxidation, defects in glycogen metabolism or gluconeogenesis, hyperinsulinemic states)
  - Adrenogenital syndrome, adrenal insufficiency, or hypopituitarism
- Intoxication
  - Accidental or intentional exposure to drugs (prescription or illicit), depressing the CNS
  - Carbon monoxide
- Trauma
  - Accidental
  - Shaken baby syndrome
  - Munchausen syndrome by proxy
  - Thermal environmental stress
- Neoplastic disease
  - CNS tumors affecting respiratory control
  - Tumors causing extrinsic or intrinsic airway compromise
- Other causes
  - Gastroesophageal reflux
  - Seizure with or without fever

WORKUP

Relevant medical testing is suggested by the carefully obtained history and physical examination.

LABORATORY TESTS

- Testing may be indicated by the history and physical examination.
  - Complete blood cell count
  - Blood chemistries, including electrolytes, glucose, calcium, phosphorous, and lactate
  - Blood gas analysis
  - Specific bacterial or viral cultures, including nasopharyngeal swabs for pertussis and bacterial culture of the urine
  - Electrocardiogram
  - Electroencephalogram
  - Polysomnography

IMAGING STUDIES

- Imaging studies may be indicated by the history and physical examination.

- Chest radiograph
- Axial or appendicular skeletal surveys in cases of suspected nonaccidental trauma
- Computed tomography of the head for suspected acute bleeding, hydrocephalus, or a space-occupying lesion
- Magnetic resonance imaging for remote trauma, gray or white matter lesions, or tumors

TREATMENT

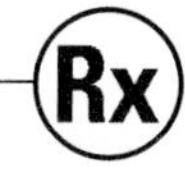

NONPHARMACOLOGIC THERAPY

- Cardiorespiratory monitoring may be indicated for those infants with documented or suspected apnea of infancy or respiratory control disorders.
- Prescriptions for event monitors should include CPR and monitor alarm training for caregivers.

ACUTE GENERAL Rx

Results of the diagnostic evaluation can suggest specific treatments, such as antibiotics for suspected sepsis, anticonvulsants for seizures, and antireflux measures for gastroesophageal reflux.

CHRONIC Rx

Results of the diagnostic evaluation can suggest specific treatments.

DISPOSITION

- In-hospital observation is suggested for most infants after an ALTE.
- Self-resolving episodes of choking or gagging in well-appearing infants may be observed through the outpatient setting if all elements of the evaluation are normal.

PEARLS & CONSIDERATIONS

COMMENTS

- Pertussis and bacterial urinary tract infections collectively account for approximately 15% to 20% of ALTEs, highlighting the importance of obtaining the appropriate diagnostic studies at the time of the initial evaluation.
- Direct ophthalmoscopic examination should be obtained for all infants for whom nonaccidental trauma is suspected. Child abuse reporting protocols should be followed.
- When in doubt regarding the cause, infants with ALTEs should be hospitalized.

PREVENTION

Evidenced-based guidelines for prevention are lacking. Immunization is logical in terms of reducing risk, although many of the pertussis-related ALTEs occur in young infants who are incompletely or not immunized.

PATIENT/FAMILY EDUCATION

- Families may harbor fears that the ALTE is a harbinger of SIDS.
- From retrospective series, only 5% of SIDS victims had a preceding ALTE.

SUGGESTED READINGS

Brooks JG: Apparent life-threatening events. *Pediatr Rev* 17:257, 1996.

Davies F et al: Apparent life threatening events in infants presenting to an emergency department. *Emerg Med J* 19:11, 2002.

Gozal D: New concepts in abnormalities of respiratory control in children. *Curr Opin Pediatr* 16:305, 2004.

Gray C et al: Apparent life-threatening events presenting to a pediatric emergency department. *Pediatr Emerg Care* 15:195, 1999.

Kiechl-Kohlendorfer U et al: Epidemiology of apparent life threatening events. *Arch Dis Child* 90:297, 2005.

Little GA et al: National Institutes of Health consensus development on infantile apnea and home monitoring. *Pediatrics* 79:292, 1987.

AUTHOR: **PATRICK L. CAROLAN, MD**

BASIC INFORMATION

DEFINITIONS

Acute appendicitis is inflammation of the vermiform appendix. Chronic appendicitis is characterized by chronic inflammatory changes of the vermiform appendix thought to be a possible factor in chronic recurrent abdominal pain, but many surgeons are unsure how often this occurs. Perforated appendicitis refers to perforation of the vermiform appendix; perforated appendicitis may result in the formation of a localized periappendiceal abscess with an appendiceal mass, or generalized peritonitis. Gangrenous appendicitis is acute appendicitis or perforated appendicitis accompanied by gangrene of the vermiform appendix.

SYNONYMS

"Appy"
Perityphlitis

ICD-9-CM CODES
540 Acute appendicitis
540.0 With generalized peritonitis
540.1 With peritoneal abscess
540.9 Without mention of peritonitis
541 Appendicitis, unqualified
542 Other appendicitis (chronic, recurrent, subacute)

EPIDEMIOLOGY & DEMOGRAPHICS

- Appendicitis accounts for 8% of emergency department visits for acute abdominal pain.
- Approximately 80,000 appendectomies are performed per year.
- There is a slight male predominance.
- Incidence is 1 to 2 cases per 10,000 children each year for children 0 to 4 years old.
- The incidence is 25:10,000 children/year for ages 10 to 19 years old
- Appendicitis is rare in infants younger than 1 year.

CLINICAL PRESENTATION

History

- The classic history of 24 to 36 hours of pain starting in the periumbilical area and localizing to the right lower quadrant is valid for less than one half of children with appendicitis.
- The child with appendicitis often has a low-grade fever and lower abdominal pain, usually greater in the right lower quadrant than in the left.
- The child is anorexic and may be nauseated or have a history of vomiting.
- A low-lying or pelvic appendix can produce diarrhea, dyschezia, or pelvic pain in female patients.
- None of these symptoms is universal or diagnostic of appendicitis.
- A history of more than a few days' duration should alert the clinician to the possibility of a perforated appendix or an appendiceal abscess.
- Children younger than 3 years often present with perforated appendicitis.

Physical Examination

- The physical examination is the most important aspect in diagnosing appendicitis, and proficiency in making this diagnosis improves with increasing experience.
- The child may be lethargic and lying on the stretcher with the knees bent in an attempt to decrease peritoneal irritation.
- Children may look well and still have appendicitis.
- Low-grade fever is common.
- A child with appendicitis has tenderness in the right lower quadrant, usually with involuntary guarding.
- Focal peritoneal signs are the hallmark of appendicitis.
  - Rovsing's sign: pain in the right lower quadrant when pressing on the patient's left and releasing suddenly
  - Obturator sign: pain with internal rotation of the flexed thigh
  - Psoas sign: pain on passive extension of the right hip
- Rectal examination may reveal inflammation in the right lower quadrant or a mass in the pelvis if the patient has a pelvic abscess low enough to be palpated.

ETIOLOGY

- Acute appendicitis is most often initiated by proximal luminal obstruction.
- Luminal obstruction is often the result of a fecalith or inspissated enteric material forming an impaction at the appendiceal orifice. Lymphoid hyperplasia is also an important cause of luminal obstruction in children.
- Obstruction of the luminal orifice leads to elevated luminal pressure, which eventually exceeds capillary venous pressure, resulting in mucosal ischemia and infarction. This also results in decreased bacterial clearance from the appendiceal lumen, with subsequent bacterial overgrowth, inflammation, infection, infarction, and pain.
- Protracted obstruction may result in perforation.
- Less common causes of appendicitis include the following:
  - Foreign bodies
  - Bacterial infections, including *Yersinia, Salmonella,* and *Shigella*
  - Parasitic infections, most commonly pinworms
  - Tumors, most commonly a mucocele or carcinoid

DIAGNOSIS

DIFFERENTIAL DIAGNOSIS

- Viral gastroenteritis
- Bacterial enterocolitis
- Constipation
- Urinary tract infection
- Ruptured ovarian cyst
- Ovarian torsion
- Pelvic inflammatory disease
- Ectopic pregnancy
- Cholecystitis
- Crohn's disease
- Meckel's diverticulitis
- Renal lithiasis
- Intussusception
- Henoch-Schönlein purpura
- Primary peritonitis
- Porphyria
- Trauma
- Pancreatitis

WORKUP

- In some centers, clinical pathways for right lower quadrant pain exist for children older than 3 years.
- Pathways attempt to minimize unnecessary laboratory and radiographic studies, and were developed to provide a unified approach to patients with suspected appendicitis.

LABORATORY TESTS

- White blood cell (WBC) count may be normal or only mildly elevated, especially in the early course of appendicitis. Neutrophilia may be more sensitive than the WBC.
- Urinalysis is often done to exclude a urinary cause of symptoms. Occasional red or white blood cells may be seen because of irritation of the ureter from an inflamed appendix.

IMAGING STUDIES

- Abdominal radiographs are normal for up to 77% of children with appendicitis.
  - They are helpful in evaluating for constipation and obstruction and for excluding free air.
  - An appendicolith may be seen in 13% to 22% of patients with appendicitis.
- Ultrasonography may be helpful in identifying an inflamed appendix.
  - Patient's body habitus, overlying gas, or abnormal appendix position all contribute to the inability to visualize the appendix and potential false-negative results.
  - In adolescent females, ultrasound may be useful in evaluating for gynecologic abnormalities.
- Computed tomography (CT) has a sensitivity and specificity of 90%. A CT scan is most useful for a child who is suspected of having perforated appendicitis or a patient whose clinical presentation may be unusual or unclear.

TREATMENT

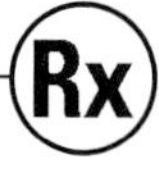

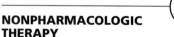

NONPHARMACOLOGIC THERAPY

- Nonperforated appendicitis
  - Acute appendicitis is best treated with prompt appendectomy. This can safely be performed with an open procedure or laparoscopically.

- Morbidity of this operation remains quite low, with wound infection and intra-abdominal abscess formation being the most common postoperative complications.
- Children are given one dose of antibiotics preoperatively, usually a second-generation cephalosporin, and one dose postoperatively. They are allowed to eat ad libitum postoperatively.
- Most patients with uncomplicated appendicitis are discharged on postoperative day 1.

- Perforated appendicitis
  - Early perforated appendicitis is treated by open surgery or laparoscopic appendectomy.
  - Postoperatively, these patients often have a prolonged ileus, requiring nasogastric tube decompression, and they can be febrile for many days.
  - Postoperative culture of the febrile patient with perforated appendicitis is unnecessary.
  - Broad-spectrum intravenous antibiotics are initiated preoperatively and continued postoperatively at least until discharge, with some physicians advocating a 7-day course and others switching the patient to oral antibiotics on discharge.
  - Persistent fever or an elevation in the WBC count beyond 7 days should raise the suspicion of an intraperitoneal abscess and may warrant a CT scan.
  - If symptoms at presentation have been present for more than 3 to 5 days, a CT scan may be helpful in determining the presence of an abscess.
  - When an abscess is present, consideration is given to percutaneous abscess drainage with interval appendectomy in 6 weeks. Antibiotics are given intravenously for a total of 7 to 10 days, similar to the approach to the patient who is treated for perforated appendicitis postoperatively. Earlier operation is considered if symptoms worsen or do not improve with drainage and antibiotics.

DISPOSITION

- There usually are no significant risks for uncomplicated appendicitis.
- Patients with perforated appendix or peritonitis have a long-term increased risk of bowel obstruction and adhesions.

REFERRAL

Appendicitis is a surgical disease, and a pediatric or general surgeon should be consulted early in the evaluation.

PEARLS & CONSIDERATIONS

COMMENTS

- A child with abdominal pain and fever should raise the suspicion for appendicitis.
- The most reliable way to diagnose appendicitis is the abdominal examination performed by an experienced physician.
- If there is any question about the diagnosis, prompt surgical consultation should be requested.

SUGGESTED READINGS

Arca MJ, Caniano DA: Acute appendicitis. *In* Mattei P (ed): *Surgical Directives: Pediatric Surgery.* Philadelphia, Lippincott Williams & Wilkins, 2003, pp 395–398.

Muehlstedt SG et al: The management of pediatric appendicitis: A survey of North American pediatric surgeons. *J Pediatr Surg* 39:875, 2004.

AUTHOR: **RICHARD A. FALCONE, JR., MD**

BASIC INFORMATION

DEFINITION

Infectious and septic arthritis refer to microbial invasion of the synovial space, typically with bacteria in acute septic arthritis and rarely with fungi or mycobacteria.

SYNONYMS

Acute septic arthritis
Acute suppurative pyoarthrosis
Infectious arthritis

ICD-9-CM CODE
711.0 Septic arthritis
711.9 Infectious arthritis

EPIDEMIOLOGY & DEMOGRAPHICS

- The incidence is estimated at 5.5 to 12 cases per 100,000 individuals.
- The peak incidence occurs in children younger than 3 years.
- There is a male-to-female ratio of 2:1.
- Lower extremities (e.g., knees, hips, ankles) account for 80% of infections.
- More than 90% of infections are monoarticular.

CLINICAL PRESENTATION

History
- Patients may have fever, malaise, and arthralgias.
- Some patients report a recent upper respiratory infection (URI) or local soft tissue infection.
- Neonates may have poor feeding, irritability, or nonmovement of limbs.
- Children usually complain of pain and limp, or they refuse to walk.
- Onset is more acute than with osteomyelitis.

Physical Examination
- Examination reveals local erythema, warmth, and swelling of affected joints.
- The patient has tenderness with passive joint motion and decreased active range of motion.
- The joint is held in a position of comfort (e.g., abduction, external rotation for hip).
    - In infants, swelling and erythema may not be present, and results of the physical examination may be remarkable only for fever and irritability.
- The patient may have decreased or absent movement (pseudoparalysis) of the affected limb or joint.

ETIOLOGY

- The synovial space may become infected by hematogenous seeding, local spread from adjacent infection, or trauma or surgical infection.
- Synovial fluid cushions and nourishes the avascular cartilage of the joint.
- The rich capillary network of the synovial membrane produces synovial fluid.
    - This network is the port of entry for bacteria.
    - Bacterial hyaluronidase decreases the viscosity and function of synovial fluid.
    - Bacterial endotoxin stimulates the release of cytokines.
    - Cytokines stimulate the release of proteolytic enzymes.
    - This eventually leads to pressure necrosis from accumulation of purulent fluid.
- Because infants have blood vessels that connect metaphysis and epiphysis, septic arthritis may be a complication of osteomyelitis.
- Hips and shoulders are at risk for extension of osteomyelitis into septic arthritis because the joint capsule overlies the metaphysis in the femur and humerus.
- Predisposing factors for infectious arthritis include the following:
    - Trauma
    - Joint surgery
    - Joint injections
    - Hemoglobinopathies
    - Immunodeficiency
    - Intravenous drug use
    - Juvenile arthritis
- Bacterial causes should be considered.
    - *Staphylococcus aureus* is the most common, followed by group A streptococci and *Streptococcus pneumoniae.*
    - Other causes include *Neisseria gonorrhoeae* (in neonates and sexually active adolescents), gram-negative bacteria, *Salmonella* (about 1% of all cases, more common with sickle cell disease), and *Kingella kingae.*
    - *Haemophilus influenzae* is becoming rare since the introduction of immunization.
    - Causes in neonates include *S. aureus,* group B streptococci, gram-negative enteric organisms, and methicillin-resistant *Staphylococcus aureus* (MRSA).

DIAGNOSIS

DIFFERENTIAL DIAGNOSIS

- Toxic synovitis
- Juvenile arthritis
- Rheumatic fever
- Leukemia
- Henoch-Schönlein purpura
- Legg-Calvé-Perthes disease
- Slipped capital femoral epiphysis
- Villonodular synovitis
- Ulcerative colitis
- Bacterial endocarditis
- Reactive arthritis from a variety of infectious agents:
    - *Borrelia burgdorferi* (Lyme disease)
    - *Chlamydia*
    - *Mycoplasma*
    - Viral hepatitis A and B, rubella, human immunodeficiency virus, mumps, parvovirus B19, enterovirus, herpes
- Sterile inflammatory arthritis in association with infection at a distant site
- Reiter's syndrome, which occurs after intestinal infection with *Salmonella, Shigella, Yersinia,* or *Campylobacter*
    - May or may not have fever; can be monoarticular or oligoarticular
    - Knees and ankles most commonly affected
    - Culture only way to differentiate between septic and reactive arthritis
    - Synovial leukocyte count may be helpful
- Gonococcal arthritis
    - Hematogenous spread of infection leads to fever, chills, maculopapular rash with petechiae, tenosynovitis, and migratory polyarthralgia.
    - Polyarthritis is seen in 50% of patients.
    - Knees, elbows, ankles, wrists, and the small joints of hands and feet all may be affected.
    - Arthritis can be reactive or septic.
    - Synovial culture is positive in 25% to 35%, blood culture is positive in 20%, and genital culture is positive in 80%.
- Lyme arthritis
    - This form of arthritis occurs several weeks to months after infection with the spirochete *B. burgdorferi.*
    - Most cases occur in the Northeast, with a lower frequency in the upper Midwest and uncommon reports from northern California.
    - Acute, oligoarticular arthritis (e.g., knees) may be seen.
        - This arthritis is episodic, lasts for days, and may occur without prior symptoms.
        - Treat with oral amoxicillin or doxycycline (for patients older than 8 years).
- Viral arthritis
    - The most common viruses are rubella, parvovirus B19, and hepatitis B.
    - Viral arthritis is more common in adults than in children.
    - There is often more arthralgia than arthritis. The disease is migratory, lasts for 1 to 2 weeks, and resolves without residual disease.
    - Symmetric joints of the hand are affected after rubella (or after rubella vaccine) and hepatitis B infection.
- Mycobacterial arthritis
    - Unusual in North America and Europe
    - Joint infection from reactivation and hematogenous spread
    - Slowly progressive monoarthritis, usually affecting the knee or hip
    - History of exposure; positive purified protein derivative
- Fungal arthritis
    - Rare
    - Risk factors: immunodeficiency, malignancy
    - Chronic monoarticular arthritis

WORKUP

- Joint aspiration should be done without delay if the diagnosis is suspected.

- The aspirate should be sent for Gram stain, aerobic and anaerobic culture, white blood cell (WBC) count with a differential cell count, synovial glucose determination and comparative blood glucose level, and a mucin clot test.
- Median synovial fluid leukocyte count is 40,000 to 50,000 WBCs/mm^3, and 75% to 90% are neutrophils.
- Sensitivity and specificity are 90% for WBC counts higher than 40,000/mm^3.
  - Glucose concentration is often decreased (30% of blood value), but this is also seen in cases of rheumatoid joints and acute rheumatic fever.
  - Joint culture is positive in 50% to 60% of cases.

LABORATORY TESTS

- Complete blood cell (CBC) count with differential cell count, which may be elevated with a left shift
- Erythrocyte sedimentation rate (ESR) (usually elevated but nonspecific; returns to normal in about 4 weeks) or C-reactive protein (CRP) level (elevated; returns to normal more quickly than ESR; secondary rise may be a warning sign of return of infection)
- Blood cultures: 30% positive

IMAGING STUDIES

- Radiograph: increased joint space or soft tissue swelling; may see subluxation of the femoral head, especially in neonates
- Ultrasound: modality of choice to identify fluid and guide aspiration
- Scintigraphy: increased tracer uptake; less focal and less intense than with osteomyelitis
- Computed tomography (CT) and magnetic resonance imaging (MRI) scans: cannot differentiate septic from nonseptic arthritis
- MRI: highly sensitive for early detection of joint fluid; superior to CT in outlining soft tissue

TREATMENT

NONPHARMACOLOGIC THERAPY

- Open drainage is indicated if the hip joints (and perhaps shoulders) are involved.
- If large amounts of fibrin, tissue debris, or loculation are present, surgical drainage is needed.
- If the patient is not improving with medical treatment in 3 days, drainage may be needed.

ACUTE GENERAL Rx

- Joint aspiration is followed by parenteral antimicrobial therapy for 3 to 4 weeks.
- Empirical coverage should include a β-lactamase–resistant penicillin or a first-generation cephalosporin.
  - Cefuroxime is a useful alternative (covers *H. influenzae*).
  - If methicillin (or oxacillin) resistant staphylococcus aureus (MRSA, ORSA) or pneumococcus is suspected or the patient has a penicillin or cephalosporin allergy, administer vancomycin.
  - For neonates, a β-lactamase–resistant penicillin in combination with an aminoglycoside or with a third-generation cephalosporin is suggested.
  - For children with sickle cell anemia, a third-generation cephalosporin (i.e., ceftriaxone or cefotaxime) and antistaphylococcal therapy (i.e., nafcillin) are used.
  - Parenteral treatment with ceftriaxone or cefotaxime for 7 to 14 days is indicated for gonococcal arthritis.
  - For immunocompromised hosts, ceftazidime or ticarcillin-clavulanate with an aminoglycoside is chosen.
- Antibiotic therapy should be narrowed after the organism and sensitivities are identified.
- Oral therapy can be instituted when the patient's condition has stabilized and Compliance can be ensured (i.e., oral antibiotics given at two to three times the usual doses).
- Direct infusion of antibiotics into the joint is not helpful; some antibiotics may even increase the inflammatory response.

DISPOSITION

- Acute treatment follow-up
  - Serial ESR, CRP, or CBC tests
  - Serial bactericidal titers of at least 1:8
  - Monitoring for adverse drug reactions
- Long-term follow-up for residual effects
  - Leg length discrepancy
  - Limitation of motion
  - Chronic pain
  - Need for secondary surgical procedures
- Important predictors of poor outcome
  - Duration of symptoms longer than 7 days before treatment
  - Age younger than 1 year
  - Infection of hip or shoulder

REFERRAL

Early orthopedic consultation is critical for diagnosis and management.

PEARLS & CONSIDERATIONS

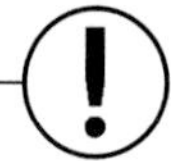

COMMENTS

- Gram stain of the joint fluid is important.
  - Joint fluid is bacteriostatic, preventing organisms from growing well in culture.
  - Approximately 30% of joint cultures are sterile despite other findings consistent with bacterial joint infection.
- A preceding URI is common in septic arthritis caused by *H. influenzae* and *K. kingae*.

PATIENT/FAMILY EDUCATION

- Stress the importance of compliance and follow-up.
- Discuss potential long-term complications.

SUGGESTED READINGS

Krogstad P, Smith AL: Osteomyelitis and septic arthritis. *In* Feigin R, Cherry J (eds): *Pediatric Infectious Diseases.* Philadelphia, WB Saunders, 1998.

Shetty AK, Gedalia A: Septic arthritis in children. *Rheumatol Clin North Am* 24:287, 1998.

Sonnen GM, Henry NK: Pediatric bone and joint infections: Diagnosis and management. *Pediatr Clin North Am* 43:933, 1996.

AUTHOR: **MEREDITH LANDORF, MD**

BASIC INFORMATION

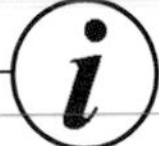

DEFINITION

Chronic arthritis in children is diagnosed when all three of the following criteria are met. 1. The age of onset is younger than 16 years; 2. Arthritis includes swelling or effusion, or presence of two or more of the following: a) limitation of range of motion; b) tenderness or pain on motion; c) increased heat in one or more joints; and 3. The duration of disease is 1½ months or longer. Based on disease charateristics in the first 6 months after onset, juvenile arthritis is classified as follows:

- System onset: arthritis with charateristic quotidian fever pattern, rash, adenopathy, hepatosplenomegly
- Polyarthritis rheumatoid factor negative: five or more inflamed joints
- Polyarthritis rheumatoid factor positive: five or more inflamed joints
- Oligoarthritis: lessthan five inflamed joints
- Exgended oligoarthritis: begins with fewer than 5 inflamed joints but progresses to polyarthritis
- Enthesitis related arthritis: sacroiliitis, enthesitis, HLA-B27
- Psoriatic arthritis

SYNONYMS

Idiopathic arthritides of childhood
Juvenile chronic arthritis
Juvenile rheumatoid arthritis
Still's disease (usually refers only to systemic onset)

ICD-9-CM CODES

713.31 Juvenile psoriatic arthritis with psoriasis
713.32 Juvenile psoriatic arthritis without psoriasis
714.30 Juvenile rheumatoid arthritis
714.31 Systemic onset
714.32 Pauciarticular (oligoarthritis)
714.33 Polyarthritis
720.01 Juvenile ankylosing spondylitis

EPIDEMIOLOGY & DEMOGRAPHICS

- The incidence is 9.2 to 19.6 cases per 100,000 children.
- Prevalence is 69.1 to 196.3 cases per 100,000 children.
- The female-to-male ratio is 3:1 for oligoarthritis, 5:1 to 6:1 if uveitis is present, 2.8:1 for polyarthritis, and 1:1 for systemic onset.
- The peak age of onset is 1 to 3 years overall and is less skewed toward younger children in cases of polyarthritis and systemic onset.

CLINICAL PRESENTATION

History

- Oligoarthritis: minimal constitutional symptoms; involved joints often not significantly painful
- Polyarthritis: mild to moderate constitutional symptoms; more pain and stiffness
- Systemic onset: prominent constitutional symptoms; patient quite ill and debilitated, especially when febrile

Physical Examination

- Oligoarthritis
  - Usual absence of fever; knee most commonly affected
  - Swelling
  - Warmth
  - Mild to moderate tenderness
  - Limitation of range of motion
  - Uveitis or iridocyclitis, especially in presence of antinuclear antibody (ANA)
- Polyarthritis
  - Mildly febrile
  - Fatigue
  - Weight loss
  - Small and large joints
  - Symmetric, especially in presence of positive rheumatoid factor (RF)
- Systemic onset
  - Daily spiking fever to higher than 39°C, usually in the afternoon or early evening
  - Irritability
  - Fatigue
  - Weight loss
  - Pale pink, macular, evanescent rash
  - Lymphadenopathy
  - Hepatosplenomegaly
  - Tends to be polyarticular but may not develop until weeks after onset of systemic features

ETIOLOGY

The cause is unknown.

DIAGNOSIS

DIFFERENTIAL DIAGNOSIS

- Infectious arthritis
- Postinfectious arthritis
- Hematologic disorders
- Hemophilic arthropathy
- Neoplasm
- Familial Mediterranean fever
- Sarcoidosis
- Other connective tissue disorders
- Vasculitis
- Inflammatory bowel disease
- Pigmented villonodular synovitis

LABORATORY TESTS

- Complete blood cell count with differential and platelet count: leukocytosis, anemia, and thrombocytosis most prominent in systemic-onset form and least likely in oligoarthritis
- Erythrocyte sedimentation rate, C-reactive protein: markedly elevated in systemic-onset form, moderately elevated in polyarthritis, mild to moderate elevation in oligoarthritis
- ANA: present in subset of oligoarthritis; marker for increased risk of uveitis
- RF: present only in small subset of patients with polyarthritis
- Liver function tests: levels elevated in systemic onset
- HLA-B27: present in juvenile ankylosing spondylitis

IMAGING STUDIES

- Joint radiographs
  - Erosions appear after persistent disease, especially in polyarthritis disease.
  - Sacroiliitis is seen in ankylosing spondylitis.
  - Cervical spine films most commonly show fusion, except in RF-positive patients.

TREATMENT

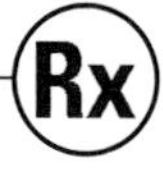

NONPHARMACOLOGIC THERAPY

- Physical therapy (PT)
- Occupational therapy (OT), including heat, ultrasound, and splinting
- Psychotherapy and counseling
- Joint replacements (should be performed at as old an age as possible to preserve long bone growth and decrease the potential number of prosthesis revisions)
- Tendon-release procedures

ACUTE GENERAL Rx

- Nonsteroidal anti-inflammatory drugs (NSAIDs)
- Disease-modifying antirheumatic drugs, initially methotrexate
- Systemic corticosteroids (typically in systemic-onset form); intra-articular corticosteroids (e.g., triamcinolone hexacetonide)
- Tumor necrosis factor-α antagonists (e.g., etanercept, infliximab)
- Other immunosuppressants

CHRONIC Rx

- Patients require multidisciplinary care with aggressive PT and OT.
- Medications may need to be manipulated according to the degree of disease activity.
- Patients may need intensive physical rehabilitation.
- Surgical consultation is necessary in long-term and persistent cases.

DISPOSITION

Information is offered in the "Treatment" and "Pearls & Considerations" sections.

REFERRAL

Rheumatologist or pediatric rheumatologist should be consulted when available for diagnosis and treatment considerations. Referrals may be needed for OT, PT, orthopedic surgery, psychology, social work, and ophthalmology.

PEARLS & CONSIDERATIONS

COMMENTS

- There are no absolutely confirmatory laboratory tests. It is a clinical diagnosis.

- Uveitis occurrence does not correlate with the level of joint inflammation.
- Peripheral, large-joint arthritis typically precedes any spine involvement in juvenile ankylosing spondylitis.
- Folic acid or folinic acid supplementation for patients receiving methotrexate can decrease side effects.

PREVENTION

- Screening slit-lamp examinations of eyes for patients at high risk for uveitis
- Monitoring for gastric erosion or ulcer disease in patients on NSAIDs or corticosteroids
- Osteoporosis prevention strategies for patients receiving long-term corticosteroids

PATIENT/FAMILY EDUCATION

- Patients follow very different disease courses; oligoarthritis tends to be least problematic.
- The adjustment to a chronic, disabling disease can be challenging.
- Nonmedical therapy is as important as medical.
- Support groups are available through organizations such as the American Juvenile Arthritis Organization (1330 W. Peachtree St., Atlanta, GA 30309; 404-872-7100).

SUGGESTED READINGS

Arthritis Foundation www.arthritis.org

Fink CW: Proposal for the development of classification criteria for idiopathic arthritides of childhood. *J Rheumatol* 22:1566, 1995.

Lovell DJ, et al: Long-term efficacy and safety of etanerapt in children with polyarticular-course juvenile rheumatoid arthritis: interim results from an ongoing multicenter, open-label, extended-treatment trial. Arthritis Rheum 48:218 2003.

Weiss JE, Ilowite NT: Juvenile idiopathic arthritis. *Pediatr Clin North Am* 52:413, 2005.

AUTHOR: **DAVID M. SIEGEL, MD, MPH**

BASIC INFORMATION

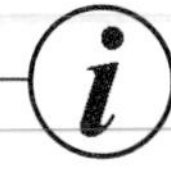

DEFINITION

Aspiration pneumonia results from aspiration of materials or chemicals foreign to the tracheobronchial tree from above (e.g., aspiration of colonized oropharyngeal materials) or from below (e.g., aspiration of gastroesophageal contents).

SYNONYMS

Aspiration lung injury
Aspiration syndromes
Chemical pneumonitis
Bacterial aspiration pneumonia

ICD-9-CM CODES
507.0 Aspiration pneumonia or pneumonitis
997.3 Acid pulmonary aspiration syndrome

EPIDEMIOLOGY & DEMOGRAPHICS

- Silent aspiration is common, even in normal individuals. However, the incidence of aspiration-related respiratory illness in infants and children is unknown.
- Between 5% and 15% of community-acquired pneumonia cases are aspiration pneumonia.
- Gastroesophageal reflux (GER) with aspiration may cause acute or chronic chemical injury to the lung.
- Craniofacial anomalies with associated swallowing dysfunction increase the risk of aspiration.
- Aspiration occurs in 16% to 80% of children who are endotracheally intubated.
- Neuromuscular deficits or weakness of bulbar musculature increases risk.
  - Depressed level of consciousness (e.g., drug overdose, general anesthesia, head trauma, seizures, central nervous system infection)
  - Immaturity or elderly age
  - Vocal cord paralysis or dysfuntion
  - Various neurologic conditions (e.g., cerebral palsy, increased intracranial pressure, strokes, muscular dystrophy, Werdnig-Hoffman disease)
- Patients with episodic or chronic airway obstruction are at increased risk for oropharyngeal aspiration.
  - Upper airway obstruction (e.g., laryngomalacia, obstructive sleep apnea)
  - Lower airway obstruction (e.g., tracheobronchomalacia, vascular ring)
- As many as 50% of cases of aspiration pneumonia are associated with subsequent bacterial infection.
- The mortality rate after aspiration of gastric contents is high.
  - Immediate death: 16%
  - Death as the disease progresses: 24%
  - Stabilization and recovery: 60%

CLINICAL PRESENTATION

History

- Irritability, colic, Sandifer syndrome, abdominal pain, or heartburn
- Nighttime or recumbent episodes of wheezing, coughing, gagging, or respiratory distress
- Frequent regurgitation or vomiting
- Coughing, gagging, or choking with feeds by mouth or by nasogastric tube
- Apnea or apparent life-threatening events
- Failure to thrive
- Recurrent pneumonias
- Stridor or hoarseness
- Anemia from hematemesis or melena

Physical Examination

- Respiratory distress (e.g., dyspnea, cyanosis, tachypnea, acute bronchospasm)
- Possible fever
- Orotracheal or endotracheal suctioning of gastric contents

ETIOLOGY

- Congenital anomalies of the palate and upper respiratory tract
- Swallowing disorders from anatomic, mechanical, or neurologic causes
- Disorders of esophageal motility
- Decreased lower esophageal sphincter (LES) pressure
- Delayed gastric emptying
- Depressed level of consciousness
- Gastrointestinal dysmotility caused by critical illness (e.g., sepsis, shock, trauma, burns, surgery)

DIAGNOSIS

DIFFERENTIAL DIAGNOSIS

- Acute or chronic sinopulmonary infections
- Airways hyperreactivity without aspiration
- Reflex laryngospasm without aspiration

LABORATORY TESTS

- Tracheal aspirate for quantitative and qualitative cultures

IMAGING STUDIES

- Chest radiograph
  - Airspace disease or interstitial infiltrates: in the basal segments of the lower lobes when upright or semirecumbent and in the posterior segments of the upper lobes or apical segments of the lower lobes when recumbent
  - Atelectasis or obstructive pneumonitis
  - Possible visible aspirated substance on the radiograph
- Upper gastrointestinal (UGI) series with fluoroscopy
  - To evaluate anatomic defects (e.g., vascular ring, tracheoesophageal fistula, pulmonary sling or gastric outlet obstruction)
  - To observe for esophageal dysmotility
- Modified barium swallowing study
  - To assess deglutition or aspiration into the larynx or trachea
  - Uses barium as contrast with different textures, including solid, soft, and liquid
- Gastroesophageal scintiscan (i.e., milk scan) with technetium 99m sulfur colloid mixed with milk or formula given orally
  - To assess gastric emptying time
  - To detect radioactivity in the lung fields, which indicates aspiration

SPECIAL TESTS

- Bronchoscopy to evaluate for erythema or inflammation of laryngeal structures or tracheobronchial tree
- Bronchoalveolar washings to detect food fibers or particles and to evaluate quantitative lipid-laden macrophages (i.e., lipid-laden macrophage index correlates with the degree of chronic microaspiration in children)
- Manometry to measure esophageal motility and sphincter pressures

TREATMENT

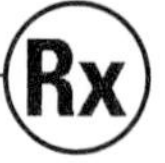

NONPHARMACOLOGIC THERAPY

- Direct therapy at the underlying condition.
- Alter feeding techniques (e.g., thickened feeds; frequent, smaller feeds; continuous tube feedings instead of bolus feedings).
- Alter the patient's position (e.g., feeding only when upright, laying down in semi-upright position, prone position for infants).
- Provide adequate oxygen and ventilatory support.
- Provide good pulmonary toilet.
- Bronchoscopy is used to remove particulate matter in the tracheobronchial tree.
- Antireflux surgery may be performed.
  - Nissen or Thal fundoplication in patients with GER alone
  - Gastrostomy tube placement with fundoplication in patients with oral or pharyngeal dysphagia and GER
  - Fundoplication and pyloroplasty in patients with GER and delayed gastric emptying

ACUTE GENERAL Rx

- The upper airway should be suctioned if aspiration is witnessed.
- Use broad-spectrum antibiotics (e.g., second- or third-generation cephalosporins, fluoroquinolones, piperacillin, clindamycin, or penicillin G) to cover gram-positive organisms (e.g., *Staphylococcus aureus, Streptococcus pneumoniae*), enteric gram-negative bacilli (e.g., *Pseudomonas*, others), *Haemophilus influenzae,* and anaerobes.

CHRONIC Rx

- Prokinetic drugs: agents with cholinergic activity that improve sphincter tone and increase esophageal motility and gastric emptying (e.g., metoclopramide, bethanechol)
- Acid modifiers: reduce gastric acidity and decrease the release of gastric secretions

- Histamine$(H)_2$-receptor antagonists: cimetidine, ranitidine, famotidine, nizatidine
- Proton pump inhibitors: omeprazole, lansoprazole, pantoprazole

DISPOSITION

- Less than one third of infants and children undergoing antireflux surgery experience side effects from the surgical procedure.
  - Inability to vomit or burp: 28%
  - Gas bloating: 36%
  - Slow eating: 32%
  - Choking on some solids: 25%
- Approximately 9% require reoperation (e.g., "slipped" wrap or disrupted fundoplication, incisional hernia or dehiscence, hiatal hernia, bowel obstruction).
- A 1.3% fatality rate results from the surgical procedure.
- Pneumonia recurs in up to 40% of patients, and the rate appears to be highest for children with profound neurologic disability.

REFERRAL

Patients should be referred to appropriate subspecialists for workup and management when necessary.

- Gastroenterologist
- Pulmonologist
- Otolaryngologist
- Pediatric surgeon
- Nutritionist
- Speech pathologist
- Respiratory therapist

PEARLS & CONSIDERATIONS

COMMENTS

- A high index of suspicion should be maintained in light of chronic cough or wheeze, nighttime symptoms, recurrent pneumonias, and failure to thrive.
- Adequate nutritional rehabilitation in malnourished patients improves the surgical outcome.
- Strict nothing-by-mouth orders and a program of respiratory care during nutritional rehabilitation before surgery prepares patients' lungs to be in best possible and healed condition; persistent cough can disrupt surgical fundoplication.

PREVENTION

- Early recognition and modification of factors that place patients at high risk are important.
- Good oral hygiene and antibiotic treatment of upper respiratory bacterial infections can decrease the risk of complications in aspiration.
- Craniofacial abnormalities, vascular ring or sling, or tracheoesophageal fistula should be surgically corrected.
- Patients scheduled for anesthesia and surgery should fast preoperatively.
- Preoperative use of H_2-blockers and prokinetic drugs may reduce the risk of aspiration pneumonitis in patients with this history.
- Oversedation, excessive analgesia, and obtundation should be avoided to help maintain the tone and function of the LES and the protective laryngeal closing reflex.
- Patients intubated with uncuffed endotracheal tubes should be suctioned frequently.
- For dysphagic patients, chin lowering as a postural technique can help eliminate aspiration resulting from delayed pharyngeal swallow or reduced airway closure.
- Maintain mechanically ventilated and bedridden patients in a semirecumbent or upright position to reduce gastric aspiration.

PATIENT/FAMILY EDUCATION

- Good oral hygiene should be encouraged, especially in neurologically disabled patients.
- Early recognition and treatment prevent progression to chronic lung disease and permanent damage, including:
  - Interstitial pulmonary fibrosis
  - Bronchiectasis
  - Bronchiolitis obliterans
  - Other complications—adult respiratory distress syndrome, hypovolemia, sepsis, or death
- The most favorable outcome and the lowest morbidity are achieved when surgery is postponed until the patient is adequately nourished.

SUGGESTED READINGS

Ahrens P et al: Antireflux surgery in children suffering from reflux-associated respiratory diseases. *Pediatr Pulmonol* 28:89, 1999.

Bauer ML, Lyrene RK: Chronic aspiration in children: evaluation of the lipid-laden macrophage index. *Pediatr Pulmonol* 28:94, 1999.

Beal M et al: A pilot study of quantitative aspiration in patients with symptoms of obstructive sleep apnea: a comparison to a historic control group. *Laryngoscope* 114:965, 2004.

Collins KA et al: The cytologic evaluation of lipid-laden alveolar macrophages as an indicator of aspiration pneumonia in young children. *Arch Pathol Lab Med* 119:229, 1995.

Marik PE: Aspiration pneumonitis and pneumonia: a clinical review. *N Engl J Med* 344:665, 2001.

Midulla F et al: Micro-aspiration in infants with laryngomalacia. *Laryngoscope* 114:1592, 2004.

Platzker AG: GER and aspiration syndromes. *In* Chernick V, Boat TF (eds): *Kendig's Disorders of the Respiratory Tract in Children,* 6th ed. Philadelphia, WB Saunders, 1998, pp 584–600.

AUTHOR: **EULALIA R. Y. CHENG, MD**

BASIC INFORMATION

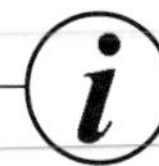

DEFINITION

Asthma is a chronic inflammatory disorder of airways leading to airway hyperresponsiveness to a variety of stimuli, including allergens, irritants, cold air, and viruses. In susceptible individuals, airway inflammation also leads to recurrent respiratory symptoms, including wheezing, breathlessness, chest tightness, and cough, particularly at night and in the early morning. These episodes are associated with widespread but variable airflow obstruction that is often reversible spontaneously or with treatment.

SYNONYMS

Reactive airway disease (RAD)
Wheezy bronchitis

ICD-9-CM CODES
493.0 Asthma with hay fever
493.1 Intrinsic asthma (late onset)
493.9 Asthma
493.91 Asthma with status asthmaticus

EPIDEMIOLOGY & DEMOGRAPHICS

- Asthma prevalence is 54 cases per 1000 children, or about 5%.
- Almost 9 million children younger than 18 years have been diagnosed with asthma.
- Approximately 30% of all children wheeze by age 3 years; only one third of these children have persistent symptoms up to age 6.
- Allergy is the major predictor of persistence.
- Ironically, exposure to indoor pets, daycare, or a farming environment in the first year of life may decrease allergen sensitization and asthma manifestations later in life.
- Sixty percent of all children with asthma have resolution by adulthood, but those with severe asthma and significant atopy are less likely to "outgrow" their asthma.
- High-risk populations include the following:
  - African Americans
  - Inner-city dwellers
  - Premature or low-birth-weight children
- Predisposing factors include the following:
  - Maternal asthma
  - Personal or family history of atopy
  - Maternal smoking
  - Male gender

CLINICAL PRESENTATION

History

- Recurrent respiratory symptoms include cough, wheeze, difficulty breathing, and chest tightness, which are often worse at night.
- Symptoms occur or worsen in the presence of the following:
  - Exercise
  - Viral infections
  - Animals with fur or feathers
  - House-dust mites
  - Molds
  - Smoke (e.g., tobacco, wood)
  - Pollen
  - Changes in weather
  - Strong emotions
  - Airborne chemicals or dusts
  - Menses

Physical Examination

- Hyperexpansion of thorax
- Wheezing during normal breathing
- Prolonged expiratory phase during forced maneuvers
- Symptomatic relief after bronchodilator use
- Alternative diagnoses (e.g., evidence of clubbing, nasal polyps, stridor)

ETIOLOGY

- Genetic predisposition
  - Genetic markers on chromosomes 5, 11, and 14 are associated with atopy and asthma.
- Structural predisposition
  - Wheezing in early life is associated with decreased measures of lung function.
- Inflammation and airway hyperresponsiveness: final pathway
  - Mast cells, eosinophils, T lymphocytes, macrophages, neutrophils, and epithelial cells all have a role in producing proinflammatory cytokines and chemokines.
  - Constituent cells of airway (i.e., fibroblasts, endothelial cells, and epithelial cells) also produce cytokines and chemokines.
  - Modulation of smooth muscle tone, vascular permeability, neuronal activity, and mucus secretion are orchestrated by cell mediators.

DIAGNOSIS

Dx

DIFFERENTIAL DIAGNOSIS

- Large airway obstruction or compression
  - Foreign body
  - Mediastinal mass
  - Laryngotracheomalacia, tracheal stenosis, or bronchostenosis
  - Vascular rings or slings
- Large and small airway involvement
  - Aspiration
  - Cystic fibrosis
  - Gastroesophageal edema
  - Pulmonary edema
- Other causes
  - Recurrent lower respiratory infection secondary to immune dysfunction
  - Vocal cord dysfunction
  - Psychogenic cough
  - Allergic rhinitis or sinusitis
  - Hyperventilation syndrome
  - Hypersensitivity pneumonitis
  - Bronchiolitis obliterans

COMPLICATING & COMORBID CONDITIONS

- Gastroesophageal reflux
- Rhinitis and sinusitis
- Allergic bronchopulmonary aspergillosis
- Exposure to inhalant allergens or irritants
- Aspirin or sulfite sensitivity

WORKUP

- Detailed medical history and physical examination
- Pulmonary function testing (e.g., spirometry, lung volumes)
  - Documentation of airflow obstruction or reversibility
  - Methacholine or exercise challenge
- History- or examination-directed evaluations
  - Chest radiograph for hyperinflation, peribronchial cuffing, patchy atelectasis
  - Allergy testing, which may identify allergens for directed environmental control or avoidance
  - A pH probe or barium swallow to rule out gastroesophageal reflux or aspiration
  - Flexible bronchoscopy to rule out structural abnormalities

TREATMENT

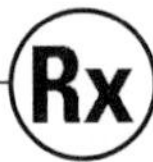

NONPHARMACOLOGIC THERAPY

- Environmental control
- Irritant and allergen avoidance

ACUTE GENERAL Rx

- Quick relief for all patients is provided with short-acting, inhaled β_2-agonists as needed for symptoms.
- For viral respiratory infections, a bronchodilator is used every 4 to 6 hours for 24 hours; longer with a physician consultation.
- Consider a systemic corticosteroid if exacerbation is severe or the patient has history of a severe exacerbation.
- In mild, intermittent asthma, use of short-acting β_2-agonists more than twice weekly may indicate the need for long-term control.

CHRONIC Rx

- Stepwise approach for management is based on severity.
- Define severity before treatment by National Asthma Education Program Expert Panel classification.
  - Step 1: mild intermittent
    - Morning symptoms $\leq$2 times/week
    - Overnight symptoms $\leq$2 times/month
    - Forced expiratory volume in 1 second (FEV_1) or peak expiratory flow (PEF) $\geq$80% predicted
    - PEF variability <20%
  - Step 2: mild persistent
    - Morning symptoms >2 times/week, but <1 time/day
    - Overnight symptoms >2 times/month
    - FEV_1 or PEF $\geq$ 80% predicted
    - PEF variability = 20% to 30%

- Step 3: moderate persistent
  - Daily symptoms
  - Nighttime symptoms >1 time/week
  - FEV_1 or PEF = 60% to 80% predicted
  - PEF variability >30%
- Step 4: severe persistent
  - Continual daily symptoms
  - Nighttime symptoms—frequency
  - FEV_1 or PEF = 60% predicted
  - PEF variability >30%
- Assign patient to most severe step in which any clinical feature occurs.
- Children younger than 6 years may not be able to perform FEV_1 or PEF maneuvers.

- Medications to maintain long-term control:
  - Step 1: mild intermittent
    - No daily medications needed
  - Step 2: mild persistent
    - Preferred treatment: low-dose inhaled corticosteroid
    - Alternate treatment: Cromolyn or leukotriene receptor antagonist
  - Step 3: moderate persistent
    - Preferred treatments: low-dose inhaled corticosteroids with long-acting inhaled β_2-agonists or medium-dose inhaled corticosteroids
    - Alternate treatment: low-dose inhaled corticosteroids and a leukotriene receptor antagonist or theophylline
  - Step 4: severe persistent
    - High-dose inhaled corticosteroids and long-acting inhaled β_2-agonists
    - If needed, long-term oral corticosteroid
  - Establish prompt control, and then step down.
- Goals of therapy for all asthmatics:
  - Prevent chronic and troublesome symptoms.
  - Maintain normal or near-normal pulmonary function.
  - Maintain normal activity levels.
  - Prevent recurrent exacerbations.
  - Minimize adverse effects from therapy.
  - Meet patient and family expectations for care.
- Notable points regarding specific therapies:
  - Inhaled corticosteroids are useful.
    - First-line therapy for patients with persistent asthma
    - Multiple strengths, formulations, and dosing schedules
    - Multiple delivery devices (e.g., metered-dose inhaler, breath-actuated)
    - Oral candidiasis: decreased with spacer use; rinse and spit following each dose
    - Altered linear growth, with catch-up growth in late puberty and no difference in adult height
    - Cataracts: rare in children
    - Adrenal suppression: not reported in children
  - Role of leukotriene-receptor antagonists as a first-line prevention agent is still unclear.
  - Immunosuppression is not indicated for most patients, but it may be useful in a subgroup with allergic rhinitis.

DISPOSITION

- Written asthma action plan for acute and chronic intervention is needed.
- Frequent follow-up is necessary until control is maintained (every 1 to 6 months).
- After asthma is under good control, semiannual visits are needed to review goals and reinforce education and to consider step-down therapy.
- Risk factors for death from asthma include the following:
  - History of sudden severe exacerbations
  - Prior intubation or intensive care unit admission for asthma
  - Two or more hospitalizations
  - Three or more emergency care visits for asthma in the past year
  - Hospitalization or emergency care visit for asthma within the past month
  - Use of more than two canisters per month of an inhaled short-acting β_2-agonist
  - Current use of systemic corticosteroids or recent withdrawal from systemic corticosteroids
  - Difficulty perceiving airflow obstruction or its severity
  - Comorbidity (e.g., cardiovascular diseases)
  - Serious psychiatric disease or psychosocial problems

REFERRAL

Referral to an asthma specialist may be needed:

- Goals of therapy not being met
- Diagnostic assistance
- Educational support
- Nonstandard or exceptional therapy indicated
- Asthma severe or life-threatening

PEARLS & CONSIDERATIONS

COMMENTS

- "Rule of twos" helps to identify persistent asthma. Anyone with symptoms more than two times per week or more than 2 nights per month has persistent asthma and should be managed accordingly.
- Chronic anti-inflammatory therapy may also be useful for patients with exercise-induced asthma that is poorly controlled with bronchodilator use before exercise.
- Action plan is based on peak flow monitoring.
  - Technique dependent
  - Need to establish personal baseline when well
  - Zones based on personal best and plan based on zone
    - Green: 80% to 100% of personal best; continue daily medication
    - Yellow: 60% to 80% of personal best; step up therapy as instructed
    - Red: < 60% of personal best; contact physician
- With acute exacerbations, patient may need to increase the dose of an inhaled short-acting β_2-agonist from 2 puffs to 4 or 6 puffs for adequate relief. Be very specific in the action plan to prevent overuse of medication.
- Tailor therapy for elective surgery.
  - Maximize control, which may include a short course of systemic corticosteroids.
  - Stress-dose hydrocortisone may be indicated for patients receiving recent systemic corticosteroids.
- After control is achieved, attempt to reduce the dose.

PATIENT/FAMILY EDUCATION

- Reinforce the therapeutic plan frequently.
- Establish partnerships among parents, patients, and provider for asthma management and role of medications.
- Develop an acute action plan.
- Ensure proper techniques for inhaled medications.
- Use of spacers should be encouraged for all age groups.
- Review techniques for self-monitoring (e.g., symptom recognition, peak flows).
- Discuss environmental control measures and precipitant avoidance.
- Review cultural beliefs and practices associated with asthma.
- Support groups are available through organizations such as the Allergy and Asthma Network/Mothers of Asthmatics (www.aanma.org) and the Asthma and Allergy Foundation of America (www.aafa.org).

SUGGESTED READINGS

1997 Expert Panel guidelines and 2002 Update on Selected Topics: www.nhlbi.nih.gov

Barnes PJ, Pedersen S, Busse WW: Efficacy and safety of inhaled corticosteroids: new developments. *Am J Respir Crit Care Med* 157:S1, 1998.

Brooks AM, McBride JT: The asthma specialist: when and why to refer the pediatric patient. *Pediatr Ann* 28:55, 1999.

Guill MF: Asthma update: clinical aspects and management. *Pediatr Rev* 25:335, 2004.

Guill MF: Asthma update: epidemiology and pathophysiology. *Pediatr Rev* 25:299, 2004.

Mannino DM et al: Surveillance for asthma—United States 1960–1995. *MMWR Morb Mortal Wkly Rep* 47:1, 1998.

National Asthma Education Program Expert Panel: *Report II. Guidelines for the Diagnosis and Management of Asthma.* NIH Publication No. 97-4051. Bethesda, MD, April 1997, National Institutes of Health, National Heart, Lung and Blood Institute.

Szilagyi PG, Kemper KJ: Management of chronic childhood asthma in the primary care office. *Pediatr Ann* 28:43, 1999.

Taylor WR, Newacheck PW: Impact of childhood asthma on health. *Pediatrics* 90:657, 1992.

Yoos HL, McMullen A: Symptom monitoring in childhood asthma: how to use a peak flow meter. *Pediatr Ann* 28:31, 1999.

AUTHOR: **BARBARA A. CHINI, MD**

BASIC INFORMATION

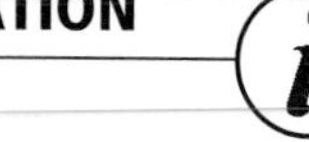

DEFINITION

Atopic dermatitis is an inherited inflammatory skin disorder often found in association with asthma or allergic rhinitis.

SYNONYM

Eczema

ICD-9-CM CODE

691.8 Atopic dermatitis and related conditions

EPIDEMIOLOGY & DEMOGRAPHICS

- Ten percent to 20% prevalence rate of atopic dermatitis (AD).
- AD has a strong genetic influence with up to 75% of all patients having a positive family history.
- Sixty percent of children with AD manifest their disease in the first year of life and 90% by 5 years.
- No racial differences are noted in children.

CLINICAL PRESENTATION

- The clinical picture varies with the age of the patient and disease severity.
- Pruritus is a hallmark of the disease.
- Associated clinical findings include xerosis, ichthyosis vulgaris, keratosis pilaris, allergic shiners (orbital hyperpigmentation), Dennie-Morgan folds (atopic pleats), hyperlinear palms or soles, and susceptibility to recurrent infections (bacterial, viral, and fungal).

Infants

- Infants usually present with acute dermatitis.
- There can be intensely pruritic erythematous papules and vesicles that become excoriated and exudative.
- Lesions are distributed over the scalp, forehead, cheeks, trunk, and extensor extremities.
- The diaper area is usually spared.

Older Children

- A more subacute presentation is common.
- Excoriated erythematous scaling papules and plaques located on the wrists, ankles, and antecubital and popliteal fossae are observed.
- The hands and feet are commonly involved, with dryness, cracking, and scaling.
- Chronic changes secondary to repeated rubbing and scratching include lichenification with skin that is thickened and has prominent skin markings.
- Perifollicular accentuation is common in patients with dark skin.

ETIOLOGY

- Although the cause is unknown, both genetic and environmental factors play a role.
- Immune dysfunction (abnormality in T2-helper cells with increased production of immunoglobulin E and interleukin-4) occurs in patients with AD, but whether it is the cause or effect of the disease has not been determined.
- Food allergens in some patients are exacerbating.
- Aeroallergens, such as trees and grass pollens, play an important role in the exacerbation of AD.
- Both immediate hypersensitivity skin tests and delayed-type hypersensitivity patch tests are often positive in patients with AD.

DIAGNOSIS

Dx

DIFFERENTIAL DIAGNOSIS

- Seborrheic dermatitis
- Psoriasis
- Tinea corporis
- Nummular dermatitis
- Irritant or allergic contact dermatitis
- Scabies (especially in infants)
- Histiocytosis X
- Wiskott-Aldrich syndrome

WORKUP

The diagnosis is usually made on the basis of a characteristic clinical picture, as well as a family and personal history of atopy.

TREATMENT

Rx

NONPHARMACOLOGIC THERAPY

- Mild soaps (e.g., Dove, Tone, Purpose, Basis) or a soap substitute (e.g., Cetaphil) should be used once or twice a day.
- Emollients (e.g., Vaseline petroleum jelly, Aquaphor ointment, Theraplex emollient, Eucerin cream) should be used two to three times per day.
  - In general, creams or ointments are preferred to lotions.
- Bathing (5 to 10 minutes in lukewarm water) is fine as long as damp skin is moisturized with creams or ointments immediately after bathing.
- Irritants such as detergents, solvents, and fabrics such as wool or nylon, should be avoided.

ACUTE GENERAL Rx

- Choose the mildest topical steroid that can control the disease.
- Most patients can be controlled with low-potency topical corticosteroids applied twice a day to individual areas for several weeks.
  - Use stronger, nonfluorinated low-potency to mid-potency ointment during flare-ups.
- Another option is a topical immune modulator (i.e., topical tacrolimus and pimecrolimus) that does not contain corticosteroid.
  - Immune modulators can be used as second-line therapy when tapering off of a topical corticosteroid or a first-line therapy in mild disease. However, recent cancer warnings have mitigated use of these medications.
- Sedating antihistamines (e.g., hydroxyzine, cyproheptadine, or diphenhydramine) may help children sleep and prevent itching during sleep.
- Secondary bacterial infection can be present during flare-ups.
  - *Staphylococcus aureus* colonizes the skin of more than 95% of patients with AD.
  - Treat superinfections with appropriate systemic antibiotics for 7 to 14 days.

CHRONIC Rx

- Reduce corticosteroid potency as the disease is controlled.
- Continue antihistamines as needed for pruritus.

REFERRAL

Patients with severe or extensive disease should be referred to a dermatologist.

PEARLS & CONSIDERATIONS

COMMENTS

More than 75% of children with AD improve by adolescence.

SUGGESTED READINGS

Abramovits W: Atopic dermatitis. *J Am Acad Dermatol* 53(1):S86, 2005.

American Academy of Dermatology. Available at www.aad.org

National Eczema Association for Science and Education. Available at www.eczema-assn.org

The National Eczema Society. Available at www.eczema.org

Simpson EL, Hanifin JM: Atopic dermatitis. *Med Clin North Am* 90(1):149, 2006.

Society for Pediatric Dermatology. Available at www.spdnet.org

Williams HC: Clinical practice. Atopic dermatitis. *N Engl J Med* 2:352(22):2314, 2005.

AUTHOR: **SUSAN HALLER PSAILA, MD**

BASIC INFORMATION

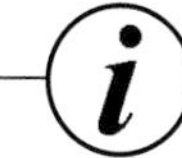

DEFINITION

Atrial septal defect is a direct communication between the right and left atria, most commonly in the region of the fossa ovalis, with normally connected pulmonary veins. Sinus venosus defects lie outside of the confines of the fossa ovalis near the superior or inferior vena cavae, and they are always associated with abnormal connection of the right pulmonary veins to the right atrium.

SYNONYMS

Fossa ovalis atrial defect
Secundum atrial septal defect

ICD-9-CM CODE
745.5 Ostium secundum-type atrial septal defect

EPIDEMIOLOGY & DEMOGRAPHICS

- Atrial septal defects are common, accounting for 7% to 10% of congenital cardiac malformations, and they occur in 1 of 1500 live births.
- The male-to-female ratio is 1:2.
- Cases are usually sporadic.
- Spontaneous closure occurs by 2 years of age in 40% to 50% of the defects detected in early infancy.
- Some cases are familial (e.g., Holt-Oram syndrome).
  - Atrial defect with upper limb deformities and cardiac conduction abnormalities
  - Autosomal-dominant inheritance
- The defect often is an integral (and sometimes necessary) component of complex congenital cardiac malformations.
- Between 25% and 30% of individuals with an otherwise normal heart have a probe-patent foramen ovale, which is not considered an atrial defect.

CLINICAL PRESENTATION

History

- The patient is usually asymptomatic, although physical endurance may be limited (in retrospect, after closure).
- Uncommonly, fatigue, dyspnea on exertion, or recurrent lower respiratory infections are reported.
- The patient is usually small in stature, but true failure to thrive is rare.
- The disease is commonly detected in early childhood but may be identified in infancy.
- In untreated patients, late atrial arrhythmias, especially atrial fibrillation, congestive heart failure, or pulmonary vascular obstructive disease, may ensue in an unpredictable fashion.

Physical Examination

- Height and weight are often below normal.
- Precordial activity is increased.
- Grade I to III/VI systolic pulmonary flow murmur is detected at the upper left sternal border.
- A persistent wide split of the second heart sound with a pulmonary closure sound of normal intensity is heard.
- If pulmonary blood flow is at least twice systemic flow, a soft mid-diastolic murmur related to relative tricuspid stenosis is audible at the lower left sternal border.

ETIOLOGY

- Secundum atrial defects are caused by defective development of the septum secundum or excessive resorption of the septum primum.
- Sinus venosus defects are caused by unroofing of the right pulmonary veins.

DIAGNOSIS

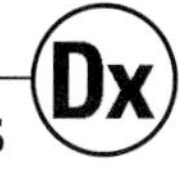

DIFFERENTIAL DIAGNOSIS

- Functional pulmonary flow murmur
- Pulmonary valve stenosis
- Primum atrial septal defect (partial a-v canal defects)

LABORATORY TESTS

- Electrocardiogram
  - Frontal plane QRS axis to the right
  - The rSR′ pattern in V_1, V_3R (right ventricular volume load)
  - Mild right atrial enlargement
  - Mild PR prolongation
  - May be normal in 5% of patients

IMAGING STUDIES

- Chest radiograph
  - Mild cardiomegaly
  - Right atrial and ventricular and main pulmonary artery enlargement
  - Increased pulmonary blood flow
- Echocardiography
  - Visualization of the defect in the region of the fossa ovalis
  - Visualization of the pulmonary venous connections
  - Color and pulsed Doppler documentation of flow across the defect, usually left to right
  - Right atrial and ventricular and main pulmonary artery enlargement
  - Exclusion of associated anomalies

TREATMENT

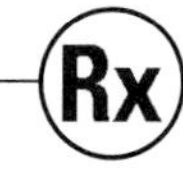

NONPHARMACOLOGIC THERAPY

- Because many atrial septal defects close spontaneously, observation alone may be sufficient.
- If a hemodynamically significant defect is present at age 2 years or older, closure should be performed at 2 to 4 years of age to prevent late problems such as arrhythmias, heart failure, or pulmonary vascular disease.
- Closure can be accomplished surgically with very low mortality and morbidity rates.
- Alternatively, closure with a catheter-inserted device may be undertaken.
- Sinus venosus defects require baffling or redirection of right pulmonary venous drainage to the left atrium on cardiopulmonary bypass.

DISPOSITION

- The outlook after closure is highly favorable, with a normal life expectancy.
- Between 2% and 7% of patients experience late atrial arrhythmias, perhaps less with earlier closure (2 to 4 years old).
- An increase in exercise endurance and growth are common after atrial defect closure.

REFERRAL

Children with a suspected atrial defect should be referred to a cardiologist.

PEARLS & CONSIDERATIONS

COMMENTS

- If the second heart sound split in a newborn or young infant is "too easy" to detect, consider an atrial defect, even in the absence of a murmur.
- For isolated atrial defects, bacterial endocarditis prophylaxis is not necessary preoperatively or more than 6 months after surgery unless a patch was used in the repair.

PATIENT/FAMILY EDUCATION

Patients and family members should be instructed to contact the cardiologist if palpitations or syncope occur.

SUGGESTED READINGS

Bricker T, et al: Dysrhythmias after atrial septal defect repair. *Tex Heart Inst J* 13:203, 1986.
Campbell M: The natural history of atrial septal defects. *Br Heart J* 32:820, 1970.
Ghisla RP, et al: Spontaneous closure of isolated secundum atrial septal defects in infants: an echocardiographic study. *Am Heart J* 109:1327, 1985.
Murphy JG, et al: Long-term outcome after surgical repair of isolated atrial septal defects. *N Engl J Med* 323:1645, 1990.
Rome JJ, et al: Double-umbrella closure of atrial septal defects. *Circulation* 82:751, 1990.

AUTHOR: **J. PETER HARRIS, MD**

BASIC INFORMATION

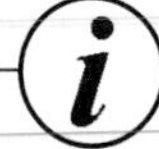

DEFINITION

Complete atrioventricular (AV) canal defect is an embryonic cardiovascular malformation caused by the failure to separate the common AV orifice into the mitral and tricuspid valves and the failure to close the atrial (primum) and ventricular (inlet) septums. Less severe variants of AV canal include a primum atrial septal defect (partial AV canal), an inlet or posterior ventricular septal defect, and an isolated cleft mitral valve. Unbalanced AV canals are developmentally related but are not discussed further here.

SYNONYMS

AV canal defects
AV septal defects
Canal defects
Endocardial cushion defects

ICD-9-CM CODE
745.69 Atrioventricular canal-type ventricular septal defect

EPIDEMIOLOGY & DEMOGRAPHICS

- Congenital cardiovascular malformations have an incidence of 8 per 1000 live births.
- This spectrum of defects accounts for 2% to 4% of all congenital cardiovascular malformations.
- Other commonly associated congenital cardiovascular lesions include:
  - Patent ductus arteriosus (PDA)
  - Secundum atrial septal defects (ASDs)
  - Ventricular septal defects (VSDs)
  - Tetralogy of Fallot (TOF)
- Approximately 40% of children born with an AV canal have trisomy 21 (Down syndrome).
  - Trisomy 21 has an incidence of approximately 1 in 700 to 800 live births.
- Approximately 40% of children with trisomy 21 have a congenital heart defect.
  - AV canal is the most common (approximately 40%) congenital heart defect in trisomy 21.
- The typical child with trisomy 21 and AV canal has a complete and balanced defect.
  - These patients are excellent candidates for complete surgical repair.
- AV canals associated with normal karyotypes (heterotaxia syndromes and non-heterotaxia)
  - More complex and often unbalanced
  - More difficult surgical repair
  - Heterotaxia syndromes include:
    - Asplenia and polysplenia
    - Right and left atrial isomerism
  - Other thoracoabdominal abnormalities, such as the number, location, and function of splenic tissue and malrotation of the gut, must be determined.
- The Ellis-van Creveld syndrome is associated with common atrium, which may be a variant of AV canal.

CLINICAL PRESENTATION

History

- The child is usually asymptomatic at birth, unless severe AV regurgitation is present.
- With the normal neonatal decrease in pulmonary vascular resistance, progressive congestive heart failure (CHF) from left to right shunt and pulmonary overcirculation is expected.
- The child has feeding difficulties and failure to thrive.
- Respiratory infections are common.
- If CHF does not develop, earlier repair is indicated to protect the pulmonary vascular bed, especially in trisomy 21 as these patients are at greater risk of pulmonary vascular disease.

Physical Examination

- Children with AV canal defects may exhibit stigmata of trisomy 21 (see Down Syndrome in Diseases and Disorders [Section I]).
- A holosystolic regurgitant murmur from AV valve regurgitation is usually present.
  - The grade of the holosystolic regurgitant murmur ranges from I to II/VI with mild AV regurgitation to III to IV/VI with severe AV regurgitation.
  - The location of the murmur depends on whether the source is right-sided AV regurgitation (most intense at the left lateral sternal border) or left-sided AV regurgitation (most intense at the apex with radiation to the back).
- With the development of CHF, the following occurs:
  - Poor weight gain, tachypnea, and tachycardia
  - Possible hyperdynamic precordium, with a thrill at the left lower sternal border
  - Possible mid-diastolic rumble and a gallop rhythm
  - Hepatomegaly

ETIOLOGY

- The developmental hallmarks of AV canal defects include the following (Figure 1-1):

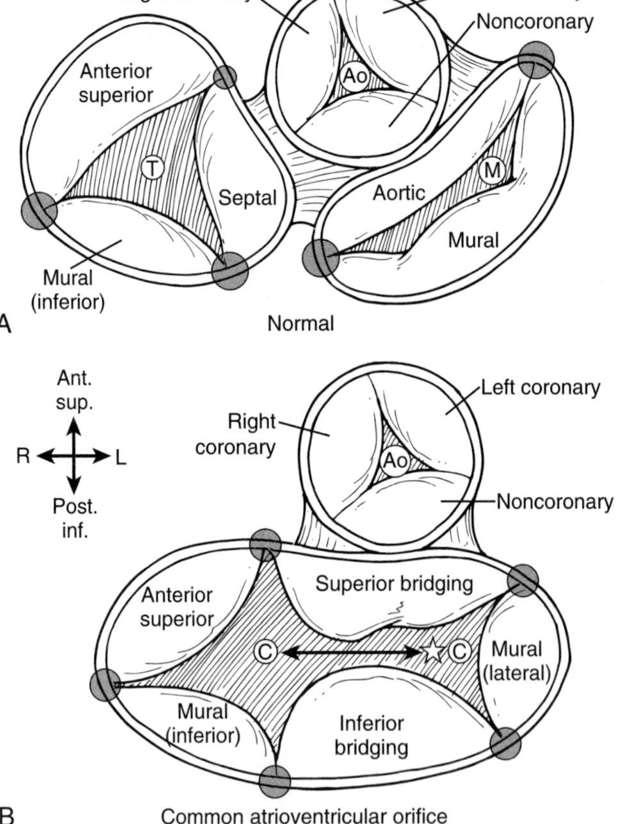

FIGURE 1-1 Anatomy of Atrioventricular Orifice. Anatomic diagram of the atrioventricular (AV) valve leaflets in normal **(A)** and complete AV canal **(B)**. The atrial defect is above the bridging leaflets and the ventricular defect is below the bridging leaflets. The bridging leaflets will be divided during the surgical repair to close the defects and create a right and left AV valve. Note the anterior displacement of the aortic valve in AV canals. Orientation: Ant. sup., anterior superior; Post. inf., posterior inferior; R, right; L, left. Abbreviations: Ao, aorta; T, tricuspid valve; M, mitral valve; C, common AV valve; ☆ location of mitral "cleft." (Adapted from Ebels T, Anderson RH: Atrioventricular septal defects. *In* Anderson RH et al (eds): *Paediatric Cardiology,* 2nd ed., Vol. 1. Edinburgh, Churchill Livingstone, 2002, p 941.)

- Maldevelopment of the endocardial cushions that guard the embryonic AV orifice
- Failure to close the atrial and ventricular septums
- Malformation of the anterior leaflet of the mitral valve

- During normal cardiac development, the endocardial cushion containing extracellular matrix is invaded by cardiac fibroblasts in response to several growth factors.
    - Cardiac fibroblasts form the AV valve leaflets via a process called *ectomesenchymal transformation.*
    - Abnormalities in the extracellular matrix are believed to be responsible for the pathogenesis of AV canal defects.
- The frequent association of trisomy 21 and AV canal defects implicates a genetic locus on chromosome 21; however, other loci are likely to be important as well.

DIAGNOSIS

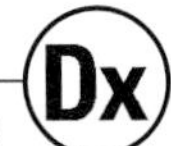

DIFFERENTIAL DIAGNOSIS

- Lesions with left-to-right shunts, such as ASD, VSD, PDA, or acyanotic TOF
- Lesions with significant AV valve regurgitation, such as Ebstein's malformation or congenital mitral regurgitation

LABORATORY TEST

Karyotype analysis for trisomy 21 if clinically suspected.

IMAGING STUDIES

- Electrocardiography
    - A right and superior (northwest) QRS frontal plane axis is characteristic of AV canal defects.
    - First-degree AV block (prolonged PR interval) is often seen.
    - Right ventricular hypertrophy or right bundle branch block is common.
- Chest radiography
    - Cardiomegaly and increased pulmonary vascular markings from CHF are seen.
- Echocardiography
    - Two-dimensional echocardiography delineates all of the critical anatomic components for the medical and surgical management of AV canals.
        - The size of the AV valve orifices and how evenly they are committed to each ventricular mass
        - Chordal insertion of the AV valves
        - Size of each ventricle
    - Color-flow Doppler echocardiography is important in quantifying AV regurgitation.
    - Prenatally, AV canals can be readily diagnosed by fetal echocardiography in the four-chamber view.
    - Prenatal genetic counseling and testing for trisomy 21 should be considered.

TREATMENT

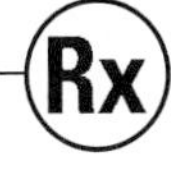

NONPHARMACOLOGIC THERAPY

- Presently, all infants with AV canal undergo repair in infancy.
- If corrective repair is not possible, palliation with a pulmonary arterial band limits CHF and protects the pulmonary bed from pulmonary hypertension.
- Unrepaired:
    - CHF can cause significant morbidity and mortality during infancy.
    - In a patient with an unrepaired AV canal, progressive pulmonary hypertension and irreversible pulmonary vascular obstructive disease (PVOD) will develop.
    - PVOD causes right-sided heart failure and polycythemia from progressive cyanosis and is invariably fatal.
- Important factors for the repair of AV canals include the following:
    - Degree of AV regurgitation
    - Relative size of the AV valves and their spatial relationship to the ventricles
    - Location of the AV valve chordae insertion into the ventricles
- With favorable anatomy, primary repair is often performed in infancy without the need for further surgery.
    - Primary repair can be achieved with either a one- or two-patch technique (Figure 1-2).
    - Children in CHF may require intubation.

ACUTE GENERAL Rx

- Most infants require CHF therapy.
    - Digitalis
    - Diuretics
    - Afterload reduction
- Potassium homeostasis must be preserved using a potassium-sparing agent or potassium or an angiotensin-converting enzyme (ACE) inhibitor.
- Increased caloric support

CHRONIC Rx

Lifelong subacute bacterial endocarditis (SBE) prophylaxis.

DISPOSITION

- Prolonged postoperative ventilation may be required.
- Resolve significant pulmonary overcirculation.

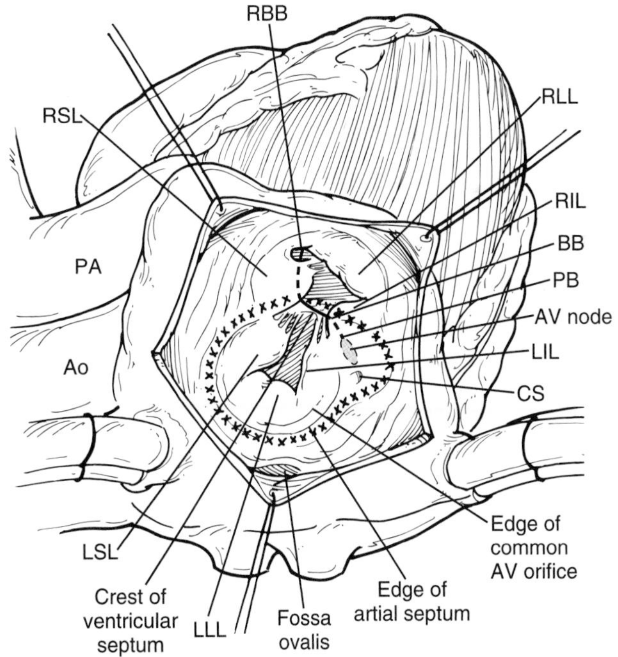

FIGURE 1-2 Surgical Approach to Complete Atrioventricular Canal. Typical operative view from a right atriotomy of a complete atrioventricular (AV) canal. The superior and inferior bridging leaflets have been divided and will create the two AV valves when sutured to the patch at the dots. The ventricular defect is closed on the RV surface of the crest of the ventricular septum from ~ 10 to 2 o'clock (demarcated by the stippled x's), avoiding the conduction system. The atrial defect is closed from ~2 to 10 o'clock and is located inferiorly from this view (demarcated by the solid x's). Abbreviations: Ao, aorta; ASD, atrial septal defect; AV, atrioventricular; BB, branching portion of the bundle of His; CS, coronary sinus ostium; LIL, left inferior leaflet; LLL, left lateral leaflet; LSL, left superior leaflet; PA, pulmonary artery; PB, penetrating portion of the bundle of His; RBB, right bundle branch; RIL, right inferior leaflet; RLL, right lateral leaflet; RSL, right superior leaflet. (Adapted from Kirklin JW, Barrett-Boyes BG (eds): Atrioventricular canal defect. *In* Cardiac Surgery, 2nd ed. New York, Churchill Livingstone, 2003, p 712.)

- Reestablish adequate calories from preoperative cachexia.
- Rarely, distortion of the AV valves from the surgical repair results in increased AV regurgitation requiring further repair of the AV valve.
  - This aspect is more critical for the newly created mitral valve because of the elevated pressures in the left ventricle compared with those of the right ventricle.
- Rarely, postoperative mitral regurgitation induces a hemolytic anemia from mechanical shearing of the regurgitant red blood cells striking the left side of the atrial patch.
- Postoperative third-degree (complete) heart block is seen less often today but may require permanent pacemaker implantation.

REFERRAL

Initial evaluation and management by a pediatric cardiologist who will refer to a pediatric cardiothoracic surgeon for repair.

PEARLS & CONSIDERATIONS

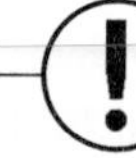

PATIENT/FAMILY EDUCATION

- With trisomy 21, appropriate genetic counseling is needed.
- Preoperative counseling includes the following:
  - Management of CHF
  - Discussion of the anatomic factors that are critical to the requisite surgical repair
  - Operative morbidity and mortality risks
  - The risks for an uncomplicated AV canal are presently quite low.
- Postoperative counseling includes the following:
  - Cessation of anticongestive (CHF) therapy
  - Potential long-term complications of arrhythmias and AV valve dysfunction

SUGGESTED READINGS

Apfel HD, Gersony WM: Clinical evaluation, medical management and outcome of atrioventricular canal defects. *Prog Pediatr Cardiol* 10:129, 1999.

Daebritz S, del Nido PJ: Surgical management of common atrioventricular canal. *Prog Pediatr Cardiol* 10:161, 1999.

Ebels T, Anderson RH: Atrioventricular septal defects. *In* Anderson RH et al (eds): *Paediatric Cardiology,* 2nd ed. Edinburgh, Churchill Livingstone, 2002, pp 939–981.

Kertesz NJ: The conduction system and arrhythmias in common atrioventricular canal. *Prog Pediatr Cardiol* 10:153, 1999.

Levine JC, Geva T: Echocardiographic assessment of common atrioventricular canal. *Prog Pediatr Cardiol* 10:137, 1999.

Loyola University, Stritch School of Medicine. Available at www.meddean.luc.edu/lumen/MedEd/GrossAnatomy/thorax0/Heart_Development/PersistentAV.html

Network Access Services. Available at www.nas.com/ downsyn/

AUTHOR: **PETER N. BOWERS, MD**

BASIC INFORMATION

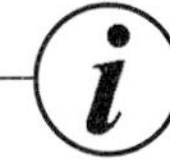

DEFINITION

Attention deficit/hyperactivity disorder (AD/HD) is a behavioral syndrome characterized by developmentally inappropriate levels of inattention or hyperactivity and impulsivity that interfere significantly with function.

SYNONYMS

AD/HD
ADD
Attention deficit disorder
Hyperactivity

ICD-9-CM CODES

314.00 AD/HD, predominately inattentive type
314.01 AD/HD, combined type
314.01 AD/HD, predominately hyperactive-impulsive type
314.9 AD/HD, not otherwise specified

EPIDEMIOLOGY & DEMOGRAPHICS

- AD/HD is the most common significant behavior disorder in children.
- Between 4% and 12% of American school-age children have AD/HD.
- The incidence is reportedly higher in lower socioeconomic status groups.
- The male-to-female ratio is approximately 3:1.
- AD/HD persists into adolescence and adulthood in up to 70% of patients.
- AD/HD has been found worldwide, with rates of 3% to 18%.

CLINICAL PRESENTATION

History

- Diagnostic criteria for AD/HD are from the *Diagnostic and Statistical Manual of Mental Disorders,* fourth edition, 1994, by the American Psychiatric Association (Table 1-2).
- Signs must occur often and be present for at least 6 months to a level that is maladaptive and inconsistent with the child's developmental level.
- Symptoms must cause impairment in social, academic, or occupational functioning.
- Some core symptoms must have been present before the child was 7 years old.
- Symptoms must be causing impairment in two or more settings.
- Symptoms do not occur exclusively as part of another disorder.

Physical Examination

- Results of the physical examination are usually normal.
- Careful assessment of developmental status should be undertaken.
- Symptoms may not be evident in medical setting.
- Attention should be paid to hearing, vision, dysmorphic features, cutaneous markers, or neurologic findings suggestive of medical or genetic disorders.
- Patients may have increased incidence of "soft" neurologic signs (e.g., synkinesia, overflow, disinhibition, motor clumsiness), but their significance is unclear.

ETIOLOGY

- Genetic causes
  - Accounts for up to 80% of the variance
  - Probably polygenic inheritance
- Medical causes
  - Many studies have shown anatomic differences in cerebral cortex, cerebellar vermis, basal ganglia, corpus callosum, and cingulate gyrus. None are conclusive.
  - AD/HD may involve neurotransmitter alterations.
- Environmental causes
  - AD/HD has been linked to prenatal exposure to alcohol and tobacco.
  - Increased lead level and exposure to environmental toxins have been suggested as causative.
- Neuropsychological causes
  - Disorder of executive function can lead to disinhibition and poor self-regulation.
- "Goodness of fit" between the environment and individual affects the severity of symptoms.

DIAGNOSIS Dx

DIFFERENTIAL DIAGNOSIS

- Table 1-2 summarizes the diagnostic criteria.
- More than 50% of individuals have comorbid conditions.
- Many other conditions may have similar behavioral manifestations (see Table 1-3).

WORKUP

- There is no single diagnostic test for AD/HD.
- The American Academy of Pediatrics and National Initiative for Children's Healthcare Quality offers a web site (www.nichq.org/resources/toolkit) with tools for assessment, guidelines, management, and education.
- The diagnosis is clinical and based on the following factors:
  - History (preferably from multiple observers)
  - Collaboration with schools to screen for learning disability or cognitive delay
  - Developmental assessment with appropriate referrals for suspected delay
  - Physical examination
  - School, parent, and student rating scales and questionnaires to document DSM-IV criteria and screen for common comorbid conditions (e.g., Vanderbilt Parent and Teacher Scales, Conners' Parent and Teacher Rating Scales–Revised–Long Form)
  - Psychosocial assessment considering comorbid conditions and differential diagnosis

LABORATORY TESTS

- Laboratory assessment is undertaken only as indicated by the history and physical examination results.
- In preschool children, check the hematocrit and lead levels.

IMAGING STUDIES

Imaging studies are not routinely indicated for AD/HD.

TABLE 1-2 Diagnostic Criteria for Attention Deficit/Hyperactivity Disorder

Inattention (Six or More of the Following)	Hyperactivity and Impulsivity (Six or More of the Following)
1. Fails to give close attention to details or makes careless mistakes in schoolwork, chores, or other tasks.	1. Fidgets with hands or feet or squirms in seat.
2. Has difficulty sustaining attention to tasks, chores, or duties.	2. Leaves seat in classroom or in other situations in which remaining seated is expected.
3. Does not seem to listen when spoken to directly.	3. Runs about or climbs excessively in situations in which it is inappropriate (in adolescents and adults may be limited to restlessness).
4. Does not follow through on instructions and fails to finish schoolwork, chores, or duties.	4. Has difficulty playing or engaging in leisure activities quietly.
5. Has difficulty organizing tasks and activities.	5. Is "on the go" or acts as if "driven by a motor."
6. Avoids, dislikes, or is reluctant to engage in tasks that require sustained mental effort.	6. Talks excessively.
7. Loses things necessary for tasks or activities.	7. Blurts out answers before questions have been completed.
8. Is easily distracted by extraneous activities.	8. Has difficulty awaiting turns.
9. Is forgetful in daily activities.	9. Interrupts or intrudes on others.

AD/HD, combined type: six or more symptoms from each list.
AD/HD, predominantly inattentive type: six or more symptoms from Inattention list.
AD/HD, predominantly hyperactive-impulse type: six or more symptoms from Hyperactivity and Impulsivity list.

TABLE 1-3 **Differential Diagnosis and Common Comorbid Conditions**

Developmental Conditions	Emotional Conditions	Environmental Conditions	Medical Conditions
Developmental delay	Anxiety	Social chaos	Seizure disorder
Mental retardation	Depression	Mental illness in family	Sensory impairment
Pervasive development disorders	Mood disorders	Substance abuse in family	Iron deficiency
Language disorders	Posttraumatic stress disorder	Violence/abuse	Hyperthyroid or hypothyroid
Giftedness	Conduct disorder	Inappropriate educational setting	Traumatic brain injury
Learning disabilities	Mania		Substance abuse
	Adjustment reaction		Medication side effect
	Bipolar disorder		Sleep disorder
			Tourette's syndrome
			Neurodegenerative disorders
			Fetal alcohol and drug exposure

TREATMENT

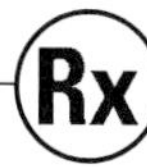

NONPHARMACOLOGIC THERAPY

- Educate the parents, teachers, and patient about the disorder.
- Parents and teachers may benefit from training in specific behavior management techniques for impulsive and inattentive children.
- School interventions are undertaken as necessary, including consideration of the 504 Accommodation Plan or Individualized Educational Plan if symptoms significantly interfere with academic progress.
- Some families may benefit from family therapy.
- Older students may benefit from "coaching" in executive function skills.
- Some children may benefit from social skills training.
- Dietary interventions are of no proven benefit.
- Intervention should be implemented for comorbid conditions.

ACUTE GENERAL Rx

No acute treatment is needed.

CHRONIC Rx

- Multiple studies overwhelmingly demonstrate that medication intervention is the single most effective strategy for managing AD/HD.
- Medication management is indicated for specific target symptoms.
- Medication management remains effective for adolescents and adults.
- Medications are listed in order of prevalence and importance:
  - Stimulant medications include methylphenidate, dextroamphetamine, and mixed amphetamine salts.
    - These are first-line medications.
    - If side effects occur with one stimulant class, try another.
    - Up to 80% of appropriately diagnosed patients have a robust response to one of the classes of stimulant medication.
    - Pemoline is not recommended for first-line therapy because of reported hepatic toxicity.
    - There are many dosage forms, including short-acting, intermediate-acting, and long-acting drugs.
  - If stimulants are unavailable or result in unacceptable side effects, atomoxetine is the second-line choice.
    - It is a noradrenergic reuptake inhibitor.
    - The U.S. Food and Drug Administration (FDA) mandated a boldface warning concerning possible hepatic toxicity.
  - α-Adrenergic agents and bupropion are occasionally used off label, but there is insufficient evidence to recommend their routine use for AD/HD.

DISPOSITION

AD/HD is a chronic disorder that requires ongoing assessment and intervention, which include the following:

- Medication management
- Monitoring of educational achievement
- Monitoring of social progress
- Monitoring of family functioning
- Ongoing surveillance for other comorbid conditions
- Referrals as indicated

REFERRAL

- Many children with AD/HD, especially those with comorbid conditions, are referred to a developmental pediatrician, child neurologist, or child psychiatrist.
- Consider referral to a clinical psychologist, educational specialist, or speech and language pathologist, as indicated.
- The primary care physician should refer the patient to a developmental pediatrician, child neurologist, or child psychiatrist when the following conditions exist:
  - There is diagnostic confusion.
  - First-line interventions are not beneficial.
  - Combinations of medications are necessary.
- For very young children with symptoms of AD/HD, a thorough developmental assessment is imperative.
- The effect of stimulant medication is not paradoxical and does not stop at puberty.
- There is no clear benefit for drug holidays or use of medication on school days only.
- As with other chronic conditions, numerous nontraditional interventions are available; many are without proven efficacy.

PEARLS & CONSIDERATIONS

PREVENTION

Environmental factors may ameliorate expression of the disorder.

PATIENT/FAMILY EDUCATION

- The most common cause of AD/HD is genetic.
- AD/HD is a lifelong condition in up to 70% of people.
- The patient and family must learn strategies to manage the symptom complex.
- Manifestations and symptoms change over time.
- The severity of symptoms varies dramatically in different environments.
- Information and support groups may be found through Children and Adults with Attention Deficit/Hyperactivity Disorder (www.chadd.org), which has many local chapters throughout the United States.
- Many communities and some schools have local support groups. School psychologists, school social workers, developmental pediatricians, child neurologists, and child psychiatrists often are aware of local resources.

SUGGESTED READINGS

American Academy of Pediatrics: Caring for children with ADHD: a resource toolkit for clinicians. Available at http://www.nichq.org/resources/toolkit

American Academy of Pediatrics: Clinical practice guidelines: diagnosis and evaluation of the child with attention deficit/hyperactivity disorder. *Pediatrics* 105:1158, 2000.

American Academy of Pediatrics: Clinical practice guidelines: treatment of the school-age child with attention deficit/hyperactivity disorder. *Pediatrics* 108:1033, 2001.

AUTHOR: **MARY ELLEN GELLERSTEDT, MD**

BASIC INFORMATION

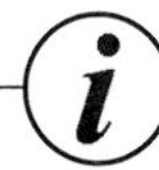

DEFINITION

A developmental disorder characterized by a qualitative impairment in social reciprocity, a qualitative impairment in communication, and repetitive behaviors. The Autism Spectrum includes five disorders:

- Autism: stringent criteria are met with symptoms in all three areas listed above.
- Asperger's syndrome: defined by normal early language, normal cognition, and symptoms related to social reciprocity and restricted interests/repetitive behaviors.
- Rett syndrome: found primarily in girls with loss of language and hand use.
- Disintegrative disorder: symptoms start later in childhood and extend to daily living and motor skills.
- Pervasive developmental disorder—not otherwise specified: when the criteria for the other disorders in this category are not met.

SYNONYMS

Autism spectrum disorders (ASDs)
Pervasive developmental disorders (PDDs)

ICD-9-CM CODES

299 Pervasive developmental disorders
299.0 Autism
299.1 Disintegrative disorder
299.8 Asperger's syndrome
330.8 Rett syndrome

EPIDEMIOLOGY & DEMOGRAPHICS

- This condition may affect as many as 1 in 166 people; older studies cite numbers of 4 to 5 in 10,000.
  - Question of increasing prevalence versus better detection and broader definition
  - Autism may have prevalence of 40:10,000; PDD/ASD overall may be as much as 60:10,000
- Male predominance of 4:1 for autistic disorder
- Up to 70% of people with autism also have mental retardation.
  - Asperger's syndrome defined by IQ in typical range.

CLINICAL PRESENTATION

- Infancy: decreased eye contact, language delays, acts as if deaf, repetitive behaviors
  - One fourth to one third of autistic children lose language skills in the second year of life.
- Early childhood: insistence on routine, lack of pretend play, repetitive behaviors
- Later childhood/adolescence: problems with peer interactions
- Generally nondysmorphic
- May be associated with tuberous sclerosis, fragile X syndrome
  - Less frequent comorbidity with Down syndrome, Möbius' syndrome, and Joubert's syndrome, among others
  - Comorbidity with neurologic symptoms like seizures (25%) or tics (9%) common
- May have clumsiness, mild hypotonia

ETIOLOGY

- The cause is unknown.
- The evidence for a genetic etiology is strong.
  - Concordance in identical twins is greater than 60% for autism and greater than 90% if symptoms, but not the complete disorder, are included.
  - Recurrence risk is 100 times the general population for families with one child with autism.
- Epidemiologic and basic science evidence does not support either measles-mumps-rubella vaccination or mercury toxicity from thimerosal as causative.
- Pathologic findings are varied but include the following:
  - Hypoplasia of cerebellar vermis
  - Decreased numbers of Purkinje cells in the cerebellum
  - Increased cell packing in the limbic system
  - Hypoplasia of cranial nerve nuclei
- This condition can be associated with fetal exposure to infectious agents (e.g., rubella) or teratogens (e.g., thalidomide, valproic acid, ethanol).
- Immunologic factors are under investigation.
- Psychological construct: Theory of Mind—cannot understand that other people have a different point of view, which is necessary for communication and social reciprocity.

DIAGNOSIS

DIFFERENTIAL DIAGNOSIS

- Mental retardation with stereotyped behaviors
- Sensory impairment
- Epileptic aphasia (Landau-Kleffner syndrome)
- Tourette's disorder
- Obsessive-compulsive illness
- Childhood schizophrenia
- (Rarely) attention deficit/hyperactivity disorder (AD/HD) or language disorders

WORKUP

- Diagnosis is made by history and clinical presentation, applying DSM-IV criteria.
- Diagnosis is supported by valid assessment measures.
  - Autism Diagnostic Interview—Revised
  - Autism Diagnostic Observation Schedule-G
  - Childhood Autism Rating Scale
  - PDD Screening Test
  - Autism Behavior Checklist
  - Gilliam's Autism or Asperger Rating Scale
- Testing should include cognitive, language, and hearing assessments.

LABORATORY TESTS

- An electroencephalogram (optional) is suggested when there has been a loss of skills, variability in behavior, or seizures.
- Assessment of the underlying cause is based on history, family history, examination, and presence or absence of mental retardation.
  - Consider fragile X testing with comorbid developmental delay or mental retardation or family history of mental retardation
  - Consider karyotype with family history of developmental disorders, dysmorphic features
- Popular complementary approaches include immune, nutritional, and allergic assessments that have not yet been scientifically investigated.

IMAGING STUDIES

- Magnetic resonance imaging is not typically diagnostically helpful although it may be recommended as part of an initial evaluation for causes of global developmental delay.

TREATMENT

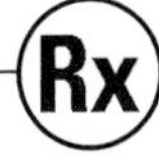

NONPHARMACOLOGIC THERAPY

- The mainstay of therapy involves educational interventions, behavioral therapy, and speech therapy.
- Multiple service models are available.
  - Little outcome data exist, though, except for strict behavioral programs.
- Children with language and higher cognitive abilities benefit from social skills and pragmatic language training in inclusive educational environments.

CHRONIC Rx

- Inattention, impulsivity, and motor hyperactivity may respond to stimulant medications or α-agonists, as in AD/HD.
- Selective serotonin reuptake inhibitors may decrease aggression, self-injury, and obsessions.
- Atypical neuroleptics (e.g., risperidone) may decrease aggression, stereotyped behaviors, and self-injury.
- Current studies are examining the use of anticonvulsants as mood stabilizers.
- Medication should be used only as an adjunct to a behavioral program.

COMPLEMENTARY & ALTERNATIVE MEDICINE

Mentioned here are a variety of complementary therapies that have been tried, with no scientific evidence yet for successful treatment of symptoms of autism:

- Casein-free and gluten-free diet
- Auditory integration training
- Vitamin B_6 with magnesium
- Dimethylglycine

- Anti-yeast agents
- Chelation
- Vitamin B_{12} injections
- Intravenous secretin: multiple double-blind controlled trials could not detect any benefit in autism.

DISPOSITION

- Medication monitoring requires input from school personnel and parents.
- The efficacy of intervention needs to be monitored. School reassessment should be conducted every 3 years for formal testing. Response to the program must be re-evaluated more often.

REFERRAL

- 0 to 3 years of age: early intervention program
- 3 to 21 years of age: school district committee on special education
- Confirmation of the diagnosis by a child psychologist, developmental/behavioral pediatrician, child neurologist, or child psychia rist familiar with the disorder

PEARLS & CONSIDERATIONS

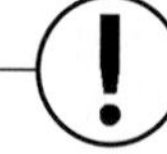

COMMENTS

- It is possible to have a few symptoms of the disorder without meeting the diagnostic criteria for a PDD. This is called the *broader autistic* phenotype.
- Symptoms in toddlers include absence of pointing to show interest, absence of pretend play, and decreased eye gaze to regulate social interaction, especially with language delays.
- Many people with PDD, and all people with Asperger's syndrome, have typical intelligence. They may seem professorial as children.

PATIENT/FAMILY EDUCATION

- The recurrence risk is 3% to 7% unless a specific cause is known.
- Cognitive assessment is difficult in very young children with PDD and may not be predictive of later intellectual potential.
- Obtaining disorder-specific educational programs may require significant advocacy efforts by the parents.

SUGGESTED READINGS

First Signs. Available at: www.firstsigns.org

Ozonoff S, et al: *A Parent's Guide to Asperger Syndrome and High Functioning Autism: How to Meet the Challenges and Help Your Child Thrive.* Guilford Publications, NY, NY, 2002.

Practice Parameters for Diagnosis and Screening of Autism, American Academy of Neurology. Available online at: http://www.aan.com/professionals/practice/pdf/g10063.pdf

Volkmar FR, Wiesner LA: *Health Care for Children on the Autism Spectrum: A Guide to Medical, Nutritional, Behavioral Issues.* 2004, Woodbine House, Inc. Bethesda, MD.

AUTHOR: **SUSAN L. HYMAN, MD**

BASIC INFORMATION

DEFINITION

- Fever: a rectal temperature of higher than 38°C
- Bacteremia: the presence of bacteria in the blood
- Sepsis: systemic inflammatory response syndrome (SIRS) associated with infection
- Fever without source: acute febrile illness without identified etiology after history and physical examination
- Serious bacterial infection (SBI): bacteremia, meningitis, pneumonia, urinary tract infection, cellulitis, bone or joint infection, and enteritis

ICD-9-CM CODES
780.6 Fever
790.7 Bacteremia
995.91 Sepsis

EPIDEMIOLOGY & DEMOGRAPHICS

- Fever is a very common reason for health care visits in the young child.
- Most febrile illnesses in young children are caused by viral infections.
- Increased hospitalization in young febrile infants corresponds with influenza and enterovirus outbreaks.
- In nontoxic-appearing febrile infants less than 3 months of age, the incidence of serious bacterial infection is about 10%. The incidence of bacteremia in this group is about 2%.
- The risk of occult bacteremia in children 3 to 36 months of age with temperature ≥39°C was about 5% but is decreased with current immunizations.

CLINICAL PRESENTATION

- It is important to do a quick assessment. If ill appearance, stabilize and obtain cultures without delaying intravenous antibiotics.
- A thorough history is important including a complete review of systems.
- Details of fever history should record how temperature was measured and height of fever and its duration.
- Obtain medication and immunization history.
- Past medical history should include premature birth, prior antibiotics, prior illness, and previous hospitalization.
- Parental medical history is important.
- Social history should include family situation, unusual exposures, and travel. This history may influence need for hospitalization.
- The physical exam includes an overall general assessment and accurate vital signs.
- A complete exam is important.

ETIOLOGY

Common Bacterial Pathogens

- *Streptococcus agalactiae* (group B streptococcus)*
- *Listeria monocytogenes**
- *Streptococcus pneumoniae*
- *Neisseria meningitidis*
- *Haemophilus influenza*
- *Enterococcus*
- *Streptococcus pyogenes*
- *Salmonella species*
- *Escherichia coli*
- *Staphylococcus* species

Common Viral Pathogens

- Enteroviruses
- Respiratory syncytial virus
- Influenza viruses
- Parainfluenza viruses
- Rotavirus
- Rhinovirus
- Human herpes virus 6, 7
- Herpes simplex virus
- Parvovirus
- Adenovirus
- Cytomegalovirus
- Varicella zoster virus

DIAGNOSIS

Dx

DIFFERENTIAL DIAGNOSIS

- Possible noninfectious etiologies of fever include:
  - Collagen vascular diseases
  - Malignancy
  - Drug reaction
  - Metabolic disorders
  - Central nervous system dysfunction

LABORATORY TESTS

- For infants who are ≤3 months of age the full evaluation for possible sepsis includes:
  - Complete blood count with differential
  - Urinalysis
  - Cerebrospinal fluid (CSF) analysis
  - Blood, urine, and CSF cultures for bacteria
  - Chest X-ray (CXR) if respiratory symptoms
  - Additional studies such as stool culture; viral studies; culture of joint, bone, skin, and so on as indicated.
- For infants who are ≤3 months of age who appear well or were previously well, no evidence of bacterial infection on exam, and normal lab evaluation [white blood cell (WBC) count 5000 to 15,000, absolute band count <1500, ≤10 WBC/high-power field (hpf) on spun urine, ≤5 WBC/hpf on stool smear if diarrhea] a lumbar puncture (LP) may not be part of the evaluation. An LP should be done if infant is to be treated with antibiotics.
- For children 3 to 36 months of age, the lab evaluation is more dependent upon the physical exam—more lab evaluation is done in ill-appearing children.
- For well-appearing children 3 to 36 months of age with temperature ≥39°C:
  - Obtain complete blood cell count (CBC) with differential. If WBC ≥15,000, obtain blood culture.
  - For boys less than 6 months of age and girls less than 2 years of age, obtain urine culture.
  - Obtain CXR if symptoms supportive of pneumonia. Consider CXR if elevated WBC.
  - Obtain stool culture if bloody diarrhea or ≥5 WBC/hpf in stool smear.
  - Consider LP, particularly in child less than 1 year of age.

*Uncommon in healthy children > 3 months of age.

TREATMENT

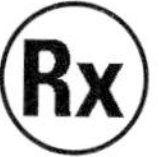

ACUTE GENERAL Rx

- Infants 3 months of age:
  - Ill-appearance or suspected bacterial infection mandate admission. Intravenous antibiotics are administered after cultures obtained.
  - Antibiotics usually given are ampicillin and ceftriaxone (cefotaxime) or ampicillin and gentamicin.
  - If pneumococcal meningitis is suspected vancomycin and ceftriaxone are recommended pending results from cultures.
  - Selected infants ≥1 month of age who appear well, were previously well, show no evidence of bacterial infection on exam, and have normal labs (WBC 5000 to 15,000, absolute band count <1500, ≤10 WBC/hpf on spun urine, ≤5 WBC/hpf on stool smear if diarrhea) may be managed as outpatients if there will be an appropriate home situation and close follow-up with physician. Ceftriaxone given intramuscularly is often administered to these infants.
  - Full evaluation for sepsis (including LP) should be performed before antibiotics are given.
- Children 3 months to 3 years of age:
  - Ill-appearing children should be hospitalized and intravenous antibiotics administered.
  - Intravenous antibiotics used are ceftriaxone (or cefotaxime). If pneumococcal meningitis or resistant *Staphylococcal aureus* is suspected, add vancomycin.
  - If child is well-appearing but has temperature of 39°C and WBC ≥15,000, ceftriaxone is often administered. An LP should be considered before giving ceftriaxone.

DISPOSITION

- Young infants who are managed as outpatients should be evaluated within 24 hours. If cultures become positive or infant looks ill, child should be admitted.
- For children 3 months to 3 years of age, managed as outpatients, there should be close follow-up.
    - If continued fever and cultures are negative, perform physical examination.
    - If urine culture is positive, complete course of antibiotics.
    - If child is febrile and has positive blood culture, repeat blood culture, perform LP, and admit for intravenous antibiotics.
    - If child is well-appearing and afebrile with blood culture suggestive of *S. pneumoniae* a second dose of ceftriaxone may be given while awaiting further results.

REFERRAL

- Consultation with an infectious disease specialist is recommended for children with unusual infections, severe infections, or clinical/laboratory findings that are difficult to interpret.

PEARLS & CONSIDERATIONS

COMMENTS

- Infants less than 3 months of age with history of a fever who are afebrile on presentation are usually evaluated as a febrile infant.
- If an infant of 3 months of age is to receive antibiotics, a full evaluation for sepsis should be done before antibiotics.

PREVENTION

- Children should be immunized as recommended by the current schedule.

PATIENT/FAMILY EDUCATION

- Parents should be educated about limiting exposures and the importance of good hand washing.
- Parents of newborns should be instructed in measurement of child's temperature. They should contact provider if there is fever or clinical instability.

SUGGESTED READINGS

Baraff LJ et al: Practice guideline for the management of infants and children 0 to 36 months of age with fever without source. *Pediatrics* 92:1, 1993.

Lorin MI, Feigin RD: Fever without source and fever of unknown origin. *In* Feigin RD et al (eds): *Textbook of Pediatric Infectious Diseases.* Philadelphia, Saunders, 2004, pp 825–836.

Shapiro ED: Fever without localizing signs. *In* Long SS et al (eds): *Principles Practice of Pediatric Infectious Diseases.* Philadelphia, Churchill Livingstone, 2003, pp 110–114.

AUTHOR: **CAROL A. MCCARTHY, MD**

BASIC INFORMATION

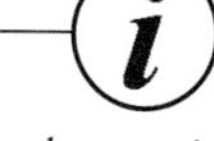

DEFINITION

Balanitis is an inflammation of the glans penis or clitoris.

SYNONYMS

Balanitis circinata: inflammation grossly appears as a reddened papular ring.

Balanitis xerotica obliterans (BXO): inflammation is characterized by submucosal edema and fibrosis, with little cellular component. This is a grossly aggressive and scarring balanitis.

Balanoposthitis: inflammation includes prepuce (foreskin).

Zoona's balanitis plasmacellularis: inflammatory cells are predominantly plasma cells.

ICD-9-CM CODE
607.1 Balanitis

EPIDEMIOLOGY & DEMOGRAPHICS

- Peak age for balanoposthitis is 2 to 4 years but 9 to 11 years when considering BXO
- Incidence: 3% balanoposthitis in uncircumcised males by age 18 years
- Diabetes: 11% of adults presenting with balanoposthitis

CLINICAL PRESENTATION

History

- Redness or swelling of the glans penis
- Pain
- Dysuria
- Preputial or urethral discharge
- Inability to retract previously reducible foreskin
- Prior episodes in less than 1%

Physical Examination

- Focal or global erythema of glans
- Discharge, swelling, erythema, or fissures of prepuce (balanoposthitis)
- Inguinal adenopathy

ETIOLOGY

- Infectious
  - *Candida albicans*
  - β-Hemolytic streptococci (groups A and B)
  - *Bacteroides* species
  - *Gardnerella vaginalis*
  - *Chlamydia trachomatis*
  - Tuberculosis
  - Herpes simplex virus
  - *Trichomonas vaginalis*
  - *Amoeba enterocolitica*
  - Scabies
- Dermatoses
  - Psoriasis
  - Lichen planus
  - Seborrheic dermatitis
  - Contact dermatitis
- Miscellaneous
  - Erythema multiforme exudativum (Stevens-Johnson syndrome)
  - Fixed drug eruption
  - Ankylosing spondylitis
  - Reiter's syndrome

DIAGNOSIS

DIFFERENTIAL DIAGNOSIS

- Reddened glans
  - Chemical burn (ammonia, detergents)
  - Trauma
  - Insect bite
  - Condyloma acuminatum
  - Erythroplasia of Queyrat
  - Chancre/chancroid
- Preputial swelling
  - Paraphimosis (prolonged retraction with subsequent swelling of an uncircumcised prepuce and distal glans)
  - Angioedema
  - Lymphedema
  - Leukemic infiltration

WORKUP

The diagnosis is made on clinical grounds and based on characteristic appearance or the presence of lesions at other sites (e.g., mouth, conjunctiva, skin, anus).

- Biopsy may be warranted in atypical, unresponsive, or persistent lesions.
  - Urethral involvement should lower the threshold for early biopsy (BXO).
- Specific testing for conditions in the differential diagnosis should be performed as warranted.

LABORATORY TESTS

- Urinalysis, including a glucose screen, is obtained.
- Cultures are done as needed.
- Gram stains of discharge or epithelial scrapings may direct therapy.
- Cultures should be sent of discharge or biopsy material to refine treatment.

TREATMENT

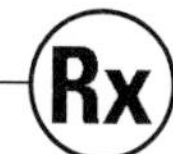

NONPHARMACOLOGIC THERAPY

- Balanitis
  - Observe the patient
  - Eliminate exposure
  - Administer sitz baths
- Balanoposthitis
  - Observe the patient
  - Eliminate exposure
  - Administer sitz baths
  - *Rare:* irrigate with saline solution between prepuce and glans
- Surgical intervention for balanoposthitis rarely indicated
  - Dorsal slit to provide drainage as adjunct to antibiotics

ACUTE GENERAL Rx

- Balanitis
  - Topical triamcinolone or nystatin, *or*
  - Oral trimethoprim-sulfamethoxazole or cephalexin
- Balanoposthitis
  - Amoxicillin-clavulanic acid

DISPOSITION

- Follow the patient for 24 to 48 hours to ensure a response in balanoposthitis.
- Remainder of follow-up depends on the cause.

REFERRAL

All lesions that persist, recur, or involve the urethra mandate evaluation by a pediatric urologist.

PEARLS & CONSIDERATIONS

COMMENTS

- Thirty percent to 40% of preputial discharge cultures are sterile.
- Oatmeal baths are a soothing adjunct and are often therapeutic.
- If infections are not congruent with the child's reported sexual activity, abuse should be considered.
- In sexually active patients, consider latex allergy or spermicidal agent as causes.

PATIENT/FAMILY EDUCATION

- Most episodes are self-limited and do not recur.
- A single episode of balanoposthitis does not warrant mandatory circumcision.
- The foreskin should never be retracted forcibly because fissures may represent portals of entry for infection.

SUGGESTED READINGS

Langer JC, Coplen DE: Circumcision and pediatric disorders of the penis. *Pediatr Clin North Am* 45:801, 1998.

Rickwood AMK: Medical indications for circumcision. *BJU Int* 83:45, 1999.

Waugh MA: Balanitis. *Dermatol Clin* 16:757, 1998.

AUTHORS: **ROBERT A. MEVORACH, MD, WILLIAM C. HULBERT, MD,** and **RONALD RABINOWITZ, MD**

BASIC INFORMATION

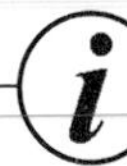

DEFINITION

A syndrome characterized by the acute onset of unilateral facial paralysis which progresses over a 2- to 5-day period.

SYNONYM(S)

Facial nerve palsy
Idiopathic facial nerve paralysis
Seventh nerve palsy

ICD-9-CM CODE
351.0 Bell's facial palsy

EPIDEMIOLOGY & DEMOGRAPHICS

- 20 to 30 cases per 100,000 people per year
- Incidence increases with age.
- Both sexes are affected equally.
- Recovery is better in children.

CLINICAL PRESENTATION

- Onset:
  - Facial paralysis of sudden onset which may progress over 3 to 72 hours
  - Pain (50%) near mastoid process
  - Poor eye closure and excessive tearing
  - Hyperacusis
  - Abnormal taste
  - Cannot keep food in mouth
- Prognosis is better if:
  - Incomplete facial nerve paralysis
  - Early improvement
  - Slow progression
  - Younger age
  - Normal salivary flow
  - Normal taste
- Improvement after onset: 10 days to 2 months
- Plateau: 6 weeks to 9 months
- Residual signs:
  - Synkinesis: 50%
  - Face weakness: 30%
  - Contracture: 20%
  - Crocodile tears: 6%

Physical Examination

- Limited to facial nerve pathology
  - Must distinguish upper motor neuron (e.g., stroke) from lower motor neuron (peripheral facial nerve) weakness
    - Unilateral
    - Degree: complete paralysis in 70%
    - Facial asymmetry
    - Eyebrow droop
    - Loss of forehead creases and nasolabial folds
    - Drooping of corner of mouth
    - Uncontrolled tearing
    - Inability to close eye
- Stapedius dysfunction (33%): hyperacusis
- Lacrimation: mild in some patients
- Taste: no clinically significant changes in most

ETIOLOGY

- Localized inflammation of cranial nerve VII (facial nerve) often presumed to be due to herpesvirus infection.
- Presumably occurs with other viral infections and may be a postinfectious symptom.
- Varicella zoster virus: (also called "Ramsay-Hunt syndrome") can infect the VII nerve or geniculate ganglion causing Bell's palsy associated with a vesicular rash of the ear.
- *Borrelia burgdorferi*: Lyme disease
- Leprosy
- Sarcoid

DIAGNOSIS

DIFFERENTIAL DIAGNOSIS

- Stroke
- Hemifacial spasm
- Neoplasms
- Trauma
- Congenital and genetic syndromes can be associated with facial nerve weakness: Möbius syndrome, Melkersson syndrome
- Guillain-Barré syndrome
- Other neuromuscular conditions: myopathies, myasthenia gravis

WORKUP

- Diagnosis can usually be made by clinical findings of facial palsy due to lower motor neuron weakness.
- Electroneurography (performed in electromyography laboratories) can be helpful in predicting long-term outcome, but should not be performed until at least 3 days after onset.
  - In general, this testing does not guide decision-making about medical management, but may influence decisions about surgery.

LABORATORY TEST

- Serologic testing for Lyme disease is useful in endemic areas.

IMAGING STUDIES

- Magnetic resonance imaging can be useful in detecting brainstem tumors.

TREATMENT

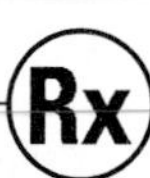

NONPHARMACOLOGIC THERAPY

- Eye care: lubricate the eye frequently with drops during the day and eye ointment at night (with patching) to prevent corneal abrasion.
- Surgical decompression is considered in severe cases.

ACUTE GENERAL Rx

- The adult literature supports the use of corticosteroids (prednisone) and acyclovir in moderate to severe facial palsy within 72 hours of onset.
- There are no studies in children to support the use of these agents, though they are generally considered safe and well-tolerated.

DISPOSITION

Patients should see a physician immediately for prompt initiation of treatment, including instructions for good eye care.

REFERRAL

- Consider referral to a neurologist if the patient is not experiencing good recovery in 2 weeks.
- Patient may benefit from having electrodiagnostic studies performed to assess facial nerve function.

PEARLS & CONSIDERATIONS

COMMENTS

In children in endemic areas, Lyme disease may be an important etiology of facial nerve weakness.

SUGGESTED READINGS

Gilden DH: Bell's palsy. *New Engl J Med* 351:1323, 2004.

Grogan PM, Gronseth GS: Practice parameter: steroids, acyclovir, surgery for Bell's palsy (an evidence-based review): report of the Quality Standards Subcommittee of the American Academy of Neurology. *Neurology* 56:830, 2001.

AUTHOR: **JENNIFER M. KWON, MD**

BASIC INFORMATION

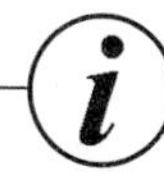

DEFINITION

Biliary atresia is a fibro-obliterative destructive process involving the extrahepatic biliary tree, which occurs in the first 2 months of life.

SYNONYM

Extrahepatic biliary atresia

ICD-9-CM CODES
576.2 Obstruction, biliary
751.61 Extrahepatic biliary atresia

EPIDEMIOLOGY & DEMOGRAPHICS

- 1 in 10,000 to 1 in 15,000 live births
- No gender predilection (some studies suggest female preponderance)
- Most common cause of neonatal cholestasis
- Typically not inherited (80% or more)

CLINICAL PRESENTATION

History

- Persistent jaundice for more than 3 weeks
- Dark urine or pale stools

Physical Examination

- Healthy infant
- Jaundice
- Typically without apparent associated malformations (more than 80% of cases)
- Hepatomegaly with or without splenomegaly
- Rectal examination reveals acholic stools
- If associated with polysplenia syndrome, the following clinical findings may also present:
  - Laterality sequence
    - Polysplenia
    - Abdominal situs inversus
    - Intestinal malrotation
    - Anomalous portal/hepatic veins (e.g., preduodenal portal vein)
    - Complex cardiac malformations
  - Nonlaterality anomalies
    - Cardiac (e.g., ventricular septal defect, common atrioventricular canal)
    - Urinary tract (e.g., solitary kidney, horseshoe kidney)
    - Gastrointestinal (e.g., Meckel's diverticulum)
    - Facial (e.g., cleft lip/palate, choanal atresia)

ETIOLOGY

Etiology, unknown but several hypotheses exist.

- Normal development and maturation of biliary tree is believed to be interrupted during a critical period in a genetically or immunologically susceptible host.
  - Perinatal (acquired): pathologic interaction between immune response and viral infection (e.g., reovirus, rotavirus)
    - Accounts for at least 80% of cases
  - Fetal (embryonic): malformation syndrome due to gene mutation(s) that regulate bile duct development
    - Accounts for fewer than 20% of cases

DIAGNOSIS

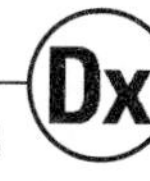

DIFFERENTIAL DIAGNOSIS

- See Jaundice/Hyperbilirubinemia in Differential Diagnosis (Section II).
- Essential diseases to exclude before surgical repair include:
  - Cystic fibrosis
  - α-Antitrypsin deficiency
  - Alagille syndrome

WORKUP

- See Jaundice/Hyperbilirubinemia in Differential Diagnosis (Section II).
- Diagnostic studies that may suggest extrahepatic biliary atresia include:
  - Liver biopsy (bile duct proliferation, portal expansion, bile duct plugs)
  - Hepatobiliary excretory scan (e.g., HIDA scan, nonexcretion)
  - Fasting abdominal ultrasound (absent or hypoplastic gallbladder, triangular cord sign, irregular gallbladder wall; *note:* finding of gallbladder or description of common bile duct does not exclude biliary atresia)
- The ultimate diagnosis is made at the time of exploratory laparotomy or laparoscopy, with demonstration of destruction of the extrahepatic biliary tree.

LABORATORY TESTS

- Chemistry panel including total and direct bilirubin and gamma-glutamyl transpeptidase (GGTP)
- Complete blood count, platelets and differential
- Urine analysis
- Sweat test
- α_1-Antritrypsin phenotype

IMAGING STUDIES

- Fasting abdominal ultrasound (absent or hypoplastic gallbladder, triangular cord sign, irregular gallbladder wall; *note:* finding of gallbladder or description of common bile duct does not exclude biliary atresia)
- Hepatobiliary excretory scan (e.g., HIDA scan, nonexcretion)

TREATMENT

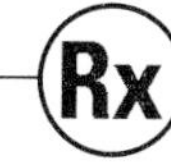

NONPHARMACOLOGIC THERAPY

- Hepatoportoenterostomy (Kasai procedure)
- Potential variants
  - Gallbladder Kasai
  - Kasai procedure with ostomy
  - Kasai procedure with intussusception antireflux valve

ACUTE GENERAL Rx

Diagnostic evaluation and surgery optimal by 60 days of age.

CHRONIC Rx

Postoperative Issues

- Cholangitis
  - Empiric prophylactic antibiotics have not been proven to be beneficial but are used by many. Prophylaxis against recurrent cholangitis with trimethoprim sulfamethoxazole is a reasonable clinical approach.
- Cholestasis
  - Poor drainage: empiric ursodeoxycholic acid and steroid boluses have been used. Ursodeoxycholic acid has not been shown to alter the outcome in biliary atresia, but its low toxicity and potential beneficial effects make it a reasonable therapy. Administration of ursodeoxycholic acid in children with total bilirubin in excess of 10 to 15 mg/dL is likely to be ineffective and there are theoretical toxicities in this setting. Recent anecdotal reports advocate high-dose corticosteroid use in the first 1 to 3 months after the Kasai procedure. This approach has not been proven to be effective and could be associated with a significant number of potential adverse events.
  - Malnutrition: formulas containing medium-chain triglycerides and fat-soluble vitamin supplementation (augmented by d-α-tocopheryl polyethylene glycol 1000 succinate vitamin E) are standard therapy. Breastfeeding needs to be monitored carefully in cholestatic infants (TB > 2.0 mg/dL) because of the risk of fat malabsorption and associated failure to thrive.
  - Pruritus: several regimens exist, including ursodeoxycholic acid, rifampin, cholestyramine, and opioid antagonists (antihistamines are commonly used and are relatively ineffective).

DISPOSITION

- Overall results
  - Complete drainage (postoperative total bilirubin <2 mg/dL): long-term palliation may result in development of biliary cirrhosis over 10 to 20 years.
  - Incomplete drainage (postoperative total bilirubin 2 to 5 mg/dL): short-term palliation may result in development of biliary cirrhosis in 2 to 10 years.
  - Failed procedure (postoperative bilirubin >8 mg/dL): liver failure in 6 to 18 months necessitates immediate liver transplant evaluation.
- Potential postoperative complications include:
  - Cholangitis
  - Cholestasis
    - Malabsorption
    - Bone disease/osteopenia
    - Pruritus
    - Xanthoma/xanthelasma
  - Failure to thrive
  - Portal hypertension
    - Ascites
    - Gastrointestinal/variceal hemorrhage
    - Hepatopulmonary syndrome
  - Synthetic liver failure

REFERRAL

- All children with clinically significant direct hyperbilirubinemia should be immediately referred to a pediatric gastroenterologist or a pediatric surgeon for evaluation.

- The following complications should initiate a referral for liver transplant evaluation:
  - Total bilirubin more than 5 mg/dL 3 months after portoenterostomy
  - Intractable cholangitis (more than two episodes in a 12-month period)
  - Failure to thrive
  - Variceal hemorrhage
  - Abdominal ascites
  - Recalcitrant pruritus
  - Liver synthetic dysfunction

PEARLS & CONSIDERATIONS

COMMENTS

- Jaundice at birth or jaundice persisting beyond 3 weeks of age requires exclusion of significant liver disease.
- The infant must be NPO (nothing by mouth) for more than 4 hours before abdominal ultrasound.
- Pigmented stools or the finding of a gallbladder or common bile duct on ultrasound does not exclude biliary atresia.
- Always exclude cystic fibrosis, α_1-antitrypsin deficiency, and Alagille's syndrome before performing a portoenterostomy.

PATIENT/FAMILY EDUCATION

- American Liver Foundation. Available online at www.liverfoundation.org
- Children's Liver Alliance. Available online at http://www.liverkids.org.au/biliary.htm
- Children's Liver Association for Support Services. Available online at http://www.classkids.org/library/biliaryatresia.htm

SUGGESTED READINGS

Balistreri WF et al: Biliary atresia: current concepts and research directions. *Hepatology* 23:1682, 1996.

Biliary Atresia Research Consortium. Available at http://www.med.umich.edu/borc/barc/

Chardot C et al: Prognosis of biliary atresia in the era of liver transplantation: French national study from 1986 to 1996. *Hepatology* 30:606, 1999.

Children's Liver Alliance. Available at http://www.liverkids.org.au/biliary.htm

Children's Liver Association for Support Services. Available at http://www.classkids.org/library/biliaryatresia.htm

Davenport M et al: Biliary atresia: the King's College Hospital experience (1974–1995). *J Pediatr Surg* 32:479, 1997.

Diem H et al: Pediatric liver transplantation for biliary atresia: results of primary graft in 328 recipients. *Transplantation* 27:1692, 2003.

Karrer FM et al: Long term results with the Kasai procedure for biliary atresia. *Arch Surg* 131:493, 1996.

Sokol RJ et al: Pathogenesis and outcome of biliary atresia: current concepts. *J Pediatr Gastroenterol Nutr* 37:4, 2003.

AUTHOR: **BENJAMIN L. SHNEIDER, MD**

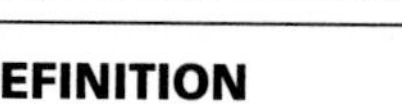

BASIC INFORMATION

DEFINITION

Blepharitis is a spectrum of acute and chronic inflammation of the eyelids.

SYNONYMS

Chalazia
Meibomitis
Seborrheic blepharitis
Staphylococcus blepharitis

ICD-9-CM CODE
373.00 Blepharitis—unspecified

EPIDEMIOLOGY & DEMOGRAPHICS

More commonly a disease of adults but can be seen in pediatric population.

CLINICAL PRESENTATION

History

- Nonspecific ocular discomfort (burning, irritation, and itching)
- Red eye
- Tearing
- Ocular discharge, which may occur in cycles

Physical Examination

- Red, thickened eyelids
- Dry crusting on the lid
- Acute hordeolum (stye)
- Occasionally conjunctivitis or corneal ulceration is seen.

ETIOLOGY

- Myriad, including acute infection with bacteria such as *Staphylococcus aureus, Propionibacterium acnes,* and *Streptococcus epidermidis.*
- *Demodex folliculorum* caused by a mite and inhabitant of human hair follicles, which may act as a vector for bacteria.
- Seborrhea

DIAGNOSIS

Dx

DIFFERENTIAL DIAGNOSIS

- Acute or chronic conjunctivitis
- Contact dermatitis
- Preseptal cellulitis
- Sebaceous cell carcinoma (usually adults)

WORKUP

The diagnosis is usually made on physical examination.

TREATMENT

Rx

NONPHARMACOLOGIC THERAPY

- Lid hygiene
- Warm compresses

ACUTE GENERAL Rx

- Topical antibiotic ointment (e.g., erythromycin) is applied to the lids.
- Topical antibiotic and a steroid combination ointment are used for resistant or severe cases.
- Oral antibiotic may be necessary.

DISPOSITION

- As needed

PEARLS & CONSIDERATIONS

!

COMMENTS

- May be seen commonly with rosacea and Down syndrome

PATIENT/FAMILY EDUCATION

Blepharitis is often a chronic disorder with periods of exacerbation requiring daily maintenance of nonpharmacologic therapy.

SUGGESTED READINGS

American Academy of Ophthalmology: *Pediatric ophthalmology and strabismus, section 6. Basic and Clinical Science Course.* American Academy of Ophthalmology, Orlando, Florida, 1998–1999.

Eliason JA: Blepharitis: overview classification. *In* Krachmer JH et al (eds): *Cornea.* St. Louis, Mosby, 1997.

AUTHOR: **ANNA F. FAKADEJ, MD, FAAO, FACS**

BASIC INFORMATION

DEFINITION

Botulism is a neuroparalytic illness characterized by symmetric, descending, flaccid paralysis of motor and autonomic nerves caused by intoxication with botulinum toxin. Three forms of the disease are recognized:

- Classic botulism or foodborne botulism is caused by the ingestion of preformed botulinum toxin in contaminated foods.
- Infant botulism is caused by colonization of the gastrointestinal (GI) tract with the organism *Clostridium botulinum,* followed by absorption of the neurotoxin produced in the GI tract.
- Wound botulism follows contamination of a wound with spores from *C. botulinum,* followed by production and absorption of the toxin from the wound.

SYNONYM

Sausage poisoning

ICD-9-CM CODE
005.1 Botulism

EPIDEMIOLOGY & DEMOGRAPHICS

- Approximately 150 cases of botulism are reported in the United States each year; 60% are infant botulism.
- Wound botulism increased in 1995 and 1996 primarily among injecting drug users (possibly associated with black tar heroin).
- Foodborne botulism outbreaks have been associated with both restaurant and home-prepared foods of all types, including the consumption of commercially prepared foods which have been stored improperly (toxin types A and B).
- Alaska has the highest incidence of foodborne botulism primarily due to the consumption of improperly prepared Alaskan native foods of fish or marine origin (toxin type E).
- Infant botulism occurs with increased frequency in California, Utah, and southern Pennsylvania (toxin types A and B).
- Most cases of infant botulism occur and between 2 and 6 months of age and equally among males and females throughout the year.

CLINICAL PRESENTATION

- Patients with foodborne botulism can present with GI disturbances such as nausea, vomiting, diarrhea, and abdominal pain, followed by neurologic symptoms.
- Common neurologic symptoms are dry mouth, blurred vision, diplopia, dysphonia, dysphagia, cranial nerve paralysis, and descending weakness, including the muscles of respiration.
- The symptoms of wound botulism are similar to foodborne botulism without GI complaints.
- Constipation, poor feeding or cry, progressive weakness or floppiness, and decreased spontaneous movements are the most common symptoms reported in infant botulism.
  - Prior ingestion of honey is reported in 15% of cases of infant botulism.
- Patients are afebrile, with diminished spontaneous movements and motor responses to stimuli.
- Ptosis, paralysis of the extraocular muscles, decreased pupillary constriction and corneal reflexes, impaired gag and swallow reflexes, and limb weakness in a proximal-to-distal pattern with decreased respiratory effort may all be present.
- Deep tendon reflexes may be decreased or absent in a descending distribution.
- Autonomic dysfunction may include dry mucous membranes, fluctuations in pulse and blood pressure, urinary retention, and alterations in skin color.

ETIOLOGY

C. botulinum is an anaerobic, spore-forming, gram-positive bacillus that produces a lethal neurotoxin. *Clostridium baratii* and *Clostridium butyricum* also can rarely be the cause of toxin production and disease.

DIAGNOSIS

DIFFERENTIAL DIAGNOSIS

- Myasthenia gravis
- Guillain-Barré syndrome
- Eaton-Lambert syndrome
- Poliomyelitis
- Stroke syndrome
- Hypothyroidism
- Drug or heavy metal poisoning
- Paralytic shellfish poisoning or puffer fish ingestion
- Wernig-Hoffmann syndrome
- Tick paralysis
- Sepsis

WORKUP

Electromyography demonstrating a pattern termed *BSAP* (brief, small, abundant motor-unit potentials) is characteristic of botulism and can be completed rapidly.

LABORATORY TESTS

The diagnosis is confirmed by detection of the neurotoxin in the serum or stool by neutralization assay or by the isolation of *C. botulinum* from feces.

TREATMENT

NONPHARMACOLOGIC THERAPY

- Meticulous supportive care, including ventilatory and nutritional support, is the mainstay of treatment.

ACUTE GENERAL Rx

- Trivalent equine antitoxin (TEAT) is not recommended for use in infants.
- Botulism immune globulin intravenous (human), trade name BabyBIG, was licensed for the treatment of infant botulism caused by Type A or B *C. botulinum* in 2003.
- If used within 3 days of hospitalization BabyBIG decreases the length of stay by more than 3 weeks, as well as decrease the length of time spent in the intensive care unit.
- TEAT use in adults has been beneficial.

DISPOSITION

- Prolonged hospitalization for supportive care is typical.
- The case:fatality ratio in infant botulism is less than 2% of hospitalized patients.
- The long-term prognosis is excellent, with gradual full recovery if the diagnosis is made promptly with institution of supportive care and complications of hospitalization avoided.

REFERRAL

Patients with botulism need to be monitored closely and transported to a pediatric center, where airway and ventilatory support can be instituted.

PEARLS & CONSIDERATIONS

COMMENTS

- With suspected botulism, use aminoglycoside antibiotics with caution because these medications can potentiate neuromuscular blockade and precipitate respiratory decompensation

PREVENTION

- Avoid feeding infants honey as this has been associated with infant botulism.
- Proper handling and storage of food to prevent spore germination and toxin production.

PATIENT/FAMILY EDUCATION

- Infants should not be fed honey because of the risk of botulism.
- There is no known person-to-person transmission of botulism.

SUGGESTED READINGS

Kalluri P et al: An outbreak of foodborne botulism associated with food sold at a salvage store in Texas. *Clin Infect Dis* 37:1490, 2003.

Long SS: Infant botulism. *Pediatr Infect Dis J* 20:707, 2001.

Reddy V et al: Infant botulism—New York City, 2001–2002. *MMWR* 52(2):21, 2003.

Sobel J et al: Foodborne botulism in the United States, 1990–2000. Emerg Infect Dis [serial on the internet, 2004]. Available at www.cdc.gov/ncidod/EID/vol10no9/03-0745.htm

U.S. Food and Drug Administration web site. Available at www.fda.gov/cber/products/igivcdhs102303.htm

AUTHOR: **MARY T. CASERTA, MD**

BASIC INFORMATION

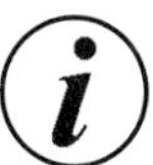

DEFINITION

Brain tumors result from an uncontrolled proliferation of cells derived from neural tissue or structural, supportive (glial) tissue within the brain. There are many types of brain tumors. Most are localized growths, but some disseminate throughout the central nervous system (CNS), and in rare instances spread outside the CNS.

SYNONYMS

Brain cancer
CNS malignancy

ICD-9-CM CODE
239.6 CNS tumor

EPIDEMIOLOGY & DEMOGRAPHICS

- The incidence is 40 cases per 1 million children per year. Approximately 3200 children younger than 19 years of age are diagnosed annually in the United States.
- The most common age at diagnosis is 5 to 10 years, but the disease can occur at any age.
- Brain tumors are the second most common pediatric malignancy; they are the most common pediatric solid tumors.
- Sixty percent are posterior fossa tumors; 40% are supratentorial (15% midline, 25% cerebral).
- Major brain tumor types include the following:
  - Astrocytoma (50%)
    - Low-grade: low-grade astrocytoma, ganglioglioma, and optic glioma
    - High-grade: brainstem glioma, anaplastic astrocytoma, and glioblastoma multiforme
  - Medulloblastoma (20%)
  - Ependymoma (10%)
  - Other (20%)
    - Low-grade: craniopharyngioma and oligodendroglioma
    - High-grade: lymphoma, supratentorial primitive neuroectodermal tumor (PNET), CNS atypical teratoid/rhabdoid tumor, choroid plexus carcinoma, and germ cell tumor

CLINICAL PRESENTATION

History

- General
  - Signs and symptoms are often related to hydrocephalus.
  - Signs and symptoms are often nonfocal.
  - Headaches, vomiting, and lethargy are common.
  - Ten percent of children present with seizures.
  - When focal findings develop in children, they are often related to balance, vision, and facial movements.
- Infants and toddlers
  - Irritability
  - Developmental delay or plateau
  - Vomiting
- School-age children and adolescents
  - Headaches
  - Vomiting
  - Double vision
  - Lethargy
  - Decline in school performance
  - Moodiness

Physical Examination

- Focal deficits uncommon, particularly in infants and toddlers
- Lethargy
- Papilledema
- Infants and toddlers
  - Widened or delayed closure of fontanelles
  - Abnormal increase in head circumference
  - Decreased upward gaze
- School-age children and adolescents
  - Poor balance and coordination
  - Dysconjugate gaze
  - Nystagmus
  - Facial weakness
  - Focal motor or sensory deficits

ETIOLOGY

- Unknown in most cases
- Increased incidence in children with neurofibromatosis types I and II, Gardener's syndrome (Turcot's syndrome), tuberous sclerosis, and Li-Fraumeni syndrome
- Increased incidence after cranial irradiation
- Environmental causes (e.g., power lines, cellular phones, chemical exposures) possible (these have been investigated, but none have been proven to cause brain tumors)

DIAGNOSIS

Dx

DIFFERENTIAL DIAGNOSIS

- Migraine headache
- Brain abscess or arteriovenous malformation
- Hydrocephalous from other causes
- Depression or other psychological disorder

WORKUP

- Lumbar puncture (LP) for cerebrospinal fluid (CSF) cytologic examination should be performed for patients with tumors that can disseminate throughout the CNS (e.g., ependymoma, medulloblastoma).
- LP should be done with caution because of the risk of herniation and should be done only after consultation with a neurosurgeon or neurologist.

LABORATORY TESTS

- Laboratory studies are generally not helpful in making the diagnosis.
- Serum and CSF β-human chorionic gonadotropin (β-hCG) and α-fetoprotein (AFP) should be obtained in patients with pineal region or suprasellar tumors to assess the possibility of a CNS germ cell tumor.

IMAGING STUDIES

- Magnetic resonance imaging (MRI) with gadolinium is the best imaging study.
- Computed tomography (CT) with contrast can be used if MRI is not available.
- MRI of the spine should be performed for patients with tumors that can disseminate throughout the CNS (e.g., ependymoma, medulloblastoma).

TREATMENT

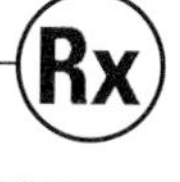

SURGERY

- A complete resection improves the prognosis for almost all types of brain tumors.
- Involvement of a skilled pediatric neurosurgeon is essential.
- Ventriculoperitoneal (VP) shunt placement is sometimes necessary.
- Children with a gross total or near gross total resection of low-grade astrocytoma, ganglioglioma, and oligodendroglioma need no further therapy.

RADIATION

- Focal external beam radiation is used for children 3 to 5 years of age or older who have brainstem glioma, anaplastic astrocytoma, glioblastoma, ependymoma, or partially resected craniopharyngioma, as well as for children with symptomatic, incompletely resected, or progressive low-grade astrocytoma.
- Craniospinal radiation is used for children with medulloblastoma, supratentorial PNET, and children with CNS germ cell tumor not receiving chemotherapy.
- Delayed or dose-reduced radiation is appropriate for children younger than 5 years of age who are being treated initially with chemotherapy.
- Stereotactic radiosurgery (or gamma knife) is focused, single-dose irradiation for previously irradiated children with local recurrences smaller than 4 cm in diameter.
- Toxicity of radiotherapy includes cognitive deficits, delayed growth and puberty, and late second malignancies.

CHEMOTHERAPY

- Chemotherapy is indicated for children with medulloblastoma, supratentorial PNET, anaplastic astrocytoma, glioblastoma multiforme, and CNS germ cell tumors.
- It is indicated for most children younger than 5 years of age who have any of the tumor types (except completely resected low-grade astrocytoma, ganglioglioma, or oligodendroglioma).
- Active agents include nitrosoureas, procarbazine, vincristine, VP-16, *cis*-platinum, carboplatin, and cyclophosphamide.
- New promising agents include temozolomide, irinotecan, and thalidomide.
- Toxicity includes hair loss, myelosuppression, hearing loss, and infertility.

DISPOSITION

- Cure rates are as follows:
  - Completely resected low-grade tumors (e.g., astrocytoma): 90% to 95%
  - Medulloblastoma, completely resected ependymoma: 70% to 80%
  - Brain tumors in children younger than 3 years of age: 20% to 60%
  - High-grade astrocytoma (e.g., anaplastic, glioblastoma): 20% to 30%
  - Brainstem glioma, atypical teratoid tumor: 0% to 20%
- Serial MRI is often performed during treatment and for several years after treatment to assess the response to therapy and the possibility of recurrence.
- The greatest likelihood of recurrence of high-grade tumors is within 2 to 3 years of diagnosis; low-grade tumors are less likely to recur but can recur at any time.
- Careful, coordinated follow-up by a team, including a pediatric neurosurgeon, radiation oncologist, pediatric oncologist, neurologist, social worker, teacher, and late-effects specialist, is essential throughout the initial evaluation, treatment, and follow-up period.
- The late effects of radiation and chemotherapy depend on the child's age and dose and location of radiation.
  - Hearing loss
  - Growth failure
  - Delayed puberty
  - Intellectual deficits

REFERRAL

- Children should be referred promptly to a pediatric neurosurgeon, pediatric radiation oncologist, and pediatric oncologist/neuro-oncologist.
- Future therapy will be directed at more selective tumor kill and less long-term toxicity and will include antiangiogenic therapy, gene therapy, and differentiation therapy.

PEARLS & CONSIDERATIONS

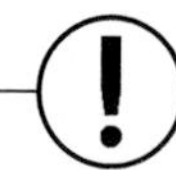

COMMENTS

The pattern of symptoms over time (e.g., headaches, poor school performance, emesis) is far more telling than the findings at a single physician visit.

PATIENT/FAMILY EDUCATION

- Brain tumors are complex diseases requiring careful, coordinated care by many subspecialists and support care personnel.
- Opinions among physicians may differ because many cases are complicated and unique.
- Most children with brain tumors are cured. The treatment strategy is designed to maximize cure rates and minimize long-term toxicity.
- There is a high likelihood of long-term toxicity.

SUGGESTED READINGS

National Brain Tumor Foundation. Available at www.braintumor.org

Pediatric Brain Tumor Foundation. Available at www.ride4kids.org

Strother DR et al: Tumors of the central nervous system. *In* Pizzo PA, Poplack DG (eds): *Principles and Practice of Pediatric Oncology.* Philadelphia, Lippincott-Raven, 2002.

AUTHOR: **DAVID N. KORONES, MD**

BASIC INFORMATION

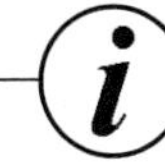

DEFINITION

- Nipple trauma: blistering, cracking, bruising, or bleeding of nipple associated with breastfeeding
- Breast infection
  - Mastitis: infection of lobule of breast and cellulitis of overlying skin
  - Monilial infection of the epidermis of the nipple and surrounding areola
- Obstructed duct: plugging of a collecting duct in the breast
- Engorgement: increased vascularity and accumulation of milk in the breast; may involve the whole breast or the areola

SYNONYMS

Monilial infection (yeast or candidal infection)
Nipple bruising
Nipple confusion
Nipple injury resulting from breastfeeding
Nipple trauma

ICD-9-CM CODES

611.0 Mastitis, breast infection, infection of nipple, yeast infection of nipple, yeast infection of breast
611.71 Sore nipple/breast pain
611.79 Engorgement of breast
675.9 Yeast infection/infection of breast with nipple
676.30 Plugged duct/absence of milk secretion

EPIDEMIOLOGY & DEMOGRAPHICS

- Nipple trauma
  - Increased prevalence is seen with flat or inverted nipples (approximately 10% of women).
  - Increased incidence occurs when infants have a short frenulum or oral motor problems.
  - Many women report some increased sensitivity of the nipples in the first 5 days of breastfeeding that occurs at the start of a feeding and lasts about 30 seconds. This normal sensitivity resolves by 1 to 2 weeks postpartum. Pain due to trauma persists or worsens throughout the feeding.
- Monilial infection risk factors: antibiotic use in infant or mother, maternal diabetes, infant thrush or monilial diaper rash
- Engorgement
  - Common day 1 to 3 postpartum
  - May occur later with milk stasis; may be generalized or limited to one lobe
  - Risk factors: skipped feedings, failure to empty the breast adequately, poor infant latch, overuse of breast pumping
- Mastitis
  - Occurs in as many as 9.5% of women, with the highest incidence in the first 6 weeks
  - Risk factors: mastitis with previous child, cracked or traumatized nipples in same week, use of a manual breast pump
  - Recurrent mastitis is often associated with delayed or inadequate treatment.
    - Sometimes associated with an area of the breast that drains poorly (e.g., previous surgery)
  - Abscess formation in a small proportion of women (approximately 5% to 11% of those with mastitis) is often associated with delayed or inadequate treatment.

CLINICAL PRESENTATION

History

- Nipple trauma
  - Nipple pain that occurs with breastfeeding, lasting throughout the entire feeding.
  - Vigorous nursing style in the infant.
    - Appropriate frequency (8 to 12 times per day in the neonate)
    - Appropriate interpretation of need to feed (Is the infant frantic by the time mother feeds?)
  - If milk transfer is affected, the infant may not gain weight appropriately.
    - Neonate should gain 15 to 30 g/day after milk increases in quantity.
    - Lactogenesis II (copious onset of milk production) usually occurs by 3 days postpartum.
    - Infant may have feeding-related jaundice.
    - Lack of urine and stool output may be seen (fewer than six to eight voids and three to four stools per day in neonate).
  - Delayed breastfeeding after birth and use of supplemental feedings
  - Exposure to artificial nipples such as pacifier use or bottle-feeding
- Breast infection
  - Yeast
    - Stinging, burning pain radiating throughout the breast during and between feedings
    - Thrush, monilial diaper rash in the infant; yeast vaginitis in the mother
    - Antibiotic use in the mother or infant
  - Mastitis
    - Fever, malaise, nausea, and flulike symptoms
    - Failure to resolve a plugged duct
    - History of breast surgery
    - Poor emptying of breast
    - Use of bras with stays
    - Engorgement
    - Refusal to nurse
- Obstructed duct
  - Soreness of breast localized to one area with a lump
  - Mother afebrile without systemic symptoms
- Engorgement
  - Generalized soreness of entire breast
  - Missed feedings
  - Breasts that are full, hard and warm to touch; shiny and transparent skin
  - Possible difficulty with latching on
  - Supplemental feeding of infant
  - Low-grade fever

Physical Examination

- Nipple trauma
  - Observation of breastfeeding to assess technique and infant attachment to the breast (see Fig. 1-3)
  - Cracked, bruised, or blistered nipples
  - Coexisting problems
    - Mastitis (see following discussion)
    - Contact dermatitis: red, irritated, dry nipple

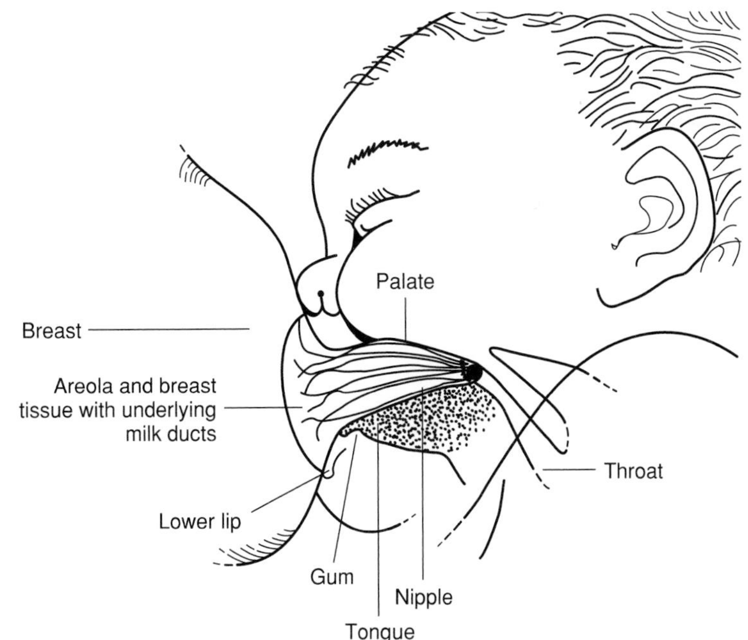

FIGURE 1-3 Infant latch.

- Engorgement: bilateral fullness of breasts with increased vascularity and warmth; skin may be transparent and shiny, and nipple may appear flat if areolar engorgement is prominent
- Tight frenulum: heart-shaped appearance of infant's tongue; with attempts to extend, tongue will not reach beyond lower alveolar ridge

- Breast infection
  - Monilial
    - Nipple may look normal or be shiny and red with satellite lesions around nipple.
    - Thrush or monilial diaper rash may be seen in the infant.
  - Mastitis
    - Wedge-shaped area of redness that is tender, firm, and warm to touch
    - Maternal fever
    - With breast abscess, fluctuant mass palpable
- Obstructed duct
  - Tender lump in breast
  - No evidence of cellulitis (area is not red, indurated, or warm to touch)
  - Mother well, afebrile without systemic symptoms
- Engorgement
  - Breasts are hard and warm to touch; skin is shiny and transparent.
  - Increased vascularity of breast is seen.
  - Low-grade fever is possible.

ETIOLOGY

- Nipple trauma
  - Improper latch (poor positioning of infant at breast) may be associated with maternal nipple abnormalities or engorgement, or short frenulum or other oral motor abnormalities in infant
  - Improper detachment techniques
  - Overly eager baby
  - Improper breast pump use
- Breast infection
  - Monilial
    - Colonization of maternal breast with yeast from infant's mouth or diaper area
    - Yeast overgrowth because of antibiotic use
  - Mastitis
    - Infection with *Staphylococcus aureus, Escherichia coli,* rarely *Streptococcus* species
    - Infection after nipple trauma
    - Associated with milk stasis, failure to resolve an obstructed duct or engorgement, or poor drainage of an area of the breast after breast biopsy or surgery
- Obstructed ducts
  - Breasts overly full
    - Early lactogenesis with missed or irregular feedings
    - Poor positioning with ineffective nursing and poor breast emptying
    - Inadequate letdown
    - Engorgement
  - Poor drainage of an area of the breast
    - External pressure on breast (poorly fitting bra)
    - Previous breast surgery

DIAGNOSIS

Dx

DIFFERENTIAL DIAGNOSIS

- Nipple trauma
  - Negative pressure on ductules with initial latch and suckling often occurs before the development of full lactogenesis II (produces temporary discomfort with attachment and initial suckling).
  - Contact dermatitis is caused by use of soaps, astringents, creams, nipple shields, or plastic bra liners.
  - Plugged duct
  - Monilial infection
  - Nipple trauma often coexists with other breastfeeding problems.
    - Mastitis may result from nipple trauma with subsequent infection.
    - In engorgement, the infant is unable to latch because of engorged areola.
    - With a short frenulum or other oral motor abnormality, the infant cannot properly position tongue.
- Breast infection
  - Monilial infection
    - Contact dermatitis
    - Other causes of nipple trauma
  - Mastitis
    - Plugged duct
    - Engorgement
    - Breast tumor (especially recurrent mastitis in same location with lack of response to antibiotics)
    - Breast abscess
- Obstructed duct
  - Mastitis
  - Engorgement
  - Breast tumor
- Engorgement
  - Mastitis
  - Plugged duct
  - Breast tumor

WORKUP

Usually not needed because diagnosis is made during observation of breastfeeding and physical examination of the mother and infant

LABORATORY TESTS

- Scrape and culture of tender or deeply cracked nipples for bacteria and yeast
  - Culture may be positive for *S. aureus*
  - Yeast culture positive, KOH prep may show hyphae indicative of *Candida albicans*
- With mastitis, a milk culture and analysis may be helpful if patient is unresponsive to 48 hours of antibiotic therapy directed against most common causal agent *S. aureus.*
  - Midstream culture, Gram stain, and white blood cell (WBC) count
    - In mastitis: more than 10^6 WBCs/mL and more than 10^3 bacteria/mL
    - In milk stasis without infection: less than 10^6 WBCs/mL and less than 10^3 bacteria/mL

IMAGING STUDIES

- Plugged ducts – unrelieved plugged ducts may lead to galactoceles or a milk retention cyst. Galactoceles may be visualized by ultrasound.

TREATMENT

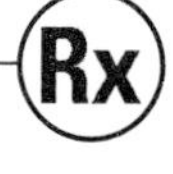

NONPHARMACOLOGIC THERAPY

- Nipple trauma
  - Ensure that positioning at breast is correct. Signs of poor latch-on include:
    - Contact of upper and lower lip at the corners of the mouth
    - Sunken or dimpled cheeks
    - Clicking sounds that correspond to breaking suction
    - Tongue not visible below the nipple when the lower lip is pulled down
    - Creased nipple following nursing
  - Instruct mother about proper detachment. Break suction with finger before removing the infant from the breast
  - Encourage short, frequent feedings (8 to 12 per day is normal in early weeks).
    - Begin with the least sore nipple to help with letdown on the more painful side.
    - If the mother is unable to put the infant to her breast because of pain, instruct her to begin breast pumping to maintain the milk supply until breastfeeding can be resumed.
  - Discontinue use of pacifier and bottle feeding. If the infant requires continued supplements, the use of a supplemental nursing system or cup feeding should be considered.
  - Discontinue use of any soaps, creams, or ointments if contact dermatitis is an aggravating factor.
  - Express milk and rub it into nipple after breastfeeding, then air dry nipples.
  - Consider referral to a community health nurse (with special training in lactation), or for infants with problems such as short frenulum or oral motor problems, suggest consultation with a lactation consultant or an occupational therapist. If ankyloglossia is present consider referral to ear, nose, throat specialist for frenuloplasty.
  - Suggest community support groups.
    - WIC (Women, Infants, and Children) peer counselors
    - La Leche League
  - If nipple trauma is associated with inverted or flat nipples, the mother may benefit from using something to draw out the nipple before attempting to attach the infant (i.e. a breast pump).

- If trauma is associated with mastitis, see following discussion.
- If trauma is associated with engorgement:
  - Milk expression (by hand or pump) before attaching the infant helps in allowing proper latch (especially if the areola is engorged).
  - Massage and application of warm packs to the breast may aid in beginning expression.
  - Frequent breastfeeding is essential to prevent re-engorgement.
  - Apply cold packs to breast after feeding.

- Breast infection
  - Monilial infection
    - Air dry nipples.
    - Avoid plastic liners on nursing pads and change pads frequently.
    - Sterilize items that come in contact with the infant's mouth (e.g., pacifiers, bottle nipples).
  - Mastitis
    - Infant may continue to nurse.
    - Begin with the least sore breast.
    - Ensure adequate emptying of the infected breast, apply warm packs, and massaging the breast before feeding.
    - Ensure that the mother rests adequately because stress and fatigue are often precipitating factors.
    - Ensure that the mother's bra does not have underwires or stays that inhibit drainage of one aspect of the breast.
- Obstructed duct
  - Begin frequent and effective nursing on the affected breast.
  - Apply moist, hot packs to the area before nursing.
  - Massage the area before nursing.
  - Alter nursing positions to encourage better drainage of the area. Position infant so that chin is directed toward the occluded duct.
- Engorgement
  - Begin frequent and effective nursing
  - Hand express or pump to relieve areola engorgement so that infant can attach
  - Massage breast before nursing
  - Apply cold compresses after nursing

ACUTE GENERAL Rx

- Nipple trauma
  - Administer a mild analgesic, such as aspirin, ibuprofen, or acetaminophen.
  - If area is dry, consider using an ointment, such as purified lanolin or A & D ointment. Routine use of ointments is not recommended.
  - Deeply cracked nipples are at risk for superficial infection that may lead to mastitis. Common causative agents are *S. aureus* and *C. albicans.* If cultures are positive for *S. aureus* treat with oral antibiotics to prevent the development of mastitis, which occurs in approximately 25% of patients.
  - After bacterial and fungal infections have been ruled out, severely affected nipples may respond to 1% cortisone ointment (2 days is usually adequate).
- Breast infection
  - Monilial infection
    - Nystatin oral suspension for the infant and nystatin cream for the mother
    - Treat for 7 to 10 days
    - For resistant cases, consider oral fluconazole in mother and baby
  - Mastitis should be treated for 10 to 14 days with antibiotics that are effective against *S. aureus.* Therapy can begin with dicloxacillin or cloxacillin (500 mg PO four times daily); if no response after 24 to 48 hours the patient can be switched to cephalexin or amoxicillin with clavulanate (Augmentin).
    - Poor compliance with the full course of antibiotics often leads to abscess formation.
    - If mastitis is bilateral, consider streptococcal infection.
- Obstructed duct or engorgement
  - Administer a mild analgesic, such as aspirin, ibuprofen, or acetaminophen

DISPOSITION

- Uncomplicated nipple trauma
- Follow-up within 2 to 3 days to assess resolution of pain, nipple healing, and infant well-being
- Condition may require more frequent visits if associated with poor weight gain in infant or feeding-related jaundice

Plugged Duct

- Follow-up by telephone within 24 hours to assess resolution
- If maternal systemic symptoms develop, consider progression to mastitis

Engorgement or Mastitis

- Follow-up within 24 hours
- Assess improvement in symptoms, response to antibiotics (mastitis), and infant well-being (hydration)

REFERRAL

- Sore nipples secondary to a short frenulum in the infant: experts increasingly recommend frenulum release in the infant to allow correct tongue positioning.
- Galactoceles that do not resolve with conservative management can be treated with needle aspiration but often refill and may require repeated aspiration or surgical removal under local anesthesia.
- Abscess formation with mastitis requires surgical drainage.

PEARLS & CONSIDERATIONS

PREVENTION

- Provide patient education in the hospital about proper attachment and detachment
- Initiate on-demand, frequent breastfeeding
- Avoid pacifiers and nonmedically indicated supplemental feedings

PATIENT/FAMILY EDUCATION

- Basic physiology of lactation:
  - Supply follows demand for milk from infant.
  - Frequent feedings are the norm (8 to 12 per day in the early weeks of breastfeeding).
  - Effective and frequent emptying of the breast is essential to maintaining the milk supply and avoiding milk stasis, which can lead to engorgement, plugged ducts, and mastitis.
- Expect six to eight wet diapers and a minimum of three to four yellow, seedy stools per day to ensure that infant is getting adequate amounts of milk after 4 to 5 days of life.
- Systemic symptoms, fever, malaise, nausea, or redness of breast indicates mastitis.

Support Groups

La Leche League International

WIC peer support programs

Both groups provide mother-to-mother support for breastfeeding women.

SUGGESTED READINGS

Academy of Breastfeeding Medicine (ABM): Provides evidenced-based clinical protocols for the management of common breastfeeding problems. Available at www.bfmed.org

American Academy of Pediatrics Breastfeeding Initiatives. Available at www.aap.org/advocacy/bf/brpromo.htm

Ballard JL et al: Ankyloglossia: assessment, incidence, and effect of frenuloplasty on the breastfeeding dyad. *Pediatrics* 110(5):e63, 2002.

Foxman B et al: Lactation mastitis: occurrence and medical management among 946 breastfeeding women in the United States. *Am J Epidemiol* 155(2):103, 2002.

Gartner LM et al: Breastfeeding and the use of human milk. *Pediatrics* 115(2):496, 2005.

Hopkinson J, Schanler RJ: Common problems of breastfeeding in the postpartum period. UpToDate online (12.3) 01-07-2005. Available at www.uptodate.com

La Leche League International (LLLI). Available at www.lalecheleague.org

Lawrence RA, Lawrence R: *Breastfeeding: a guide for the medical profession,* 6th ed. St. Louis, Mosby, 2005.

Protocol Committee Academy of Breastfeeding Medicine, J. L. Ballard et al: ABM Clinical Protocol Number 11: Guidelines for the Evaluation and Management of Neonatal Ankyloglossia and Its Complications in the Breastfeeding Dyad. Academy of Breastfeeding Medicine Mar 3, 2005. Available at http//www.bfmed.org/protos.html

San Diego County Breastfeeding Coalition: Provides an updated list of Internet sites with breastfeeding information. Available at www.breastfeeding.org

AUTHOR: **CYNTHIA R. HOWARD, MD, MPH, FAAP**

BASIC INFORMATION

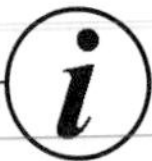

DEFINITION

- **Breastfeeding jaundice** is an abnormal unconjugated hyperbilirubinemia during the first week of life resulting from decreased enteral intake and increased enterohepatic circulation of bilirubin. There is no associated increase in bilirubin production. It is a sign of failure to establish adequate breastfeeding.
- **Breastmilk jaundice** is a normal extension of physiologic jaundice of the newborn (normally occurring unconjugated hyperbilirubinemia in the first week of life). It begins after the fifth day of life and continues for several weeks. It is believed to be caused by an inhibitor of bilirubin conjugation present in human milk.

SYNONYM

Breastfeeding jaundice is also termed *lack of breastmilk jaundice.* Infants, whether breastfed or formula fed, will become jaundiced with inadequate caloric intake.

ICD-9-CM CODES
774.2 Breastfeeding jaundice (physiologic jaundice) in preterm infants
774.6 Breastfeeding jaundice (physiologic jaundice) in term infants
774.39 Breastmilk jaundice

EPIDEMIOLOGY & DEMOGRAPHICS

- Physiologic jaundice
  - Occurs in 65% of newborns.
  - Classically, bilirubin rises from 1.5 mg/dL in cord serum to 5 to 6 mg/dL on the third day of life, declining to normal levels by the second week of life. Asian infants have a more rapid rise in bilirubin levels, with peak values of 8 to 12 mg/dL on days 4 to 5. Approximately 2% of term Asian newborns attain levels of more than 20 mg/dL in contrast to 1% in white and black infants during the first week of life.
- Breastfeeding jaundice
  - Breastfed infants (9%) are more likely than formula-fed infants (2%) to have a bilirubin level greater than 13 mg/dL (224 μmol/L) and are more likely (2% versus 0.3%) to attain levels greater than 15 mg/dL (258 μmol/L).
  - The pathogenesis appears to be decreased enteral intake and increased enterohepatic circulation.
  - Under normal circumstances, with optimal breastfeeding initiation, frequency, and support, there are no significant differences in the serum bilirubin concentrations of breastfed and artificially fed infants during the first 4 to 5 days of life (Fig. 1-4).
  - A breastfed infant with a high bilirubin level caused by breastfeeding jaundice may go on to have breastmilk jaundice.
- Breastmilk jaundice
  - At 5 to 6 days of age, bilirubin concentrations decline more rapidly in artificially fed infants than in breastfed infants (see Fig. 1-6).
  - In breastfed infants, concentrations either rise, remain stable for several days, or gradually decline.
  - Previously believed to affect less than 1% of all breastfed infants, breastmilk jaundice has now been shown to affect 10% to 30% of infants during the second to sixth week of life. One study demonstrated that one third of 12- to 21-day-old healthy, thriving breastfed infants had bilirubin levels higher than 1.5 mg/dL and another one third had levels higher than 5 mg/dL and were clinically icteric. Two thirds of normal breastfed infants may be expected to have prolonged indirect hyperbilirubinemia up to 12 weeks of age.
  - Maximal bilirubin levels vary from 10 to 30 mg/dL (172 to 516 μmol/L).
  - If nursing is interrupted for 24 to 48 hours, the bilirubin level falls precipitously and will not rebound to the same level when nursing is resumed.

CLINICAL PRESENTATION

History

- Pregnancy information
  - Blood group and type
  - Serology
  - Race and ethnic origin
  - Illness during pregnancy
  - Medications during pregnancy
  - History of anemia or jaundice in family; previous siblings with jaundice
- Birth history
  - Premature rupture of membranes
  - Vacuum extraction or forceps delivery
  - Type of delivery—vaginal versus cesarean section
  - Oxytocin induction
  - Medications or anesthetics for labor
  - Apgar score
  - Age when jaundice first noted
  - Vomiting
  - Frequency, volume, and type of feeding
  - Number of stools and voids noted
  - Drugs given to the infant
- Breastfeeding jaundice
  - The role of inadequate caloric intake makes assessment of breastfeeding adequacy essential.
  - Breastfeeding jaundice may be associated with the following:
    - Delayed initiation of feedings
    - Exposure to pacifiers (substitution of sucking on pacifier for need to feed)
    - Insufficient maternal milk supply (e.g., inadequate glandular tissue, breast-reduction surgery, maternal thyroid disease, Sheehan's syndrome)
    - Excessive infant weight loss (more than 7% from birth)
    - Poor latch and ineffective suckling
    - Associated maternal nipple trauma
    - Fussy, irritable, hungry infant
    - Decreased output, fewer than six to eight voids per day, fewer than three to four stools per day (may report continued meconium stools on days 4 to 5)
    - Inadequate suckling in premature infant or infant with another condition that inhibits ability to suckle (e.g., poor tone in infant with Down syndrome).
    - The relative risk of a bilirubin level in excess of 13 mg/dL (224 μmol/L) is four times higher in an infant of 37 weeks gestation as compared with an infant of 40 weeks gestation.

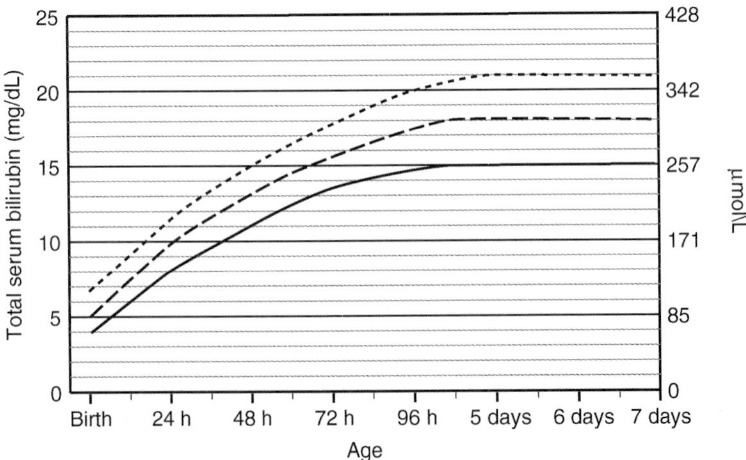

FIGURE 1-4 Phototherapy initiation by serum bilirubin, age, and risk factors.

- Breastmilk jaundice
  - Infants are well and have successfully established breastfeeding.
  - At 5 to 7 days of age, the following should be positive:
    - Weight loss from birth less than 5% to 7%
    - Mother reports that breastmilk supply has increased in quantity (leaking, breast fullness, audible swallowing during feeds)
    - Infant weight gain should be 15 to 30 g/day.
    - Feeding 8 to 12 times per day.
    - No water or formula supplements
    - Adequate time at breast (untimed on-demand feedings, of sufficient length that baby is satisfied)
    - Satisfied baby (feedings often terminated by sleep)
    - Adequate hydration, voids (six to eight per day) and stools (yellow and seedy, minimum of three to four per day)

Physical Examination

- General assessment
  - In breastfeeding jaundice, the infant may be irritable and difficult to console or sleepy and difficult to arouse.
  - In breastmilk jaundice, the infant should be well-appearing, have normal activity, and be alert.
- Infant weight
  - In breastfeeding jaundice, weight loss from birth may be more than 7% or weight gain is inadequate (less than 15 to 30 g/day after 5 days of age).
  - In breastmilk jaundice, weight gain is adequate (15 to 30 g/day).
- Hydration
  - Infants with breastfeeding jaundice may be dehydrated.
    - Dry mucous membranes, sunken fontanelle, poor skin turgor, and tenting
  - Infants with breastmilk jaundice should be well hydrated.
    - Moist mucous membranes, normal fontanelle, and normal skin turgor
- Assessment of jaundice
  - Clinical progression of jaundice from face to trunk to extremities with increasing levels of bilirubin; facial jaundice appreciated at bilirubin levels of approximately 5 mg/dL (86 μmol/L), abdominal at approximately 10 mg/dL, and distal extremities at approximately 15 mg/dL.
- Breastfeeding assessment
  - Direct observation of breastfeeding is essential.
    - Proper positioning and attachment at the breast (see Fig. 1-3).
    - Audible swallowing
    - Adequate time at breast
    - Pre-feeding and post-feeding weight to determine milk intake (1 cc of milk equal to 1 g of weight gain)
- Other pertinent aspects of examination:
  - No hepatosplenomegaly is present.
  - The infant has normal color and lack of ruddiness or paleness (rule out polycythemia or anemia associated with hemolysis).
  - Both breastfeeding and breastmilk jaundice may be worsened by other causes of exaggerated physiologic jaundice in the newborn.
    - Bruising or cephalohematoma
    - Prematurity

ETIOLOGY

- Breastfeeding jaundice
  - Lack of adequate caloric intake (lack of breastmilk)
  - Increased enterohepatic circulation of bilirubin because of lack of stool volume
- Breastmilk jaundice is believed to be caused by an inhibitor of conjugation present in human milk. Suggested substances include the following:
  - β-Glucuronidase
  - Pregnanediol
  - Free fatty acids
  - Steroids

DIAGNOSIS Dx

LABORATORY TESTS

- Bilirubin—direct and indirect
  - Indirect hyperbilirubinemia is present in both breastfeeding and breastmilk jaundice.
- Mother and infant blood type (to rule out ABO disease), direct and indirect Coombs test
- Maternal prenatal antibody screen (to rule out Rh disease and other blood group sensitization)
- Syphilis serology of cord blood
- Urine for reducing substances (to rule out galactosemia)
- Hemoglobin, blood smear, reticulocyte count (to rule out polycythemia and hemolysis, as well as red blood cell membrane abnormalities)
- Consideration of assay (if indicated by history) to rule out enzyme deficiencies such as glucose–6-phosphate dehydrogenase deficiencies (G6PD) and pyruvate kinase
- Consideration of serum electrolytes if infant appears dehydrated
  - Potential hypernatremia, elevated blood urea nitrogen (BUN), and creatinine in breastfeeding jaundice
- Consideration of need to evaluate for sepsis
- Consideration of need to evaluate electrolytes on maternal milk
  - Sodium may be elevated in breastfeeding jaundice if milk volume has decreased because of poor removal (involution of glandular tissue) or in cases of insufficient glandular tissue (normal 7 mEq/L or 16 mg/dL)

TREATMENT

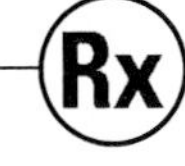

NONPHARMACOLOGIC THERAPY

- Breastfeeding jaundice
  - Ensure adequate breastmilk intake (observation of nursing is essential, see "Physical Examination").
  - If milk transfer is inadequate, infant should be supplemented.
  - Use a supplemental nursing system for best results.
  - Supplement preferably with pumped breastmilk and alternatively with formula.
  - Pump every 2 to 3 hours to maintain or enhance breastmilk supply until infant can be fully breastfed.

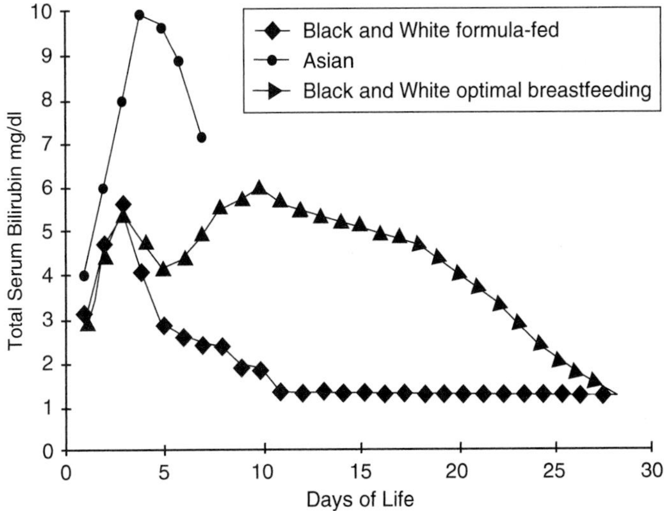

FIGURE 1-5 A synthesized representation of the typical patterns of neonatal jaundice in black and white formula-fed infants (◆), black and white optimally breastfed infants (▸) during the first 28 days of life, and Asian infants, both breastfed and formul-fed (•) during the first 7 days of life. (From Gartner LM: Pediatr Rev 15:423, 1994.)

- Begin frequent breastfeeding (every 2 to 2.5 hours, 8 to 12 times per day).
- Consider consultation with a certified lactation specialist.
- Close follow-up is important to ensure correction of hyperbilirubinemia and successful establishment of lactation.

- Breastmilk jaundice
  - Do *not* discontinue breastfeeding.
  - Management options include:
    - Continue breastfeeding with observation
    - Supplement breastfeeding with formula
    - Temporarily interrupt breastfeeding for 24 to 36 hours, with formula substitution
    - If breastfeeding is interrupted, be sure to have mother pump her breasts to maintain milk supply. Bilirubin will decrease and will not attain previous values with the reinstitution of breastfeeding.

ACUTE GENERAL Rx

- Consider phototherapy (refer to Hyperbilirubinemia in Differential Diagnosis [Section II])
- Management options, depending on the level of bilirubin, include:
  - Continue breastfeeding and administer phototherapy
  - Supplement breastfeeding with formula and administer phototherapy
  - Temporarily interrupt breastfeeding for 24 to 36 hours with formula substitution and phototherapy
  - If breastfeeding interrupted, have mother pump breast to maintain milk supply
- Follow closely to assess bilirubin levels, hydration, adequate feeding, and weight gain.

DISPOSITION

- Breastfeeding jaundice
  - If phototherapy is not indicated, the infant should be followed every 1 to 2 days, depending on level of bilirubin, to assess jaundice, hydration, adequate feeding, and weight gain.
- Breastmilk jaundice
  - After bilirubin has peaked and infant is otherwise well (with bilirubin less than 12 mg/dL), infant can be followed per usual well-child routine.

REFERRAL

- Lactation consultants (certified by the International Board of Lactation Consultants [IBCLC]) can be helpful in managing lactation problems that may lead to breastfeeding jaundice.
- Consider early referral for the following problems:
  - Maternal nipple or breast abnormalities
  - Maternal illness, stress, or fatigue
  - Maternal anxiety about breastfeeding
  - Multiple births
  - Infants with special needs (e.g., premature infants, those with Down syndrome)

PEARLS & CONSIDERATIONS

COMMENTS

- Infant bruising at birth, gestational age less than 37 weeks, maternal illness, maternal operative or difficult delivery, or breast and nipple abnormalities may increase the risk of exaggerated physiologic hyperbilirubinemia.
- In these mother-infant dyads, attention to breastfeeding management, including early consultation with a lactation consultant, may help prevent breastfeeding jaundice.
- Bilirubin at the usual physiologic levels is a potent antioxidant and peroxyl scavenger that may help the newborn avoid oxygen toxicity.
- Clinical assessment of jaundice may be less reliable in infants with darker skin pigmentation.

PREVENTION

- Breastfeeding jaundice
  - Provide patient education in the hospital about proper positioning, attachment, and detachment.
  - Encourage early initiation (within 1 hour of birth) and frequent opportunities to breastfeed (e.g., rooming-in).
  - Avoid nonmedically indicated supplemental feedings. Keep medically indicated supplements small (10 to 15 cc). Supplement with pumped breastmilk if available.
  - Avoid pacifiers.
  - Ensure adequate follow-up. Neonates should be seen for first outpatient visit and weight and jaundice check at 3 to 5 days of life.

PATIENT/FAMILY EDUCATION

- Basic physiology of lactation
  - Ensure proper positioning, attachment, and detachment
  - Breastmilk supply follows demand; encourage on-demand, frequent breastfeedings (8 to 12 per day)
  - Avoid pacifiers and nonmedically indicated supplemental feedings
  - Expect six to eight wet diapers and three to four yellow, seedy stools per day to ensure that infant is getting adequate amounts of milk
  - Refer to community sources of support (e.g., WIC [Women, Infants, and Children] peer counselors; La Leche; hospital warm line, a hospital line answered by nurses who offer advice to mothers with breastfeeding questions). Both WIC and La Leche League offer peer mother to mother support for breast-feeding.

SUGGESTED READINGS

Academy of Breastfeeding Medicine (ABM): Provides evidenced-based clinical protocols for the management of common breastfeeding problems. Available at www.bfmed.org

American Academy of Pediatrics: Provides family information about jaundice. Available at http://www.aap.org/family/jaundicefaq.htm

American Academy of Pediatrics Breastfeeding Initiatives. Available at www.aap.org/advocacy/bf/brpromo.htm

De Carvalho M et al: Fecal bilirubin excretion and serum bilirubin concentrations in breastfed and bottle-fed infants. *J Pediatr* 107:786, 1985.

De Carvalho M et al: Frequency of breastfeeding and serum bilirubin concentration. *Am J Dis Child* 136:737, 1982.

Gartner LM et al: Breastfeeding and the use of human milk. *Pediatrics* 115(2):496, 2005.

La Leche League International (LLLI). Available at www.lalecheleague.org

Lawrence RA, Lawrence R: Breastfeeding: A Guide for the Medical Profession, 6th ed. St. Louis, Mosby, 2005.

Maisels MJ, Newman TB: Kernicterus in otherwise healthy, breastfed term newborns. *Pediatrics* 95:730, 1995.

Management of hyperbilirubinemia in the newborn infant 35 or more weeks of gestation. *Pediatrics* 114(1):297, 2004.

San Diego County Breastfeeding Coalition: Provides an updated list of Internet sites with breastfeeding information. Available at www.breastfeeding.org

AUTHOR: **CYNTHIA R. HOWARD, MD, MPH, FAAP**

BASIC INFORMATION

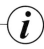

DEFINITION

Bulimia nervosa is a disorder which consists of episodic binges (large amounts of food and drink ingested in a brief period) followed by self-deprecating thoughts and a fear of gaining weight. This results in behaviors intended to rid the body of the effects of the binge, including fasting or exercising (nonpurging subtype) or vomiting, laxative, or diuretic use (purging subtype).

SYNONYM

Bulimia, although the term strictly applies to binge eating/drinking

ICD-9-CM CODES
307.51 Bulimia
783.6 Polyphagia

EPIDEMIOLOGY & DEMOGRAPHICS

- Prevalence of bulimia nervosa in adolescents has increased during the past 50 years.
- Between 2% and 5% of adolescent females and males meet criteria for bulimia nervosa.
- Approximately 90% to 95% of patients affected are female. Males are more likely to have bulimia nervosa than anorexia nervosa.
- Bulimia is more likely to develop in the late teens and early 20s, slightly later than anorexia nervosa.
- It is estimated that bulimia occurs in 1% to 2% of adolescents and young women, although various symptoms and a milder version of the disorder occur in 5% to 10% of young women.
- Most girls and women with eating disorders are white, although in recent years, the disorder has been increasing in women of color.

CLINICAL PRESENTATION

- Medical disorders or syndromes associated with weight fluctuation or vomiting can usually be ruled out by taking a detailed history focused on weight control methods (e.g., binge eating, fasting, vomiting, laxative or diuretic use, exercise).
- Psychiatric disorders should also be ruled out (e.g., depression, schizophrenia).
- A detailed physical examination is required, with special emphasis on cardiovascular stability and electrolyte status.
- The following physical signs should be examined:
  - Salivary gland enlargement
  - Subcutaneous and subconjunctival hemorrhage
  - Chronic throat irritation
  - Fatigue and muscular pain
  - Loss of dental enamel without apparent cause on inner surfaces of teeth
  - Weight variations (as much as 10-kg fluctuation)
  - Mallory-Weiss tears
  - Gastric rupture
  - Esophageal irritation and bleeding
  - Large bowel abnormalities
  - Calluses and scars over the proximal interphalangeal joint (Russell sign) as a result of repetitive stimulation of the gag reflex
  - Serious cardiac or skeletal muscle problems possible in individuals who regularly use syrup of ipecac to induce vomiting
  - Menstrual irregularity or amenorrhea

Affective Signs
- Change in mood (depressive symptoms or depression)
- Severe self-criticism
- Strong need for approval from others
- Self-esteem related closely to body weight
- Interpersonal relationship difficulties (either too close or too distant) and impulsivity
- Suicidal ideation and suicide attempts

ETIOLOGY

- Specific etiologic source is unknown; triggers vary for individual patients.
- Several risk factors may play a role in the onset of bulimia nervosa. These factors can include, but are not limited by, the following:
  - Being female; if male, more likely athletic
  - Familial predisposition, may be partially genetic
  - Individual personality ("borderline") traits
  - Societal thin ideal
  - History of sexual abuse
  - History of parental neglect
  - Overweight

DIAGNOSIS (Dx)

DIFFERENTIAL DIAGNOSIS

- Anorexia nervosa
- Eating disorder
- Kleine-Levin syndrome
- Depressive disorders
- Borderline personality disorder

LABORATORY TESTS

- No single diagnostic lab study exists for bulimia.
- A chemistry panel may be ordered if dehydration or electrolyte imbalances are suspected.
  - Hypochloremic, hypokalemic metabolic alkalosis

IMAGING STUDIES

- Imaging studies are not warranted.

TREATMENT (Rx)

NONPHARMACOLOGIC THERAPY

- Psychotherapy
  - Cognitive-behavioral therapy is the most effective mode of treatment.
  - It incorporates food diaries, self-control techniques, self-edification of affect and situations that provoke bingeing behavior, and positive reinforcement.
  - This treatment also focuses on assisting the patient in changing his or her thoughts about eating, self-perceptions, and weight gain.
  - Group, family, interpersonal, and insight-oriented therapies may also be useful.
- Highly structured meal plans with regularly scheduled times to eat three to five times daily
- Medical monitoring of physical health to validate seriousness of the condition and to enable early treatment of medical complications

ACUTE GENERAL Rx

- Treatment as described.
- Fluid and electrolyte management may be required.
- Most selective serotonin reuptake inhibitors (SSRIs) reduce the symptoms of bulimia nervosa, including in those who are not depressed clinically.
- SSRIs may be especially helpful for patients who have major depression, those who have significant obsessive-compulsive or anxiety symptoms, or patients who do not respond to other treatments.
- Due to concerns regarding SSRI use and an increase in suicidal behavior in adolescents, close monitoring of patients participating in this form of treatment is warranted.

CHRONIC Rx

- Long term psychotherapy is warranted.

REFERRAL

- Referral to a mental health provider is imperative.
- Patients with eating disorders require an interdisciplinary approach to health care.
  - The primary members of the team should include the primary care provider, an eating disorder specialist, a dietitian, and a counselor or therapist.
  - Additional team members could include a social worker and necessary medical consultants (e.g., dentist, gastroenterologist, cardiologist).

PEARLS & CONSIDERATIONS

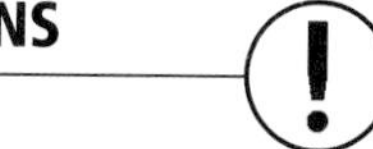

COMMENTS

- Patients with bulimia nervosa often have an overwhelming sense of shame and guilt in addition to low self-esteem. Therefore, they need an unusual amount of nonjudgmental support and encouragement from the professionals working with them.

- Focusing on the immediate medical consequences of their weight-control methods may help patients change their behaviors, especially if engaging in healthy alternative behaviors causes them to feel better (e.g., less tired, less cold, less weak, less fatigued).

PREVENTION

- Participation in programs that promote healthy eating and activity habits, as well as positive self-esteem and weight acceptance

PATIENT/FAMILY EDUCATION

- Biological and emotional consequences of the disorder, as well as benefits from establishing a highly structured daily schedule, should be discussed.
- Patients and their families should be given realistic information regarding treatment, resolution, and relapse.

SUGGESTED READINGS

American Academy of Child and Adolescent Psychiatry. Available at www.aacap.org

Gowers S, Bryant-Waugh R Management of child and adolescent eating disorders: the current evidence base and future directions. *J Child Psychol Psychiatry* 45:1, 2004.

Grange DL et al: Family-based therapy for adolescents with bulimia nervosa. *Am J Psychotherapy* 57:2, 2003.

National Eating Disorders Organization. Available at www.laureate.com

National Institute of Mental Health. Available at www.nimh.nih.gov/home.htm

Steiner H, Lock J Anorexia nervosa and bulimia nervosa in children and adolescents: a review of the past 10 years. *J Am Acad Child Adolesc Psychol* 37:352, 1998.

Wilson GT et al: Cognitive-behavioral therapy for bulimia nervosa: time course and mechanisms of change. *J Consult Clin Psychol* 70:2, 2002.

Wolraich MI et al (eds): *The Classification and Adolescents Mental Diagnoses in Primary Care, Diagnostic and Statistical Manual for Primary Care (DSM-PC), Child and Adolescent Version.* Elk Grove Village, IL, American Academy of Pediatrics, 1996.

Zaider TI et al: Psychiatric disorders associated with the onset and persistence of bulimia nervosa and binge eating disorder during adolescence. *Journal Youth Adolesc* 31:5, 2002.

AUTHORS: **KATHRYN CASTLE, PhD** and **RICHARD KREIPE, MD**

BASIC INFORMATION

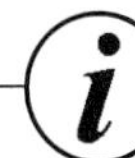

DEFINITION

Illness caused by *Campylobacter jejuni,* which includes diarrhea, extraintestinal manifestations (e.g., pancreatitis, cholecystitis, ileocecitis), and systemic illnesses.

SYNONYMS

Bacterial enterocolitis
Gastroenteritis

ICD-9-CM CODE

008.5 Bacterial enterocolitis

EPIDEMIOLOGY & DEMOGRAPHICS

- *C. jejuni* is the most common cause of bacterial diarrhea worldwide.
- In the United States:
  - The peak ages of illness occur in children younger than 5 years old and in individuals 15 to 29 years old.
  - *Campylobacter* infection occurs throughout the year, with outbreaks common in summer and early fall.
  - Fluoroquinolone resistance among *Campylobacter* species was identified in 1990, and has increased in prevalence since then. The prevalence of ciprofloxacin-resistant *Campylobacter* in 2001 was 19% (75 of 384 isolates).
- Sources of *C. jejuni* are undercooked poultry (e.g., chicken, turkey), unpasteurized milk, unchlorinated water, and young household pets with diarrhea (e.g., puppies, kittens, hamsters, birds).
- Transmission occurs via the fecal-oral route, through contaminated foods or water, or by direct contact with contaminated feces and subsequent person-to-person spread.

CLINICAL PRESENTATION

The clinical presentation of *Campylobacter* enteritis is similar to that caused by other enteric pathogens.

History

- The incubation period is 1 to 7 days.
- Acute onset of enteric illness usually occurs 2 to 4 days after exposure.
- Diarrhea can be watery, have occult blood, or be frank dysentery.
- Crampy abdominal pain, malaise, and fever are also common.
- Associated symptoms include vomiting, myalgia, and headache.
- Bacteremia is uncommon and occurs primarily in immunocompromised children.
- Neonatal infection caused by *C. jejuni,* acquired perinatally, is rare and presents as sepsis or meningitis.

Physical Examination

- Abdominal tenderness in any quadrant
- Blood-streaked stools or hematochezia

ETIOLOGY

- Aerobic, motile, curve-shaped gram-negative rod

DIAGNOSIS

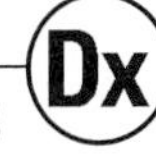

DIFFERENTIAL DIAGNOSIS

- Bacterial diarrhea caused by *Salmonella, Shigella, Vibrio parahaemolyticus,* or *Escherichia coli* 0157:H7, and *Yersinia enterocolitica.*
- The clinical presentation may mimic appendicitis, ulcerative colitis, or Crohn's disease.

LABORATORY TESTS

- In some clinical laboratories, identification of *C. jejuni* is not included when a routine stool culture is requested. A specific request to isolate *C. jejuni* is then needed. Growth of this organism requires selective media and different incubation conditions, compared to other enteric bacteria.
- The white blood cell (WBC) count can be normal or elevated, and the differential shows a left shift.
- A mild elevation in alanine aminotransferase and alkaline phosphatase is present in 25% of patients.
- *Campylobacter* grows more slowly relative to other enteric bacteria. Thus, isolation of this organism from a blood culture may not be reported for 5 to 14 days following inoculation.

TREATMENT

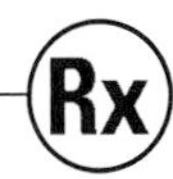

NONPHARMACOLOGIC THERAPY

In general, diarrheal episodes are mild and self-limited. The main treatment is fluid replacement, given by mouth, or intravenously if necessary.

ACUTE GENERAL Rx

- Antibiotic treatment shortens the convalescent period from 2 to 3 weeks to 2 to 3 days and helps prevent relapse of infection.
- A macrolide is the drug of choice. Erythromycin, azithromycin, and clarithromycin are all acceptable choices. The duration of treatment is 5 to 7 days. An alternative oral antibiotic choice is clindamycin.
- Emerging quinolone- and tetracycline-resistant *Campylobacter* are thought to be related to the prophylactic use of these antibiotics in animal feed, and subsequent human consumption of poultry colonized with an antibiotic-resistant *Campylobacter* strain.
- If systemic illness or extraintestinal infection is present, gentamicin, imipenem, or both, should be administered pending antibiotic-susceptibility results.

Control Measures

- Exclusion from child care/preschool:
  - Children should be kept home until 2 days after beginning antibiotic treatment or until they are asymptomatic, whichever is shorter.
  - Because asymptomatic carriage is uncommon, a stool culture is not necessary unless a child is symptomatic.
- Hospitalized persons:
  - For non–toilet-trained children, implement contact precautions for the duration of the illness.
- Occupational precautions:
  - Exclude symptomatic food handlers, hospital employees, and child care personnel until symptoms resolve completely.
  - Infected individuals may return to work as long as they are asymptomatic. Specific guidelines regarding the duration of an asymptomatic period before returning to work have not been outlined. A symptom-free period for 24 hours occurring after the start of antibiotic treatment is a reasonable time frame.
  - Erythromycin eradicates *C. jejuni* from the stool within 2 days. Complete resolution of symptoms might not occur until 3 to 4 days after beginning treatment with this antibiotic.

DISPOSITION

- Children are contagious for 2 to 3 days after antibiotic treatment is administered. Children not treated with antibiotics can shed *C. jejuni* in the stool for up to 5 to 7 weeks.
- Immunocompromised children may have prolonged relapsing diarrheal episodes, extraintestinal infections (e.g., cholecystitis, pancreatitis), and meningitis.
- Complications are reported mainly in adolescents and young adults:
  - *Guillain-Barré syndrome* results in neurologic symptoms that occur 1 to 3 weeks after diarrheal illness.
  - *Reactive arthritis* is reported in 2% to 3% of individuals with *C. jejuni* enteritis. Of these individuals, approximately 50% are positive for HLA-B27.
    - Arthritis is typically migratory and involves large joints.
    - Onset of arthritis ranges from 3 to 40 days after diarrhea occurs. Joint symptoms usually resolve after 1 to 21 days without sequelae.
    - An erythrocyte sedimentation rate (ESR) is elevated, but fever and leukocytosis are not usually present.
    - Synovial fluid is always sterile.
  - Reiter's syndrome is reported in 2% to 3% of individuals with *C. jejuni* enteritis.
  - Erythema nodosum is rare, but a few case reports have been noted in the literature.
  - Septic arthritis is rare and is reported mainly in immunocompromised persons.

REFERRAL

- If complications occur, refer to an appropriate specialist

PEARLS & CONSIDERATIONS

COMMENTS

- Onset of diarrhea less than 16 hours after food exposure is more likely caused by *Staphylococcus aureus, Bacillus cereus,* or *Clostridium perfringens.*
- In developing countries, secretory diarrhea caused by *C. jejuni* is a more common presentation than inflammatory diarrhea.

PREVENTION

- Advise careful hand washing, especially after changing diapers, disposing of animal feces, and prior to food preparation.
- Cook all poultry thoroughly. Internal meat temperature should reach 170°F for breast meat and 180°F for thigh meat.

PATIENT/FAMILY EDUCATION

- See "Control Measures"

SUGGESTED READINGS

Blaser MJ: *Campylobacter jejuni* related species. *In* Mandell GL et al (eds): *Principles and Practices of Infectious Diseases,* 5th ed. Philadelphia, Churchill Livingstone, 2000, pp 2276–2283.

Campylobacter infections: *In* Pickering LK (ed): *Red Book: 2003 Report of the Committee on Infectious Diseases,* 26th ed. Elk Grove Village, IL, American Academy of Pediatrics, 2003, pp 227–229.

Foodborne Diseases Active Surveillance Network. Available at http://www.cdc.gov/foodnet

Gupta A et al: Antimicrobial resistance among *Campylobacter* strains, United States, 1997–2001. *Emerg Infect Dis* 10(6):1102, 2004.

Heresi GP et al: *Campylobacter jejuni. In* Feigin RD (ed): *Textbook of Pediatric Infectious Diseases,* 5th ed. Philadelphia, Elsevier Science, 2004, pp 1612–1617.

Iovine NM et al: Antibiotics in animal feed and spread of resistant *Campylobacter* from poultry to humans. *Emerg Infect Dis* 10(6):1158, 2004.

AUTHOR: **LUCIA H. LEE, MD**

BASIC INFORMATION

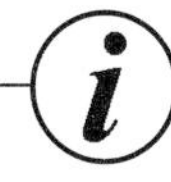

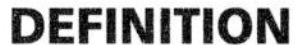

DEFINITION

Diaper dermatitis is a term used to describe an acute inflammatory skin reaction in the perineal area. It results from a reaction to friction, dampness, maceration, urine, or feces. The skin breakdown from these irritants often predisposes to infection with *Candida albicans.*

SYNONYMS

Monilia diaper rash
Napkin thrush
Skin thrush

ICD-9-CM CODES
112.1 Candidiasis of vulva/vagina
112.2 Candidiasis of other urogenital sites
691.0 Diaper dermatitis

EPIDEMIOLOGY & DEMOGRAPHICS

- This is a common infection in the immunocompetent host.
- The peak incidence occurs in the second to fourth months of life.
- It is equally common in males and females.
- The use of antibiotics and skin breakdown are risk factors for *Candida* infection.

CLINICAL PRESENTATION

- Erythematous rash in the diaper area, usually unresponsive to barrier or lubricant ointments.
  - The rash spreads to involve the perineum.
  - Maceration of the anal mucosa and perianal skin may be the first clinical sign.
- In severe cases, may involve the upper thighs, the lower abdomen, and the lower back.
  - May be more impressive in skin folds.
- Perineal skin examination reveals pale pink to bright red papules often with peripheral scale.
- May coalesce to characteristic well-defined weeping, eroded lesions with a scalloped border.
- The rash is evident in the intertriginous folds.
- Additional satellite lesions: vesicopustules or papules with collarette of scale extend beyond the intertriginous fold.
- Darker skinned infants may exhibit hypopigmented lesions.

ETIOLOGY

- *C. albicans* is the predominant fungus responsible for candidal dermatitis.
- Acquisition occurs when the neonate contacts infected vaginal mucosa during passage through the birth canal.
- Gastrointestinal and fecal colonization occur as a result of transmission and lead to skin infection in the perineal area.
- Oropharyngeal candidiasis is often seen before or concurrently with the development of candidal diaper dermatitis (see *Candida,* Oropharyngeal chapter in Diseases and Disorders [Section I]).

DIAGNOSIS

Dx

DIFFERENTIAL DIAGNOSIS

The diagnosis is usually obvious, especially if intertriginous involvement and satellite lesions are evident; however, the differential diagnosis for this rash is extensive and includes the following:

- Irritant dermatitis
- Psoriasis
- Seborrhea dermatitis
- Histiocytosis X (Letterer-Siwe disease)
- Nutritional abnormalities (zinc and biotin deficiencies)
- Secondary staphylococcal dermatitis

LABORATORY TESTS

- Routine use of laboratory tests is generally unnecessary in typical cases of candidal diaper dermatitis.
- KOH (potassium hydroxide) preparation of a lesion may reveal classic budding yeast with hyphae or pseudohypha.
- Stool culture will be positive for *C. albicans* in 90% of patients with candidal diaper dermatitis.

TREATMENT

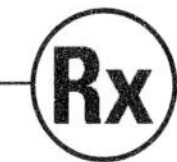

NONPHARMACOLOGIC THERAPY

- Prevention of moist, macerated skin
- Barrier creams (zinc oxide, petrolatum) to prevent skin breakdown
- Frequent diaper changes with superabsorbent disposable diapers
- Air drying of infected perineal skin
- Avoidance of soap or alcohol-containing preparations in the perineal area (these damage barrier properties of skin)

ACUTE GENERAL Rx

- Topical antifungal therapy is indicated for candidal diaper dermatitis.
- All agents are at least 80% to 90% effective.
- Nystatin is the most commonly prescribed topical antifungal for candidal diaper dermatitis. It should be applied to the affected area at least three to four times per day and continued for 1 to 2 days after the rash has cleared.
- Clotrimazole (1% cream) is the second most common topical antifungal for candidal diaper dermatitis. It should be applied twice daily for 5 to 10 days.
- Other topical antifungals include miconazole and amphotericin B.
- Combination products of an antifungal and a potent steroid are generally not recommended due to potential local and systemic steroid reactions.
  - If symptomatic relief is necessary, 1% hydrocortisone cream is an option (two times per day for a few days only).
- The concomitant use of an oral antifungal may eradicate oral and gastrointestinal colonization. Supportive evidence for this approach is limited.

DISPOSITION

- Most infections heal without complication.
- Usually managed as an outpatient.

REFERRAL

- No reason to refer for usual manifestations of this infection.

PEARLS & CONSIDERATIONS

COMMENTS

- Cornstarch powder should be avoided because it is an excellent medium for *Candida.*
- Living *C. albicans* does not penetrate healthy tissues. Candidal diaper dermatitis is caused by irritant yeast products and toxins that filter into inflamed skin after the organisms die and disintegrate. Once the inflammation has reached a peak, the KOH preparation will not reveal the organism.
- *C. albicans* is a normal constituent of the intestinal flora.

PREVENTION

- Maintaining a dry diaper area, monitoring skin breakdown, and avoiding antibiotics are the keys to prevention.

SUGGESTED READINGS

Hoppe JE: Treatment of oropharyngeal candidiasis and candidal diaper dermatitis in neonates and infants: review and reappraisal. *Pediatr Infect Dis J* 16:885, 1997.

Sánchez P: *Candida* infections. *In* Feign RD, Cherry JD (eds): *Textbook of Pediatric Infectious Diseases.* Philadelphia, WB Saunders, 2003, pp 919–924.

Ward D et al: Characterization of diaper dermatitis in the United States. *Arch Pediatr Adolesc Med* 154:943, 2000.

AUTHOR: **DANIEL YAWMAN, MD**

BASIC INFORMATION

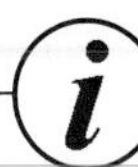

DEFINITION

Oropharyngeal *Candida* is an infection of the oral mucosal surfaces secondary to *Candida albicans,* a fungus.

SYNONYMS

Thrush

ICD-9-CM CODES

112.0 Thrush (oral)
771.7 Neonatal *Candida* infection

EPIDEMIOLOGY & DEMOGRAPHICS

- The overall incidence among immunocompetent infants is high.
- Oral *Candida* infection is 35 times more common in neonates of infected than noninfected mothers.
- Oropharyngeal candidiasis is rare in the first week of life, peak prevalence of disease occurs in the fourth week of life.
- The incubation period is 4 to 13 days.
- Transmission can occur from the skin of the mother who is nursing or from imperfect sterilization of bottles.
- Infection occurs due to immaturity of both the host defenses and normal orointestinal flora.
- Thrush is uncommon after 12 months of age, but antibiotic use predisposes to infection.

CLINICAL PRESENTATION

- Pearly white, irregular patches are seen on the mucosal surfaces, including the buccal mucosa, tongue, gums, and inner lips.
- The soft palate, uvula, and tonsils are less commonly involved.
- Candidal diaper dermatitis.

ETIOLOGY

- *Candida* species, especially *C. albicans,* are responsible for oropharyngeal candidiasis.

DIAGNOSIS

DIFFERENTIAL DIAGNOSIS

- The diagnosis is usually clinically apparent.
- The white plaques are generally not found on erythematous base.
- Occasionally formula or breastmilk is deposited on the tongue.
    - Milk deposition is transient and easily scraped off.
    - *Candida* can affect many areas of the oral mucosa and is not easily removed.
- The white plaques of thrush do not resemble vesicles or ulcers.

LABORATORY TESTS

- Routine fungal cultures are not indicated.
- Persistent thrush that is unresponsive to appropriately administered therapy should prompt consideration of immunosuppression (e.g., human immunodeficiency virus [HIV] infection, congenital T-cell abnormalities, chemotherapy [including prednisone, cancer treatment]).

TREATMENT

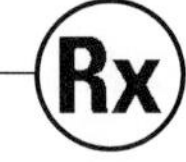

NONPHARMACOLOGIC THERAPY

- Sterilization of all nipples and pacifiers is required to eliminate colonization with *C. albicans.*
- Careful handwashing is necessary to decrease transmission between mother and infant as well as to decrease nosocomial transmission.
- Enact simultaneous treatment of maternal breast and infant's mouth to avoid recontamination.

ACUTE GENERAL Rx

- Treatment modalities include oral antifungal agents with limited or no absorption from the gastrointestinal tract (i.e., nystatin, gentian violet, amphotericin B, clotrimazole, and miconazole) and agents that are readily absorbed (i.e., fluconazole, ketoconazole, and itraconazole).
- Treatment in infants without an underlying medical condition is with nonabsorbed drugs.
    - Nystatin is a polyene antifungal agent with broad antifungal activity. It is fungicidal at very high doses, but fungistatic at typical doses.
        - Generally, safe prolonged oral use may lead to nausea and vomiting. The suspension has high osmolality, which limiting use in premature neonates.
        - Use oral suspension four times/day for one week.
        - Failure of cure may be due to inability of infant to keep the agent in the mouth, consider direct application to affected areas with a cotton swab.
        - Alternatively, a vaginal suppository may be held in the mouth until dissolved every 4 hours.
        - Reported clinical cure rates from 29% to 85%.
    - Gentian violet (methylrosaniline) has moderate efficacy.
        - Used twice daily it is to be well tolerated, but prolonged use results in mucosal irritation and ulceration.
        - It stains clothing and tissues.
        - It does not eliminate *C. albicans* from the bowel.
    - Amphotericin B is an additional polyene with broad-spectrum antifungal activity.
        - More active than nystatin against *C. albicans* in vitro
        - Suspension (100 mg = 1 mL) used orally four times daily
        - Has a very high osmolality
        - Cure rates as good as nystatin
    - Clotrimazole is a first-generation imidazole derivative.
        - It is given as a 10-mg dissolvable troche five or six times daily.
        - The troche is held in the mouth until completely dissolved.
        - Clinical studies on this form of administration are lacking.
    - Miconazole is a first-generation imidazole derivative.
        - More active than nystatin in vitro
        - Gel form of this medication not currently available in the United States
    - Fluconazole is an oral fungistatic agent.
        - Superior to nystatin in immunocompromised patients.
        - 6 mg/kg single dose followed by 3 mg/kg daily for 13 days.
        - A small study showed that 3 mg/kg daily for 7 days was superior to nystatin in immunocompetent infants.
        - It is costly; and there is potential for the emergence of resistant non-*albicans Candida.*

DISPOSITION

This condition can be managed on an outpatient basis in an immunocompetent host.

PEARLS & CONSIDERATIONS

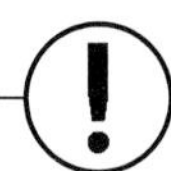

COMMENTS

- Use topical antifungal therapy on the breasts of mothers who are nursing an infant with oropharyngeal candidiasis.
- For recalcitrant thrush, consider the possibility of an immune deficiency.

PREVENTION

- Avoid unnecessary antibiotic exposure and maintain proper hygiene; however this condition commonly occurs despite these precautions.

SUGGESTED READINGS

Goins R et al: Comparison of fluconazole and nystatin oral suspensions for treatment of oral candidiasis in infants. *Pediatr Infect Dis J* 21:1165, 2002.

Rowen J: Mucocutaneous candidiasis. *Semin Perinatol* 27:406, 2003.

Sánchez P: *Candida* infections. *In* Feign RD, Cherry JD (eds): *Textbook of Pediatric Infectious Diseases.* Philadelphia, WB Saunders, 2003, pp 919–924.

AUTHOR: **DANIEL YAWMAN, MD**

BASIC INFORMATION

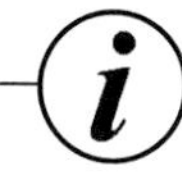

DEFINITION

Dilated cardiomyopathy is an abnormality of cardiac muscle characterized by increased ventricular, and sometimes atrial, chamber size with decreased pumping ability.

SYNONYMS

Cardiomyopathy
Dilated cardiomyopathy
Idiopathic dilated cardiomyopathy
Left ventricular noncompaction (LVNC)

ICD-9-CM CODE
425.4 Idiopathic cardiomyopathy

EPIDEMIOLOGY & DEMOGRAPHICS

- The annual incidence of cardiomyopathy in infants and children in the United States is 1.13/100,000.
  - 51% of the total incidence represents dilated cardiomyopathy
  - 42% of the total incidence represents hypertrophic cardiomyopathy
  - The remaining 7% is comprised of restrictive and mixed forms of cardiomyopathy
- It is now known that this disease can and does present in children less than 1 year of age. There should be a high index of suspicion for an infant who presents with congestive heart failure (CHF) or cardiomegaly.
  - Incidence is lower among white children
  - Predisposition for boys
  - Incidence varies by geographic regions
- Overall incidence of these diseases is likely underestimated because of the number of asymptomatic cases.
- Disease may be autosomal dominant, autosomal recessive, X-linked, mitochondrial, or sporadic.

CLINICAL PRESENTATION

- Common signs and symptoms are those of CHF:
  - Tachypnea
  - Dyspnea
  - Recurrent respiratory infections or wheezing
  - Diaphoresis with eating or with very little exertion
  - Poor weight gain
  - Recurrent emesis and abdominal pain (from organomegaly), pallor or cyanosis
  - Rarely, presentation is arrhythmia or sudden death

ETIOLOGY

- Labeled "idiopathic" because, for many years, the causes of these diseases of the cardiac myocyte were unknown.
- Cardiomyopathy has now been divided into specifically known abnormalities of the cardiomyocyte, which are genetically heterogeneous, causing force transmission or energy abnormalities (weakening of the functional myocytes) because of abnormalities of:
  - Actin
  - Desmin
  - Cardiac troponin T
  - *B*-Myosin heavy chain
  - *a*-Tropomyosin
  - Mitochondria
- There are genetic predispositions for these cytoskeletal protein/energy abnormalities, which certain toxins (such as Adriamycin) and infectious agents (such as coxsackie B19 or adenovirus) may unmask.

DIAGNOSIS

DIFFERENTIAL DIAGNOSIS

- Myocarditis
- Chronic respiratory illnesses such as asthma
- Chronic gastrointestinal abnormalities
- Pericarditis
- Structural heart disease such as anomalous left coronary artery (ALCA)
- Previously undiagnosed Kawasaki or coronary artery disease

WORKUP

- A high index of suspicion is necessary.
- It is important to distinguish between a chronic process and myocarditis, if at all possible, as this affects the treatment plan and prognosis.
- A thorough history of present illness focusing on any recent viral prodromes, past medical history and review of systems, are necessary. Long-term developmental, neuro/musculoskeletal abnormalities should be sought.
- Family history is mandatory.

LABORATORY TESTS

- 12-lead electrocardiogram (ECG) may reveal high- or low-grade rhythm abnormalities, atrial/ventricular enlargement, nonspecific ST T-wave changes, prolongation of PR and corrected QT intervals.
- Brain and atrial natriuretic peptides are elevated in CHF, but also may be elevated in certain pulmonary and renal diseases. They may be used to track patient response to therapy.
- In the future, the more sensitive biomarkers endothelin (ET)-1 and Big ET-1 may be followed.
- Troponin I and C may help distinguish between acute myocarditis (where they should be elevated) and a more chronic dilated cardiomyopathy (where they should not be elevated).
- Nonspecific markers such as the sedimentation rate and C reactive proteins may help distinguish between myocarditis and dilated cardiomyopathy.
- Baseline complete blood count (CBC) with differential (cyclic neutropenia with Barth's syndrome) and metabolic, liver, and coagulation profiles will be important in medically managing the patient and in determining chronicity of disease.
- Ammonia, carnitine levels, serum amino acids, and urine organic acids may help distinguish metabolic/mitochondrial etiologies of disease.
- Thyroid function studies
- Human immunodeficiency virus (HIV) studies
- Vitamin B and selenium studies
- Skin biopsy if mitochondrial or storage (Pompe's) disease is suspected.
- 24-hour Holter monitor: to assess for high-grade arrhythmia
- Occasionally an exercise stress test is helpful, particularly if there is difficulty in distinguishing between cardiac and pulmonary disease components.

IMAGING STUDIES

- Chest radiograph will reveal cardiomegaly and pulmonary edema.
- Two-dimensional (2D) echocardiography is the "gold standard."
  - In the hands of an experienced echocardiographer, evaluation for structural anomalies and measurements of ventricular dimensions and systolic and diastolic function can be made.
  - Assessment of myocardial and endocardial characteristics such as deep left ventricular trabeculations seen in LVNC, or endocardial fibroelastosis may give clues to the etiology of the disease.
- Cardiac magnetic resonance imaging (MRI): may yield dimensions, systolic and diastolic function, particularly in patients who are difficult to image with conventional echocardiography (e.g., obese patients, those with Duchenne's muscular dystrophy). It can also distinguish coronary anomalies such ALCA.
- Cardiac catheterization may be necessary for hemodynamic data in preparation for cardiac transplant.
  - Coronary arteries may be imaged for evidence of ALCA or history of Kawasaki disease.
  - If patient is hemodynamically stable, endomyocardial biopsies may be taken and sent for hematoxylin and eosin staining to evaluate for lymphocytic infiltration, identification of viral infiltration through polymerase chain reaction (PCR), and electron microscopy for mitochondrial abnormalities.

TREATMENT

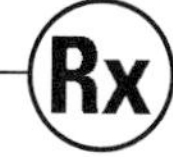

NONPHARMACOLOGIC THERAPY

- Families must be educated regarding the implications of the abnormality.
- Emotional support is a must, either through social work or parent support groups.

- The Family Leave Act should be addressed, as well as supportive communication to patient/parent employers.
- As soon as possible, arrangements should be made for homebound schooling, if the child is of appropriate age.
- Occupational and physical therapy should be implemented as soon as the patient is stable enough to tolerate therapy, in order to avoid further loss of developmental milestones.
- Please refer to treatment section in Congestive Heart Failure chapter in Diseases and Disorders (Section I).
- The ABCs (stable airway, breathing, and circulation) must be addressed first.
- Venous access is crucial.
- Acute evaluation and treatment of this subgroup of patients should occur at a tertiary care center. Appropriate, safe pediatric transportation should be arranged.
- Any acid-base or electrolyte abnormalities should be corrected if possible, but should not delay transport.
- The patient may require support of a left ventricular assist device (LVAD), or extracorporeal membrane oxygenation (ECMO), which has been proven to afford ventricular remodeling, as well as being a bridge for transplantation.
- A presentation of aborted sudden death necessitates consideration of an implantable defibrillator.
- Consideration of permanent pacing if necessary.
- Cardiac transplantation is a life-saving measure.

ACUTE GENERAL Rx

- Conditions of anemia may be addressed with transfusion.
    - Administration of large fluid boluses is to be avoided or compensated by judicious use of diuretic therapy.
- Any high-grade arrhythmias will need to be addressed urgently with a pediatric cardiologist.
    - These rhythm disturbances may need to be addressed prior to patient transport.
    - Management strategies may include adenosine (only if the patient is hemodynamically stable), electrocardioversion, amiodarone, lidocaine, esmolol, sotalol, flecainide, and temporary pacemakers.
- Consideration of myocarditis as an etiology of disease necessitates the administration of intravenous gamma globulin.
- Treat any evidence of intracardiac thrombi with appropriate anticoagulation.
- Refer to "Treatment" section in Congestive Heart Failure chapter in Diseases and Disorders (Section I).

CHRONIC Rx

- Future treatment modalities will be aimed at rectification of the etiology of the disease. For example, if the disease is proven to be due to an abnormality of dystrophin, appropriate genetic treatment will be implemented.
- In cases where metabolic or mitochondrial abnormalities are thought to play a role in the cardiomyopathies, carnitine or a form of "vitamin cocktail" (B vitamins and carnitine) may be helpful.
- Patients require subacute bacterial endocarditis prophylaxis.
- Patients with LVNC or those with known thrombi should be anticoagulated at least with low-dose aspirin therapy.
- Consider administration of Synagis for RSV prophylaxis in those children less than 2 years.
- These patients should also receive annual influenza vaccinations.

DISPOSITION

- There is a 50% five-year survival if left untreated.
- Overall prognosis is dependent upon etiology of disease. This is still frequently unknown.
- Transplantation has improved survival overall.

REFERRAL

- Refer patients and families to large, experienced centers with pediatric cardiology subspecialists who have access to geneticists and cardiovascular surgeons.

PEARLS & CONSIDERATIONS

COMMENTS

- Be aware and suspicious of any family history of sudden death, heart transplantation, known heart enlargement, and CHF.
- Be suspicious of the child who has recurrent wheezing, particularly if there is failure to thrive.

PATIENT/FAMILY EDUCATION

- There are many local family support groups for cardiomyopathy and transplant, most of which are run through large children's hospitals.

SUGGESTED READINGS

Denfield SW et al: Cardiomyopathies. *In* Garson A et al (eds): *The Science and Practice of Pediatric Cardiology.* Baltimore, Williams and Wilkins, 1998, pp 1851–1884.

Lipshultz SE et al: The incidence of pediatric cardiomyopathy in two regions of the United States. *N Engl J Med* 348:1647, 2003.

Towbin JA et al: The failing heart. *Nature* 415:227, 2002.

AUTHOR: **MICHELLE A. GRENIER, MD**

BASIC INFORMATION

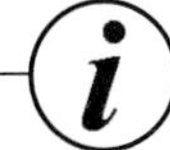

DEFINITION

Hypertrophic cardiomyopathy is excessive cardiomyocyte hypertrophy without appropriate stimulus, resulting in a thick heart with exaggerated pump function (hypercontractile systolic function) and poor relaxation (diastolic dysfunction).

SYNONYMS

Asymmetric septal hypertrophy (ASH)
Hypertrophic obstructive cardiomyopathy (HOCM/HCM)
Idiopathic hypertrophic subaortic stenosis (IHSS)
Left ventricular noncompaction (LVNC)

ICD-9-CM CODES

425.1 Obstructive hypertrophic cardiomyopathy
425.4 Nonobstructive hypertrophic cardiomyopathy

EPIDEMIOLOGY & DEMOGRAPHICS

- Overall annual incidence is reported to be 1.13 cases per 100,000 children in the United States.
- 42% of those diagnosed with cardiomyopathy have the hypertrophic form.
- There appears to be a triphasic presentation of HOCM by age: infants to 1 year, ages to 25 years, beyond 40 years. **Note:** Young onset may represent a separate disease entity.
- The incidence is lower among white children and higher among boys.
- The incidence also varies by region of the United States.

Although considered relatively uncommon, the true incidence is probably underestimated due to the number of asymptomatic cases which go unrecognized.

CLINICAL PRESENTATION

- This is a complex heart disease with unique pathophysiology characterized by many morphologic, functional, and clinical features.
- HPI common symptoms include: near syncope or syncope ("seizure disorder"), chest pain, shortness of breath, dyspnea on exertion, easy fatigability, excessive sweating/flushing for level of exertion, palpitations, and sudden death.
- Previous medical history: there may be evidence of previous neuromuscular abnormalities, abnormal developmental milestones, and failure to thrive.
- Family history: any family history of sudden death ("early heart attacks"), enlarged hearts, rhythm abnormalities, orthotopic heart transplant, or syndromes, is suspect.
- Physical examination: beware any evidence of dysmorphia (Noonan's facies), neuromuscular abnormality (Friedreich's ataxia/Pompe's disease/mitochondrial diseases), skin abnormalities (lentigines in LEOPARD syndrome), or organomegaly (storage syndromes).
- The cardiac exam may be remarkable for:
  - Displaced or hyperdynamic point of maximal impulse
  - Brisk carotid upstroke
  - Murmurs may be systolic ejection or regurgitant, and may be increased by Valsalva maneuver.
- Left ventricular noncompaction (LVNC), presentation in this particular disease is extremely variable, and may be quite confusing.

ETIOLOGY

- In familial hypertrophic cardiomyopathy (FHC), there are abnormalities of the genes that encode proteins that are part of the sarcomere. The sarcomere is a complex structure with an exact stoichiometry and several sites of protein-protein interactions.
  - Three myofilament proteins are affected:
    - B myosin heavy chain (ventricular myosin essential and regulatory light chains)
    - Four different myofilament proteins (cardiac actin, cardiac troponin T and I and α-tropomyosin)
    - One myosin binding protein (protein C and titin)
  - Each of these proteins is encoded by multigene families that show tissue-specific, developmental, and physiologically regulated patterns of expression.
- In HOCM/Wolf-Parkinson-White (WPW) syndrome there are mutations in the mitochondrial DNA which cause sarcomeric dysfunction.
- In X-linked HOCM, there are dystrophin abnormalities. This is commonly seen in the muscular dystrophies. (Dystrophin maintains structural integrity.)

DIAGNOSIS

DIFFERENTIAL DIAGNOSIS

- Dilated cardiomyopathy
- Structural heart disease/valvular heart disease
- Athletic heart
- Obesity
- Systemic hypertension
- Steroid or growth-hormone–induced left ventricular hypertrophy
- Infant of a diabetic mother

Note: Possibly the most important entity to exclude is left ventricular hypertrophy induced by systemic hypertension (blood pressure [BP] taken on physical exam) or elite athleticism (HPI and social history).

- A thorough assessment to exclude these two entities requires rigorous treatment of systemic hypertension and restriction from athletic participation for a period of 3 months, with reassessment by two-dimensional (2D) echocardiogram upon completion of the rest period/control of BP.
- The aforementioned is difficult to achieve in competitive athletes, but is absolutely mandatory in order to exclude a potentially lethal disease such as HOCM.

WORKUP

A complete and accurate family history is crucial. Any family history of sudden death requires thorough investigation.

LABORATORY TESTS

- Complete blood count (CBC) with differential may reveal chronicity of disease, or in such mitochondrial abnormalities as Barth's syndrome, may reveal cyclic neutropenia.
- Blood chemistry/ammonia may reveal metabolic, renal, or storage abnormalities.
- Urine amino acids
- Serum organic acids
- Thyroid studies
- Carnitine
- Biomarkers such as troponins, brain natriuretic peptides may be useful to follow at baseline, and then to track changes over time.
- Electrocardiogram (ECG): may be particularly useful in evaluating for such entities as LVNC, Pompe's disease, HOCM/WPW syndrome, interventricular conduction delay, assessment of ischemic changes, degree of ventricular hypertrophy, evaluation associated corrected long QT interval, or assessment for atrioventricular arrhythmias which may be characteristic of HOCM.
- 24-hour Holter monitor to assess for occult dysrhythmia.
- Exercise stress test: may show characteristics of HOCM, including outflow tract obstruction, ischemic changes, ectopy, and BP "blunting" at peak activity.

IMAGING STUDIES

- Chest radiograph is nonspecific and may not exclude HOCM if there is no evidence of cardiomegaly.
- The 2D echocardiogram remains the gold standard. An experienced sonographer can assess for structural heart disease, chamber dimensions in 2D and m-mode, and assessment of systolic and diastolic function. It is important to assess the ventricular geometry, degree of outflow tract obstruction, and systolic anterior motion of the mitral valve.
- Cardiac magnetic resonance imaging (MRI) allows for accurate estimation of chamber size, cardiac mass, and systolic and diastolic function. It may also allow accurate assessment of coronary arteries.

TREATMENT

NONPHARMACOLOGIC THERAPY

- Restriction from competitive athletics and isometric exercise, with degree of restriction correlated with disease severity, may prevent sudden death.

- The risk of sudden death must be ascertained from symptoms, family history, and diagnostic testing (Holter and exercise stress test) in order to determine necessity of implantable defibrillator (AICD).
- Pacemakers have been used to treat intractable rhythm disturbance. In some patients, pacemakers have been shown to alleviate severe ventricular outflow tract obstruction by regulating the diastolic time interval.
- Surgical intervention in the form of myectomy and mitral valve annuloplasty has been successful palliation, but does not alleviate the underlying condition.
- Alcohol ablation has been used successfully in adults, but is not generally accepted therapy in children.
- Transplantation has been used as a last resort, with good outcome. Frequently, the end stages of this disease involve systolic as well as diastolic dysfunction (a "burned-out cardiomyopathy"), resulting in congestive heart failure (CHF).

ACUTE GENERAL Rx

- Pharmacologic treatment modalities focus on improvement of the diastolic function, with arrest of further ventricular growth, if possible.
- β-Blockade is the therapy of choice, due to its reported success in decreasing the incidence of sudden death, and the known properties of affecting ventricular remodeling.
  - Commonly used β-blockers are propranolol, atenolol, nadolol.
- In cases of intolerance to or maximization of β-blockade therapy, calcium channel blockers may be used or added.
- If a patient presents with CHF, see "Treatment" section, in chapter on Congestive Heart Failure in Diseases and Disorders (Section I).
- Avoid intravascular space depletion and severe inotropy/tachycardia.

CHRONIC Rx

- Chronic treatment modalities are similar to what is recommended in the "Acute General Rx" section. Patients must be made aware that this is a chronic condition, and these therapies are "lifetime" and "lifesaving."
- Subacute bacterial endocarditis prophylaxis is recommended.
- Particularly in cases of LVNC, where there are deep trabeculations, anticoagulation in the form of low-dose aspirin therapy is recommended.
- Annual influenza vaccination is recommended.

DISPOSITION

- In cases of aborted sudden death or syncope with exertion, especially if there is a strong family history of sudden death, the prognosis is generally not good.
- Factors such as degree of hypertrophy, ventricular outflow tract obstruction, and systolic anterior motion of the mitral valve, have not been particularly predictable of sudden death in children.

REFERRAL

Patients must be actively involved with the primary care provider as well as the pediatric cardiologist and any subspecialist necessary in managing associated syndromes.

PEARLS & CONSIDERATIONS

COMMENTS

- Avoidance of dehydration and extreme weather conditions; extreme exertion should be avoided.
- Beware any strong family history of sudden death or "early heart attacks," enlarged hearts, or family syndromes.
- It is crucial to make an accurate diagnosis.
- In very athletic children, or in those who are hypertensive, these stimulants for ventricular hypertrophy must be eliminated.
- The diagnostic tools involve appropriate treatment of systemic hypertension and restriction from rigorous training with reassessment after a 3-month period of rest. This is not negotiable.

PREVENTION

Patients with this type of cardiomyopathy should try to avoid excessive weight gain, which may be a further stimulant of ventricular hypertrophy.

PATIENT/FAMILY EDUCATION

In and around tertiary care centers, there are resources for families with hypertrophic cardiomyopathy as well as other forms of pediatric cardiac disease.

SUGGESTED READINGS

Denfield SW et al: Cardiomyopathies. *In* Garson A et al (eds): *Science and Practice of Pediatric Cardiology.* Baltimore, Williams and Wilkins, 1998, pp 1851–1884.

Lipshultz SE et al: The incidence of pediatric cardiomyopathy in two regions of the United States. *N Engl J Med* 348:1647, 2003.

Towbin JA et al: The failing heart. *Nature* 414:227, 2002.

AUTHOR: **MICHELLE A. GRENIER, MD**

BASIC INFORMATION

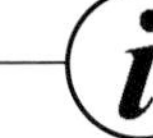

DEFINITION

A cataract is an opacity of the lens, which may be present at birth or evolve over time.

ICD-9-CM CODE
743.30 Cataract—congenital, unspecified

EPIDEMIOLOGY & DEMOGRAPHICS

- One third of bilateral cateracts are inherited, usually in an autosomal dominant fashion but can be autosomal recessive or X-linked.
- One third are associated with other disorders, either chromosomal abnormalities or metabolic disorders.
- One third have an unknown cause.

CLINICAL PRESENTATION

History

- Visual function
  - Does infant turn to face?
  - Does infant track?
  - Do eyes move together?
  - Do eyes align?
  - Are eyes symmetric?
- Family history of cataracts in childhood
- Medications or illegal substances used during pregnancy
- Infections during pregnancy

Physical Examination

- Assess visual function
  - Test tracking and fixation if nonverbal
  - If older and verbal, use acuity testing
  - *Test each eye separately,* and be diligent to observe for peeking
- Observe alignment. If any abnormality is present, suspect visual impairment.
- A thorough newborn examination may lead to a constellation of physical findings that suggest a chromosomal abnormality or metabolic disorder.
- Development of cataracts during childhood may be familial, and examination of parents and siblings may be helpful.
  - Look for a familial pattern or physical findings such as aniridia.
  - Childhood cataracts may be associated with use of medications (e.g., corticosteroids) or systemic diseases of childhood (e.g., juvenile rheumatoid arthritis).

ETIOLOGY

- In an otherwise healthy child, a cause may be elusive.
- Common causes include the following:
  - Intrauterine infection
    - TORCH (toxoplasmosis, rubella, cytomegalovirus, or herpes)
    - Varicella zoster virus
  - Chromosomal abnormalities
    - Hereditary: autosomal dominant is most common
    - Down syndrome, trisomy 13, trisomy 15, Lowe syndrome, Marfan's syndrome
  - Metabolic syndromes
    - Galactosemia, Fabry's disease, homocystinuria

DIAGNOSIS

WORKUP

- The diagnosis is usually made on physical examination, often seen during well-child examinations. Shining a bright direct ophthalmoscope into both eyes:
  - Look for bright symmetric red reflex
  - Any shadow or dark spot in the red reflex suggests a cataract or other lens abnormality
- Look for associated physical findings of various genetic syndromes and metabolic disorders

TREATMENT

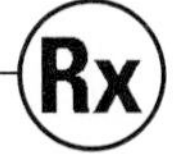

NONPHARMACOLOGIC THERAPY

- Treatment for visually significant cataracts is surgical removal of the lens and sometimes implantation of an intraocular lens.
- Surgical intervention should be undertaken within the first 6 to 8 weeks of life for congenital cataracts.
- Visual rehabilitation may include use of aphakic spectacles or contact lenses.
- Diligent evaluation of visual acuity should be continued.
- Management of amblyopia should be initiated, if necessary.

DISPOSITION

- Infants and children who are believed to have decreased vision or a cataract should be immediately referred to an ophthalmologist for a complete evaluation.
- Children with a history of cataracts should have follow-up by an ophthalmologist for amblyopia and the development of other ocular disorders, such as glaucoma.

REFERRAL

- Opthalmologist

PEARLS & CONSIDERATIONS

COMMENTS

Cataracts can occasionally be caused by trauma, and in children with other signs of trauma, child abuse should be suspected.

PATIENT/FAMILY EDUCATION

- Family members must be informed that visual prognosis is guarded, even if the cataract is successfully removed. They must be involved with careful follow-up and management of visual development.
- Development of amblyopia is a real concern until at least 8 or 9 years of age.
- Other ocular disorders, such as glaucoma, occur with greater frequency in children with cataracts.

Support Groups

- National Association of Parents of the Visually Impaired, 800-562-6265
- National Association for the Visually Handicapped, 22 West 21 St., New York, NY 10010, 212-889-3141

SUGGESTED READINGS

Childhood cataracts and other pediatric lens disorders. *In Pediatric Ophthalmology and Strabismus.* Basic and Clinical Science Course. American Academy of Ophthalmology, San Francisco, 1998-1999.

Lambert S: Lens. *In* Taylor D (ed): *Pediatric Ophthalmology,* 2nd ed. Boston, Blackwell Science, 1997.

Robb RM: Congenital childhood cataracts. *In* Albert DM, Jakobiec FA (eds): *Principles and Practice of Ophthalmology.* Philadelphia, WB Saunders, 1994.

AUTHOR: **ANNA F. FAKADEJ, MD, FAAO, FACS**

BASIC INFORMATION

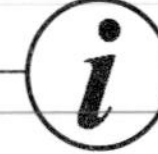

DEFINITION

Cat-scratch disease (CSD) is a subacute to chronic regional lymphadenitis syndrome that occurs after cutaneous, ocular, or mucous membrane inoculation in a person who has contact with a cat.

SYNONYM

Cat-scratch fever

ICD-9-CM CODE

078.3 Cat-scratch disease

EPIDEMIOLOGY & DEMOGRAPHICS

- There are 22,000 to 24,000 cases per year of CSD in the United States (9.3 per 100,000 population).
- Approximately 2000 patients are hospitalized per year in the United States (0.77 to 0.86 per 100,000 hospital discharges).
- Distribution is worldwide, but it is most prevalent in warm and humid climates.
- The incidence is more common in fall and winter (60% of cases identified from September to January).
- 50% of patients are younger than 15 years of age.
- A zoonotic disease of cats, especially kittens. Asymptomatic cats may be persistently bacteremic with the causative organism for long periods of time.
- Fleas maintain the zoonotic infection among cats.

CLINICAL PRESENTATION

- A papule or pustule at the site of the scratch precedes the appearance of regional lymphadenopathy by 1 to 6 weeks in 60% to 93% of patients.
- Gradual enlargement of a single, tender lymph node is observed in 80% of patients (20% have multiple node enlargements clinically, but up to 90% have multiple enlarged nodes in one site by ultrasonography).
- Most nodes (80%) are 1 to 5 cm in size and appear on the axilla, head, neck, or upper extremity.
- A papule or pustule at a distal site is drained by the enlarged node.
- Fever is usually absent or low-grade (10% with temperature higher than 39°C).
- From 10% to 30% of nodes spontaneously suppurate, but most resolve over 2 to 6 months.
- Atypical presentations include encephalopathy with seizures, hepatosplenic granulomas, multiple bone lesions, Parinaud's oculoglandular syndrome (conjunctival granuloma with ipsilateral preauricular adenopathy), neuroretinitis, endocarditis, or a prolonged febrile illness, seen in 10% to 25% of infections.
- Patients may have constitutional symptoms, including fatigue (30%), headache (14%), anorexia or weight loss (15%), or sore throat (9%) with regional lymphadenitis.
- Immunocompromised children may develop more severe manifestations of infection and should always receive antimicrobial treatment.

ETIOLOGY

- *Bartonella henselae,* a fastidious, pleomorphic, gram-negative bacillus

DIAGNOSIS (Dx)

DIFFERENTIAL DIAGNOSIS

- Bacterial adenitis
- Infectious mononucleosis
- Toxoplasmosis
- *Mycobacteria* infection
- Cytomegalovirus infection
- Lymphoma/malignancy
- Histoplasmosis

WORKUP

Initially, a clinical diagnosis is based on appropriate symptoms and a history of exposure to a cat or kitten and confirmed by serology.

LABORATORY TESTS

- Serologic diagnosis is the test of choice (indirect immunofluorescence assay or enzyme immunoassay) with a positive titer of more than 1:64 for immunoglobulin G (IgG) or more than 1:20 for immunoglobulin M (IgM).
- Lymph node biopsy reveals scattered granulomas with necrosis and abscess formation.
- Culture and Gram stain of *B. henselae* are technically very difficult.
- Polymerase chain reaction test is available at reference laboratories.

IMAGING STUDIES

- Ultrasonography demonstrates enlarged hypoechoic lymph nodes with increased vascularity on Doppler images.
- May also see hypoechoic nodules in the liver or spleen by ultrasonography in approximately 30% of patients with CSD without abdominal discomfort.

TREATMENT (Rx)

NONPHARMACOLOGIC THERAPY

- Local care, including the application of moist heat to an enlarged node or nodes

ACUTE GENERAL Rx

- Azithromycin 10 mg/kg on day 1 then 5 mg/kg on days 2 through 5 decreases lymph node size faster than placebo.

CHRONIC Rx

- A few patients require needle aspiration for drainage and relief of symptoms or complete removal of the involved node or nodes.

DISPOSITION

- Gradual and spontaneous resolution of lymphadenopathy over 2 to 6 months is the rule.

REFERRAL

- Children can be cared for by their primary care pediatrician or a pediatric infectious diseases expert.

PEARLS & CONSIDERATIONS (!)

COMMENTS

- Examine the web spaces between the fingers for an inoculation papule in a patient with lymphadenopathy of the upper extremity.
- Always consider CSD in the differential diagnosis of seizures, encephalopathy, or combative behavior and inquire about a history of cat contact while examining the patient closely for an inoculation papule or lymphadenopathy.
- Remember to think of atypical CSD in a patient with fever of unknown origin.

PREVENTION

- Avoidance of scratches or bites from cats and kittens will prevent infection.

PATIENT/FAMILY EDUCATION

- Approximately 28% of cats have evidence of past or present infection with *B. henselae.*
- Cat infection with *B. henselae* is correlated with fleas.
- There is no known person-to-person transmission of CSD.

SUGGESTED READINGS

Bass JW et al: The expanding spectrum of *Bartonella* infections: II, cat-scratch disease. *Pediatr Infect Dis J* 16:163, 1997.

Bass JW et al: Prospective randomized double blind placebo-controlled evaluation of azithromycin for treatment of cat-scratch disease. *Pediatr Infect Dis J* 17:447, 1998.

Carithers HA: Cat-scratch disease: an overview based on a study of 1,200 patients. *Am J Dis Child* 139:1124, 1985.

Garcia CJ et al: Regional lymphadenopathy in cat-scratch disease: ultrasonographic findings. *Pediatr Radiol* 30:640, 2000.

Jackson LA et al: Cat scratch disease in the United States: an analysis of three national databases. *Am J Public Health* 12:1707, 1993.

Metzkor-Cotter E et al: Long-term serological analysis and clinical follow-up of patients with cat scratch disease. *Clin Infect Dis* 37:1149, 2003.

AUTHOR: **MARY T. CASERTA, MD**

BASIC INFORMATION

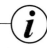

DEFINITION

Celiac disease is permanent intestinal intolerance to dietary gluten (wheat gliadin and related proteins), which produces a characteristic mucosal lesion in the proximal small bowel in genetically susceptible individuals.

SYNONYMS

Celiac sprue
Gluten-sensitive enteropathy
Nontropical sprue

ICD-9-CM CODE
579 Celiac disease

EPIDEMIOLOGY & DEMOGRAPHICS

- With the availability of sensitive screening tests for celiac disease (see "Workup") estimates of the prevalence of this disease have changed.
- Susceptibility is determined in part by a common human leukocyte antigen (HLA) association: the major histocompatibility complex class II antigens, HLA-DQ2 and HLA-DQ8.
- Environmental factors such as infant feeding practices, lower antigenicity of formulas, and later introduction of gluten may also be important in geographic and age-related prevalence rates.
- The prevalence of celiac disease in children between 2.5 and 15 years of age in the general population is 3 to 13 per 1000 (1:300 to 1:80).
- Celiac disease can be clinically silent; therefore the prevalence may have previously been underestimated.
- The incidence is now believed to be similar in Europe and in the United States.
- The prevalence is lower in Hispanics and in East Asian populations owing, in part, to lower frequency of the HLA-DQ genotypes.
- In the classic form of celiac disease, symptoms usually present between 1 and 5 years of age, but there is considerable variation in the age of onset.
- Conditions associated with an increased prevalence of celiac disease (frequency in %):
    - Type 1 diabetes mellitus (~4%)
    - Autoimmune thyroiditis (~3%)
    - Down syndrome (5% to 10%)
    - Turner syndrome (5% to 10%)
    - Williams syndrome (5% to 10%)
    - Selective IgA deficiency (~2%)
- First-degree relatives of individuals with celiac disease also have an increased risk (~2%).
- A higher frequency of other autoimmune disorders occurs in individuals with celiac disease.
- Celiac disease is associated with an increased risk of small bowel lymphomas.

CLINICAL PRESENTATION

History

- The presentation varies considerably and the disease can be clinically silent.
- The classic history in an infant or toddler is onset of diarrhea (malabsorptive stools), irritability, anorexia, and poor weight gain after the introduction of cereals into the diet.
    - Malabsorptive stools (steatorrhea) are bulky, foul smelling, greasy, "float in toilet."
- History in childhood is that of intermittent abdominal discomfort, variable stool pattern (from diarrhea to constipation), short stature, joint pains, and delayed puberty.
- A family history of celiac disease may be reported.
- For associated conditions with an increased incidence of celiac disease, see "Epidemiology & Demographics."

Physical Examination

- Examination may be normal
- Evidence of malnutrition
    - Crossing weight and then height percentiles
    - Muscle wasting in the extremities and buttocks
    - Abdominal distension
    - Finger clubbing
- Short stature
- Non-gastrointestinal manifestations of celiac disease may include:
    - Dermatitis herpetiformis
    - Enamel hypoplasia of permanent teeth
    - Osteopenia/osteoporosis
    - Delayed puberty
    - Iron deficiency anemia refractory to therapy

ETIOLOGY

- Environmental trigger in a genetically susceptible host results in chronic inflammation in the small intestinal mucosa.
- Genetically, the strongest association of celiac disease is with the HLA class II D region markers (chromosome 6).
- The environmental trigger is interaction with gluten in cereal proteins, including wheat, rye, and barley.
    - The toxicity of oats is controversial. Toxicity may be related to contamination with gluten during harvesting and processing.
- Other environmental factors may play a role.
    - Breastfeeding (has protective effect)
    - Type and amount of cereals introduced
    - Infective (particularly viral) factors
- The result of interaction of the toxic proteins in susceptible individuals is immunologically mediated damage to the small bowel mucosa, resulting in malabsorption.
- The target antigen has been identified as tissue transglutaminase (TTG), which is also the endomysial antigen recognized by the anti-endomysial IgA antibody (see "Workup").

DIAGNOSIS

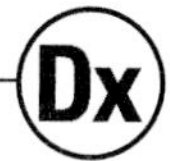

DIFFERENTIAL DIAGNOSIS

- The differential diagnosis depends on the age and signs and symptoms at the time of evaluation. There may be no gastrointestinal symptoms and a normal physical examination in the setting of silent disease.
- The differential diagnosis for the classic presentation in childhood includes:
    - Cystic fibrosis
    - Postenteritis enteropathy
    - Food protein allergies (milk, soy, wheat)
    - Chronic giardiasis

WORKUP

- Serologic studies are excellent screening tests for celiac disease (see "Laboratory Tests"):
    - Must be performed while ingesting wheat
- Small bowel biopsy is still required to confirm the diagnosis:
    - Villous atrophy, crypt hyperplasia, inflammatory cell infiltration of the lamina propria, intraepithelial lymphocytes
    - Must be performed while ingesting wheat
- A typical biopsy, along with a clinical response to a gluten-free diet, is required to make the diagnosis of celiac disease.
- Repeat biopsy after initiating a gluten-free diet is considered necessary only if complete clinical remission does not occur.
- Positive serology with normal small intestinal biopsy may represent either:
    - A false-positive test
    - Latent disease in an individual with an HLA-predisposing genotype suggesting the potential to develop gluten-induced enteropathy later in life.
- Currently recommended diagnostic strategies:
    - Symptomatic child: history and examination suggestive of celiac disease
        - Quantitative immunoglobulin A (IgA), anti-TTG IgA antibody
        - If positive, refer for endoscopic small intestinal biopsy
        - If negative, consider other diagnoses
    - Asymptomatic child but at-risk (first-degree relative, diabetes mellitus, thyroiditis, Down syndrome, Turner syndrome, Williams syndrome, IgA deficiency)
        - Anti-TTG IgA antibody (IgG antibody if known IgA deficiency)
        - If positive, refer for endoscopic small intestinal biopsy

LABORATORY TESTS

- A number of serologic studies are available.
    - Antigliadin antibodies (IgA, IgG)
    - Antireticulin antibodies (IgA)
    - Antiendomysial (EM) antibodies (IgA)

- Antitissue transglutaminase (anti-TTG) antibodies (IgA, IgG)
- The most sensitive and specific are the anti-EM and anti-TTG IgA serologies.
- A combination of the anti-TTG and anti-EM antibodies may have the highest sensitivity and specificity.
- The IgG antigliadin antibody is very sensitive but not specific (too many false positives) and is therefore not considered to be a good screening test.
- Quantitative IgA should also be obtained.
  - There is an increased incidence of IgA deficiency in association with celiac disease.
  - IgA antibodies are the most specific serologic test and coincident IgA deficiency would invalidate these tests.
- Other potential laboratory abnormalities include the following:
  - Iron deficiency anemia
  - Low-serum carotene
  - Elevated transaminases
  - Increased fecal fat (qualitative and quantitative)

TREATMENT

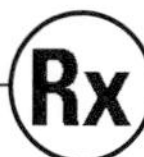

NONPHARMACOLOGIC THERAPY

- Gluten-free diet is essential (lifelong).
- Some children may have other secondary dietary protein intolerances (e.g., to milk or soy) or be lactose intolerant. If so, then milk or soy products may need to be restricted for a period as well.
- Attention must be paid to the child's overall nutritional state until the intestinal mucosa has healed and malabsorption has been corrected.
  - Fat-soluble vitamins
  - Calcium
  - Iron

DISPOSITION

- Strict adherence to a gluten-free diet will correct and prevent nutritional deficiencies and their consequences.
- Poor adherence may result not only in nutritional deficiencies but also in an increased risk for other autoimmune disorders and small bowel lymphomas over time.
- The mortality rate for individuals diagnosed with celiac disease in childhood and who adhere to appropriate dietary restrictions appears to be similar to the general population.

REFERRAL

- All patients should be referred to a (pediatric) gastroenterologist to confirm the diagnosis with an endoscopic small intestinal biopsy.
- Seeking a nutritionist with experience in gluten-free diets as a resource to families is recommended.

PEARLS & CONSIDERATIONS

COMMENTS

- This is a lifelong condition, and strict adherence to a gluten-free diet is recommended even when the patient is asymptomatic.
- An empiric trial of a gluten-free diet without serologic testing and confirmation with a small intestinal biopsy is not recommended.
- Celiac disease may be clinically silent and it is important to recognize the clinical settings in which the prevalence of celiac disease is increased in order to initiate appropriate screening.
  - Children with non-gastrointestinal manifestations (see "Clinical Presentation")
  - Children who are at-risk (see "Work-up")

PATIENT/FAMILY EDUCATION

- Dietary restrictions are strict and lifelong.
- Maintaining a gluten-free diet in children can be challenging.
- A number of organizational web sites provide educational, dietary, and support group information. There are many local and regional support groups as well.
  - Celiac Sprue Association/USA: www.csaceliacs.org
  - Celiac Disease Foundation: www.celiac.org
  - North American Society for Pediatric Gastroenterology, Hepatology and Nutrition: www.naspghan.org

SUGGESTED READINGS

Fasano A: Clinical presentation of celiac disease in the pediatric population. *Gastroenterology* 128: s68, 2005.

Hill ID et al: Guidelines for the diagnosis and treatment of celiac disease: recommendations of the North American Society for Pediatric Gastroenterology, Hepatology and Nutrition. *J Pediatr Gastroenterol Nutr* 40:1, 2005.

North American Society for Pediatric Gastroenterology, Hepatology and Nutrition. Available at www.naspghan.org

AUTHOR: **M. SUSAN MOYER, MD**

BASIC INFORMATION

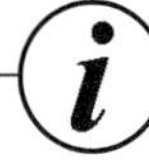

DEFINITION

Cellulitis is an acute infection of the dermis and subcutaneous tissues resulting in local pain, edema, warmth, and erythema. Periorbital or preseptal cellulitis is a specific type of cellulitis that results in an infection of the soft tissues superficial to the orbital septum. It does not involve the eye or the orbital contents. In contrast, orbital or postseptal cellulitis involves the orbit and usually is the result of disease extension from an underlying sinus infection. Erysipelas is a rapidly progressive form of superficial cellulitis usually caused by group A β-hemolytic streptococci.

SYNONYMS

Cellulitis
Periorbital or preseptal cellulitis

ICD-9-CM CODES
373.13 Eyelid cellulitis
376.01 Orbital cellulitis
682.9 Cellulitis

EPIDEMIOLOGY & DEMOGRAPHICS

- Cellulitis is common in pediatrics.
- Cellulitis was ranked as the 28th most common diagnosis in hospitalized patients.
- Cellulitis accounts for more than 2% of office visits.
- Cellulitis occurs equally in males and females.
- There are no age predictors.
- Facial cellulitis, including periorbital cellulitis, typically occurs in children younger than 6 years.
- Cellulitis is common in children between 6 months and 3 years old.
- Risks for cellulitis include the following: chronic disease, diabetes mellitus, immunodeficiency, current varicella infection, tinea pedis infection, chronic corticosteroid use, impaired peripheral circulation (e.g., venous compromise, arterial insufficiency, lymphatic compromise), underlying skin condition (e.g., atopic dermatitis), trauma-induced skin lesion, unvaccinated children (*Haemophilus influenzae* type B).

CLINICAL PRESENTATION

History

- Local trauma can cause a break in the integrity of the skin.
  - Insect bite, scratch, abrasion, laceration, animal bite
  - Surgical wound
  - Can occur at sites with normal skin integrity
- Within 1 to 3 days, development of warmth, redness, pain, and swelling.
- Without medical intervention, the area of involvement expands.
- Without erythema, warmth, swelling, and local tenderness, reconsider diagnosis.
- Systemic symptoms may include fevers, chills, malaise, and myalgias.

Physical Examination

- Confluent macular erythema with generalized edema, warmth, and tenderness.
- Margins are indistinct and not palpable.
- Lymphangitic streaking may extend from a distal extremity, proximal to the area of cellulitis.
- Regional lymphadenopathy may be appreciated.
- With a possible periorbital cellulitis, a thorough physical examination to distinguish from orbital cellulitis is neccessary.
  - A patient with periorbital cellulitis may have a history of trauma to the affected eye, with or without evidence of a local wound infection.
  - With periorbital cellulitis, the eyelid is swollen, red, and tender. A violaceous hue may exist if *H. influenzae* type B or *Streptococcus pneumoniae* are the responsible organisms.
  - The eyelid should be retracted to exclude the presence of a foreign body.
  - Proptosis, ophthalmoplegia, decreased visual acuity, and pain on eye movement must be absent for the diagnosis of periorbital cellulitis.
  - Fever is present in 75% of cases. Among children younger than 2 years, 25% have simultaneous otitis media.

ETIOLOGY

- Cellulitis is associated with previous skin trauma, but the inoculation site may be trivial.
- Because the bacterial density in tissue is low, development of disease may result from bacterial exotoxins that invoke local cytokine release.
- The most common etiologic agents are *Staphylococcus aureus, Streptococcus pyogenes* (group A β-hemolytic *Streptococcus*), *S. pneumoniae,* and *H. influenzae* type B. Non–group A β-hemolytic streptococci (groups B, C, and G) are other known pathogens.
- *Pseudomonas aeruginosa* and other gram-negative bacilli may be present in immunocompromised patients. *P. aeruginosa* infection should be suspected after a puncture wound through a sneaker.
- *H. influenzae* type B (HIB) was the predominant cause of facial cellulitis before initiation of the HIB vaccine in 1990.
  - *H. influenzae* type B was the cause of bacteremic periorbital cellulitis in 80% of cases before the era of universal immunization.
  - The other 20% of cases were a result of *S. pneumoniae* infection.
- Specific risk factors such as age, concurrent disease, exposures, and location may help establish the cause:
  - Neonates: group B *Streptococcus*
  - Diabetes mellitus: *S. aureus,* streptococci, Enterobacteriaceae, anaerobes
  - Nephrotic syndrome: *Escherichia coli*
  - Immunocompromised state
    - Bacteria: *Serratia, Proteus,* and other Enterobacteriaceae
    - Fungi: *Cryptococcus neoformans*
    - Atypical mycobacteria
  - Specific exposures
    - Human bites: *Eikenella corrodens*
    - Animal (dog and cat) bites: staphylococci, *Pasteurella multocida*
    - Puncture wound through sneaker sole: *P. aeruginosa*
    - Environmental and occupational exposures: *Erysipelothrix rhusiopathiae, Vibrio* species, *Aeromonas hydrophilia*
  - Site-specific cellulitis
    - Cellulitis of the extremities: group A streptococci, *S. aureus*
    - Recurrent cellulitis of the leg: non–group A β-hemolytic streptococci (groups C, G, B)
    - Dissecting cellulitis of the scalp: *S. aureus.* This is a rare but chronic suppurative disease of the scalp, usually seen in young adults, particularly males, and marked by numerous follicular and perifollicular reactions. Nodules develop that eventually become fluctuant and subsequently rupture, producing intercommunicating draining sinuses. Ultimately, healing occurs but results in severe scarring and alopecia.
    - Facial cellulitis: *H. influenzae* type B or *S. pneumoniae*; infects children more than 3 years old by portal of entry; consider staphylococcal and streptococcal involvement
    - Perianal cellulites: *S. pyogenes*
    - Buccal cellulitis in neonates: *H. influenzae* or group B streptococci
- Group B streptococci may cause a facial cellulitis in infants. Concomitant sepsis may be present.
- Periorbital cellulitis may arise as the result of localized infection or inflammation of the conjunctiva, eyelids, or adjacent structures; hematogenous dissemination of nasopharyngeal pathogens to the periorbital tissue; or acute sinusitis with inflammatory edema in the periorbital tissue.
  - Common pathogens include *H. influenzae* type B, *S. pneumoniae, S. aureus, S. pyogenes,* and anaerobes. *Staphylococcus epidermidis* and *Streptococcus agalactiae* have been reported.
  - When periorbital cellulitis results from dacryocystitis or dacryoadenitis, *Chlamydia trachomatis* and *Neisseria gonorrhoeae* are the likely organisms.
- Intravenous drug users may have a cellulitis due to *S. aureus,* streptococci, Enterobacteriaceae, *Pseudomonas,* and fungi.
- Rare causes include the following:
  - Anaerobic organisms
  - *Clostridium perfringens* (gas-forming)
  - Tuberculosis

- Syphilitic gumma
- Mucormycosis, aspergillosis

DIAGNOSIS

Dx

DIFFERENTIAL DIAGNOSIS

- Dermatologic conditions
  - Angioedema or allergic swelling
  - Atopic dermatitis
  - Chemical burns
  - Contact dermatitis
  - Eosinophilic cellulitis (i.e., Well's syndrome)
  - Erythema multiforme
  - Exfoliative dermatitis
  - Popsicle or cold panniculitis
  - Stevens-Johnson syndrome
  - Toxic epidermal necrolysis
  - Toxicodendron or plant poison
  - Venomous insect bite or sting with local reaction
- Infectious conditions
  - Cutaneous fungal infection
  - Erysipelas (i.e., rapidly spreading cellulitis due to *S. pyogenes*)
  - Folliculitis
  - Gas gangrene
  - Hidradenitis
  - Impetigo
  - Nontuberculous mycobacteria soft tissue infection
  - Staphylococcal scaled skin syndrome
  - Septic arthritis or osteomyelitis
  - Septic emboli
- Miscellaneous conditions
  - Traumatic contusions
- Differential diagnosis of periorbital cellulitis should include
  - Orbital cellulites
  - Blunt trauma
  - Conjunctivitis
  - Hordeolum
  - Dacryocystitis
  - Dacryoadenitis
  - Periorbital swelling associated with retinoblastoma
  - Metastatic neuroblastoma
  - Rhabdomyosarcoma
  - Rupture of a dermoid cyst
  - Systemic disease such as allergy
  - Hypoproteinemia
  - Congestive heart failure

WORKUP

- Cellulitis is primarily a clinical diagnosis.
- Complicated cases, when the patient is systemically ill or has concerning risk factors (e.g., young age, large area of involvement, chronic illness), may necessitate laboratory testing.

LABORATORY TESTS

- Complete blood cell count with a differential cell count may demonstrate an elevated white blood cell count with a left shift.
- Blood cultures may be useful.
  - Consider reserving cultures for those who are systemically ill, have recurrent episodes, have unusual exposures, or are not responding to treatment.
  - In the post-HIB vaccine era only 2% (5 of 243) of patients yield a true pathogen.
  - Other sources report positive blood cultures in 25% of all cases of cellulitis.
- Consider needle aspiration from the edge of infection.
  - Pathogen yeild in less than 33%.
  - Yield increases to 90% if bullae or abscess is present with cellulitis.
- Toe web swab culture could be considered for those with tinea pedis–related lower extremity cellulitis.
- Streptococci serology (e.g., ASO, antideoxyribonuclease B test, antihyaluronidase, Streptozyme antibody assay) can be used to support diagnosis of cellulitis caused by group A β-hemolytic streptococci.
- Lumbar puncture (LP) must be considered in a young child with periorbital cellulitis. Consider LP if meningitis is suspected or if inadequate HIB vaccine status.

IMAGING STUDIES

- Obtain radiographs if concerned to investigate for osteomyelitis or septic arthritis.
- Crepitus revealed on physical examination, warrant radiographs that may reveal gas in the affected tissue.
- Computed tomography of the orbits can confirm suspected orbital cellulitis.

TREATMENT

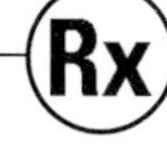

NONPHARMACOLOGIC THERAPY

- Outline the border of the involved area with a durable pen to follow progression or regression of cellulitis.
- Warm, moist compresses applied to the area provide relief and may expedite healing.
- Elevation of the affected limb above the level of the heart reduces swelling.
- Tetanus immunization if needed.
- Deep infections, those with necrosis, suspected abscesses, or rapidly spreading may need surgical débridement or drainage.

ACUTE GENERAL Rx

- Analgesics may be used to alleviate the pain and tenderness associated with cellulitis.
- Before initiating treatment in a patient with cellulitis, decide whether to hospitalize or treat as an outpatient.
  - The typical nontoxic patient may be treated with outpatient enteral therapy.
  - If there is a rapidly spreading infection, parenteral treatment should be considered.
- Treatment should be directed against the most common pathogens: *S. aureus* and β-hemolytic group A streptococci.
- Treatment for the uncomplicated patient: penicillinase-resistant antistaphylococcal synthetic penicillin or a first-generation cephalosporin for a 10- to 14-day course.
- First-line enteral coverage usually consists of the following:
  - Cephalexin (25 to 100 mg/kg/24 hours PO, divided every 6 hours) *or*
  - Dicloxacillin sodium (for mild or moderate infections: 12.5 to 25 mg/kg/24 hours PO, divided every 6 hours; for severe infections: 50 to 100 mg/kg/24 hours PO, divided every 6 hours)
    - This regimen provides better coverage for staphylococcal species than for streptococcal species.
    - This approach should not to be used for erysipelas.
- Alternative treatment options for penicillin-allergic patients include the following:
  - Clindamycin
  - Macrolides
    - Erythromycin has been used extensively in the past with success in the treatment of uncomplicated cellulitis.
    - Newer macrolides, such as azithromycin and clarithromycin, should be used if there is concern about *H. influenzae.*
    - Vigilant use of macrolides for erysipelas is warranted because of the growing resistance by streptococcal species.
  - Fluoroquinolones provide a reasonable choice for gram-negative infections. Consider additional gram-positive coverage such as clindamycin to provide adequate empirical coverage against *S. aureus* and streptococcal species. Efficacy and safety not established in patients younger than 18 years old.
- If *H. influenzae* infection is suspected, consider cefuroxime, cefotaxime, or ceftriaxone.
- Treatment for complicated patients, includes empirical therapy parenterally until improvement, followed by enteral treatment for a total of 10 to 14 days.
- No strict guidelines exist about the transition from intravenous to oral antibiotics. Most clinicians change to oral therapy after defervescence and evidence of improved local findings. This typically takes 2 to 5 days.
- Empirical antibiotic parenteral treatment options include the following:
  - Ceftriaxone (50 to 75 mg/kg/24 hours IV or IM divided every 12 to 24 hours)
  - Nafcillin (50 to 100 mg/kg/24 hours IV or IM divided every 6 hours, not to exceed 12 g/24 hours)
  - Cefazolin (50 to 100 mg/kg/24 hours IV or IM divided every 8 hours, maximum 6 g/24 hours)
- For those with a penicillin allergy, clindamycin is an appropriate alternative.
  - Vancomycin should be reserved for those with a severe penicillin allergy or in

those patients with possible methicillin-resistant *Staphylococcus aureus* (MRSA).
  - Erysipelas requiring intravenous antibiotics can be treated with penicillin G.
  - Because of the increasing resistance of *S. pneumoniae* to penicillins, consider a fluoroquinolone or vancomycin.
- The efficacy and safety of fluoroquinolones has not been established in patients younger than 18 years old.
- Several approaches are used for facial cellulitis (including periorbital cellulitis):
  - Use a β-lactamase-resistant antibiotic that also covers *H. influenzae, Staphylococcus,* and *Streptococcus.*
  - For *H. influenzae,* consider cefotaxime or cefuroxime.
  - Ceftriaxone is another option. However, if *S. aureus* is a potential pathogen, adequate coverage will not be provided.
  - Treatment on an outpatient basis is possible if the patient is nontoxic and there is no possibility of orbital involvement.
  - Ensure follow-up within 24 to 48 hours. Consider hospitalization if there is no improvement or if follow-up cannot be guaranteed.
- Special situations demand tailored therapy:
  - For MRSA, use parenteral vancomycin.
  - In fresh water exposure, when *Aeromonas* infection is a risk, consider fluoroquinolone and cefazolin until the organism is identified.
  - In salt water exposure, there is a risk of *Vibrio vulnificus* infection, and tetracycline is the treatment of choice.
  - Hot tub exposure should raise concern about *P. aeruginosa* infection. Folliculitis is more common in these cases.
  - After animal bites, there is a high likelihood of *P. multocida* infection, but infection may be polymicrobial (e.g., gram-negative organisms, *S. aureus,* streptococcal species). Use penicillin with a β-lactamase inhibitor such as amoxicillin-clavulanic acid.
  - For immunocompromised patients, given the risk of infection by atypical organisms, choose broad-spectrum antibiotics with gram-positive and gram-negative coverage. An aminoglycoside and a third-generation cephalosporin can be effective. Clindamycin, ceftriaxone, or nafcillin and a fluoroquinolone can be used, although the efficacy and safety of fluoroquinolones has not been established in patients younger than 18 years. Special attention should be paid to the risk of *P. aeruginosa.*

DISPOSITION

- Reevaluated within 24 to 48 hours.
- Improvement should occur within the first 1 to 2 days of treatment.
- Complete resolution is more gradual.
  - Symptoms resolve over 7 to 14 days.
  - Local desquamation may occur.
- Prognosis is generally excellent with early detection and treatment.
  - There is increased risk of hematogenous or lymphatic spread with late recognition of disease.
- Complications include bacteremia, sepsis, local abscess, lymphangitis, superinfection, thrombophlebitis, osteomyelitis, arthritis, and gangrene. Staphylococcal scalded skin syndrome and toxic shock syndrome are toxin-related complications. Meningitis is a potential sequelae of facial cellulitis.

REFERRAL

- Gangrene or fascitis are considered surgical emergencies and need an emergent surgical evaluation.
- Complicated or refractory cases may benefit from an infectious disease consultation.

PEARLS & CONSIDERATIONS

COMMENTS

- Perianal dermatitis or disease is sometimes classified as a specific type of cellulitis, but the nomenclature is controversial.
- Cellulitis is typically caused by group A β-hemolytic streptococci and primarily affects younger children.
  - The mean age is 4.25 years.
  - Ninety percent of patients present with localized dermatitis. Other complaints include perianal pruritus, rectal pain, and blood-streaked stools.
  - Treatment consists of 10 days of oral amoxicillin or penicillin.
  - Recurrence rates may be as high as 39%.
- Erysipelas (St. Anthony's fire) is a distinct type of cellulitis that most commonly affects the face or leg.
  - β-Hemolytic streptococci, primarily group A, cause most cases.
  - Characterized by an intensely erythematous and rapidly expanding cellulitis with clearly demarcated, raised margins.
  - The sharp demarcation between the involved and uninvolved tissues distinguishes erysipelas from typical cellulitis.
  - Marked edema of the superficial dermis without subcutaneous involvement.
  - Treatment consists of penicillin.

PREVENTION

- Protective equipment should be worn when participating in activities that could predispose the child to scrapes or lacerations.
- Proper local wound care for skin abrasions and injuries can prevent many cases of cellulitis. All wounds should be cleansed with soap and water and covered with a clean, dry cloth or bandage.
- Consider topical antibiotic ointment.
- If skin injuries are extensive due to a deep puncture wound or from an animal bite, the patient should be evaluated by a clinician.
- Patients should be brought to a clinician as early as possible for a suspected cellulitis.
- Parents should be encouraged to immunize their children based on the American Academy of Pediatrics' immunization guidelines.

PATIENT/FAMILY EDUCATION

- Improvement should occur in 24 to 48 hours after treatment.
- After the diagnosis of cellulitis is established, patient and family should be advised to observe the area for worsening symptoms, lymphangitic streaking, and development of fever or chills.
- Patients and families can be reassured that cellulitis is not contagious.

SUGGESTED READINGS

Cutis DL: Cellulitis: Emergency Medicine [serial outline]. Available at: http://www.emedicine.com/emerg/topic88.htm

Fisher RG et al: Facial cellulitis in childhood: a changing spectrum. *South Med J* 95:672, 2002.

Givner LB et al: Pneumococcal facial cellulitis in children. *Pediatrics* 106:61, 2000.

Kane KS et al: Cellulitis. *In Color Atlas and Synopsis of Pediatric Dermatology.* New York, McGraw-Hill, 2002, pp 464–466.

Powell KR: Orbital and periorbital cellulitis. *Pediatr Rev* 16:163, 1995.

Sadow KB et al: Blood cultures in the evaluation of children with cellulitis. *Pediatrics* 101:4, 1998.

Semel JD et al: Association of athlete's foot with cellulitis of the lower extremities: diagnostic value of bacterial cultures of ipsilateral interdigital space samples. *Clin Infect Dis* 24:1162, 1996.

Stulberg DL et al: Common bacterial skin infections. *Am Fam Physician* 66:119, 2002.

Wald ER: Periorbital and orbital infections. *Pediatr Rev* 25:312, 2004.

AUTHOR: **BRITTANNY LIAM BOULANGER, MD**

BASIC INFORMATION

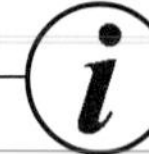

DEFINITION

Cerebral palsy (CP) is a group of disorders of movement and posture caused by a nonprogressive lesion of the developing brain (Table 1-4). Clinical features such as spasticity change over time. Classification of CP identifies the location of motor concerns; it is not related to prognosis and usually not to an underlying cause.

SYNONYM

Static encephalopathy

ICD-9-CM CODES

343.0 Diplegic cerebral palsy
343.1 Hemiplegic cerebral palsy
343.2 Quadriplegic cerebral palsy
343.3 Monoplegic cerebral palsy
343.4 Infantile cerebral palsy, hemiplegia (postnatal)
343.8 Other specified infantile cerebral palsy
343.9 Infantile cerebral palsy, unspecified

EPIDEMIOLOGY & DEMOGRAPHICS

- Prevalence: 1.5 to 2.5 cases per 1000 live births
- Incidence: up to 5 cases per 1000 children
- Risk factors
  - Unknown in many cases
  - Low birth weight: less than 2001 g
  - Preterm delivery: less than 32 weeks
  - Intraventricular hemorrhage or periventricular leukomalacia
  - Perinatal asphyxia: only 15- or 20-minute Apgar scores show correlation
  - Infection: TORCH (**to**xoplasmosis, **ru**bella, **c**ytomegalovirus, or **h**erpes); neonatal or childhood meningitis
  - Multiple gestation
  - Genetic predisposition
  - Hyperbilirubinemia (historically, this was more common)
- Certain genetic disorders with such significant hypotonia or motor concerns that a clinical diagnosis of cerebral palsy is made (e.g., Angelman's syndrome).

CLINICAL PRESENTATION

- Early diagnostic symptoms
  - Delayed or deviant acquisition of motor milestones (corrected for gestational age)
  - Standing skills better than sitting
  - Particular difficulty in the development of transitional skills
  - Handedness before 12 months (infants do not typically cross the midline to reach for an object before 12 months)
  - Toe walking
  - Abnormal movements: ataxia, significant balance issues, athetoid movements
  - Typically, no regression of milestones
  - Parental concern typically about motor delay
  - History of a risk factor
- Early diagnostic signs
  - Asymmetry revealed in the neurologic examination
  - Tone: increased, decreased anterior scarf sign; lead pipe rigidity
  - Tone that fluctuates in the first year of life
  - Deep tendon reflexes (DTRs): if brisk, indicative of upper motor neuron (long tract) dysfunction; may not be increased at a young age, even with upper motor neuron disorders
  - Toe walking
  - Persistent fisting after 3 months of age
  - Log roll (babies should roll segmentally)
  - Scissoring of the lower extremities after 2 months of age
  - Persistence of primitive neurologic reflexes (Table 1-5)
- Cerebral palsy may be difficult to diagnose before 1 year of age and, in some children, prior to 2 years.
- See Table 1-6 for associated findings.

ETIOLOGY

- Unknown in many cases
- Preterm delivery
- In utero or neonatal birth asphyxia
- Congenital infections
- Infarction (consider this in cases with hemiplegia)
- Traumatic brain injury

DIAGNOSIS

DIFFERENTIAL DIAGNOSIS

- A progressive disorder of the neurologic system
- Normal variant (e.g., toe walking)

WORKUP

- Complete physical and neurologic evaluation should include primitive reflexes.
- Because of many other comorbid conditions, consider the following:
  - Ophthalmology examination
  - Audiology evaluation
  - Identify growth and feeding issues
- Obtain an electroencephalogram if the history indicates possible seizures.

LABORATORY TESTS

- It may or may not be necessary to obtain any of the following evaluations:
  - Consider blood and urine metabolic evaluations if there is regression in abilities or if significant hypotonia or ataxia exists and *there are no critical findings* on magnetic resonance imaging (MRI) to explain the motor concerns.
  - Consider a TORCH evaluation if calcifications are found on head computed tomography (CT) and if there is a potential risk. Urinary test for cytomegalovirus can be positive for months after birth in cases of congenital infection.
  - Consider high-resolution chromosomal studies in children with dysmorphic features, structural malformations, or familial forms of cerebral palsy. Consider referral for genetics evaluation and counseling.
  - For brain infarction, consider coagulopathy evaluation.

IMAGING STUDIES

- The diagnostic hallmark in many instances is the brain MRI.
- Consider skull radiograph or CT for microcephalic children to look for calcifications.

TREATMENT

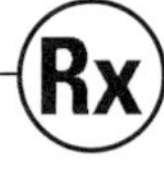

NONPHARMACOLOGIC THERAPY

- Physical and occupational therapy can address movement patterns, spasticity, bracing options for mobility, and functional skills.
- Surgical procedures can address spasticity and can include tendon releases, dorsal rhizotomy, or insertion of a baclofen pump.
- For those with strabismus, patching, eye drops, glasses, or surgery may be needed to avoid amblyopia.
- Children with developmental and learning issues benefit from early intervention, preschool, and special education with an individualized education plan (IEP).
- Children with communication difficulties may benefit from speech therapy and

TABLE 1-4 **Types of Cerebral Palsy**

Pyramidal (motor cortex, internal capsule, cortical spinal tract)	Extrapyramidal (basal ganglia, thalamus, subthalamic nucleus, cervellum)
spastic diplegia: LE involvement greater than UE	athetoid: slow writhing movements
spastic hemiplegia: unilateral involvement	chorea: quick jerky movements
spastic paraplegia: LE only	choreoathetoid: combination of above
spastic quadriplegia: all extremities involved	ataxic: tremor, wide-based gait
	hypotonic: floppy
	dystonic: lead pipe rigidity with movement

LE, lower extremity; UE, upper extremity

TABLE 1-5 Normal Primitive Reflex Development and Loss

Reflex	1mo.	2mo.	3mo.	4mo.	6mo.	9mo.	12mo.	15mo.	18mo.	24mo.	36mo.
Palmar Grasp	+	+	+/−	+/−	o	o	o	o	o	o	o
ATNR	+	+	+/−	+/−	o	o	o	o	o	o	o
Moro	+	+	+/−	+/−	o	o	o	o	o	o	o
Rooting	+	+	+	+	+	+/−	o	o	o	o	o
Neck Righting	o	o	o	+/−	+/−	+	+	+	+	+	+
Parachute	o	o	o	o	+/−	+	+	+	+	+	+
Landau	o	o	o	o	o	+	+	+	+	+/−	o

ATNR, atonic neck reflex

TABLE 1-6 Associated Complications and Management by System for Patients with Cerebral Palsy

System	Complications	Treatment	Follow-up/Referral
Musculoskeletal	Subluxed/dislocated hips	Surgical	Orthopedic surgeon
	Spasticity/contractures/pain	ROM, casting, orthotics, appropriate seating devices, surgical tendon releases, antispasticity medications, including Botox, baclofen pump, dorsal rhizotomy	Physical therapy, occupational therapy
	Scoliosis	Bracing, surgical intervention	Orthopedic surgeon
	Mobility issues	Bracing, wheelchair	Physiatrist, neurosurgeon, orthopedic surgeon, physical therapist
Ophthalmologic	Strabismus, refractive errors	Patching, eye drops, glasses, surgery	Ophthalmologist
	Visual field defects, cortical visual impairment	Therapy through Early Intervention for Visual Impairments	Local association for the blind
Gastrointestinal	GER with or without recurrent aspiration pneumonia	Acid reduction and promotility agents, surgical antireflux surgery is sometimes needed	Gastroenterologist or pediatric surgeon if needed
	Constipation	Dietary fiber, bowel program, laxatives, suppositories, enemas	Gastroenterologist if needed
	Growth and nutrition (feeding difficulties, poor suck/swallow coordination, tonic bite, hyperactive gag, tongue thrust)	Follow growth on CP grid, dietary supplements, sometimes G-tube feeds	Occupational therapy, nutritionist if needed
Neurologic	Seizures (30–50% in hemiplegic CP)	Antiepileptic medications, seizure precautions	Pediatric neurologist
	Learning disabilities (motor planning, visuospatial difficulties)	Educational interventions	Multifactored developmental evaluation, IEP
	AD/HD	Behavioral modification, medication management	Developmental pediatrician, pediatric psychologist, IEP
	Mental retardation	Educational interventions	Multifactored developmental evaluation, IEP
	Communication disorders	Augmentative communication devices, signing, picture boards	Speech and language therapist knowledgeable in CP
	Oral-Motor apraxia and/or dysarthria (affects communication and drooling)	Anti-drooling medications, anti-drooling surgical procedures	Pediatric ear, nose, and throat specialist for surgical intervention Speech and language therapy
Dental	Malocclusion, caries; exacerbated by pharmacologic or surgical attempts to decrease drooling	Regular brushing and flossing	Dentist
Hearing	Hearing loss in 10%	Aggressive treatment of hearing, hearing aids, FM systems, cochlear implant if severe to profound sensorineural hearing loss	Audiologist, speech and language pathologist, pediatric otolaryngologist
Skin	Skin breakdown if poor nutrition, unable to shift weight	Prevention! Improve nutrition, frequent turning, well fitted wheelchair, cushion for areas of pressure, appropriate bedding	If severe, plastic surgeon
Social	Family adjustments to a child with a disability, financial burdens, estate planning, advocacy for child and family, minimal respite services, peer interactions, independent living options	Multidisciplinary approach to maximize functional and independent outcomes	Counseling, SSI, MCH funding, early intervention, preschool disabilities, BVR, County Board of MRDD, local parent support groups, therapeutic recreation program

AD/HD, Attention deficit hyperactivity disorder; BVR, bureau of vocational rehabilitation; IEP, individualized education plan; MCH, maternal child health; MRDD, mental retardation and developmental disabilities; ROM, range of motion; SSI, supplemental security income.

sometimes from augmentative communication devices.
- For associated hearing concerns, hearing aids or other appropriate devices should be used based on the brain injury pattern.

ACUTE GENERAL Rx

- If seizures occur, appropriate treatment with anticonvulsants and monitoring is needed.
- For constipation, the use of fiber or stool softeners and laxatives should be considered.

CHRONIC Rx

- Treat as previously described for constipation or seizures.
- Drooling may be managed with oral medication such as glycopyrrolate (Robinul), transdermal scopolamine, or behavioral management or surgical ligation of some of the salivary ducts.
- Table 1-6 delineates management based on the system involved.

COMPLEMENTARY & ALTERNATIVE MEDICINE

Hyperbaric oxygen has been attempted, but studies in Canada demonstrated that this was not successful in improving the long-term outcome.

DISPOSITION

Disposition is shown in Table 1-6.

REFERRAL

- Consult Table 1-6.
- The primary care physician manages many children with cerebral palsy. Typically, diagnosis is made by consultations to subspecialists such as a neurologist, physiatrist, orthopedic surgeon, and neurodevelopmental or developmental and behavioral pediatricians.
- Clinics for individuals with cerebral palsy are available in many areas.
- Begin transition planning at age 16 to address adult issues such as education, employment, accessible housing, mobility, and finances. These areas are significantly affected by the overall cognitive ability of the individual and the extent of motor disability.

PEARLS & CONSIDERATIONS

COMMENTS

- Diagnosis may be difficult in the first 1 to 2 years of life, because muscular tone can fluctuate.
- Categorization as mild, moderate, or severe is based on functional limitations, not MRI abnormalities.
- Individuals with significant motor involvement can have normal cognition.
- Children who have sustained a global insult are more likely to have global developmental concerns compared with those with a more discreet insult.

PREVENTION

- Prevent preterm delivery and low-birth-weight outcomes.
- Continue efforts to vaccinate against infection and prenatally acquired infections.
- Continue to monitor and intervene for jaundice.
- Because the cause is unknown in most cases and the prevalence in the past few decades has remained largely unchanged, other preventive strategies are needed.

PATIENT/FAMILY EDUCATION

- National Institutes of Health, cerebral palsy information page: www.ninds.nih.gov/disorders/cerebralpalsy/cerebralpalsy.htm
- United Cerebral Palsy: www.ucp.org

SUGGESTED READINGS

American Academy for Cerebral Palsy and Developmental Medicine. Available at www.aacpdm.org

American Academy of Neurology and Child Neurology Society: Practice Parameter: Diagnostic Assessment of the Child with Cerebral Palsy. AAN Guideline Summary for Clinicians. Available at www.aan.com

Cooley WC, the Committee on Children with Disabilities: Providing a primary care medical home for children and youth with cerebral palsy. *Pediatrics* 114:1106, 2004.

Kuba KCK, Leviton A: Cerebral palsy. *N Engl J Med* 330:188, 1994.

Murphy N, Such-Neibar T: Cerebral palsy diagnosis and management: the state of the art. *Curr Probl Pediatr Adolesc Health Care* 33:146, 2003.

Taft L: Cerebral palsy. *Pediatr Rev* 16:411, 1995.

United Cerebral Palsy. Available at www.UCPA.org/

AUTHORS: **SUSAN WILEY, MD** and **NANCY E. LANPHEAR, MD**

BASIC INFORMATION

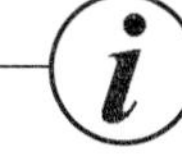

DEFINITION

A cerebrovascular accident (CVA), or stroke, is a syndrome characterized by the rapid onset (minutes to hours) of neurologic symptoms such as hemiparesis, sensory abnormalities, and aphasia. Any vascular insult resulting in a focal neurologic deficit lasting longer than 24 hours constitutes a CVA. Subtypes of CVA include hemorrhagic and ischemic stroke.

SYNONYMS

Hypoxic-ischemic brain injury
Stroke

ICD-9-CM CODE
436 Acute, but ill-defined, cerebrovascular disease (includes CVA and stroke)

EPIDEMIOLOGY & DEMOGRAPHICS

- The incidence each year is 2.5 cases per 100,000 in children between birth and 14 years old.
- Infants are disproportionately affected because of congenital heart disease and neonatal asphyxia.
- If infants are excluded, the annual incidence is 1.25 cases per 100,000 children between 1 and 14 years.
- The male-to-female ratio is 1:1.
- Approximately 45% of CVAs in children are hemorrhagic, and 55% are ischemic.
- The incidence among African-American populations is increased because of sickle cell disease (10%) and hemoglobin SC disease (2% to 5%).

CLINICAL PRESENTATION

History

- The clinical presentation varies because of the wide range of causes of CVA in children.
- Ischemic stroke typically manifests with focal neurologic deficits, such as hemiparesis or hemiplegia.
- Hemorrhagic stroke typically manifests with a more generalized change in mental status or with headache.
- The history should include questions about headaches (i.e., chronic or new); changes in vision, school performance, or motor activity (e.g., new clumsiness); new paresthesias or anesthesia; recent febrile illness; and history of bleeding or clotting disorders, trauma, hypertension, kidney disease, heart disease, metabolic disease, or drug use.

Physical Examination

- Examination of the head and neck for a possible nidus of infection.
- The heart examination is conducted with an emphasis on the source of potential paradoxical embolus.
- Examination of the looks for manifestations of neurocutaneous disorders, vasculitides, or evidence of trauma.
- Neurologic examination can help localize the lesion.
- Pupillary examination to look for miotic pupil and ptosis on contralateral side of hemiparesis, suggestive of Horner's syndrome.

ETIOLOGY

- Causes of CVA include hemorrhage and focal or diffuse ischemia.
- All types of CVAs result in inadequate delivery of glucose and oxygen to neurons, with resultant neuronal cell death.
- Multiple conditions in children can predispose them to CVA; a cause is eventually established in approximately 75% of cases:
  - Hemorrhagic stroke
  - Vascular malformations
  - Arteriovenous malformation (AVM)
  - Galen's vein aneurysm
  - Hereditary hemorrhagic telangiectasia
  - von Hippel-Lindau disease
  - Intracranial aneurysms
  - Moyamoya disease
  - Sturge-Weber syndrome
  - Brain tumors
  - Leukemia
  - Neoplasm
  - Head trauma
  - Coagulopathy
    - Disseminated intravascular coagulation
    - Idiopathic thrombocytopenic purpura
    - Clotting factor deficiencies
    - Afibrinogenemia
    - Vitamin K deficiency
    - Anticoagulation therapy (e.g., heparin, warfarin)
    - Platelet defects
    - Hemolytic uremic syndrome (HUS)
  - Herpes simplex encephalitis
  - Mycotic aneurysm
  - Bacterial or mycotic meningoencephalitis
  - Tuberculous meningitis
  - Systemic disorders
    - Hypertension
    - Hepatic failure
    - Aplastic anemia
  - Genetic disorders
    - Ehlers-Danlos syndrome (type IV)
    - Neurofibromatosis
    - Tuberous sclerosis
    - Polycystic kidney disease (adult type)
    - Hereditary neurocutaneous angiomatosis
    - Fabry's disease (e.g., ischemic stroke)
  - Cardiac disease
    - Congenital heart disease with right-to-left shunt
    - Cardiopulmonary bypass surgery or extracorporeal membrane oxygenation
    - Rheumatic heart disease
    - Prosthetic heart valve
    - Cardiac tumors (e.g., atrial myxoma)
    - Cardiomyopathy
    - Myocardial infarct
    - Arrhythmia
  - Infection
    - Meningitis
    - Encephalitis
    - Systemic: rubella, mycoplasma
  - Inflammatory conditions
    - Systemic lupus erythematosus (SLE)
    - Polyarteritis nodosa (PAN)
    - Takayasu's disease
    - Inflammatory bowel disease
    - Wegener's granulomatosis
    - Sarcoidosis
    - Behçet's disease
    - Vasculopathy
  - Migraine
  - Subarachnoid hemorrhage
  - Trauma
  - Hematologic disorders or hypercoagulable states
    - Sickle cell disease, hemoglobin SC disease
    - Protein C or S deficiency
    - Antithrombin III deficiency
    - Prothrombin A^{20210} mutation
    - Factor V Leiden deficiency
    - Hyperhomocystinemia (e.g., arterial strokes)
    - Dysfibrinogenemia
    - Antiphospholipid antibodies
    - Polycythemia
    - Thrombotic thrombocytopenic purpura (TTP)
    - HUS
  - Metabolic conditions
    - Homocystinuria
    - Fabry's disease
    - Mitochondrial encephalomyelopathies (MELAS)
    - Organic acidemias
    - Glutaric aciduria type II
    - Sulfite oxidase deficiency
    - Hypoglycemia
    - Familial lipid disorders
  - Drugs and toxins
    - Cocaine
    - Amphetamines
    - Oral contraceptives
    - Radiation therapy
    - L-asparaginase
    - Aminocaproic acid (Amicar)
  - Other systemic disorders
    - Dehydration
    - Nephrotic syndrome
    - Pregnancy and postpartum state

DIAGNOSIS

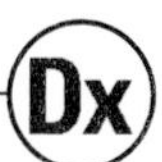

DIFFERENTIAL DIAGNOSIS

- Hemiplegic migraine
- Many types of CVA listed in the "Etiology" section

LABORATORY TESTS

- Complete blood cell count (CBC)
- Erythrocyte sedimentation rate (ESR) and C-reactive protein (CRP) level

- Coagulation studies: prothrombin time, partial thromboplastin time, bleeding time, protein C and S, fibrinogen, antithrombin III, factor V Leiden, prothrombin mutation factor 20210, factors VIII and XI, lupus anticoagulant, anticardiolipin, and homocysteine concentration
- Blood glucose level
- Electrolytes and blood urea nitrogen (BUN) determinations
- Remainder of the diagnostic evaluation undertaken after a detailed history and physical examination focusing on the more likely causes

IMAGING STUDIES

- Computed tomography (CT)
  - Detects hemorrhagic infarct immediately
  - May miss ischemic stroke in the first 12 hours
- Magnetic resonance imaging (MRI)
  - Detects ischemic or hemorrhagic stroke within minutes of symptom onset
  - Necessary for diagnosis of brainstem and cerebellar infarcts
- Echocardiogram to rule out structural heart disease
- Electrocardiogram to evaluate for arrhythmia or underlying conduction defects

TREATMENT

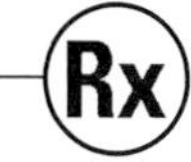

NONPHARMACOLOGIC THERAPY

- Supportive care is needed, paying close attention to airway, breathing, and circulation (ABCs).
  - Airway: If the CVA involves the brainstem or a large part of the cortex, airway protective reflexes may be impaired or lost, requiring endotracheal intubation
  - Breathing: The patient may have significant respiratory depression.
  - Circulation: Special attention should be paid to avoid frank hypotension or rapid changes in blood pressure; avoid hyperglycemia in fluid resuscitation.
  - Avoid hyperthermia.
- Surgical intervention is rarely required.
  - Evacuation of large hemorrhagic infarct that causes a midline shift
  - Tumor debulking if associated with increased intracranial pressure or a mass effect

ACUTE GENERAL Rx

- The approach depends on the cause of the CVA.
- Patients may need antihypertensives, antibiotics, blood transfusion or exchange, clotting factor, or platelet replacement.
- Heparin or enoxaparin may be used in acute, nonhemorrhagic ischemic stroke.

CHRONIC Rx

- There is some evidence in adults that daily aspirin use decreases the risk of recurrence.
- Patients with sickle cell disease may also benefit from daily aspirin use.

DISPOSITION

After an initial hospital stay and rehabilitation, the remainder of follow-up is specific to the cause of the CVA.

REFERRAL

- Pediatric neurology and neurosurgery consultations may be needed.
- Other referrals depend on the cause of the stroke.

PEARLS & CONSIDERATIONS

COMMENTS

- Overall, childhood stroke is an infrequent occurrence.
- Stroke in children is commonly associated with a combination of multiple genetic and acquired risk factors.
- Children with sickle cell disease and congenital heart disease are particularly vulnerable to CVA.
- CVA recurrence is most likely in children with inherited risk factors.

PREVENTION

- Doppler echo imaging of the brain in patients with sickle cell disease is used to assess the risk of stroke. Early and recurrent exchange transfusion is provided for those at risk of stroke.
- Other means of prevention are determined by identifying the underlying risk factors and treating accordingly.

PATIENT/FAMILY EDUCATION

More information is available from the National Institute of Neurological Disorders and Stroke (www.ninds.nih.gov/patients/stroke).

SUGGESTED READINGS

Barreirinho S et al: Inherited and acquired risk factors and their combined effects in pediatric stroke. *Pediatr Neurol* 28:134, 2003.

Burak CR et al: The use of enoxaparin in children with acute, nonhemorrhagic ischemic stroke. *Pediatr Neurol* 29:295, 2003.

Carlin TM, Chanmugam A: Stroke in children. *Emerg Med Clin North Am* 20:671, 2002.

Pavlakis SG et al: Stroke in children. *Adv Pediatr* 38:151, 1991.

Trescher WH: Ischemic stroke syndromes in childhood. *Pediatr Ann* 21:374, 1992.

AUTHOR: **ELLIOTT L. CROW, MD, FPCC**

BASIC INFORMATION

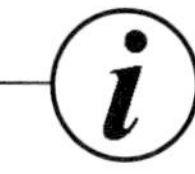

DEFINITION

Mucopurulent cervicitis (MPC) is a syndrome that is characterized by a mucopurulent discharge visible in the endocervical canal or in an endocervical swab specimen.

SYNONYMS

Cervicitis
Endocervicitis
MPC
Sexually transmitted disease (STD)
Sexually transmitted infection (STI)

ICD-9-CM CODES
098.15 Gonococcal cervicitis
098.35 Chronic cervicitis
099.53 Chlamydial cervicitis
616.0 Nonspecific cervicitis

EPIDEMIOLOGY & DEMOGRAPHICS

- MPC can be asymptomatic.
- Sexual abuse is a consideration for young adolescents and prepubertal girls.

CLINICAL PRESENTATION

History
- Vaginal discharge
- Irregular vaginal bleeding, especially after sexual intercourse
- Dyspareunia
- Lower abdominal pain; must consider pelvic infection

Physical Examination
- Visualization of purulent or mucopurulent discharge from the cervical os
- Easily induced endocervical bleeding (i.e., friability)
- Edema and erythema of the zone of ectopy on the cervix
- Signs of possible upper genital tract or pelvic infection: lower abdominal tenderness, cervical motion tenderness, and adnexal tenderness
- Right upper quadrant tenderness; consider perihepatitis

ETIOLOGY

- Commonly, no infectious cause is identified.
- Several pathogens can be identified:
  - *Chlamydia trachomatis* or *Neisseria gonorrhoeae* can cause MPC.
  - Herpes simplex virus can cause MPC.
  - *Trichomonas vaginalis* can cause ectocervicitis (i.e., strawberry cervix) (see Vaginitis chapter in Diseases and Disorders [Section I]).
- Persistent cases during adolescence may be the result of noncompliance with treatment (especially for a multiple-dose treatment regimen), reinfection from an untreated partner, or treatment failure (up to 5% failure rate for azithromycin and doxycycline treatment).

DIAGNOSIS

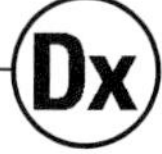

DIFFERENTIAL DIAGNOSIS

- Vaginitis
- Endometritis
- Pelvic inflammatory disease
- Inflamed ectropion-columnar epithelial cells on area surrounding the cervical os
- Foreign body

WORKUP

- Obtain a confidential sexual history, including questions about sexual activity, a new sex partner, the number of lifetime sex partners, possible exposure to an STD-infected partner, and the presence of STD symptoms.
- The adolescent must be provided the opportunity to be interviewed confidentially without parent present in the examination room.
- Perform a genital examination to evaluate for signs of infection (see "Clinical Presentation" section).
  - In girls, evaluate for pelvic inflammatory disease (PID) (see Pelvic Inflammatory Disease chapter).
  - Visualization of purulent or mucopurulent endocervical discharge from the cervical os is diagnostic.
  - The swab test result is positive if yellow cervical exudate is visualized on a white cotton-tipped swab specimen.

LABORATORY TESTS

- The most sensitive test available for *C. trachomatis* and *N. gonorrhoeae* should be performed (see *Chlamydia trachomatis* Infections and *Neisseria gonorrhoeae* chapters in Diseases and Disorders [Section I]).
- Tests for *Trichomonas vaginalis,* bacterial vaginosis, and vulvovaginal candidiasis are done to rule out vaginitis (see Vaginitis chapter in Diseases and Disorders [Section I]).
- Additional tests may be done to rule out syphilis and human immunodeficiency virus (HIV) coinfection.
- Consider Gram stain of the endocervical mucous specimen to evaluate for an increased number of polymorphonuclear leukocytes. However, this test has not been standardized, has a low positive-predictive value, and is not available in many clinical settings.

TREATMENT

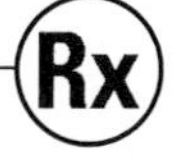

ACUTE GENERAL Rx

- Empirical treatment for *C. trachomatis* and *N. gonorrhoeae* infection is recommended by the Centers for Disease Control and Prevention (CDC) in populations at high risk for infection, treatment noncompliance, and poor follow-up, such as adolescents (see chapters on *Chlamydia trachomatis* Genital Infections and *Neisseria gonorrhoeae* Infections).
- The CDC recommends use of one of the following regimens for *C. trachomatis*:
  - Azithromycin, 1 g orally in a single dose *or*
  - Doxycycline, 100 mg orally given twice a day for 7 days
- The CDC recommends use of one of the following regimens for *N. gonorrhoeae* (plus treatment for *C. trachomatis*):
  - Cefixime, 400 mg orally in a single dose (limited availability) *or*
  - Ceftriaxone, 125 mg intramuscularly in a single dose* *or*
  - Ciprofloxacin, 500 mg orally in a single dose* *or*
  - Ofloxacin, 400 mg orally in a single dose* or
  - Levofloxacin, 250 mg orally in a single dose*

DISPOSITION

- Follow-up and management of sex partners should be appropriate for the identified or suspected STD (see *Chlamydia trachomatis* Infections and *Neisseria Gonorrhoeae* chapters in Diseases and Disorders [Section I]).
- Patients should return for diagnostic laboratory test results.
- Abstinence from sexual intercourse is recommended until therapy is completed.
- If symptoms persist after treatment, the patient should return for reevaluation. Relapse, reinfection, and nonmicrobiologic causes should be considered (e.g., inflamed zone of ectopy).
- Complications include the following:
  - PID and its sequelae (see Pelvic Inflammatory Disease chapter in Diseases and Disorders [Section I])
  - Chronic pelvic pain
  - Perihepatitis (i.e., Fitz-Hugh-Curtis syndrome)
  - Increased risk of HIV transmission and infection

REFERRAL

Gynecologic referral is recommended for persistent MPC.

PEARLS & CONSIDERATIONS

COMMENTS

- Providers need to perform a confidential sexual risk assessment for all adolescent patients.
- Providers should know state laws regarding minors' right to consent for confidential STD services.

*Because of the prevalence of quinolone-resistant *N. gonorrhoeae* [QRNG], quinolones should not be used for infections acquired in California, Asia, the Pacific islands, including Hawaii, and other areas such as England and Wales with increased prevalence, or in young men who have sex with men in the United States.

- HIV-infected patients should receive standard treatment.
- Counseling for STD prevention should be provided.

PREVENTION

- The most reliable way to avoid STD infection is to abstain from sexual intercourse (i.e., oral, vaginal, or anal sex) or to be in a long-term, mutually monogamous relationship with an uninfected partner.
- When used consistently and correctly, male latex condoms can reduce the risk of gonorrheal, chlamydial, and trichomonal infection.
- Vaginal spermicides containing nonoxynol-9 are not effective in preventing cervical gonorrhea, *Chlamydia*, or HIV infection.
- Contraceptive methods other than male or female condoms do not provide protection against STDs.

PATIENT/FAMILY EDUCATION

- Adolescent- and parent-appropriate STD information is available from several web sites (www.iwannaknow.org; www.itsyoursexlife.com; www.kidshealth.org).
- The American Social Health Association (ASHA) provides patient information brochures and online STD information (www.ashastd.org).
- Information can be obtained from the Centers for Disease Control and Prevention, Division of STD Prevention (www.cdc.gov/std/).
  - Disease facts and information: www.cdc.gov/nchstp/dstd/disease_info.htm
  - Personal health questions: www.cdc.gov/nchstp/dstd/personal_Health_Questions.htm
- Information brochures can be ordered from ETR Associates (www.pub.etr.org; 831-438-4060).
- Trained health professionals at the National STD Hotline (800-227-8922) are available to answer questions and provide referrals 24 hours each day, 7 days each week. All calls are private, personal, and confidential.

SUGGESTED READINGS

Alan Guttmacher Institute information on minors' rights to access STD services. Available at www.guttmacher.org/statecenter/spibs/spib_MASS.pdf/ Accessed January 24, 2005.

Bachmann LH et al: Measured versus self-reported compliance with doxycycline therapy for chlamydia-associated syndromes: high therapeutic success rates despite poor compliance. *Sex Transm Dis* 26:272, 1999.

Centers for Disease Control and Prevention: Sexually transmitted disease guidelines, 2002. *MMWR Morb Mortal Wkly Rep* 51(RR-6):32, 2002. Available at www.cdc.gov/STD/treatment/ Accessed January 24, 2005.

Falk L et al: Signs and symptoms of urethritis and cervicitis among women with or without *Mycoplasma genitalium* or *Chlamydia trachomatis* infection. *Sex Transm Infect* 81:73, 2005.

Holmes KK, Stamm WE: Lower genital tract infections in women. *In* Holmes KK et al (eds): *Sexually transmitted diseases,* 3rd ed. New York, McGraw-Hill, 1999, pp 761–782.

Lau CY et al: Azithromycin versus doxycycline for genital chlamydial infections: a meta-analysis of randomized clinical trials. *Sex Transm Dis* 29:497, 2002.

Magid D et al: Doxycycline compared with azithromycin for treating women with genital *Chlamydia trachomatis* infections: an incremental cost-effectiveness analysis. *Ann Intern Med* 124:389, 1996.

Tan HH et al: An open label comparative study of azithromycin and doxycycline in the treatment of non-gonococcal urethritis in males and *Chlamydia trachomatis* cervicitis in female sex workers in an STD clinic in Singapore. *Singapore Med J* 40:519, 1999.

Thorpe EM et al: Chlamydial cervicitis and urethritis: single dose treatment compared with doxycycline for seven days in community based practices. *Genitourin Med* 72:93, 1996.

AUTHORS: **GALE R. BURSTEIN, MD, MPH, SHERYL A. RYAN, MD,** and **KIMBERLY A. WORKOWSKI, MD, FACP**

BASIC INFORMATION

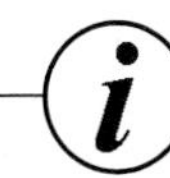

DEFINITION

Child physical abuse is the nonaccidental injury of a child. Many states add other factors to the legal definition, such as the age of the abuser and the nature of the injury. Injuries include bruises, lacerations, blunt trauma, fractures, head trauma, shaking, burns, and poisoning. Complex syndromes, such as pediatric falsification syndrome (Munchausen syndrome by proxy), may be included.

SYNONYMS

Abusive head trauma
Battered child syndrome
Child maltreatment
Shaken baby syndrome

ICD-9-CM CODES
995.50 General abuse
995.51 Emotional, psychological abuse
995.52 Neglect, nutritional abuse
995.53 Sexual abuse
995.54 Physical abuse
995.55 Shaken infant syndrome
995.59 Multiple forms of abuse
V codes may be added to indicate the perpetrator
V61.22 Parent
V62.83 Nonparent

EPIDEMIOLOGY & DEMOGRAPHICS

- Between 2000 and 2003, the annual rate of child physical abuse in the United States was 2.3 to 2.4 cases per 1000 children.
- Children are at highest risk of physical abuse during the first year of life.
- The rate of fatal child abuse in 2003 was 2.0 cases per 100,000 children, with 44% of these cases occurring in the first year of life.
- Child abuse is a complex psychosocial problem. Include characteristics of the caretaker and the child.
  - Caretaker risk factors include the following:
    - Being abused as a child
    - Domestic violence
    - Economic stress
    - Lack of social or emotional support
    - Low socioeconomic status
    - Poor impulse control
    - Single status
    - Substance abuse
    - Young age
  - Child risk factors include the following:
    - Attention deficit/hyperactivity disorder
    - Autism
    - Chronic medical condition
    - Colic
    - Developmental delay
    - Emotional problems
    - Physical disability
    - Prematurity

CLINICAL PRESENTATION

History

- There are a variety of possible clinical presentations of child abuse. Because suspicion of child abuse often begins when the history does not fit the medical findings, it is important for the medical provider to take a complete and detailed history as part of the medical evaluation.
- Infants who have been shaken often present with altered mental status, sometimes with significant respiratory and circulatory symptoms, including respiratory and cardiopulmonary arrest.
- The history is often vague.
  - Typical histories in severe cases include the caretaker having just fed the baby, noticing a choking spell with cyanosis that led to a 911 call.
  - Sometimes, the caretaker says the baby was accidentally dropped and stopped breathing, turned blue, or vomited.
  - Many babies that have been shaken or had some type of head injury present with more subtle signs and symptoms, such as fussiness, apparent feeding intolerance, or vomiting. These cases are initially missed and recognized when the infant returns with more significant symptoms, prompting head imaging.
- Older children (>1 year) often present with a history of an injury, such as falling from a bed or down stairs.
  - The diagnosis is made only if the medical provider recognizes that the injury is inconsistent with the history.
- Child victims of pediatric falsification syndrome (i.e., Munchausen syndrome by proxy) may present with a variety of symptoms.
  - Common presentations of this uncommon syndrome:
    - Apnea
    - Apparent life-threatening event (ALTE)
    - Fevers
    - Metabolic disturbances
    - Rashes
    - Seizures
    - Sepsis
    - Unusual bleeding reported in the child's emesis, urine, stool, or sputum
    - Vomiting
  - The perpetrator is most often the mother. It usually takes several interactions with the health care system for medical providers to suspect the mother is fabricating or causing the symptoms.
  - Once suspected, the diagnosis may be difficult to confirm.
- Signs and symptoms of child abuse
  - Bruises that are highly suspicious for child abuse include the following areas:
    - Abdomen
    - Bruise with a pattern
    - Cheeks
    - Chest
    - Ears
    - Genital or anal areas
    - Inner surfaces of arms and legs
    - Neck
  - The following types of burns in young children may indicate abuse:
    - Contact burns showing the shape of an object
    - Full-thickness burns
    - Immersion burns with a stocking-glove pattern
  - The following types of fractures are often caused by abuse:
    - Fracture in a nonambulatory child
    - Fracture inconsistent with the history provided
    - Metaphyseal fractures (i.e., corner, chip, or bucket-handle fractures)
    - Rib fractures
    - Scapular fractures
    - Sternum fractures
    - Vertebral body fractures
  - There are several types of head, eyes, ears, nose, and throat (HEENT) injuries:
    - Cuts or bruises in the mouth in a child with no teeth
    - Frenulum tears
    - Intracranial injury without a history of significant trauma or period of hypoxia
    - Retinal hemorrhages
    - Skull fracture from a short-distance or low-velocity fall
    - Subdural hematoma
  - Internal organ injuries in the absence of a high-velocity injury or long-distance fall may indicate abuse:
    - Duodenal hematoma
    - Esophageal or pharyngeal tear
    - Liver laceration
    - Mesenteric tear
    - Pancreatic injury
    - Pulmonary contusion
    - Splenic laceration
  - In shaken baby syndrome, the examiner may see some or all of the following:
    - Intracranial injury, usually a subdural hematoma
    - Metaphyseal fractures
    - Retinal hemorrhages
    - Rib fractures
- In cases of suspected child abuse, a complete physical examination should focus attention on the oropharynx, posterior aurielilar area, inner surfaces of extremities, external anal and genital areas.

ETIOLOGY

- The cause of child abuse is not completely understood.
- Sleep-deprived and stressed caretakers, especially those with the risk factors outlined previously, may hurt the infant or child.
- Mothers, boyfriends, and fathers are the most common perpetrators of child abuse, followed by other caretakers.

- It is unknown why some fatigued caretakers recognize their frustration with the infant or child and remain in control while others lose control and injure the child.

DIAGNOSIS

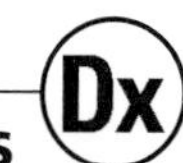

DIFFERENTIAL DIAGNOSIS

- The differential diagnosis of child abuse varies according to the age of the child and type of signs and symptoms present.
- Careful history, physical examination, and appropriate laboratory and radiographic studies can rule out most unusual entities:
  - Bruises differential:
    - Birthmarks, coagulation factor deficiencies, Ehlers-Danlos syndrome, Henoch-Schönlein purpura, Phytophotodermatitis, Rocky Mountain spotted fever, sepsis with disseminated intravascular coagulation, syphilis, Thrombocytopenia, Traditional healing practices (e.g., coining), vitamin K deficiency, von Willebrand syndrome.
  - Burns differential:
    - Bullous impetigo, cellulitis, diaper dermatitis, epidermolysis bullosa, Erysipelas, herpes simplex infection, staphylococcal scaled skin syndrome, traditional healing (e.g., cupping).
  - Fractures differential:
    - Accidental trauma, Caffey's disease, hyperparathyroidism, Jansen-type metaphyseal dysostosis, malignancy, Menkes' syndrome, osteogenesis imperfecta, ricketts, Schmidt and Schmidt-like metaphyseal chondroplasia, scurvy, syphilis, Toxicity from medications (e.g., methotrexate).
  - Subdural hematomas:
    - Accidental trauma, coagulation disorder, glutaric aciduria.

WORKUP

- The radiographic and laboratory studies recommended vary with the type of abuse and age of the child, but there are some general guidelines:
  - Children younger than 1 year usually should have a skeletal survey, retinal examination (by an ophthalmologist), and head imaging study (i.e., computed tomography [CT] or magnetic resonance imaging [MRI]).
  - If bruises or bleeding are present, a coagulation evaluation is appropriate.
- For all children suspected of being significantly physically abused, a trauma evaluation should be done.
  - Laboratory studies and radiographs are appropriate for the type of trauma suspected and may include the studies mentioned earlier with the addition of studies such as chest or abdominal CT and laboratory tests to evaluate the possibility of injury to internal organs such as liver function screening, amylase and lipase levels, and urinalysis.
- Additional studies may be appropriate. In cases of pediatric falsification syndrome, toxicology testing, careful observation by medical staff, and even covert video surveillance may be necessary to make the diagnosis.

LABORATORY TESTS

- The laboratory tests recommended depend on the clinical presentation.
- A complete blood cell count, coagulation studies, and urinalysis are recommended.

IMAGING STUDIES

Specific recommendations for imaging studies depend on the clinical presentation and the age of the child, but there are general guidelines:

- Birth to 12 months
  - Head imaging study (CT or MRI)
  - Skeletal survey (may need to repeat in 14 days)
- 12 to 24 months
  - Skeletal survey (may need to repeat in 14 days) *or*
  - Scintigraphy or bone scan (depends on timing and services available)
- 2 to 5 years
  - Skeletal survey or scintigraphy in selected cases
  - Radiographs as clinically indicated
- 5 years and older
  - Radiographs as clinically indicated

TREATMENT

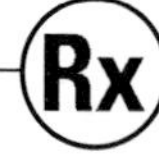

NONPHARMACOLOGIC THERAPY

- Children must be placed in a safe environment.
- Treatment may include age-appropriate counseling for the child and counseling for the parent, parenting classes, and monitoring the family.
- The criminal justice system has a role in cases when a crime has been committed.

ACUTE GENERAL Rx

Treatment depends on the child's injuries.

CHRONIC Rx

Treatment depends on the child's injuries.

DISPOSITION

- Abused children often require hospital admission for initial evaluation and treatment.
- Disposition depends on input from the medical team, but it is usually determined by appropriate child protection and social service agencies and by the Family Court System.

REFERRAL

- A team of consultants, such as a child neurologist, neurosurgeon, neuroradiologist, pediatric orthopedic surgeon, pediatric ophthalmologist, pediatric radiologist, pediatric hematologist, genetic or metabolic specialist, and pediatric radiologist, may be consulted in complex cases.
- The child abuse specialist may have several roles:
  - To determine which consultants to involve
  - To coordinate and organize medical information
  - To communicate with child protective and law enforcement agencies
- Abused children may need long-term follow-up for their medical and mental health issues, and they may require involvement of social service agencies.

PEARLS & CONSIDERATIONS

COMMENTS

- Child abuse is a complex problem that requires cooperation among medical, social service, and legal agencies.
- The medical aspects of child abuse are sufficiently complex that consultation with a child abuse specialist should be considered.

PREVENTION

- Refer new parents for appropriate counseling and instruction about dealing with the stress of caring for infants and the danger of shaking a baby.
- Screen for family violence in the primary health care setting.
- Report suspected abuse; most abuse-related child fatalities had prior social or safety concerns.

PATIENT/FAMILY EDUCATION

More information is available from the Children's Advocate, Action Alliance of Children (www.4children.org), the National Center on Shaken Baby Syndrome (www.dontshake.com), the National Conference on Shaken Baby Syndrome (www.shakenbaby.com), and the National Shaken Baby Syndrome Campaign (www.preventchildabuse.com).

SUGGESTED READINGS

American Medical Association: *International Classification of Diseases, 9th rev, clinical modification,* vol 2. Chicago, AMA Press, 2003, p 8.

Child Abuse Provider. Available at www.ChildAbuseMD.com

Jenny C et al: Analysis of missed cases of abusive head trauma. *JAMA* 281:621, 1999.

Nimkin K, Kleinman PK: Imaging of child abuse. *Radiol Clin North Am* 39:843, 2001.

Reece RM, Ludwig S: *Child Abuse Medical Diagnosis and Management,* 2nd ed. Philadelphia, Lippincott Williams & Wilkins, 2001.

US Department of Health and Human Services, Administration on Children, Youth, and Families: *Child Maltreatment 2003.* Washington, DC, U.S., Government Printing Office, 2005.

AUTHOR: **ANN M. LENANE, MD**

BASIC INFORMATION

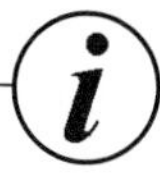

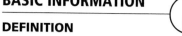

DEFINITION

Chlamydia trachomatis is a sexually transmitted infection caused by an obligate intracellular parasite.

SYNONYM

Chlamydia

ICD-9-CM CODES

099.5 *Chlamydia trachomatis* venereal disease

099.41 *Chlamydia trachomatis* urethritis

EPIDEMIOLOGY & DEMOGRAPHICS

- *C. trachomatis* infections are the most common bacterial sexually transmitted diseases (STDs) occurring during adolescence.
- Sexual abuse is a consideration for transmission in girls 12 years old or younger.
- The disease is asymptomatic in boys and girls in many cases.
- Reported rates of infection are highest among African Americans compared with white non-Hispanic and Hispanic adolescents.
- Reported rates of infection are higher among girls than boys. Higher rates among girls may reflect more screening and diagnostic testing of girls than boys.
- High positivity rates have been found for adolescent patients in diverse health settings, including public health and private practice office settings.

CLINICAL PRESENTATION

History

- Most *Chlamydia*-infected adolescents have no symptoms of genital or rectal infection.
- History may include the following:
  - Mucopurulent cervicitis (MPC), including vaginal discharge or pruritus, irregular vaginal bleeding, and dyspareunia (see Cervicitis in Diseases and Disorders [Section I])
  - Urethritis, including urethral discharge or pruritus, dysuria, urinary frequency, and burning with urination (see Urethritis in Diseases and Disorders [Section I])
  - Endometritis or salpingitis, including lower abdominal pain (see Pelvic Inflammatory Disease in Diseases and Disorders [Section I])
  - Proctitis, including anorectal pain, tenesmus, and rectal discharge
  - Neonatal conjunctivitis, which typically manifests in the second week of life as a result of vertical transmission
  - Newborn child with pneumonitis presenting in the 3rd to 16th week of life with afebrile cough, difficulty breathing, or tachypnea

Physical Examination

- Signs of MPC, such as mucopurulent cervical discharge and cervical friability (see Cervicitis in Diseases and Disorders [Section I])
- Signs of urethritis, including mucoid or purulent urethral discharge (see Urethritis in Diseases and Disorders [Section I])
- Signs of endometritis or salpingitis, including cervical motion, adnexal, and uterine tenderness (see Pelvic Inflammatory Disease in Diseases and Disorders [Section I])
- Signs of proctitis, including rectal discharge and rectal examination tenderness
- Signs of conjunctivitis, including conjunctival erythema and discharge
- Signs of pneumonitis, including tachypnea, cough, rales, wheezing, and respiratory distress, typically afebrile

ETIOLOGY

- A sexually transmitted infection during adolescence
- Vertical transmission from mother to newborn during passage through infected cervix

DIAGNOSIS

Dx

DIFFERENTIAL DIAGNOSIS

- Genital infection by another sexually transmitted pathogen, especially *Neisseria gonorrhoeae* and herpes simplex virus (see Cervicitis and Urethritis in Diseases and Disorders [Section I])
- Vaginal foreign body
- Other infectious and inflammatory causes of proctitis
- Differential diagnosis for conjunctivitis in the perinatal period: *N. gonorrhoeae*; other bacteria, such as *Staphylococcus* or *Streptococcus* species; chemical conjunctivitis in reaction to silver nitrate drops
- Differential diagnosis for pneumonia for infants of infected mothers: other bacteria and viruses

WORKUP

- Obtain confidential sexual history, including questions about sexual activity, a new sex partner, the lifetime number of sex partners, possible exposure to an STD-infected partner, and presence of STD symptoms.
- The adolescent must be provided the opportunity to be interviewed confidentially without parent present.
- Perform a genital examination to evaluate for signs of infection:
  - In girls and young women, evaluate for pelvic inflammatory disease (PID).
  - In young men who have sex with men, evaluate for signs of proctitis.

LABORATORY TESTS

- Nucleic acid amplification test (NAAT) is the most sensitive (85% to 95%) *C. trachomatis* diagnostic laboratory test (Table 1-7):
  - NAAT can be performed on cervical, urethral, vaginal, or urine specimens, but the manufacturer's instructions must be consulted for the specimen type approved for use. Table 1-4 describes available amplification tests and approved specimen types.
- Cell culture for *C. trachomatis*:
  - Cervical, urethral, conjunctival, and rectal specimens can be cultured.
  - Previously the gold standard, this test is technically cumbersome and costly, with relatively low sensitivity.
- Nonculture chlamydial tests:
  - Cervical and urethral specimens.
  - These tests are less sensitive than NAAT.
  - Several types of tests are available:
    - Enzyme immunoassay
    - Direct fluorescent antibody
    - DNA probe (Pace 2C System for *C. trachomatis* [Gen-Probe, San Diego, CA])
- The most sensitive test for *C. trachomatis* should be performed if available and affordable.
- Urine leukesterase test on first-void urine and serologic tests are not recommended for screening or diagnosis of *C. trachomatis* because of poor test performance.
- Tests for *Trichomonas vaginalis* and bacterial vaginosis should be performed to rule out vaginitis coinfection.
- The test for gonorrheal genital infection and the serologic test for syphilis should be considered because of the risk of coinfection.
- Human immunodeficiency virus (HIV) antibody test should be offered because of the risk of coinfection.

TABLE 1-7 Licensed Amplification Tests for *Chlamydia Trachomatis*

Test Type	Brand Name	Manufacturer	Specimen Type
Polymerase chain reaction (PCR)	AMPLICOR CT/NG Test	Roche Molecular System (Branchburg, NJ)	Cervical, urethral, first-void urine
Strand displacement amplification (SDA)	BD Probe-Tec ET CT/GC Test	Becton Dickenson (Sparks, MD)	Cervical, urethral, first-void urine
Transcription medicated amplification (TMA)	APTIMA Combo 2 Assay	Gen-Probe (San Diego, CA)	Cervical, urethral, first-void urine, vaginal swab*
Signal amplification assay	Hybrid Capture 2 CT/GC Test	Digene (Gaithersburg, MD)	Cervical

*Patient-collected vaginal swab specimens are an option for screening women when a pelvic exam is not otherwise indicated. The vaginal swab specimen collection kit is not for home use.

TREATMENT

ACUTE GENERAL Rx

- The Centers for Disease Control and Prevention (CDC) recommends use of one of the following standard regimens for uncomplicated genital chlamydial infection:
  - Azithromycin, 1 g orally in a single dose *or*
  - Doxycycline, 100 mg orally twice a day for 7 days
- The CDC recommends use of one of the following alternative regimens for uncomplicated genital chlamydial infection:
  - Erythromycin base, 500 mg orally four times each day for 7 days *or*
  - Erythromycin ethylsuccinate, 800 mg orally four times each day for 7 days *or*
  - Ofloxacin, 300 mg orally twice each day for 7 days *or*
  - Levofloxacin, 500 mg orally for 7 days
- The CDC recommends use of one of the following regimens in pregnancy:
  - Erythromycin base, 500 mg orally four times each day for 7 days *or*
  - Amoxicillin, 500 mg orally three times each day for 7 days
  - Alternative regimens during pregnancy include azithromycin (1 g PO in a single dose). Although azithromycin safety and efficacy in pregnant and lactating women is not established, preliminary data indicate that it may be safe and effective.
- Indications for children include:
  - Weight less than 45 kg: erythromycin base or ethylsuccinate, 50 mg/kg/day orally, divided into four doses daily for 10 to 14 days
  - Weight 45 kg or more but age younger than 8 years: azithromycin, 1g orally in a single dose
  - Age 8 years or older: azithromycin, 1g orally in a single dose, or doxycycline, 100 mg orally twice each day for 7 days
- Indications for infants include:
  - Ophthalmia neonatorum: erythromycin base or ethylsuccinate, 50 mg/kg/day orally, divided into four doses daily for 14 days (Because of the strong association between erythromycin and a subsequent increased incidence of infantile hypertrophic pyloric stenosis, monitoring at delivery rather than prophylactic treatment is recommended for infants born to women with known *C. trachomatis* infection.)
  - Infant pneumonia caused by *C. trachomatis*: erythromycin base or ethylsuccinate, 50 mg/kg/day orally, divided in four doses daily for 14 days

DISPOSITION

- Rescreening for repeat genital tract infection 3 to 4 months after treatment is recommended for adolescents.
- "Test of cure" 3 weeks after treatment with doxycycline or azithromycin therapy is not recommended.
- Management of sex partners:
  - Notification, examination, and treatment of sex partners are essential.
  - Partner notification often becomes the provider or patient's responsibility because of a lack of resources at health departments.
- Complications can include the following:
  - Pelvic inflammatory disease and its sequelae, chronic pelvic pain and perihepatitis (i.e., Fitz-Hugh-Curtis syndrome) in female patients
  - Epididymitis in male patients
  - Reiter's syndrome and increased risk of HIV transmission and infection
  - Proctitis in male patients engaging in anal intercourse
  - Conjunctivitis from autoinoculation and vertically transmitted infection
  - Pneumonitis in infants from vertically transmitted infection

REFERRAL

- Ensure that cases of reportable STDs that you diagnose are reported to the health department.
- Reporting may initiate a referral to a health department disease intervention specialist, who can assist patients in obtaining treatment and counseling and notification of sex partners for clinical evaluation referral.

PEARLS & CONSIDERATIONS

COMMENTS

- Providers need to perform a confidential sexual risk assessment on all adolescent patients.
- Providers need to know state laws regarding minors' rights to consent for confidential STD services.
- *Chlamydia* treatment for patients who are HIV infected or have other causes of immunocompromise is the same as for immunocompetent persons.
- Monitor for evidence of *Chlamydia* infection in infants born to *Chlamydia*-infected mothers.
- Consider child abuse in a young adolescent or prepubertal child.
- Any change in menses (i.e., heavier or lighter menstrual flow, worse cramping, or a change in the timing of menses, occurring earlier or later in the expected cycle) may indicate STD infection in the sexually active girl and should prompt the clinician to perform STD screening tests.

PREVENTION

- The most reliable way to avoid an STD infection is to abstain from sexual intercourse (i.e., oral, vaginal, or anal sex) or to be in a long-term, mutually monogamous relationship with an uninfected partner.
- When used consistently and correctly, male latex condoms can reduce risk of STDs.
- Vaginal spermicides containing nonoxynol-9 are not effective in preventing cervical gonorrheal, chlamydial, or HIV infection.
- Contraceptive methods other than male or female condoms do not provide protection against STDs.

PATIENT/FAMILY EDUCATION

- Adolescent and parent-appropriate STD information is available from several web sites (www.iwannaknow.org; www.itsyoursexlife.com; www.kidshealth.org).
- The American Social Health Association (ASHA) provides patient information brochures and online STD information (www.ashastd.org).
- STD information is available from the Centers for Disease Control and Prevention, Division of STD Prevention (www.cdc.gov/std/).
- Disease facts and information and answers to personal health questions are available from other CDC web sites (www.cdc.gov/nchstp/dstd/disease_info.htm; www.cdc.gov/nchstp/dstd/personal_Health_Questions.htm).
- Patient information brochures are provided by ETR Associates (pubetr.org; 831-438-4060).
- Patients can access the National STD Hotline (800-227-8922), and trained health professionals are available to answer questions and provide referrals 24 hours each day, 7 days each week. All calls are private, personal, and confidential.

SUGGESTED READINGS

Alan Guttmacher Institute information on minors' rights to access STD services. Available at www.guttmacher.org/statecenter/spibs/spib_MASS.pdf/ Accessed January 24, 2005.

American Academy of Pediatrics. Chlamydial infections. *In* Pickering LK, Baker CJ, Long SS, McMillan JA (eds): *Red Book: 2006 Report of the committee on infections Diseases,* 27th ed. Elk Grove Village, IL, American Academy of Pediatrics, 2006, pp 249–251.

Burstein GR et al: Sexually transmitted disease screening practices and diagnosed infections in a large managed care organization. *Sex Transm Dis* 28:477, 2001.

California STD/HIV Prevention Training Center Online *Chlamydia* Course and Tool-kits. Available at www.stdhivtraining.org/educ/training_module/tools.html/ Accessed January 24, 2005.

Centers for Disease Control and Prevention: Sexually transmitted disease guidelines, 2002. *MMWR Morb Mortal Wkly Rep* 51(RR-6):32, 2002. Available at www.cdc.gov/STD/treatment/ Accessed January 24, 2005.

Geisler WM et al: Epidemiological and genetic correlates of incident *Chlamydia trachomatis* infection in North American adolescents. *J Infect Dis* 190:1723, 2004.

Hollblad-Fadiman K et al: American College of Preventive Medicine practice policy statement: Screening for *Chlamydia trachomatis. Am J Prev Med* 24:287, 2003.

Massachusetts STD/HIV Prevention Training Center Online *Chlamydia* Course and Tool-kits. Available at http://www.mass.gov/dph/cdc/std/guidelines/chlamydia_toolkit.pdf/ Accessed January 24, 2005.

Peipert JF: Genital chlamydial infections. *N Engl J Med* 349:2424, 2003.

Stamm WE: *Chlamydia trachomatis*—the persistent pathogen: Thomas Parran award lecture. *Sex Transm Dis* 28:684, 2001.

AUTHORS: **GALE R. BURSTEIN, MD, MPH, SHERYL A. RYAN, MD,** and **KIMBERLY A. WORKOWSKI, MD, FACP**

BASIC INFORMATION

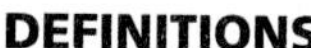
 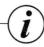

DEFINITIONS

Gallstones (i.e., cholelithiasis) are made of various combinations of cholesterol, calcium salts, and protein. Stones may be found in the gallbladder or in the cystic, common, or intrahepatic bile ducts. Cholecystitis, or inflammation of the gallbladder, may be chronic or acute, acalculous or result from obstruction caused by stones in the neck of the gallbladder or in the cystic or common bile duct. Hydrops of the gallbladder is acute distention without gallstones or inflammation. Choledochal cysts are congenital cystic dilations of the extrahepatic biliary tract. Cholangitis is inflammation or infection of the bile ducts.

SYNONYMS

Choledocholithiasis (common duct stones, usually seen with gallstones)
Gallbladder stones
Gallstones

ICD-9-CM CODES
574.2 Cholelithiasis
574.5 Choledocholithiasis
575.10 Cholecystitis
576.1 Cholangitis
751.69 Choledochal cyst
782.3 Hydrops

EPIDEMIOLOGY & DEMOGRAPHICS

- Cholelithiasis is often seen with underlying conditions.
  - Black pigment stones are associated with the following conditions:
    - Congenital heart disease
    - Gastrointestinal disorders
    - Hemolytic diseases (40% to 50%)
    - Hepatobiliary diseases
    - Malabsorption, ileal diseases, previous intestinal resection
    - Necrotizing enterocolitis
    - Sepsis
    - Serious medical illness with biliary stasis
    - Total parenteral nutrition (TPN) in premature infants or chronic TPN in older patients
  - Brown pigment stones are seen predominantly in Asia. They are associated with infections and more likely to form in cystic duct than gallbladder.
  - Cholesterol stones are usually associated with obesity and pregnancy.
- Spontaneous resolution of stones in infants has been reported.
- Obese female patients with a family history of gallstones are more likely to have cholesterol stones.
  - Small bile acid pool size is related to and may be causative in cholesterol stone development.
  - The Pima Indian population has a very high incidence of gallstones.
- Between 10% and 15% of patients with cholelithiasis will develop pancreatitis.
- Cholecystitis in children is often chronic and may not be a complication of cholelithiasis.
- Choledochal cysts occur in 1 of 13,000 to 15,000 people.
  - Females outnumber males.
  - Two thirds of patients present before 10 years of age.
- Primary sclerosing cholangitis is a rare, progressive disorder with inflammation and fibrosis of the biliary duct and eventual cirrhosis. (This is not further discussed here.)

CLINICAL PRESENTATION

History

- Cholelithiasis
  - Usually asymptomatic
  - Colicky, recurrent abdominal pain
  - Right upper quadrant abdominal pain
  - Irritability in infants
  - Jaundice
  - Acholic stools
  - Fatty food intolerance
  - Personal history positive for hemolytic anemia, malabsorption or bowel stasis, or systemic illness
  - Family history positive for gallstones, especially in obese female patients with no other predisposing factors
  - Pregnancy or recent childbirth
- Cholecystitis
  - Right upper quadrant pain
  - Nausea, vomiting
  - Fever
  - In chronic cholecystitis, possible intolerance to fatty foods
- Hydrops of the gallbladder
  - Crampy abdominal pain
  - Nausea, vomiting
  - Fever
  - Jaundice
- Choledochal cyst
  - Acholic stools
  - Jaundice
  - Epigastric or right-sided abdominal pain
  - Vomiting
  - Failure to thrive
  - Irritability

Physical Examination

- Cholelithiasis
  - Physical examination usually normal.
  - Jaundice occurs if there is obstruction or hemolysis.
  - Tender right upper quadrant may be appreciated, especially if infection is present.
  - Obesity is a factor.
- Cholecystitis
  - Shallow breathing.
  - Tenderness or a mass is detected in the right upper quadrant.
  - Positive Murphy's sign. The inflamed gallbladder is palpated by pressing the fingers under the rib cage; deep inspiration causes pain when the gallbladder is forced down to touch the fingers.
  - Jaundice is possible.
  - The patient may have fever.
- Hydrops of the gallbladder
  - A distended gallbladder may be palpable.
- Choledochal cyst
  - Infants often present with jaundice.
  - Hepatomegaly.
  - Less than one third of patients have a palpable abdominal mass.
  - The classic triad of abdominal pain, jaundice, and a palpable mass is seen in less than 20% of patients.
  - Portal hypertension and ascites may be found in the presence of underlying cirrhosis from chronic obstruction.

ETIOLOGY

- Two major classifications of cholelithiasis—predominantly pigment stones and predominantly cholesterol stones.
- Pigment stones are found in 70% to 80% of pediatric cases.
  - Black pigment stones are predominantly composed of pigment polymer and calcium salts, with less than 10% cholesterol.
    - Found in patients with hemolytic diseases
    - Develop in up to 60% of patients with sickle cell disease
  - Brown pigment stones are predominately composed of calcium bilirubinate, calcium fatty acid soaps, and up to 30% cholesterol (more calcium and more cholesterol than in black pigment stones).
    - Stone formation is associated with infections, especially with *Escherichia coli* or other β-glucuronidase–producing strains.
    - Cholelithiasis is reported more often in Asia.
  - Cholesterol stones are found in 15% of pediatric patients with cholelithiasis.
    - Content generally more than 50% cholesterol
    - Caused by a relative imbalance of too little bile salt and lecithin with too much cholesterol
  - Other or unknown types affect 10% to 20% of the Asian population.
- Acalculous cholecystitis is uncommon.
  - Associated with infection or other systemic illness:
    - Streptococci: groups A and B
    - Gram-negative organisms: *E. coli, Salmonella, Shigella*
    - *Leptospira interrogans*
    - Parasites: ascaris, *Giardia*
  - May be associated with trauma.
  - Associated with systemic vasculitis: Kawasaki disease, periarteritis nodosa, and others.
- Cholecystitis may result from obstruction by gallstones (i.e., calculous cholecystitis) in the neck of the gallbladder or in the cystic or common bile duct.
- Hydrops of the gallbladder may be temporally associated with infections such as

scarlet fever and leptospirosis and with Kawasaki disease.
- The cause of choledochal cyst is unknown.

DIAGNOSIS

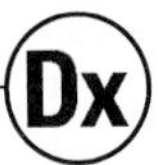

DIFFERENTIAL DIAGNOSIS

Aside from differentiating the various disorders from each other, the differential diagnosis for right upper quadrant pain and jaundice includes other liver and biliary tract diseases and other abdominal processes:

- Acute gastroenteritis
- Biliary atresia, paucity of bile ducts (e.g., syndromic, nonsyndromic)
- Biliary duct obstruction (e.g., idiopathic, post-traumatic, pancreatic compression)
- Caroli's disease
- Cirrhosis
- Fitz-Hugh-Curtis syndrome (i.e., perihepatitis associated with sexually transmitted pelvic inflammatory disease)
- Hepatitis
- Hepatocellular tumor, other primary or metastatic liver tumors
- Peptic ulcer disease
- Pneumonia or empyema

LABORATORY TESTS

- Mildly elevated levels of bilirubin, alkaline phosphatase, and transaminases are common with symptomatic stones, cholecystitis, and choledochal cysts.
- Complete blood cell count demonstrates leukocytosis with cholecystitis.

IMAGING STUDIES

- Ultrasound is the single best test for helping to define gallbladder and bile duct abnormalities.
  - Stones are easily visualized, with and without dilation of the bile ducts; ultrasound is the most sensitive and specific test for cholelithiasis and bile duct dilatation.
  - A thick-walled gallbladder is seen with cholecystitis.
  - Ultrasound confirms a large gallbladder in hydrops.
  - Choledochal cysts are easily visualized.
- Inability to visualize the gallbladder with hepatobiliary scintigraphy suggests acute cholecystitis.
- A cholangiogram (usually endoscopic retrograde cholangiopancreatography [ERCP]) is often used to localize an obstruction and stones and to define the anatomy and extent of cysts. Stones in the common bile duct can be removed endoscopically.

TREATMENT

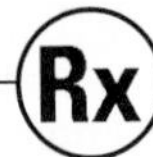

NONPHARMACOLOGIC THERAPY

- Patients with symptomatic cholelithiasis and cholecystitis usually require cholecystectomy.
  - Performance of non-emergent cholecystectomy is encouraged.
  - Morbidity and mortality are higher with emergent than with elective surgery.
  - Most procedures can be done laparoscopically.
- Children with stones from an underlying hemolytic disorder (e.g., sickle cell disease) should undergo cholecystectomy, even if they are asymptomatic.
  - Risk of developing symptomatic stones is high in this population.
- Patients with asymptomatic stones or hydrops may not need surgery.
  - Treatment of the underlying disease usually leads to resolution of hydrops of the gallbladder.
  - If stones become symptomatic, cholecystectomy is indicated.
- A choledochal cyst requires excision.
  - Roux-en-Y hepaticojejunostomy is usually done.
  - The abnormal ducts may have malignant potential.

ACUTE GENERAL Rx

- The treatment for most gallbladder disease in children is surgery.
- Lithotripsy or dissolution therapy can be tried for those at high surgical risk.
  - Dissolution therapy is not effective with pigment stones.
- Antibiotic coverage, especially for acalculous cholecystitis, is recommended. Use piperacillin plus an aminoglycoside *or* Unasyn.
- Anti-inflammatory therapy for the primary disorder presumably resolves noninfectious forms of acalculous cholecystitis.

DISPOSITION

Patients with underlying disorders need to be followed closely for complications and for recurrences.

REFERRAL

- Involvement of a pediatric gastroenterologist is imperative.
- Surgeons need to be consulted for cholecystectomy or choledochal cyst excision and repair.

PEARLS & CONSIDERATIONS

COMMENTS

- Gallbladder disease is uncommon in children but should be considered in the appropriate clinical setting.
- Ultrasound is the diagnostic screening test of choice for gallbladder disease.
- The pathogenesis of cholelithiasis in pediatrics is evolving; a smaller percentage of stones is related to hemolysis.

PREVENTION

- Cholecystectomy should be performed in patients with hemolytic diseases and stones before symptoms or cholecystitis occur.
- Encourage maintenance of appropriate weight, especially in postpartum adolescents with a positive family history.

SUGGESTED READINGS

Heubi JE et al: Diseases of the gallbladder in infancy, childhood, and adolescence. *In* Such FJ et al (eds): *Liver Disease in Children.* Philadelphia, Lippincott Williams & Wilkins, 2001.

McEvoy C, Suchy F: Biliary tract disease in children. *Pediatr Clin North Am* 43:75, 1996.

Miyano T, Yamataka A: Choledochal cysts. *Curr Opin Pediatr* 9:283, 1997.

Shaffer EA: Gallbladder disease. *In* Walker WA et al (eds): *Pediatric Gastrointestinal Disease: Pathophysiology, Diagnosis, Management,* 3rd ed. Philadelphia, BC Decker, 2000.

AUTHOR: **LYNN C. GARFUNKEL, MD**

BASIC INFORMATION

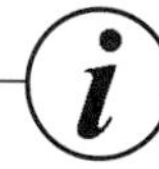

DEFINITION

Chronic fatigue syndrome (CFS) is profound fatigue of more than 6 months' duration that causes significant functional disability and that remains unexplained after a comprehensive medical and psychological evaluation. The 1994 revised Centers for Disease Control and Prevention case definition allows the coexistence of nonmelancholic depression and anxiety disorders and requires a minimum of four additional physical symptoms.

SYNONYMS

Akureyri disease
Chronic Epstein-Barr virus syndrome
Chronic fatigue and immune dysfunction syndrome
Myalgic encephalomyelitis
Neuromyasthenia
Postviral fatigue syndrome
Royal free disease

ICD-9-CM CODE
780.71 Chronic fatigue syndrome

EPIDEMIOLOGY & DEMOGRAPHICS

- Scant pediatric data exist.
- Adult population-based studies estimate the prevalence of CFS-like illness at 200 to 2800 cases per 100,000 people, with a 3:1 female-to-male ratio.
- CFS appears to be rare in childhood, with increasing prevalence in adolescence, which is estimated at 23 to 116 cases per 100,000, with a 2.5:1 female-to-male ratio.
- Studies in referred populations suggest that CFS is increased in the white population, with no consistent trend in socioeconomic status.

CLINICAL PRESENTATION

- In approximately two thirds of cases, onset follows an apparent acute viral illness; one third of cases develop insidiously.
- The clinical course is persistent in approximately one half of cases and intermittent in the other half, with remissions and relapses of several months' duration.
- In addition to profound, disabling fatigue, common symptoms include, in descending order, exercise intolerance, sore throat, difficulty concentrating, insomnia, hypersomnia, myalgia, generalized weakness, and arthralgia.
- Functional disability usually impairs all spheres of activity, and decreased school performance and marked absenteeism are often dramatic.
- Results of the initial examination are generally unremarkable.
- Growth and development, as well as pubertal progression, are unaffected.
- Although common in adults with CFS, more than a few fibromyalgia tender points are not usually found in adolescents.
- Despite the reported sensation of cervical adenopathy and sore throat, otolaryngologic examination results usually are normal.
- Supine-to-standing blood pressure measurements usually do not reveal significant orthostatic changes.
- The mental status examination is normal.

ETIOLOGY

- The cause of CFS is unknown.
- Prominent theories include the following:
  - Persistent, latent viral infection
  - Subtle immune system activation
  - Orthostatic intolerance
  - Impairment of the hypothalamic-pituitary-adrenal axis
  - Sleep disorder
  - Atypical depression
  - Somatoform disorder

DIAGNOSIS

Dx

DIFFERENTIAL DIAGNOSIS

- The revised case definition of the International Chronic Fatigue Syndrome Study Group (1994) calls for clinically evaluated, unexplained, persistent, or relapsing fatigue that meets the following criteria:
  - Of new or definite onset
  - Associated with a substantial reduction in previous levels of occupational, educational, social, or personal activities
  - Not the result of ongoing exertion
  - Not substantially reduced by bed rest
- Concurrent occurrence of four or more of the following symptoms, all of which must have persisted or recurred for at least 6 months and must not have predated the fatigue:
  - Substantially impaired short-term memory or concentration
  - Sore throat
  - Tender cervical or axillary adenopathy
  - Myalgias
  - Polyarthralgias
  - Headache of a new type, pattern, or severity
  - Unrefreshing sleep
  - Postexertional malaise lasting longer than 24 hours
- The following conditions exclude an individual from the diagnosis:
  - Any active medical condition that may explain symptoms
  - Any past or current diagnosis of a major depressive disorder with psychotic or melancholic features, bipolar affective disorders, schizophrenia, delusional disorders, dementias, anorexia nervosa, and bulimia nervosa
  - Alcohol or substance abuse
  - Severe obesity
- Any condition defined primarily by symptoms that cannot be confirmed by laboratory tests, including the following, do not exclude the diagnosis:
  - Anxiety disorders
  - Fibromyalgia
  - Multiple chemical sensitivity disorder
  - Neurasthenia
  - Nonpsychotic or nonmelancholic depression
  - Somatoform disorders
- The differential diagnosis includes the following diseases and conditions:
  - Occult systemic disease (e.g., cardiopulmonary disorder, hypothyroidism, Addison's disease, connective tissue disease, neoplasm, renal failure, inflammatory bowel disease)
  - Significant psychosocial stress in family, peer, school, or community relationships
  - Depression, anxiety, or somatoform disorder
  - Drug or alcohol abuse
  - Sleep disorder
  - Malingering (appears to be unusual)

WORKUP

- Conduct a comprehensive history, review of systems, and physical examination.
- Obtain a confidential psychosocial history from the adolescent and parent separately.

LABORATORY TESTS

- Complete a selected laboratory evaluation, including a complete blood cell count and determinations of acute-phase reactant, thyroid-stimulating hormone, electrolytes, blood urea nitrogen, creatinine, lactate dehydrogenase, alanine aminotransferase (ALT), aspartate aminotransferase (AST), and urinalysis.
- Unless specifically suggested by the history and physical examination, other laboratory studies, such as antinuclear antibodies, viral titers, immunoglobulins, and cortisol, are rarely useful in establishing the diagnosis of CFS in adolescence.
- Cardiovascular tilt-table testing may be useful in patients with symptoms suggesting orthostatic intolerance.

TREATMENT

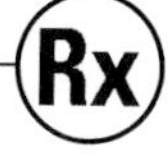

NONPHARMACOLOGIC THERAPY

- Cognitive-behavioral therapy may improve coping and decrease functional disability.
- Sleep hygiene (i.e., routine, consistent sleep rituals) to minimize napping and normalize sleep-wake cycles is important.
- A graduated exercise program may enhance the activity level.
- A gradual return to normal activity and school attendance is indicated.

ACUTE GENERAL Rx

- Analgesics and anti-inflammatory agents may be useful for headache, arthralgia, and myalgia.
- Salt, mineralocorticoids, peripheral vasoconstrictors, and selective serotonin reuptake inhibitors may ameliorate symptoms of orthostatic intolerance.
- Antidepressants may be indicated for associated anxiety and depression.

CHRONIC Rx

Continue the therapies discussed in the "Acute General Rx" section.

DISPOSITION

- Treatment should be aimed at target symptoms.
- Regular follow-up is needed to monitor functional status and promote a return to normal activity.

REFERRAL

- Unless there is evidence of a specific disorder, multiple medical subspecialty consultations are rarely useful.
- With symptoms suggesting orthostatic intolerance, a cardiology consultation may be useful.
- With significant functional disability and associated anxiety or depressive symptoms, a mental health consultation is indicated.

PEARLS & CONSIDERATIONS

COMMENTS

- Although fatigue is a common complaint of patients with anxiety and depression, many adolescents with CFS do not meet the criteria for psychiatric disorders.
- When present with CFS, it may be difficult to ascertain whether anxiety and depression are primary or secondary conditions.
- Many adolescents with CFS and their parents believe that the disorder is often not validated by others as a true medical condition, and they may be defensive and resist discussion regarding the role of psychosocial factors and stress.
- Nevertheless, psychological factors are common in adolescent CFS and may play an important role in precipitation or maintenance of the disorder.

PATIENT/FAMILY EDUCATION

- There is no evidence that the disorder is progressive or degenerative.
- Although prospective studies are few, it appears that most adolescents with CFS improve within 6 months to 2 years.

SUGGESTED READINGS

Afari N, Buchwald D: Chronic fatigue syndrome: A review. *Am J Psychiatry* 160:221, 2003.

Carter BD et al: Psychological symptoms in chronic fatigue and juvenile rheumatoid arthritis. *Pediatrics* 103:975, 1999.

Centers for Disease Control and Prevention. Available at www.cdc.gov/ncidod/diseases/cfs/cfshome.htm

Chronic Fatigue and Immune Dysfunction Syndrome (CFIDS) Association of America. Available at www.cfids.org

Jason LA et al: *Handbook of Chronic Fatigue Syndrome.* Hoboken, NJ, John Wiley & Sons, 2003.

Jordan KM et al: Chronic fatigue syndrome in children and adolescents: A review. *J Adolesc Health* 22:4, 1998.

Marshall GS: Report of a workshop on the epidemiology, natural history, and pathogenesis of chronic fatigue syndrome in adolescents. *J Pediatr* 134:395, 1999.

AUTHOR: **MARK SCOTT SMITH, MD**

BASIC INFORMATION

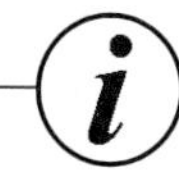

DEFINITIONS

Cleft lip is the incomplete closure of the lip. Cleft palate is the incomplete closure of the palate. Cleft lips and cleft palates may be unilateral or bilateral, complete or incomplete.

SYNONYMS

Cleft lip: cheiloschisis
Congenital fissure of lip
Harelip
Labium leporinum

ICD-9-CM CODES
749.0 Cleft palate
749.1 Cleft lip
749.2 Cleft palate with cleft lip, unspecified

EPIDEMIOLOGY & DEMOGRAPHICS

- The incidence in the United States is about 1 in 500 in Asians, 1 in 700 in whites, and 1 in 2500 in blacks.
- Cleft lip occurs more frequently in males than in females (3:2).
- Minor variations exist among different races.
- Isolated cleft palate does not have gender or ethnic predilection.
- See "Patient/Family Education."

CLINICAL PRESENTATION

History
- Usually recognized at birth
- May be prenatally diagnosed by ultrasound (>21 weeks gestation)
- Occasionally family history of clefting

Physical Examination
- Cleft lip can be unilateral or bilateral, complete or incomplete, and it is usually accompanied by nasal and maxillary flattening of the affected side.
- Cleft palate is broadly classified into V-shaped or U-shaped cleft, affecting the soft or hard palate.
  - V-shaped clefts generally represent primary malformation.
  - U-shaped clefts represent interference with palatal closure by the tongue.
- Seen in Pierre Robin sequence.
- Micrognathia and retrognathia are common.
- The extent of palatal clefting can vary between complete clefting of palate, alveolar ridge and lip, to that involving the secondary palate only.
- Bifid uvula, submucous cleft palate, and midline furrowing of the palate are the mildest but most common manifestations of palatal clefting.
- Notching of vermilion with lip crease is a mild form of cleft lip.
- Hypernasal speech is caused by velopharyngeal insufficiency.
- Multiple dental abnormalities occur, such as malocclusion, inhibition of tooth eruption, and absent teeth.
- Because clefting may be associated with a genetic syndrome, a careful, comprehensive physical examination should be performed, looking for other minor anomalies.
  - Lip-pits seen in patients with cleft lip suggest the Van der Woude's syndrome, an autosomal dominant trait.
  - The velocardiofacial syndrome, which consists of a conotruncal heart defect, velopharyngeal insufficiency or clefting, facial characteristics, long tapering fingers, and behavioral abnormalities, is often caused by a deletion of chromosome 22q.

ETIOLOGY

- Both cleft lip and cleft palate are associated with genetic syndromes (approximately 30% to 40%).
- Nonsyndromic cleft lips and palates are multifactorial in cause.
- Approximately 10% of isolated cleft palates are associated with chromosome 22q11 deletion.
- Pedigree analysis suggests two genetic forms of nonsyndromic palatal clefting:
  - Cleft lip with or without cleft palate
  - Cleft palate only

DIAGNOSIS

Dx

DIFFERENTIAL DIAGNOSIS

- Amniotic band disruption sequence can cause facial clefting that does not follow the usual landmarks of labial or palatal fusion.
- Pseudo-cleft of the upper lip, which is seen in some genetic syndromes (e.g., orofacio-digital syndromes), is a slight median indentation or clefting of the upper lip that usually does not extend beyond the vermilion border.
- For clefting in patients with a high likelihood of a syndrome association (presence of other congenital anomalies), the differential diagnosis should be considered within the context of these other anomalies.

WORKUP

- Evaluation of feeding and respiratory competence: primary concern in the newborn
- A cleft-craniofacial team evaluative approach for future surgical and nonsurgical interventions within the first week of life
- Speech and language evaluation
- Hearing evaluation
- Genetic evaluation for a possible syndrome association as indicated

LABORATORY TEST

Chromosomal analysis is indicated if other congenital anomalies are identified.

TREATMENT

Rx

NONPHARMACOLOGIC THERAPY

- Special nipples are available to help with feeding.
  - Children with cleft palate are not able to achieve a negative-pressure suck.
  - Special squeeze bottles help manually dispense milk or formula intraorally.
- Infants with the Pierre Robin sequence may have respiratory obstruction caused by micrognathia and glossoptosis. Prone positioning often helps alleviate this difficulty.
- All children with cleft lip or palate can benefit from nasoalveolar molding—a type of early orthodontics—which helps align the lip, nose, and alveolar elements before surgical correction of the clefts.
- Staged correction of clefts can be managed by plastic surgery, with cleft lip repair occurring at 3 months of age and cleft palate repair at 9 months.
- Most patients with cleft palate will have persistent serous otitis media secondary to eustachian tube dysfunction requiring myringotomy tube placement.
- Children with severe Pierre Robin sequence and respiratory obstruction can benefit from tongue-lip adhesion surgery or mandibular distraction and lengthening.

DISPOSITION

- Monitor growth and development for late-developing signs of a genetic syndrome (e.g., retinal detachment or degenerative arthritis in Stickler's syndrome).
- Monitor for conductive hearing loss caused by recurrent otitis media or chronic serious otitis.
- Ongoing speech and language evaluation and therapy.
- Monitor for multiple dental and orthodontic problems caused by inherent midface growth deficiency.

REFERRAL

- All patients should be referred to a craniofacial team consisting of the following specialists:
  - Plastic surgeon
  - Otolaryngologist
  - Speech pathologist
  - Dentist, orthodontist, oral surgeon, and prosthodontist
  - Geneticist
  - Pediatrician
- Craniofacial teams certified by the American Cleft Palate Association can be found on their web site.

PEARLS & CONSIDERATIONS

COMMENTS

- The presence of lip-pits suggests Van der Woude's syndrome, which has an autosomal dominant pattern of inheritance.
- Growth hormone deficiency is sometimes seen in children with cleft lip or palate and may require growth hormone replacement therapy.
- Cleft lip or palate seen in individuals with hypertelorism or hypotelorism suggests a

more extensive midline defect (e.g., Opitz syndrome or holoprosencephaly, respectively).

- Hypernasal voice, with or without obvious palatal cleft, should raise the suspicion of velocardiofacial syndrome, and a fluorescence in situ hybridization study for a chromosome 22q deletion should be considered.

PREVENTION

- Several prenatal environmental exposures, such as alcohol, cigarette smoking, or valproate, are associated with an increased risk for clefting, but in no case is the risk greater than 5%.
- Some reports suggest an association between poor prenatal nutrition (e.g., folate deficiency) and increased risk of clefting, but these theories are difficult to prove. Good prenatal care should be provided to all pregnant women.
- Prenatal diagnosis for some forms of syndromic cleft lip or palate is available.

PATIENT/FAMILY EDUCATION

- For nonsyndromic cleft lip or palate, the chance for the parents who have one affected child to have additional children with clefting is on the order of 3% to 5% for each pregnancy.
  - This recurrence risk is higher for families in which the affected child has a more severe manifestation (e.g., recurrence risk is higher for families with bilateral cleft lip versus unilateral cleft lip).
  - The recurrence risk increases significantly to 10% to 15% if the parents have two affected children.
- For syndromic clefting, the recurrence risk depends on the pattern of inheritance for the particular syndrome.

SUGGESTED READINGS

American Cleft Palate-Craniofacial Association. Available at www.acpa-cpf.org

Cleft.com. Available at www.cleft.com/cpf/cpffrm.html

Wyszynski DF: Cleft Lip and Palate: From Origin to Treatment. Boston, Oxford University Press, 2002.

AUTHORS: **JOHN GIROTTO, MD** and **CHIN-TO FONG, MD**

BASIC INFORMATION

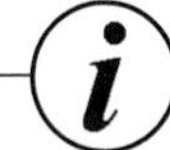

DEFINITION

Clubfoot is a complex deformity of the foot with hindfoot equinus (i.e., plantar-flexion) and varus (i.e., turned inward), cavus of the midfoot, and forefoot adduction of varying severity.

SYNONYM

Talipes equinovarus

ICD-9-CM CODE
754.51 Clubfoot

EPIDEMIOLOGY & DEMOGRAPHICS

- The incidence is 1 case in 1000 whites and higher for Pacific Islanders.
- The male-to-female incidence is 2:1.
- The disease is bilateral in 30% to 50% of cases.
- Multifactorial inheritance characterizes clubfoot:
  - The risk of having a subsequent child with a clubfoot if the first child was a boy is 1 in 40; if the first child was a girl, the risk is 1 in 16.
  - The risk of having a subsequent child with a clubfoot if a parent has a clubfoot is 1 in 4.

CLINICAL PRESENTATION

Physical Examination

- The deformity is evident at the time of the neonatal examination; occasionally, the diagnosis is suggested by prenatal ultrasound.
- Careful examination of the entire child is necessary to rule out syndromic or neurologic feet.
- The clubfoot is smaller than its counterpart and cannot be held in a corrected position.
- The ankle and hindfoot is in equinus (i.e., plantar-flexion) and varus, and the Achilles tendon is contracted.
- Clubfoot consists of forefoot supination, metatarsus adductus, and a cavus component. A medial midfoot crease is evident; its depth depends on the severity and rigidity of the deformity.
- The calf is atrophic.
- Leg length discrepancy is often identified.

ETIOLOGY

- Postural clubfoot: caused by intrauterine molding ("cramped quarters")
- Idiopathic clubfoot: most common
- Neurogenic clubfoot: spina bifida, tethered spinal cord, arthrogryposis
- Syndromic clubfoot: diastrophic dwarfism, Freeman-Sheldon syndrome, Smith-Lemli-Opitz syndrome

DIAGNOSIS

Dx

DIFFERENTIAL DIAGNOSIS

The differential diagnosis is not in doubt, except to rule out neurologic or syndromic clubfeet.

IMAGING STUDIES

- Radiographs are of limited value early.
  - Ossification of tarsal bones may be delayed.
  - Ossification centers may be eccentrically positioned.
- Anteroposterior, lateral, and dorsiflexion lateral radiographs measure residual deformity.
- Ultrasound, computed tomography, and magnetic resonance imaging have limited use.

TREATMENT

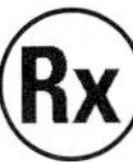

NONPHARMACOLOGIC THERAPY

- The goal is to obtain a normal-looking, painless, flexible, plantigrade foot.
- Nonoperative techniques have largely replaced the need for extensive surgical procedures.
- Serial manipulation with immobilization in a long leg cast.
- Percutaneous Achilles tendon lengthening is performed early, after correction of forefoot and midfoot deformities.
- Prolonged bracing is used to minimize the risk of recurrence.
- Recurrent deformity may be corrected by repeat casting.
- Residual deformity or recurrence may require more intensive surgery (e.g., tendon transfers, posteromedial release).

DISPOSITION

Periodic examinations and radiographs are necessary to follow growth and development.

SUGGESTED READINGS

Carroll NC: Clubfoot: what have we learned in the last quarter century? *J Pediatr Orthop* 17:1, 1997.

Cooper DM, Dietz FR: Treatment of idiopathic clubfoot: a thirty-year follow-up note. *J Bone Joint Surg Am* 77:1477, 1995.

Morcuende JA et al: Radical reduction in the rate of extensive corrective surgery for clubfoot using the Ponsetti method. *Pediatrics* 113:376, 2004.

Pediatric Orthopaedic Society of North America. Available at www.posna.org

Virtual Children's Hospital, Treatment of Congenital Clubfoot. Available at www.vh.org/pediatric/orivuder/orthopaedics/Clubfoot/Clubfoot.html

AUTHOR: **DENNIS ROY, MD**

BASIC INFORMATION

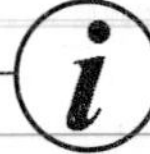

DEFINITION

Coarctation of the aorta is an obstructing shelf-like lesion arising from the posterolateral aortic wall opposite the aortic end of the ductus arteriosus or ligamentum arteriosum as a result of localized thickening of the aortic media protruding into the vessel lumen. It is often associated with narrowing of the distal transverse and proximal descending thoracic aorta with poststenotic dilation of the descending thoracic aorta immediately distal to the coarctation.

SYNONYMS

Aortic coarctation
Coarc
Tubular or isthmus hypoplasia, stenosis, or narrowing

ICD-9-CM CODE
747.1 Coarctation of the aorta (preductal or postductal)

EPIDEMIOLOGY & DEMOGRAPHICS

- The disease accounts for approximately 8% of congenital heart disease malformations.
- The incidence is 15 cases per 100,000 live births.
- Male predominance is seen.
- It is the most common cause of congestive heart failure in acyanotic infants in the first 2 weeks of life.
- Associated lesions include bicuspid aortic valve in 50% to 85% of patients and distal aortic arch hypoplasia, ventricular septal defects, and mitral valve anomalies in more complex coarctation malformations.
- Coarctation is found in 15% of patients with Turner syndrome.
- Berry aneurysms in the circle of Willis may occur in up to 10% of patients, with the greatest risk of rupture in late adulthood.
- Without treatment, patients with aortic coarctation have a mortality rate of 90% by age 50 due to cardiogenic shock in early infancy and later deaths from aortic rupture or dissection, endocarditis, congestive heart failure, and intracranial hemorrhage.

CLINICAL PRESENTATION

History

- Two presentations are common:
  - Congestive heart failure and cardiogenic shock in the neonatal period
  - Heart murmur, systemic hypertension, and decreased lower extremity pulses in later infancy or childhood
- In the early presentation, infants usually have a history of progressively worsening feeding, tachypnea, pallor, diaphoresis, lethargy, diminishing urine output, and grunting.
- Rarely, young infants may be asymptomatic.
- Older infants and children are usually asymptomatic, but complaints of leg discomfort with running (possible claudication variant), headaches, and epistaxis may be elicited.

Physical Examination

- Symptomatic neonates commonly exhibit signs of congestive heart failure, including tachypnea, retractions, grunting, pallor, diaphoresis, tender hepatomegaly, a gallop rhythm, and a single accentuated second heart sound.
- If cardiogenic shock is present, all of the pulses are diminished, with lower and upper extremity hypotension.
- If right-to-left ductal shunting is present, mild desaturation of the lower one half of the body may be noticed.
- Physical findings in older infants and children are more characteristic, with a clear-cut disparity between upper and lower extremity pulses and blood pressures.
  - Blood pressure in the legs is often unobtainable.
  - Distal lower extremity pulses are commonly absent, and diminished femoral pulses lag behind the brachial pulses.
  - Upper extremity pulses are vigorous. However, if the coarctation involves the origin of the left subclavian artery, the left arm pulse will also be diminished.
- If a bicuspid aortic valve is present, an ejection click is heard between the lower left sternal border and the apex.
  - Typically, a systolic bruit is audible over the middle left back and the upper left sternal border.
  - If a systolic ejection murmur is heard at the upper right sternal border, aortic stenosis is present on the basis of a bicuspid aortic valve.
- Collateral vessels (i.e., branches off the subclavian arteries feeding the intercostal arteries in a retrograde direction, thereby enhancing aortic flow below the coarctation) are often palpable along the inferior border of the scapulas in children but not in young infants.
- Short stature, webbed neck, shield chest, cubitus valgus, and neonatal nonpitting edema of the dorsa of the hands and feet suggest Turner syndrome.

ETIOLOGY

- The cause is unknown but attributed to perturbed prenatal arterial flow patterns at the junction of the proximal descending thoracic aorta (isthmus), patent ductus arteriosus, and postductal descending thoracic aorta.
- There is often a relatively rapid obstructive exacerbation as the ductus arteriosus closes in the neonatal period.

DIAGNOSIS

DIFFERENTIAL DIAGNOSIS

- Early presentation: other causes of cardiogenic shock in the neonatal period
  - Hypoplastic left heart syndrome
  - Interrupted aortic arch
  - Critical aortic stenosis
  - Myocarditis
  - Cardiomyopathies
- Older infant or child: abdominal coarctation

LABORATORY TESTS

- An electrocardiogram is useful for the following assessments:
  - Right ventricular (RV) hypertrophy or RV dominance in neonates
  - Normal or left ventricular (LV) hypertrophy in children
  - Occasionally, left atrial enlargement

IMAGING STUDIES

- Chest radiograph
  - Cardiomegaly, pulmonary venous congestion in neonates
  - Normal or LV enlargement in children
  - The 3 sign (i.e., prestenotic and poststenotic dilation of the descending aorta, producing the reversed E or 3 sign): may be seen in the upper left mediastinum in children
  - Rib notching: rare in children younger than 5 years old
- Echocardiography: useful for identifying the coarctation, ductus arteriosus, associated lesions, and ventricular function
- Cardiac catheterization: usually unnecessary unless atypical features are present or a balloon angioplasty is being considered

TREATMENT

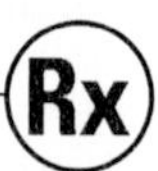

NONPHARMACOLOGIC THERAPY

- Surgery provides the definitive intervention.
- After initial stabilization, symptomatic neonates should undergo repair within 2 to 3 days.
- Asymptomatic infants and children should undergo repair by 4 years of age.
- If upper extremity hypertension persists or if LV dysfunction or severe ventricular hypertrophy develops, repair should be undertaken immediately.
- Types of repair include the following:
  - Infants and neonates: subclavian flap (i.e., patch aortoplasty or extended aortic arch anastomoses)
  - Older children: end-to-end beveled anastomoses
- At some centers, balloon aortoplasty of the native coarctation is undertaken, but there is a definite risk of recoarctation.

ACUTE GENERAL Rx

- Prostaglandin E_1 infusion maintains ductal patency, which reduces LV afterload and improves subdiaphragmatic blood flow.
- Dopamine or dobutamine improve LV function, which may enhance the upper-lower extremity pulse discrepancy.

BASIC INFORMATION

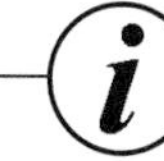

DEFINITION

Conjunctivitis is any inflammatory condition of the columnar epithelial membranes that line the eyelids (i.e., tarsal or palpebral conjunctiva) or exposed surface of the sclera (i.e., bulbar conjunctiva). The corneal surface is composed of squamous epithelium, and inflammation of the cornea is called keratitis.

SYNONYMS

Pink eye
Red eye

ICD-9-CM CODES
077.98 Chlamydial conjunctivitis
077.99 Viral conjunctivitis
098.40 Neonatal conjunctivitis
372.0 Acute or allergic conjunctivitis
372.01 Chronic conjunctivitis

EPIDEMIOLOGY & DEMOGRAPHICS

- Most common acute condition of the eye seen by pediatricians
- Neonate
  - Occurs in 1.6% to 12% of all newborns
  - Acute causes of ophthalmia neonatorum: chemical (e.g., silver nitrate), chlamydial, bacterial (including gonococcal), or rarely, viral (without other nonocular manifestations)
- Infants
  - Chlamydial, bacterial causes
  - Obstructed lacrimal duct
- Children
  - Bacterial pathogen twice as likely as viral
  - *Haemophilus influenzae:* 40% to 50% of cases
  - *Streptococcus pneumoniae:* 10% to 15% of cases
  - *Moraxella Catarrhalis:* 8% of cases
  - Adenovirus: 20% to 30% of cases
- Allergic
  - Hay fever conjunctivitis
  - Vernal conjunctivitis

CLINICAL PRESENTATION

History

- Viral: acute onset; may be associated with upper respiratory symptoms (i.e., fever and sore throat); unilateral but usually becomes bilateral within 24 to 48 hours; associated with gritty or sandy or burning feeling; associated with watery or mucoid discharge; some morning crusting common
- Bacterial: acute or hyperacute onset; significant crusting common; unilateral or bilateral; green, yellow, or white profuse discharge
- Allergic: usually bilateral; itching is hallmark
  - Hay fever conjunctivitis: acute onset, short duration, and many recurrences
  - Vernal conjunctivitis: onset at age 3 to 12 years, onset usually in spring, more common in warm climates, more common in boys than girls, often associated with history of atopy, rhinitis, or sinusitis
  - Atopic keratitis
  - Giant papillary conjunctivitis
- Chemical or toxic cause: medication history, work-related exposures, cosmetics
- Dry eyes: antidepressant use, collagen vascular diseases
- Foreign body: unilateral (may be bilateral in contact lens wearers)
- Time of onset: especially important in neonatal conjunctivitis
  - In first 24 hours of life: chemical most likely
  - Between 2 and 5 days of life: gonococcal (later onset if prophylaxis given)
  - Between 5 and 23 days of life: chlamydial

Physical Examination

- Pattern of the conjunctivitis
  - Papillary: allergic or contact irritant
    - Large papules
    - Tarsal conjunctiva, especially upper lids
    - Not specific
  - Follicular
    - Lower lid lymphoid follicles
    - Seen with adenoviral, chlamydial, topical medication, herpes simplex virus (HSV)
- Viral forms
  - Conjunctival injection
  - Watery, serous, or mucoid discharge
  - Preauricular adenopathy
  - Bilateral or unilateral
  - Associated rashes
  - If associated with pharyngitis, adenovirus likely
  - If vesicles or corneal ulceration, HSV keratoconjunctivitis likely
- Bacterial forms
  - Conjunctival injection
  - Chemosis
  - Mucopurulent or purulent discharge (green, white, or yellow)
  - If associated with otitis media, *H. influenzae* likely
- Allergic forms
  - Serous or mucoid discharge, often very stringy
  - Prominent ocular itching
  - Conjunctival injection
  - Occurs with or without photophobia
  - Hay fever conjunctivitis: mild conjunctival swelling, upper more than lower eyelid
  - Vernal conjunctivitis: more severe infection than hay fever conjunctivitis
    - Large papillary response of upper lid or perilimbal (i.e., margin between scleral and cornea)
    - Keratitis: painful inflammation of the corneal surface
    - Corneal opacification
  - Atopic keratoconjunctivitis: lower lid papillary response more than upper lid and with associated keratitis
- Examination of ears to look for otitis media
- Physical examination to look for systemic disorders

ETIOLOGY

- Infectious causes
  - Viral: adenovirus (most common viral cause), Coxsackievirus, HSV, varicella-zoster virus, Epstein-Barr virus, rubeola, rubella, mumps, enteroviral
  - Bacterial: *H. influenzae* (most common bacterial cause), streptococcal, *Moraxella,* staphylococcal (including *Staphylococcus epidermitis), Neisseria gonorrhoeae, Pseudomonas*
  - Chlamydial: *Chlamydia trachomatis*
- Allergic: hay fever conjunctivitis (e.g., pollens, molds, fungi, dust, foods), vernal conjunctivitis
- Chemical or toxic: ophthalmologic medications, work or environmental exposures, cosmetics
- Foreign body: contact lenses, other foreign bodies
- Idiopathic
- Other: graft-versus-host disease, Stevens-Johnson syndrome, Reiter's syndrome, Kawasaki disease

DIAGNOSIS

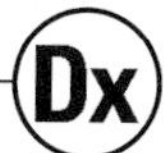

DIFFERENTIAL DIAGNOSIS

- Keratitis: inflammation of the cornea caused by infection, trauma (contact lens use), ultraviolet radiation exposure
- Uveitis, anterior uveitis (e.g., iritis, iridocyclitis): inflammation of iris and ciliary muscle, usually an autoimmune reaction
- Scleritis: focal or diffuse scleral inflammation, usually autoimmune
- Episcleritis: focal inflammation of deep subconjunctival (episcleral) tissues, autoimmune
- Acute angle-closure glaucoma: medical emergency caused by blockage of aqueous humor outflow leading to a sudden elevation in intraocular pressure; uncommon in pediatrics
- Corneal abrasion
- Styes (hordeolum): may irritate conjunctivae

WORKUP

- The diagnosis is usually made based on history and physical examination.
- Conjunctival culture and scraping with Gram stain is done for neonates to diagnose gonococcal and chlamydial disease.
- Culture and Gram stain may be helpful in other selected individuals.
- Many eosinophils (Giemsa stain) in eye discharge may indicate allergic cause.
- High serum and tear immunoglobulin E (IgE) levels are seen in vernal conjunctivitis and atopic keratitis.

TREATMENT

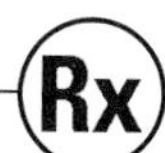

NONPHARMACOLOGIC THERAPY

- Most cases of acute conjunctivitis are benign and self-limited.

- Apply warm or cool compresses to eyes.
- Avoid the irritant or allergen.

ACUTE GENERAL Rx

- Antibiotic therapy is necessary to help prevent the sight-threatening complications of gonococcal and chlamydial conjunctivitis.
- For other bacterial causes, topical antibiotic treatment hastens resolution of symptoms and prevents secondary cases, although most cases resolve without specific antibiotic therapy.
  - Staphylococcal and streptococcal causes: topical ophthalmologic antibiotic preparation (drops or ointment)
- If systemic antibiotic treatment is used, topical treatment is not necessary.
- In neonates, the specific antibiotic is based on culture results and clinical suspicion.
  - Gonococcal cause: ceftriaxone or cefotaxime for 1 to 7 days
  - Chlamydial cause: systemically administered erythromycin (eliminates nasopharyngeal carriage and possibly subsequent pneumonia)
- Allergic conjunctivitis is treated with a topical ophthalmologic antihistamine or mast cell stabilizer.

CHRONIC Rx

Oral antihistamine may be helpful in chronic allergic diatheses.

REFERRAL

- Referral to a pediatric ophthalmologist should be considered if the patient has severe pain, photophobia, or blurred vision that does not improve with blinking.
- Patients with HSV infections or other agents that produce corneal ulcerations should also be referred to a pediatric ophthalmologist.
- If other causes of pink eye are strongly considered (i.e., iritis, acute angle-closure glaucoma), ophthalmology referral is indicated.

PEARLS & CONSIDERATIONS

COMMENTS

- One fourth of patients have associated otitis media at the time of diagnosis, and another one fourth develop otitis media if treated with a topical antibiotic.
- Outside the neonatal period, conjunctivitis is often self-limited (7 to 10 days); antibiotic therapy helps hasten the amelioration of symptoms and prevents secondary cases caused by spread.

PREVENTION

- Neonatal prophylaxis: 1% silver nitrate, 0.5% erythromycin, or 1% tetracycline
  - All are equally effective for prophylaxis of gonorrheal eye infections.
  - The regimens are helpful in reducing chlamydial ophthalmic infections.
- Good hand-washing practice in families, in daycare settings, and for individuals with upper respiratory infections

PATIENT/FAMILY EDUCATION

- Good hand-washing technique should be taught and used in family and daycare settings.
- The rapid spread and extreme contagiousness of infective conjunctivitis should be explained and understood.
- Known irritants or allergens should be avoided, if possible.

SUGGESTED READINGS

Alessandrini EA: The case of the red eye. *Pediatr Ann* 29:112, 2000.

Gigliotti F: Acute conjunctivitis. *Pediatr Rev* 16:203, 1995.

Gigliotti F et al: Efficacy of topical therapy in acute conjunctivitis in children. *J Pediatr* 104:623, 1984.

Jacobs DS: Conjunctivitis. UpToDate Online 13:3, 2005. Available at http://www.utdop.com

Silverman MA, Bessman E: Conjunctivitis. *E Medicine Instant Access to the Minds of Medicine.* Available at http://www.emedicine.com/EMERG/topic110.htm Accessed March 3, 2005.

Weber CM, Eichenbaum JW: The red eye: differentiating viral conjunctivitis from other, common causes. *Postgrad Med* 101:185, 1997.

AUTHOR: **LYNN C. GARFUNKEL, MD**

BASIC INFORMATION

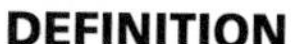

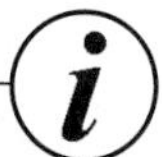

DEFINITION

Constipation definitions include a hard, infrequent (more than three times per week) stool that is usually painful to pass; failure to empty the lower colon with each bowel movement; and delay or difficulty in defecation, present for 2 weeks or more and sufficient to cause significant distress to the patient. Encopresis is fecal soiling as a result of stool leaking around a distended rectum that has decreased sensation.

SYNONYMS

Constipation
- Fecal withholding
- Functional fecal retention
- Idiopathic constipation

Encopresis
- Fecal soiling
- Soiling

ICD-9-CM CODES
306.4 Constipation, psychogenic
564.0 Constipation, neurogenic
787.6 Encopresis

EPIDEMIOLOGY & DEMOGRAPHICS

- Constipation accounts for 3% of general pediatric and 25% of pediatric gastroenterologist visits.
- Twenty-five percent of patients present before 1 year of age.
- Prevalence of constipation in children varies between 0.3% and 28%, with a peak between 2 and 4 years. The male-to-female ratio is 2:1.
- The prevalence is increased among patients with cerebral palsy or autism and those born at very low birth weight (<750 g).
- Encopresis occurs in 2% of children and is six to nine times more common in boys.

CLINICAL PRESENTATION

History
- If late, meconium passage may indicate a primary colonic problem (i.e., Hirschsprung's disease).
- Perinatal illnesses, especially necrotizing enterocolitis (NEC), may lead to stricture development.
- Character of stools, including consistency, caliber, volume, and frequency, should be assessed.
    - Stool patterns should be assessed at birth and in the first 24 hours, early infancy, later infancy, and childhood.
    - Small pellets indicate incomplete evacuation.
    - Massive stools indicate infrequent stooling with functional retention.
    - Narrow-caliber stools, especially with abdominal distention, may indicate Hirschsprung's disease, stenosis, or ectopic anus.
- Perianal disorders (e.g., fissure, dermatitis, abscess) cause pain that may lead to stooling avoidance (i.e., withholding).
- Obtain a history to determine the following:
    - Sexual or physical abuse
    - Prior surgery
    - Laxative use or abuse
    - Tolerance of early feeding
- Assess transitions and bowel habits.
    - Change may be caused by a transition from breast milk or formula to cow's milk; introduction of cow's milk is the most common cause of constipation.
    - The transition from strained foods to table foods may change the stool.
    - A transition from home care to daycare may change the stool.
    - The transition from diapers to toilet training is the most common time for withholding.
- Other medical issues should be assessed.
    - Hospitalizations (i.e., acute and chronic illnesses)
    - Allergies
    - Coarse, dry hair (i.e., hypothyroidism)
    - Cold or heat sensitivity (i.e., thyroid disease)
    - Recurrent otitis
- Assess relevant components of the history
    - Developmental history
    - Social history
    - Family history of bowel habits and patterns and of evacuation difficulties
    - Family history of thyroid disease, myopathies, Hirschsprung's disease, or cystic fibrosis
    - History of encopresis; fecal soiling or overflow diarrhea occurs from leakage around formed stool in the dilated, insensitive rectum and may be the first recognized symptom of chronic constipation.
    - History of abdominal pain
    - History of rectal bleeding

Physical Examination
- Fever, anorexia, nausea, vomiting, poor weight gain, and weight loss indicate an organic disorder.
- Growth parameters and velocity must be measured (e.g., short stature may indicate hypothyroidism).
- A thorough neurologic examination should be conducted because children with neurologic abnormalities (e.g., cerebral palsy, diskitis) or myopathy (e.g., muscular dystrophy) may have abnormal stools.
    - Cremasteric reflex
    - Anal wink
    - Tone, strength, and deep tendon reflexes
- Abdominal distention and bowel sounds should be assessed.
- The perineal examination looks for acute infections (e.g., candidal, group A streptococcal), anal tags, fissures, and anal placement. Ectopic anterior displacement of anus is one of the most common and under diagnosed anatomic causes of constipation.
    - A ratio of the female anus-fourchette to the coccyx-fourchette measurement of less than 0.34 is abnormal.
    - A ratio of the male anus-scrotum to the coccyx-scrotum measurement of less than 0.46 is abnormal.
- Rectal examination includes the following:
    - The anal canal should relax, although it may be initially tight on examination.
    - A dilated ampulla, especially if filled with stool, indicates retention.
    - Assess for fecal and other masses.
    - Hemorrhoids are rare in children.
    - Perirectal ulcers, fistulas, abscess, and strictures are associated with Crohn's disease.
    - Palpate internal fissures.
    - Rectal prolapse should be identified.
- Examine the back and spine.
    - Dimple
    - Hair tufts

Common Clinical Presentations
- Soiling or encopresis
- Infrequent (less than three times per week) stool
- Large stool
- Straining and pain with defecation
- Retentive posturing
- Abdominal distention

Other Clinical Presentations
- Megacolon
- Urinary tract infection
- Enuresis
- Renal caliceal dilation
- Behavioral problems
    - Anxiety
    - Attention deficit/hyperactivity disorder
    - Depression
    - Developmental delay or mental retardation
    - Low or poor self-esteem
    - Obsessive-compulsive disorder
    - Oppositional defiant disorder

ETIOLOGY

- Constipation may be functional or organic (organic in less than 5% of cases, with a large differential diagnosis).
- Several theories exist for functional constipation.
    - Diminished relaxation of internal anal sphincter and active contraction of external anal sphincter during defecation
    - Decreased awareness of rectal distention
    - Increased threshold volume of distention
    - Decreased ability to evacuate rectal content
    - Possible right-sided colonic dysfunction in severe constipation
- No data are available to confirm or refute that these dysfunctions predate clinical findings.
- Usually, no underlying organic or psychiatric problem is present.
- Constipation is a symptom, not a disease, with contributions from the following:
    - Transition from human to cow's milk
    - Low-fiber diet or inadequate food intake

- Decreased fluid intake
- Medication (e.g., anticholinergics, opiates, antidepressants)
- Diabetes mellitus, hypothyroidism, hypercalcemia
- Withholding (i.e., not wanting to defecate at school)
- Anal fissure or anal rectal malformations
- Inappropriate toilet training

DIAGNOSIS

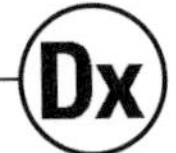

DIFFERENTIAL DIAGNOSIS

- Loening-Barcke diagnostic criteria for pediatric constipation call for at least two of the following:
  - Defecation less than three times per week
  - Two or more episodes of encopresis per week
  - Periodic passage of very large stool (7 to 30 days)
  - Palpable abdomen or rectal mass
- Rome II diagnostic criteria for functional defecation disorders in childhood include the following:
  - Infant dyschezia: at least 10 minutes of straining and crying before successful passage of soft stool
  - Functional constipation for infants and preschool children
  - Pebble-like, hard stool for most stools *or* firm stool two or fewer times per week *and* no evidence of structural, endocrine, or metabolic disease
- Functional fecal retention for infants to children 16 years old is defined by the following:
  - At least 12 weeks' duration
  - Passage of large-diameter stools at intervals of less than two times per week
  - Retentive posturing, avoiding defecation by contracting pelvic floor and gluteal muscles
- Functional nonretentive fecal soiling in children older than 4 years is defined by the following:
  - At least one episode per week for 12 weeks
  - Defecation into places and at times inappropriate to the social context
- In the absence of structural or inflammatory disease and the absence of signs of fecal retention, the differential diagnosis should include the following:
  - Chronic intestinal pseudo-obstruction
    - Diarrhea is more common because of bacterial overgrowth.
    - Pseudo-obstruction is divided into two main types: neuropathic and myopathic
  - Cow's milk protein reaction (questionably an allergic reaction)
  - Cystic fibrosis
  - Dehydration
  - Diabetes mellitus (DM), with neuropathy of colon seen as a late complication of DM
  - Electrolyte abnormality: hyponatremia, hypercalcemia, or hypokalemia
  - Hirschsprung's disease
  - Hypothyroidism
  - Malnutrition
  - Medications:
    - Anticholinergics (e.g., atropine, scopolamine, hyoscyamine)
    - Anticonvulsants
    - Antidiarrheal agents (e.g., diphenoxylate, loperamide, paregoric)
    - Antihistamines
    - Bismuth
    - Calcium channel blockers
    - Chemotherapeutic agents (some)
    - Cholestyramine
    - Iron supplements
    - Nonsteroidal anti-inflammatory drugs
    - Opiate narcotics
    - Tricyclic antidepressants
  - Neuromuscular disease with constipation as a common feature:
    - Cerebral palsy
    - Muscular dystrophy
    - Multiple sclerosis
    - Myelomeningocele
  - Structural abnormality:
    - Anterior ectopic anus
    - Perianal abscess, fistula, hemorrhoid
    - Rectal ectasia
    - Rectal prolapse: rule out cystic fibrosis

WORKUP

- Most children without suspicious findings in the history or physical examination do not need an extensive workup, but a symptom diary, diet diary, and stool diary may be helpful.
- Perianal injury caused by sexual abuse leads to pain on defecation and constipation.
- Organic causes must be excluded.
- Patients rarely need the following:
  - Anorectal manometry: may be useful, requires gastroenterology referral
  - Rectal biopsy: in patients suspected of having Hirschsprung's disease

LABORATORY TESTS

- Determinations of electrolytes, calcium, and magnesium to rule out abnormalities
- Urinalysis and urine culture
- For suggestive history or physical examination findings, thyroid studies to look for hypothyroidism

IMAGING STUDIES

- Abdominal flat plate radiograph can show excessive stool or obstruction.
- Consider barium enema to rule out Hirschsprung's disease and strictures or stenosis (especially after NEC).
- Consider lumbosacral spine imaging to rule out tumor, diskitis, or other spinal or canal abnormalities.

TREATMENT

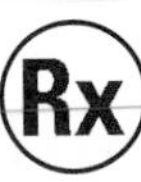

NONPHARMACOLOGIC THERAPY

- Explain to parents that their child is experiencing pain with defecation; this is usually not willful misbehavior.
- The goal of therapy is to remove the association of pain, anxiety, and negative attributes with stooling and soiling.
- Provide diet guidelines.
  - Good fluid intake, especially juices with high osmotic load
    - Absorbable and nonabsorbable carbohydrates soften stool.
    - Sorbitol (in prune, pear, and apple juices) increases the frequency and water content of the stool.
  - High-fiber diet for children older than 2 years according to the following formula:
    - Age (in years) + 5 (or 6) = Number of grams of fiber per day
- Behavioral modification and calendars or stickers are useful adjuncts.
  - Regular, unhurried time on the toilet (more than three times per day for 5 minutes after meals)
  - Stooling pattern and consistency diary
  - Reward system
- Try relaxation and biofeedback.
  - Must be at least 5 years old to participate and cooperate effectively
  - Painless and risk free approach

ACUTE GENERAL Rx

- The three phases of constipation care are as follows:
  - Empty the rectum thoroughly.
  - Sustain rectal clearing and restore normal tone.
  - Wean from medical interventions.
- Disimpaction may be required before initiation of maintenance therapy.
  - Any one of the following types of enemas can be used, if necessary, every 6 to 12 hours for 1 or 2 days or two to four times every 24 hours:
    - Saline
    - Mineral oil
    - Phosphate
    - Phosphate and mineral oil (3:1)
    - Milk and molasses (3 ounces of milk, 3 ounces of molasses, 1 to 2 ounces of mineral oil)
  - Oral disimpaction is also possible:
    - Mineral oil (for those older than 2 years and without risk for aspiration): 1 ounce per year of age (up to 8) twice each day for 2 to 3 days; maximum of 8 ounces per dose *or*
    - Polyethylene glycol (PEG, MiraLax): 1.5 g/kg/day for 3 to 4 days
- Disimpaction should be followed immediately by the maintenance phase, which may need to continue for months. Daily soft stool is the goal.

- Stool should be loose enough so that defecation occurs without pain.
- Stool should be loose to prevent withholding and ensure complete rectal emptying.
- Osmotic cathartics or lubricants alone or in combination may be used.
  - PEG, a non-absorbable, high molecular weight compound that is not metabolized by colonic bacteria, is easy to use at recommended doses by age (0.1–0.8 g/kg/day in 8 ounces of fluid once per day). It is only approved for 2 week course, however many physicians use PEG for months if needed. Recommended daily doses follow:
    - <18 months - 0.5–1 tsp once per day
    - 1½–3 years - 1–2 tsp once per day
    - >3 years - 2–4 tsp once per day
    - Teen/adult - 17 g (1 capful) per day
  - Lactulose: 1–3 mL/kg/day, one to two times per day
  - Milk of magnesia: 1–2 mL/kg/day, one to two times per day
    - May mix with juice, milk, cereal, or any other drinks
  - Sorbitol: 1–3 mL/kg/day
  - Mineral oil: 1–4 mL/kg, one to two times per day (for older child and those not at risk for aspiration)
    - Less palatable; mix with juice
    - Lipoid pneumonia if aspiration occurs
- If cathartics or lubricants are not successful, may add or substitute with bulk agents or stimulants.
  - Bulk-forming agents increase the nonabsorbable contents and increase movement through the gastrointestinal tract. This approach may also be used as maintenance.
    - Psyllium, age-based dosing: 1.25 to 7.5 g/dose, taken orally one to three times per day
    - Malt soup extract: 0.5 to 2 teaspoons per 8 ounces of liquid, one or two times per day
  - Stimulants or irritants allow the gastrointestinal tract to respond to distention more quickly. Use as rescue agents for 2 to 4 days when necessary.
    - Senna: 10 to 20 mg/kg/dose at bedtime
    - Bisacodyl: one to three 5-mg tablets per day (0.3 mg/kg/day) or one half to one 10-mg suppository per day
    - Mineral oil: a stimulant and a lubricant; contraindicated in infants younger than 12 months or those at risk for aspiration
  - Emollients soften feces.
    - Docusate: 40 to 50 mg per day, divided for one to four doses per day
  - Hyperosmotic agents increase volume and thereby stimulate emptying.
    - Glycerin suppository
    - Lactulose
    - Magnesium (hydroxide or citrate): age-based dosing

CHRONIC Rx

- After normal, soft stools are achieved daily for 1 month, the patient may decrease the laxative dose by 25% monthly for several months.
- If defecation continues without constipation, continue to decrease the dose.
- If constipation recurs, return to previous dose that led to a soft, daily stool.

DISPOSITION

Significant involvement by phone or in the office is needed to ascertain success and compliance with therapy.

REFERRAL

- Refer to a pediatric gastroenterologist if treatment is unsuccessful or there is a question about other causes.
- Refer to a pediatric surgeon if the cause is not a functional problem.

PEARLS & CONSIDERATIONS

COMMENTS

- Discuss with parents (and with child if old enough) to explain pain and long-term therapy.
- Often, parents use too little medication for too short a time.

PREVENTION

- Appropriate guidance for diet
- Appropriate guidance for toilet training
- Early treatment for new-onset constipation

PATIENT/FAMILY EDUCATION

- If the stool is hard, it hurts to defecate, and it is important to explain this to the parents and the patient.
- The patient needs to achieve soft to runny stools daily to twice daily to avoid pain association.
- *Short term* means months of therapy, especially for a toddler.
- More information is available from the International Foundation for Functional Gastrointestinal Disorders (P.O. Box 1786, Milwaukee, WI 53217; 414-964-1799).

SUGGESTED READINGS

Baker S et al: Constipation in infants and children: evaluation and management. *J Pediatr Gastroenterol Nutr* 29:612, 1999.

Benninga MA et al: Childhood constipation: is there new light in the tunnel? *J Pediatr Gastroenterol Nutr* 39:448, 2004.

Ferry GD: Prevention and treatment of acute constipation in infants and children. UpToDate Pediatrics 2005. Available at http://www.uptodate.com/physicians/pediatrics_toclist.asp

Guerrero RA, Cavender CP: Constipation: physical and psychological sequelae. *Pediatr Ann* 28:312, 1999.

Love JR, Parks BR: Movers and shakers: a clinician's guide to laxatives. *Pediatr Ann* 28:307, 1999.

Medinfo. Available at medinfo.co.uk/conditions/constipation.html

National Institute of Digestive Disorders. Available at www.niddk.nih.gov/health/digest/pubs/whyconstr/whyconst.htm

Nowicki MJ, Bishop PR: Organic causes of constipation in infants and children. *Pediatr Ann* 28:293, 1999.

Parker PH: To do or not to do? That is the question. *Pediatr Ann* 28:280, 1999.

Wellness Web. Available at www.wellweb.com/index/qconstip.htm

AUTHOR: **LYNN C. GARFUNKEL, MD**

BASIC INFORMATION

DEFINITION

Contact dermatitis is an acute or relapsing skin disorder whose hallmarks are pruritus and skin inflammation caused by some offending agent. The two subtypes are primary irritant and allergic dermatitis.

SYNONYMS

Diaper dermatitis
Rhus dermatitis

ICD-9-CM CODE
692.9 Contact dermatitis

EPIDEMIOLOGY & DEMOGRAPHICS

- The incidence in children is unknown, but contact dermatitis represents approximately 20% of all dermatitis in children.
- Almost 50% of all infants have diaper dermatitis at some point; onset is usually between 9 and 12 months of age.
- For irritant dermatitis, common offending agents include saliva, urine, and feces.
- For the allergic subtype, common offending agents are poison ivy and oak (i.e., *Rhus* dermatitis). Other agents include nickel, topical medications, soaps, and latex.
- Allergic reactions occur about 1 week after the primary exposure (i.e., sensitization phase). Reactions after subsequent exposures may occur within hours.

CLINICAL PRESENTATION

History

- History taking should be guided by the age of patient and location of the rash.
- A history of known exposure is often difficult to elicit and requires thoughtful questioning.

Physical Examination

- Discrete areas of erythema correspond to the areas of skin exposed to the irritant or allergen.
- Vesiculation, oozing, and erythematous papules may be present, particularly in acute allergic dermatitis.
- In diaper dermatitis, confluent erythema is present on maximal exposure areas, sparing the inguinal folds. More severe forms may be associated with erosions and blister formation and possibly with secondary infection.
- Chronic exposure in allergic and irritant contact reactions leads to lichenification (i.e., thickening) of the skin.
- Id reaction is a secondary, generalized pruritic eruption consisting of fine, erythematous papules and caused by a generalized sensitivity in a person with a localized allergic contact reaction.
- Phytophotodermatitis results from exposure to lime or lemon juice, carrot, or celery followed by exposure to sunlight, and it is characterized by redness, blistering, or hyperpigmentation (may be confused with abuse).

ETIOLOGY

- Irritant dermatitis
  - There is a direct toxic effect to the skin.
  - The reaction is related to the concentration and duration of the exposure and to the underlying skin integrity.
  - No immune response is involved.
- Allergic dermatitis
  - Exposure to a particular antigen mediates a delayed hypersensitivity (type IV) immunologic response.
  - The antigen penetrates the skin, is processed by cutaneous (Langerhans) macrophages, and is presented to circulating T lymphocytes.

DIAGNOSIS

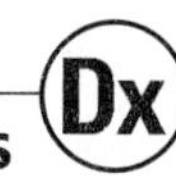

DIFFERENTIAL DIAGNOSIS

- Atopic dermatitis
- Herpes simplex
- Impetigo
- Monilial dermatitis
- Nummular dermatitis
- Psoriasis
- Seborrheic dermatitis
- Tinea corporis

WORKUP

- The workup is based on clinical presentation, with particular attention to distribution of rash (e.g., chronic erythema of the lips and perioral area indicates lip licker's dermatitis, a form of irritant dermatitis).
- Patch testing may be done.
  - Prepackaged antigens are applied to skin's surface, which is reexamined in 48 to 72 hours for inflammation.
  - Adult testing reagents are used, and there is a high false-positive rate for children with active lesions.
- Indications for patch testing include the following:
  - Refractory atopic dermatitis
  - Recurrence of contact dermatitis after response to steroid therapy
  - Atopic dermatitis requiring systemic therapy
  - Worsening contact dermatitis in potential sites for contact allergen

TREATMENT

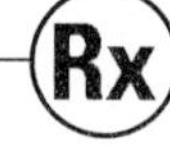

NONPHARMACOLOGIC THERAPY

- Removal of offending agent, if possible
- Cool compresses
- Diaper dermatitis
  - Keep diaper area dry with diaper changes every several hours.
  - Use an occlusive barrier, such as zinc oxide, to protect the skin.
  - Avoid use of plastic or rubber pants.
  - When the child is soiled, rinse the skin with warm water but minimize soap and diaper wipe use. Some caregivers find that a spray bottle works well to minimize the insult to the skin.

ACUTE GENERAL Rx

- Topical corticosteroids
  - Middle to high potency usually required.
  - Low potency is indicated for the face, axilla, and groin.
  - Apply twice each day for 5 to 7 days.
- Oral diphenhydramine used for its antipruritic effect and comfort management
- Systemic steroids
  - May be required for more than 10% to 15% involvement of the body surface
  - Prednisone, 2 mg/kg/day for 7 days, followed by a 7-day taper
- Longer courses (2 to 3 weeks) of systemic therapy often required for allergic *(Rhus)* dermatitis because of persistence of the immunologic response
- Increased incidence of relapse occurs with short courses of therapy
- Diaper dermatitis
  - Apply low-potency hydrocortisone (1%) cream twice each day for only a few days.
  - Use a generous amount of antifungal cream if the rash persists for more than 3 days because candidal colonization is common.

DISPOSITION

Schedule a follow-up visit in 1 to 2 weeks to assess the child's response to therapy.

REFERRAL

Refer the patient to an allergist or a dermatologist if patch testing is necessary.

PEARLS & CONSIDERATIONS

COMMENTS

- Consider a contact reaction whenever a rash is localized to the face, hands, or feet.
- With diaper dermatitis, consider the possibility of superinfection with *Candida,* and consider nystatin or clotrimazole cream for treatment.
- Cloth diapers (versus disposable) may increase the severity of the dermatitis.
- For topical therapy suggest creams on wet lesions, gels on the scalp, and ointments on dry lesions.

PATIENT/FAMILY EDUCATION

- For diaper dermatitis, emphasize the importance of therapeutic measures and the to decrease contact of urine and feces with the skin.
- Use of topical steroids for short periods (<2 weeks) for contact dermatitis.

SUGGESTED READINGS

Eichenfield LF, Friedlander SF: Coping with chronic dermatitis. *Contemp Pediatr* 15:53, 1998.
Friedlander SF: Contact dermatitis. *Pediatr Rev* 19:166, 1998.
Weston WL et al: *Color Textbook of Pediatric Dermatology.* St. Louis, Mosby, 1996.

AUTHOR: **KRISTEN SMITH DANIELSON, MD**

BASIC INFORMATION

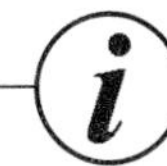

DEFINITION

Cor pulmonale is right-sided heart failure or significant right ventricular hypertrophy (RVH) resulting from pulmonary hypertension. It usually implies that the pulmonary hypertension is caused by pulmonary parenchymal disease, airway obstruction, or hypoventilation syndromes rather than by left-sided heart failure, congenital heart disease, or primary pulmonary hypertension syndromes (see the Pulmonary Hypertension chapter in Diseases and Disorders [Section I] for descriptions of pediatric pulmonary hypertension).

ICD-9-CM CODE
416.9 Cor pulmonale

EPIDEMIOLOGY & DEMOGRAPHICS

Cor pulmonale is much less common in children than in adults, in whom chronic obstructive pulmonary disease and emphysema are common causes.

CLINICAL PRESENTATION

History

- Underlying disease history (see "Etiology")
- Dyspnea
- Fatigue and exercise intolerance
- Syncope

Physical Examination

- Prominent right ventricular impulse on precordial palpation
- Loud, narrowly split or single second heart sound
- Pulmonary artery ejection click
- Jugular venous distention
- Edema or ascites (rare)
- Cyanosis and clubbing in severely hypoxemic patients (e.g., cystic fibrosis)

ETIOLOGY

- Bronchopulmonary dysplasia or chronic lung disease after prematurity
- Chronic interstitial pneumonitis, including human immunodeficiency virus (HIV) infection
- Cystic fibrosis
- Muscular dystrophies
- Obstructive apnea
- Primary hypoventilation
- Sickle cell anemia with recurrent pulmonary infarction
- Thoracic dystrophies
- Obstructive apnea and hypoventilation are common in children with syndromic diagnoses in which midfacial hypoplasia and other abnormalities in the growth and development of the facial, oral, pharyngeal, and hypopharyngeal structures may be present.
- Examples of associated abnormalities include the following:
  - Trisomy 21 (midfacial hypoplasia)
  - Marfan syndrome (palatal abnormality)
  - Pierre-Robin sequence (retrognathia)
  - Prader-Willi syndrome (severe obesity)

DIAGNOSIS

Dx

DIFFERENTIAL DIAGNOSIS

- Chronic lung disease may cause similar symptoms even without pulmonary hypertension or its secondary cardiac effects.
- Primary cardiac disorders, especially right-sided congenital heart disease or unrepaired cyanotic heart disease, may have similar clinical signs and symptoms.
  - Severe RVH from untreated pulmonary valve stenosis
  - Eisenmenger complex from unrepaired intracardiac shunts

WORKUP

- Electrocardiogram usually shows RVH.
- Neurologic examination or consultation may demonstrate muscular or skeletal dystrophies.
- Cardiac catheterization is rarely required to demonstrate pulmonary hypertension or RVH, but it may be needed to test the efficacy of vasodilators when there is severe pulmonary hypertension

LABORATORY TESTS

- Pulmonary function testing and oximetry may show abnormalities of primary lung disease.
- Polysomnography may diagnose sleep apnea or obstructive apnea.

IMAGING STUDIES

- Echocardiogram confirms RVH and may demonstrate pulmonary hypertension without congenital heart disease. Doppler velocities of tricuspid or pulmonary valve regurgitation allow semiquantitative assessment of pulmonary arterial pressures.
- Chest radiography may suggest RVH or show enlarged central pulmonary arteries.
- Chronic pulmonary parenchymal disease may be diagnosed by standard radiography or by chest computed tomography (CT).

TREATMENT

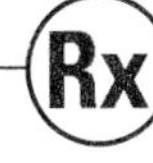

NONPHARMACOLOGIC THERAPY

- Therapy is for primary lung disease.
- Supplemental oxygen to correct hypoxia can decrease pulmonary hypertension and allow abnormal RVH to regress.
- Tonsillectomy and adenoidectomy are helpful in treating obstructive forms.
- Hypoventilation from obstructive apnea must be effectively treated even if a tracheostomy is necessary.
- Aggressive pulmonary toilet and antibiotics may improve right-sided heart failure in serious, chronic parenchymal disease, such as cystic fibrosis.
- Home ventilator treatment needed by some with muscular or thoracic dystrophies when signs of right heart failure occur.
- Bilevel positive airway pressure (BiPap) devices may alleviate obstructive hypoventilation during sleep.

ACUTE GENERAL Rx

Diuretics are adjunctive therapy when edema results from right heart failure.

CHRONIC Rx

- Primary cardiac medication, such as digoxin, is often prescribed, but studies proving its benefit are lacking.
- Vasodilator drugs may have limited use in the pulmonary diseases listed here (see the Pulmonary Hypertension chapter in Diseases and Disorders [Section I]).

DISPOSITION

- Periodic echocardiography for changes in pulmonary hypertension or RV size and function after treatment of pulmonary disease or airway obstruction.
- Follow-up polysomnogram after surgical intervention or adding ventilatory support.

REFERRAL

- Pediatric pulmonology referral is necessary for most children, with otolaryngologic consultation if there is obstructive apnea, neurologic consultation if there is muscular dystrophy, and hematologic consultation for sickle cell disease.
- Physicians with dedicated experience in sleep disorders may be consulted.

PEARLS & CONSIDERATIONS

COMMENTS

- Adenotonsillar hypertrophy and sleep obstruction should be investigated even in patients who may have another reason for pulmonary hypertension (e.g., sickle cell patients with previous pulmonary infarctions).
- Sleep obstruction is common, can coexist with other diseases, and is additive in its deleterious effect on pulmonary vascular resistance.

PREVENTION

- Early diagnosis and treatment of obstruction may prevent cor pulmonale.

PATIENT/FAMILY EDUCATION

American Sleep Apnea Association (www.sleepapnea.org/info/practitioner/pediatrics.html).

SUGGESTED READINGS

American Academy of Pediatrics, Section on Pediatric Pulmonology: Clinical practice guidelines: Diagnosis and management of childhood obstructive sleep apnea syndrome. *Pediatrics* 109:704, 2002.

Chan J et al: Obstructive sleep apnea in children. *Am Fam Physician* 6:1147, 2004. Available at www.aafp.org/afp/20040301/1147.html

Perkin RM et al: Sleep-disordered breathing in infants and children. *Respir Care Clin North Am* 5:395, 1999.

AUTHOR: **DAVID W. HANNON, MD**

BASIC INFORMATION

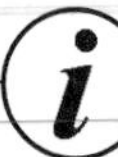

DEFINITION

A corneal abrasion is a superficial de-epithelialization of the cornea, usually caused by trauma or by chemical, thermal, or ultraviolet light exposure.

ICD-9-CM CODE
918.1 Corneal abrasion

EPIDEMIOLOGY & DEMOGRAPHICS

- Corneal abrasions account for 10% of new patients seeking medical attention in emergency departments for eye problems.
- Corneal abrasions are common in young adults, especially in those who work on cars.

CLINICAL PRESENTATION

History

- There is usually a history of exposure with at least one of the following:
  - Intense ocular pain
  - Redness
  - Light sensitivity
  - Copious tearing
- In nonverbal children, the only history may be inconsolable irritability.

Physical Examination

- Relief is obtained with topical anesthesia.
- Irregular epithelium is identified by slit-lamp examination.
- Fluorescein dye may stain the abraded area, which can be seen with cobalt blue light or Wood's lamp.

ETIOLOGY

- Trauma
  - Young children: sand, dirt, or other foreign bodies
  - Teens: sports impact, contact lens wear, or foreign bodies
- Chemical: contact lens solution, permanent hair solution
- Ultraviolet radiation: exposure to welding arc
- Thermal
  - Young children: cigarette burns
  - Teens: curling iron burns

DIAGNOSIS

Dx

DIFFERENTIAL DIAGNOSIS

- Congenital glaucoma
- Corneal ulcer
- Occult ruptured globe
- Uveitis

WORKUP

Perform a thorough physical examination, including visual acuity testing.

TREATMENT

Rx

NONPHARMACOLOGIC THERAPY

- Patch the affected eye. Small abrasions may not require patching.
- Maintaining a patch is a challenge.
- There is a risk of deprivation amblyopia.

ACUTE GENERAL Rx

- Broad-spectrum antibiotic solution or ointment
- Artificial tears
- Topical nonsteroidal anti-inflammatory eye drops

DISPOSITION

- The abrasions should heal within 2 to 3 days.
- The patient should be followed until corneal abrasion heals and visual acuity returns to baseline.

REFERRAL

- Referral is indicated if visual acuity does not return to baseline or if healing is not seen within 4 to 5 days.
- An uncommon complication is recurrent erosion syndrome, which is an intermittent de-epithelization of a previously abraded area.

PEARLS & CONSIDERATIONS

COMMENTS

Corneal abrasion is in the differential diagnosis of the inconsolable child.

SUGGESTED READINGS

Hamill MB: Corneal injury. *In* Krachmer JH et al (eds): *Cornea.* St. Louis, Mosby, 1997.

Wilson ME et al: Ocular trauma in childhood. *In Pediatric Ophthalmology and Strabismus.* San Francisco, American Academy of Ophthalmology, 1998–1999.

AUTHOR: **ANNA F. FAKADEJ, MD, FAAO, FACS**

BASIC INFORMATION

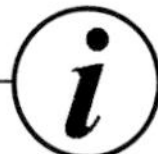

DEFINITION

Costochondritis is a syndrome of diffuse inflammation involving the costal cartilage, typically at the costochondral or costosternal junctions. It is associated with pain and reproducible tenderness on palpation.

SYNONYMS

Anterior chest wall syndrome
Costosternal syndrome
Fibrositis (misnomer because this is a separate entity)
Tietze's syndrome (misnomer because this is a separate entity)

ICD-9-CM CODE
733.6 Costochondritis

EPIDEMIOLOGY & DEMOGRAPHICS

- Chest pain in pediatrics is common.
- Although usually benign, the potential implications of this complaint may lead to significant anxiety.
- 21% to 45% of cases are idiopathic.
- Conditions affecting the musculoskeletal system are identified as the cause of chest pain in 15% to 31% of cases. Among these musculoskeletal conditions is the diagnosis of costochondritis.
- The incidence of costochondritis is approximately 4% among children and adolescents.
- The prevalence of costochondritis ranges from 14% to 30%. One report revealed that 79 of 100 adolescents presenting with chest and upper abdominal pain were ultimately diagnosed with costochondritis.
- Girls are diagnosed with costochondritis more often than boys (2:1 ratio).
- Heavy lifting and exercise may be risk factors. Reports of costochondritis have been linked to muscular and ligamentous strain from carrying heavy school bags, especially over one shoulder.

CLINICAL PRESENTATION

History

- Costochondritis is characterized by pain in the anterior chest wall that may radiate to the back or upper abdomen.
- Symptoms typically are short-lived, although they can last for several months. The onset is most commonly insidious, developing over several days or weeks.
- Discomfort varies in intensity and quality.
  - Usually sharp and stabbing but can be dull.
  - May be pleuritic in nature.
  - Intensity can range from mild to severe.
- Costochondritis is typically unilateral, affecting the left side most frequently, but it can be bilateral.
  - Any of the seven costochondral junctions can be affected.
  - The left second through fifth costochondral cartilages are most commonly involved.
  - Some sources state that the left fourth sternocostal cartilage is the most common site of involvement.
- The patient may have many areas of tenderness. In 90% of cases, more than one site is painful.
- Exacerbating factors include coughing, sneezing, inspiration, upper body movement.
- Antecedent upper respiratory illness or recent participation in exercise.
- While obtaining the history, eliminate red flags for systemic disease.
  - Diffuse pain, fatigue, and altered sleep may raise the possibility of fibromyalgia.
  - With chronic low back pain consider ankylosing spondylarthritis.
- Constitutional symptoms and other worrisome symptoms that may indicate a non-musculoskeletal cause of complaints. Inquire about fever, chills, cough, dyspnea, pain with exertion and radiation of pain, or associated numbness in the arm and neck.

Physical Examination

- Vital signs, including pulse oximetry, should be within normal limits for the patient's age.
- Alterations in vital signs may depend on the level of the patient's pain and anxiety.
- Assessment of symmetry should be included with inspection of the chest wall.
- Confirmation of normal pulmonary, cardiac, and abdominal examinations is essential for the diagnosis of costochondritis.
- Palpate all costochondral junctions, the inframammary region, and the origin of the pectoralis muscle group. Single-digit palpation of the involved area is the preferred method of examination.
- Palpate articulations at both ends of the clavicle (i.e., acromioclavicular and sternoclavicular joints).
- The entire length of the sternum should be examined to rule out tenderness of the sternalis muscle, the manubriosternal and xiphisternal joints, and the xiphoid process.
- Various musculoskeletal maneuvers may be helpful in differentiating costochondritis from other musculoskeletal disorders of the chest wall. As with focal palpation, these maneuvers are considered diagnostic if pain is reproduced.
  - The crowing rooster maneuver involves the examiner standing behind and patient and exerting traction on the patient's upper arms by pulling them backward and slightly superiorly.
  - In horizontal arm flexion, the arm is adducted across the anterior chest, and while the arm remains steady, prolonged traction is applied in a horizontal direction.
  - The hooking maneuver, a test to exclude slipping rib syndrome, is performed by hooking the examiner's fingers under the anterior lower costal margins. This test is considered positive if pain is elicited while the rib cage is pulled anteriorly.
- The diagnosis of costochondritis is confirmed by the reproduction of pain on palpation of the local site.

ETIOLOGY

- Most cases are considered idiopathic.
- The presumed pathophysiology of costochondritis is inflamed or irritated cartilage from various causes.
- Several possible causes have been identified.
  - Repeated trauma to the chest wall resulting in local irritation
  - Excessive exercise leading to stretching and straining of costochondral junction
  - Repeated straining of costochondral junction from significant coughing
  - Infection
    - Viral: direct inflammation of the costochondral junctions
    - Bacterial: more likely in intravenous drug user or after upper chest surgery
    - Fungal: rarely causes costochondritis

DIAGNOSIS

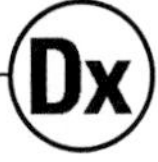

DIFFERENTIAL DIAGNOSIS

- Chest wall
  - Breast development and disease
    - Fibrocystic disease
    - Gynecomastia
    - Mastitis
    - Thelarche
  - Fibrositis
  - Herpes zoster and postherpetic neuralgia
  - Intercostal neuritis
  - Lower rib pain syndromes
    - Clicking rib syndrome
    - Rib-tip syndrome
    - Slipping rib syndrome
    - Twelfth rib syndrome
  - Malignancy
    - Primary or secondary: rare in children
  - Muscular strain
  - Myositis
  - Neurofibroma of intercostal nerve
  - Osteomyelitis or infectious arthritis of chest wall
  - Posterior chest wall syndrome
    - Costovertebral joint dysfunction
    - Thoracic disk herniation
  - Precordial catch; Texidor's twinge
  - Rheumatic disease
    - Rheumatoid arthritis
    - Ankylosing spondylitis
    - Fibromyalgia
    - Psoriatic arthritis
    - SAPHO syndrome (i.e., synovitis, acne, pustulosis, hyperostosis, osteomyelitis)
    - Relapsing polychondritis
  - Rib fracture
  - Rib infarction (i.e., proposed with sickle cell disease)
  - Spontaneous sternocostal subluxation
  - Sternalis syndrome
  - Stress fracture of rib or rib cage
  - Tietze's syndrome

- Trauma
- Xiphoidalgia

- Cardiac conditions
  - Aortic root dissection
  - Coronary artery anomalies
  - Mitral valve prolapse
  - Myocarditis
  - Myocardial infarction
  - Myocardial ischemia or coronary vasospasm
  - Pericarditis
  - Tachyarrhythmia or palpitations
- Gastrointestinal conditions
  - Esophagitis
  - Foreign body
  - Gastroesophageal reflux
  - Motility disorder (e.g., diffuse esophageal spasm, achalasia)
  - Stricture
- Pulmonary
  - Acute chest syndrome
  - Asthma
  - Bronchitis
  - Exercise-induced bronchospasm
  - Pleural effusion
  - Pleuritis
  - Pleurodynia
  - Pneumonia
  - Pneumomediastinum
  - Pneumonitis
  - Pneumothorax
  - Pulmonary embolism
  - Pulmonary hypertension
- Miscellaneous conditions
  - Anxiety disorder; panic attack
  - Hyperventilation
  - Psychogenic causes

WORKUP

- The diagnosis is established by the history and physical examination.
- If symptoms are of recent onset in an otherwise healthy patient, it is unlikely that the symptoms have a nonmusculoskeletal cause, and there are few roles for laboratory testing or imaging studies.
- However, if the patient has atypical pain, persistent pain, or signs and symptoms of a chronic illness or constitutional symptoms such as fever, chills, and weight loss, consider further evaluation.

IMAGING STUDIES

- Imaging studies have no role in the diagnosis of costochondritis. If concerned about trauma-associated rib fracture, malignancy, or systemic disease exists, consider a chest radiograph or axial computed tomography (CT) of the chest.
  - The diagnostic yield of chest radiographs is less than 2% for isolated costochondritis.
  - Axial CT of the chest is a more valuable diagnostic tool because costal cartilage swelling can be seen.

TREATMENT

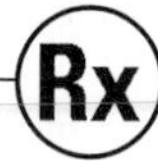

NONPHARMACOLOGIC THERAPY

- Rest
- Reassurance, especially in view of the anxiety of the patient and family
- Avoidance of activities that trigger or worsen pain
- Application of ice to the affected area at 20-minute intervals

ACUTE GENERAL Rx

- For mild to moderate pain, use nonsteroidal anti-inflammatory drugs (NSAIDs) or other analgesics.
  - Ibuprofen
  - Naprosyn
  - Acetaminophen
- Severe symptoms are not a common problem during a typical course of costochondritis in children. The physician should consider administration of injectable treatments only if comfortable with performing such procedures.
  - Intramuscular injection of ketorolac tromethamine is followed by a several-day oral course, not to exceed 5 days of use. Because the safety and efficacy in children younger than 16 years of age have not been established, this approach is not recommended for children.
  - Local injection of corticosteroid and anesthetic must be done cautiously because of the risk of pneumothorax and laceration of local blood vessels. Narcotics should be avoided.

CHRONIC Rx

- Use of tricyclic antidepressants may play a role in the treatment of chronic costochondritis.
  - These drugs are not routinely used.
  - The physician and family must be cognizant of the risk of nonaccidental and accidental ingestion.

DISPOSITION

- Costochondritis usually has a self-limited course.
- Some patients may suffer from an exacerbation.
- Consider a follow-up appointment in 4 to 6 weeks after the initial presentation.

REFERRAL

If the clinical scenario is atypical for costochondritis, if symptoms are remitting and persistent, or if there is concern about systemic disease, consider referral to appropriate specialist such as a pediatric rheumatologist or orthopedic surgeon.

PEARLS & CONSIDERATIONS

COMMENTS

- Tietze's syndrome should be on the differential diagnosis list for suspected costochondritis. Controversy exists about whether Tietze's syndrome and costochondritis are distinct entities or represent variations along a spectrum of one disorder.
- Tietze's syndrome is a rare and benign but painful, nonsuppurative, localized swelling of the costosternal, sternoclavicular, or costochondral joints.
  - It can be distinguished from costochondritis by the presence of swelling.
  - It most commonly affects adolescents and young adults but has been reported in young children.
  - It usually involves the second and third ribs.
  - Treatment consists of NSAIDs or local corticosteroid injections.
  - Typically, it has a self-limited course. Pain often subsides within several weeks, but local swelling can persist for much longer.

PREVENTION

Encourage children to use school bags appropriately.

PATIENT/FAMILY EDUCATION

- Reassure patient and family that costochondritis is usually a benign, self-limited entity.
- Avoid contact sports until the patient can perform related activity without discomfort.
- Return to exacerbating activities before pain resolution may evoke relapse of costochondritis.

SUGGESTED READINGS

Anzai AK et al: Adolescent chest pain. *Am Fam Physician* 53:1682, 1996.

Brown RT: Costochondritis in adolescents. *J Adolesc Health Care* 1:198, 1981.

Disla E et al: Costochondritis: a prospective analysis in an emergency department setting. *Arch Intern Med* 154:2466, 1994.

Garry JP et al: Costochondritis. *eMedicine: Emergency Medicine [serial outline]*, 2004. Available at http://www.emedicine.com/ped/topic487.htm

Gregory PL et al: Musculoskeletal problems of the chest wall in athletes. *Sports Med* 32:235, 2002.

Selbst SM: Chest pain in children. *Am Fam Physician* 41:179, 1990.

Selbst SM: Consultation with the specialist: chest pain in children. *Pediatr Rev* 18:169, 1997.

Selbst SM: Evaluation of chest pain in children. *Pediatr Rev* 8:56, 1986.

Selbst SM et al: Pediatric chest pain: a prospective study. *Pediatrics* 82:319, 1988.

AUTHOR: **BRITTANNY LIAM BOULANGER, MD**

BASIC INFORMATION

DEFINITION

Croup is a syndrome of respiratory distress caused by subglottic narrowing. It is characterized by hoarseness, inspiratory stridor, and a barklike cough.

SYNONYMS

Acute laryngotracheitis
Laryngotracheobronchitis

ICD-9-CM CODE
464.4 Croup

EPIDEMIOLOGY & DEMOGRAPHICS

- Primarily affects children between the ages of 6 months and 3 years
- Peaks at age 2 years, with a mean age of 18 months
- Accounts for 15% of respiratory disease in children
- Predominance in fall and winter; may occur in spring or summer in more temperate climates
- Spread by person-to-person contact or by large droplets and contaminated nasopharyngeal secretions
- Incubation period of 2 to 6 days
- Affects boys more than girls

CLINICAL PRESENTATION

History

- Prodrome of upper respiratory tract symptoms for 1 to 2 days
- Hoarse voice and cry
- "Barky" cough, often described as a seal-like noise
- Respiratory difficulty and noisy breathing
- Fever, but usually less than 39°C
- Thorough history needed to narrow diagnosis
  - History of trauma
  - Previous intubation history
  - Cough with oral intake
  - Cough or choking after playing with small toys

Physical Examination

- General examination
  - The patient usually has a nontoxic appearance. If severe airway narrowing is present, however, the child may be in significant respiratory distress.
  - If patient is in the tripod or "sniffing dog" position, be aware of imminent airway obstruction. This is more common with epiglottitis.
- Vital signs
  - Increased respiratory rate
  - Increased heart rate
  - Increased temperature
- Respiratory conditions
  - Stridor
  - Sternal retractions
  - Dyspnea
  - Tachypnea
  - Cyanosis
- Degrees of croup (many croup scoring systems are available):
  - Mild croup: normal color, normal mental state, air entry with stridor audible only with stethoscope, and no retractions
  - Moderate croup: normal color, audible stridor, mild to moderate retractions, and slightly diminished air entry in an anxious child
  - Severe croup: cyanotic, loud stridor, significant decrease in air entry, and marked retractions in a highly anxious child
  - Imminent respiratory failure: disappearance of retractions and stridor in a child with severe croup

ETIOLOGY

- Parainfluenza type 1 (most common)
- Parainfluenza types 2, 3, and 4
- Human metapneumovirus
- Respiratory syncytial virus
- Influenza A and influenza B
- Adenovirus types 1 through 4, 7, 8, 11, 14, and 21
- Rhinovirus
- Coxsackievirus types A9 and B4
- Echovirus types 4, 11, and 21
- Rarely, *Mycoplasma pneumoniae* and rubeola

DIAGNOSIS

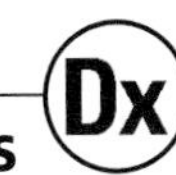

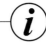

DIFFERENTIAL DIAGNOSIS

- Spasmodic croup
  - Usually age 3 months to 3 years
  - Primarily at night
  - No fever
- Foreign body
- Epiglottitis
  - Rare now because of immunizations
  - Toxic and very anxious child
  - Muffled voice or not talking; often drooling
- Bacterial tracheitis
  - High fever and toxic appearance.
  - May follow irritation of trachea or occur in immunocompromised patients.
  - Caused by secondary infection with bacteria (e.g., *Staphylococcus aureus, Haemophilus influenza, Streptococcus pneumoniae, Moraxella*).
  - Often manifests with increasing toxicity, drooling, and increased respiratory effort after several days of croup symptoms.
- Peritonsillar or retropharyngeal abscess
- Vocal cord dysfunction
  - Acute onset
  - Lasts minutes to hours
  - Usually in older children and adolescents
- Tracheomalacia
- Subglottic stenosis (if prior history of intubation)
- Gastroesophageal reflux
- Trauma (e.g., burns, laryngeal fracture)
- Neoplasm
- Vascular ring
- Angioneurotic edema (often associated with hives or a generalized allergic reaction)
- Tracheal hemangioma or vocal cord papilloma
- Psychogenic stridor
- Hypocalcemic tetany and laryngospasm
- Diphtheria
  - Rare
  - Virtually excluded if patient had prior diphtheria vaccine
  - Primarily in foreign-born patients

WORKUP

Croup is primarily a clinical diagnosis.

LABORATORY TESTS

Specific viral causes can be diagnosed by culture or antigen detection.

IMAGING STUDIES

- Radiographs of the neck can be a diagnostic aid.
  - Classic steeple sign is found in 50% of patients. It is narrowing of the laryngeal air column 5 to 10 mm below the vocal cords.
  - Sensitivity is 93%, and specificity is 92% for the diagnosis of viral croup.
  - Airway management should never be delayed for the sake of obtaining a radiographic study.
- Endoscopy can be used in children with an atypical course or when an underlying anatomic abnormality or foreign body is suspected. It can also be used in controlled conditions if bacterial tracheitis or epiglottitis is suspected.
- Magnetic resonance imagine (MRI) or computed tomography (CT) may be required if noninfectious causes of croup are possible.

TREATMENT

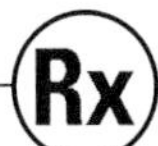

NONPHARMACOLOGIC THERAPY

- There is no substitute for close observation, frequent reassessment, and appropriate airway management.
- The child should be kept calm and comfortable.
- Cool mist tents are not recommended because they can increase anxiety. Cool night air or steam from a shower may be effective because they may decrease the viscosity of secretions.

ACUTE GENERAL Rx

- Nebulized epinephrine (0.5 mL of a 2.25% solution in normal saline) is given to patients with stridor at rest or respiratory distress. Patients should be observed for at least 2 hours after treatment to monitor for recurrent symptoms.
- Dexamethasone (0.6 mg/kg) may be given orally or intramuscularly as a single dose. It may also be given every 8 to 12 hours for three

doses if preferred. This has resulted in a shorter duration of symptoms, fewer hospitalizations, and decreased severity of symptoms.
  - A single oral dose of dexamethasone is as effective as a single intramuscular dose.
  - Nebulized budesonide also is equally effective, but the cost may be prohibitive.
- Droplet isolation should be maintained in the hospital setting.
- Oxygen for hypoxemia and intubation for respiratory failure may be needed.

DISPOSITION

- Most patients recover completely within 2 to 4 days and do not require hospitalization.
- Children should be hospitalized in the following circumstances:
  - Significant respiratory distress is unresponsive to nebulized epinephrine. Admission can be considered if more than two treatments are required.
  - The patient has severe symptoms, including hypoxia and fatigue.
  - The patient lives a long distance from the clinical setting or emergency room.
  - There is a lack of an appropriate home setting for outpatient management. This includes a lack of transportation and lack of telephone.

PEARLS & CONSIDERATIONS

COMMENTS

- Croup is the most common cause of stridor in children.
- In children younger than 2 years, rule out foreign body aspiration.

PREVENTION

- No croup-specific vaccine is available.
- Influenza vaccine may prevent some cases.
- Antiviral therapy can be administered for acute influenza.
  - Amantadine and rimantadine are effective only for influenza A.
  - Oseltamivir is effective for influenza A and B.
- Good hand-washing techniques should be practiced.

PATIENT/FAMILY EDUCATION

- Review the signs and symptoms of respiratory distress.
- Remind parents that symptoms may continue to flare at night for 2 to 3 days after initiating acute management.
- The benefits of cool night air or shower steam, as well as the importance of adequate hydration, should be emphasized.

SUGGESTED READINGS

American Academy of Pediatrics. Available at www.aap.org/healthtopics/commonillness.cfm

Bjornson CL et al: A randomised trial of a single dose of oral dexamethasone for mild croup. *N Engl J Med* 351:1306, 2004.

Cetinkaya F et al: A comparison of nebulized budesonide, and intramuscular, and oral dexamethasone for treatment of croup. *Int J Pediatr Otorhinolaryngol* 68:453, 2004.

Hay W et al: Croup syndrome. *In* Hay W et al (eds): *Current Pediatric Diagnosis and Treatment.* New York, McGraw-Hill, 2005, pp 513–515.

Kaditis AG, Wald ER: Viral croup: current diagnosis and treatment. *Pediatr Infect Dis J* 17:827, 1998.

KidsHealth. Available at www.kidshealth.org/parent/infections/lung/croup.html

Malhotra A, Krilov LR: Viral croup. *Pediatr Rev* 22:5, 2001.

Osmond M: Croup. *In* Barton S (ed): *Clinical Evidence Pediatrics.* London, BMJ Publishing Group, 2002, pp 71–80.

Rittichier KK, Ledwith CA: Outpatient treatment of moderate croup with dexamethasone: intramuscular versus oral dosing. *Pediatrics* 106:1344, 2000.

Schwartz RH: Laryngeal subglottic infections. *In* Long SS et al (eds): *Principals and Practice of Pediatric Infectious Diseases.* New York, Churchill Livingstone, 2003, pp 210–211.

AUTHORS: **MARY ANNE JACKSON, MD** and **J. BRYAN WOHLWEND, MD**

BASIC INFORMATION

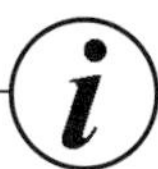

DEFINITION

Cryptorchidism is failure of the testis to completely descend into the scrotum. The term is derived from the Greek words *kryptos* and *orchis,* meaning "hidden testis."

SYNONYMS

Incompletely descended testis
Undescended testis

ICD-9-CM CODE
752.51 Undescended testis

EPIDEMIOLOGY & DEMOGRAPHICS

- Incidence is related to gestational age because testes descend late in fetal growth.
  - Cryptorchidism occurs in up to 30% of preterm infants.
  - The incidence is 1 (3%) in 33 term newborns.
  - A less than 1% incidence is seen after age 6 months.
- Five percent of cases are nonpalpable.
- Distribution is 65% right, 25% left, and 10% bilateral.
- Approximately 80% of cases are identified at birth, whereas 20% manifest later in childhood.
- Cryptorchidism is associated with many central nervous system anomalies, including the following:
  - Myelomeningocele
  - Hydrocephalus
  - Anencephaly
  - Hypopituitarism
- It is associated with abdominal wall defects such as prune-belly syndrome and gastroschisis.
- The incidence is increased among premature infants and small-for-gestational-age (SGA) infants.
- Increased familial incidence (10% of siblings) is observed.
- There is an increased incidence of testicular malignancy in maldescended testes.
- The risk for impaired fertility is increased for those with undescended testes.
- Increased incidence of cryptorchidism is associated with multiple malformation syndromes, including chromosomal anomalies and single-gene defects.

CLINICAL PRESENTATION

History

- Cryptorchidism is usually identified on physical examination.
- It is not associated with pain, tenderness, or discomfort in most cases.
- Many malformation syndromes, chromosomal abnormalities, and neurologic defects are associated with maldescended testes, including the following:
  - Aarskog syndrome
  - de Lange's syndrome
  - Kallmann's syndrome
  - Klinefelter syndrome
  - Laurence-Moon-Biedl syndrome
  - Noonan-Opitz-Frias syndrome
  - Prader-Willi syndrome
  - Robinow's syndrome
  - Rubinstein-Taybi syndrome
  - Smith-Lemli-Opitz syndrome
  - Trisomy 21

Physical Examination

- The following conditions are important during the examination:
  - Warm environment
  - Relaxed patient in the frog-leg position
  - Warm examiner's hands
  - Abdominal examination preceding inguinal-scrotal palpation
- Examine patients carefully, especially those with the risk factors listed in "Epidemiology & Demographics."
- Examine genitalia for other abnormalities (e.g., hypospadias).

ETIOLOGY

- The cause is uncertain, but cryptorchidism probably results from multiple factors, including the following:
  - Improper traction of the gubernacular (i. e., fetal cord that attaches to the testis)
  - Abnormal intra-abdominal pressure
  - Epididymal differentiation and maturation abnormalities
  - Improper attachment of gubernaculum testis
  - Hormonal impairment (e.g., androgen deficiency, decreased luteinizing hormone–releasing hormone)
- Traumatic dislocation of the testis (e.g., straddle injury) may cause incomplete descent.
- Surgical dislocation of testis (e.g., snagged spermatic cord during hernia repair, surgeon does not position testis correctly) may affect later development and movement.

DIAGNOSIS Dx

DIFFERENTIAL DIAGNOSIS

- Ectopic testes (i.e., never descend)
- Retractile testes
- Anorchia (i.e., lack of testes)
- Atrophic testis
- Ambiguous genitalia
  - Genetic female with androgen excess
  - Genetic male with androgen insensitivity

WORKUP

- The diagnosis is based on findings of the physical examination.
- Ultrasonography is rarely helpful in localizing the testes.
- Computed tomography can help localize testes and evaluate testes, but it is rarely necessary.

LABORATORY TESTS

- Endocrine evaluation (i.e., testosterone, dihydrotestosterone, luteinizing hormone [LH], and follicle-stimulating hormone [FSH]) should be performed for patients with bilateral, nonpalpable testes who are chromosomal males.
  - Elevated LH and FSH levels with absent or low testosterone levels indicate nonfunctioning or absent testes or an intersex disorder.
  - Elevated testosterone levels occur with androgen insensitivity.
- A human chorionic gonadotropin (hCG) stimulation study should be conducted for bilateral, nonpalpable testes; after stimulation, measure testosterone, LH, and FSH levels.
  - If the testosterone level is elevated, testes are present.
  - If no testosterone is detected and LH and FSH levels are elevated, no functioning testes exist.
- Test inhibin, which may be a more sensitive marker than testosterone.
  - This test is not widely available.
  - A lack of inhibin indicates no functioning testes.
  - Inhibin presence indicates functional testicular tissue.

IMAGING STUDIES

- Ultrasonography is rarely helpful in localizing the testes (less helpful than physical examination).
- Computed tomography can help localize testes, but it is rarely necessary.

TREATMENT

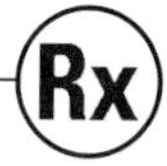

NONPHARMACOLOGIC THERAPY

- Open inguinal and abdominal incisions are used to manage most undescended testes.
- Laparoscopy is used in selected instances of older boys with nonpalpable, undescended testes.

ACUTE GENERAL Rx

- Therapeutic hCG stimulation is used for bilateral, nonpalpable testes.
  - To bring testes down and potentially avoid surgery
  - To stretch cord structure in preparation for surgery

DISPOSITION

- The primary care physician should perform interval physical examinations throughout childhood and puberty.
- Follow pubertal testicular growth for possible atrophy.
- Instruct the patient to conduct monthly testicular self-examinations beginning in teens to look for malignancy.

REFERRAL

- All boys with cryptorchidism should be referred to a pediatric urologist.
    - If the patient has bilateral, nonpalpable testes, refer at birth.
    - If the patient has unilateral cryptorchidism at birth, refer at 3 to 5 months.
    - If the patient has highly retractile or late presentation of cryptorchidism, refer at that time.
- Endocrinologists are usually involved in cases that are complicated by ambiguous genitalia or micropenis to rule out and manage enzyme defects and hormonal deficiencies.

PEARLS & CONSIDERATIONS

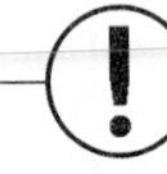

COMMENTS

- Ultrasound is rarely helpful for this condition.
- Because of the potential for late presentation of cryptorchidism, all boys should have confirmation of testicular location at intervals throughout childhood and puberty.

PATIENT/FAMILY EDUCATION

- Pubertal testicular self-examination
- Pubertal education regarding fertility potential
- Pubertal education regarding malignant potential

SUGGESTED READINGS

Bogaert GA et al: Therapeutic laparoscopy for intra-abdominal testes. *Urology* 42:182, 1993.

Elder JS: Ultrasonography is unnecessary in evaluating boys with a nonpalpable testis. *Pediatrics* 110:748, 2002.

Rabinowitz R, Hulbert WC: Late presentation of cryptorchidism: the etiology of testicular re-ascent. *J Urol* 157:1892, 1997.

Rajfer J et al: Hormonal therapy of cryptorchidism. *N Engl J Med* 314:466, 1986.

Scorer CG: The descent of the testis. *Arch Dis Child* 39:605, 1964.

AUTHORS: **RONALD RABINOWITZ, MD, WILLIAM C. HULBERT, MD,** and **ROBERT A. MEVORACH, MD**

BASIC INFORMATION

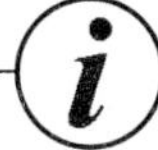

DEFINITION

Cystic fibrosis (CF) is an inherited, multisystem disease of exocrine gland function that is primarily characterized by diffuse obstruction and chronic infection of the airways and poor digestion resulting from exocrine pancreatic insufficiency. Although multiple organ systems are affected, progressive lung destruction (i.e., bronchiectasis) is the major cause of morbidity and mortality in those affected with CF.

SYNONYM

Mucoviscidosis

ICD-9-CM CODES
277.00 Cystic fibrosis, pancreatic
518.89 Cystic fibrosis, pulmonary

EPIDEMIOLOGY & DEMOGRAPHICS

- One of the most common fatal genetic disorders among whites
- Autosomal recessive inheritance
- Estimated incidence: 1 case per 3200 whites; 1 case per 15,000 blacks; 1 case per 11,000 Native Americans; 1 case per 31,000 Asian Americans; 1 case per 9500 Hispanics
- Carrier frequency: 1 in 32 overall in the United States

CLINICAL PRESENTATION

History

- A family history of CF may be reported (16%).
- Multiple organ systems are affected, most commonly the sweat ducts, pancreas, and airways.
- CF most often manifests in early childhood with persistent respiratory illness (50%), malnutrition and poor growth (34%), abnormal stools (26%), or a combination of these features.
- Signs and symptoms may vary widely by age:
  - Neonate: meconium ileus or peritonitis (15%)
  - Infancy: obstructive jaundice, hypochloremic alkalosis, hyponatremic dehydration, heat prostration, steatorrhea, hypoproteinemia, edema, salty taste
  - Infancy and childhood: failure to thrive, bronchiolitis, recurrent wheezing
  - Childhood and older: rectal prolapse, nasal polyposis, panopacification of sinuses, pancreatitis, unexplained cirrhosis, gallstones, allergic bronchopulmonary aspergillosis
  - Adolescence and adulthood: cor pulmonale, glucose intolerance, diabetes mellitus, biliary cirrhosis, hemoptysis
  - Any age: absence of the vas deferens, azoospermia, recurrent pneumonia or wheezing, chronic cough (often productive), staphylococcal pneumonia, mucoid pseudomonas in lung, bronchiectasis, digital clubbing

Physical Examination

- Respiratory system
  - Chronic productive cough
  - Recurrent or persistent crackles or wheezing
  - Diminished breath sounds
  - Barrel chest deformity, hyperinflation
  - Use of accessory muscles of respiration; tachypnea
  - Chronic sinusitis, nasal polyps, widening of the nasal bridge
- Gastrointestinal system
  - Poor weight gain
  - Rectal prolapse
  - Abdominal distention
  - Loss of subcutaneous fat and muscle
  - Edema, hepatomegaly
- Reproductive system
  - Absence or atresia of vas deferens
  - Testicular hernia, hydrocele, undescended testes
  - Delayed puberty
- Skeletal system
  - Hypertrophic osteoarthropathy
  - Digital clubbing
- Other difficulties
  - Acrodermatitis enteropathica
  - Enlarged submaxillary glands
  - Bulging fontanelle (i.e., vitamin A deficiency)

ETIOLOGY

- The basic defect is an abnormality of chloride transport in apical membrane epithelial cells.
- The responsible gene is on the long arm of chromosome 7, and it codes for the CF transmembrane conductance regulator (CFTR protein).
- More than 800 gene mutations are known.
- The most prevalent mutation of CFTR is the deletion of one phenylalanine residue at amino acid 508 (ΔF508).
- Genetic heterogenicity occurs and may partially account for the wide spectrum of disease severity and rate of progression.
  - An individual genotype poorly predicts pulmonary disease progression.
- The patient is unable to clear mucous secretions easily.
  - Inadequate water in mucous secretions ("sticky mucous")
  - Persistent infection of the lower respiratory airways

DIAGNOSIS

Dx

DIFFERENTIAL DIAGNOSIS

- Bronchiectasis
- Chronic reactive airways disease
- Immotile cilia syndrome
- Immunodeficiency
- Malabsorption syndromes
- Protein-calorie malnutrition

WORKUP

The diagnosis of CF is suspected on clinical grounds or from the family history.

LABORATORY TESTS

- Newborn screening: A few U.S. states screen newborns for CF by measuring immunoreactive trypsin (IRT) in blood. Most infants who have CF have elevated IRT levels, but there are many false-positive results. The diagnosis must be confirmed by sweat test or by genotyping.
- Genotyping: There are commercial genotyping tests for about 100 specific mutations in the *CFTR* gene.
  - Genotyping identifies about 95% of all CF alleles.
  - A patient in whom two alleles are not identified by commercial genotyping still can have CF because there are more than 800 mutations.
- Sweat chloride test: The diagnosis of CF can be confirmed by a sweat chloride concentration greater than 60 mEq/L in the presence of appropriate clinical manifestations (i.e., chronic pulmonary disease or pancreatic insufficiency, or both) or an appropriate family history.
  - The test should be performed in an experienced, reliable laboratory.
  - A positive result must always be confirmed by a second test.
  - False-positive results are few, but they may be caused by untreated Addison's disease, ectodermal dysplasia, glycogen storage diseases, or untreated hypothyroidism.
- Pulmonary function testing: Tests offer evidence of obstruction, flow limitation, or air trapping.
- Sputum culture: *Staphylococcus aureus* or mucoid forms of *Pseudomonas aeruginosa* from sputum strongly suggest CF.

IMAGING STUDIES

- Chest radiograph: peribronchial cuffing, mucous plugging, infiltrates, atelectasis, fibrosis, bronchiectasis, hyperinflation
- Sinus films: panopacification of sinuses
- Computed tomography of the chest: can demonstrate air trapping and bronchiectasis long before radiographs show changes

TREATMENT

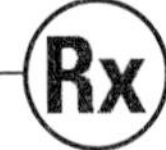

NONPHARMACOLOGIC THERAPY

- There is no cure for CF, but the significantly increasing life span appears to be linked to early and aggressive management of the disease.
- Treatment plans must be individualized to account for age and for type and severity of symptoms.
- Hospitalize all newly diagnosed patients to facilitate verification of the diagnosis, to provide education for the family, and to determine the baseline disease status.

- A multidisciplinary team should include a nurse, respiratory therapist, social services advisor, dietitian, psychologist, and physician.
- Maintain hydration, particularly in a hot environment and during ongoing losses.
- Perform airway clearance techniques daily to assist with clearing of mucus.
- Neonates with CF may present with meconium ileus or meconium peritonitis, requiring immediate surgical intervention (15% of CF patients).
- MediPort placement may be required for frequent intravenous administration of antibiotics.
- A gastrostomy tube and fundoplication may be required to optimize the patient's nutritional status.
- Complications of progressive CF may require surgical intervention.
  - Lobectomy for chronic, recalcitrant atelectasis (controversial) or recurrent hemoptysis
  - Bronchial artery embolization for recurrent hemoptysis
  - Chest tube for pneumothorax
  - Pleurodesis for recurrent pneumothorax
  - Lung transplantation for end-stage lung disease

ACUTE GENERAL Rx

- Primarily directed at respiratory and nutritional support
- Inhalation therapies: bronchodilators aid daily airway clearance of mucus, aerosolized antibiotics, human recombinant DNAase
- Antibiotics
  - Oral: Use at first sign of increasing lower respiratory tract symptoms to cover *S. aureus*, nontypable *H. influenzae*, and *P. aeruginosa* (e.g., amoxicillin, ciprofloxacin, clindamycin).
  - Intravenous: Use when limited response to oral and inhalation therapy and when symptoms are worsening. Usually, two antibiotics are necessary to cover suspected pathogens.

CHRONIC Rx

- Primarily directed at respiratory and nutrition support
- Inhalation therapies: bronchodilators aid daily airway clearance of mucus, aerosolized antibiotics, human recombinant DNAase
- Anti-inflammatory drugs (i.e., corticosteroids): for chronic reactive airways disease and allergic bronchopulmonary aspergillosis
- Nutrition
  - Pancreatic enzymes are replaced.
  - Fat-soluble vitamin deficiencies: Replace vitamins A, D, E, and K by supplementation.
  - Increased caloric need requires increased intake of high-calorie foods.
- Immunizations: maintain schedule, with special attention to pertussis and yearly influenza vaccinations

DISPOSITION

- Frequent outpatient visits after an initial diagnosis and hospitalization are essential.
- Patients should be seen by the multidisciplinary CF team every 3 or 4 months. As the disease progresses, more frequent appointments may be necessary.

REFERRAL

- All patients with CF should be referred to a CF care center accredited by the Cystic Fibrosis Foundation for coordinated care by a multidisciplinary CF team.
- In addition to the multidisciplinary CF team, patients may require consultation with experts in endocrinology, gastroenterology, rheumatology, and surgery.

PEARLS & CONSIDERATIONS

COMMENTS

- Although most common in whites, CF is also seen in blacks and Native Americans.
- Patients may present with predominantly respiratory or gastrointestinal symptoms.
- Patients may present with right upper lung collapse, failure to thrive, or hyponatremic dehydration.

PATIENT/FAMILY EDUCATION

Information is available from the Cystic Fibrosis Foundation (www.cff.org).

SUGGESTED READINGS

Boat TF: Cystic fibrosis. *In* Behrman RE (ed): *Nelson Textbook of Pediatrics,* 16th ed. Philadelphia, WB Saunders, 2000, pp 1315–1327.

Davis PB: Cystic fibrosis. *Pediatr Rev* 22:257, 2001.

Gibson RL et al: State of the art: pathophysiology and management of pulmonary infections in cystic fibrosis. *Am J Respir Crit Care Med* 168:918, 2003.

MacLusky I: Cystic fibrosis for the primary care pediatrician. *Pediatr Ann* 22:541, 1993.

Wilmott RW, Fiedler MA: Recent advances in the treatment of cystic fibrosis. *Pediatr Clin North Am* 41:431, 1994.

AUTHOR: **BARBARA A. CHINI, MD**

BASIC INFORMATION

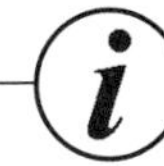

DEFINITION

Cytomegalovirus (CMV) infections are ubiquitous. Most primary CMV infections are asymptomatic, particularly in children. Primary CMV infections can be symptomatic in the congenitally infected neonate and may manifest as infectious mononucleosis (i.e., heterophile negative) in children and adults or as multiorgan disease in the immunocompromised host. Reactivation of latent CMV in immunocompromised individuals most commonly results in retinitis or pneumonitis.

SYNONYMS

Blueberry muffin baby (not specific for congenital CMV infection)
CMV mono
Cytomegalic inclusion disease (CID)

ICD-9-CM CODE
078.5 Cytomegaloviral disease

EPIDEMIOLOGY & DEMOGRAPHICS

- The prevalence of CMV antibody increases with age but varies widely based on geographic, socioeconomic, and ethnic backgrounds and on child-rearing practices such as breast-feeding and use of day-care facilities.
- For neonatal infections, transmission rates are 30% to 50% when the primary infection occurs during pregnancy.
- Transmission rates are approximately 1% among seropositive or immune pregnant women.
- The congenitally infected neonate is likely to be symptomatic.
- Perinatal and early childhood infections occur.
  - Infectious cervicovaginal secretions around the time of delivery transmit infection in more than 50% of patients.
  - Approximately 50% of infants fed with infectious breast milk become infected.
  - Shedding rates of 30% to 80% from children in day-care facilities have been documented.
- Most infected babies are asymptomatic.
- Between 10% and 20% develop sensorineural deafness or mental retardation.
- Children who are shedding CMV can infect other children and adults in day-care facilities and in the home.
- Transmission can occur by blood products that contain leukocytes.
  - In premature infants, infection by blood products may cause shock, lymphocytosis, and pneumonitis.
  - Infection may hasten the progression of bronchopulmonary dysplasia.
  - In those who receive large volumes of blood, transfusion may cause CMV mononucleosis or hepatitis.
- Sexual transmission accounts for the increase in seroprevalence during adolescence and early adulthood.
- Transmission affects immunosuppressed patients.
  - Infection can occur by CMV-infected blood products, transplanted bone marrow, or organs.
  - It may cause a primary infection, reactivation, or reinfection.
- The highest risk is in CMV-seronegative recipients of latently CMV-infected blood products or organs.
- Manifestations of infection include pneumonitis, retinitis, hepatitis, gastrointestinal disease, and CMV syndrome.

CLINICAL PRESENTATION

History

- Congenital infections
  - Maternal CMV status
  - Route of infection: transplacental versus exposure to cervicovaginal secretions
- Other infections
  - Previous serostatus
  - Exposure to potentially infectious persons or infected blood products
  - Presence and severity of immunosuppression
  - Duration of immunosuppression

Physical Examination

- Severe congenital CMV disease
  - Intrauterine growth retardation (50%)
  - Microcephaly (53%)
  - Chorioretinitis (17% to 41%)
  - Sensorineural deafness (58%)
  - Jaundice (67%)
  - Hepatosplenomegaly (60%)
  - Petechiae (76%)
  - Pneumonitis: increased respiratory rate, rales, and cough
- CMV mononucleosis
  - Fever
  - Tender hepatomegaly
  - Tonsillopharyngitis and splenomegaly rare compared with Epstein-Barr virus (EBV) mononucleosis
- Immunocompromised patients
  - Asymptomatic or produce a variety of manifestations
  - Interstitial pneumonia: fever and dry cough
  - Progresses to hypoxia
  - May require assisted ventilation
  - Occurs most often 1 to 3 months after transplantation
- Retinitis
  - Decreased vision or visual field defect
  - Fluffy white perivascular infiltrates and hemorrhage
- CMV syndrome
  - Fever without other explanation
  - CMV cultured in blood

ETIOLOGY

- CMV is an enveloped DNA herpesvirus.
- Horizontal transmission occurs by direct person-to-person contact through saliva, seminal and cervicovaginal fluids, breast milk, and urine or by latently infected blood and organs.
- Vertical transmission is mother-to-child infection that occurs in utero, and it may occur during primary and recurrent infections.
- Incubation periods are as follows:
  - Household by horizontal transmission: unknown
  - After blood transfusion: 4 to 12 weeks
  - After tissue transplantation: 4 to 16 weeks
- Viral shedding may continue for years after the primary infection.
- The infection persists in the latent state in blood and organs.
- Presence of CMV immunoglobulin G (IgG) indicates past infection but is not protective against infection.
- Humoral immunity modifies the severity of disease.
  - Primary infections are more likely to be symptomatic.
  - Neonatal infections occurring as a result of maternal reactivation are rarely symptomatic.

DIAGNOSIS

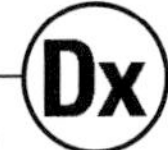

DIFFERENTIAL DIAGNOSIS

- Congenital infections
  - Toxoplasmosis
  - Rubella
  - Herpes simplex
  - Syphilis
- CMV mononucleosis
  - EBV
  - *Toxoplasma gondii*
  - Viral hepatitis
  - Acute human immunodeficiency virus (HIV) infection
  - Lymphoma, leukemia
- CMV infections in immunocompromised patients
  - Pneumonitis: *Pneumocystis jiroveci* (formerly designated *Pneumocystis carinii*), any interstitial pneumonitis
  - Retinitis: cotton-wool spots, *T. gondii*, syphilis, herpes simplex, varicella-zoster virus
  - CMV syndrome: entire spectrum of causes of fever in immunocompromised patients must be considered

WORKUP

The presence of clinical manifestations of congenital infection (e.g., intracerebral calcifications, chorioretinitis, ventriculitis) may assist in differentiation of congenital (intrauterine) from perinatal infections

LABORATORY TESTS

- Congenital infections: Infants who have isolation of CMV by culture or detection by electron microscopy from urine within the first 2 weeks of life have congenital CMV infection, regardless of symptoms.
- Viral nucleic acid detection methods in this situation are less sensitive.

- Negative results for CMV IgG in cord blood rule out congenital infection. Positive results for CMV IgG in cord blood may result from passive transfer of maternal antibodies.
- Immunoglobulin M (IgM) antibody assays may vary in accuracy for diagnosing primary infection. Serial IgG testing at 1, 3, and 6 months is performed to determine resolution or persistence of CMV IgG.
- Perinatal infections have the following diagnostic characteristics:
  - Negative viral culture at birth
  - Positive viral culture at 2 to 4 months
  - Persistence of CMV IgG
- Primary infection (beyond perinatal period) has the following diagnostic characteristics:
  - Positive CMV IgG and IgM
  - Positive viral culture in a previously seronegative individual
- Recurrent infection or reinfection in immunocompromised patients has the following diagnostic characteristics:
  - Because viral shedding may not correlate with clinically significant disease, the diagnosis requires detection of productive infection in the suspected organ.
  - Detection of CMV in bronchoalveolar lavage (BAL) specimen is achieved by cytologic examination.
  - A positive viral culture result is needed to diagnose pneumonitis: detection of pp65 antigen in white blood cells or detection of viral DNA.
  - Prospective evaluation of those at high risk is recommended and requires serial testing of blood, urine, and BAL specimens.
- Other potential abnormal laboratory tests include the following:
  - Elevated alanine aminotransferase (ALT) level (83%)
  - Thrombocytopenia (77%)
  - Mononucleosis on complete blood count

IMAGING STUDIES

Computed tomography of the head can be used to identify intracerebral calcification.

TREATMENT

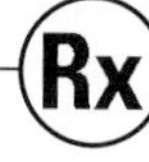

NONPHARMACOLOGIC THERAPY

Therapy is principally supportive.

ACUTE GENERAL Rx

- Insufficient data are available to support the routine use of ganciclovir for congenital CMV infections.
- Treatment of CMV infections in immunocompromised patients includes the following:
  - Pneumonitis: Ganciclovir can be given, but the role of CMV hyperimmune globulin is uncertain.
  - Retinitis: Ganciclovir, valganciclovir, or foscarnet can be given.
  - Prophylactic or preemptive therapies: Acyclovir, ganciclovir, and CMV hyperimmune globulin have been used with variable or uncertain efficacy.
  - Toxicities of ganciclovir include granulocytopenia, anemia, and thrombocytopenia. In animal studies, ganciclovir was carcinogenic and teratogenic, and it caused aspermatogenesis.
  - Foscarnet deposits in bone, teeth, and cartilage.

CHRONIC Rx

Ganciclovir is virostatic, and maintenance therapy is required for the duration of the immunocompromised state.

DISPOSITION

Asymptomatic infected infants (i.e., congenitally acquired CMV) require close follow-up to detect sensorineural deafness and learning problems.

PEARLS & CONSIDERATIONS

PREVENTION

- Use good hand-washing practices in the home, day-care setting, and hospital setting.
- Identify seronegative women early in pregnancy, and provide appropriate education.

PATIENT/FAMILY EDUCATION

- Seronegative pregnant women should be taught about the possibility of transmission from children and should be educated regarding the following:
  - Good hand-washing practices
  - Avoidance of sharing utensils or glassware and kissing on the mouth
- Information and support groups are available through the National Congenital CMV Disease Registry (Texas Children's Hospital, MC3-2371, 6621 Fannin Street, Houston, TX 77030-2399; phone: 713-770-4387; fax: 713-770-4330).

SUGGESTED READINGS

American Academy of Pediatrics: Cytomegalovirus infection. *In* Pickering LK (ed): *2003 Red Book: Report of the Committee on Infectious Diseases,* 26th ed. Elk Grove Village, IL, American Academy of Pediatrics, 2003.

Razonable RR, Paya CV: Herpesvirus infections in transplant recipients: current challenges in the clinical management of cytomegalovirus and Epstein-Barr virus infections. *Herpes* 10:3, 2003.

Ross SA, Boppana SB: Congenital cytomegalovirus infection: outcome diagnosis. *Semin Pediatr Infect Dis* 16:1, 2005.

AUTHOR: **THERESE CVETKOVICH, MD**

BASIC INFORMATION

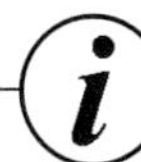

DEFINITION

Deep venous thrombosis (DVT) is the presence of thrombus within a deep vein, most commonly the iliac, femoral, or popliteal.

SYNONYMS

DVT
Thromboembolism

ICD-9-CM CODE
671.4 Deep venous thrombosis

EPIDEMIOLOGY & DEMOGRAPHICS

- DVT is the third most common cardiovascular disease after acute coronary syndromes and stroke.
- It affects approximately 2 million Americans per year.
- Almost 40% of patients with DVT without symptoms of pulmonary embolism (PE) have signs of PE on lung scanning.
- Risk factors include underlying hypercoagulable state, trauma, or immobilization.

CLINICAL PRESENTATION

- The patient may have subacute onset of pain, swelling, and erythema of the affected limb.
- Trauma or immobility of the affected extremity (e.g., fracture with casting)
- Underlying hypercoagulable state
- Trauma to the vein, including venous catheterization

Physical Examination

- The most trustworthy of signs and symptoms include the following:
  - Localized tenderness along the distribution of the deep venous system
  - Thigh and calf swollen (should be measured)
  - Calf swelling by more than 3 cm compared with the asymptomatic leg (measured 10 cm below the tibial tuberosity)
  - Pitting edema in the symptomatic leg only
  - Dilated superficial veins (nonvaricose) in the symptomatic leg only
  - Erythema

DIAGNOSIS

DIFFERENTIAL DIAGNOSIS

- Cellulitis
- Myositis
- Ruptured Baker's cyst
- Septic arthritis

LABORATORY TESTS

- Activated protein C resistance (i.e., factor V Leiden)
- Antithrombin III
- Lupus anticoagulant
- Partial thromboplastin time (PTT)
- Protein C
- Protein S
- Prothrombin gene mutation
- Prothrombin time (PT)

IMAGING STUDIES

- Doppler ultrasound of the affected limb is virtually diagnostic.
- Venogram is the gold standard and is reserved for discordance between pretest probability and the ultrasound results.

TREATMENT

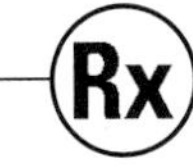

NONPHARMACOLOGIC THERAPY

- The affected limb should be elevated.
- Placement of a venacaval (Greenfield) filter should be reserved for patients with contraindications to anticoagulation or with clot extension or pulmonary embolism despite full anticoagulation.

ACUTE GENERAL Rx

- After DVT is confirmed, immediate anticoagulation with heparin is indicated to prevent extension or PE.
- Twice-daily, subcutaneous, low-molecular-weight heparin has outcomes comparable to those of intravenous, unfractionated heparin administered by drip.

CHRONIC Rx

- Oral anticoagulation is indicated for at least 1 year.
- If an irreversible underlying hypercoagulable state is found, lifelong oral anticoagulation is indicated.

DISPOSITION

- Resolution of the acute clot can be expected within 7 to 14 days.
- Ambulation should be avoided for the first 24 to 48 hours to prevent PE.

REFERRAL

- If an underlying hypercoagulable state is found, referral to a hematologist is helpful.
- If an inferior vena cava filter is indicated, referral to a vascular surgeon or interventional radiologist is indicated.

PEARLS & CONSIDERATIONS

COMMENTS

- Treatment with subcutaneous, low-molecular-weight heparin is equally as effective as intravenous, unfractionated heparin, and it does not require monitoring of the activated PTT. It can also be given on an outpatient basis, avoiding hospitalization for appropriate patients.
- DVT of the arm can occur, usually in association with venous catheters, and it should be approached in the same manner as that for the leg, because it also increases the risk for PE.
- DVT of the leg below the knee is associated with a very low risk of PE. Anticoagulation is reasonable and prevents extension into the proximal leg, which has a much higher risk of PE. Alternatively, serial Doppler ultrasound scans of the leg to monitor for extension without anticoagulation is a reasonable clinical approach in the patient at high risk for bleeding on anticoagulants.

PREVENTION

- Prophylactic, low-dose, subcutaneous heparin is indicated for prolonged immobility such as hospitalization or postoperatively
- Begin early ambulation after surgery.

PATIENT/FAMILY EDUCATION

- Treatment with anticoagulants reduces the incidence of PE to less than 1%.
- The risk of warfarin therapy is major bleeding, with an incidence of 5% per year.
- For those with no risk factors or those not in a hypercoagulable state, the recurrence rate is very low.
- Treatment with oral warfarin necessitates intense education about the risks of bleeding and dietary restrictions.

SUGGESTED READINGS

Kearon C et al: The role of venous ultrasonography in the diagnosis of suspected deep venous thrombosis and pulmonary embolism. *Ann Intern Med* 129:1044, 1998.
Kearon C et al: Noninvasive diagnosis of deep venous thrombosis. *Ann Intern Med* 128:663, 1998.

AUTHOR: **BRETT ROBBINS, MD**

BASIC INFORMATION

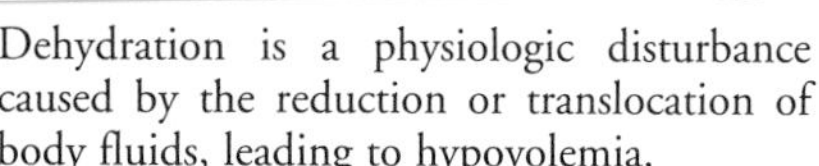

DEFINITION

Dehydration is a physiologic disturbance caused by the reduction or translocation of body fluids, leading to hypovolemia.

- Isonatremic or isotonic dehydration
  - Serum osmolarity of 270 to 300 mOsm/L
  - Serum sodium level of 130 to 150 mEq/L
- Hyponatremic or hypotonic dehydration
  - Serum osmolarity of less than 270 mOsm/L
  - Serum sodium level of less than 130 mEq/L
- Hypernatremic or hypertonic dehydration
  - Serum osmolarity of more than 300 mOsm/L
  - Serum sodium level of more than 150 mEq/L
- Severity
  - Mild: less than 50 mL/kg body fluid loss or less than 5% weight loss
  - Moderate: 50 to 100 mL/kg body fluid loss or 5% to 10% weight loss
  - Severe: more than 100 mL/kg body fluid loss or more than 10% weight loss

SYNONYMS

Hypovolemia
Hypovolemic shock

ICD-9-CM CODES
276.5 Volume depletion
785.59 Hypovolemic shock

EPIDEMIOLOGY & DEMOGRAPHICS

- Diarrhea is the most common cause of dehydration in infants and children and is the leading cause of death worldwide in children younger than 4 years of age.
- In the United States, an average of 300 children die of diarrhea annually.
- Another 200,000 children are hospitalized per year in the United States because of diarrheal illnesses with dehydration.
- Other common causes of dehydration include vomiting, stomatitis or pharyngitis with poor intake, febrile illnesses with increased insensible losses and decreased intake, and diabetic ketoacidosis.
- Among patients with hypernatremic dehydration, there is a 10% mortality rate. Between 40% and 50% of survivors have neurologic sequelae, and 5% to 10% are severely affected.
  - Learning disabilities
  - Cognitive deficits, motor deficits
  - Behavioral changes

CLINICAL PRESENTATION

History

- Because gastrointestinal losses from diarrhea and vomiting are the most common causes, information regarding the amount and character of losses is needed.
- Consider any underlying disease such as cystic fibrosis, diabetes, hyperthyroidism, or renal disease.
- Assess for weight loss caused by dehydration.
- Urine output may diminish, as evidenced by a decrease in the number and degree of wet diapers.
- Absence of tears may indicate dehydration.
- The character and amount of ingested fluids should be assessed.

Physical Examination

- Vital signs
  - Tachycardia: first sign of mild dehydration
  - Respiratory rate and pattern: with increasing acidosis, an increased respiratory rate and hyperpneic pattern
  - Orthostatic changes in older children
  - Hypotension: late sign of uncompensated severe dehydration
- Weight loss
- Sunken eyes and fontanelle
- Dry lips and mucous membranes, absence of tears
- Prolonged capillary refill, cool extremities
- Tenting of skin, except in hypernatremic dehydration
- Older children: signs of dehydration shown earlier than babies because of their decreased extracellular water
- Hyponatremic dehydration: earlier and more pronounced signs of dehydration
  - Seizures, especially with a rapid decrease in the sodium concentration
- Hypernatremic dehydration: later and more subtle signs of dehydration
  - Lethargic, but excessive irritability when stimulated
  - Increased muscle tone
  - Doughy or smooth, velvety skin turgor
  - Intracranial hemorrhage in 10%
  - Possible thrombosis of dural sinus
  - Possible signs of intracranial swelling and seizures with too-rapid rehydration

ETIOLOGY

- Decreased intake
  - Physical restriction
  - Anorexia
  - Voluntary cessation: pharyngitis, stomatitis, respiratory distress
- Increased output
  - Insensible losses: fever, sweating, heat prostration, high ambient temperature, hyperventilation, cystic fibrosis, thyrotoxicosis
  - Renal losses
    - Osmotic: diabetic ketoacidosis, acute tubular necrosis, high-protein diet, mannitol administration
    - Non-osmotic: diabetes insipidus (DI), sustained hypokalemia or hypercalcemia, sickle cell disease, chronic renal disease, Bartter's syndrome
    - Sodium losing: congenital adrenal hypoplasia, diuretic use, sodium-losing nephropathy, pseudohypoaldosteronism
  - Gastrointestinal losses
    - Diarrhea: secretory or nonsecretory
    - Vomiting: obstructive or nonobstructive
- Translocation of fluids
  - Burns
  - Ascites
  - Intestinal: paralytic ileus, after abdominal surgery
- Hyponatremic dehydration
  - This is typically seen with diarrhea and vomiting, especially with inappropriate (hypotonic) fluid replacement.
  - It also occurrs with excessive salt loss, as in congenital adrenal hyperplasia.
  - The degree of total body dehydration may be overestimated. For example, the patient may be in shock although only 10% dehydrated because of the relative increase in intravascular depletion.
  - These patients are the most likely to need immediate circulatory support.
- Hypernatremic dehydration
  - This is usually associated with winter diarrhea.
  - The sodium level is more than 150 mEq/L, but the total-body level of sodium is depleted.
  - Hypernatremic dehydration must be distinguished from salt poisoning with dehydration, in which the total-body sodium level is increased.
  - This condition is rarely seen in children older than 2 years.

DIAGNOSIS

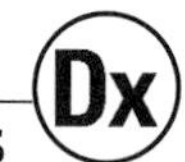

DIFFERENTIAL DIAGNOSIS

Information about the differential diagnosis can be found in the "Etiology" section.

WORKUP

An initial clinical assessment should be made to determine the degree of volume depletion using weight loss and clinical signs, especially to determine whether the patient is in shock.

LABORATORY TESTS

- Hemoconcentration: elevated hemoglobin, hematocrit, plasma proteins (hemoglobin and hematocrit may be normal with underlying anemia)
- Serum sodium level: isonatremic, hyponatremic, hypernatremic
- Alteration in measured or calculated serum osmolarity: isotonic, hypotonic, or hypertonic
- Serum potassium level: hypokalemia with significant stool or gastric losses; hyperkalemia with acidosis or diminished renal function
- Serum bicarbonate or blood gas determinations
  - Acidosis occurs with stool losses, tissue catabolism, and diminished renal function.
  - Alkalosis occurs with protracted vomiting or nasogastric drainage.
- Low glucose level, especially in a young infant who has been poorly tolerating feedings
- Elevated levels of blood urea nitrogen and serum creatinine

- Increased urine specific gravity and osmolarity increased (except with DI)

TREATMENT

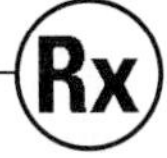

NONPHARMACOLOGIC THERAPY

- The goal of therapy is to replace the deficit, provide maintenance fluids, and continue to replace ongoing losses.
- Consider oral rehydration in patients with mild to moderate dehydration who do not have severe vomiting, who do not have high stool output (>20 mL/kg/hr), or who can adhere to instructions (Table 1-8).
  - Initial rehydration fluid should contain 75 to 90 mEq/L of sodium. Give a volume equal to the estimated fluid deficit to drink over 4 to 6 hours.
  - Maintenance solutions should contain 40 to 60 mEq/L of sodium.
  - Both solutions should have approximately 20 mEq/L of potassium and 2% to 2.5% glucose.

ACUTE GENERAL Rx

- Patients with moderate or severe dehydration or uncompensated shock require intravascular therapy.
  - For initial therapy, restore the intravascular volume, regardless of serum osmolarity or the cause of dehydration.
  - Administer 20 mL/kg of isotonic fluid (normal saline or Ringer's lactate) as a rapid intravenous bolus; reassess and repeat until heart rate, perfusion, and blood pressure are improved.
- Deficit water losses are based on the following criteria:
  - Weight loss: 1 g of water for each gram of weight loss *or*
  - Physical guidelines: 3% to 5% = dry mucous membranes; 5% to 7% = sunken fontanelle, decreased skin turgor; 7% to 10% = sunken eyes, skin tenting, tachycardia; 10% to 15% = shock
- Deficit acute electrolyte losses are 60% of extracellular fluid and 40% of intracellular fluid. For every 100 mL of water lost, the following are also lost:
  - Sodium: 8.4 mEq/100 mL
  - Potassium: 6.0 mEq/100 mL
  - Chlorine: 6.0 mEq/100 mL
- Maintenance water needs reflect the following values:
  - 100 mL/kg for the first 10 kg
  - 50 mL/kg for the second 10 kg
  - 20 mL/kg for each 1 kg over 20 kg
- Maintenance electrolyte needs are based on the following criteria:
  - Sodium: approximately 3.0 mEq/100 mL
  - Potassium: approximately 2.0 mEq/100 mL
- Base calculations for deficit replacement and maintenance fluids on the original "wet" weight.
- Replacement of ongoing losses are based on the following criteria:
  - Replace gastric losses with one-half normal saline ({1/2}NS = 0.45%) plus 10 to 15 mEq/L of potassium chloride.
  - Add bicarbonate with stool or small-bowel losses.
  - Replace cerebrospinal fluid with normal (0.9%) saline.
- Isotonic dehydration is treated as follows:
  - If indicated, give 20 mL/kg of isotonic fluid as a bolus.
  - Calculate maintenance needs.
  - Calculate deficit needs (minus fluid and electrolytes given with the bolus).
  - Administer maintenance plus deficit needs over 24 hours (some physicians suggest giving one half of the deficit over 8 hours and the other half over the remaining 16 hours). Fluid (water plus electrolytes) often calculates to D_5{1/3} NS + 40 mEq/L of KCl.
- Hypotonic dehydration is addressed as follows:
  - The degree of total body dehydration may be overestimated, but the patient can be in shock although only 10% dehydrated.
  - These patients are most likely to need immediate circulatory support.
  - Calculate fluid losses the same as with isotonic dehydration.
  - Calculate the electrolyte deficit, and add it to the maintenance needs (remember to subtract fluid and electrolytes from the bolus).
    - Correct sodium to 130 mEq/L using the following formula: desired Na level − measured Na) × (0.6) × (weight in kg) = mEq Na deficit.
    - If losses are acute, replace over 24 hours.
- Hypertonic dehydration is addressed as follows:
  - Bolus with normal saline or Ringer's lactate as needed.
  - Avoid electrolyte-free solutions.
  - Calculate water maintenance and the free water deficit using 4 mL/kg for every 1 mEq of Na more than 145 mEq.
  - Electrolyte replacement is accomplished as follows:
    - Total cation (Na or Na + K) concentration should be approximately one half of the normal solution (70 to 80 mEq/L) initially.
    - A significant potassium deficit usually exists; add potassium after the patient voids.
    - Generally, start with something similar to $D_5$0.2% NS + 40 mEq/L of KCl.
  - Replace the deficit *slowly* over 48 hours: rate/hr = (maintenance × 2) + (deficit ÷ 48 hours).
  - Monitor sodium every 2 to 4 hours, and adjust fluids accordingly.
    - Do not correct sodium faster than 10 to 12 mEq/L/day (0.5 mEq/L/hr).
    - Change fluids to D_5W + K if correcting too slowly.
    - Change fluids to $D_5$0.45% NS + K if correcting too quickly.
- If seizures or signs of intracranial swelling occur, treat with 0.5 to 1.0 g/kg of mannitol over 20 minutes.

CHRONIC Rx

For patients with hyponatremic or hypernatremic dehydration, to rule out ongoing losses or a chronic condition, reevaluate sodium levels after the sodium concentration is corrected and the patient has resumed a normal diet.

REFERRAL

Consider neuropsychiatric testing or neurologic follow-up after hypernatremic dehydration.

TABLE 1-8 **Guide for Oral Rehydration**

	DEHYDRATION OF 3% TO 5%		DEHYDRATION OF 6% TO 9%	
Weight (kg)	**First 6 hours (mL/hr)**	**Next 18 hours (mL/hr)**	**First 6 hours (mL/hr)**	**Next 18 hours (mL/hr)**
5	45	35	60	35
10	80	55	125	55
15	125	70	190	70
20	140	85	200	85
25	170	90	250	90
30	200	95	300	95
40	250	110	400	110

PEARLS & CONSIDERATIONS

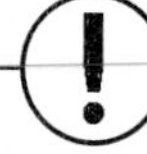

PREVENTION

- Encourage fluids during exercise, in high ambient temperatures, and with vomiting and diarrheal illnesses.
- Advise prompt therapy when the underlying disorder (e.g., congenital adrenal hyperplasia [CAH], diabetes mellitus [DM], DI, cystic fibrosis [CF]) is known.

PATIENT/FAMILY EDUCATION

Provide parents with written instructions about the signs and symptoms, home treatment, and when to seek medical attention, especially during the gastroenteritis season and for those with known underlying disorder (e.g., CF, CAH, DM, DI).

SUGGESTED READINGS

Adelman RD, Solhaug MJ: Fluid and electrolyte treatment of specific disorders. *In* Nelson WE et al (eds): *Textbook of Pediatrics,* 15th ed. Philadelphia, WB Saunders, 1996.

Adelman RD, Solhaug MJ: Fluid therapy. *In* Nelson WE et al (eds): *Textbook of Pediatrics,* 15th ed. Philadelphia, WB Saunders, 1996.

Adelman RD, Solhaug MJ: Principles of therapy. *In* Nelson WE et al (eds): *Textbook of Pediatrics,* 15th ed. Philadelphia, WB Saunders, 1996.

Cronan KM, Norman ME: Renal and electrolyte emergencies. *In* Fleisher GR, Ludwig S (eds): *Textbook of Pediatric Emergency Medicine,* 3rd ed. Baltimore, Williams & Wilkins, 1993.

Dalby-Payne J, Elliott E: Acute gastroenteritis in children. (Update in *Clin Evid* 10:386, 2003, update of *Clin Evid* 7:227, 2002). *Clin Evid* 8:242, 2002.

Dale J: Oral rehydration solutions in the management of acute gastroenteritis among children. *J Pediatr Health Care* 18:211, 2004.

Drkoop.com. Available at http://drkoop.com/conditions/encyclopedia/articles/004000a/00400025.html

Health-Center.com. Available at www.healthguide.com/english/family/infant/medicalconcepdehydr.htm.

On health. Available at http://www.onhealth.com/ch1/resource/conditions/item.48191.asp

Roberts KB: Fluid and electrolytes: parenteral fluid therapy. *Pediatr Rev* 22:380, 2001.

Steiner MJ et al: Is this child dehydrated? *JAMA* 291:2746, 2004.

UpToDate Online. Available at http://www.utdol.com/application/topic.asp?file=pedineph/17080;http://www.utdol.com/application/topic.asp?file=pedineph/6086

AUTHOR: **KAREN S. POWERS, MD**

BASIC INFORMATION

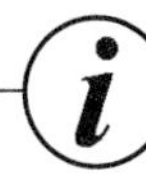

DEFINITION

Puberty is delayed if there is a lack of secondary sexual characteristics by age 14 years in boys or age 13 in girls.

SYNONYMS

Constitutional growth delay
Late bloomer

ICD-9-CM CODE
259.0 Delayed puberty

EPIDEMIOLOGY & DEMOGRAPHICS

- Delayed puberty is more often a complaint in boys.
- About 2% of boys are not in puberty by age 14 years.
- By age 15 years, 0.4% of boys are not in puberty.
- Approximately 50% of patients with delayed puberty have a family history of a first- or second-degree relative with late puberty.

CLINICAL PRESENTATION

History

- With constitutional growth delay (i.e., simple delayed puberty)
  - The chief complaint or associated complaint may be short stature (see Short Stature in Diseases and Disorders [Section I]).
  - Growth curves show a period of decreased growth in the first or second year of life.
  - The history does not suggest chronic systemic illness, gastrointestinal disease, intracranial mass, or hypothyroidism.
  - The patient has a history of little or no pubertal development.
- Delayed puberty may be associated with a history of excessive exercise or with an eating disorder, especially in girls.

Physical Examination

- Delay or lack of secondary sex characteristics is the hallmark (see Breast Development, Pubic Hair (Male and Female), Genital Development (Male), and Early Adolescence Through Young Adults: Pubertal Events and Tanner stages pictures and text in Charts, Formulas, Laboratory Tests and values [Section IV]).
  - Girls have delayed or absent breast development.
  - Boys have a lack of testicular enlargement (<4 mL testicular volume *or* testicular length <2.2 cm).
  - In both sexes, there is no pubic hair and no growth acceleration.
- In constitutional growth delay, no signs of chronic systemic illness, gastrointestinal disease, intracranial mass, or hypothyroidism exist on physical examination.

ETIOLOGY

- Constitutional growth delay (i.e., simple delayed puberty) is a normal variant with unknown cause.
- There are many pathologic causes (see "Differential Diagnosis").

DIAGNOSIS

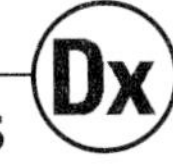

DIFFERENTIAL DIAGNOSIS

- Permanent hypogonadotropic hypogonadism (i.e., permanent lack of gonadotropins)
  - Isolated gonadotropin deficiency, partial or complete
  - Kallmann's syndrome with associated anosmia
  - Gonadotropin deficiency associated with other central nervous system and hypothalamic or pituitary abnormalities, such as congenital hypopituitarism, craniopharyngioma, or histiocytosis
- Functional hypogonadotropic hypogonadism (i.e., transient lack of gonadotropins)
  - Hypothyroidism
  - Weight loss
- Chronic illness
- Purposeful dieting
- Anorexia nervosa
- Increased physical activity (especially when combined with weight restriction)
- Chronic disease
  - Hypergonadotropic hypogonadism: gonadal failure associated with elevated gonadotropins
  - Turner syndrome (i.e., XO karyotype, girls only): other phenotypic features (see Turner Syndrome in Diseases and Disorders [Section I] and Turner Syndrome Growth Chart in Charts, Formulas, Laboratory Tests and values [Section IV])
  - Klinefelter syndrome (i.e., XXY karyotype, boys only): usually have normal start of puberty but may not complete puberty because of testicular fibrosis (see Klinefelter Syndrome in Diseases and Disorders [Section I])
  - Other forms of gonadal failure (rare)

LABORATORY TESTS

- Screening tests are aimed at ruling out occult disease or conditions.
- All screening test results should be normal for age for children with constitutional growth delay, except possibly hematocrit, insulin-like grow factor-1 (IGF-1), and testosterone levels.
  - The hematocrit value is in the prepubertal to early pubertal range; results of the complete blood cell count (CBC) and sedimentation rate should otherwise be normal.
  - Results of the urinalysis, electrolyte determinations, and renal function tests should be normal.
- Thyroid function tests (free thyroxine [T_4] and thyroid-stimulating hormone [TSH])
  - Normal thyroid test results are expected for children with constitutional delay.
  - A low free T_4 level with an elevated TSH level indicates primary hypothyroidism.
- IGF-1 level may be abnormal (screen for growth hormone deficiency).
  - Abnormally low free T_4 and IGF-1 (adjusted for pubertal stage) may indicate pituitary or hypothalamic abnormalities.
  - It may be very difficult to differentiate true isolated growth hormone insufficiency from constitutional growth delay.
- Check morning testosterone levels (in boys).
  - Testosterone levels should be in the prepubertal to early pubertal range.
  - A morning testosterone level of more than 20 ng/dL indicates a good probability of the onset of puberty in the next year.
- Assess gonadotropins (luteinizing hormone [LH] and follicle-stimulating hormone [FSH]).
  - Low (i.e., prepubertal) gonadotropin levels are expected in constitutional delay when measured in standard assays.
  - New ultrasensitive (third-generation) LH assays can detect the small amount of LH present in very early puberty in children with constitutional growth delay. Near zero levels are found in cases of hypogonadotropic hypogonadism.
  - Elevated gonadotropin levels indicate gonadal failure, and in girls, this should prompt chromosomal analysis for Turner syndrome.
- Abnormality of any screening test (except those mentioned) should direct evaluation toward the specific system.

IMAGING STUDIES

- Bone age
  - Bone age should be delayed proportional to height.
  - Bone and height age are both delayed compared with chronologic age.
- A 13-year-old boy with the height of an average 10-year-old and a bone age of 10 years is typical for constitutional delay.

TREATMENT

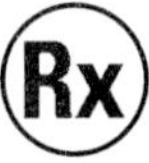

NONPHARMACOLOGIC THERAPY

- Weight gain is important for those with anorexia nervosa or excessive dieting.
- Encourage the patient to decrease extreme exercise routines.

CHRONIC Rx

Low-dose testosterone (50 to 100 mg intramuscularly every month for 3 to 6 months) may stimulate start of puberty in boys who are prepubertal.

DISPOSITION

- Clinical follow-up is needed every 3 to 6 months to document normal height velocity (>5 cm/year) and pubertal progression.
  - Increase in testicular size is most important.
  - Penis size does not increase significantly in early puberty.
  - Pubic hair growth is also influenced by adrenal androgens.

REFERRAL

Refer the patient to a pediatric endocrinologist if bone age and height age are not proportional or if growth velocity falls below 4 to 5 cm per year.

PEARLS & CONSIDERATIONS

COMMENTS

- Boys often seek evaluation at the time they are in early puberty (determined by testicular size) but do not yet have obvious secondary sex characteristics such as pubic hair.
- Delayed puberty is often associated with a transient pause in linear growth just before commencement of puberty.

PREVENTION

Bone age in a child at risk for delayed puberty may allow anticipatory guidance.

SUGGESTED READINGS

De Luca F et al: Management of puberty in constitutional delay of growth and puberty. *J Pediatr Endocrinol Metab* 14(Suppl 2):953, 2001.

McKeever MO: Delayed puberty. *Pediatr Rev* 21:250, 2000.

Rosen DS, Foster C: Delayed puberty. *Pediatr Rev* 22:309, 2001.

Saenger P, Sandberg DE: Delayed puberty: when to wake the bugler. *J Pediatr* 133:724, 1998.

AUTHOR: **CRAIG ORLOWSKI, MD**

BASIC INFORMATION

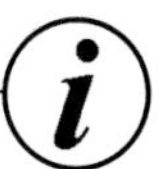

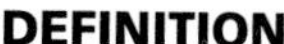

DEFINITION

Depression is a disorder of mood, characterized by pervasive feelings of sadness and often accompanied by feelings of helplessness, hopelessness, and irritability; loss of interest in people; and loss of enjoyment in previously enjoyed activities. Depression often includes loss of motivation; indecisiveness; withdrawal; passivity; disturbances in appetite, weight, and sleep; and other physical symptoms.

SYNONYMS

Adjustment disorder with depressed mood
Affective mood disorder
Bereavement
Bipolar disorder, depressed; manic depressive disorder, depressed
Depressive disorder not otherwise specified; minor, recurrent, brief depression
Dysthymia: neurotic depression, chronic depression (at least 1 year in children)
Major depressive disorder: biologic or psychotic depression
Posttraumatic stress disorder (PTSD)

ICD-9-CM CODES
296.2 Major depressive disorder
296.5 Bipolar disorder I, depressed
300.4 Dysthymia
311 Depressive disorder not otherwise specified

EPIDEMIOLOGY & DEMOGRAPHICS

- Prevalence is 1% among preschoolers, 2% among school-aged children, 4.7% among adolescents, but 7% among patients in the general pediatric population.
- Depression is unrecognized and untreated in more than 50% of pediatric cases.
- Depression affects boys and girls equally in childhood; after puberty, it is more common in females.
- There are no reported racial or ethnic variations, but it may be underdiagnosed in minority patients.
- A family history of depression, bipolar disorder, or substance abuse is common.

CLINICAL PRESENTATION

- Early abuse may be precursor.
- Family conflict often triggers a mood change.
- Anxiety tends to precede depression in children.
- Oppositional behavior or conduct disorder in a previously well-behaved child may signal the onset of depression.
- Substance abuse in adolescents may represent self-medication.
- Mood cycling or volatility before the onset of depression may suggest bipolar disorder, especially if there is a positive family history for the disorder.
- Symptoms may include the following:
  - Depressed mood: feeling bored, irritable, lonely, touchy, dysphoric, tearful
  - Poor self-esteem, worthlessness, inappropriate shame and guilt, feeling rejection by others (e.g., peers, schoolmates)
  - Oppositionality: conduct disturbance that resolves with treatment
  - Sleep disturbances: early morning awakening (less common than in adults), early or middle-of-night sleeplessness, prolonged sleep (adolescents)
  - Appetite changes: failure to gain rather than lose weight or impressive gain from overeating
  - Academic difficulty from poor concentration and poor motivation
  - Social isolation or new association with "troubled" children
  - Complaints of headache, stomachache, sleepiness, no energy
  - Classic melancholia occasionally in older adolescents
  - Preoccupation with suicide (increases with age)

ETIOLOGY

- The cause of depression is unknown, but many theories exist. It is likely that genetic susceptibility and environmental or social stressors overlap.
- Genetic risks include a family history of mood disorders (e.g., depression, bipolar disorder, especially if early onset) and substance abuse.
- Biologic markers include the hypothalamic-pituitary-adrenal stress response with neuroamine depletion, which may be initiated by physical causes.
  - Drugs
  - Infections
  - Neoplasms
  - Irradiation
- Social and environment factors may contribute.
  - Losses: rejection, death, separation
  - Stressors: family conflict, abuse
  - Emotional trauma, particularly to self-esteem
  - Maladaptive coping style and communication difficulties
  - Low self-esteem

DIAGNOSIS

Dx

DIFFERENTIAL DIAGNOSIS

- Fifty percent of depressed children and adolescents have other physical and psychiatric disorders.
- Symptoms of anxiety are common and often precede depression.
- Refusal to attend school may be more evident than the underlying dysphonic mood.
- The comorbidity of attention deficit/hyperactivity disorder (AD/HD) is common, especially in patients with the depressed form of bipolar disorder.
- Oppositional defiant disorder may divert attention from depression.
- When depression results from conduct disorder and punishment, there is usually less family history of mood disorder than when conduct problems are triggered by underlying depression.
- Several other conditions should be ruled out.
  - Personality disorder
  - Learning disorder
  - Eating disorder
  - Seasonal affective disorder

WORKUP

- Family history of mood disorders, especially depression, bipolar disorder, and substance abuse, must be sought.
- Parents notice signs of depression, and the patient can relate symptoms.
- Instruments used to screen for depression include the Reynolds Child Depression Scale, the Children's Depression Scale, and the Beck Depression Inventory.
- Teacher reports and psychological test results may be helpful.
- The risk of suicide should be assessed.
- Growth delay may occur, especially in younger children, and failure to thrive may be caused by depression.
- The causes of weight gain or loss and of bruising (in abuse, as parent's response to child's irritability) should be sought.

LABORATORY TESTS

Although the dexamethasone suppression test, thyroid-stimulating hormone suppression, and rapid eye movement delay may be used to rule out other disorders, no laboratory tests are diagnostic for depression.

IMAGING STUDIES

Positron emission tomography (PET) scanning, not available for clinical use, can demonstrate diminished prefrontal density.

TREATMENT

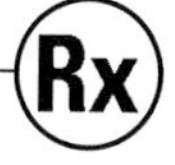

NONPHARMACOLOGIC THERAPY

- Seek appropriate environmental, family, and school changes.
- Energetic supportive interventions are usually most effective.
- Use cognitive-behavioral therapy, if available and the patient is willing.
- Avoid extensive revisiting of symptoms and psychodynamics.
- Psychotherapy or medication alone is usually less successful than both together.

ACUTE GENERAL Rx

- Using medication necessitates close follow-up, because the response may be slow, and irritability and suicidality may supervene.

- Fluoxetine is the most researched and most accepted drug; other selective serotonin reuptake inhibitors have been questioned.
  - Begin fluoxetine at 5 to 10 mg for children and 10 to 20 mg for larger adolescents.
  - The patient should be seen weekly to assess side effects.
  - Administer medication in the morning, and increase the dose if no response is seen in 3 to 4 weeks.
- Tricyclic antidepressants are not indicated because of cardiac conduction delays and suicidal risk from overdose.
- Venlafaxine may be useful if AD/HD is a comorbidity.
- Augmentation with lithium, levothyroxine, or a second antidepressant may be required.
- Electroconvulsive therapy may be lifesaving.
- Light therapy may help seasonal affective disorder.

CHRONIC Rx

- Authorities differ on the duration of treatment. After good response over 6 to 8 months, a trial off medication may be appropriate. Many physicians recommend treatment for 1 year.
- When medication is discontinued, ensure close follow-up.
- Recurrence of depression may be delayed. Inform the patient and family that it may occur, with reassurance that resumption of previously effective treatment is usually successful.
- Stressing the biologic basis of depression allays shame and blame.

COMPLEMENTARY & ALTERNATIVE MEDICINE

- At least 30 minutes of aerobic exercise daily may be helpful.
- Promotion of socialization and pleasurable activities is useful.
- Emphasize structure. A regular schedule (especially bedtime) and school or summertime employment may be productive.

DISPOSITION

Patients should be seen regularly, with follow-up arranged in advance.

REFERRAL

- When response to treatment is poor, consult with a child psychiatrist skilled in multimodal (including psychopharmacologic) treatment.
- Consider telephone or video conferencing if there is no local consultant.
- Continue to support the patient and family after referral to avoid a perception of abandonment, particularly until a good response to treatment occurs.

PEARLS & CONSIDERATIONS

COMMENTS

- Always ask about suicidality if depression is suspected.
- Use the antidepressant that worked in a previous episode or an antidepressant that has worked for a close relative.
- Placebo responses are common, especially in children.
- Direct questions about symptoms and suicidality are effective and therapeutic; not asking them can be risky.
- Bipolar disorder frequently begins with depression and can be provoked by antidepressants. A complete family history is essential.

PATIENT/FAMILY EDUCATION

Patient and family education about current concepts of depression and its treatment should be a part of any effective treatment, including the possibility of recurrence and the effectiveness of repeated treatment.

SUGGESTED READINGS

American Academy of Child & Adolescent Psychiatry. Available at www.aacap.org

American Psychiatric Association: *Diagnostic & Statistical Manual of Mental Disorders,* 4th ed, text revision. Washington, DC, American Psychiatric Association, 2000.

Emslie GJ et al: Fluoxetine for acute treatment of depression in children and adolescents: a placebo-controlled, randomized clinical trial. *J Am Acad Child Adolesc Psychiatry* 41:1205, 2002.

Findling RL et al: Somatic treatment for depressive illness in children and adolescents. *Psychiatr Clin North Am* 27:113, 2004.

AUTHOR: **CHRISTOPHER H. HODGMAN, MD**

BASIC INFORMATION

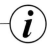

DEFINITION

Dermatomyositis is a multisystem disorder characterized by vascular inflammation, primarily involving skin and muscle and producing rash and proximal muscle weakness. Additional manifestations of the vasculitis can include esophageal and intestinal dysmotility, myocarditis, conduction abnormalities, alveolitis, interstitial lung disease, arthralgias, arthritis, cutaneous ulcerations, peripheral edema, and calcinosis.

SYNONYMS

Inflammatory myopathy
Inflammatory myositis
Juvenile dermatomyositis

ICD-9-CM CODE
710.3 Dermatomyositis

EPIDEMIOLOGY & DEMOGRAPHICS

- Three or four cases of inflammatory myopathy per 1 million children occur each year in the United States.
- Peak childhood incidence is between the ages of 5 and 9 years.
- Seventeen percent of cases occur before adulthood.
- The incidence is similar for males and females and across racial groups.
- Dermatomyositis is the most common inflammatory myopathy of childhood (85% of cases).
- Polymyositis accounts for an additional 8% of childhood cases.
- Case studies suggest that an amyopathic dermatomyositis (skin findings only) may exist as separate entity.
- Malignancy-associated disease occurs primarily in adults.
- The presence of calcinosis is related to the severity of disease and delay in initiation of therapy.

CLINICAL PRESENTATION

History

- Rapid onset of muscle weakness is reported in one half of cases, whereas insidious progression occurs in others.
- Muscle weakness in the proximal extremities and trunk manifests as difficulty climbing stairs, difficulty rising from the floor, and awkward gait.
- Rash is seen predominantly on the face and hands.
- Photosensitivity is common, with sun exposure producing exacerbation of muscle weakness and rash.
- Other clinical features include the following:
  - Raynaud's phenomenon
  - Arthralgias
  - Dysphagia
  - Extremity swelling

Physical Examination

- Heliotropic rash: violaceous or erythematous rash involving the periorbital area, especially the upper lid
- Scaling or edema of the face
- Gottron's papules: erythematous, scaly eruptions involving the extensor surfaces of joints, particularly the small joints of hands
- Erythema: on the malar area, bridge of the nose, and sun-exposed V area of the upper chest and back
- Proximal muscle weakness
- Nailbed capillary telangiectasias
- Peripheral edema
- Calcinosis: small superficial plaques or nodules on extremities or deep intramuscular deposits that can be painful and limit range of motion

ETIOLOGY

- Dermatomyositis is probably an autoimmune disorder.
- The cause is unknown but is likely multifactorial.
  - Genetic origins: increased incidence in twins and first-degree relatives; association with some human leukocyte antigen (HLA) types (e.g., B8, DR3, DQA1) and polymorphism in the tumor necrosis factor-α (TNF-α) gene (TNF-α–308A allele)
  - Infectious origins: evidence for antigen-driven pathogenesis through molecular mimicry; influenza, parainfluenza, hepatitis B, and group A streptococci have been implicated.
  - Environmental origins: increased incidence in spring and summer; sunlight may increase TNF-α production in those with the allele.
  - Evidence for autoimmune activity: complement-mediated vessel injury and increased levels of soluble adhesion molecules (e.g., ICAM-1, VCAM-1, L-selectin)

DIAGNOSIS (Dx)

DIFFERENTIAL DIAGNOSIS

- Amyopathic dermatomyositis
- Drug-induced myositis
- Graft-versus-host disease
- Mixed connective tissue disease
- Muscular dystrophy
- Myasthenia gravis
- Polymyositis
- Postviral myositis (e.g., influenza B, parainfluenza)
- Systemic lupus erythematosus

WORKUP

The diagnosis usually made clinically in the setting of characteristic skin and muscle findings.

LABORATORY TESTS

- Supportive data include elevated levels of creatinine kinase, aspartate aminotransferase (AST), aldolase, erythrocyte sedimentation rate (ESR), and von Willebrand factor antigen.
- Autoantibodies are uncommon in children (20%); anti-Mi-2 and anti-nRNP each present in 5% of cases.
- Electromyography reveals nonspecific proximal myopathy.
- Muscle biopsy provides the definitive diagnosis.

IMAGING STUDIES

- Magnetic resonance imaging (MRI) reveals increased signal intensity on T2-weighted images of affected muscles and may have role in monitoring disease activity.
- Chest radiographic findings may indicate interstitial lung disease, and there may be electrocardiographic evidence of conduction abnormalities in selected cases.

TREATMENT

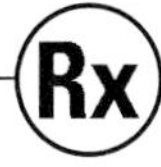

NONPHARMACOLOGIC THERAPY

- Sunscreen use and sun avoidance to prevent exacerbation of cutaneous manifestations
- Aggressive physical therapy, using range-of-motion exercises initially and strengthening later
- Aggressive skin care to avoid decubitus ulcers

ACUTE GENERAL Rx

- Corticosteroids are the first-line therapy.
  - Initially administer methylprednisolone (30 mg/kg, maximum of 1g/day) intravenously every 48 hours until evidence of improvement appears (i.e., normalization of creatinine kinase).
  - Then administer oral prednisone (2 mg/kg daily). In some cases of mild or moderate disease, initiate therapy with oral prednisone.
  - Use high-dose, intravenous immunoglobulin for refractory cases.

CHRONIC Rx

- Multiple steroid-sparing agents are available for nonresponders or patients with steroid-related toxicities: methotrexate, cyclosporine, cyclophosphamide, or azathioprine.
- Hydroxychloroquine can be used for cutaneous disease. Topical tacrolimus may also have role.

DISPOSITION

Patients are monitored for response to therapy by improvement in muscle weakness and dermatologic findings and by reductions in muscle enzyme levels.

REFERRAL

Referral to a rheumatologist is advised for diagnostic questions and for long-term management.

PEARLS & CONSIDERATIONS

COMMENTS

- Do not forget about bone health (i.e., calcium and vitamin D supplementation) for patients on chronic steroids.
- Nailbed capillary changes can be visualized with immersion oil and an ophthalmoscope at 40+ diopters.

PREVENTION

Early therapy has been shown to decrease the incidence and severity of calcinosis.

PATIENT/FAMILY EDUCATION

- The clinical courses are variable for monocyclic (lasting up to 2 years), polycyclic, and chronic cases.
- Relapse is uncommon after complete remission.
- Approximately 25% of patients do not respond to steroids, and up to 50% develop significant steroid-related toxicities.

SUGGESTED READINGS

Ansell BM: Juvenile dermatomyositis. *Rheumatol Dis Clin North Am* 17:931, 1991.

Arthritis Foundation. Available at www.arthritis.org

Callen JP: Dermatomyositis. *Lancet* 355:53, 2000.

Cawkwell GM: Inflammatory myositis in children, including differential diagnosis. *Curr Opin Rheumatol* 12:430, 2000.

Klippel JH, Dieppe PA: Rheumatology, 2nd ed. St. Louis, Mosby, 1998.

Miller ML: Clinical manifestations and diagnosis of juvenile dermatomyositis and polymyositis. UpToDate version 12.3. Available at www.UpToDate.com

Myositis Association of America. Available at www.myositis.org

Rider LG, Miller FW: Classification and treatment of the juvenile idiopathic inflammatory myopathies. *Rheumatol Dis Clin North Am* 23:619, 1997.

Wargula JC: Update on juvenile dermatomyositis: new advances in understanding its etiopathogenesis. *Curr Opin Rheumatol* 15:595, 2003.

AUTHOR: **JONATHAN F. NASSER, MD**

BASIC INFORMATION

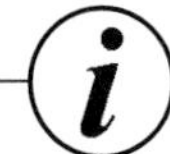

DEFINITION

Developmental dysplasia of the hip (DDH) is an abnormal formation of the hip joint, which may occur prenatally or within the first year of life. Teratologic dysplasia occurs early in utero (12 to 18 weeks) and is associated with neuromuscular disorders such as myelodysplasias and arthrogryposis. Typical DDH, which occurs in the last 4 weeks of gestation or within the first year, is the focus of this chapter.

SYNONYMS

The following terms were used in the past but are no longer considered appropriate:

- Congenital disease of the hip
- Congenital dislocation of the hip
- Congenital dysplasia of the hip

ICD-9-CM CODES
754.30 Dislocation
755.63 Dysplasia

EPIDEMIOLOGY & DEMOGRAPHICS

- The overall risk of DDH is 11.5 cases per 1000 newborns (4.1 cases/1000 boys, 19 cases/1000 girls).
- Risk is significantly increased by breech presentation (29 cases/1000 boys, 133 cases/1000 girls).
- Patients with positive family history have an increased risk (6.4 cases/1000 boys, 32 cases/1000 girls).
- A displaced left hip is three times more common than a displaced right hip. The left occiput anterior position of a non-breech infant causes the left hip to reside posteriorly against the spine in utero.
  - Left: 60%
  - Right: 20%
  - Bilateral: 20%
- The risk for DDH is increased for Native Americans and Lapps; it is decreased for African Americans, Koreans, and Chinese.
- Other factors include associated with increased risks for DDH:
  - Older, primiparous mother
  - First-born females
  - Oligohydramnios
- The risk is increased for patients with metatarsus adductus, clubfoot, hyperextended or dislocated knees, and congenital muscular torticollis.

CLINICAL PRESENTATION

History

- In infancy, the diagnosis is based on the physical examination findings.
- Breech (20% of frank breech, 2% footling breech, 0.7% of cephalic presentations) birth is associated with DDH.
- A family history of DDH (6% risk if one sibling, 12% risk if one parent, 36% risk if one parent and a sibling) increases the risk of DDH for the infant.
- Parents may report difficulty changing diapers.
- If missed in infancy, DDH may manifest with gait abnormalities or pain in the second to fourth decades of life.

Physical Examination

- Inner thigh skin fold asymmetry, buttocks skin fold asymmetry
- Knee height difference (i.e., Allis' or Galeazzi sign) or leg length discrepancy
- Abduction limitation
  - Normally, hips can be adducted to 30 degrees and abducted through 75 to 80 degrees.
  - Less than 50 to 60 degrees of abduction (or adduction asymmetry) is considered abnormal.
  - In a 3-month-old child, limitation of abduction is the most reliable sign.
- Dynamic instability: maneuvers for Barlow and Ortolani signs
  - Barlow sign
    - With the infant supine on a firm surface, flex the hips 90 degrees.
    - Hold the thigh in adduction, and apply gentle downward force on the femur at the flexed knee.
    - Posterior displacement of the femur out of the acetabular head is appreciated as a palpable click by the examiner's hand.
  - Ortolani sign
    - With hips flexed at 90 degrees as previously described, abduct the femur.
    - The femoral head relocating back into the acetabulum is appreciated as a palpable click as the femur is abducted.

ETIOLOGY

- The femoral head is aligned inappropriately within the acetabulum.
- These changes in alignment lead to bony abnormalities (e.g., flattening of the acetabulum, deformation of femoral head) and contractures of hip muscles.
- The hormone relaxin, associated with *in utero* malposition is believed to be causative.

DIAGNOSIS

DIFFERENTIAL DIAGNOSIS

- The diagnosis is based on the physical examination findings.
- Exclude the following conditions:
  - Abnormal joint laxity (e.g., trisomy 21)
  - Cerebral palsy
  - Congenital coxa vera
  - Tight hip adductors

IMAGING STUDIES

- Ultrasound before 3 to 4 months is associated with a high false-positive rate.
  - Abnormal angles between the acetabulum and ileum on static imaging
  - Demonstration of hip instability (femoral head moving in and out of acetabular cup) in real time
- Anteroposterior radiograph of hip can be helpful after ossification of femoral head (by 4 to 6 months).
  - Elevation and lateral displacement of femur
  - Delayed ossification of femoral head
  - Increased angle between a line that runs through the top of the triradiate cartilages (Hilgenreiner's line) and its intersection with a line that runs parallel to the acetabulum

TREATMENT

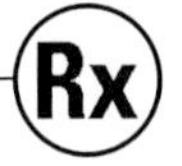

NONPHARMACOLOGIC THERAPY

- All patients with positive physical examination findings should be referred to a pediatric orthopedic surgeon for management.
- A Pavlik harness is used for infants younger than 6 months.
  - Holds hip in more than 90 degrees of flexion and 45 to 60 degrees of abduction, allowing movement in the "safe zone."
  - Use prohibits dislocation and avoids adduction and hyperabduction. Extreme abduction leads to increased risk of avascular necrosis.
  - It is worn constantly for 1 to 3 weeks, with weekly orthopedic evaluations.
  - Use is continued for 6 weeks to 9 months.
- A spica cast is used for closed reduction and immobilization for 6 to 18 months.
  - The cast is changed every 4 to 6 weeks for two or three times.
  - If unsuccessful, open reduction may be necessary.
- Open surgical reduction is used for those older than 18 months.
  - Pelvic and femoral osteotomies are commonly needed to obtain a stable femoral-acetabular relationship.
  - Rehabilitation takes a long time.
  - Imperfect repair is common.

DISPOSITION

- All newborns should be screened by physical examination for DDH.
- The 2000 American Academy of Pediatrics (AAP) clinical guidelines suggest screening all breech births with ultrasound at 6 weeks or radiography at 4 months, even in absence of abnormal examination findings.
- These guidelines also suggest imaging for girls with positive family history.
- Patients with positive physical examination findings suggesting DDH should be referred to a pediatric orthopedic surgeon for definitive diagnosis and treatment.

REFERRAL

All patients with DDH or suggestive findings on physical examination, ultrasound scans, or radiographs should be referred to a pediatric orthopedic surgeon, who can decide on therapy and maintain follow-up.

PEARLS & CONSIDERATIONS

COMMENTS

- Ideally, the infant is relaxed and on a firm surface during the examination.
- Postive Barlow and Ortolani sign may only be present in the first few months of life with DDH; by 3 to 4 months, abduction limitation and knee height asymmetry will predominate the clinical picture.
- Bilateral DDH may be very difficult to diagnose because of the symmetry.

PATIENT/FAMILY EDUCATION

- A success rate of 80% to 95% is achieved for normal hip development when repair is prompt and early.
- The incidence of avascular necrosis of the femoral head despite appropriate treatment is 2%.
- Long-term results of untreated or unsuccessfully treated DDH include the following:
  - Early degenerative joint disease or osteoarthritis
  - Functional disability by the third to fifth decade of life
  - Pain
  - Abnormal gait
  - Leg length discrepancy
  - Decreased agility
- For parents, information about DDH and the Pavlik harness is available on the Internet (www.childhosp.bc.ca/childrens/ortho/pavlikharness.html; www.childhosp.bc.ca/childrens/ortho/CDH.html).

SUGGESTED READINGS

Aronsson DD et al: Developmental dysplasia of the hip. *Pediatrics* 94:201, 1994.

Ballock RT, Richards BS: Hip dysplasia: early diagnosis makes a difference. *Contemp Pediatr* 14:108, 1997.

Committee on Quality Improvement, Subcommittee on Developmental Dysplasia of the Hip: Clinical practice guidelines: early detection of developmental dysplasia of the hip. *Pediatrics* 105:896, 2000.

Donaldson JS, Feinstein KA: Imaging of developmental dysplasia of the hip. *Pediatr Clin North Am* 44:591, 1997.

Mooney JF, Emans JB: DDH: a clinical overview. *Pediatr Rev* 16:229, 1995.

Novacheck TE: Developmental dysplasia of the hip. *Pediatr Clin North Am* 43:829, 1996.

AUTHOR: **LYNN C. GARFUNKEL, MD**

BASIC INFORMATION

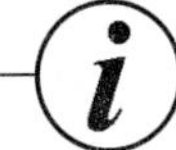

DEFINITION

Diabetes insipidus (DI) is the inability to concentrate urine, resulting in polyuria (i.e., excretion of abnormally large volumes of dilute urine) and polydipsia (i.e., large volume of water intake). There are four categories of DI: central (CDI), congenital or acquired nephrogenic (NDI), primary polydipsia, and gestational.

SYNONYMS

Central diabetes insipidus
- Antidiuretic hormone (ADH)-responsive diabetes
- Hypothalamic diabetes
- Neurogenic diabetes insipidus
- Neurohypophyseal diabetes

Gestational diabetes insipidus
- Gestagenic diabetes

Nephrogenic diabetes insipidus
- Vasopressin-resistant diabetes

Primary polydipsia
- Dipsogenic diabetes

ICD-9-CM CODES

253.5 Diabetes insipidus
253.55 Pituitary diabetes insipidus
588.1 Nephrogenic, vasopressin-resistant diabetes insipidus

EPIDEMIOLOGY & DEMOGRAPHICS

- The estimated incidence of DI is 3 cases per 100,000 people in the general population.
- CDI is the most common type.
- The nephrogenic type has a genetic basis and is rare.
  - The X-linked form accounts for approximately 90% of cases, and the estimated incidence is 4 cases in 1 million people.
  - Autosomal dominant and recessive forms also exist.
  - The acquired form is more common than genetic forms.

CLINICAL PRESENTATION

History

- CDI has several symptoms.
  - Often abrupt onset of polydipsia and polyuria
  - Associated symptoms can include:
    - Failure to thrive
    - Fatigue
    - Growth retardation
    - Headache
    - Visual defect
  - Can be associated with syndromes
    - Holoprosencephaly
    - Kabuki syndrome
    - Septio-optic dysplasia
    - Wolfram syndrome
- Symptoms of congenital NDI can occur within the first few weeks of life.
  - Polydipsia
  - Polyuria (i.e., represents an excessive volume of urine output and must be differentiated from urinary frequency, in which the total urine output is not increased)
  - Failure to thrive
  - Irritability
  - Constipation
  - Anorexia
  - Vomiting
  - Fever (e.g., from dehydration)
  - Seizures (i.e., rarely may occur during treatment if rehydration occurs too quickly, with sodium concentrations falling too rapidly)
- Symptoms of NDI occurring later in childhood:
  - Nocturia
  - Enuresis
  - Poor growth, especially if untreated
  - Malnutrition (e.g., anorexia, emesis resulting from high volumes of water ingestion)
  - Developmental delay (e.g., result of repeated bouts of hypernatremic dehydration with or without cerebral edema caused by overaggressive rehydration)
  - Possible influence on psychosocial development (e.g., competing demands for drinking and voiding and for playing and learning, hyperactivity, short-term memory problems)

Physical Examination

- Growth failure (i.e., poor weight gain and poor height velocity)
- Irritability
- Signs of dehydration: dry skin, loss of normal skin turgor, sunken fontanelle, dry mucous membranes, scaphoid abdomen
- Dysmorphic features

ETIOLOGY

- CDI (i.e., inadequate secretion of vasopressin)
  - Idiopathic
  - Pituitary surgery
  - Head trauma
  - Tumor (e.g., craniopharyngioma, lymphoma)
  - Infiltrative disease (e.g., histiocytosis, sarcoidosis)
  - Infection (e.g., meningitis)
  - Cerebral anoxia
- Nephrogenic DI (i.e., renal insensitivity to vasopressin)
  - Congenital form
    - X-linked form: mutation in the V_2 receptor gene
    - Autosomal dominant or recessive forms: mutation in the aquaporin-2 gene
  - Acquired form
    - Downregulation of aquaporin-2 expression
    - Medications: lithium, gentamicin
    - Systemic diseases: sickle cell anemia or trait, chronic kidney disease, sarcoidosis
    - Kidney disease: dysplasia, obstructive uropathy
    - Electrolyte abnormalities: hypocalcemia, hypokalemia
- Polydipsic DI (i.e., excessive fluid ingestion suppresses vasopressin release)
  - Abnormal thirst
  - Psychological dysfunction
  - Iatrogenic
- Gestational DI (i.e., increased metabolism of vasopressin during pregnancy)

DIAGNOSIS

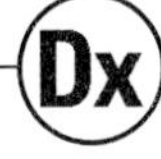

DIFFERENTIAL DIAGNOSIS

- Diabetes mellitus
- Primary polydipsia
- Other acquired forms of concentrating defects or polyuria

WORKUP

- Diagnosis suggested by the following:
  - Polyuria
  - Specific gravity on first-morning urine of less than 1.010
  - High serum osmolality associated with low urine osmolality
- Evaluation
  - Blood tests: ADH level, chemistries (e.g., sodium, potassium, calcium, glucose), blood urea nitrogen (BUN) concentration, creatinine level, osmolality
  - Urine tests: urine osmolality, urine volume, urine glucose concentration
  - Head magnetic resonance imaging (MRI)
  - Therapeutic trial of 1-deamino–8-D-arginine-vasopressin (DDAVP) with close monitoring of serum electrolytes and osmolality, urine osmolality, and urine volume
  - Water deprivation test: should be performed under the supervision of a pediatric endocrinologist or pediatric nephrologist
  - Genetic testing for NDI (*AVPR2* gene mutation)

LABORATORY TESTS

- ADH levels
- Serum chemistries, BUN, creatinine level, osmolality
- Urine osmolality and volume

IMAGING STUDIES

- Head MRI
- Renal ultrasound: to assess acquired forms of nephrogenic DI such as renal dysplasia

TREATMENT

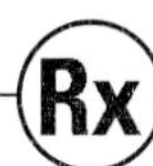

NONPHARMACOLOGIC THERAPY

- Easy, unlimited access to water
- Salt (solute) restriction

ACUTE GENERAL Rx

- During an episode of dehydration:

- Institute fluid resuscitation with normal saline and then switch to a hypotonic fluid. Monitor for possible hemolysis caused by administration of large volumes of hypotonic fluid.
- The patient may require central line placement to keep up with ongoing urine losses and to replace the deficit.
- Closely monitor the blood glucose level, and consider a change to 2.5% to 3% dextrose because patients can become hyperglycemic on 5% dextrose (D_5) solutions because of the high rates needed to keep up with volume losses.
- Glycosuria can exacerbate the situation by inducing an osmotic diuresis.

- If treating CDI, consider administration of DDAVP.
- If DI is acquired and results from a medication, remove the offending agent (e.g., lithium); if it is caused by an electrolyte abnormality, make the appropriate correction.

CHRONIC Rx

- CDI
  - DDAVP (oral or intranasal)
- NDI
  - Thiazides with or without amiloride (potassium-sparing diuretic) can reduce the volume of urine output by inducing mild intravascular volume contraction.
    - Hydrochlorothiazide: 2 to 4 mg/kg/day, divided for twice-daily doses
    - Amiloride: up to 20 mg/1.73 m^2/day, divided for twice-daily doses
  - Indomethacin can reduce the glomerular filtration rate.
    - 2 mg/kg/day, divided for twice-daily doses
  - Easy, unlimited access to water and solute restriction may be adequate therapy for adolescents.
- Primary polydipsia
  - Gradual reduction in oral intake reestablishes the medullary concentration gradient.

DISPOSITION

- Closely monitor electrolytes.
  - Risk for hypokalemia with thiazide
  - Risk for hyponatremia with DDAVP
- Monitor for side effects of indomethacin: gastrointestinal upset and bleeding; renal function.
- Monitor growth and development.
- Monitor anterior pituitary function if CDI.

REFERRAL

Most children are referred to a pediatric nephrologist or endocrinologist for evaluation and ongoing therapy.

PEARLS & CONSIDERATIONS

COMMENTS

- A high serum sodium level associated with polyuria in a dehydrated infant suggests a renal concentrating defect.
- Seizures, when they occur, usually occur during too-rapid rehydration.
- Early diagnosis, treatment, and careful rehydration have resulted in a decrease in frequency of mental retardation.

PATIENT/FAMILY EDUCATION

- Review the genetics of the disease with the parents. Explain that perinatal testing for carrier status is available.
- Severe dehydration can occur quickly, particularly with illnesses associated with vomiting and diarrhea.
- Neurologic sequelae typically result from repeated bouts of dehydration and overly aggressive rehydration.
- Solute restriction is important in decreasing obligatory water loss.
- Support groups are available through the Diabetes Insipidus and Related Disorders (DIARD) Network (535 Echo Court, Saline, MI 48176-1270); the Nephrogenic Diabetes Insipidus Foundation (Main Street, P.O. Box 1390, Eastsound, WA 98245; http://www.ndif.org); and the National Organization for Rare Disorders (55 Kenosia Avenue, P.O. Box 1968, Danbury, CT 06813-1968; www.rarediseases.org).

SUGGESTED READINGS

Berl T, Kumar S: Disorders of water metabolism. *In* Johnson RJ, Feehally J (eds): *Comprehensive Clinical Nephrology*. London, Mosby, 2000.

Maghnie M et al: Central diabetes insipidus in children and young adults. *N Engl J Med* 343:998, 2000, pp 232–236.

Online Mendelian Inheritance in Man (OMIM). Available at http://www.ncbi.nlm.nih.gov/omim

Saborio P et al: Diabetes insipidus. *Pediatr Rev* 21:122, 2000.

AUTHOR: **AYESA N. MIAN, MD**

BASIC INFORMATION

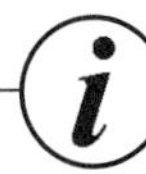

DEFINITION

Diabetes mellitus (DM) type 1 is an autoimmune disorder characterized by insulin deficiency resulting from progressive destruction of the insulin-producing β cells of the pancreas. This insulin deficiency leads to hyperglycemia and ketosis. Chronic hyperglycemia is associated with long-term damage, leading to dysfunction of the kidney, eyes, nerves, heart, and blood vessels.

SYNONYMS

Insulin-dependent diabetes mellitus (IDDM)
Juvenile-onset diabetes mellitus (JODM)
Type 1 DM

ICD-9-CM CODES

250.01	Diabetes mellitus type 1
250.03	Diabetes mellitus type 1 uncontrolled
250.10	Diabetic ketoacidosis
250.73	Diabetes mellitus type 1 with peripheral vascular disease
250.91	Diabetes mellitus type 1 with complications

EPIDEMIOLOGY & DEMOGRAPHICS

- An incidence of 1.7 (1.2 to 3.5 depending on geography) affected individuals per 1000 people younger than 20 years has been reported. It appears to be increasing slowly.
- The incidence of type 1 DM is higher in whites than blacks and lowest in Asians.
- Diabetes is more prevalent in northern than southern climates.
- Approximately 13,000 new cases in the United States are diagnosed annually in children.
- Approximately 150,000 individuals younger than 19 years of age have diabetes.
- The genetics are multifactorial and include the effects of many genes interacting with many unknown environmental agents.

CLINICAL PRESENTATION

- The presentation may be acute with diabetic ketoacidosis (see Diabetic Ketoacidosis in Diseases and Disorders [Section I]).
- The presentation may follow 1 to 3 weeks of polyuria, polydipsia, or polyphagia.
- DM may present with new-onset enuresis in a previously continent child.
- The presentation may be an incidental laboratory finding of glucosuria or hyperglycemia.

ETIOLOGY

- Relative or absolute insulin deficiency, from autoimmune destruction of the β cells of the pancreas.

DIAGNOSIS

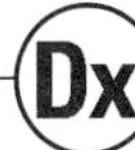

DIFFERENTIAL DIAGNOSIS

- Urinary tract infection
- Diabetes insipidus
- Type 2 diabetes mellitus
- Stress hyperglycemia
- Neurogenic bladder

WORKUP

Usually not required, laboratory tests are confirmatory.

LABORATORY TESTS

- Fasting blood glucose is higher than 126 mg/dL.
- Two-hour post-oral glucose test is higher than 200 mg/dL or random glucose higher than 200 mg/dL and symptoms.
- Glycosylated hemoglobin is higher than normal.
- Antibodies to islet cells, glutamate acid decarboxylase, insulin, islet-related autoantigens, and others; these antibodies not used in routine diagnosis of diabetes.
- Thyroid-stimulating hormone and celiac antibodies should be obtained at baseline.

IMAGING STUDIES

- Not required

TREATMENT

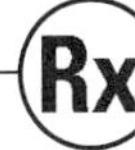

NONPHARMACOLOGIC THERAPY

- Begin a diabetic meal plan based preferably on the carbohydrate counting system rather than the diabetic exchange system. The carbohydrate counting system is based on the carbohydrate content of all foods.
  - The goal is to eat a consistent amount of carbohydrates at each meal regardless of the food group. The carbohydrate counting system requires more guidance to balance protein, carbohydrate, and fat ratios. The carbohydrate counting system allows more flexibility.
  - The exchange system is based on the American Diabetes Association and American Dietetic Association guidelines for food groups; portion sizes; and carbohydrate, protein, and fat distribution. The exchange system assigns all foods to one of nine groups. Carbohydrate, protein, and fat caloric content are given for portion size. The meal plan is designed for the patient to eat the same number of exchanges from day to day at each meal and snack. This plan provides consistent carbohydrate, protein, and fat content from day to day.
- Psychological support should be available for the patient and family.

ACUTE GENERAL Rx

- Insulin: the usual regimen consists of a total daily dose of 0.7 to 1.0 U/kg/day, in divided doses using either a mixed-split twice-a-day regimen or multiple daily injections.
- With the mixed-split twice-a-day regimen, the usual distribution is two thirds of the total daily dose given in the morning, distributed as two-thirds intermediate insulin (NPH) and one-third short-acting insulin (LysPro or Aspart). The remaining one third of the total daily dose is taken in the evening. It is divided as one-half long-acting and one-half short-acting insulin. The evening dose may be split by giving the short-acting insulin before dinner and the long-acting insulin before bedtime.
- With multiple daily injections, approximately half of the total daily insulin, using Glargine insulin, is given once a day either consistently in the evening or consistently in the morning. The remaining half is given as short-acting insulin (LysPro or Aspart) in three divided doses with breakfast, lunch, and dinner.
- Home blood glucose monitoring is done, with determinations before each meal and at bedtime.
- Urine ketone determination during acute illnesses and with blood sugars higher than 300 mg/dL.

DISPOSITION

- Initial education should be provided regarding diabetes, insulin adjustment, blood glucose, urine ketone monitoring, and meal planning.
- Frequent phone management should occur to review the patient's glucose log and recommend insulin adjustments.
- Usual follow-up is maintained through visits to an outpatient pediatric diabetes center four times per year.
- At each visit, the glucose log is reviewed and recommendations are made for insulin adjustments if needed.
- Glycosylated hemoglobin levels should be checked three to four times per year to assess chronic control.
- Phone contact should be maintained for illness management.

REFERRAL

- An ophthalmologic examination should be performed yearly.
- Thyroid function tests should be performed at the onset of disease and every 2 to 3 years thereafter.
- Urine for microalbuminuria should be checked annually 3 to 5 years after the onset of diabetes.

PEARLS & CONSIDERATIONS

COMMENTS

- Tight glycemic control significantly reduces the rate of complications.
- During puberty, increases in total daily insulin up to 1.5 U/kg/day are often needed.
- Psychosocial issues of dealing with a chronic disease are the most common cause of difficulties with diabetes care.

PREVENTION

- Experimental only

PATIENT/FAMILY EDUCATION

- The major component of diabetes management is education of patients and their families.
- School personnel (e.g., teachers, nurses, day-care providers) should also be educated regarding diabetes.
- Psychological support should be promptly provided upon identification of need.

Support Groups

- American Diabetes Association: www.diabetes.org
- Juvenile Diabetes Research Foundation International: www.jdf.org/index.html

SUGGESTED READINGS

American Diabetes Association. Available at www.diabetes.org

American Diabetes Association: Practice guidelines. *Diabetes Care* 28:186, 2005.

Children with Diabetes. Available at www.childrenwithdiabetes.org

Diabetes Control and Complications Research Group: The effect of intensive diabetes treatment on the development and progression of long-term complications in adolescents with insulin-dependent diabetes mellitus. *J Pediatr* 125:177, 1994.

The effect of intensive treatment of diabetes on the development and progression of long-term complications in insulin-dependent diabetes mellitus. *N Engl J Med* 329:977, 1993.

Insulin-Free World Foundation. Available at www.insulin-free.org/main/htm

Juvenile Diabetes Research Foundation International. Available at www.jdf.org/index.html

Kaufman FR: Diabetes mellitus. *Pediatr Rev* 18:383, 1997.

AUTHOR: **NICHOLAS JOSPE, MD**

BASIC INFORMATION

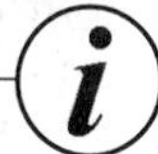

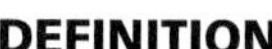

DEFINITION

Diabetes mellitus (DM) type 2 is a combination of resistance to insulin action and defective glucose-mediated insulin secretion. Patients are not prone to ketosis under basal conditions, and exogenous insulin is not required for short-term survival.

SYNONYMS

Non–insulin-dependent diabetes mellitus (NIDDM)
Type 2 DM
Old-term: adult-onset diabetes mellitus (AODM)

ICD-9-CM CODES

250.00 Diabetes mellitus type 2 uncomplicated
250.02 Diabetes mellitus type 2 uncontrolled
250.20 Diabetic hyperglycemic hyperosmolar nonketotic state with coma
250.92 Diabetes mellitus type 2 uncontrolled with complications
648.83 Gestational diabetes antepartum
790.29 Oral glucose tolerance test 2-hour level between 140 and 200

EPIDEMIOLOGY & DEMOGRAPHICS

- The incidence of type 2 DM is increasing in parallel with the increased prevalence of exogenous obesity. Nearly all of that increase is due to obesity. More than 17 million Americans of all ages have diabetes, and currently one fourth to more than one half of all new diabetes cases in children are type 2 diabetes, depending on geography.
- Type 2 DM is a polygenic disorder and the pattern is complex, since both impaired β-cell function and insulin resistance are involved.
  - Certain minority populations are at a higher risk of both obesity and type 2 DM.
  - African Americans, Pima Indians, and Mexican Americans are at high risk for type 2 DM.
- Environmental factors are highly associated with type 2 DM.
  - Increase in sedentary lifestyles
  - Increased access to high-calorie, high-fat foods

CLINICAL PRESENTATION

- Symptoms of type 2 DM are subtle because the disease develops and progresses slowly.
- The presentation may follow weeks of polyuria, polydipsia, and polyphagia.
- The presentation may be incidental documentation of glucosuria or hyperglycemia.
- The presentation can be diabetic ketoacidosis (DKA).
- In women, vaginal yeast infections or fungal infections may be present.
- Adolescent females may have oligomenorrhea and polycystic ovary syndrome.
- Strong family history for DM and obesity may be reported.

ETIOLOGY

- In type 2 DM, there is primary insulin resistance with relative insulin deficiency or a predominant secretory defect with insulin resistance.
- Variable interplay exists between genetic and environmental factors.
- The precise genetic factors are unknown and vary among population groups.
- Increasingly, sedentary lifestyles and dietary changes contribute to the increasing prevalence of obesity and type 2 DM.

DIAGNOSIS

Dx

DIFFERENTIAL DIAGNOSIS

- Type 1 DM
- Stress hyperglycemia

LABORATORY TESTS

- Glycosuria without ketonuria is demonstrated on urinalysis.
- Hyperglycemia is present.
  - Fasting blood glucose is more than 126 mg/dL.
  - DKA is possible but much less common than in type 1 DM.
  - Random glucose is more than 200 mg/dL and symptoms are present.
  - Two-hour post-oral glucose test is higher than 200 mg/dL.
- Glycosylated hemoglobin is higher than normal.
- Insulin or C-peptide levels are useful when elevated above normal, indicative of insulin resistance.
- Family history of type 2 DM is reported.

TREATMENT

Rx

NONPHARMACOLOGIC THERAPY

- Diet to induce weight loss
  - Even mild weight loss is beneficial for glucose control.
  - Caloric restriction even before weight loss is beneficial for glucose control.
- Modification of lifestyle to increase exercise

ACUTE GENERAL Rx

Insulin therapy may be needed in early stages, until reduction in glucose is achieved and oral medications have the chance to reach therapeutic levels.

CHRONIC Rx

- Oral agents: these are used in early stages when insulin secretion is still present and may be used alone, in combination, or with insulin. Long-term safety and efficacy have not been well established in children.
  - Sulfonylureas stimulate pancreatic insulin secretion and have a direct insulin-sensitizing effect. They may cause hypoglycemia and weight gain. Second-generation sulfonylureas, glipizide, glyburide, and glimepiride may be less associated with weight gain.
  - Biguanides (metformin) inhibit hepatic glucose output. These enhance insulin sensitivity in liver and muscle but are not associated with hypoglycemia. They may also cause some weight loss and gastrointestinal side effects. They are synergistic as glycemic control when used in combination with sulfonylureas.
  - Glucosidase inhibitors (e.g., acarbose) delay digestion of complex carbohydrates. They decrease the rise in postprandial plasma glucose. Significant gastrointestinal side effects such as diarrhea, flatulence, and abdominal distension occur.
  - Thiazolidinediones (pioglitazone and rosiglitazone) are insulin sensitizers, and decrease insulin resistance. These agents improve cholesterol levels, including high-density lipoprotein levels. They can cause swelling from fluid buildup and weight gain.
  - Insulin therapy may be needed in later stages, when β-cell function is lost.
- See Diabetes Mellitus Type 1 in Diseases and Disorders (Section I).
- Satisfactory glycemic control is best obtained with mixed short-acting intermediate insulin.

COMPLEMENTARY & ALTERNATIVE MEDICINE

- Education is not the same as in type 1 DM.
- Emphasis is on caloric restriction and lifestyle changes. The recommendations regarding the diabetic diet are evolving, and at present, no single diet meets all the needs of everyone with type 2 DM. Nonetheless, patients and families should meet with a dietitian to plan a diet that aims to limit fats (particularly saturated fats and trans fatty acids) and cholesterol, encourages plenty of fiber-rich foods (whole grains and fresh fruits and vegetables), and not limit protein. Reduced salt is advised as a first line of therapy for high blood pressure in this setting.

PEARLS & CONSIDERATIONS

COMMENTS

- Aggressive intervention with oral agents or insulin is necessary.
  - Delays complications
  - Significantly improves outcome
- It may be difficult to establish whether a child with new-onset DM has type 1 or type 2. This distinction may be helped by measuring islet cell antibodies that are

present only in type 1 DM and measuring c-peptide, which is low to absent in type 1 DM.
  - It is safe to start these patients on insulin. Switch to oral agents if appropriate.

PREVENTION

- Weight loss, through lifestyle modifications, including reduced caloric intake and increased activity and behavior modification can prevent type 2 DM.
- Either biguanides or thiazolidinediones can prevent the onset of type 2 DM in a patient at risk.
- Atypical antipsychotics differ in potential to cause metabolic disturbances: obesity, diabetes, dyslipidemia, and metabolic syndrome.
  - Clozapine and olanzapine: greatest risks
  - Risperidone and quetiapine: lower risks
  - Ziprasidone and aripiprazole: minimal metabolic risks

SUGGESTED READINGS

American Diabetes Association. Available at http://diabetes.org

American Diabetes Association: Practice guidelines. *Diabetes Care* 22(Suppl 1, Clinical Practice Recommendations), 1999.

Dean H: Diagnostic criteria for non-insulin dependent diabetes in youth (NIDDM-Y). *Clin Pediatr* 37:67, 1998.

Jones KL: Non-insulin dependent diabetes in children and adolescents: the therapeutic challenge. *Clin Pediatr* 37:103, 1998.

AUTHOR: **NICHOLAS JOSPE, MD**

BASIC INFORMATION

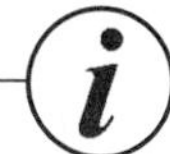

DEFINITION

Diabetic ketoacidosis (DKA) is dehydration and acidosis resulting from insulin deficiency (relative or absolute) in a patient with diabetes mellitus type 1 or 2.

ICD-9-CM CODE
250.13 Diabetic ketoacidosis

EPIDEMIOLOGY & DEMOGRAPHICS

- DKA is three to four times more common in patients with known diabetes than in patients with new-onset diabetes.
- The mortality rate for DKA ranges from 2% to 5% in developed countries.

CLINICAL PRESENTATION

- DKA may be a presentation of new-onset type 1 diabetes mellitus and, more rarely, type 2 diabetes mellitus.
- DKA ensues after omission of insulin for 24 to 48 hours in a patient with type 1 diabetes mellitus.
- DKA occurs in conjunction with illness and relative under insulinization.
- Polyuria and polydipsia are seen.
- Abdominal pain is common.
- Vomiting may occur.
- Increasing polyuria and polydipsia, variable weight loss, weakness, then drowsiness, decreased consciousness, and eventually coma may occur.
- Dehydration and hypovolemia (reduced skin turgor, hypotension, and tachycardia) may occur.
- Fruity odor may be evident.
- Kussmaul respirations may be noted.
- Hyperpnea may be present.

ETIOLOGY

- Relative or absolute deficiency of insulin, resulting in uncontrolled hyperglycemia and thus osmotic diuresis with electrolyte, glucose, ketone, and fluid losses
- Hyperglycemia as a result of hepatic and renal overproduction of glucose and muscle under utilization of glucose; ketoacidosis parallels hyperglycemia and is also caused by insulin deficiency
- Increased counter-regulatory hormones (e.g., cortisol, catecholamines, glucagon, growth hormone)

DIAGNOSIS

DIFFERENTIAL DIAGNOSIS

- No other metabolic abnormality can account for laboratory and physical examination findings.
- Initial presentation with polyuria or polydipsia may suggest diabetes insipidus.
- Other causes of dehydration and vomiting may be entertained (gastritis, gastroenteritis, pancreatitis, hepatitis, urinary tract infection) until laboratory values are known.
- Abdominal pain mimics an acute abdomen.
- Other causes of mental status abnormalities may be suggested (encephalitis, drug ingestion or overdose, alcohol intoxication) until laboratory results are known.

WORKUP

- Hyperglycemia (normal glucose uncommon but does not rule out DKA)
- Acidosis: venous blood gas with pH less than 7.2 and PCO_2 less than 15 mEq/L
- Ketonemia, ketonuria (urine ketotest)
- Hyperosmolarity mostly caused by hyperglycemia
- Hyperlipidemia
- Electrolyte disturbances
    - Sodium loss of approximately 10 to 15 mEq/kg body weight. Expect a 1.6 mEq/L decrease in serum sodium for every 100 mg/dL increase of glucose concentration
    - Chloride loss of 4 mEq/kg
    - Potassium loss of 5 mEq/kg—usual deficit is 3 to 5 mEq/kg, but therapy and continued losses may exacerbate hypokalemia (nadir at 4 to 12 hours)
- Urinary ketones correlate poorly with degree of serum ketonemia. Ketonuria remains positive up to 2 days after successful treatment of DKA.
    - Not useful as a monitor of ongoing therapy

LABORATORY TESTS

- Venous blood gas with pH less than 7.2 and PCO_2 less than 15 mEq/L
- Glucose should be taken hourly at the bedside.
- Electrolytes and pH followed at admission and at 2, 6, 9, 12, 18, and 24 hours.

IMAGING STUDIES

- Head computed tomography (CT) scan only if cerebral edema is suspected

TREATMENT

NONPHARMACOLOGIC THERAPY

- Clinical monitoring should be maintained every 30 to 60 minutes.
- Keep a good flow sheet which includes, minimally: time, IV and oral intake, amount of insulin given, urine and other output, glucose, pH, PCO_2, Na, H_2CO_3, chloride, blood urea nitrogen (BUN), creatinine, magnesium, phosphate, calcium

ACUTE GENERAL Rx

- Fluids: bolus with 10 to 20 mL/kg normal saline over 1 hour and repeat only if hypotensive
- Insulin: 0.1 U/kg/hour using regular insulin or lispro insulin by continuous intravenous infusion. Alternative is 0.3 U/kg intramuscularly every 3 hours. Avoid the subcutaneous route. The infusion rate may be doubled if the pH fails to rise within 4 to 6 hours.
- If the glucose falls by more than 100 mg/dL/hour, the insulin infusion may be decreased by 30% to 50% and glucose is added to the intravenous fluid.
- Replace fluid over 24 to 48 hours using one-half normal saline, combining deficit plus daily maintenance:
    - Fluid deficit (usually 7% to 10%) = body weight × estimated deficit × 1000 mL
    - Daily maintenance = 100 mL/kg for first 10 kg body weight, 50 mL/kg for next 10 kg, and 20 mL/kg over 20 kg
- Do not give more than 4 L/m^2 over first 24 hours.
- Add potassium to the intravenous fluid only after urine output is confirmed and based on potassium in the following ranges:
    - If serum [K] = 3 to 4 mEq/L, add 40 mEq/L of potassium (as KCl plus KPO_4)
    - If [K] = 4.0 to 5.5, add 20 mEq/L of potassium
    - If [K] = 5.5 to 6.0, add 10 mEq/L of potassium
    - If [K] is greater than 6, add no potassium to the intravenous fluids
- Routine use of phosphate supplementation is not recommended.
- Add 5% dextrose when serum glucose falls to 250 to 300 mg/dL.
- Bicarbonate therapy is not recommended, except possibly with circulatory collapse.

CHRONIC Rx

- Patients may begin eating when no longer vomiting or complaining of abdominal pain or anorexia.
- Transition by administering appropriate subcutaneous insulin and, 30 minutes later, discontinue intravenous insulin.
- Do transition around meal time, using established insulin dose.
- Begin new patient on appropriate insulin dose (see chapter on Diabetes Mellitus Type 1 in Diseases and Disorders [Section I]).

PEARLS & CONSIDERATIONS

COMMENTS

- Persistent acidosis: if [HCO_3] fails to rise after 6 hours, increase the insulin infusion rate
- Cerebral edema
    - Cerebral edema is marked by sudden headache and pupillary, mental status, or vital signs changes.
    - Complicates about 0.7% to 1.0% of cases of DKA in children.
    - Lethal in 20% to 50%.
    - Recovery without permanent impairment of function is only 7% to 14%.

- Occurs hours into treatment and is not heralded by specific signs or symptoms.
- Mannitol (0.5 to 2.0 g/kg repeated as necessary) is the treatment of choice.

- DKA is in the differential diagnosis of nonsurgical acute abdomen.
- Amylase may be elevated in DKA and is not specific for pancreatitis.
  - Lipase is more specific for pancreatitis.
- Abdominal pain should dissipate as acidosis resolves; if it does not, suspect an intra-abdominal problem.
- A significant proportion of DKA occurs in patients with type 2 diabetes mellitus. Therapy for DKA with intravenous insulin addition of intravenous glucose as the plasma glucose level decreases, sufficient fluid and electrolyte replacement, and attention to associated problems is standard of care, regardless of the type of diabetes.
- High-dose glucocorticoids, atypical antipsychotics, diazoxide, and some immunosuppressive drugs have been reported to precipitate DKA in individuals not previously diagnosed with type 1 diabetes mellitus.

PREVENTION

- Rapid attention to rising blood sugar and verification of urine ketones

SUGGESTED READINGS

American Diabetes Association. Available at www.diabetes.org

Children with Diabetes. Available at www.childrenwithdiabetes.org

Duck SC, Wyatt DT: Factors associated with brain herniation in the treatment of diabetic ketoacidosis. *J Pediatr* 113:10, 1988.

Dunger DB et al: ESPE/LWPES consensus statement on diabetic ketoacidosis in children and adolescents. *Arch Dis Childhood* 89:188, 2004.

Harris GD et al: Minimizing the risk of brain herniation during treatment of diabetic ketoacidemia: a retrospective and prospective study. *J Pediatr* 117:22, 1990.

Insulin-Free World Foundation. Available at www.insulin-free.org

Juvenile Diabetes Foundation International. Available at www.jdf.org

Newton CA, Raskin P: Diabetic ketoacidosis in type 1 and type 2 diabetes mellitus: clinical and biochemical differences. *Arch Intern Med* 164:1925, 2004.

Rosenbloom AL, Hanas R: Diabetic ketoacidosis (DKA): treatment guidelines. *Clin Pediatr* 35:261, 1996.

Rosenbloom AL, Schatz DA: Diabetic ketoacidosis in childhood. *Pediatr Ann* 23:284, 1994.

AUTHOR: **NICHOLAS JOSPE, MD**

BASIC INFORMATION

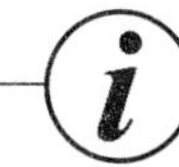

DEFINITION

Antibiotic-associated diarrhea is the presence of diarrhea (defined as three mushy or watery stools per day or a significant increase in the frequency or looseness of stools above baseline) either during or after the administration of antibiotics.

SYNONYMS

Antibiotic-associated colitis
Clostridium difficile-associated diarrhea/colitis
Pseudomembranous colitis

ICD-9-CM CODE

008.45 Pseudomembranous colitis

EPIDEMIOLOGY & DEMOGRAPHICS

- Diarrhea is often associated with antibiotic use and can develop anywhere from 2 hours to 8 to 10 weeks after antibiotic use (usually 4 to 9 days).
- The incidence differs with antibiotics and ranges from 5% to 38%.
  - The most commonly associated antibiotics are ampicillin (amoxicillin), clindamycin, and cephalosporins.
- Approximately 10% to 20% of cases of antibiotic-associated diarrhea are related to toxigenic *C. difficile.*
  - It is acquired by the oral-fecal route.
  - From 1% to 3% of healthy adults are asymptomatic carriers compared with 25% to 60% of healthy neonates and infants (up to 12 months of age).
    - Infants may lack the intestinal membrane receptor for the toxin.
  - It may occur without antibiotic exposure in immunosuppressed or immunocompromised patients and patients with inflammatory bowel disease.
  - It is one of the most common nosocomial infections in hospital practice.
  - It is isolated in 95% to 100% of patients with pseudomembranous colitis.
  - The risk is related to the type of antibiotic, length of treatment, and number of antibiotics used.

CLINICAL PRESENTATION

- History of exposure to antibiotics (within 2 hours to 2 to 3 months)
- Other symptoms vary.
  - Simple antibiotic-associated diarrhea
    - Mild watery diarrhea with mucus but no blood
    - Mild crampy abdominal pain
  - Non-pseudomembranous antibiotic-associated colitis (often *C. difficile*)
    - Watery diarrhea with or without visible blood
    - Malaise, nausea, and anorexia
    - Possible low-grade fever
  - Pseudomembranous colitis (*C. difficile*)
    - Similar but more severe symptoms
    - Diarrhea usually bloody and may contain pseudomembranes
  - Fulminant colitis/toxic megacolon (*C. difficile*)
    - Severe and diffuse abdominal pain
    - Bloody diarrhea
    - If an ileus develops, may have no stool output
    - Systemic symptoms including chills
- Physical findings also vary.
  - Simple antibiotic-associated diarrhea
    - May have mild abdominal tenderness
  - Non-pseudomembranous antibiotic-associated colitis
    - Abdominal tenderness
    - Low-grade fever
    - Hemoccult-positive stools
  - Pseudomembranous colitis
    - Similar findings but abdominal tenderness may be more pronounced
    - Fever generally higher
  - Fulminant colitis/toxic megacolon
    - Toxic-appearing with high fever, evidence of dehydration or shock
    - Abdominal distension with significant tenderness with or without peritoneal signs
    - Hemoccult-positive stools

ETIOLOGY

- Antibiotic-associated diarrhea can be related to a number of factors.
  - Suppression or altered composition of normal intestinal flora
    - Functional disturbances
      - Colonic carbohydrate metabolism defect, which can result in an osmotic diarrhea.
      - Abnormal metabolism and malabsorption of bile acids, which are potent secretory agents in the colon.
    - Overgrowth of pathogenic microorganisms, including:
      - *C. difficile*
      - Other potential pathogens (rarely) such as toxin-producing, gram-negative organisms; *Candida;* and *Staphylococcus aureus*
  - Direct effects of the antibiotic include the following:
    - Allergic and toxic effects on intestinal mucosa
      - Neomycin directly damages small bowel mucosa.
    - Pharmacologic effects on motility
      - Erythromycin acts as a motilin receptor agonist and stimulates gastroduodenal contractions.
- The predominant cause is overgrowth of *C. difficile.*
  - Gram-positive, anaerobic, spore-forming bacterium
    - Spores allow the organism to survive for weeks to months and make it difficult to eradicate.
  - Produces an enterotoxin (toxin A) and a cytotoxin (toxin B), which cause mucosal damage and inflammation in the colon.
  - Can cause a spectrum of disease ranging from mild (diarrhea) to severe (pseudomembranous colitis and toxic megacolon).
  - Antimicrobial agents that predispose to *C. difficile* diarrhea and colitis:
    - Frequent: cephalosporins, penicillins (amoxicillin, ampicillin), and clindamycin
    - Infrequent: tetracyclines, sulfonamides, erythromycin, chloramphenicol, trimethoprim, and quinolones
    - Rarely: parenteral aminoglycosides, bacitracin, metronidazole, and vancomycin

DIAGNOSIS

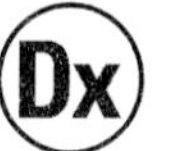

DIFFERENTIAL DIAGNOSIS

- Simple antibiotic-associated diarrhea
  - Infectious diarrhea
    - Bacterial
    - Viral
    - Parasitic (*Giardia*)
  - Lactose intolerance
  - Food protein sensitivity (infants and toddlers)
  - Postenteritis enteropathy
  - Chronic nonspecific diarrhea (toddler's diarrhea)
  - Celiac disease
- Colitis (mild to severe)
  - Infectious diarrhea
    - Bacterial (enteric pathogens): *Salmonella, Shigella, Yersinia, Campylobacter, Escherichia coli* O157:H7
    - Parasites (*Entamoeba histolytica*)
  - Inflammatory bowel disease
  - Henoch-Schönlein purpura
  - Hirschsprung's enterocolitis (usually infants)
  - Allergic colitis (infants)

WORKUP

Stool studies can establish the presence of *C. difficile* and the absence of other enteric pathogens (see "Laboratory Tests").

- Negative stool studies do not necessarily rule out the association of symptoms with antibiotic use.
- Sigmoidoscopy/colonoscopy may be indicated in the presence of persistent symptoms with negative stool studies.
  - Can address other diseases in the differential diagnosis (inflammatory bowel disease, allergic colitis) and make the diagnosis of pseudomembranous colitis
    - Raised yellow plaques from 2 to 10 mm in size scattered over colorectal mucosa, usually in the rectosigmoid, although may be limited to the proximal colon
  - Perform with extreme caution in cases of toxic megacolon and fulminant colitis

LABORATORY TESTS

- Stool studies should include the following:
  - Stool hemoccult
  - *C. difficile* toxin, preferably both A and B
  - Stool culture for enteric pathogens (bacterial and viral)
  - Stool for *E. coli* O157:H7 in the appropriate setting
  - Stool for ova and parasites
- Stool test for *C. difficile*
  - Stool culture for *C. difficile* is not a reliable test.
  - Toxin assays are currently the diagnostic test of choice to detect the presence of *C. difficile.*
    - Enzyme immunoassays to toxin A and B are fairly sensitive (70% to 90%) and very specific (99% to 100%). False-negative results do occur.
  - Studies in children suggest that assay for only one of the two toxins can result in a missed diagnosis.
- Other studies as clinically indicated:
  - Use the lactose breath hydrogen test to assess for underlying lactose intolerance if stool studies are unrevealing in the setting of mild diarrhea without evidence of colitis.
  - Complete blood count with differential, erythrocyte sedimentation rate, and albumin in the clinical setting is suggestive of underlying colitis (gross or occult blood in stool).

IMAGING STUDIES

- A kidney, ureter, and bladder study (KUB) can identify the presence of toxic megacolon in the patient with severe colitis.
  - Colon dilated more than 7 cm in greatest diameter

TREATMENT

Rx

NONPHARMACOLOGIC THERAPY

- General measures (simple antibiotic-associated diarrhea)
  - If the child is still taking the antibiotic, discontinue the medication or change to an antibiotic less likely to cause diarrhea if possible.
  - Avoid lactose, poorly soluble carbohydrates (e.g., fructose, sorbitol), and dietary fibers (vegetables such as cabbage, carrots, peas) while symptomatic.
    - These contribute to the functional disturbances related to antibiotic use which are usually self-limited.
  - Avoid antimotility agents.
- Toxic megacolon or fulminant colitis may require surgical intervention.
  - Subtotal colectomy with temporary ileostomy is performed in the setting of perforation or persistent toxicity despite aggressive medical therapy.

ACUTE GENERAL Rx

- If *C. difficile*-positive diarrhea persists after the antibiotic is discontinued or symptoms are moderate to severe, consider the following:
  - Metronidazole 20 to 30 mg/kg/day (up to 500 mg/dose) orally divided three or four times daily for 7 to 14 days
    - First-line treatment of choice (inexpensive, effective)
    - Side effects: nausea, vomiting, metallic taste, alcohol intolerance
    - Secreted in bile and colon, so can be used intravenously (although not as effective as orally)
  - Vancomycin 20 to 40 mg/kg/day (up to 2 g/day) orally divided four times daily for 7 to 14 days
    - May be slightly more effective than metronidazole but is significantly more expensive
    - Side effects: few
    - Indicated for patients who are intolerant or fail to respond to metronidazole and those with severe pseudomembranous colitis
    - Not as effective as metronidazole intravenously
    - Can predispose to development of vancomycin-resistant enterococcus
  - Bacitracin (up to 25,000 U/dose) divided four times daily for 7 to 14 days is another alternative but is expensive and less effective than metronidazole or vancomycin.
- Overgrowth of other organisms
  - Whether overgrowth of an organism other than *C. difficile* can be pathogenic is controversial.
  - If no other cause for the diarrhea is identified an empiric trial of metronidazole may be considered.

CHRONIC Rx

- Recurrent (relapsing) *C. difficile* infection
  - First relapse: repeat 10- to 14-day course of initial antibiotic used (development of antibiotic resistance in *C. difficile* has not been demonstrated)
    - This can be followed with a course of lactobacillus GG.
  - Second relapse: vancomycin for 7 to 14 days, followed by a taper over 2 to 3 weeks

COMPLEMENTARY & ALTERNATIVE MEDICINE

- Probiotics have been used both during and after antibiotic use to prevent or ameliorate antibiotic-associated diarrhea.
  - Lactobacillus GG 1 to 2 capsules daily (1 capsule = 10 billion colony-forming units)
  - Live culture yogurt (if tolerated); not always tolerated by lactose-deficient children

DISPOSITION

Antibiotic-associated diarrhea and colitis resolve with appropriate therapy in the majority of cases.

REFERRAL

- Infants and children should be referred to a gastroenterologist for the following:
  - Evidence of moderate-to-severe colitis (systemic signs and symptoms)
  - Chronic or recurrent *C. difficile*
  - Persistent diarrhea with negative stool studies. If symptoms are mild, consider the following prior to referral:
    - Dietary manipulation to address chronic nonspecific diarrhea
    - Trial of a lactose-free diet
    - Empiric trial of metronidazole

PEARLS & CONSIDERATIONS

COMMENTS

- Avoid unnecessary use of antibiotics, particularly in children with a history of antibiotic-associated diarrhea.
- Use the antibiotic with the narrowest spectrum or those less frequently associated with diarrhea.
- Consider using probiotics (lactobacillus GG) in patients with a history of antibiotic-associated diarrhea.
- The diagnosis of *C. difficile* may be missed in children if the laboratory does not measure both toxin A and B. If the index of suspicion is high enough and other causes have been ruled out, consider an empiric trial of metronidazole.
- *C. difficile* may be present in neonates and infants up to 1 year of age without causing disease.

PREVENTION

- Antibiotics should be used judiciously.
- Universal precautions should be followed with hospitalized/institutionalized patients.
- Lactobacillus GG during antibiotic use may decrease the incidence.

PATIENT/FAMILY EDUCATION

- Avoid unnecessary use of antibiotics.
- Mild diarrhea during and after antibiotic exposure may respond to simple dietary manipulations or use of probiotics.
  - Avoid excessive lactose, juices, and some fiber-containing foods while symptomatic
- Avoid alcohol while taking metronidazole.

SUGGESTED READINGS

Beaugerie L, Petit JC: Microbial-gut interactions in health and disease: antibiotic-associated diarrhea. *Best Pract Res Clin Gastroenterol* 18:337, 2004.

Brook I: Pseudomembranous colitis in children. *J Gastroenterol Hepatol* 20:182, 2005.

D'Souza AL et al: Probiotics in prevention of antibiotic associated diarrhea: meta-analysis. *BMJ* 324:1361, 2002.

Turk D et al: Incidence and risk factors of oral antibiotic-associated diarrhea in an outpatient pediatric population. *J Pediatr Gastroenterol Nutr* 37:22, 2003.

AUTHOR: **M. SUSAN MOYER, MD**

BASIC INFORMATION

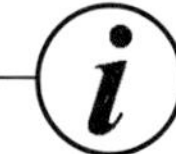

DEFINITION

Toddler's diarrhea is a common benign diarrheal disorder that presents in the toddler with three to six large, loose, watery stools per day for more than 3 weeks, but without evidence of systemic illness, failure to thrive, or other gastrointestinal disorder. Diarrhea should be present for at least 3 weeks (and preferably 4 weeks) to be considered "chronic" and may be episodic rather than continuous.

SYNONYMS

Chronic nonspecific diarrhea (CNSD)
Irritable colon of childhood
Sloppy stool syndrome

ICD-9-CM CODE
787.91 Diarrhea

EPIDEMIOLOGY & DEMOGRAPHICS

- Toddler's diarrhea is thought to be common, but the exact prevalence is unknown.
- It is the most common type of chronic diarrhea referred to pediatric gastroenterologists.
- Typical age is 12 to 36 months (range 6 months to 5 years).
- Symptoms resolve in 90% of children by 40 months of age.
- May be a variant of irritable bowel syndrome.

CLINICAL PRESENTATION

History

- Recent travel, drinking water sources, antecedent illness, infectious contacts, day care, new foods
- Use of antibiotics, laxatives, prescribed or over-the-counter drugs that may contain sorbitol, home remedies, alternative therapies
- Family history of gastrointestinal diseases
- An accurate description of the stool appearance and pattern
- Dietary history to ascertain total calories and fat consumed daily, quantities of milk and juice consumed daily, and any trials of elimination diets or currently eliminated foods
  - It is possible for a child to have toddler's diarrhea and have poor weight gain merely because he or she was placed on a hypercaloric diet by the caretakers in an attempt to control the diarrhea.
- Specifically, with toddler's diarrhea, the history will reveal the following:
  - Onset is at 6 months or later.
  - No stools occur overnight.
  - Stooling is most common in the morning.
  - There may be oscillation between normal and watery stools.
  - Stools are sloppy—generally watery but occasionally with mucus.
  - Stools often contain recognizable undigested food particles.
  - There is no associated nausea, vomiting, abdominal pain, flatulence, blood in the stool, fevers, weakness, decreased activity, anorexia, dermatologic problems, weight loss, poor growth, or other symptoms of systemic disease.
  - Although there may have been an antecedent illness, children with toddler's diarrhea exhibit no evidence of current enteric infection or malabsorption.
  - They continue to show normal growth and development unless caloric intake has been inadequate.

Physical Examination

- The physical examination and growth parameters are normal with toddler's diarrhea.
- The single most important aspect of the physical examination is accurate measurement of weight, height, and head circumference. Serial plots are needed.
- Abdominal and rectal examinations are entirely normal.
- Look for signs of dehydration—none are present in toddler's diarrhea.
- Check for evidence of malnutrition or malabsorption—none of the following are present in toddler's diarrhea:
  - Lack of subcutaneous fat
  - Eczematous rash of essential fatty acid deficiency and zinc deficiency
  - Glossitis
  - Easy bruising
  - Skin, hair, or nail abnormalities
  - Tired or ill-appearing
  - Decreased reflexes
- Examine the perianal area—there may be evidence of irritation from toddler's diarrhea, but true perianal disease, abscesses, fistulas, or rectal prolapse would indicate another disorder.

ETIOLOGY

- Toddler's diarrhea is a multifactorial problem. The following are contributing factors:
  - Excessive fluid intake
  - Disordered intestinal motility—resulting in rapid transit time
  - Carbohydrate malabsorption from excessive fruit and fruit juice consumption
  - Sorbitol
  - Fructose, when the concentration exceeds glucose concentration
  - Dietary fat restriction
  - Elevated colonic bile salts concentration

DIAGNOSIS (Dx)

DIFFERENTIAL DIAGNOSIS

- Enteric infection
  - Parasite
  - Protracted viral gastroenteritis (several viruses can rarely promote chronic diarrhea)
  - Rare for any bacterial infection to be chronic but has been reported (usually in younger infants with *Salmonella, Shigella, Yersinia, Campylobacter, Aeromonas,* and *Plesiomonas*)
- Intestinal malabsorption
  - Postviral enteritis (caused by flattened villi after an infection with rotavirus, adenovirus, astrovirus, or coronavirus)
  - Inflammatory bowel disease
  - Celiac disease
- History of onset or change in bowel habits; diarrhea present before 3 months of age, including the following:
  - Congenital microvillous atrophy
  - Disaccharidase abnormalities
  - Milk and soy allergies
  - Hollow visceral myopathy
- Protein intolerance: usually unknown mechanism (e.g., animal proteins, soy proteins)
- Food allergy: will usually have other gastrointestinal symptoms, such as oral pruritus, vomiting, or abdominal pain, in addition to diarrhea; may also have systemic symptoms such as skin rash, bronchospasm, or anaphylaxis
- Lactose intolerance
  - Primary acquired (late onset): lactase levels decrease through late childhood
  - Secondary acquired: caused by mucosal injury
  - Congenital: exceedingly rare
- Medication-induced
- Encopresis
- Immune system disorders: eosinophilic enteritis, acquired immunodeficiency syndrome, immunoglobulin A (IgA) deficiency, autoimmune enteropathy
- Acrodermatitis enteropathica (zinc deficiency)
- Anatomic abnormalities: short intestine, malrotation
- Fat malabsorption: cystic fibrosis, Shwachman-Diamond syndrome, pancreatitis
- Endocrine disorders: hyperthyroidism, diabetes
- Hormone-secreting tumors
  - APUDomas: These tumors originate in the APUD cells (amine precursor uptake and decarboxylation of amino acids) of the gastroenteropancreatic endocrine system.
  - Cell origin is adrenal or extra-adrenal neurogenic sites.
- Hirschsprung's disease
- Vasculitis: hemolytic uremic syndrome, Henoch-Schönlein purpura
- Pseudoobstruction
- Appendicitis
- Munchausen syndrome by proxy

LABORATORY TESTS

- A fresh stool sample may be the only body fluid needed and can be examined.
  - pH, reducing substances, neutral fat, occult blood
  - Ova and parasites, *Giardia* antigen
  - Leukocytes, eosinophils
  - *Clostridium difficile* toxin

- All of these stool studies are normal in toddler's diarrhea.
  - Occult blood could be present if there is a perianal rash or excoriation from the frequent stools.
- Other laboratory tests should be done only if indicated because of an abnormality found on fresh stool sample or because a different diagnosis is suspected based on history or physical examination.

TREATMENT

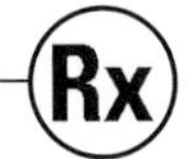

NONPHARMACOLOGIC THERAPY

- Provide parental reassurance
- Reduce juice consumption
- Eliminate soda and non-juice sweet drinks
- Normalize fluid consumption (to about 100 mL/kg/day)
- Reduce dietary sorbitol and free fructose
- Normalize diet (especially fats) if parents are restricting
- Increase dietary fat content to 35% to 40% of total calories (usually more than 4 g/kg/day)
- Increase dietary fiber

ACUTE GENERAL Rx

- Usually, no medical treatment is needed; resist the temptation and parental pressure to use medication.
- Green stools may contain abnormally high quantities of bile acid.
  - Treatment with the bile salt-binding medications cholestyramine and bismuth subsalicylate has reduced stool frequency and water content in some patients.
- Psyllium (2 to 3 g twice daily for 2 weeks) or Citrucel (1 to 2 tsp/day) may offer some cohesiveness to stools.
- Metronidazole will help the patient with undetected *Giardia.*
- Do not prescribe antispasmodic agents or antidiarrheal agents (e.g., loperamide) because these are not helpful.

COMPLEMENTARY & ALTERNATIVE MEDICINE

One study suggests that ingestion of yeast can benefit some patients with toddler's diarrhea by altering the intestinal microflora and thereby decreasing the chance of bacterial overgrowth.

DISPOSITION

- Although an extensive workup is not necessary, these children should be followed at least three times a year.
- If any additional signs or symptoms of gastrointestinal disease occur, or if the child has poor weight gain or weight loss, further evaluation will be necessary.

PEARLS & CONSIDERATIONS

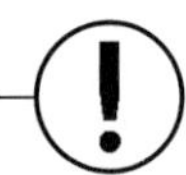

COMMENTS

- Normally, postprandial activity interrupts and replaces the migrating motor complex (MMC) the moment food enters the digestive system, slowing the transit of food through the intestine and allowing more time for the absorption of fluid, electrolytes, and nutrients. In children with toddler's diarrhea, food may fail to interrupt MMC activity, perhaps because of delayed gut motor development.
- Excess bile salts can enter the colon from rapid transit time and are thought to contribute to diarrhea because bacterial degradation of the salts produces bile acids and hydroxylated fatty acids, which may act as secretogogues in the colon.

PREVENTION

See "Nonpharmacologic Therapy."

PATIENT/FAMILY EDUCATION

- Explain the common nature and cause
- Show parents the child's normal growth parameters
- Provide a list of fruits (and juices) low in sorbitol and low in free fructose (equal concentrations of fructose and glucose or more glucose)
  - Several fruits (and juices) have no sorbitol and also have a favorable fructose: glucose ratio; examples include:
    - Citrus fruits
    - Cranberries
    - Grapes
    - Pineapples
    - Raspberries
    - Blackberries
    - Strawberries

SUGGESTED READINGS

Judd RH: Chronic nonspecific diarrhea. *Pediatr Rev* 17:379, 1996.

Kleinman RE (ed): *Pediatric Nutrition Handbook,* 5th ed. Elk Grove Village, IL, American Academy of Pediatrics, 2004.

Liacouras CA, Baldassano RN: Is it toddler's diarrhea? *Contemp Pediatr* 15:131, 1998.

Walker WA et al: *Pediatric Gastrointestinal Disease,* 3rd ed. London, BC Decker, 2000.

Wyllie R, Hyams JS: *Pediatric Gastrointestinal Disease: Pathophysiology, Diagnosis, Management,* 2nd ed. Philadelphia, WB Saunders, 1999.

AUTHOR: **LARRY DENK, MD**

BASIC INFORMATION

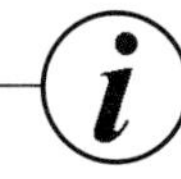

DEFINITION

Diskitis is an inflammatory process involving the intervertebral disks and adjacent vertebral bodies.

SYNONYMS

Acute osteitis of the spine
Benign osteomyelitis of the spine
Intervertebral disk space infection
Nontuberculous spondylodiscitis
Pyogenic infectious spondylitis
Spondylodiscitis

ICD-9-CM CODES
722.91 Cervical
722.92 Thoracic
722.93 Lumbar

EPIDEMIOLOGY & DEMOGRAPHICS

- Diskitis is uncommon—the exact incidence is unknown, but diskitis may account for 1 in 30,000 clinic visits.
- Diskitis is very rare in children older than 6 years of age.
- There is no sex predilection.
- Diskitis is not associated with trauma or osteomyelitis or septic arthritis elsewhere in body.
- Diskitis most commonly involves the lumbar spine.

CLINICAL PRESENTATION

History

- Presenting complaints are age-specific.
- Younger children refuse to bear weight, walk, or maintain a seated posture.
- Older children complain of back pain, hip pain, or pain with walking.
- Patients are most comfortable lying down.
- As many as 15% of children have abdominal pain.
- Changes in bowel or bladder patterns (e.g., new onset constipation) may be reported.

Physical Examination

- Affected children are usually irritable, but not acutely ill.
- Low-grade fever is often present.
- Range of motion of the spine is limited; pain occurs with any motion of the spine.
- Paravertebral muscle spasm may occur.
- Gower sign may be present.
- Neurologic findings are very uncommon and should prompt a thorough evaluation for alternative etiologies.

ETIOLOGY

- The pathophysiology of diskitis is controversial.
  - Diskitis may represent a low-grade bacterial infection or an inflammatory process.
- Blood cultures are positive in less than 30% of patients; disk aspiration cultures are positive in less than 50% of patients.
  - *Staphylococcus aureus* is the usual causative agent.
  - *Kingella kingae*, anaerobes, gram-negative enteric organisms, and *Streptococcus pneumoniae* have been isolated.
- In children, unlike adults, there are widespread vascular anastomoses between the vertebral bodies and disk tissues, accounting for the observed involvement of a disk and the adjacent vertebral end plates.
  - These anastomoses regress as children age, which likely accounts for the lack of diskitis in older children and adults.

DIAGNOSIS

DIFFERENTIAL DIAGNOSIS

- Vertebral osteomyelitis
- Osteomyelitis of the pelvis
- Septic arthritis of the hip or sacroiliac joint
- Psoas muscle or pelvic abscess
- Spinal epidural abscess
- Meningitis
- Appendicitis
- Malignancy
- Pyelonephritis
- Tuberculous spondylitis

LABORATORY TESTS

- Elevated erythrocyte sedimentation rate (ESR) common, but the level is rarely more than 60 mm/hour.
- Mild leukocytosis may occur.
- Although often negative, blood cultures should be obtained as positive culture results are important for guiding therapy.
- Disk aspiration cultures may only be necessary in patients who fail to improve or who have atypical presentations.

IMAGING STUDIES

- Conventional radiographs: normal until 2 to 4 weeks after onset, then narrow disk space with irregular or demineralized vertebral end plates. Sclerotic changes may occur in vertebral end plates 2 to 3 months after onset.
- Computed tomography (CT) demonstrates disk space narrowing and vertebral involvement early in the course of disease. False-negative CT scans have been reported.
- Magnetic resonance imaging (MRI) may be the most helpful imaging modality for confirming the diagnosis and identifying alternative diagnoses.
- Technetium-99 bone scans demonstrate increased uptake at the level of disk space involvement.

TREATMENT

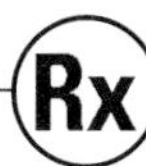

NONPHARMACOLOGIC THERAPY

- Most children respond to bed rest within 48 hours.
- Immobilization of the spine is sometimes required.
  - Optimal duration of immobilization has not been determined.
- Lack of rapid response should prompt further investigation.

ACUTE GENERAL Rx

- Nonsteroidal anti-inflammatory drugs can be given.
- Antibiotics may not be necessary for cure but may result in more rapid improvement in symptoms.
  - Patients who are systemically ill or who have positive culture results should definitely be treated with antibiotics.
  - In culture-negative patients, empiric antistaphylococcal antibiotic use is reasonable.
  - Antibiotics can be given intravenously until the patient has significant improvement in pain, fever, and ESR, after which oral therapy is sufficient.
  - Optimal duration of therapy is unknown.
  - Treatment is often continued until the ESR normalizes.

DISPOSITION

- Healing generally occurs by 8 weeks.
- Disk space narrowing may be permanent or may proceed to intervertebral fusion.
- Observation for possible spinal deformity is necessary for several years.
- Most patients have complete resolution without residual restrictions. Some patients have mild chronic back pain.

REFERRAL

Refer patients with suspected diskitis to a pediatric orthopedist if possible.

PEARLS & CONSIDERATIONS

COMMENTS

Variability of clinical presentation is related to age.

SUGGESTED READING

Gutierrez KM: Diskitis. *In* Long SS et al (eds): *Principles and Practice of Pediatric Infectious Disease.* New York, Churchill Livingstone, 2003, pp 481–484.

AUTHOR: **MELANIE WELLINGTON, MD**

BASIC INFORMATION

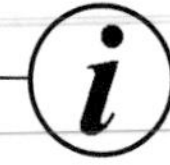

DEFINITION

Disseminated intravascular coagulation (DIC) is an acute or chronic disorder causing thrombosis or hemorrhage, which occurs as a secondary complication of an underlying disease. It is characterized by consumption of coagulation factors caused by intravascular activation of the coagulation sequence, which leads to the formation of thrombi throughout the microcirculation of the body, and secondarily, activation of fibrinolysis.

SYNONYMS

Consumption coagulopathy
Defibrination syndrome
DIC

ICD-9-CM CODE
286.6 Disseminated intravascular coagulation (DIC)

EPIDEMIOLOGY & DEMOGRAPHICS

- The most common underlying cause is sepsis.
- Estimates in patients with gram-negative sepsis range from 10% to 50%.

CLINICAL PRESENTATION

- Hemorrhage is the most common presentation, but microvascular thrombosis is the primary mechanism. The clinician must be attentive to the possibility of DIC as the cause of severe bleeding, thrombosis, or both.
- Manifestations of hemorrhage caused by plasmin generation include the following:
  - Spontaneous bruising
  - Petechiae
  - Gastrointestinal bleeding
  - Respiratory tract bleeding
  - Persistent bleeding at venipuncture sites
  - Bleeding at surgical wounds
  - Intracranial bleed
  - Hematuria
- Manifestations of thrombosis caused by thrombin generation include the following:
  - Renal failure
  - Coma
  - Liver failure
  - Respiratory failure
  - Skin necrosis
  - Gangrene
  - Venous thromboembolism
- Manifestations of cytokine generation include the following:
  - Tachycardia
  - Hypotension
  - Edema

ETIOLOGY

- Thrombin production is a normal response to tissue damage.
  - Multiple illnesses result in unregulated thrombin production, which leads to widespread microvascular thrombosis.
  - Thrombin is produced in sepsis and other inflammatory illnesses via cytokines.
- Cytokines (e.g., tissue necrotic factor-α [TNF-α]) are generated in response to endotoxin.
- Cytokines induce the extrinsic pathway, which results in thrombin production.
  - Excess plasmin production is a compensatory mechanism to maintain vascular patency.
- Acute presentation
  - Infection: gram-negative sepsis; gram-positive sepsis, especially with hyposplenism; systemic fungal infection; malaria; viral infections; rickettsial infections
  - Obstetric: placental separation, amniotic fluid embolism
  - Trauma: head trauma; burns, heat stroke, lightning strike
  - Other: transfusion of ABO-incompatible red blood cells, liver disease, snake bites, malignant hypertension
- Chronic presentation
  - Malignancy: adenocarcinoma, acute promyelocytic leukemia
  - Obstetric: retained dead fetus syndrome, toxemia
  - Vascular disease: aortic aneurysm, giant hemangioma, vasculitis

DIAGNOSIS

DIFFERENTIAL DIAGNOSIS

- Thrombotic thrombocytopenic purpura
- Hemolytic uremic syndrome
- Paroxysmal nocturnal hemoglobinuria
- Heparin-induced thrombocytopenia
- Liver disease
- Vitamin K deficiency

LABORATORY TESTS

- Expected results include the following:
  - Thrombocytopenia
  - Prolonged prothrombin time
  - Prolonged activated partial thromboplastin time
  - Decreased fibrinogen
  - Elevated fibrin degradation products
- Other laboratory results include red blood cell fragmentation.
  - Other tests should be used to determine the degree of renal, liver, and pulmonary involvement.

ACUTE GENERAL Rx

- Treatment of the underlying process that initiated DIC is essential. Infection, shock, acidosis, and hypoxia require immediate attention.
- Blood components are used if the patient is bleeding or if an invasive procedure is indicated.
- Platelets: give 1 donor unit per 10 kg of body weight when the platelet count is below 50,000.
- Fresh frozen plasma (FFP) has more fibrinogen than cryoprecipitate.
  - Give 15 mL of FFP per kg of body weight.
- Cryoprecipitate may be given when FFP cannot maintain fibrinogen concentration.
- Heparin has been effective in children with DIC associated with purpura fulminans and promyelocytic leukemia. Considerable debate exists regarding the use of heparin.
- Infusions of antithrombin and activated protein C are being studied.

DISPOSITION

DIC increases organ failure and mortality compared to the underlying diseases without DIC.

REFERRAL

Hematology referral is recommended for all patients.

PEARLS & CONSIDERATIONS

COMMENTS

- Platelet counts and fibrinogen may be elevated initially in DIC because of inflammation.
- Vitamin K and folate deficiencies may accompany DIC and should be corrected.

SUGGESTED READING

Bick RL: DIC current concepts of etiology, pathophysiology, diagnosis, and treatment. *Hematol Oncol Clin North Am* 17(1):149, 2003.

AUTHOR: **EDGARD A. SEGURA, MD**

BASIC INFORMATION

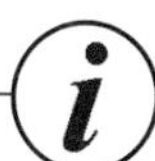

DEFINITION

Down syndrome is a chromosomal disorder characterized by recognizable facial features, multiple malformations, and mental impairment. Historically, it was one of the first known chromosomal causes of mental retardation and developmental disability.

SYNONYM

Trisomy 21

ICD-9-CM CODE
758.0 Down syndrome

EPIDEMIOLOGY & DEMOGRAPHICS

- Down syndrome is the most common chromosomal anomaly associated with mental retardation.
- The prevalence is approximately 1 in 800 live births.
- The risk of having a child with Down syndrome increases with increasing maternal age.
  - Most infants with Down syndrome, however, are born to women younger than 35 because of a higher rate of pregnancy in this age group.
- There is an increased incidence in the Latino population in the United States compared to other ethnic groups.

CLINICAL PRESENTATION

A combination of the following features is found, but not all features are present in each individual.

- Hypotonia
- Hypermobility of joints
- Microcephaly
- Excess skin at the back of the neck
- Flat facial profile
- Up-slanting of the palpebral fissures
- Epicanthal folds
- Brushfield spots or speckling of the irides
- Ears and mouth may appear small
- Wide gap between first and second toes with a deep fissure line
- Fifth finger clinodactyly with dysplasia of the midphalanx
- Single palmar crease
- Short and broad hands and feet
- Widely spaced nipples
- Cutis marmorata (lacy pattern to skin)

Associated Medical Complications

- Congenital heart disease (seen in 40% to 60% of infants with Down syndrome)
  - Endocardial cushion defect (atrioventricular septal defect), ventricular septal defect, and atrial septal defect are the three most common defects. Other defects do occur.
  - Valvular heart disease can occur after 18 years of age.
- Ophthalmologic disorders
  - Congenital cataracts
  - Refractive errors, strabismus, nystagmus, blepharitis, and nasolacrimal duct obstruction are most common.
- Ear, nose, and throat problems
  - Hearing loss, including congenital and acquired with conductive, mixed, and sensorineural etiologies
  - Chronic middle ear fluid—may be difficult to visualize because of narrow ear canals
  - Recurrent sinusitis and upper respiratory infections
  - Tracheomalacia
  - Obstructive sleep apnea
- Gastrointestinal
  - Feeding difficulties, secondary to decreased tone and poor coordination of suck/swallow
  - Gastrointestinal malformations, including atresias, Hirschsprung's disease, annular pancreas, and imperforate anus
  - Constipation
  - Gastroesophageal reflux
  - Celiac disease
- Dermatologic
  - Atopic dermatitis and seborrheic dermatitis
  - Vitiligo
- Dental
  - Malocclusion and periodontal disease
- Endocrine and growth issues
  - Hypothyroidism (may be clinically silent)
  - Short stature and obesity (specific growth charts have been developed for individuals with Down syndrome)
  - Type I diabetes mellitus
  - Primary gonadal deficiency
- Orthopedic
  - Joint laxity
  - Atlantoaxial instability
- Neurodevelopmental issues
  - Hypotonia with associated gross motor delays; typical age of walking is 2 years.
  - Developmental disability with mental retardation.
- Mild to moderate mental retardation is most common.
  - Patients can have dual diagnoses with other developmental disorders, such as attention deficit/hyperactivity disorder, oppositional and aggressive behavior, and autism spectrum disorders.
  - Plaques and neurofibrillary tangles are seen in the brains of adults with Down syndrome, similar to individuals with Alzheimer's disease. The exact risk for individuals with Down syndrome to develop Alzheimer's disease is still unclear, but the prevalence is higher than in the general population.
- Hematologic
  - Leukemia occurs at a higher rate than in the general population.
  - Leukemoid reactions are common.
- Infectious disease
  - Immunoglobulin G (IgG) subclass deficiencies

ETIOLOGY

- Approximately 95% of cases are secondary to nondisjunction during meiosis, leading to the presence of an extra chromosome 21.
- Approximately 3% to 4% of cases are secondary to translocation of a critical portion of an extra chromosome 21 to another chromosome (usually 14 or 21).
- Approximately 1% to 2% of cases show mosaicism, in which some, but not all, of cells have an extra chromosome 21. This occurs after fertilization during mitosis.

DIAGNOSIS

Dx

DIFFERENTIAL DIAGNOSIS

- Little else is considered when many of the distinguishing features are present, but isolated features can be present in individuals without chromosomal disorder.

WORKUP

- Growth velocity on standard and syndrome specific charts (available on web sites listed in "Suggested Readings", also see Down Syndrome Growth Chart in Section IV)
- Sleep study if clinically indicated for sleep disruption, apnea, or snoring
- Audiologic evaluation at birth, every 6 months until 3 years, then annually
- Ophthalmologic evaluation by 6 months and then annually

LABORATORY TESTS

- Prenatal
  - Screening: "triple" or "quadruple" screen. The triple screen includes α-fetoprotein, human chorionic gonadotropin, and estriol. The quadruple screen also includes inhibin-A.
  - Diagnostic: chromosome analysis via chorionic villus sampling or amniocentesis.
- Karyotype
- Thyroid screening (thyroid-stimulating hormone and thyroxine) at 6 months, 12 months, and then annually
  - Screen for celiac disease between 2 and 3 years of age. New guidelines are under consideration.

IMAGING STUDIES

- Prenatal ultrasound with characteristic findings, including nuchal translucency
- Echocardiogram at birth or at time of diagnosis
- Cervical spine roentgenogram once at 3 to 5 years of age and then as needed

TREATMENT

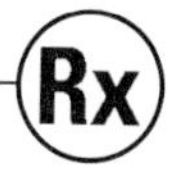

NONPHARMACOLOGIC THERAPY

- Early intervention educational programs beginning in the newborn to 3-year-old population have been shown to improve motor and developmental functioning. Therapy and school programs often include physical, occupational, and speech therapy.

- Preschool programs and individualized educational plans for preschool and school-age children are helpful. Many children with Down syndrome can be integrated into regular education programs with modifications and support.
- Refer for Supplemental Security Income.
- Diet and exercise for weight control.

ACUTE GENERAL Rx

- There is no cure for Down syndrome and few prospects exist to treat with gene therapy.
- SBE prophylaxis is recommended for children with cardiac defects (See SBE Prophylaxis Table in Prevention [Section V]).
- When making a neonatal or prenatal diagnosis, physicians should provide up-to-date materials and contact numbers.
- Talk with family members about the positive aspects of Down syndrome.
- Ensure that information presented is accurate and unbiased by own beliefs in developmental delays and mental retardation.
- Discuss sensitive issues with both parents present, particularly at initial disclosure.

CHRONIC Rx

- Aggressive management of treatable causes of hearing loss
- If change in functional level at any age, investigation for a treatable cause such as hypothyroid, sleep apnea, depression, or adjustment reaction should be sought.

COMPLEMENTARY & ALTERNATIVE MEDICINE

- Because of the chronic and incurable nature of Down syndrome, families are especially vulnerable to trying unproven alternative therapies.
- Scientific studies to date have shown no benefit from vitamin or mineral supplements, hormonal injections, or cell therapy.
- The primary care physician should carefully weigh the risks and benefits with family of all proposed therapeutic suggestions.

DISPOSITION

- Specific follow-up based on secondary medical problems (hypothyroidism, cardiac anomalies, and so forth)
- Begin transition planning at age 16 to address adult issues such as employment, housing, and finances

REFERRAL

- The primary care physician manages many children with Down syndrome with consultations to such individuals as cardiologists, otolaryngologists, geneticists, gastroenterologists, oncologists, and dentists.
- A consultative clinic for individuals with Down syndrome is available in many areas.
- Problematic behavior at times can warrant a referral to a behavioral specialist.

PEARLS & CONSIDERATIONS

COMMENTS

- A balanced translocation must be excluded in both parents if the child has a translocation.
- Individuals with Down syndrome function like those without Down syndrome in many ways.

PATIENT/FAMILY EDUCATION

- Regional Down Syndrome associations

SUGGESTED READINGS

American Academy of Pediatrics: Committee on Genetics: Health supervision for children with Down syndrome. *Pediatrics* 107(2):442, 2001.

Cohen W: Health care guidelines for individuals with Down syndrome. *Down Syndrome Quarterly* 4:3, 1999.

Down Syndrome Health Issues. Available at www.ds-health.com

Eberly S et al: Medical & Surgical Care for Children with Down Syndrome: A Guide for Parents. Woodbine House, 1994.

National Down Syndrome Congress. Available at www.ndsccenter.org

National Down Syndrome Society. Available at www.ndss.org

AUTHORS: **NANCY E. LANPHEAR, MD** and **HEIDI A. CASTILLO, MD**

BASIC INFORMATION

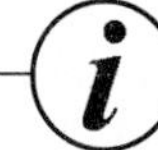

DEFINITION

Dysfunctional uterine bleeding (DUB) is excessive (>80 mL or a significant decrease in hemoglobin), prolonged (flow duration >7 to 10 days), or unpatterned (<21 days or >40 to 45 days in an adolescent) endometrial bleeding unrelated to structural or systemic disease. It may be described as ovulatory (e.g., heavy, cyclical bleeding) or anovulatory (e.g., irregular bleeding).

SYNONYMS

Abnormal uterine bleeding
Anovulatory bleeding

ICD-9-CM CODE
626.8 Dysfunctional uterine bleeding

EPIDEMIOLOGY & DEMOGRAPHICS

- Up to 95% of cases of abnormal vaginal bleeding in adolescents are caused by DUB due to anovulation.
- Although many adolescents are anovulatory, most do not develop DUB.

CLINICAL PRESENTATION

History

- Age at menarche
- Detailed menstrual history (e.g., duration, frequency, regularity of menses, dysmenorrhea) and menstrual calendar (calendar with days of spotting and bleeding)
- Characteristics of first menses
- History of sexual activity, contraceptive use, pregnancies, and sexually transmitted infections (obtained without parental presence)
- Review of systems (e.g., easy bruising)
- Family history (e.g., polycystic ovary syndrome, bleeding disorders)

Physical Examination

- Include a search for other causes of menstrual abnormalities such as adrenal disorders, thyroid disorders, prolactinoma, bleeding disorders, pregnancy, abdominal and pelvic masses
- Vital signs including height, weight, orthostatic pulse, and blood pressure
- General assessment including sexual maturity
- Pelvic examination with bimanual digital examination (alternatively, if accepted, rectoabdominal examination for nonsexually active adolescent). Speculum exam to assess vagina and cervix.
    - Expect a normal exam
    - Rule out foreign body, trauma, infection (including pelvic inflammatory disease [PID]), ovarian or uterine mass, and partial obstruction of the genital tract

ETIOLOGY

- Ovulatory DUB occurs with loss of local endometrial hemostasis leading to cyclical, heavy bleeding.
- Anovulatory DUB often is caused by impairment of the hypothalamic-pituitary-ovarian axis.
    - Failure of the negative feedback system (follicle-stimulating hormone [FSH] and estrogen) occurs during the follicular phase of the menstrual cycle.
    - Failure of FSH levels to decline occurs as a result of continued estrogen secretion.
    - Persistent unopposed estrogen secretion produces an excessively thickened, unstable endometrium with subsequent uncoordinated, painless sloughing.
- Structural pathology occurs in less than 10% of adolescent girls

DIAGNOSIS

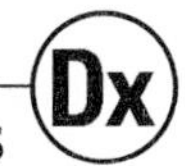

DIFFERENTIAL DIAGNOSIS

- Pregnancy
    - Ectopic pregnancy
    - Spontaneous, threatened, and incomplete abortion
- Hormonal
    - Immaturity of the hypothalamic-pituitary-ovarian axis causes anovulation in pubertal girls (50% to 80% in first 2 years, 30% to 55% years 2 to 4 postmenarche, 20% years 4 and 5 postmenarche).
    - Adrenal disease with androgen excess (e.g., late-onset congenital adrenal hyperplasia [CAH])
    - Polycystic ovary syndrome (PCOS)
    - Hyper- and hypothyroidism
    - Hyperprolactinemia
- Infections
    - Endometritis (rare in adolescent)
    - Endocervicitis (*Chlamydia trachomatis, Neisseria gonorrhea*)
    - Vaginitis
    - PID
- Mechanical
    - Endometriosis
    - Endometrial or cervical polyps
    - Fibroids
    - Arteriovenous malformation
    - Intrauterine device
    - Trauma
    - Foreign body (e.g., retained tampon)
- Medications
    - Oral contraceptive pills (OCPs)
    - Depomedroxyprogesterone acetate (Depo-Provera)
    - Anticoagulants
    - Platelet inhibitors
    - Anticonvulsants
- Cancer
- Uterine cancer (rare in adolescents)
- Vaginal neoplasm
- Other
    - Blood dyscrasias (e.g., thrombocytopenia, von Willebrand disease, and other clotting disorders)
    - Systemic illness (e.g., diabetes mellitus, cystic fibrosis SLE)
    - Stress and excessive exercise
    - Poor nutritional status (e.g., anorexia nervosa)

WORKUP

- Diagnosis of exclusion

LABORATORY TESTS

- Complete blood count with platelet count
- Pregnancy test
- Sexually transmitted infection screening
- Thyroid function tests
- Remainder of workup guided by history and physical examination to rule out other suspected causes. Examples include:
    - Pelvic ultrasound to rule out a structural abnormality or confirm pregnancy
    - Coagulopathy workup based upon clinical history or suspicion
    - Antinuclear antibody (ANA) to rule out autoimmune disease
    - Erythrocyte sedimentation rate (ESR) to investigate inflammatory process
    - Androgen and 17-hydroxyprogesterone (17-OHP) to investigate late-onset CAH and PCOS

IMAGING STUDIES

- Pelvic ultrasound as needed to rule out structural abnormality or confirm pregnancy

TREATMENT

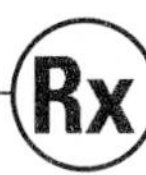

NONPHARMACOLOGIC THERAPY

- Menstrual calendar (days of bleeding and spotting)

ACUTE GENERAL Rx

- Guided by hemoglobin and hematocrit and presence of active bleeding
- Hemoglobin 12 mg/dL or greater
    - Menstrual calendar
    - Iron supplementation
    - Reassurance
    - Re-evaluation in 3 to 6 months
    - Consider nonsteroidal anti-inflammatory drugs (NSAIDs) which may decrease bleeding
    - If irregular menses are bothersome to the patient, consider once-daily monophasic intermediate-dose (30 to 35 μg ethinyl estradiol) combined OCP. Estrogen provides hemostasis and progesterone provides endometrial stabilization.
- Hemoglobin 10 to 12 mg/dL
    - Menstrual calendar
    - Iron supplementation
    - Consider addition of NSAID
    - Hormonal therapy
        - Once-daily monophasic intermediate-dose combined OCP
        - If unable or unwilling to take OCPs or not sexually active, cyclic progesterone may be used starting on the first calendar day or the 14th day of the menstrual cycle.

    - Medroxyprogesterone acetate 10 mg for 10 to 14 days every month for 3 to 6 cycles, or norethindrone acetate 2.5 to 10 mg daily for 10 to 14 days every month for 3 to 6 cycles
  - Re-evaluation in 3 months with continued, regular follow-up
- Hemoglobin less than 10 mg/dL; patient asymptomatic with no active bleeding
  - Menstrual calendar
  - Iron supplementation
  - Hormonal therapy (as above)
  - Frequent follow-up until hemoglobin and hematocrit normalize, then every 3 to 6 months
- Hemoglobin less than 10 mg/dL; patient symptomatic (orthostatic, fatigue, syncopal, dizzy, or light-headed) or actively bleeding
  - Hospital/Emergency room evaluation
  - Fluids
  - Intravenous estrogen (see below)
  - Blood transfusion (rarely necessary)
  - Hormonal therapy: acute treatment (either oral or intravenous)
    - Oral: intermediate- or high-dose monophasic combined OCP and antiemetic
      - One 30 to 50 μg ethinyl estradiol combined OCP every 4 hours until bleeding slows or stops, then taper to one pill four times a day for 2 to 4 days, then 3 times a day for 3 days, then twice a day for 2 weeks
    - Following acute management, a once-daily monophasic intermediate-dose combined OCP for 3 to 6 months until the hematocrit is increased. If the patient is very anemic, avoid the withdrawal (placebo) week by continuous use of the oral contraceptive.
    - Intravenous: conjugated estrogen if unable to tolerate oral medication; give with an antiemetic
      - Give 25 mg conjugated estrogen intravenously every 4 hours for two to three doses until bleeding stops.
      - To stabilize the endometrium, add an oral progesterone for 5 to 7 days. A progesterone withdrawal bleed is expected. Alternatively, a combined OCP may be initiated within 24 to 48 hours after intravenous conjugated estrogen.
  - Hormonal therapy: maintenance
    - Once-daily monophasic intermediate-dose combined OCP should be continued daily for 3 to 6 months. Cyclic medroxyprogesterone for 3 to 6 months may also be given, but is less effective.
    - If the patient is unable or unwilling to take OCPs or medroxyprogesterone, and iron stores are normal, therapy may be discontinued and the patient's menstrual calendar followed.
    - If the patient has more than 6 weeks without menses, give oral medroxyprogesterone acetate 10 mg daily for 10 to 14 days to induce a withdrawal bleed (consider a pregnancy test as well).
  - Iron supplementation
  - Frequent follow-up
  - Imaging and surgery may be necessary when hemostasis cannot be achieved medically. Obstetric/gynecologic consultation is mandatory.

CHRONIC Rx

- Treatment of underlying cause of abnormal uterine bleeding
- Prevention of endometrial hyperplasia and endometrial stabilization with combined OCPs

DISPOSITION

See individual treatment plans above.

REFERRAL

- Obstetrician/gynecologist consult for patients with hemoglobin level of 10 mg/dL who are symptomatic or for further management of persistent or symptomatic DUB
- Hematology consult if coagulopathy is suspected

PEARLS & CONSIDERATIONS

COMMENTS

- DUB is a diagnosis of exclusion.
- Vaginal bleeding in a premenarchal girl is abnormal (outside the physiologic, self-limited withdrawal bleeding in some female newborns) and warrants further investigation.
- The longer the period of anovulation for an adolescent, the higher the risk for DUB.
- Patients with a long history of anovulatory cycles and dysfunctional uterine bleeding have an increased risk of later infertility and endometrial carcinoma.
- Patient estimations of menstrual flow tend to be inaccurate.

PREVENTION

- Treatment of underlying cause of abnormal uterine bleeding
- Prevention of endometrial hyperplasia and endometrial stabilization with combined OCPs

PATIENT/FAMILY EDUCATION

- Explain cause of DUB.
- Adolescents have more variation in menstrual cycle length, with normal menstrual bleeding from 2 to 7 days in 80% to 90% of adolescent girls and normal blood loss less than 80 mL (average 30 to 40 mL).
- The interval between menarche and regular, ovulatory periods is associated with age at menarche:
  - Younger than 12 years at menarche: 50% of menstrual cycles will be ovulatory by 1 year.
  - Between 12 and 13 years: 50% of menstrual cycles will be ovulatory by 3 years.
  - Older than 13 years: 50% of menstrual cycles will be ovulatory by 4.5 years.
- Most adolescents respond well to treatment, with half of patients having regular menstrual patterns within 4 years of menarche.

SUGGESTED READINGS

Emans SJ: Dysfunctional uterine bleeding. *In* Emans SJ et al: *Pediatric & Adolescent Gynecology,* 5th ed. Philadelphia, Lippincott Williams & Wilkins, 2005, pp 270–286.

Hillard PJ: Menstruation in young girls: A clinical perspective. *Obstet Gynecol* 99:655, 2002.

London SN: Abnormal uterine bleeding. *In* Scott JR et al (eds): *Danforth's Obstetrics and Gynecology.* Philadelphia, Lippincott Williams & Wilkins, 2003, pp 643–651.

Mitan LA, Slap GB: Dysfunctional uterine bleeding. *In* Neinstein LS (ed): *Adolescent Health Care: A Practical Guide.* Philadelphia, Lippincott Williams & Wilkins, 2002, pp 966–972.

AUTHOR: **PONRAT PAKPREO, MD**

BASIC INFORMATION

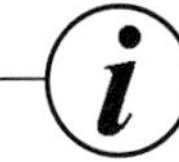

DEFINITION

Primary dysmenorrhea is pain with menses in the absence of a secondary cause. Secondary dysmenorrhea is pain with menses that is secondary to other pelvic disease.

SYNONYM

Menstrual cramps

ICD-9-CM CODES
306.52 Psychogenic dysmenorrhea
625.3 Dysmenorrhea

EPIDEMIOLOGY & DEMOGRAPHICS

- Primary dysmenorrhea occurs in 50% to 80% of menstruating females.
- Prevalence in adolescent girls ranges from 20% to 90%.
- Prevalence is higher with increasing Tanner stage and increasing age, until 20 years.
- Onset of symptoms occurs within 6 months to 2 years of menarche.
- Secondary dysmenorrhea occurs later in the reproductive years of women and it is associated with other pathologic conditions.

CLINICAL PRESENTATION

History

- The most common symptom is crampy lower abdominal pain that may radiate to the back and thighs and that ensues with the onset of menses.
- Other symptoms include dizziness, nausea, vomiting, diarrhea, fatigue, and headache.
- Obtain a careful menstrual history to characterize symptoms.
  - Onset and frequency of menses
  - Length and quality of flow
  - Timing of symptoms with respect to cycle
  - Degree of impairment of daily activities (absenteeism from school or work)

Physical Examination

- The physical examination is tailored to identify causes of secondary dysmenorrhea.
  - In absence of physical findings, a diagnosis of primary dysmenorrhea may be made with a consistent history.
- For sexually active adolescents and adolescents 18 years or older, a pelvic examination with speculum is indicated.
- Evaluate for sexually transmitted diseases (*Chlamydia,* gonorrhea, pelvic inflammatory disease [PID]).
- Assess the anatomy of the external and internal genitalia.
- Bimanual examination is indicated to evaluate for the following:
  - Uterine anomalies
  - Size and quality of adnexa
  - Specific areas of tenderness
- In the adolescent who is younger than 18 years and not sexually active, the history is sufficient to try therapy.
- If the patient is unresponsive to therapy, an external genital examination with rectoabdominal bimanual examination should be performed.
  - Palpate the uterus and adnexa to evaluate for tenderness, masses, and congenital anomalies.

ETIOLOGY

- There is an association of increased prostaglandin F_2 (PGF_2) and E_2 (PGE_2) levels with symptoms of dysmenorrhea.
- Under the influence of progesterone, PGE_2 and PGF_2 are produced and act locally to cause increased myometrial tone and contractions, vasoconstriction, and then ischemia of the uterine lining.
- PGE_2 also causes hypersensitivity of pain nerve terminals in the myometrium.

DIAGNOSIS

DIFFERENTIAL DIAGNOSIS

- Sexually transmitted diseases (*Chlamydia,* gonorrhea, PID)
- Endometriosis
- Genital tract cysts and neoplasms
- Pelvic adhesions
- Obstructing malformations of the uterus or vagina
- Complications of pregnancy
- Intrauterine device

LABORATORY TESTS

- Erythrocyte sedimentation rate to evaluate for malignancy or PID.
- Cervical cultures to rule out infection.

IMAGING STUDIES

Endovaginal or transabdominal ultrasonography or magnetic resonance imaging is indicated if the history is atypical and further evaluation of anatomic structures is indicated.

TREATMENT

NONPHARMACOLOGIC THERAPY

- Education and reassurance
- Well-balanced diet

Surgical

- Laparoscopy or laparotomy is indicated either when pain persists despite interventions or when the history suggests the need for further evaluation of pelvic anatomy

ACUTE GENERAL Rx

- Nonsteroidal anti-inflammatory drugs (NSAIDs) are used at the onset of menses and continued for the first 1 to 2 days of the cycle or for duration of cramps. They inhibit the conversion of arachidonic acid to prostaglandins via the enzyme cyclooxygenase, thereby preventing the production of PGF_2 and PGE_2.
  - Ibuprofen 400 mg orally three to four times per day
  - Naproxen 500 mg orally, then 250 mg orally every 12 hours
  - Naproxen sodium 550 mg orally, then 275 mg orally every 12 hours
  - Mefenamic acid 500 mg orally, then 250 mg orally every 4 to 6 hours

CHRONIC Rx

- Oral contraceptives if NSAID regimen is insufficient to control symptoms.
- Depomedroxyprogesterone acetate or implantable levonorgestrel if oral contraceptives are unrealistic.
- Calcium channel blockers have been tried with some success.

DISPOSITION

- Primary dysmenorrhea: Follow-up after another menstrual cycle has passed to see how effective intervention has been.
- Secondary dysmenorrhea: Follow-up is indicated based on the nature of the primary diagnosis.

REFERRAL

For patients who are unresponsive to standard approaches, referral to a gynecologist who is familiar with the comprehensive evaluation and treatment of pelvic pain is indicated.

PEARLS & CONSIDERATIONS

COMMENTS

- A monthly pain calendar may identify the cyclic and recurrent nature of pain.
- Well-documented menstrual history is important for diagnosis and management.

PREVENTION

Omega-3-fatty acids, which are found in fish oil supplements (1080 mg eicosapentaenoic acid, 720 mg docosapentaenoic acid, 1.5 mg of vitamin E) should be administered in two divided doses per day. Taken daily, this diminishes symptoms compared to placebo.

PATIENT/FAMILY EDUCATION

- NSAIDs should be started at initiation of pain, before it becomes severe.
- NSAIDs are often associated with decreased menstrual flow.
- The benefits of oral contraceptives may not be noticed for two to three cycles.

SUGGESTED READINGS

Braverman PK, Neinstein L: Dysmenorrhea and premenstrual syndrome. *In* Neinstein LS (ed): *Adolescent Health Care: A Practical Guide.* Philadelphia, Williams & Wilkins, 2002, pp 952–965.

Dysmenorrhea. Available at www.emedicine.com/emerg/topic156.htm

Laugher M, Goldstein D: Dysmenorrhea, pelvic pain, premenstrual syndrome. *In* Emans SJH et al (eds): *Pediatric and Adolescent Gynecology.* Philadelphia, Lippincott Williams, & Wilkins, 2005.

AUTHOR: **CAROLYN JACOBS PARKS, MD**

BASIC INFORMATION

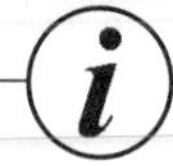

DEFINITION

An ectopic pregnancy is a fertilized ovum implanted anywhere other that the endometrial lining of the uterine cavity. Implantation usually occurs in the fallopian tubes.

SYNONYM

Tubal pregnancy

ICD-9-CM CODE

633.9 Ectopic pregnancy

EPIDEMIOLOGY & DEMOGRAPHICS

- Incidence: 19 cases per 1000 pregnancies
- Fatality rate: 4 cases per 10,000 ectopic pregnancies
- Ruptured ectopic is leading cause of maternal death, accounts for 10% to 15% of maternal deaths.
- Sites of ectopic pregnancies
  - Tubal: less than 95%
  - Cornual, interstitial: 2%
  - Ovarian: 1 case per 7000 pregnancies
  - Cervical: 1 case per 9000 pregnancies
  - Abdominal: 1 case per 5000 pregnancies
- Risk factors
  - History of an ectopic pregnancy; recurring ectopic pregnancy in 15% to 25% of presentations
  - History of pelvic infections: *Chlamydia*, gonorrhea, pelvic inflammatory disease (PID), or nonspecific salpingitis
  - Tubal surgery
  - Tubal ligation: increased risk of pregnancy during the first 2 years after sterilization
  - Abdominal surgery
  - Use of intrauterine device (IUD)
  - Infertility
  - Cigarette smoking: increases risk almost twofold
  - Diethylstilbestrol (DES) exposure: increases risk more than twofold
  - Increasing maternal age

CLINICAL PRESENTATION

- Often symptomatic
- Lower abdominal pain
- Absent or irregular bleeding
  - Vaginal bleeding in 80% of patients
  - Presentation usually between 6 to 10 weeks after last menstrual period (LMP)
- Shoulder pain
- Dizziness, syncope, shock
- Urge to defecate
- Breast tenderness
- Nausea

ETIOLOGY

- Tubal damage from inflammation
- Contraception: IUD, progesterone therapies
- Prior tubal or abdominal surgeries, including tubal ligation
- Advanced reproductive technologies (interfere with embryo migration)
- Developmental abnormalities: DES exposure

DIAGNOSIS

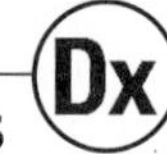

DIFFERENTIAL DIAGNOSIS

- Normal uterine pregnancy
- Abortion
- Rupture, torsion, or bleeding from an ovarian cyst
- Appendicitis
- PID
- Urinary tract infection or calculi
- Diverticulitis
- Degenerating uterine leiomyoma
- Endometriosis
- Dysfunctional uterine bleeding

WORKUP

- The diagnosis is complicated by the wide spectrum of patient presentations, ranging from vaginal spotting to shock.
- Major advances in early detection include β-human chorionic gonadotropin (β-hCG), ultrasound, and laparoscopy.
- Culdocentesis and curettage can be useful but are second-line approaches compared with β-hCG and ultrasound.
  - Culdocentesis confirms the presence of intra-abdominal bleeding.
  - Dilation of the cervical os and curettage of the endometrial lining can be used to establish the diagnosis of ectopic pregnancy if no chorionic villi are found. If decidua without chorionic villi is found, it may indicate an ectopic pregnancy. A completed spontaneous abortion may also have decidua only.

LABORATORY TESTS

- β-hCG determination
  - An abnormal pregnancy is identified by the level of β-hCG not doubling in 48 hours; a 66% rise in the β-hCG level over 48 hours represents the lower limit of normal for a viable intrauterine pregnancy (IUP).
  - Fifteen percent of viable IUPs have a less than 66% increase in β-hGC in 48 hours.
  - Fifteen percent of ectopic pregnancies do have more than a 66% increase in β-hCG.
  - The β-hCG determination is best used early in pregnancy; it is less reliable after 6 to 7 weeks.
  - The β-hCG level alone does not help distinguish between an ectopic and an abnormal uterine pregnancy.
- The progesterone level is another diagnostic tool and an adjunct to β-hCG and ultrasound.
  - The progesterone level cannot necessarily distinguish an IUP from a spontaneous abortion (SAB) or an ectopic pregnancy.
  - A level less than 5 ng/mL indicates a nonviable pregnancy.
  - A level greater than 25 ng/ml indicates a normal pregnancy.
  - A level between 10 and 20 ng/mL is not diagnostic.

IMAGING STUDIES

- Ultrasound detects an IUP within 5 to 6 weeks of the LMP.
- An IUP can be visualized by transabdominal ultrasound at a β-hCG level above 6500 mIU/mL and by transvaginal ultrasound at levels above 1000 to 2000 mIU/mL.

TREATMENT

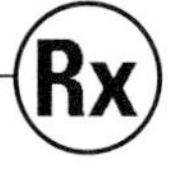

NONPHARMACOLOGIC THERAPY

- Less than 25% of ectopic pregnancies resolve without treatment.
- Expectant management is restricted to the following:
  - Falling β-hCG titers
  - Ectopic pregnancy in the fallopian tube, not the cervix, abdomen, or ovary
  - No bleeding
  - No evidence of rupture

ACUTE GENERAL Rx

- Methotrexate (MTX), a folic acid antagonist, is used, with a success rate between 67% and 100%.
- MTX is used for small, unruptured ectopic pregnancies.
  - It inhibits dihydrofolic acid reductase and interrupts DNA synthesis.
  - A complete blood cell count and platelet count, liver function test, and levels of creatinine and β-hCG are obtained on day zero as a baseline.
  - Intramuscular MTX (50 mg/m^2) is given.
  - RhoGAM is given to Rh-negative women.
  - The β-hCG determination is repeated on days 4 and 7.
  - If there is less than a 15% decrease from day 4 to 7, a second dose of MTX (50 mg/m^2) is given.
  - If there is more than a 15% decrease, continue monitoring the β-hCG level every 3 to 4 days.
- Fifty percent of patients have abdominal pain with treatment.
- Evaluate for a ruptured ectopic pregnancy if the patient has abdominal pain.
- Patients are eligible for medical treatment if the following criteria are met:
  - Hemodynamically stable
  - Agree to close outpatient follow-up
  - Have a small, unruptured ectopic pregnancy (presence of a fetal heart is not a definitive exclusion criteria)
  - Level of β-hCG is not decreasing 12 to 24 hours after curettage
  - No evidence of liver or renal disease (levels of transaminases less than twice normal and creatinine less than 1.5 mg/dL)

- Contraindications to MTX: breastfeeding, liver disease, overt immunodeficiency, significant anemia, and peptic ulcer disease

CHRONIC Rx

- For tubal pregnancy
  - Laparoscopic salpingostomy or salpingectomy is done.
  - Laparotomy may be necessary.
- For ovarian ectopics
  - A wedge resection is indicated.
  - Removal of the entire ovary may be unavoidable.
- For cervical ectopic pregnancies, the management is controversial.
  - Dilation plus curettage is contraindicated.
  - MTX can be given systemically or locally.
  - Uterine artery embolization is often successful and useful for management of hemorrhage.
  - Hysterectomy is often indicated.

REFERRAL

All patients with a suspected ectopic pregnancy should be referred to an obstetrician or gynecologist emergently.

PEARLS & CONSIDERATIONS

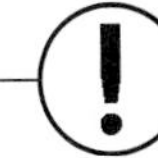

COMMENTS

- In general, a complete abortion has a rapidly falling β-hCG level, usually about 50% over 48 hours.
- The β-hCG levels during an ectopic pregnancy rise or plateau.
  - Most ectopic pregnancies have β-hCG levels of less than 6500 mIU/mL.
  - In IUPs, the β-hCG level is approximately 100 mIU/mL at the time of a missed menses, and it peaks at 100,000 mIU/mL at 10 weeks.
- When waiting for the 48 hours between β-hCG levels to determine the status of the pregnancy, the patient should be given information regarding possible ectopic rupture and spontaneous abortion precautions. Reasons to seek urgent care include the following:
  - Increasing abdominal pain
  - Dizziness or light-headedness
  - Shoulder pain
  - Increasing vaginal bleeding
- If MTX is given, the patient should stop prenatal vitamins, decrease foods high in folic acid, and abstain from alcohol.

PREVENTION

- Avoid conditions that scar the fallopian tubes.
- Provide early treatment for sexually transmitted diseases.
- Avoid risk factors for sexually transmitted diseases.
  - Multiple partners
  - Intercourse without a condom

PATIENT/FAMILY EDUCATION

Support groups are available: www.Ectopic.org

SUGGESTED READINGS

ACOG Practice Bullet in: Medical management of tubal pregnancy, No.3. *Int J Gynaecol Obstet* 65:97, 1999.

Rock J, Damario M: Ectopic Pregnancy. *In* The Linde RW, Thompson JD (eds): Te Lindes operative gynecology, 9th ed. Philadelphia, Lippincott Williams & Wilkins, 2003.

Stenchever M: Ectopic Pregnancy. *In* William Droegemuller: *Comprehensive Gynecology*, 4th ed. St Louis, Mosby, 2001.

AUTHOR: **ELIZABETH K. CHEROT, MD**

BASIC INFORMATION

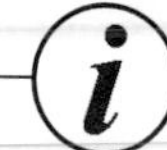

DEFINITION

Human granulocytic ehrlichiosis (HGE) is an acute, febrile, nonspecific illness occurring through the bite of *Ixodes* ticks, which can result in hospitalization and death, particularly in the elderly.

ICD-9-CM CODE
288.0 Human granulocytic ehrlichiosis (HGE)

EPIDEMIOLOGY & DEMOGRAPHICS

- Transmitted by a tick vector, predominantly *Ixodes scapularis* (dammini), in the northeastern and southeastern United States and *Ixodes pacificus* in western states.
- Peak incidence is from May to July but occurs year-round.
- The incubation period is 5 to 10 days after a tick bite.
- Approximately 75% of cases occur in the upper midwestern and northeastern United States.
- Most cases are sporadic.
- Perinatal transmission has been documented.

CLINICAL PRESENTATION

History

- The patient may report history of tick bite or potential tick exposure.
- Abrupt onset of fever (often higher than 39°C) is accompanied by headache, malaise, and myalgia.
- Nausea, vomiting, and anorexia are common.
- Less common are diarrhea, cough, and abdominal pain.

Physical Examination

- Fever
- Rash in less than 10% of patients
  - Is pleomorphic, variable in appearance, and commonly involves the trunk
  - Spares the hands and feet
  - Is more common in pediatric patients
- Central nervous system: photophobia, lethargy, confusion

ETIOLOGY

- "Agent of HGE" is a still unnamed *Ehrlichia* species related to *E. phagocytophila* and *E. equi.*
- Genus *Ehrlichia* consists of small, gram-negative, obligate intracellular organisms within the rickettsial family.
- Organisms form microcolonies of elementary bodies (morulae) within the leukocyte, which rupture into the circulation to infect other leukocytes.

DIAGNOSIS

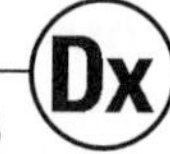

DIFFERENTIAL DIAGNOSIS

- Extensive and varies according to organ systems most affected
- Other tick-borne diseases: Rocky Mountain spotted fever, babesiosis, Lyme disease
- Human monocytic ehrlichiosis
- Viral hepatitis
- Epstein-Barr virus
- Tularemia
- Murine typhus
- Leptospirosis
- Viral meningitis
- Gastroenteritis

LABORATORY TESTS

- Complete blood count (CBC)
  - Leukopenia and thrombocytopenia (70% to 80%)
  - Mild anemia (50%)
- Mildly elevated erythrocyte sedimentation rate and lactic dehydrogenase
- Elevated hepatic transaminases
- Cerebral spinal fluid: lymphocytic or neutrophilic pleocytosis
- Blood smears: examination of peripheral blood smears for morulae; insensitive
- Fourfold change in antibody titer between acute and convalescent sera, obtained 3 to 6 weeks apart. Obtained via indirect immunofluorescent antibody detection using *E. equi* antigen.
- Polymerase chain reaction: sensitive and facilitates early confirmation of acute illness, but not yet widely available for clinical purposes

TREATMENT

NONPHARMACOLOGIC THERAPY

Supportive care and adequate hydration should be maintained.

ACUTE GENERAL Rx

- Doxycycline is the drug of choice.
  - 4 mg/kg/day in two divided doses (maximum, 100 mg)
  - Continue for 3 days after defervescence, with a 5- to 7-day minimum duration of therapy.
- Doxycycline is even recommended for children less than 9 years old due to the potentially life-threatening nature of the illness.
- Rifampin has been used in pregnancy.
- Parenteral nutrition may be necessary.
- Pain management should be initiated as needed.

DISPOSITION

- Repeat CBC to make sure values are normalizing.
- Obtain convalescent antibody titers approximately 3 to 6 weeks after acute illness.

REFERRAL

Infectious disease specialist may be helpful as the diagnosis is difficult to confirm.

PEARLS & CONSIDERATIONS

COMMENTS

- Tick should be saved for county health department for appropriate identification.
- Very little is known about this disease in children; most information is based on adult patients who required hospitalization.

PREVENTION

- Prevention is directed primarily at minimizing the risk of tick bites.
- Preventive clothing includes long pants tucked into socks, long sleeves, and shoes (not sandals).
- Insect repellents containing N,N diethyl-m-toluamide (DEET) and permethrin are available as a repellent for shoes and clothes and should not be applied to skin.

PATIENT/FAMILY EDUCATION

- The mean duration of illness is 3 weeks; recovery without sequelae usually occurs.
- Inform parents of strategies for preventing tick bites.

SUGGESTED READINGS

American Academy of Pediatrics: Human granulocytic ehrlichiosis. *In* Pickering LK (ed): *2003 Red Book: Report of the Committee on Infectious Diseases,* 26th ed. Elk Grove Village, IL, American Academy of Pediatrics, 2003.

Centers for Disease Control and Prevention. Available at www.cdc.gov

Fritz CL, Glaser CA: Ehrlichiosis. *Infect Dis Clin North Am* 12:123, 1998.

Horowitz HW et al: Perinatal transmission of the agent of human granulocytic ehrlichiosis. *N Engl J Med* 339:375, 1998.

Jacobs RF, Schutze GE: Ehrlichiosis in children. *J Pediatr* 131:184, 1997.

AUTHOR: **KRISTEN SMITH DANIELSON, MD**

BASIC INFORMATION

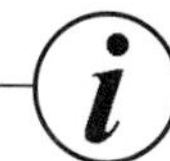

DEFINITION

Acute viral encephalitis is a virally induced inflammation of the brain parenchyma that develops over a period of hours to days. It is often accompanied by changes in the meninges as well, leading to meningoencephalitis.

SYNONYM

Acute viral meningoencephalitis

ICD-9-CM CODES

049.0 Lymphocytic meningoencephalitis
049.8 Epidemic encephalitis
049.9 Viral encephalitis NOS
054.3 Herpes encephalitis
055.0 Post-measles encephalitis
056.01 Progressive rubella panencephalitis
062 Mosquito-borne viral encephalitis
062.0 Japanese B encephalitis
062.1 Western equine encephalitis
062.2 Eastern equine encephalitis
062.3 St. Louis encephalitis
062.5 California encephalitis
062.5 La Crosse encephalitis
062.8 Other mosquito-borne viral encephalitis
062.9 Mosquito-borne viral encephalitis NOS
064 Arbovirus encephalitis NOS
066.2 Venezuelan equine encephalitis
066.41 West Nile fever with encephalitis
072.2 Mumps encephalitis

EPIDEMIOLOGY & DEMOGRAPHICS

- Neonates have the highest incidence, about 17 cases/100,000 population
  - HSV
    - HSV encephalitis most common in second week of life
    - Less than half of the mothers of infected neonates have no history of lesions
    - Highest risk when delivered during primary outbreak in mother
  - Enterovirus can be severe disease accompanied by sepsis and liver failure
- Children/adolescents have lower incidence, about 0.5 cases/100,000 population
  - Human transmission
    - Acute
    - Enterovirus family tends to occur in epidemics, summer
    - Adenovirus is epidemic
    - Epstein-Barr virus (EBV), cytomegalovirus (CMV)—sporadic cases throughout the year
    - HSV is most common cause of sporadic disease in developed world. Can be prevented with vaccine.
    - Measles, mumps, influenza, polio, varicella—highest risk when unvaccinated
    - Japanese encephalitis B is most common epidemic cause outside United States
    - Reactivation of latent virus
    - HSV types 1 and 2—prior history of oral or facial herpes
    - Human herpes virus 6 (HHV6)—almost all children between 6 to 18 months of age get primary infection
  - Zoonotic
    - Lymphocytic choriomeningitis virus—rodents
    - Rabies—bats, skunks, carnivorous mammals; rodents unlikely
  - Arthropod-borne
    - Mosquitoes—Japanese B, West Nile, La Crosse, St. Louis, eastern/western/Venezuelan equine
    - Tick-borne—Colorado tick fever virus
    - Most common in summer, fall

CLINICAL PRESENTATION

- Alteration of mental status is universal in all forms.
  - Infants—poor feeding, lethargy or irritability, seizures
  - Children—lethargy, pseudo-psychosis, complex partial seizures, tonic-clonic seizures, emotional lability, stupor, coma
- Neurologic findings are variable.
  - Headaches
  - Seizures
  - Cranial nerve palsies
  - Flaccid paralysis
  - Ataxia/movement disorders
- Fever is almost universal. It differentiates from toxic/metabolic causes.
- Meningitis can occur with encephalitis.
  - Headache, stiff neck, photophobia
- Rash
  - Vesicles—HSV, varicella, Enterovirus family
  - Macular/maculopapular—measles, West Nile virus, HHV6, Enterovirus family
- Lymphadenopathy
  - West Nile virus, EBV, CMV
- Travel
  - Japanese encephalitis—epidemic
  - Rabies, Nipah virus—animal-associated
- Animal contact
  - Bats—rabies
  - Rodents—lymphocytic choriomeningitis virus

ETIOLOGY

- Common viral causes of acute encephalitis include:
  - Herpesviridae: HSV1, HSV2, varicella zoster virus (VZV), EBV, CMV, HHV6
  - Arboviruses: Japanese B, West Nile, St. Louis, eastern/western/Venezuelan equine, LaCrosse/California
  - Others:
    - Enterovirus (71), poliovirus
    - Colorado tick fever virus
    - Human immunodeficiency virus
    - Measles, mumps, rubella
    - Influenza A, adenovirus
    - Lymphocytic choriomeningitis virus
    - Rabies, Nipah virus
  - Postinfectious encephalitis
    - Occurs acutely 1 or more weeks after viral infection
      - VZV, measles, mumps, rubella, influenza are most common triggers

DIAGNOSIS

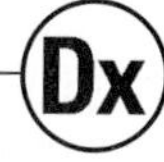

DIFFERENTIAL DIAGNOSIS

- Metabolic diseases: hypoglycemia, uremia, hepatic failure
- Toxic disorders: drug ingestion, Reye's syndrome
- Central nervous system mass lesions: tumor and abscess
- Intracerebral or subarachnoid hemorrhage
- Demyelinating disorders: multiple sclerosis
- Seizure conditions: postictal, nonconvulsive seizure
- Psychiatric illness: schizophrenia
- Bacterial infections: meningitis, abscess, tuberculosis

LABORATORY TESTS

- Cerebrospinal fluid (CSF) analysis if no mass or no increased intracranial pressure or no thrombocytopenia
  - Routine analysis: cell count, differential, protein, glucose, culture, AFB stain, tuberulosis culture, opening pressure
    - Expect lymphocytic pleocytosis, elevated protein, normal glucose
    - Xanthochromic fluid and red cells in HSV
  - Viral culture—HSV, CMV, measles, enterovirus may grow
  - Polymerase chain reaction (PCR) to detect viral nucleic acids
    - Most sensitive test for HSV
    - May be available for enterovirus, EBV, CMV, West Nile, others
  - Antibody testing often used for arboviruses
- Serology—acute and convalescent titers for suspected etiologies
- Viral cultures—consider nasopharynx, rectal, and/or skin lesion swabs
- EEG
  - May show seizures, global slowing
  - Periodic lateralized epileptiform discharges (PLEDs)
    - Seen in temporal region with HSV
    - Neonates with more diffuse disease
- CBC—frequently shows leukocytosis
  - Leukopenia or lymphopenia seen with West Nile Virus
  - Atypical lymphocytes seen in EBV infections

IMAGING STUDIES

- Computed tomography (CT scan) is used to quickly rule out hemorrhage, mass, elevated intracranial pressure.
- Magnetic resonance imaging (MRI) is most sensitive for early changes in encephalitis.
  - Diffuse hyperintensity on T2
  - Temporal involvement with HSV in children and adults

TREATMENT

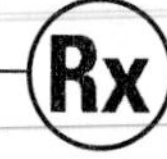

ACUTE GENERAL Rx

- Acyclovir for any case that could be HSV
  - 60 mg/kg/day, divided every 8 hours intravenously for neonatal disease
  - 30 mg/kg/day, divided every 8 hours intravenously for older children and adolescents
- No specific antiviral therapy for most other causes
- Anticonvulsant medications
- May need to treat other etiologies until they are ruled out (i.e., bacterial meningitis)

CHRONIC Rx

Suppressive acyclovir therapy for neonatal herpes disease is being studied but is associated with neutropenia.

DISPOSITION

- Often need neurologic rehabilitation but outcome varies widely based on agent involved
- Neurodevelopmental follow-up
- Hearing screening

REFERRAL

- Neurology
- Infectious diseases
- Rehabilitation medicine

PEARLS & CONSIDERATIONS

COMMENTS

Even without a bite, any bat exposure to a young child should be considered for rabies prophylaxis.

PREVENTION

- Arthropod-borne disease: use N,N diethyl-m-toluamide (DEET) and permethrin as insect repellents.
- The following are preventable with vaccine: influenza, Japanese B, measles, mumps, rubella, varicella, rabies.

PATIENT/FAMILY EDUCATION

For information on enterovirus infections:
Centers for Disease Control (CDC) National Center for Infectious Diseases, Respiratory and Enteric Viruses Branch. Web site: www.cdc.gov/ncidod/dvrd/revb/index.htm

For information on West Nile Virus and other types of arboviral encephalitis:
Centers for Disease Control (CDC) Division of Vector-Borne Infectious Diseases. Web site: www.cdc.gov/ncidod/dvbid/arbor/index.htm

SUGGESTED READINGS

Centers for Disease Control (CDC) Division of Vector-Borne Infectious Diseases. Available at www.cdc.gov/ncidod/dvbid/arbor/index.htm

Kimberlin DW et al: Natural history of neonatal herpes simplex virus infections in the acyclovir era. *Pediatrics* 108:223, 2001.

Petersen LR, Marfin AA: West Nile virus: a primer for the clinician. *Ann Intern Med* 137:173, 2002.

AUTHOR: **CHRISTOPHER E. BELCHER, MD, FAAP**

BASIC INFORMATION

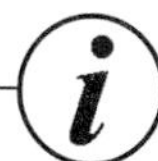

DEFINITION

Infective endocarditis (IE) is an intravascular infection of the endocardium, including valvular structures, or an infection of the endothelium of large blood vessels (endarteritis).

SYNONYMS

Acute bacterial endocarditis
Bacterial endocarditis
Subacute bacterial endocarditis

ICD-9-CM CODE

421.0 Infective endocarditis

EPIDEMIOLOGY & DEMOGRAPHICS

- *Staphylococcus aureus* and *Streptococcus* species are the most common pathogens.
- Other infective organisms include *Staphylococcus epidermidis,* enterococci, *Candida,* HACEK bacteria (***H**aemophilus parainfluenzae, aphrophilus, and paraphrophilus;* ***A**ctinobacillus;* ***C**ardiobacterium;* ***E**ikenella;* and ***K**ingella), Coxiella,* and *Brucella.*
- Culture-negative endocarditis occurs in 5% to 7% of patients, related to prior antibiotic therapy or fastidious and slow-growing organisms.
- In newborn infants, *S. aureus,* coagulase-negative staphylococci and *Candida* are the most common etiologies.
- Pediatric hospital admissions for IE have declined recently.
- Substrates:
  - Most common
    - Prosthetic cardiac valves and conduits
    - Repaired or palliated complex cyanotic congenital cardiac malformations
    - Systemic-to-pulmonary artery shunts
  - Less common
    - Unrepaired congenital malformations
    - Mitral valve prolapse
    - Rarely rheumatic heart disease
- In infancy and in immunocompromised patients, venous catheters are a common predisposing factor.
- Minimal to no risk is present in patients with an atrial septal defect or mild pulmonary valve stenosis.

CLINICAL PRESENTATION

History

- Underlying congenital or acquired cardiovascular lesion or surgery with a predisposition to the formation of a nonbacterial thrombotic vegetation
- Central venous catheter
- Recent procedure or infection associated with bacteremia
- Fever
- Malaise, weakness, fatigue, poor appetite, weight loss, night sweats, rigors, arthralgias, and myalgias
- Insidious or rapidly progressive onset

Physical Examination

- Fever: 95% or more
- Splenomegaly: 50%
- Congestive heart failure: 30% to 40%
- Petechiae: 10% to 25%
- Splinter hemorrhages: 10%
- Osler's nodes, Janeway lesions: less than 5%
- Roth spots: very rare
- Major systemic emboli: 15% to 25%
- New or changed murmur: incidence difficult to define
  - New aortic or mitral insufficiency is significant.
  - Louder preexisting murmur is not sufficient.

ETIOLOGY

- Endocardial or endothelial injury is caused by the following:
  - A jet lesion from a ventricular septal defect, valvular insufficiency, systemic-to-pulmonary artery shunt, valvular or vascular stenosis
    - Fifty percent of IE occurs in children after cardiac surgery.
  - An intravascular catheter (8% to 10%, especially in neonates)
- These injuries lead to platelet and fibrin deposition to form a nonbacterial thrombotic vegetation (NBTV).
- Circulating microorganisms then adhere to the NBTV, initiating IE and propagation of the vegetation, followed by local invasive damage and distal embolic events.

DIAGNOSIS

DIFFERENTIAL DIAGNOSIS

- Acute rheumatic fever
- Rheumatoid diseases
- Collagen vascular disease
- Kawasaki disease
- Sepsis or other infections
- Cardiac myxoma

LABORATORY TESTS

- Blood cultures, three or more (prior antibiotic therapy reduces the recovery rate of bacteria by 35% to 40%)
- Electrocardiogram
- Complete blood count, sedimentation rate, circulating immune complexes
- Urinalysis
- Duke clinical criteria
  - Definite IE
    - Pathologic criteria:
      - Microorganisms: demonstrated by culture or histology in a vegetation or in a vegetation that has embolized, or in an intracardiac abscess *or*
      - Pathologic lesions: vegetations or intracardiac abscess present, confirmed by histology showing active endocarditis
    - Clinical criteria using the following definitions:
      - Two major criteria, *or*
      - One major criterion and three minor criteria, *or*
      - Five minor criteria
  - Possible IE
    - Findings consistent with IE that fall short of "definite" but not "rejected"
  - Rejected
    - Firm alternative diagnosis for manifestations of endocarditis, *or*
    - Resolution of manifestations of endocarditis with antibiotic therapy for 4 days or less, *or*
    - No pathologic evidence of IE at surgery or autopsy, after antibiotic therapy for 4 days or less
- Definition of terms used in the Duke criteria:
  - Major criteria:
    - Positive blood culture for IE; typical microorganisms consistent with IE from two separate blood cultures
      - *Viridans streptococci,* * *Streptococcus bovis,* or HACEK group, or community-acquired *S. aureus* or enterococci, in the absence of a primary focus, *or*
      - Microorganisms consistent with IE from "persistently positive blood cultures," defined as two or more positive cultures of blood samples drawn more than 12 hours apart, *or*
      - All three or a majority of four or more separate cultures of blood with first and last sample drawn 1 hour or more apart
  - Evidence of endocardial involvement:
    - Positive echocardiogram for IE defined as oscillating intracardiac mass, on valve or supporting structures, or in the path of regurgitant jets, or on implanted material in the absence of an alternative anatomic explanation, *or*
    - Abscess, *or*
    - New partial dehiscence of prosthetic valve, *or*
    - New valvular regurgitation (worsening or changing of preexisting murmur not sufficient)
  - Minor criteria:
    - Predisposing heart condition or intravenous drug use
    - Temperature 38°C or higher
    - Vascular phenomena: major arterial emboli, septic pulmonary infarcts, mycotic aneurysm, intracranial hemorrhage, conjunctival hemorrhages, and Janeway lesions
    - Immunologic phenomena: glomerulonephritis, Osler's nodes, Roth spots, and rheumatoid factor
    - Microbiologic evidence: positive blood culture, but does not meet a major criterion as noted previously* or serologic

*Includes nutritionally variant strains (abiotrophic species).

evidence of active infection with organism consistent with IE
- Echocardiographic findings: consistent with IE but do not meet a major criterion as noted previously

IMAGING STUDIES

- Transthoracic echocardiography (TTE) (sensitivity, 80%)
- Transesophageal echocardiography (TEE) if TTE is negative and endocarditis is strongly considered
- Chest radiograph

TREATMENT

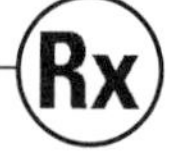

NONPHARMACOLOGIC THERAPY

Indications for surgery include the following:

- Congestive heart failure unresponsive to medical therapy
- Valvular obstruction
- Prosthetic valve dehiscence
- Graft or conduit obstruction
- Uncontrollable infection or relapse
- Fungal endocarditis
- Emboli
- Local invasion/periannular extension
  - Purulent pericarditis
  - Papillary muscle/chordal rupture
  - Sinus of Valsalva rupture
  - Ventricular septal rupture
  - Heart block

ACUTE GENERAL Rx

- Prolonged parenteral therapy with bactericidal antibiotics is necessary for complete eradication of the infecting organism.
- Antibiotic sensitivity information (minimum inhibitory concentration) is essential for guiding therapy.
- Antibiotic combinations may be synergistic, allowing smaller doses of each drug to be used, thereby reducing toxicity.
- Repeat blood cultures are done after therapy is initiated to document vascular cleansing.
- For acutely ill patients, in whom waiting for culture data before initiating therapy may be very hazardous, an appropriate starting regimen would be penicillinase-resistant penicillin and an aminoglycoside.
- Early consultation with the pediatric infectious disease service is recommended to determine and guide antibiotic therapy.

DISPOSITION

- Although home therapy has been proposed for IE, this approach should be reserved for uncomplicated infections with common and sensitive organisms and only after observation in the hospital because of the risk of serious complications.
- Potential complications:
  - Congestive heart failure, usually related to valvular destruction
  - Localized suppuration leading to abscess formation or periannular extension
  - A ventricular septal defect or creation of a fistula
  - Emboli
  - Mycotic aneurysms
  - Conduction and rhythm abnormalities
  - Purulent pericarditis or myocarditis
  - Prosthetic device (valve, graft, conduit) dysfunction
  - Glomerulonephritis/renal failure

REFERRAL

All patients with unexplained fever and cardiac lesions, or central venous catheters, which place them at high risk for IE, should be referred back to their cardiologist.

PEARLS & CONSIDERATIONS

COMMENTS

- Rarely, patients may be afebrile, especially with prior antibiotic therapy.
- The risk of IE in patients with aortic stenosis increases over time.
- Consider taking blood cultures (1 to 3 mL in young infants, 5 to 7 mL in older children) in febrile patients with high-risk lesions (prosthetic valves, shunts, complex congenital malformations, aortic stenosis) before initiating antibiotic therapy, even if the source of fever is apparent.
- The absence of vegetations does not rule out IE.

PREVENTION

- Prophylaxis
  - Prophylaxis is indicated for dental, respiratory, gastrointestinal, and genitourinary procedures associated with important bacteremias to kill circulating or adhered bacteria (see Endocarditis Prophylaxis in Prevention [Section V]).
  - Only 5% to 20% of IE can be related to prior procedures.
  - Prophylaxis is generally administered 30 to 60 minutes before a procedure but may be effective up to 2 hours after a procedure.
  - The regimen for dental or respiratory procedures consists of amoxicillin or clindamycin/azithromycin for patients allergic to penicillin.
  - Ampicillin plus gentamicin is used for gastrointestinal or genitourinary procedures in high-risk patients (vancomycin plus gentamicin in penicillin-allergic individuals). Moderate-risk patients are given amoxicillin or ampicillin (vancomycin, alternatively).
- Lesions not requiring prophylaxis:
  - Native secundum atrial defects
  - More than 6 months after repair of atrial and ventricular defects and ductus arteriosis without residua
  - Mitral valve prolapse without regurgitation
  - Previous Kawasaki disease or rheumatic fever without valvular involvement
- Consultation with the patient's pediatric cardiologist is always appropriate if questions arise concerning prophylaxis.

PATIENT/FAMILY EDUCATION

Parents should contact their pediatric practitioner and cardiologist in the presence of persistent fever, even if low grade, and constitutional symptoms. Establish and maintain the best possible oral health.

SUGGESTED READINGS

Bayer AS et al: Diagnosis and management of infective endocarditis and its complications. *Circulation* 98:2936, 1998.

Ferrieri P et al: Unique features of infective endocarditis in childhood. *Circulation* 105:2115, 2002.

Morris CD et al: Thirty-year incidence of infective endocarditis after surgery for congenital heart defect. *JAMA* 279:599, 1998.

Pajani AS et al: Prevention of bacterial endocarditis: recommendations by the American Heart Association. *JAMA* 277:1794, 1997.

AUTHOR: **J. PETER HARRIS, MD**

BASIC INFORMATION

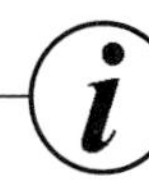

DEFINITION

The presence and growth of endometrial stroma and glands in locations other than the uterine cavity and muscle.

ICD-9-CM CODES

617.0 Endometriosis uterus, cervix
617.2 Endometriosis of fallopian tube
617.3 Endometriosis of pelvic peritoneum
617.8 Endometriosis—site specified (lung, bladder, umbilicus, vulva)
617.9 Endometriosis—site unspecified

EPIDEMIOLOGY & DEMOGRAPHICS

- Prevalence is approximately 10% of menstruating adolescents and women.
- Prevalence in adolescents with chronic pelvic pain is approximately 45% to 65%.
- The average age of diagnosis is 25 to 29 years.
- Familial predisposition is recognized.
- Incidence is increased in patients with reproductive tract anomalies, such as müllerian duct abnormalities, or cervical or vaginal obstruction.

CLINICAL PRESENTATION

History

- Cyclic pelvic pain
- Abnormal uterine bleeding
- Pain with defecation
- Rectal pain with bleeding
- Dyspareunia
- Infertility

Physical Examination

- Tenderness of pelvic structures
- Tender lymph nodes in the cul-de-sac
- Tender uterosacral ligaments
- Tender, enlarged adnexa with ovary involvement
- Fixed and retroverted uterus

ETIOLOGY

- Most widely proposed and accepted mechanism
  - Transplanted endometrium by retrograde menstruation
  - Risk increases in the presence of genital tract obstructions.
- Theory of deficient cell-mediated immunity
  - Inability of the immune system to remove refluxed menstrual debris.
  - Leukocytic cytokines may stimulate initiation and growth of endometrial implants.
- Other theories
  - Coelomic metaplasia
  - Transplanted endometrium by vascular, lymphatic, or iatrogenic spread of endometrial cells
  - Embryologically multipotent cells undergo metaplastic transformation into functioning endometrium.
  - Induction theory: shed endometrium releases substances that induce undifferentiated mesenchyma to form endometriotic tissue.

DIAGNOSIS

DIFFERENTIAL DIAGNOSIS

- Primary dysmenorrhea
- Pelvic inflammatory disease
- Pelvic masses, including fibroids and ovarian neoplasms
- Bowel neoplasm
- Anatomic abnormalities

WORKUP

- Gold standard for diagnosis: laparoscopy or laparotomy for definitive diagnosis and staging
  - Findings include "powder burn" or "chocolate cyst" implants (8 mm to 8 cm) located in the dependent portions of the female pelvis.
  - Less common sites include, but are not limited to, the rectosigmoid, umbilicus, and areas of previous surgery.
- Ovarian endometriosis may be accurately diagnosed noninvasively, based on symptoms, signs, and ultrasound.

LABORATORY TESTS

Measurements of serum proteins: CA-125 is neither sensitive nor specific but may be used to follow response to therapy and progression of disease.

IMAGING STUDIES

- Magnetic resonance imaging is not diagnostic but gives detailed confirmatory information.
- Pelvic ultrasonography is not diagnostic but may help distinguish solid from cystic lesions.

TREATMENT

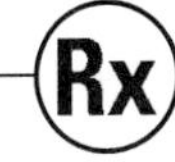

NONPHARMACOLOGIC THERAPY

- Conservative: laparoscopy or laparotomy to relieve pain and ameliorate infertility
  - Implants are removed by coagulating, vaporizing, or resecting the lesions while preserving reproductive capacity.
  - Length of time of symptom improvement varies.
  - Approximately 25% of patients return for subsequent laparoscopy.
- Definitive: total abdominal hysterectomy, bilateral salpingo-oophorectomy, and removal of endometriosis lesions may be performed
  - This procedure is reserved for advanced and burdensome disease.

ACUTE GENERAL Rx

Analgesics: naproxen sodium was found to be more helpful than placebo.

CHRONIC Rx

- Most widely used medications: gonadotropin-releasing hormone (GnRH) agonists and oral contraceptives
- GnRH agonists do the following:
  - Produce a state of medical oophorectomy
  - Reduce pain
  - Have unknown effect on fertility
  - Can be given as one of the following:
    - Leuprolide 3.75 mg intramuscularly every 28 days up to 6 months
    - Leuprolide 1 mg subcutaneously daily
    - Leuprolide causes reversible bone loss.
      - "Add-back" norethindrone 10 mg orally daily or combination norethindrone 2.5 mg plus sodium etidronate 400 mg plus calcium carbonate 500 mg orally daily to prevent bone loss.
    - Goserelin 3.6 mg subcutaneously every 28 days for 6 months
    - Nafarelin 200 to 400 mg intranasally two times daily for 6 months
    - Buserelin 300 to 400 μg intranasally three times daily
- Danazol is a synthetic steroid with mild androgenic effects (weight gain, muscle cramps, decreased breast size, hirsutism, acne, decreased high-density lipoprotein [HDL], elevated liver transaminases, hot flashes, and mood changes) that does the following:
  - Suppresses the pituitary-ovarian axis and may result in the resolution of implants
  - Causes anovulation
  - Causes androgenic side effects, of which deepening of the voice may be irreversible
  - Reduces pain up to 6 months after discontinuation of therapy
  - Does not appear to affect fertility
  - Usual dosage is 100 to 400 mg orally two times per day or 200 to 800 mg orally once daily for approximately 6 months.
- Continuous combination estrogen/progestogen oral contraceptives:
  - Produce amenorrhea
  - May reduce symptoms by approximately 80%
  - Dosage is 30 to 35 μg ethinyl estradiol plus a progestogen daily for 4 to 6 months.
  - The dosage is increased to manage breakthrough bleeding.
- Progestogens:
  - Provide effective treatment in approximately 75% of women with endometriosis
  - Cause prolonged amenorrhea
  - Do not appear to affect fertility, although contraceptive effectiveness limits its use to women who do not wish to become pregnant in the short term
  - Reduce pain
  - Must be given for a prolonged period of time

- Can be given as one of the following:
  - Medroxyprogesterone acetate 20 to 30 mg orally daily for 6 months then depomedroxyprogesterone acetate 100 mg intramuscularly every 2 weeks for 2 months, then 200 mg intramuscularly monthly for 4 months
  - Norethindrone acetate 5 mg orally daily for 2 weeks then increase by 2.5 mg per day every 2 weeks until a goal of 15 mg daily is reached
- New therapies will target various molecular receptors, factors, and enzymes.

DISPOSITION

Patients require close follow-up to ensure proper monitoring of the progression of disease and response to treatment, as well as to ensure appropriate education.

REFERRAL

Patients with suspected endometriosis must be managed by practitioners who are familiar with techniques to definitively diagnose and treat this disorder.

PEARLS & CONSIDERATIONS

COMMENTS

- The stage of disease (i.e., the number and extent of lesions) is not related to the severity of symptoms.
- Medical therapy used for pain relief does not address infertility.
- The risks and benefits of surgical treatment in patients with infertility should be carefully weighed as it may cause early menopause.

PREVENTION

When the presentation of endometriosis occurs in adolescence, the practitioner should evaluate for congenital outflow obstruction, which may be corrected and allow for less severe disease.

PATIENT/FAMILY EDUCATION

- A monthly pain calendar may be useful to identify the cyclic nature of pain.
- Danazol may cause virilization of a developing fetus, resulting in female pseudohermaphroditism.

SUGGESTED READINGS

Emans SJ: Dysmenorrhea, pelvic pain and premenstrual syndrome. *In* Emans SJH et al (eds): *Pediatric and Adolescent Gynecology.* Philadelphia, Lippincott-Raven, 1998.

Endometriosis Association. Available at www.endometriosis.org.au/teen.htm

Eskenazi B et al: Validation study of nonsurgical diagnosis of endometriosis. *Fertil & Steril* 76:929, 2001.

Giudice LC et al: Endometriosis. *Lancet* 364:1789, 2004.

OBGYN.net. Available at www.obgyn.net

Schenken RS: Endometriosis. *In* Scott JR et al (eds): *Danforth's Obstetrics and Gynecology,* 9th ed. Philadelphia, Lippincott Williams & Wilkins, 2003.

Vercellini P et al: Progestogens for endometriosis: forward to the past. *Hum Reprod Update* 9:387, 2001.

AUTHOR: **NICOLE L. MIHALOPOULOS, MD, MPH**

BASIC INFORMATION

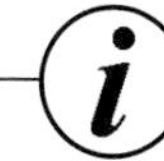

DEFINITION

The term *enuresis* is of Greek etymology and means "to urinate in." Nocturnal enuresis, or enuresis, denotes bed wetting only. Enuresis refers to the involuntary passage of urine during sleep in children older than age 5. Day wetting is referred to as urinary incontinence. Primary enuresis occurs in a child who has had no period of dryness for at least 6 months. Secondary enuresis occurs in a child who has already had a period of dryness for at least 6 months. Polysymptomatic nocturnal enuresis (PNE) is bed wetting associated with severe urgency, severe frequency, or other signs of an unstable bladder. Monosymptomatic nocturnal enuresis (MNE) is bed wetting with normal daytime urination.

SYNONYMS

Bed wetting
Nocturnal enuresis

ICD-9-CM CODE
788.30 Enuresis

EPIDEMIOLOGY & DEMOGRAPHICS

- Ninety percent of enuretic children have MNE.
- For enuretic children, males outnumber females by a ratio of 3:2.
- The overall prevalence of enuresis decreases with age—spontaneous cure rates of 15% per annum have been reported.
- Studies have estimated that:
  - Twenty percent to 25% of children at age 4 are bed wetters.
  - Five percent to 10% of child at age 7 are bed wetters.
  - Enuresis persists in 0.5% to 3.0% of adults ages 18 to 64.
- As age advances, bed wetters with more severe symptoms are more likely to have persistent problems into adult life.
- Numerous studies report varying but generally high prevalence of enuresis in other family members.
- The family history of nocturnal enuresis gives an indication of the age at which dryness will be achieved.
- Several chromosomes (including 8, 12, 13, 16, and 22) have been reported to be linked to enuresis.
- Studies offer conflicting results regardingthe association of enuresis with delayedsomatic and psychological development.

CLINICAL PRESENTATION

- Primary and secondary enuresis may be associated with the following medical conditions: cystitis, constipation, fecal impaction, neurogenic bladder, urethral obstruction, ectopic ureter, dysfunctional voiding, seizures, sleep apnea, diabetes mellitus, diabetes insipidus, hyperthyroidism, and heart block.
- Enuresis may also be associated with psychological stresses, including parental divorce, birth of a new sibling, hospitalization, school trauma, neglect, and abuse.
- In a majority of cases, enuresis creates secondary psychological problems, including negative self-esteem.
- Obtaining the enuresis history can be divided into four parts:
  - Eliciting the type and severity of enuresis
  - Identifying the specifics of fluid intake
  - Clarifying the voiding and sleep history
  - Thoroughly investigating the patient's medical, social, and family history
- The enuresis history addresses the number of bed wetting episodes per week and per night, and the time at which they occur.
- Fluid intake history includes the amount and types of fluids ingested daily, and the timing of ingestion.
- The voiding history addresses whether there are any daytime wetting episodes, daytime voiding frequency, voiding characteristics, and void volumes. Characteristics include identifying whether the patient needs to push to void or needs to wait before initiating a stream, or if there is an interruption in the stream.
- The sleep history addresses the presence or absence of nocturnal arousals, sleep walking, sleep terrors, and nightmares.
- The medical history elicits any signs of illness (e.g., fever, dysuria, urgency, stooling history, polydipsia, developmental delays, seizures, weight loss).
- The social history addresses family stress associated with the enuresis, other family stressors, accessibility of laundry facilities, already attempted interventions, and consequences for the patient (e.g., is the child kept from participating in peer or family activities because of enuresis).
- The family history identifies whether other family members have been enuretic, to what degree, and until what age.
- The physical exam focuses on behavioral observations, blood pressure, presence or absence of nasal obstruction and tonsillar hypertrophy, thyromegaly, abdominal masses, urogenital anomalies, cutaneous abnormalities in the lumbar and sacral areas, rectal masses, and a thorough neurologic exam including observation of gait, muscle power, tone, sensation, and reflexes.

ETIOLOGY

- Enuresis is thought to be a heterogeneous disorder with various underlying mechanisms.
- Primary and secondary enuresis can be caused by:
  - A mismatch between nocturnal bladder capacity and the amount of urine produced during sleep
  - A disorder of sleep arousal
  - Multiple medical and social conditions (see "Clinical Presentation")
  - Possibly insufficient antidiuretic hormone during sleep
- In an attempt to understand enuresis more fully, recent research has also investigated mechanisms by which the bladder communicates with the kidney to regulate urine production.

DIAGNOSIS

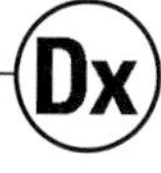

DIFFERENTIAL DIAGNOSIS

- Urinary incontinence—wetting both day and night
- See also medical and social conditions listed in "Clinical Presentation"

LABORATORY TESTS

- Urinalysis
- Urine culture

IMAGING STUDIES

- If daytime wetting is present or cannot be excluded:
  - Voiding cystourethrogram
  - Renal/bladder ultrasound
- If lumbar or sacral anomalies are present:
  - Lumbosacral spine films

TREATMENT

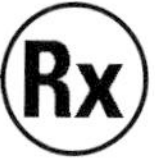

NONPHARMACOLOGIC THERAPY

- General considerations:
  - Convey a sense of understanding to the child and family
  - Educate families regarding prognosis, including the 15% per annum spontaneous remission rate
- Behavioral counseling (see "Prevention")
- Bed wetting alarms:
  - Current alarms consist of a small sponge pad that is worn inside night clothes and to which an electric sensor is clipped. Urine leakage completes an electrical circuit and sounds an alarm.
  - Alarms are indicated as first-line treatment for children with MNE or in patients with severe symptoms refractory to desmopressin.
  - Current evidence suggests that conditioning (alarm therapy) gives the best long-term outcome.
  - Alarm therapy requires a minimum of 6 to 8 weeks of continuous use before its effect will appear.
  - Efficacy increases with duration of therapy.
  - Optimal results require a motivated child and family, and a significant commitment of effort and time.
  - Consideration needs to be given to whether a family is willing to make the time commitment necessary, and to the impact of disrupted sleep on other family members.

ACUTE GENERAL Rx

- Treat underlying acute conditions, such as urinary tract infections
- Address chronic underlying conditions such as sleep apnea, and constipation and encopresis before initiating enuresis-specific therapy
- Ensure optimal treatment of chronic conditions such as diabetes mellitus and seizure disorders
- Pharmacologic treatment includes:
  - DDAVP or desmopressin—comes in nasal spray or tablet
    - Is indicated when enuresis is presenting a significant problem for the patient and family, and when there is a need for a rapid response
    - Functions as an analog of antidiuretic hormone, enhancing increased urine concentration by reabsorption of water in the kidney
    - Initial doses include 10 μg per spray, one spray in each nostril before bedtime (up to 20 μg per nostril maximum) or 0.2 mg orally before bedtime (up to 0.6 mg maximum).
    - Is generally well tolerated for long-term treatment (1 year or more) and is associated with a low incidence of adverse effects. There is a potential risk for water intoxication if a patient ingests large fluid volumes. The medication also should not be administered at times of illness when fluids are to be encouraged.
    - Occasionally produces delayed responses: treatment for at least 2 to 3 months is recommended before noting unresponsiveness.
    - One week interruptions in treatment are recommended every 3 months to see if the enuresis has resolved.
    - May also be used intermittently (if works) for sleepovers or special occasions when child wants to be dry all night
  - Imipramine
    - This medication is a second choice when compared to alarms or desmopressin due to potential cardiotoxic effects.
    - A suggested mechanism of action is reduced detrusor activity and increased bladder capacity caused by anticholinergic and smooth muscle relaxant effects.
    - The starting dose is 10 mg at bedtime, with a maximum of 50 mg daily for children 8 to 12 years old.
  - Oxybutynin has anticholinergic and smooth muscle relaxant properties
    - This may be of use in a subset of patients with detrusor overactivity at night. These patients usually present with daytime frequency, urgency, or incontinence.
    - Side effects include constipation, which may counteract beneficial effects.

DISPOSITION

- Enuretic children and their families require consistent follow-up, initially every 2 to 3 weeks, to provide support and to address any problems that may arise.
- Initial success is defined as 14 consecutive dry nights within a 16-week treatment period.
- Nearly all relapses, defined as more than two wet nights in 2 weeks, occur within the first 6 months of treatment.

REFERRAL

- Referral to the following specialties may be indicated:
  - Neurology—for any neurologic abnormalities or seizure history
  - Otolaryngology—if nasal obstruction or adenotonsillar hypertrophy is suspected
  - Psychiatry or counseling—in cases of abuse or psychiatric disorders
  - Sleep disorders—for suspected sleep apnea
  - Urology—for any anatomic anomalies or unresponsiveness to the above therapies

PEARLS & CONSIDERATIONS

COMMENTS

- Enuresis is often discovered as a problem when a family is specifically questioned regarding sleep and urination issues. Families may be reluctant to initiate a conversation about enuresis.
- Wetting occurs in all stages of sleep.
- Almost all patients with MNE have normal functioning bladder capacity.
- Seventy-eight percent of children with PNE have functional bladder abnormalities.

PREVENTION

- Maintain consistent schedules regarding sleeping, eating, and drinking
- Promote a high-fiber diet, regular daytime toileting, and regular exercise
- Avoid excessive dairy and refined carbohydrate ingestion
- Avoid caffeinated beverages
- Address constipation issues promptly
- Be compliant with therapies for other chronic disorders

PATIENT/FAMILY EDUCATION

- Provide reassurance about the prevalence of the problem and its eventual likely resolution
- Inform parents that enuresis is not volitional or from laziness
- Encourage parents to have patients avoid drinking large amounts of fluid before bed and to use the toilet just before bed
- Encourage older children to help change wet sheets and clean up
- Suggest protecting beds with rubber or plastic covers
- Have parents contact the pediatrician for any new symptoms
- Offer a lot of emotional support to patients and parents until bed wetting resolves

Resources

American Foundation for Urologic Disease web site. Available at www.afud.org

Bedwetting Store web site. Available at www.bedwettingstore.com. Also available by phone at: 1-800-214-9605.

National Kidney Foundation web site. Available at www.kidney.org. Also available by phone at: 1-800-622-9010.

Web Sites of Interest

KidsHealth for Parents. What Parents Need to Know about Bedwetting. Available at kidshealth.org/parent/general/sleep/enuresis.html

National Kidney and Urologic Diseases Information Clearinghouse. Available at kidney.niddk.nih.gov/kudiseases/pubs/uichildren/

NotMyKid.org. Bedwetting: You Are Not Alone. Available at notmykid.org/parentArticles/Bedwetting/default.asp

SUGGESTED READINGS

Cossio SE: Enuresis. *South Med J* 95(2): 2002.

Emedicine: "Enuresis." Available at www.emedicine.com/ped/topic689.htm

Fritz G et al: Practice parameter for the assessment and treatment of children and adolescents with enuresis. *J Am Acad Child Adolesc Psychiatry* 43:12, 2004.

Hjalmas K et al: Nocturnal enuresis: an international evidence based management strategy. *J Urol* 171:6, 2004.

AUTHOR: **ANDREE JACOBS-PERKINS, MD**

BASIC INFORMATION

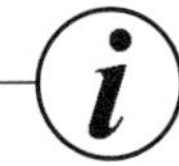

DEFINITION

Inflammation of the epididymis, the coiled tubular structure adjacent and posterior to the testis, which is essential for sperm transport and maturation.

SYNONYM

Epididymo-orchitis

ICD-9-CM CODE

604.90 Orchitis and epididymitis, unspecified

EPIDEMIOLOGY & DEMOGRAPHICS

- Nonsexually active males:
  - Rare in prepubertal boys
  - Twenty percent to 60% of cases are associated with urinary tract infection (UTI).
  - Up to 50% of cases associated with urologic or anorectal structural abnormality.
  - May be associated with dysfunctional voiding or infrequent voiding
- Sexually active males: most common cause of acute scrotum.

CLINICAL PRESENTATION

- Scrotal pain with gradual onset
- May have referred pain to the ipsilateral inguinal canal or abdomen
- May have fever, dysuria, urgency, and urinary frequency
- Rarely, nausea and vomiting
- Urethral discharge possible in sexually active adolescents
- Ask about urethral instrumentation, catheterization, and trauma
- Elicit history of hypospadias, previous anorectal abnormalities, bowel or bladder elimination problems
- Examine uninvolved testis first to compare.
- Unilateral epididymal/testicular tenderness
- Early: epididymis is tender and swollen, normal testis; later: intrascrotal landmarks obliterated by swelling, tenderness throughout.
- Testis, if discernable, has a normal vertical axis
- Cremasteric reflex usually present early on
- Secondary hydrocele formation possible
- Examine spine for occult spinal dysraphism
- Examine the anus for signs of an abnormality

ETIOLOGY

- Bacterial
  - Prepubertal/nonsexually active: gram-negative coliforms, usually *Escherichia coli*
  - Sexually active: *Chlamydia trachomatis, Neisseria gonorrhoeae*
  - Less common: *Mycobacterium tuberculosis, Haemophilus influenzae, Brucella,* cytomegalovirus
  - Sickle cell disease: *Salmonella*
  - Cystic fibrosis: *Staphylococcus aureus*
- Nonbacterial
  - Trauma
  - Chemical—intrusion of sterile urine, retrograde, into ejaculatory ducts, vas deferens, and thus to epididymis
    - High-pressure bladder storage or emptying, as in neurogenic or non-neurogenic dysfunctional voiding, and some types of reflux in boys
    - Bladder outlet obstruction such as posterior urethral valves, anterior urethral valves, urethral stricture
    - Straining or lifting with a full bladder
  - Autoimmune disease/vasculitis
  - Viral—primarily mumps orchitis or epididymo-orchitis

DIAGNOSIS

DIFFERENTIAL DIAGNOSIS

- Torsion of spermatic cord/testis (must be eliminated as a possible diagnosis)
- Torsion of testicular or epididymal appendage
- Orchitis
- Testis neoplasm, with or without hemorrhage
- Testicular abscess
- Traumatic hydrocele/hematocele
- Henoch-Schönlein purpura
- Idiopathic scrotal edema
- Scrotal fat necrosis
- Scrotal skin infection or inflammation: cellulitis; infected sebaceous cyst
- Incarcerated scrotal hernia
- Other intraperitoneal process manifesting in scrotum (e.g., meconium scrotitis)

WORKUP

Rarely, aspiration of an intrascrotal collection or abscess for culture. If the physical examination does not rule out testis torsion, *immediate urologic consultation* is imperative.

LABORATORY TESTS

- Urinalysis for pyuria and bacteria
- Urine for culture and sensitivity
- If urethral exudate: gram stain; culture for *C. trachomatis* and *N. gonorrhea*; serum for syphilis and HIV; counseling

IMAGING STUDIES

- The goal is to rule out testis torsion.
  - Color Doppler ultrasound; the affected epididymis usually shows increased blood flow and the ipsilateral testis has normal or increased blood flow.
  - In a prepubertal child without fever and with a normal urinalysis, increased blood flow probably represents a torsed appendage of the testis or epididymis with a surrounding inflammatory response, rather than a true epididymitis.
- In the prepubertal child with UTI, and in others with recurrent episodes: contrast voiding cystourethrogram to evaluate the urethra; upper tract study such as ultrasound or intravenous urogram may be important following acute treatment.

TREATMENT

NONPHARMACOLOGIC THERAPY

If uncertain about testis torsion, proceed to scrotal exploration; scrotal elevation, bed rest; scrotal support may help; timed voiding

ACUTE GENERAL Rx

- Anti-inflammatories and analgesics
- Not sexually active: treat for gram-negative UTI empirically and adjust by culture results
- Sexually active: treat empirically according to CDC guidelines (2002) and encourage referral and treatment of partners
  - Ceftriaxone 250 mg intramuscularly × 1, plus doxycycline 100 mg orally twice a day × 10 days
  - For those allergic to cephalosporins or tetracyclines, use ofloxacin 300 mg orally twice a day × 10 days or levofloxacin 500 mg orally once a day × 10 days.
  - Systemically ill patients: parenteral antibiotics and analgesics

CHRONIC Rx

Suppressive antibiotics for recurrent problems; vasectomy in some cases; continued timed voiding for chemical epididymitis

DISPOSITION

- Follow up positive urine culture for cure
- Prophylactic antibiotics in nonsexually active boy with UTI until structural imaging completed
- Scrotal edema and tenderness resolve in several days, but palpable epididymal induration can persist for several weeks.

REFERRAL

Pediatric urology for acute scrotum of uncertain etiology or surgical diagnosis

PEARLS & CONSIDERATIONS

COMMENTS

- Prehn's sign (lifting the scrotum to modify testicular position and assess change in pain) is nonspecific and not helpful in differentiating torsion from epididymitis.
- Urethral swabbing may be traumatic and is rarely helpful with diagnosis in the absence of other findings.

PREVENTION

Evaluate prepubertal epididymitis associated with UTI for structural abnormality.

SUGGESTED READINGS

American Urologic Association. Available at www.urologyhealth.org

Centers for Disease Control and Prevention. Available at www.cdc.gov

Merlini E et al: Acute epididymitis and urinary tract anomalies in children. *Scand J Urol Nephrol* 32:273, 1998.

Rabinowitz R, Hulbert WC: Acute scrotal swelling. *Urol Clin North Am* 22:101, 1995.

AUTHORS: **WILLIAM C. HULBERT, MD, ROBERT A. MEVORACH, MD,** and **RONALD RABINOWITZ, MD**

BASIC INFORMATION

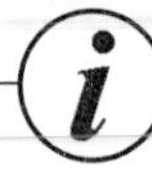

DEFINITION

Epistaxis is hemorrhage from the nose.

SYNONYMS

Bloody nose
Nosebleed

ICD-9-CM CODE
784.7 Epistaxis

EPIDEMIOLOGY & DEMOGRAPHICS

- Epistaxis occurs most commonly in the winter months (dry air).
- Children ages 2 to 10 are more commonly affected than adults.
- It may be a presentation of coagulopathy (e.g., von Willebrand disease).

CLINICAL PRESENTATION

History

- Frequency of occurrence
- Bleeding from one or both nostrils
- Amount and duration of bleeding; ability to stop bleeding with home first aid
- What type of first aid was done prior to presenting? Was it done correctly?
- Sensation of blood in back of throat as first awareness of bleeding (more suggestive of posterior bleeding)
- Trauma
- Nose picking
- History of upper respiratory infections and sinusitis
- Allergic rhinitis or chronic nasal discharge
- Bleeding disorder (e.g., easy bruising, bleeding) or family history of bleeding disorder
- Recent surgery
- Nasal obstructive symptoms; progressing obstructive symptoms after trauma or surgery
- Medications
- Exposure to airborne irritants and toxic chemicals, including cigarette smoke
- Substance abuse such as cocaine, or other drugs that may be abused nasally such as heroin or methamphetamine

Physical Examination

- Vital signs (blood pressure to look at hypo- or hypertension and heart rate)
- Airway
- Mental status
- Inspection of the nose with nasal speculum for discharge, trauma, or evidence of foreign body and identifying source of bleeding (anterior versus posterior, right versus left)
- Posterior bleeding usually seen as bleeding along the posterior pharynx
- Nasal septum exam for septal hematoma (a large, soft, red or bluish mass, obstructing one or both nares)
- Evidence of other hematologic disease (e.g., petechiae, purpura, pallor, hepatosplenomegaly, lymphadenopathy)

ETIOLOGY

- The nose is a common site for recurrent minor trauma.
- Small vessels that supply the nasal mucosa have little structural support; contraction and hemostasis for an injured vessel are thus limited.
- Nasal mucosa has a rich vascular supply (terminal branches from the internal and external carotid arteries) that forms multiple anastomoses.
- The anterior portion of the nose is the most common site of bleeding in children.
  - Kiesselbach's plexus in Little's area of the anterior nasal septum, approximately 0.5 cm from the tip of the nose, is a common site of anterior bleeding.
  - This area is easily irritated by finger manipulation and drying effects of the air.
- Posterior bleeding is more common in the elderly.

DIAGNOSIS

DIFFERENTIAL DIAGNOSIS

- Trauma
  - Nose picking
  - Facial trauma
  - Perforation of septum: usually as a result of chronic erosion, but must consider vasculitis, granulomatous disorder, or lymphoma; cocaine use should be considered in older children
  - After facial surgery
- Inflammation
  - Acute respiratory infection, sinusitis, allergic rhinitis; cause nasal lining inflammation
  - Foreign body: unilateral, foul-smelling discharge typical
- Tumor
  - Juvenile nasopharyngeal angiofibroma: benign vascular neoplasm in lateral nasopharynx
  - Malignant neoplasms: rhabdomyosarcoma, lymphoma, midline reticuloses, olfactory neuroblastoma
  - Polyps (uncommon except in cystic fibrosis)
  - Meningocele or encephalocele
- Chemical
  - Airborne irritants and toxic chemicals can cause epistaxis.
  - Primary or secondary exposure to cigarette smoke can cause epistaxis.
- Blood disorders
  - von Willebrand disease
  - Hemophilia
  - Thrombocytopenia
  - Leukemia
  - Sickle cell anemia
  - Osler-Weber-Rendu disease (hereditary telangiectasis)
  - Platelet aggregation disorders
  - Bernard-Soulier syndrome
- Other
  - Hypertension: very rare in children with malignant hypertension
  - Vicarious menstruation: monthly epistaxis related to monthly vascular congestion coinciding with menses; related to monthly hormonal changes
  - Septal deviation: nasal dryness and crusting in area of deflection
  - Septal hematoma: hematoma separates perichondrium from septal cartilage; vascular supply compromised; can progress to necrosis, abscess
  - Medications: aspirin, nonsteroidal anti-inflammatory drugs (NSAIDs), warfarin, steroid nasal sprays

LABORATORY TESTS

- Children with no evidence of significant blood loss, no evidence of systemic disease by history and physical examination, and anterior epistaxis that is easily stopped by local pressure require no laboratory workup.
- Consider coagulation disorder workup for patients with pertinent findings on personal or family history or physical examination. Workup to begin with the following:
  - Complete blood count and platelet count are obtained to look for anemia.
  - Prothrombin time, partial thromboplastin time, closure (bleeding) time may require further workup pending results.

IMAGING STUDIES

Not routinely done unless findings on exam suggest need, such as if a mass is seen.

TREATMENT

NONPHARMACOLOGIC THERAPY

- Exert digital compression over the nasal alar and anterior septal area for at least 5 minutes.
- Bend forward at the waist, allowing blood to flow out of nostrils rather than into the back of the throat.
- Cauterize with silver nitrate.
  - Both sides of septum should not be cauterized at the same time because of the risk of septal perforation.
- Apply anterior nasal packing when local measures are unsuccessful at controlling bleeding.
  - Petroleum gauze impregnated with antibiotic ointment is inserted into the nares.
  - It is removed by 72 hours.
  - Synthetic sponge packs (tampons) may also be used. If minimal pressure needed may consider use of hemostatic agent such as Gelfoam packing.
  - There is a risk of toxic shock syndrome with nasal packing.
  - Patients should receive prophylactic oral antibiotics because of the risk of sinusitis.

- Oral antibiotics do not affect the risk of toxic shock syndrome.
- Posterior nasal packing is rarely needed in children.
- Remove foreign body if present.
- Septal hematoma: simple aspiration for small hematoma; may require more complicated surgical drainage.
- Endoscopic cauterization under general anesthesia:
  - Nasal cavity cleansed and endoscopically examined
  - Source of bleeding identified
  - Electrocauterization to appropriate area
- Arterial ligation is used to decrease arterial blood flow to the bleeding area.

ACUTE GENERAL Rx

- At home patients can use one spray of oxymetazoline (Afrin) or Neo-Synephrine (0.25% to 1%) in the nostril and then place a piece of cotton with spray of the same medication into the nostril for 10 minutes.
- Remove clots and apply topical oxymetazoline hydrochloride (Afrin), epinephrine (1:1000), or 4% cocaine to the involved area with a cotton pledget. This is done before cautery.
  - Local vasoconstrictors are usually combined with an anesthetic, such as tetracaine or lidocaine.
- Apply antibiotic cream or ointment to the cauterized area twice daily for 5 days to prevent crusting and infection.

DISPOSITION

- Usually managed in outpatient setting
- If significant bleeding with hemodynamic instability or surgery required, patient would be admitted to hospital

REFERRAL

Referral to an otolaryngologist should be considered for the following:

- Patients with specific local abnormalities, such as tumors, polyps, telangiectasias
- Patients with severe, recurrent, or posterior nasal bleeding

PEARLS & CONSIDERATIONS

COMMENTS

- Nose picking is the most common cause of epistaxis in children.
- Juvenile nasopharyngeal angiofibromas are found only in pubescent males and are hormonally sensitive.

PREVENTION

- Nose picking: apply antibiotic ointment to inside of nose daily to decrease crust build-up and itching.
- Use buffered nasal saline regularly during transitional weather times (fall to winter, winter to spring).
- Apply petroleum jelly to the inside of the nares twice daily to help maintain moisture of nasal mucosa.
- Use a cool mist vaporizer during the winter, especially with forced-air heating.
- In allergic rhinitis, treatment with an antihistamine-decongestant may be indicated; however, overuse may cause over-drying of the mucosa.

PATIENT/FAMILY EDUCATION

Important to review home first aid treatment.

SUGGESTED READINGS

Alvi A, Joyner-Triplett N: Acute epistaxis: how to spot the source and stop the flow. *Postgrad Med* 99:83, 1996.

Avigdor N: Index of suspicion case 3. *Pediatr Review* 25:177, 2004.

Culbertson MC et al (eds): *Pediatric Otolaryngology*. Philadelphia, WB Saunders, 1990.

Emanuel J: Epistaxis. *In* Cummings CW et al (eds): *Otolaryngology: Head & Neck Surgery*. St. Louis, Mosby, 1998.

Henretig F: Epistaxis. *In* Fleisher GR, Ludwig S (eds): *Textbook of Pediatric Emergency Medicine*. Baltimore, Williams & Wilkins, 1993.

Mulbury P: Recurrent epistaxis. *Pediatr Rev* 12:213, 1991.

Sandoval C, Dong S: Clinical and laboratory features of 178 children with recurrent epistaxis. *J Pediatr Hematol Oncol* 24:47, 2002.

Sparacino L: Epistaxis management: what's new & what's noteworthy. *Primary Care Pract* 4(5):498, 2000.

Tan LK, Calhoun KH: Epistaxis. *Med Clin North Am* 83:43, 1999.

AUTHOR: **DIANA BARNETT KUDES, MD**

BASIC INFORMATION

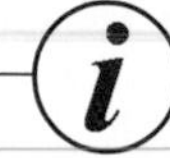

DEFINITION

In the normal host, the most common manifestation of Epstein-Barr virus (EBV) infection is infectious mononucleosis (IM). IM is an acute multisystem illness, which is usually self-limited, with systemic signs of acute and subacute infection. Acute neurologic disorders may be associated with IM or as a manifestation of primary EBV infection without IM. These disorders include Bell's palsy, aseptic meningitis, encephalitis, Guillain-Barré syndrome, and transverse myelitis.

- Diseases caused by EBV associated with immunodeficiency include the X-linked lymphoproliferative syndrome, post-transplant lymphoproliferative disorders, B-cell lymphomas, and severe atypical EBV infections.
- Burkitt lymphoma (in Central Africa and Papua New Guinea) and nasopharyngeal carcinoma (in Southeast Asia) are important EBV-associated diseases outside the United States.

SYNONYMS

EBV infections
Infectious mononucleosis
Mono

ICD-9-CM CODE
075 Epstein-Barr virus infection

EPIDEMIOLOGY & DEMOGRAPHICS

- In lower socioeconomic communities, primary infection occurs early in life.
  - Approximately 80% to 100% of people are seropositive by 3 to 6 years of age.
  - In this setting, most infections are asymptomatic or produce mildly symptomatic disease (tonsillitis).
- In developed countries, primary infection occurs between the ages of 10 and 30 (particularly among college students). They most often manifest as acute IM.
- There is no seasonal pattern.

CLINICAL PRESENTATION

History

- IM
  - Prodrome of fatigue, malaise, myalgia, and headache may last 7 to 14 days.
  - Acute onset of high fever in some.
  - Common symptoms of IM indicate the following:
    - Fever
    - Sore throat, swallowing difficulty
    - Malaise
    - Headache
    - Myalgia
    - Sweats
    - Anorexia
    - Abdominal pain
    - Chest pain
    - Cough
  - Onset may be insidious
- Reactivation diseases/syndromes—congenital or acquired immunodeficiency

Physical Examination

- Fever is present in more than 90% of cases.
- Lymphadenopathy is present in more than 90% of cases.
- Tonsillopharyngitis is present in 70% of cases.
- Splenomegaly is present in 75% of cases.
- Hepatomegaly is present in 50% of cases.
- Petechial enanthem may occur.
- Lymphadenopathy involves the anterior and posterior cervical chains but may be generalized.
- Traumatic palpation of the spleen must be avoided because of the risk of splenic rupture.
- Maculopapular rashes occur rarely; however, almost all patients given ampicillin develop such rashes.

ETIOLOGY

- EBV is an enveloped DNA herpesvirus.
- It is transmitted via saliva, requiring close personal contact.
- The incubation period for IM is 30 to 45 days.
- IM persists in a latent state in B lymphocytes after primary infection.

DIAGNOSIS

DIFFERENTIAL DIAGNOSIS

- Streptococcal pharyngitis
- Adenoviral pharyngitis
- Cytomegalovirus
- *Toxoplasma* gondii
- Viral hepatitis
- Leptospirosis
- Rubella
- Acute human immunodeficiency virus (HIV) infection
- Lymphoma or leukemia

LABORATORY TESTS

- Lymphocytosis, both relative (>50% lymphocytes) and absolute (>4500/mm^3)
- Atypical lymphocytes (Downey cell) on smear
- Hemolytic anemia (rare)
- Abnormal liver function tests (predominantly elevated transaminases) in 80% of cases
- Heterophile antibody testing
  - Paul-Bunnell test and slide agglutination (Monospot) may be positive.
  - Heterophile antibodies are a nonspecific serologic response to EBV infection.
  - Repeat testing may be necessary.
  - Forty percent are positive in the first week.
  - Eighty percent to 90% are positive by the third week.
  - These tests are usually negative in infants and children younger than 4 years of age.
- Specific tests for EBV antibodies (i.e., anti-VCA immunoglobulin G [IgG], anti-VCA immunoglobulin M [IgM], anti-EA, and anti-EBNA) are not usually necessary to diagnose typical IM.
  - Useful in the diagnosis of heterophile-negative IM, severe or atypical disease, or lymphoproliferative disease
- Rapid test or throat culture for group A β-hemolytic streptococci (GABS) should be obtained. This test is positive in 5% to 25% of patients with IM.

TREATMENT

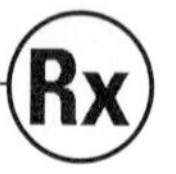

NONPHARMACOLOGIC THERAPY

- Symptomatic therapy
- Bed rest and limited activity
- Fluids
- No contact sports with splenomegaly

ACUTE GENERAL Rx

- Antipyretics and analgesics are given for comfort.
- Corticosteroids: prednisone 1 mg/kg/day for 7 days is indicated for the following:
  - Severe tonsillitis to prevent of airway obstruction caused by pharyngeal or laryngeal edema
  - Acute hemolytic anemia
  - Neurologic complications
- Antiviral agents such as acyclovir have not demonstrated a clinical benefit in otherwise healthy children.
- Appropriate treatment for GABS when throat culture is positive.

DISPOSITION

- Symptoms of IM usually last 2 to 4 weeks.
- Organomegaly resolves within 1 to 3 months.
- Several months may be required for patient to return to normal sense of wellness.

PEARLS & CONSIDERATIONS

PREVENTION

- Kissing is thought to be one mechanism of transmission.
- No specific isolation precautions are necessary other than handwashing and careful handling of oral secretions.
- Blood donation should be deferred in those with recent IM or IM-like illness.

PATIENT/FAMILY EDUCATION

Avoid contact sports until splenomegaly has resolved.

SUGGESTED READINGS

American Academy of Pediatrics: Epstein-Barr infections. *In* Pickering LK (ed): *2003 Red Book: Report of the Committee on Infectious Diseases,* 26th ed. Elk Grove Village, IL, American Academy of Pediatrics, 2003.

Razonable RR, Paya CV: Herpesvirus infections in transplant recipients: current challenges in the clinical management of cytomegalovirus and Epstein-Barr virus infections. *Herpes* 10:3, 2003.

AUTHOR: **THERESE CVETKOVICH, MD**

BASIC INFORMATION

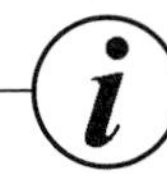

DEFINITION

Erythema multiforme is an acute hypersensitivity reaction characterized by distinctive, target-shaped skin lesions.

SYNONYMS

EM
Erythema multiforme minor

ICD-9-CM CODE
695.1 Erythema multiforme

EPIDEMIOLOGY & DEMOGRAPHICS

- Incidence is unknown but rare in children.
- Of all cases of erythema multiforme, approximately 20% occur in childhood.

CLINICAL PRESENTATION

- Acute onset of multiple lesions is typical, with most appearing in a 24-hour period.
- Lesions may itch or burn.
- The disease is self-limited, lasting approximately 2 weeks.
- Heals without scarring.
- Herpes simplex virus (HSV) lesion usually precedes the onset of erythema multiforme by 3 to 14 days.
- One or two recurrences per year are common.
- Initial lesions are dusky red macules or erythematous wheals.
- They progress into target-shaped lesions of concentric zones of color, with duskier areas more centrally located.
    - Target lesions have a central dusky or purple zone surrounded by a pale edematous ring with a peripheral erythematous margin.
- The lesions are symmetric.
    - Most common locations are the dorsum of hands and forearms.
    - Often found on palms, trunk, neck, and face.
- Lesions tend to be grouped, especially around elbows and knees.
- Any part of the lesion may develop vesicles or bullae.
- Discrete oral lesions are present in more than 50% of children with erythema multiforme.
    - Oral lesions may begin as vesicles or bullae but rapidly become painful superficial erythematous erosions, often with yellowish-white pseudomembrane formation.

ETIOLOGY

- Most children with erythema multiforme have preceding HSV infection.
- Up to 50% have noted herpes labialis infection.
- Controversy exists regarding the role of medications and *Mycoplasma pneumoniae* infection.

DIAGNOSIS (Dx)

DIFFERENTIAL DIAGNOSIS

- Giant urticaria (lesions < 24 hours at any one site)
- Vasculitis
- Systemic lupus erythematosus
- Fixed drug eruptions

WORKUP

- Diagnosis is usually made on the basis of a characteristic clinical picture.

TREATMENT (Rx)

NONPHARMACOLOGIC THERAPY

- Because the disease is self-limiting, one may simply follow course without intervention.
- Biopsy is rarely needed to confirm the diagnosis.
- No therapeutic surgical procedure is available.

ACUTE GENERAL Rx

- Symptomatic therapy is initiated, with oral antihistamines for burning or itching.
- Recurrent HSV-associated erythema multiforme may benefit from acyclovir prophylaxis (10 mg/kg/day) for 6 to 12 months.
- No studies support the use of oral steroids.

PEARLS & CONSIDERATIONS

COMMENTS

- Target lesions appear predominately on upper extremities.
- Individual lesions appear fixed at the same skin site for 7 days or more.
    - Multiforme applies to each lesion.
    - Lesions do not migrate like they do with urticaria.

SUGGESTED READINGS

American Academy of Dermatology. Available at www.aad.org

Carder KR: Hypersensitivity reactions in neonates and infants. *Dermatol Ther* 18(2):160, 2005.

Shin HT, Chang MW: Drug eruptions in children. *Curr Probl Pediatr* 31(7):207, 2001.

Society for Pediatric Dermatology. Available at www.spdnet.org

Yeung AK, Goldman RD: Use of steroids for erythema multiforme in children. *Can Fam Physician* 51:1481, 2005.

AUTHOR: **SUSAN HALLER PSAILA, MD**

BASIC INFORMATION

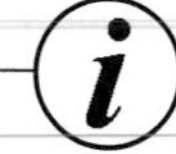

DEFINITION

Erythema nodosum is an inflammatory reaction pattern in the skin to several inciting factors; it is the most common type of panniculitis.

ICD-9-CM CODE
695.2 Erythema nodosum

EPIDEMIOLOGY & DEMOGRAPHICS

- The greatest incidence occurs during spring and fall; it is less common during summer.
- It can occur at any age.
- Male:female ratio is approximately equal in children.
- Racial and geographic incidences vary, depending on prevalence of diseases that are etiologic factors.

CLINICAL PRESENTATION

- Cutaneous eruption is sometimes associated with low-grade fever, malaise, fatigue, cough, arthralgia, headache, and conjunctivitis.
- Abdominal pain, vomiting, and diarrhea may also appear with the skin findings.
- Symmetric, tender, erythematous, warm nodules and plaques are present.
- Lesions range in size from 1 to 15 cm and may number from 1 to 10.
- The lesions usually manifest bilaterally, on distal anterior lower extremities.
- More extensive cases can involve the thighs, arms, neck, and rarely, the face.
- Ulceration is not seen, and nodules heal without atrophy or scarring.
- Eruptions last 3 to 6 weeks on average; lesions flatten and become less erythematous during this time.
- Lesions may recur, and some patients may develop chronic and persistent forms.

ETIOLOGY

- Numerous causes exist, including infections, medications, malignant diseases, and a wide group of miscellaneous conditions.
- Streptococcal and respiratory infections are the most common etiologies in children.
- In young adult women, birth control pills are a common cause of this condition.
- In the past, primary tuberculosis was a common cause.
- The cause is unknown in up to 20% of cases.

DIAGNOSIS

DIFFERENTIAL DIAGNOSIS

- Common bruises
- Cellulitis/erysipelas
- Deep fungal infections
- Insect bites
- Deep thrombophlebitis
- Angiitis
- Erythema induratum
- Fat-destructive panniculitis

WORKUP

- The diagnosis is usually made on the basis of the characteristic clinical picture.
- If in doubt, bacterial and fungal cultures and skin biopsy may help clarify the diagnosis.

TREATMENT

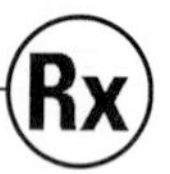

NONPHARMACOLOGIC THERAPY

- The lesions usually regress spontaneously.
- Identification and treatment of underlying cause is necessary.
- Bed rest with leg elevation is useful in patients who are experiencing severe discomfort.

ACUTE GENERAL Rx

- Nonsteroidal anti-inflammatory drugs are helpful when pain, inflammation, or arthralgia is prominent.
- Intralesional corticosteroids often cause rapid involution of lesions.
- Systemic corticosteroids are not indicated, especially if an underlying infectious cause has not been ruled out.

SUGGESTED READINGS

American Academy of Dermatology. Available at www.aad.org

Callen JP: Neutrophilic dermatoses. *Dermatol Clin* 20(3):409, 2002.

Society for Pediatric Dermatology. Available at www.spdnet.org

Sutra-Loubet C et al: Neutrophilic panniculitis. *J Am Acad Dermatol* 50(2):280, 2004.

Ter Poorten MC, Thiers BH: Panniculitis. *Dermatol Clin* 20(3):421, 2002.

AUTHOR: **SUSAN HALLER PSAILA, MD**

BASIC INFORMATION

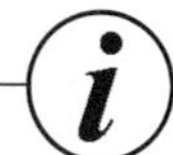

DEFINITIONS

Esophageal atresia is a congenital interruption or discontinuity of the esophagus resulting in esophageal obstruction. Tracheoesophageal fistula (TEF) is an abnormal communication (i.e., fistula) between the esophagus and trachea. Atresia or fistula can occur alone (8% and 4%, respectively), but in 86% of patients, both abnormalities are present, with an upper esophageal pouch and a fistula from the trachea to the lower esophageal segment.

SYNONYMS

Esophageal atresia
Tracheoesophageal fistula

ICD-9-CM CODE

750.3 Congenital esophageal atresia with or without tracheoesophageal fistula

EPIDEMIOLOGY & DEMOGRAPHICS

- The incidence is 1 case in 4500 live births.
- The male-to-female ratio is 1.26:1.
- Chromosomal anomalies (i.e., trisomy 13 or 18) occur in 6.6% of patients.
- Polyhydramnios is common.
- Associated anomalies include the following and occur in 50% to 70% of patients
    - Most common in pure EA and least common in TEF without atresia
    - VACTERL (**v**ertebral, **a**norectal, **c**ardiac, **t**racheal, **e**sophageal, **r**enal, **l**imb) association
    - Cardiac abnormalities most common (approximately 35%) and account for most deaths
    - Pure EA associated with the CHARGE syndrome (**c**oloboma, **h**eart defects, **a**tresia choanae, developmental **r**etardation, **g**enital hypoplasia, **e**ar deformities)

CLINICAL PRESENTATION

History

- Prenatal ultrasound may demonstrate a small fetal stomach with polyhydramnios.
- Most infants are symptomatic in the first few hours of life.
- EA results in pooling of oral secretions and feedings into a blind upper esophageal pouch, causing excessive drooling, coughing, choking, and regurgitation.
- TEF results in spillage of gastrointestinal secretions into the trachea, causing cyanosis, coughing, tachypnea, chemical pneumonitis, and wheezing.
- In patients with pure TEF but without EA, symptoms are less evident at birth. They usually have repeated episodes of aspiration or pneumonia associated with feeding.

Physical Examination

- Associated VACTERL abnormalities
    - **V**ertebral: meningocele, myelomeningocele
    - **A**norectal: imperforate or anteriorly displaced anus, anal stenosis
    - Abnormal **c**ardiac examination
    - **L**imb abnormalities: absent radius, thumb
- Inability to pass a nasogastric tube into the stomach
- Stigmata of chromosomal abnormalities: trisomy 13, trisomy 18
- Wheezing or diminished breath sounds

ETIOLOGY

- Abnormal embryogenesis of the esophagus and trachea is caused by unknown factors.
- The condition results from alteration of the rate and timing of cell proliferation and differentiation during the separation of the esophagus and developing lung bud.
- Environmental teratogens may have a role: prolonged maternal exposure to contraceptives, exposure to progesterone and estrogens during pregnancy, infants of diabetic mothers, and infants exposed to thalidomide.

DIAGNOSIS

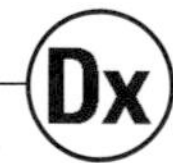

DIFFERENTIAL DIAGNOSIS

- Gastroesophageal reflux (GER)
- Laryngotracheoesophageal cleft
- Tracheomalacia
- Premature (surfactant-deficient) lungs
- Vascular ring

IMAGING STUDIES

- Plain chest and abdominal radiographs
    - It is important to exclude congenital heart disease.
    - Confirm the inability to pass a nasogastric tube into the stomach, and evaluate how far the nasoesophageal tube is able to be passed into the thorax (i.e., how close to the carina).
    - Evaluate the ribs and vertebrae.
    - Look for a gasless abdomen; the combination of a gasless abdomen and the inability to pass a nasogastric tube into the stomach is diagnostic of pure EA without fistula.
- Echocardiogram
    - Use echocardiography to exclude intracardiac abnormalities.
    - Determine which side the aortic arch is on; this finding dictates on which side to perform a thoracotomy.
- Ultrasound of spine to exclude tethered cord, occult myelomeningocele
- Esophagogram to look for a TEF
    - This study should be done only after EA has been excluded by passage of the nasogastric tube into the stomach.
    - Study is not necessary if EA has already been demonstrated.

TREATMENT

Rx

NONPHARMACOLOGIC THERAPY

Minimize the aspiration of gastrointestinal and salivary secretions by using a nasoesophageal tube to suction secretions and by placing the infant in an upright position.

ACUTE GENERAL Rx

- The specific surgical approach is dictated by patient presentation.
    - In an otherwise healthy child with the most common anomaly (i.e., EA with distal TEF), thoracotomy is performed with division of the fistula and primary end-to-end esophageal reanastomosis.
    - In a premature child with respiratory distress syndrome and an inability to ventilate, emergent thoracotomy is performed with division of TEF only. No attempt is made to reestablish esophageal continuity initially. The resistance to air inflation of the lungs is high; the positive-pressure air preferentially goes down the trachea, across the fistula, and into the stomach. This causes gastric distention, with a greater risk for aspiration of gastrointestinal secretions and more difficulty with diaphragm movement.
    - In an older infant with TEF and without EA, neck incision is performed with division and repair of the fistula (thoracotomy is not usually necessary).
    - Placement of a gastrostomy tube only is indicated for palliation for an infant with complex congenital heart disease or extreme low birth weight (<1000 g) who does not have significant respiratory difficulty; the gastrostomy helps prevent the spillover of gastric contents into the trachea during the period required for care of the cardiac lesion or prematurity.
    - Placement of a gastrostomy tube only is indicated in a patient with pure EA and without a fistula (i.e., gasless abdomen). The distance between the upper and lower esophageal segments is usually too great to allow for repair in the newborn period. A gastrostomy in this case allows feeding until the patient is of sufficient size (approximately 20 pounds) to reestablish esophageal continuity using a colon interposition or a tubularized portion of stomach to form a neoesophagus.

CHRONIC Rx

- Esophageal stricture may develop with onset of dysphagia or foreign body obstruction of the esophagus (i.e., meat or vegetable). Treatment is esophageal dilation.
- Gastroesophageal reflux is common.
    - Treatment with gastric neutralizing medications, positioning, and thickened, smaller-volume feeding
    - May require antireflux surgery if symptoms are severe or a cause of esophageal stricture
- Recurrent TEF has symptoms of coughing with feeding and recurrent pneumonias. Repeat surgery is required.

DISPOSITION

Patient outcome is most influenced by the presence and the severity of associated anomalies. In patients with the most common anomaly, oral feedings are begun after a water-soluble contrast study has excluded a leak or stricture at the site of the EA. This study is usually performed 5 to 10 days postoperatively.

REFERRAL

A board-certified pediatric surgeon should manage all infants and children with this anomaly, with the ready availability of pediatric subspecialists, including those from neonatology, anesthesia, urology, neurosurgery, gastroenterology, and cardiology.

PEARLS & CONSIDERATIONS

PATIENT/FAMILY EDUCATION

- American Academy of Family Physicians: www.aafp.org/afp/990215ap/910.html
- Family support groups: EA/TEF (www.eatef.org), www.familyvillage.org, and www.wisc.edu/libea-tef.html

SUGGESTED READINGS

Dillon PW, Cilley RE: Newborn surgical emergencies: gastrointestinal anomalies, abdominal wall defects. *Pediatr Clin North Am* 40:1289, 1993.

Engum SA et al: Analysis of morbidity and mortality in 227 cases of esophageal atresia and/or tracheoesophageal fistula over two decades. *Arch Surg* 130:502, 1995.

Foglia RP: Esophageal disease in the pediatric age group. *Chest Surg Clin North Am* 4:785, 1994.

Martin LW, Alexander F: Esophageal atresia. *Surg Clin North Am* 65:1099, 1985.

Spitz L: Esophageal atresia: past, present, and future. *J Pediatr Surg* 31:19, 1996.

Spitz L et al: Oesophageal atresia: at-risk groups for the 1990s. *J Pediatr Surg* 29:723, 1994.

AUTHOR: **BRAD W. WARNER, MD**

BASIC INFORMATION

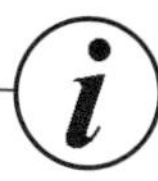

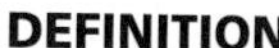

DEFINITION

The Ewing's sarcoma family of tumors consists of malignancies of neural origin that arise from postganglionic parasympathetic cholinergic neurons and that usually occur in bone. This family of tumors includes Ewing's tumor of bone (87%), extraosseous Ewing's tumor (8%), and peripheral primitive neuroectodermal tumors (PNETs) (5%). A PNET of the chest wall is known as Askin's tumor. Ewing's sarcoma and peripheral PNET are related but not identical tumors.

ICD-9-CM CODE

170.9 Malignant neoplasm of bone and articular cartilage

EPIDEMIOLOGY & DEMOGRAPHICS

- Ewing's sarcoma and PNET represent approximately 3% of pediatric cancers.
- Ewing's sarcoma is the most common malignant bone tumor in children younger than 10 years.
- The incidence is 2 to 3 cases per 1 million whites per year; it is rare in patients of African or Asian descent. There are approximately 200 new cases each year in the United States.
- Approximately 27% of patients are diagnosed in the first decade of life, 64% in the second decade, and 9% in the third decade.
- The incidence is slightly greater in males than in females.
- Primary sites are as follows:
    - Central (overall): 47%
        - Pelvis: 45%
        - Chest wall: 34%
        - Spine and paravertebral: 12%
        - Head and neck: 9%
    - Extremity (overall): 53%
        - Distal: 52%
        - Proximal: 48%

CLINICAL PRESENTATION

History

- Pain
- Mass lesion
- Limited range of motion
- Pathologic fracture
- Systemic symptoms, including fever and fatigue
- Respiratory distress caused by chest tumor or pleural effusion

Physical Examination

- A mass may be palpable, or tenderness may be associated with a site of pain.
- Central axis lesions, such as pelvic primaries, may not be palpable.
- Decreased breath sounds may be heard in patients with Askin's tumor.

ETIOLOGY

- No environmental risk factors are identified.
- Reports of Ewing's tumors in patients with congenital abnormalities, constitutional chromosomal abnormalities, or skeletal abnormalities are probably the result of chance.

DIAGNOSIS

Dx

DIFFERENTIAL DIAGNOSIS

- Osteosarcoma, but Ewing's sarcoma more likely for a central axis or diaphyseal lesion
- Other primary or metastatic malignancy, including rhabdomyosarcoma and other soft tissue sarcomas, lymphoma, and neuroblastoma
- Benign bone tumors
- Infection
- Traumatic lesions

WORKUP

- Biopsy of primary lesion (initial resection usually not possible or recommended)
- Bilateral bone marrow aspirates and biopsies as part of the metastatic evaluation (11% of metastases)
- Pathology
    - The neoplasm is one of the small, blue-cell tumors of childhood.
    - Peripheral PNET is the more differentiated form in this family of tumors.
    - A characteristic chromosomal translocation t(11;22) is present in 90% to 95% of tumors in the Ewing's family, and t(21;22) occurs in 5% to 10% of tumors, both resulting in related aberrant transcription factors. The specific fusion transcripts are independently associated with stage of disease and survival. These translocations occur rarely in other tumors.

LABORATORY TESTS

No diagnostic laboratory tests are available.

IMAGING STUDIES

- Obtain plain x-ray films of the symptomatic area ("onion peel" appearance of bone lesions is not sensitive or specific).
- Magnetic resonance imaging (MRI) of the primary lesion is useful.
- Metastatic evaluation includes the following:
    - Chest radiograph
    - Computed tomography (CT) of the chest (38% of metastases)
    - Bone scan (31% of metastases)
- There is no commonly used staging system. Patients are stratified by the presence or absence of detectable metastases. Approximately 25% of patients have detectable metastases at diagnosis, although more than 80% have at least microscopic metastases.

TREATMENT

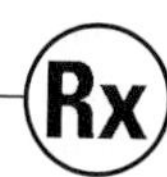

NONPHARMACOLOGIC THERAPY

- Surgical removal may be considered if the lesion is resectable without resulting in unacceptable cosmetic or functional impairment.
- Radiation may be used in place of surgery for unresectable tumors or in addition to surgery if the resection is not complete or tumor is found too close to the margins of resection.

ACUTE GENERAL Rx

- The current standard is alternating cycles of vincristine, doxorubicin, and cyclophosphamide plus ifosfamide or VP-16. Investigations are studying the benefits of cycles of chemotherapy every 2 weeks versus every 3 weeks.
- Chemotherapy is given neoadjuvantly, before radiation therapy or surgery for local control, and after radiation therapy or surgery.
- Another active agent is topotecan.
- Role of myeloablative therapy with hematopoietic stem cell rescue may be considered for metastatic or recurrent disease, but it remains under investigation.

DISPOSITION

- The most significant adverse prognostic factor is the presence of metastatic disease.
- Response to treatment correlates with survival.
- Current prognosis is as follows:
    - Approximately 70% rate of 5-year survival for localized disease
    - Less than 30% rate of 5-year survival for patients with metastatic disease
- MRI or CT scans of the primary lesion, a chest radiograph, CT scan of the chest, and a bone scan usually are obtained every 3 months for 1 year after completion of therapy, then every 4 to 6 months for 2 years, and then up to every year until 10 years off therapy.
- The late effects of chemotherapy may include renal tubular dysfunction, cardiomyopathy, infertility or early menopause, and secondary malignancies, including leukemia and bladder cancer.
- The late effects of irradiation depend on the radiation field but may include hypoplasia, leg length discrepancy, hair loss, gonadal failure, and secondary malignancy.
- Patients with limb-salvage surgery for local control may experience infectious, traumatic, or other complications, and they need long-term follow-up by the orthopedic surgeon.

REFERRAL

Patients, including adults younger than 30 years of age, should be referred to pediatric oncologists and treated on formal protocol therapy, if available. Treatment decisions should be made in conjunction with radiation oncologists and surgeons with the appropriate oncologic expertise.

PEARLS & CONSIDERATIONS

COMMENTS

- Persistent pain, even after trauma, or pain associated with a mass lesion should be evaluated with a plain x-ray film of the involved area.
- Even bone tumors with a benign appearance should be evaluated by an experienced orthopedic surgeon.
- Because medical oncologists rarely see patients with Ewing's sarcoma, young adults with this disease should be referred to pediatric oncologists. Referral should take place at the same time as referral to orthopedic surgeon for suspicious lesions.

PREVENTION

No preventive interventions are available for Ewing's sarcomas.

PATIENT/FAMILY EDUCATION

- Although treatment is difficult, the benefits of chemotherapy, radiation therapy, and surgery are significant.
- Pediatric oncologists can refer patients and parents to local and national organizations for children with cancer and their families. National organizations include the American Cancer Society and CureSearch, a component of the Children's Oncology Group.
- More information is available on the Internet (www.curesearch.org, www.cancer.org).

SUGGESTED READINGS

Ginsberg JP et al: Ewing's sarcoma family of tumors: Ewing's sarcoma of bone and soft tissue and the peripheral primitive neuroectodermal tumors. *In* Pizzo PA, Poplack DG (eds): *Principles and Practice of Pediatric Oncology,* 4th ed. Philadelphia, Lippincott Williams & Wilkins, 2002, pp 972–1016.

Marcus KJ, Tarbell NJ: Ewing's sarcoma. *In* Halperin EC et al (eds): *Pediatric Radiation Oncology,* 4th ed. Philadelphia, Lippincott Williams & Wilkins, 2005, pp 271–290.

Rodriguez-Galindo C et al: Treatment of Ewing sarcoma family of tumors: Current status and outlook for the future. *Med Pediatr Oncol* 40:276, 2003.

AUTHOR: **ANDREA S. HINKLE, MD**

BASIC INFORMATION

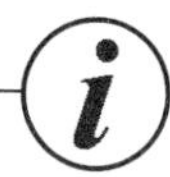

DEFINITION

Failure to thrive (FTT) refers to subnormal growth in a young child that is not caused by known hormonal or genetic syndromes. There is no agreement on a single criterion. Weight gain is lower than expected for age, and the growth curve may cross major percentile lines; weight-for-age and weight-for-height values are typically below the 5th (or 3rd) percentile on Centers for Disease Control and Prevention (CDC) growth charts. FTT is a clinical sign, not a specific diagnosis. The causes are often nonorganic (e.g., neglect, abnormal dietary practices, psychological distress) and organic (e.g., gastroesophageal reflux, oral-motor incoordination, food intolerance). Uncorrected, FTT is associated with long-term cognitive and behavioral impairment.

SYNONYMS

Growth delay or growth failure
Stunting (i.e., below-normal height-for-age)
Wasting (i.e., below-normal weight-for-height)

ICD-9-CM CODE

783.4 Failure to thrive

EPIDEMIOLOGY & DEMOGRAPHICS

- FFT affects 1% to 2% of hospitalized children.
- FFT affects 5% to 10% of children in poverty.
- FFT typically affects children between birth and 5 years old.
- The incidence is equal for boys and girls.

CLINICAL PRESENTATION

- FTT is most accurately detected using standard growth charts. Mild FTT may not be apparent on casual inspection, because the cheeks often remain chubby even with moderate wasting.
- Look for signs of moderate to severe malnutrition: decreased energy, thin arms and legs, dry skin, and sparse or lanugo hair.
- Look for abnormal posture and behavior: lying on back, elbows flexed with hands at the sides of the head, and more eye contact with distant than near adults.
- In taking the medical history, assess the following:
  - Prenatal care, infections, exposures, labor and delivery course
  - Early growth pattern and age of onset of delays (best seen on growth charts)
  - Central nervous system: swallowing difficulty (i.e., choking), tactile hypersensitivity
  - Respiratory system: snoring, shortness of breath, chronic cough
  - Cardiovascular system: exercise or feeding intolerance
  - Gastrointestinal tract: choking, spitting, vomiting, constipation, greasy or pale stools, excessive gas, distention
  - Infectious diseases: travel, exposures (e.g., living in a shelter), recurrent infections
  - Allergy: food, environmental reactions, atopy
  - Family history: genetic diseases, atopy, immune deficiency; parental heights and weights
- The nutritional assessment should include the following:
  - Twenty-four-hour diet recall
  - Determining who is responsible for feeding and food preparation
  - Formula preparation (mixed correctly?), intake of juice, milk, water
  - Introduction of solids, timing, any special reaction
  - Feeding pattern, feeding behaviors, feeding environment (e.g., highchair, TV, others at table, typical events surrounding mealtime)
- The developmental assessment should include the following:
  - Milestones, especially gross motor, fine motor, language, self-care, autonomy
  - Family history of developmental delays
  - Services in place (e.g., early intervention)
  - Results of screening questionnaires or tests
- The social and emotional assessment should include the following:
  - Family, home constellation, child care (i.e., center-based versus family child care)
  - Financial status, food availability
  - Separations, trauma (e.g., physical or emotional injury, family or neighborhood violence, deaths)
  - Parental mental health: depression, substance abuse, parents' early childhood experiences
- A thorough physical examination should look especially for neurologic abnormalities, adenoidal facies, dental lesions, heart murmur, clubbing, abdominal distention, surgical scars, and signs of abuse.

ETIOLOGY

- Multiple causal factors are common.
- Inadequate intake occurs in approximately 80% of cases. Food may not be available, not offered, or refused, or there may be excessive intake of low-calorie food (e.g., excessive juice). Causes include psychosocial and family stressors (e.g., poverty), subtle oral-motor deficits, parent-child relationship problems, an acquired food aversion, and neglect or abuse.
- Excessive losses may occur through vomiting (e.g., pyloric stenosis, gastroesophageal reflux), chronic diarrhea, malabsorption (e.g., cystic fibrosis, short-gut syndrome, gluten enteropathy).
- Inefficient metabolism may be caused by hypothyroidism, cyanotic heart disease, genetic syndromes, or psychosocial dwarfism (rare).
- Increased needs may reflect congenital heart disease, hyperthyroidism, immunodeficiency, other chronic illnesses, and underheated homes in cold climates.

DIAGNOSIS

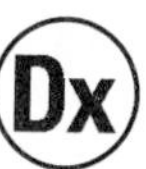

DIFFERENTIAL DIAGNOSIS

Consider a broad differential diagnosis in medical, nutritional, developmental, and social areas.

WORKUP

- Limit screening laboratory tests to a few common ones.
  - Complete blood cell count and differential cell count (i.e., anemia and decreased lymphocytes as sign of malnutrition and an elevated white blood cell count as sign of chronic infection)
  - Electrolytes (i.e., metabolic acidosis as cause or complication)
  - Urinalysis and culture (i.e., chronic infection)
  - Purified protein derivative (i.e., tuberculosis) and controls (i.e., anergy is likely with malnutrition)
  - Lead (if exposure possible)
- Other investigations as indicated by history (see Table 1-9)
- The best index of acute malnutrition is the patient's weight as a percentage of the ideal weight (fiftieth percentile) on the weight-for-height curve (see Table 1-10).

LABORATORY TESTS

Other than screening, test only as suggested by the history or physical examination results. For example, consider stool ova and parasites if there is a history of travel or residence in a shelter or if the patient has abdominal distention or cramping.

IMAGING STUDIES

No imaging is indicated for screening purposes. Use imaging studies as dictated by the clinical presentation.

TREATMENT

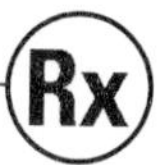

NONPHARMACOLOGIC THERAPY

- Treat underlying medical diagnoses.
- Intensity of therapy is tied to the severity of undernutrition.
- Level I care: primary provider alone
  - Nutritional counseling to increase caloric density of feedings (e.g., mix formula with less water; use whole milk, cream, and added fats and oils; restrict lower-calorie beverages)
  - Daily multivitamin with zinc and iron (i.e., zinc deficiency, a result of undernutrition, causes taste bud dysfunction)
  - Guidance to improve mealtime structure and behaviors: three meals and three snacks without "grazing" in between, highchair, turn off the television, mild approval for eating, no forced feedings
  - Close monitoring; if no catch-up, move to level II

TABLE 1-9 Historical Clues

History	Diagnostic Consideration	Investigation
Spitting, vomiting	Gastroesophogeal reflux	Upper gastrointestinal series, pH probe, esophagoscopy
Abdominal distention	Malabsorption (e.g., cystic fibrosis, celiac disease, lactase deficiency)	D-Xylose test, stool fat, antigliadin titer or biopsy, sweat chloride*
Travel to or from developing country; homeless, overcrowded, or living in shelter	Parasitosis (especially *Giardia*), tuberculosis, inadequate access to cooking facility and refrigeration	Stool O & P, duodenal biopsy, string test, PPD
Snoring, periodic breathing during sleep, restless sleep, noisy or mouth breathing	Adenoid hypertrophy	Lateral neck film (soft tissues and airway)
"Asthma"	Chronic aspiration, cystic fibrosis	Chest film, milk scan, sweat chloride*
Frequent (minor) infections	HIV, other immune deficiency	Serologic tests, immunoglobulins,* PPD with control for anergy*

HIV, Human immunodeficiency virus; O & P, stool for ova and parasites; PPD, purified protein derivative.
*May be abnormal secondary to malnutrition.

TABLE 1-10 Grading Severity of Failure to Thrive

Weight-for-Height Percentage	Grade of Undernutrition	Severity	Level of Care
Ideal			
≥90	0	Pre-FTT or normal	I: Outpatient management by primary physician
≥80 to <90	1	Mild	I or II: Consider adding home visiting, social work
≥70 to <80	2	Moderate	II or III: Consider hospitilization
<70	3	Severe	III: Hospitalize immediately

FTT, Failure to thrive.

- Level II care: outpatient team
  - Home visits by nutritionist and social worker to assess mealtime interactions and environment and to intervene in the patient's environment
  - Referral for developmental and behavioral intervention (e.g., center- or home-based early intervention program)
  - Recruitment of community supports as needed (e.g., parent support groups, respite, mental health treatment for parents)
  - Continued close monitoring; if no catch-up, consider moving to level III care
- Level III care: multidisciplinary in-hospital team or day hospital
  - Intensive feeding therapy
  - Intensive parent support, parent training, and family intervention
  - Consider referral to a tertiary care facility with an established FTT team
- Move more quickly to higher levels of care depending on child's age and grade of undernutrition (see Table 1-9).

ACUTE GENERAL Rx

- For severe, acute nutritional rehabilitation, limit feeds initially to prevent overfeeding.
- Cyproheptadine as an adjunct to nutritional therapy may facilitate catch-up by reducing satiation.

CHRONIC Rx

- Depending on age and size, full catch-up may require months.
- Educational interventions, parent training, social support networks are all important in the long-term care of a child with FTT.

DISPOSITION

Most children with FTT can be cared for as outpatients. Hospitalize only severe, recalcitrant cases.

REFERRAL

Refer moderate to severe cases to multidisciplinary teams.

PEARLS & CONSIDERATIONS

COMMENTS

- The term *failure to thrive* puts parents on the defensive; they tend to see it as their own failure. The term *growth deficiency* is less stigmatizing.
- Multimodal, coordinated team management works better for established FTT.
- Avoid the temptation to order "shotgun" testing, but aggressively follow-up on any hint from the history or physical examination results.
- Remember to work simultaneously in four areas: medical, nutritional, developmental, and social.
- Use a flowchart to track weight and weight gain in grams per day to avoid under-detection and under-treating.

PREVENTION

- Plot weight on growth curves at every routine infant and toddler visit.
- Pay special attention to children at risk because of single parenting or low income; however, FTT can affect children with no identified risks.

PATIENT/FAMILY EDUCATION

Empathy from treating physicians gives the parents crucial support. Otherwise, parents who feel guilty and defensive will not feed effectively and may be unable to attend to professional suggestions.

SUGGESTED READINGS

Drotar D: Failure to thrive. *In* Routh D (eds): *Handbook of Pediatric Psychology.* New York, Guildford Press, 1988.

Frank DA, Zeisel SH: Failure to thrive. *Pediatr Clin North Am* 35:1187, 1988.

Kessler D, Dawson P (eds): *Failure to Thrive and Pediatric Undernutrition: A Transdisciplinary Approach.* Philadelphia, Paul H. Brookes, 1999.

AUTHOR: **ROBERT NEEDLMAN, MD**

BASIC INFORMATION

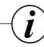

DEFINITION

A febrile seizure is one occurring in the presence of fever higher than 38.0°C in a child between the ages of 6 months and 6 years of age. Excluded are patients with a history of afebrile seizures, electrolyte abnormality, or central nervous system (CNS) infection. Simple febrile seizures last less than 15 minutes, are generalized, and if occurring in a series, have a total duration less than 30 minutes. Complex febrile seizures last more than 15 minutes, are focal, or occur in a series with total duration longer than 30 minutes.

SYNONYM

Febrile convulsions

ICD-9-CM CODE
780.31 Febrile seizure

EPIDEMIOLOGY & DEMOGRAPHICS

- Occur in 2% to 4% of children
- Two and a half times higher incidence in first-degree relatives compared with the population at large

CLINICAL PRESENTATION

History

- Most febrile seizures occur on the first day of illness.
- The seizure is often the presenting symptom.
- Most febrile seizures are of the simple type (90%), with brief bilateral clonic or tonicoclonic movements and no postictal paralysis or prolonged somnolence.

Physical Examination

- Temperature $\geq$ 38.0°C
- Examination may demonstrate a focus of infection.
- Assess neurologic examination carefully:
  - Mental status
  - Meningeal signs
  - Focal neurologic deficits

ETIOLOGY

- Genetic factors play a role in expression.
  - Single febrile seizure: polygenic model
  - Multiple episodes: dominant with incomplete penetrance
  - Specific genetic loci have been identified on several chromosomes from different families associated with susceptibility to febrile seizures.
- Risk factors
  - Primary human herpesvirus 6 (HHV6) infection is associated with febrile seizures, particularly complex types.
  - Increased risk noted after immunization with pertussis and measles-mumps-rubella (MMR) vaccines.
- Pertussis vaccine increases risk on first day after immunization and only when whole cell pertussis is used (acellular pertussis risk is much less).
- MMR vaccine increases risk of febrile seizure 8 to 14 days after vaccination.
- Vaccine-associated febrile seizures are not linked to risk of developing epilepsy, learning, behavioral, or psychiatric disorders.

DIAGNOSIS

DIFFERENTIAL DIAGNOSIS

- Most important differential diagnosis is meningitis or encephalitis.
- Chills are fine, rhythmic, oscillatory movements about a joint, not clonic in nature.
- Focal febrile seizures may need to be differentiated from seizures caused by CNS mass lesions (e.g., tumor, intracranial bleeding).

LABORATORY TESTS

- Routine laboratory studies (including neuroimaging and electroencephalogram [EEG]) are not indicated in most cases of simple febrile seizures.
- Examination of cerebrospinal fluid should be carried out according to the following:
  - Lumbar puncture should be strongly considered in any infant younger than 12 months of age because clinical signs of meningitis are not reliable in this age group.
  - Between 12 and 18 months of age, lumbar puncture should be considered.
  - Older than 18 months of age, lumbar puncture is indicated only when meningeal signs are present or if an adequate neurologic examination cannot be performed.
- If clinically indicated, obtain a complete blood count and blood and urine cultures (to rule out bacteremia and urinary tract infection).
- Complex febrile seizures may warrant further investigation when indicated.
  - Stat blood glucose, electrolytes, Ca^{2+}, Mg^{2+} if prolonged seizure or postictal somnolence
- EEG or computed tomography/magnetic resonance imaging scan of the head if a focal seizure or persistent neurologic deficit is detected with a complex febrile seizure.

TREATMENT

NONPHARMACOLOGIC THERAPY

- Protection of the airway is the most important therapeutic intervention in the seizing child.
  - Provide oxygen
  - Position the head

ACUTE GENERAL Rx

- Administer antipyretics, such as acetaminophen 15 mg/kg orally or rectally; ibuprofen 8 to 10 mg/kg orally.
- Any patient with a seizure lasting more than 15 minutes should be treated with midazolam 0.1 mg/kg intravenously or rectally; the dose may be repeated two more times in 5-minute intervals if the seizure persists.
- Diazepam (Valium®) rectal gel (0.5 mg/kg) may also be used.
- Administer Phenytoin (Dilantin) 15 to 20 mg/kg intravenously slow load if midazolam is ineffective.
- Administer phenobarbital 15 to 20 mg/kg intravenously slow load for recalcitrant seizures.

DISPOSITION

- The child should be observed until both the health care provider and parents are satisfied with the child's appearance after the temperature is reduced.
- Follow-up may be needed if blood and urine cultures are obtained.

REFERRAL

- Consultation with a pediatric neurologist is recommended in the following cases:
  - Complex febrile seizures
  - When considering use of prophylactic anticonvulsant for recurrent febrile seizures

PEARLS & CONSIDERATIONS

COMMENTS

- A brief, generalized seizure from which the child recovers quickly to baseline neurologic status is unlikely to be caused by meningitis.

PREVENTION

- Early administration of antipyretics during febrile illnesses is advocated; however, their efficacy is limited.
- Daily prophylactic use of anticonvulsants has a very limited role.
  - Modest efficacy (66% reduction in recurrence) must be weighed against adverse effects on behavior and sleep patterns.
  - Patients with simple febrile seizures are not candidates for prophylactic anticonvulsants.
  - Appropriate candidates are those with prolonged and frequent seizures.
  - Prophylactic anticonvulsant treatment does not appear to reduce the sequelae of prolonged seizures or subsequent development of epilepsy.
  - The first-line prophylactic anticonvulsant is phenobarbital.
- Rectal administration of diazepam at the time of febrile illness is also a treatment option.

PATIENT/FAMILY EDUCATION

- For simple febrile seizures, there is no risk of brain injury.
- Most simple febrile seizures do not indicate any underlying brain abnormality.

- Overall, the risk of recurrence of febrile seizures is 30%.
- Increased incidence of recurrence associated with independent risk factors:
  - Early age of first seizure
  - History of febrile seizures in first-degree relative
  - Low degree of fever in outpatient setting (emergency department, office)
  - Brief duration between onset of fever and initial seizure
- The incidence of subsequent epilepsy in children having a febrile seizure is increased (1%) compared with the incidence of epilepsy in the general population (0.5%).
- The risks of recurrence of febrile seizures or development of subsequent epilepsy are increased in children with a history of developmental delay or complex febrile seizures.

SUGGESTED READINGS

Barlow WE et al: The risk of seizures after receipt of whole-cell pertussis or measles, mumps, and rubella vaccine. *N Engl J Med* 345:656, 2001.

Berg AT et al: Predictors of recurrent febrile seizures. A prospective cohort study. *Arch Pediatr Adolesc Med* 151:371, 1997.

Epilepsy Foundation of America. Available at www.efa.org/news/fever.html

Fenichel GM: Paroxysmal disorders. *In Clinical Pediatric Neurology: A Signs Symptoms Approach,* 5th ed. Philadelphia, Elsevier Saunders, 2005, pp 17–18.

Fishman AF: Febrile seizures. *In* McMillan JA et al (eds): *Oski's Pediatrics.* Philadelphia, Lippincott Williams & Wilkins, 2005, pp 1949–1952.

Suga S et al: Clinical characteristics of febrile convulsions during primary HHV-6 infection. *Arch Dis Child* 82:62, 2000.

AUTHOR: **PAUL LEHOULLIER, MD**

BASIC INFORMATION

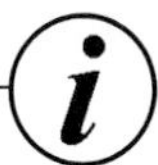

DEFINITION

Fibroadenoma is a benign neoplasm of the breast that is characterized by localized proliferation of breast ducts and stroma.

SYNONYM

Biphasic tumor (i.e., tumor involving epithelial and stromal elements)

ICD-9-CM CODE
217.00 Fibroadenoma of breast

EPIDEMIOLOGY & DEMOGRAPHICS

- Fibroadenomas account for 70% to 95% of biopsied breast masses in adolescents.
- These neoplasms are uncommon in males.
- The incidence tends to peak in late adolescence (17 to 20 years), but fibroadenomas can occur up to 2 years before menarche.

CLINICAL PRESENTATION

- Usually, the fibroadenoma is identified as an asymptomatic, incidental breast mass on examination by the patient or examiner. It is a nontender, rubbery mass, and it enlarges over several weeks or months.
- The mass does not vary significantly in size during menstrual cycles, but it can grow significantly with large fluctuations in estrogen, especially during pregnancy.
- Nipple discharge does not occur.
- The fibroadenoma usually slips easily under examining fingers.
- It is usually unilateral; 25% of cases are bilateral or multiple growths.
- Large lesions can produce symptoms that are associated with malignancy, including peau d'orange and enlarged superficial veins.
- Can be 3 to 4 cm at the time of discovery, and if not removed, it can grow up to 15 cm in diameter.
- It can be found in any quadrant, but it is more common in the upper, outer quadrants.
- It is more common in black girls.

ETIOLOGY

- Fibroadenoma is likely a hormonally dependent form of nodular hyperplasia.
- The histologic similarity to male gynecomastia and virginal hyperplasia suggests an exaggerated response of localized tissue to estrogen.
- The tumor has estrogen receptors, and timing of growth is likely related to prolonged exposure to estrogen.

DIAGNOSIS

Dx

DIFFERENTIAL DIAGNOSIS

- Cystic breast disease
- Giant or juvenile fibroadenoma (i.e., fibroadenoma >5 cm in diameter and can double in 3 to 6 months)
- Cystosarcoma phyllodes (i.e., rare in adolescents but the most common malignant breast tumor in this age group)
- Virginal (juvenile) hypertrophy (i.e., idiopathic breast hypertrophy): extremely rapid, unilateral or bilateral growth of a breast immediately after thelarche
- Breast cancers (1% of all cancers in those younger than 20 years old and only 1% of breast cancers occur in those younger than 20 years old)
- Abscesses

WORKUP

- A small, well-defined, nontender, rubbery lesion in an adolescent or child can be expectantly observed over 2 to 4 months. Slow growth and no changes in symptoms are consistent with a fibroadenoma, which does not necessarily require additional workup.
- A conservative approach includes triple assessment (i.e., clinical surveillance, ultrasound, and cytology). Conservative measures need to be reassessed if the tumor increases in size.

LABORATORY TESTS

Core biopsy is the definitive evaluation of a solid breast mass.

IMAGING STUDIES

- Ultrasound can identify cystic lesions but cannot differentiate types of solid lesions (i.e., fibroadenomas versus cystosarcoma phyllodes).
- Ultrasound can identify multiple fibroadenomas, which can be useful in developing a treatment plan.
- Mammography is rarely useful in defining growths in women younger than 25 years.

TREATMENT

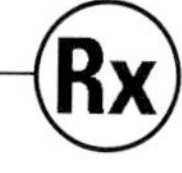

NONPHARMACOLOGIC THERAPY

Total excision is the most definitive treatment for single or enlarging masses.

ACUTE GENERAL Rx

- There is no standard approved or recommended pharmacotherapeutic treatment for fibroadenomas.
- Progestin therapy (i.e., 19-nortestosterone derivatives, used 15 to 20 days per cycle) can be considered.
- Estrogen antagonists (i.e., Tamoxifen) have been studied.

DISPOSITION

Triple evaluation (i.e., physical examination, ultrasound, and fine-needle aspiration [FNA]) can be used to classify the lesion as a fibroadenoma, and if it remains stable or regresses after 6 months, the patient can be discharged to clinical follow-up only.

REFERRAL

Refer the patient to a breast (surgical) specialist for definitive excision of breast mass and for diagnostic evaluation (i.e., FNA or core biopsy).

PEARLS & CONSIDERATIONS

!

COMMENTS

- Watchful waiting may not be prudent if the fibroadenoma is large, because excision may make cosmetic results less satisfactory.
- The patient and parents may opt for complete excision rather than face the anxiety of repeated clinical visits or diagnostic follow-up methods.

PATIENT/FAMILY EDUCATION

- Reassure the patient and parents that small masses with slow growth are commonly fibroadenomas and rarely breast cancer.
- Web sites provide more information: http://www.keepkidshealthy.com/

SUGGESTED READINGS

Duflos C et al: Breast diseases in adolescents. *Endocr Dev Basel* 7:183, 2004.

Greydanus DE et al: Breast disorders in children and adolescents. *Pediatr Clin North Am* 36:601, 1989.

AUTHOR: **GUS GIBBONS EMMICK, MD**

BASIC INFORMATION

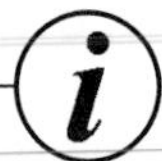

DEFINITION

Patients with fibromyalgia experience diffuse pain, have tender points demonstrated on physical examination, and have other symptoms but no inflammatory process or other diseases that can account for the discomfort.

SYNONYMS

Fibromyositis
Fibrositis
Juvenile primary fibromyalgia

ICD-9-CM CODE
729.0 Fibromyalgia syndrome

EPIDEMIOLOGY & DEMOGRAPHICS

- Fibromyalgia predominantly affects adolescent and adult white women.
- There have been few studies of the prevalence in children.
  - One cross-sectional analysis of 338 schoolchildren between the ages of 9 and 15 years yielded a prevalence of 6%.
  - Other studies have suggested a lower prevalence of 2%.

CLINICAL PRESENTATION

History

At diagnosis, patients typically describe a gradual accumulation of signs and symptoms.

- Widespread pain (above and below the waist and on both the right and left sides of the body) of the soft tissues, muscles, and tendons
- Fatigue
- Restless or nonrestorative sleep
- Headache
- Depressed mood
- Dizziness
- Abdominal pain and irritable bowel-like symptoms
- Dysmenorrhea
- Subjective swelling of hands
- Paresthesias in extremities

Physical Examination

- Tender points may occur in any of the 18 symmetric and characteristic sites (see Figure 1-6).
- Diagnostic criteria for fibromyalgia in adults stipulate at least 11 of 18 tender points (see Table 1-11).
- In adolescents, fewer points are more common.
- Examination technique: palpation of tender point with 4 kg of pressure

DIAGNOSIS

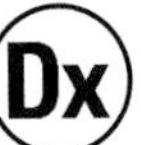

DIFFERENTIAL DIAGNOSIS

- Myofascial pain syndrome
- Chronic fatigue syndrome
- Depression
- Thyroid disease
- Hypermobility syndrome
- Somatization disorder

WORKUP

- Laboratory study results are normal, including a complete blood cell count with a differential cell count, erythrocyte sedimentation rate, and creatine phosphokinase level.
- Radiographs are normal.
- Muscle biopsy (not typically obtained) reveals no signs of inflammation.

TREATMENT

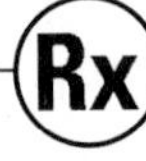

NONPHARMACOLOGIC THERAPY

- Initiate a consistent sleep-wake schedule (i.e., good sleep hygiene).
- Encourage regular, moderate exercise.
- Explore psychotherapy options.
- Reinstitute a daily routine, school attendance, and other regular schedules and activities.

ACUTE GENERAL Rx

- Consider low-dose tricyclic medication 1 to 2 hours before bedtime to restore restful sleep.
- Consider a low-dose selective serotonin reuptake inhibitor, particularly if fibromyalgia is associated with significant depression.
- Nonsteroidal anti-inflammatory drugs are not usually beneficial but are sometimes useful.

DISPOSITION

- Patients require regular contact with health care providers; improvement occurs gradually.
- Despite attainment of remission, recurrence of symptoms is common, particularly in times of stress or with erratic sleep-wake schedules.

REFERRAL

Referral to a physical therapist, occupational therapist, or psychotherapist/counselor may be necessary.

PEARLS & CONSIDERATIONS

COMMENTS

- Adolescents may have only a few tender points.
- Palpation of tender points requires significant pressure (4 kg).
- A consistent sleep-wake schedule (even on weekends) is important.
- Every effort should be made to have the patient attend school.

PREVENTION

Anticipation of stressful events or disruption of the sleep-wake schedule is a time to intensify therapy, which can decrease the severity and duration of the disease flare.

TABLE 1-11 1990 Criteria for the Classification of Fibromyalgia

History of widespread pain*

Definition: Pain is considered widespread when all of the following are present:

- Pain exists in the left side of the body, pain in the right side of the body, pain above the waist, and pain below the waist.
- Axial skeletal pain (cervical spine or anterior chest or thoracic spine or low back) also must be present.
- Shoulder and buttock pain is considered as pain for each involved site.
- Low back pain is considered lower segment pain.

Pain in 11 of 18 tender point sites on digital palpation*

Definition: Pain on digital palpation must be present in at least 11 of the following 18 sites:

- Occiput: bilateral, at the suboccipital muscle insertions
- Low cervical: bilateral, at the anterior aspects of the intertransverse spaces at C5 to C7
- Trapezius: bilateral, two sets, one above the scapula spine near the medial border the other at the midportion of the spinous process of the scapula (see Figure 1-6)
- Second rib: bilateral, at the second costochondral junctions, just lateral to the junctions on the upper surfaces
- Lateral epicondyle: bilateral, 1 cm distal to the epicondyles
- Gluteal: bilateral, in upper outer quadrants of buttocks in anterior fold of muscle
- Great trochanter: bilateral, posterior to the trochanteric prominence
- Knee: bilateral, at the medial fat pad proximal to the joint line

Digital palpation should be performed with an approximate force of 4 kg.

For a tender point to be considered positive for pain, the subject must state that the palpation was painful. *Tender* is not considered *painful*.

*For classification purposes, patients are said to have fibromyalgia if both criteria are satisfied. Widespread pain must be present for at least 3 months. The presence of a second clinical disorder does not exclude the diagnosis of fibromyalgia.

From Wolf F et al: The American College of Rheumatology 1990 criteria for the classification of fibromyalgia: report of the multicenter criteria committee. *Arthritis Rheum* 33:160, 1990.

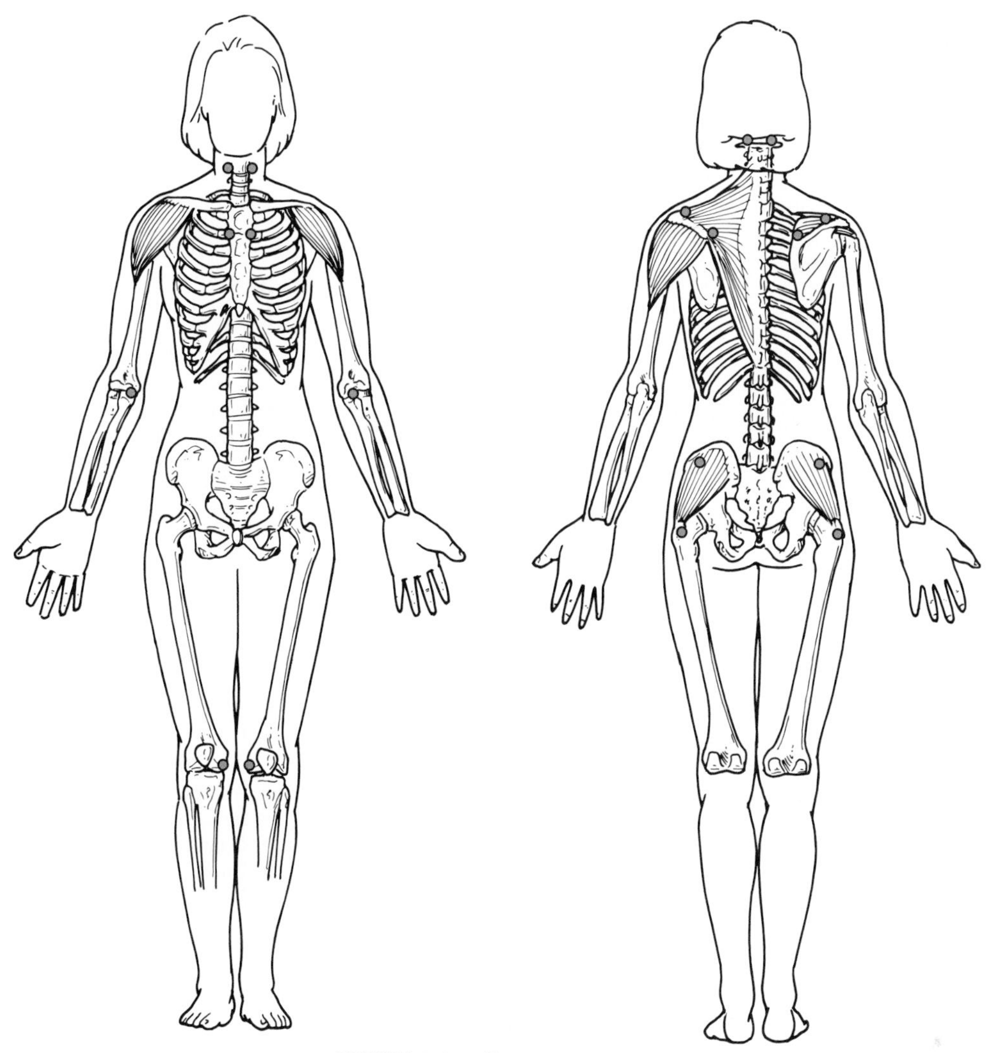

FIGURE 1-6 Fibro pain points.

PATIENT/FAMILY EDUCATION

- Point out that the response to treatment and prognosis for adolescents tends to be better than it is for adults.
- Beware of unsubstantiated, non–peer-reviewed information.
- Involvement of family in the treatment plan is helpful.

SUGGESTED READINGS

Arthritis Foundation. Available at www.arthritis.org

Goldenbert DL et al: Management of fibromyalgia syndrome. *JAMA* 292:2388, 2004.

Siegel DM et al: Fibromyalgia syndrome in children and adolescents: clinical features, a presentation, and status at follow-up. *Pediatrics* 101:377, 1998.

Wolfe F et al: The American College of Rheumatology 1990 criteria for the classification of fibromyalgia. *Arthritis Rheum* 33:160, 1990.

AUTHOR: **DAVID M. SIEGEL, MD, MPH**

BASIC INFORMATION

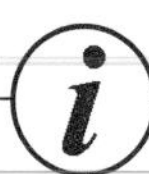

DEFINITION

Folliculitis is superficial or deep inflammation of the hair follicle. It is usually caused by an infection (e.g., pyoderma localized to hair follicles), but it may be the result of physical injury or chemical injury. Furuncles (i.e., boils) represent deep bacterial folliculitis. They may originate from a preceding folliculitis or may arise initially as a deep-seated perifollicular nodule. They are painful, circumscribed, perifollicular abscesses that have a tendency for central necrosis and suppuration. Carbuncles are large, deep-seated abscesses made up of aggregates of interconnected furuncles that drain at multiple points on the cutaneous surface.

SYNONYMS

Bockhart's impetigo (i.e., superficial folliculitis)

Sycosis barbae (i.e., folliculitis barbae when in the bearded area)

ICD-9-CM CODES

680.9 Furunculosis (deep folliculitis)

680.9 Carbuncle

704.8 Folliculitis

EPIDEMIOLOGY & DEMOGRAPHICS

- Folliculitis, furuncles, and carbuncles occur most commonly on hair-bearing areas of the skin that are subject to friction, perspiration, and maceration.
  - Particularly affect the face, scalp, back of the neck, axillae, buttocks, and perineum
  - Other predisposing factors: hyperhidrosis, preexisting dermatitis, and low serum iron levels
  - Reduced host resistance also a risk factor, as seen in cases of diabetes mellitus, immunodeficiencies, impaired circulation, and malnutrition
- The incidence is not known.
  - Some forms, such as folliculitis barbae, are thought to be extremely common.
  - Other forms seem rare (e.g., following epilation methods).
- Demodex mites are an extremely common infestation in humans.
  - Some studies have shown a clear association with histologic and clinical folliculitis.
  - It is not clear whether the *Demodex* organism is causative or preferentially selects follicles with inflammation.

CLINICAL PRESENTATION

History

- *Pseudomonas* folliculitis occurs after exposure to whirlpools, hot tubs, and less commonly, community swimming pools and water slides.
- Poor hygiene, maceration, and drainage from wounds and abscesses can be provocative factors.
- Cases have been reported after use of contaminated recreational diving suits, synthetic and loofah sponges, and skin epilation.
- Antibiotic administration and corticosteroid therapy can predispose to *Candida* folliculitis.

Physical Examination

- The manifestations of infection of the hair follicle vary clinically with the location and depth of follicular involvement.
  - Superficial folliculitis (i.e., Bockhart's impetigo) is an infection at the follicular orifice characterized by tiny, discrete, superficial, red papules or dome-shaped, thin-walled yellow pustules 1 to 2 mm in diameter.
    - It is painless but may be pruritic.
    - Papules and pustules occur in crops.
    - Favored sites include the scalp, buttocks, and extremities.
    - Heals in 7 to 10 days without scarring.
  - *Pseudomonas* folliculitis is characterized by discrete pruritic papules and erythematous to violaceous papulopustular lesions.
    - Lesions usually develop within 1 to 2 days of exposure (8 to 48 hours).
    - The greatest density is on areas of the body covered by bathing suits.
    - Associated conjunctivitis and external otitis are seen in some cases when infection is caused by *P. aeruginosa.*
- Furunculosis appears as a tender, erythematous nodule.
  - Furunculosis is a group of circumscribed, perifollicular abscesses.
  - The overlying skin becomes thin and tense.
  - The abscess tends to become centrally necrotic, leaving a core of pus.
  - Healing often results in a slightly depressed scar.
- Confluence of two or more adjacent areas of furunculosis produces a tender erythematous tumor called a *carbuncle,* which becomes soft and fluctuant after several days.

ETIOLOGY

- Superficial infectious folliculitis
  - Bacterial
    - Often found to contain normal skin flora
    - *Staphylococcus aureus*
    - *P. aeruginosa* ("hot tub folliculitis"): usually caused by serotype O-11
    - Others (rare): *Streptococcus, Proteus,* coliform bacteria
  - Fungal
    - *Pityrosporum ovalis* (i.e., *Malassezia ovalis*)
    - *Candida albicans* (in immunocompromised patients)
  - Viral
    - Herpes simplex viruses types 1 and 2
    - Varicella zoster virus
- Superficial noninfectious folliculitis
  - Caused by obstruction of pilosebaceous follicles, resulting in follicular plugging and inflammation (may become secondarily infected)
  - Steroid acne (often caused by *Malassezia ovalis*)
  - Occlusive dressings with polyethylene or adhesive
  - Occupational contact with oils
  - Occupational or therapeutic contact with tars
  - Complication of any epilation method (e.g., shaving, waxing, depilatory creams, electrolysis, electric rotating coil devices)
- Deep folliculitis (furunculosis)
  - *S. aureus*
  - Gram-negative organisms (rare)
  - Eosinophilic pustular folliculitis (i.e., Ofuji disease) in immunocompromised patients and rarely infants

DIAGNOSIS

DIFFERENTIAL DIAGNOSIS

- Fungal infections
- Molluscum contagiosum
- Varicella (i.e., chickenpox) or zoster (i.e., shingles)
- Scabies
- Insect bites
- Contact dermatitis
- Papular atopic dermatitis
- Miliaria
- Steroid acne
- Pruritic folliculitis of pregnancy
- If localized to the face or neck: acne vulgaris or pseudofolliculitis barbae (ingrown hair)
  - A common inflammatory disorder of the pilosebaceous follicles of the beard
  - Shaved hairs curve inward, with resultant penetration of the skin on reentry into the epidermis, when the hairs grow in a curved or arcuate path
  - Creates an inflammatory foreign body reaction
- Folliculitis keloidalis nuchae (i.e., acne keloidalis nuchae)
  - Chronic perifollicular inflammation with scar and keloid formation
  - Nape of the neck
  - Seen in males after onset of puberty
- Herpetic sycosis: folliculitis in the beard area caused by herpes simplex virus

WORKUP

The history and physical examination are often sufficient to form a diagnosis.

LABORATORY TESTS

Gram stain or culture of a lesion is occasionally helpful.

TREATMENT

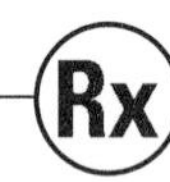

NONPHARMACOLOGIC THERAPY

- The treatment of choice for superficial folliculitis, including cases caused by

Pseudomonas, is good personal hygiene, including frequent, thorough hand washing and daily skin cleansing with soap and warm water.
- Patients should wear loose-fitting clothing.
- Patients should avoid offending agents.
- Patients should shave with a clean razor.
- For early lesions in deep folliculitis, warm compresses can be used to promote drainage.

ACUTE GENERAL Rx

- Superficial folliculitis
  - Topical antibiotics, such as mupirocin (Bactroban) or fusidic acid, are helpful.
  - Topical keratolytics, such as the benzoyl peroxide gels, should be applied twice daily for 4 to 5 days.
  - Systemic antibiotics are rarely required.
  - For *Pityrosporum (Malassezia)* folliculitis, an oral imidazole antifungal drug, such as itraconazole or ketoconazole, should be used.
- Deep folliculitis
  - If severe, widespread, or persistent, use systemic antibiotics with good antistaphylococcal coverage for 10 days.
  - If lesions are large and fluctuant, incision and drainage are indicated.
- Recurrences of staphylococcal infections: consideration of elimination of possible *S. aureus* carriage in the anterior nares
  - Mupirocin nasal ointment is applied to the anterior nares twice daily for 4 weeks. *Or*
  - Mupirocin nasal ointment is applied to the anterior nares twice daily for 5 consecutive days every month. *Or*
  - Rifampin is taken orally for 5 to 10 days.
- The administration of vitamin C (1 g/day for 4 to 6 weeks) can prevent recurrent furunculosis in patients with impaired neutrophil function.

DISPOSITION

- Emphasize proper hygiene and prevention measures at follow-up visits.
- Evaluation for diabetes and immunodeficiencies is not warranted until there are recurrences or concomitant systemic infections.

REFERRAL

Referral to a dermatologist is recommended if the diagnosis is uncertain, if the condition does not respond to usual therapy, or if steroid acne or Ofuji disease are being considered.

PEARLS & CONSIDERATIONS

COMMENTS

- *Pityrosporum (Malassezia)* folliculitis is an entity different from tinea versicolor, even though it is caused by the same organism.
  - Patients with this form of folliculitis often have concomitant tinea versicolor, seborrheic dermatitis, and acne vulgaris.
  - The predisposing factors of *Pityrosporum* folliculitis are similar to those of tinea versicolor.
    - A history of treatment with corticosteroids or antibiotics (e.g., tetracycline)
    - Diabetes mellitus
    - Possibly Cushing's syndrome
  - Many cases of presumed steroid acne are *Pityrosporum* folliculitis.
  - A histopathologic diagnosis is essential for appropriate therapy.
- Patients with Behçet's disease often present with papulopustular lesions that are sterile folliculitis or acne-like lesions on an erythematous base, which appear as a papule and in 1 to 2 days become pustular.

PREVENTION

- Avoid using sponges for the bath or shower (i.e., use washcloths).
- Avoid sharing razors, towels, and washcloths.
- Ensure proper chlorination of public swimming facilities, hot tubs, spas, and similar facilities.
- Follow the advice of local health departments regarding the avoidance of streams and lakes at times of high bacterial counts or chemical residues.

SUGGESTED READINGS

Feigin RD, Cherry JD (eds): *Textbook of Pediatric Infectious Diseases,* 5th ed. Philadelphia, WB Saunders, 2004.

Hurwitz S: *Clinical Pediatric Dermatology,* 2nd ed. Philadelphia, WB Saunders, 1993.

Weston WL et al: *Color Textbook of Pediatric Dermatology,* 2nd ed. St Louis, Mosby, 1996.

AUTHOR: **LARRY DENK, MD**

BASIC INFORMATION

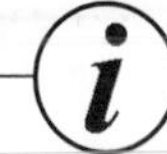

DEFINITION

Bacterial food poisoning is a gastrointestinal illness caused by ingestion of food contaminated with bacteria or bacterial toxins.

ICD-9-CM CODE
005.9 Food poisoning

EPIDEMIOLOGY & DEMOGRAPHICS

- The estimated incidence in the United States is 6 to 81 million cases per year.
- Most identifiable cases and deaths are caused by bacteria.
- Peak incidence varies seasonally by the specific organism.
  - Summer: *Staphylococcus aureus, Salmonella, Shigella*
  - Summer and fall: *Clostridium botulinum, Vibrio parahaemolyticus*
  - Spring and fall: *Campylobacter jejuni*
  - Winter: *Clostridium perfringens, Yersinia*

CLINICAL PRESENTATION

- What is the patient's recent travel history?
- What foods were eaten at the suspected meal?
- What was the incubation period of the illness?
- What are the presenting signs and symptoms?
- Any combination of gastrointestinal signs and symptoms with or without fever is suspect.
- The cause should be suspected on basis of the incubation period and major symptoms.
- A short incubation period (1 to 16 hours) is the result of ingestion of a preformed toxin and is noninvasive.
  - *S. aureus:* within 30 minutes to 6 hours; severe abdominal cramps, nausea, vomiting, diarrhea, occasionally low-grade fever; caused by enterotoxins, associated with ingestion of contaminated meats, filled pastries, and egg and potato salads
  - *Bacillus cereus:* a short incubation (emetic) form, characterized by vomiting, abdominal cramps, and 33% with diarrhea, and a long incubation (diarrheal) form, characterized by abdominal cramps and watery diarrhea. The illness is usually mild. Fever is unusual and resolves within 12 to 24 hours. The most likely food is unrefrigerated rice.
  - *C. perfringens:* severe, crampy, midepigastric pain with watery diarrhea. Fever and vomiting are unlikely. Symptoms usually resolve in 24 hours. Food poisoning is caused by a heat-labile toxin. Implicated foods include beef, poultry, gravies, and Mexican-style foods. Outbreaks are related to cooked meat or poultry that is allowed to cool without refrigeration.
- The moderate incubation period is 16 to 48 hours for toxin-mediated and invasive sources.
- Toxin producers include the following:
  - *C. botulinum:* diarrhea with or before paralysis, with severity related to amount of toxin ingested; unusual nerve palsies with descending paralysis; associated with home-canned foods
  - Enterotoxigenic *Escherichia coli* (ETEC): most common cause of traveler's diarrhea; after 1- to 2-day incubation period, abdominal cramps and diarrhea; resolves in 3 or 4 days; associated with contaminated water, salad, or rice
  - Enterohemorrhagic *E. coli* (EHEC): severe abdominal cramps, watery diarrhea, bloody diarrhea possible (O157: H7); noninvasive and no fever; complications include hemolytic uremic syndrome (HUS); associated with contaminated beef (especially hamburger), water, salad dressings, and raw milk
  - *Vibrio cholerae:* varies from a mild to life-threatening illness associated with voluminous, painless diarrhea, nausea, and vomiting; hypovolemic shock possible in 4 to 12 hours if fluid losses exceed intake; recovery within 1 week; associated with ingestion of contaminated water or food (especially raw or undercooked shellfish), moist grains, or dried or raw fish
- Invasive organisms include the following:
  - *Salmonella:* incubation period of 12 to 48 hours followed by nausea, vomiting, diarrhea, and abdominal cramps typical; fever possible; outbreaks associated with contaminated poultry, beef, pork, eggs, dairy products, vegetables, and fruits
  - *Shigella:* asymptomatic infection possible, but some with fever, watery diarrhea; may progress to bloody diarrhea and dysentery; usually self-limited, resolving in a few days; with severe illness, complications (e.g., bacteremia, HUS, seizures, colonic perforation) possible; transmission usually person to person but can occur by fecal contamination of food or water; associated with contaminated lettuce and egg salads
  - *Campylobacter jejuni:* incubation period of about 24 hours; prodrome of fever, headaches, and myalgias, followed by diarrhea with fever and abdominal pain; diarrhea mild to profuse and bloody; resolves in 1 week; associated with undercooked poultry, unpasteurized milk, drinking from freshwater streams
- Longer incubation periods are possible.
- *Yersinia enterocolitica* and *Yersinia pseudotuberculosis* infections are characterized by the following:
  - Incubation period is usually 4 to 6 days.
  - Manifests with fever, diarrhea, and abdominal pain lasting 1 to 3 weeks.
  - Mesenteric adenitis syndrome can mimic acute appendicitis.
  - It is associated with uncooked pork (i.e., chitterlings or raw pork intestines), unpasteurized milk, contaminated water, and tofu.
  - Stools often contain leukocytes, blood, and mucus.
- *Vibrio parahaemolyticus* infection is characterized by the following.
  - Incubation period is 15 hours (range, 4 to 96 hours).
  - It is associated with coastal or cruise ship outbreaks during the summer months.
  - Symptoms include explosive, watery diarrhea; nausea; vomiting; abdominal cramps; and headache.
  - Symptoms resolve in 1 week.
  - Associated with contaminated seafood that is eaten raw or not thoroughly cooked, such as crab, shrimp, and oysters.
- Enteroinvasive *E. coli* (EIEC) infection is rare in the United States, and infection is characterized by fever and bloody diarrhea.
- *Listeria* has an incubation period of 2 to 8 weeks.
  - Infection is rare in healthy people; it is more likely in pregnant women, newborns, and immunocompromised patients.
  - It manifests with fever, flulike illness, and headaches.
  - Implicated foods are unpasteurized milk; soft cheeses; undercooked poultry; pâté; and unwashed, raw vegetables.

ETIOLOGY

- Categorized as invasive (i.e., inflammatory) or noninvasive (i.e., noninflammatory)
- Invasive forms: *Campylobacter,* EIEC, *Salmonella, Shigella, V. parahaemolyticus,* and *Yersinia;* intestinal tissue invaded; fecal leukocytes present
- Noninvasive: *B. cereus, S. aureus, C. botulinum, C. perfringens,* ETEC, EHEC; no fecal leukocytes

DIAGNOSIS

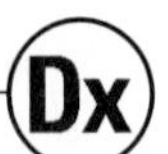

DIFFERENTIAL DIAGNOSIS

- Viruses (e.g., Norwalk, rotavirus)
- Parasites (e.g., *Entamoeba histolytica, Giardia lamblia*)
- Toxins (e.g., ciguatoxins, scombroid toxin, mushrooms)
- Heavy metals (e.g., copper, cadmium, tin, zinc)

WORKUP

- Test stool for fecal leukocytes and blood.
- Cultures should be obtained. Some organisms have special culture requirements, and the laboratory should be notified if the following are suspected: *Yersinia, C. botulinum, Vibrio* species, *E. coli* O157:H7.
- Examine stool for ova and parasites.
- Examine stool for *Clostridium difficile* toxin if current or recent antibiotic use is reported.

- If botulism is suspected, send food, serum, and stool for a toxin assay.
- Obtain blood cultures for febrile, toxic patients.

TREATMENT

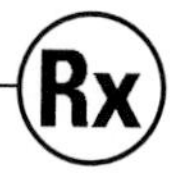

NONPHARMACOLOGIC THERAPY

Supportive therapy and rehydration constitute the primary treatment.

ACUTE GENERAL Rx

- No antimicrobial agents are needed for noninvasive organisms: *B. cereus, S. aureus, C. perfringens, V. parahaemolyticus, Yersinia,* and EHEC.
- For ETEC, use trimethoprim-sulfamethoxazole (TMP-SMX) for 3 days (10 mg/kg/day TMP component, divided every 12 hours).
- For *Salmonella,* treatment is as follows:
  - No antimicrobial treatment is available for gastroenteritis.
  - Consider antimicrobial therapy for patients with an increased risk of invasive disease, such as infants younger than 3 months and immunocompromised patients.
  - Consider therapy for invasive disease (e.g., bacteremia, osteomyelitis).
  - The drug chosen should be based on susceptibilities.
- For shigellosis, antibiotics (i.e., ampicillin or TMP-SMX, based on susceptibility testing) shorten the duration of disease and eliminate organisms from stool. Duration of treatment is 5 days.
- For *Campylobacter,* erythromycin shortens the duration of illness and prevents relapse. Duration of treatment is 5 to 7 days.

DISPOSITION

- Most infections are self-limited and do not require therapy.
- Serious complications are possible in an immunocompromised host.
- Postinfectious syndromes include the following:
  - Reiter's syndrome: *Salmonella,* shigellosis, *Campylobacter, Yersinia,* HLA-B27 positive individuals
  - Guillain-Barré syndrome: *Campylobacter*

REFERRAL

Hospitalize the patient if severe illness or complications develop, and consider consultation with a pediatric infectious disease specialist or pediatric gastroenterologist.

PEARLS & CONSIDERATIONS

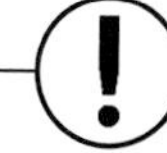

COMMENTS

- Food poisoning is often underreported and underdiagnosed.
- All cases should be reported to the local health department.

SUGGESTED READINGS

American Academy of Pediatrics: Food poisoning. *In* Pickering LK (ed): *Red Book 2003: Report of the Committee on Infectious Diseases,* 26th ed. Elk Grove Village, IL, American Academy of Pediatrics, 2003, pp 810–813.

Centers for Disease Control and Prevention. Available at www.cdc.gov

Cleary TG: Bacillus cereus. *In* Long SS et al (eds): *Principles and Practice of Pediatric Infectious Diseas.* Philadelphia, Churchill Livingstone, 2003, pp 1318–1324.

AUTHOR: **CYNTHIA CHRISTY, MD**

BASIC INFORMATION

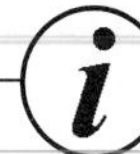

DEFINITIONS

A superficial ocular foreign body is a foreign body on the cornea, conjunctiva, or lid. An intraocular foreign body is a foreign body that penetrates the eye. An intraorbital foreign body is a foreign body that penetrates the orbit.

ICD-9-CM CODES
360.64 Retina foreign body
374.86 Foreign body, lid retained
871.6 Vitreous foreign body
930.0 Foreign body, corneal
930.1 Foreign body, conjunctival

CLINICAL PRESENTATION

History

- Usually, there is a history of trauma, but in younger children, there may only be a history of a red eye, tearing, light sensitivity, and irritability.
- Common circumstances are playing in sand, working around cars, and playing with pellet guns.

Physical Examination

- Inspect for the presence of a life-threatening injury.
- Assess the patient's visual acuity.
- Perform a slit-lamp examination and ophthalmoscopy to differentiate a superficial from an intraocular foreign body.

DIAGNOSIS

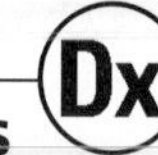

DIFFERENTIAL DIAGNOSIS

- Superficial corneal foreign body
  - Corneal abrasion
  - Acute conjunctivitis
  - Uveitis
  - Congenital glaucoma
- Intraocular foreign body
  - Uveitis
  - Intraocular foreign body
  - Retinal detachment
  - Vitreous hemorrhage
- Intraorbital foreign body
  - Orbital cellulitis

WORKUP

- The physical examination is key.
- Rule out an intraocular foreign body.
- If there is a suspicion of an intraocular or intraorbital foreign body, a computed tomography (CT) scan should be ordered. A CT scan is often better for evaluation of trauma, and it can identify metallic and organic foreign bodies.

TREATMENT

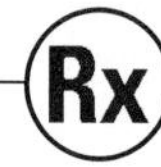

NONPHARMACOLOGIC THERAPY

- Some superficial foreign bodies may be rinsed out with water or with normal saline or tearing.
- A foreign body in or around the eye must be removed.
- If the foreign body is superficial, it may be removed with a cotton-tipped applicator under topical anesthesia.
  - Use of a forceps or other ophthalmic instruments, particularly with metallic foreign bodies, may be needed.
  - Remove the entire foreign body.
  - Use of a slit lamp is often required.
- For a young child, even a superficial foreign body may need to be removed in the operating room with sedation or general anesthesia.
- Organic foreign bodies should be evaluated by an ophthalmologist because there is a greater likelihood of infection from bacterial or fungal organisms.

DISPOSITION

Continue to monitor the patient until the injury has healed.

REFERRAL

- Ophthalmologic evaluation is needed for any suspected foreign body not easily removed in the office or to rule out other damage to the eye.
- For intraocular or intraorbital foreign bodies, consult an ophthalmologist.

SUGGESTED READINGS

Hamill MB: Corneal injury. In Krachmer JH et al (eds): *Cornea.* St. Louis, Mosby, 1997.

AUTHOR: **ANNA F. FAKADEJ, MD, FAAO, FACS**

BASIC INFORMATION

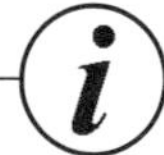

DEFINITION

Peptic acid disease includes diffuse compromise or inflammation of the gastric (i.e., gastritis) and duodenal mucosa (i.e., duodenitis). It may lead to discrete, superficial lesions (i.e., erosions) or deep lesions (i.e., ulcers).

SYNONYMS

Duodenal ulcers
Duodenitis
Gastric ulcers
Gastritis
Peptic acid diseases
Peptic ulcer disease (PUD)

ICD-9-CM CODES

531.3 Acute gastric ulcer
531.9 Gastric ulcers
533.4 Peptic ulcer with hemorrhage
533.9 Peptic ulcer
535.5 Gastritis
535.50 Gastritis without hemorrhage
535.51 Gastritis with hemorrhage
535.60 Duodenitis
535.61 Duodenitis with hemorrhage

EPIDEMIOLOGY & DEMOGRAPHICS

- The prevalence among infants and children is not well defined.
- Peptic acid–related diseases, particularly gastritis, are an important cause of abdominal pain and upper gastrointestinal symptoms.
- Primary ulcer disease is much less prevalent among infants and young children than adults because of the lower prevalence of *Helicobacter pylori.*
- Seroprevalence of *H. pylori* among children in the United States by age 10 years is about 10%.
- *H. pylori* acquisition increases with age. The prevalence of related diseases is therefore higher among adolescents.
- Other factors that increase the prevalence of *H. pylori* are poor socioeconomic environment (including adoptees from developing countries and immigrants) and living with other household members with *H. pylori* disease.
- Methods of transmission include fecal-oral, oral-oral, and gastric-oral routes.
- *H. pylori* infection has been associated with the development of gastric adenocarcinoma (1% to 2%) and mucosa-associated lymphoid tissue (MALT) lymphomas (rare in children).
- Increased incidence of peptic acid disease is seen in settings that predispose to secondary gastritis or ulcer disease.
    - Hospitalized patients (particularly in intensive care units)
    - Children taking certain medications (e.g., nonsteroidal anti-inflammatory drugs [NSAIDs], steroids, chemotherapy)
    - After viral illnesses (e.g., postviral gastritis)

CLINICAL PRESENTATION

- Symptoms vary with age.
    - Infants may present with irritability, vomiting, and failure to thrive.
    - School-aged children are more likely to present with abdominal pain.
- Characteristics of pain are as follows:
    - Epigastric (i.e., above the umbilicus)
    - Awakening at night with pain
    - May be worse with meals
    - Exacerbated by acidic foods
    - Relieved with antacids
- Associated symptoms include the following:
    - Nausea
    - Vomiting
    - Early satiety
- A precipitating event may be identified:
    - Viral illness
    - Medication
    - Hospitalization or surgery
- History that may be suggestive of risk factors for *H. pylori* includes the following:
    - Lower socioeconomic environment
    - Other household members with *H. pylori* disease
    - Immigrant or adopted child from a developing country
- Physical examination results may be normal.
- Physical findings suggestive of peptic acid disease include the following:
    - Epigastric or right upper quadrant tenderness
    - Hemoccult-positive stools
    - Weight loss if intake has been compromised
    - Tachycardia or pallor if there has been significant gastrointestinal blood loss

ETIOLOGY

- Peptic acid disease (e.g., gastritis, duodenitis, ulcers) results from an imbalance between the protective mechanisms and aggressive factors in the upper gastrointestinal tract.
- Protective measures include the following:
    - Mucous-bicarbonate barrier
    - Prostaglandins
    - Growth factors
    - Cell turnover
    - Microcirculation
- Aggressive factors include the following:
    - Excess acid
    - Excess pepsin
    - Ischemia or hypoxia
    - Bile acids, drugs, caustic agents, ethanol
    - Infections (e.g., viruses, *H. pylori*)
- Acid is required for development or perpetuation of mucosal damage.
- Traditionally, gastritis and peptic ulcer disease are classified as primary (i.e., no specific cause could be identified) or secondary.
    - Most primary disease is believed to be related to *H. pylori* infection.
    - *H. pylori* is a gram-negative, spiral-shaped organism that colonizes gastric epithelium and that can cause gastritis and peptic ulcer disease.
- Causes of secondary gastritis and ulcers compromise mucosal barrier function or enhance acid production or other aggressive factors and include the following:
    - Physiologic stress (e.g., burns, head injury, sepsis, shock, trauma)
    - Drug-related (e.g., NSAIDs, aspirin, corticosteroids, chemotherapy, ethanol)
    - Caustic substances
    - Viral infections (i.e., compromising the gastric mucosa and resulting in a postviral gastritis)
    - Excessive acid production (e.g., Zollinger-Ellison syndrome, renal failure, hyperparathyroidism)
    - Other causes (e.g., eosinophilic gastroenteritis, Crohn's disease, Ménétrier's disease)

DIAGNOSIS

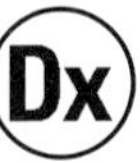

DIFFERENTIAL DIAGNOSIS

- Functional abdominal pain
- Esophagitis, GERD
- Nonulcer dyspepsia
- Crohn's disease involving the upper gastrointestinal tract
- Hepatobiliary disease
- Pancreatic disease
- Eosinophilic (allergic) gastroenteritis

WORKUP

- The diagnosis can be made with a careful history and physical examination, followed by a clinical response to a trial of acid suppression.
- Acid suppression is the therapy of choice for any peptic acid–related disorder (other than *H. pylori*); therefore, differentiating among the different conditions is not necessary to initiate therapy.
- If the diagnosis is unclear or the response to acid suppression is questionable, further evaluation can be pursued, including laboratory tests (see "Laboratory Tests") and endoscopy.
- Endoscopy (esophagogastroduodenoscopy [EGD]) is part of the examination.
    - This is the most sensitive and specific diagnostic test.
    - It should be performed if presenting symptoms are severe or empiric therapy fails.
    - It is the diagnostic test of choice for children with suspected *H. pylori*–related disease.
    - This test can determine the location, severity, and cause of disease, as well as verify the presence of *H. pylori* by histology or a rapid urease test.

LABORATORY TESTS

- Nonspecific tests: used to exclude other causes and assess complications of mucosal irritation
    - Complete blood count to identify iron deficiency anemia

- Erythrocyte sedimentation rate to evaluate for IBD
- Liver profile to evaluate for hepatobiliary disease
- Amylase and lipase levels to evaluate for pancreatic disease
- Noninvasive screening for *H. pylori*
  - Serology: IgG *H. pylori* titers. Children have reduced antibody levels; therefore, this test is not as sensitive or specific in children younger than 7 to 9 years. The test is not reliable for following response to therapy or recurrent disease.
  - Urea breath test (UBT): ^{13}C-labeled UBT (i.e., a stable isotope used in children). This is the most sensitive and specific noninvasive test, and it can be used to follow the response to therapy and for recurrence in adults. The ability to physically perform the test and lack of rigorous validation in children limits usefulness in pediatric patients.
  - Stool antigen test: Initial studies suggest that this may be a sensitive and specific test in children and adults for diagnosis and for demonstrating eradication.
- Because these noninvasive tests have not been fully validated in children, EGD with gastric biopsy is the diagnostic strategy of choice for a child with suspected *H. pylori* infection.
- No association has been found between *H. pylori* and chronic, recurrent abdominal pain. These children should not be routinely tested.

IMAGING STUDIES

- Upper gastrointestinal (UGI) series
  - UGI is fairly insensitive for superficial mucosal inflammation (e.g., gastritis, duodenitis) and for gastric ulcers.
  - An air-contrast UGI series can identify approximately 90% of duodenal ulcers.
  - Nonspecific findings include antral spasm and a thickened proximal duodenal fold.
  - In the child with significant vomiting, a UGI series is the study of choice to rule out a structural abnormality, but it otherwise does not contribute to the diagnostic workup of peptic acid disease in children.
- Abdominal ultrasound may be used to rule out other causes of abdominal pain (i.e., hepatobiliary and pancreatic disease).

TREATMENT

Rx

NONPHARMACOLOGIC THERAPY

- Apply general therapeutic measures.
  - Avoid acidic foods if they increase symptoms. They do not cause irritation but may exacerbate symptoms before the mucosa has healed.
  - Avoid smoking and alcohol.
- Discontinue medications that may be mucosal irritants, if possible.
- Management of a child with suspected gastritis or peptic ulcer disease integrates diagnostic studies with response to therapy.

ACUTE GENERAL Rx

- For history and examination results consistent with gastritis or peptic acid disease, use the following:
  - Treat with acid suppression (i.e., H_2-blocker), and discontinue use of potential causes (e.g., NSAIDs). Unless symptoms increase, allow at least 2 weeks on therapy to assess response.
  - After a response, continue treatment for 6 to 8 weeks.
  - For a partial response, change to a proton pump inhibitor (PPI) or refer the patient to a gastroenterologist.
  - There may be no response to the PPI or a recurrence of symptoms after treatment. For an adolescent, consider screening for *H. pylori* in the appropriate setting or refer to a gastroenterologist (i.e., endoscopy). For a child, refer to a gastroenterologist for further evaluation (i.e., endoscopy).
- Medications most frequently used for acid suppression are H_2-blockers and PPIs.
- H_2-blockers block histamine-stimulated acid secretion and are first-line medications for gastritis or peptic acid disease (i.e., non-*H. pylori* diseases). Doses are given up to the maximum adult dose.
  - Cimetidine (Tagamet): 20 to 40 mg/kg/day, divided two to four times daily
  - Ranitidine (Zantac): 1 to 2 mg/kg/dose given twice daily (three times daily for infants and toddlers)
  - Famotidine (Pepcid): 0.5 to 1 mg/kg/dose given twice daily
  - Nizatidine (Axid) (limited information): 5 to 10 mg/kg/day, divided two times daily
- PPIs block the gastric proton pump itself and are recommended for severe or refractory disease and for the treatment of *H. pylori.* Doses are given to maximum of the adult dose. Doses are not well established for all preparations.
  - Omeprazole (Prilosec): 0.7 to 3.5 mg/kg/day as a single dose or divided twice daily; available over the counter
  - Lansoprazole (Prevacid): available as a suspension and as soluble tablets, 0.5 to 1.6 mg/kg/day or dosages by weight:
    - $<$10 kg: 7.5 mg once daily
    - 10 to 30 kg: 15 mg once or twice daily
    - $>$30 kg: 30 mg once or twice daily
  - Pantoprazole (Protonix): 0.5 to 1 mg/kg/day; available as an intravenous preparation
  - Rabeprazole (AcipHex): dose not established
  - Esomeprazole (Nexium): dose not established
- Crushing or chewing the tablets (other than lansoprazole soluble tablets) or granules results in inactivation of the medication in the stomach. Liquid preparations can be compounded using a bicarbonate solution to avoid activation.
- Side effects of medications include headaches, abdominal cramping, and diarrhea.
- Combination therapies used for eradication of *H. pylori* include a strong acid suppressor (PPI) and *two* antibiotics effective against *H. pylori.*
  - Duration of treatment is 10 to 14 days. A twice-daily regimen (adult dose) enhances compliance.
    - PPI: 1 to 2 mg/kg/day, divided twice daily (i.e., 20 mg twice daily), plus two of the following:
    - Clarithromycin: 15 mg/kg/day, divided twice daily (i.e., 500 mg twice daily)
    - Amoxicillin: 50 mg/kg/day, divided twice daily (i.e., 1 g twice daily)
    - Metronidazole: 20 mg/kg/day, divided twice daily (i.e., 500 mg twice daily)
  - Whether asymptomatic individuals with *H. pylori* should be treated to reduce the long-term risk for gastric cancer is controversial.
- Sucralfate binds to damaged mucosa and provides a protective barrier against peptic acid injury.
  - Sucralfate should not be given with meals or other medications and should be used with caution in patients with renal disease.
  - Dosages for pediatric patients are not well established: 125 to 250 mg/dose four times daily in infants or toddlers; 0.5 to 1 g in older children and adolescents.
- Antacids buffer acid and provide fairly immediate relief when used as an adjunct to acid suppression (0.5 mL/kg/dose).

DISPOSITION

- Acid suppression therapy is effective in resolving peptic acid disease in the absence of ongoing aggressive factors.
- Regimens for eradication of *H. pylori* are also effective.
- Persistent *H. pylori* infection is related to poor compliance with the drug regimen and to development of antibiotic-resistant strains.

REFERRAL

- Patients should be referred to a gastroenterologist based on the pediatrician's comfort level with the acid suppression medications and treatment regimens for *H. pylori.*
  - Patients may be referred after a failed response to an empirical trial of acid suppression therapy (i.e., H_2-blockers or PPIs) or recurrent symptoms after treatment.
  - Children who are suspected of having *H. pylori* infection and have failed acid suppression therapy should be referred to a gastroenterologist for endoscopy. Adolescents should be referred to a

gastroenterologist for further evaluation or screen with noninvasive tests for *H. pylori* (i.e., serologies or UBT) before referral.

- A gastroenterologist may be consulted for any child with severe symptoms.
  - Vomiting suggesting gastric outlet obstruction
  - Hematemesis or other evidence of significant gastrointestinal bleeding
  - Significant anorexia and weight loss
- Severe pain and peritoneal signs on examination suggesting perforation (rare) require emergency evaluation by a surgeon and a gastroenterologist.

PEARLS & CONSIDERATIONS

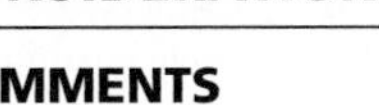
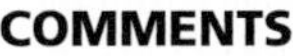

COMMENTS

- Medications that suppress acid do not primarily heal the mucosa; they minimize perpetuation of injury by acid and allow the body to repair the damage. It may take a few weeks before a child's symptoms improve significantly, and an empirical trial should not be deemed a failure until the medication has been taken as prescribed for at least 2 weeks.
- Infants and younger children tend to present with complications of peptic ulcer disease.
- The index of suspicion for *H. pylori*–related disease should be higher for children who are from a lower socioeconomic background, adopted or immigrated from developing countries, or live in households where other members have *H. pylori.*
- The comfort level with the clinical diagnosis and medications should dictate referral to a gastroenterologist.

PREVENTION

- When possible, avoid medications that can cause mucosal damage or co-administer acid suppression therapy.
- Initiate acid suppression therapy in the setting of significant physiologic stress (e.g., intensive care unit).

PATIENT/FAMILY EDUCATION

- Children should complete the 6- to 8-week course of medication even if they are asymptomatic.
- Foods that are spicy or acidic do not cause peptic acid disease but may aggravate symptoms before mucosal healing is complete.
- Mental and emotional stress does not cause gastritis or ulcers but may exacerbate symptoms.
- More information on acid suppression therapy is available from the North American Society for Pediatric Gastroenterology, Hepatology and Nutrition (www.naspghan.org).

SUGGESTED READINGS

Chelimsky G, Czinn S: Peptic ulcer disease in children. *Pediatr Rev* 22:349, 2001.

Czinn SJ: *Helicobacter pylori* infection: detection, investigation, and management. *J Pediatr* 146: S21, 2005.

Gold BD et al: *Helicobacter pylori* infection in children: recommendations for diagnosis and treatment. *J Pediatr Gastroenterol Nutr* 31:490, 2000.

North American Society for Pediatric Gastroenterology, Hepatology and Nutrition. Available at www.naspghan.org

AUTHOR: **M. SUSAN MOYER, MD**

BASIC INFORMATION

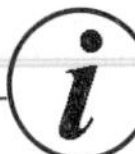

DEFINITION

Gastroesophageal reflux (GER) describes the effortless retrograde movement of gastric contents into the esophagus. The passage of refluxed gastric contents into the oral pharynx is known as regurgitation. Gastroesophageal reflux disease (GERD) is any symptom or tissue damage secondary to reflux of gastric contents. GERD is a clinical diagnosis that may be objectively confirmed by several diagnostic tests. It may manifest without the concomitant findings of erosions in the esophagus, just as tissue damage may be identified in the absence of typical symptoms. Infantile reflux becomes symptomatic during the first months after birth and resolves by 1 to 2 years of age in at least 80% of patients. Adult-type reflux may develop against a background of infantile reflux in some children, but it often appears in children beyond infancy, and it tends to persist, waxing and waning symptomatically.

SYNONYMS

GER
GERD
Reflux esophagitis

ICD-9-CM CODES
530.11 Gastroesophageal reflux, gastroesophageal reflux disease
530.81 Esophageal reflux

EPIDEMIOLOGY & DEMOGRAPHICS

- Mildly symptomatic reflux is extremely common and may be so benign as to be considered virtually normal.
- Twenty percent of otherwise normal infants regurgitate to an extent that their parents consider it a problem.
- Seven percent of infants have severe enough symptoms to come to medical attention; less than 2% of them require investigation.
- Less than 0.5% of infants have GERD severe enough to warrant fundoplication.
- Very-low-birth-weight infants are more likely to have GERD, and up to 10% have reflux-associated apnea, bradycardia, or bronchopulmonary dysplasia exacerbations.
- Significant reflux disease occurs in 2% to 8% of older children.
- Children with neurologic disease, chronic respiratory disease, increased abdominal pressure or distention, or vagal dysfunction or injury are at increased risk for GERD.

CLINICAL PRESENTATION

History

- Infantile regurgitation is the most common and obvious presentation of GERD, but it may not require further investigation if no other symptoms are present.
- When regurgitation is associated with weight loss, irritability, or ill appearance, a thorough evaluation is warranted.
- Infants may present with extraesophageal manifestations, including recurrent pneumonia, wheezing or asthma, stridor or hoarseness, apnea, apparent life-threatening event (ALTE), and sandifer syndrome (i.e., dystonic posturing or arching resulting from reflux).
- Older children may mention the following more common symptoms:
  - Heartburn or chest pain
  - Epigastric pain
  - Bilious taste in the mouth
  - Dysphagia or odynophagia in more severe cases
- Hoarseness, nocturnal cough, wheezing or asthma, hematemesis, otitis media, recurrent sinus infection, and dental erosions may be attributable to GERD in children.

Physical Examination

- The physical examination in an infant or child with GERD is usually normal.
- Possible physical findings include irritability, ill appearance, pallor, weight loss, posturing and twisting of the head and neck, stridor or wheezing, and epigastric tenderness.

ETIOLOGY

- GERD is a multifactorial disorder, but the key event in the pathogenesis is the movement of acid or other noxious substances from the stomach into the esophagus.
- Under normal circumstances, GER is prevented by an antireflux barrier consisting of the lower esophageal sphincter (LES) and the crural diaphragm and located at the gastroesophageal junction.
- The increased frequency of reflux in infants younger than 4 months may reflect the developmental immaturity of the LES, which is innervated by the vagus nerve and regulated by a variety of neurotransmitters, as well as a shorter esophagus with small capacity and increased time spent in the recumbent position.
- Transient LES relaxation (TLESR) is an abrupt decrease in pressure across the sphincter, which is part of the reflex that normally permits gas to escape from the stomach and is unrelated to swallowing or peristalsis. In children and adults with GER, the frequency and duration of TLESRs are increased.
- Impaired luminal clearance of gastric acid, caused by esophageal dysmotility and delayed gastric emptying, is another factor in the pathogenesis of GERD.
- Patients with hiatal hernia can have progressive disruption of the diaphragmatic sphincter, depending on the extent of axial herniation, and they may experience GER.
- GERD commonly occurs in patients who have had an esophageal operation (especially repair of esophageal atresia) and in those who are neurologically disabled.

DIAGNOSIS (Dx)

DIFFERENTIAL DIAGNOSIS

- Gastrointestinal obstruction: pyloric stenosis, malrotation, intermittent volvulus
- Allergic (eosinophilic) esophagitis or gastroenteritis
- Esophageal or gastroduodenal dysmotility
- Pseudo-obstruction
- Gastritis or duodenitis
  - *Helicobacter pylori*
  - Nonsteroidal anti-inflammatory drug induced
  - *Giardia*
- Inborn errors of metabolism: galactosemia, fructose intolerance, urea cycle defects
- Drugs or toxins (ipecac, lead poisoning, vitamin A toxicity)
- Infections: sepsis, meningitis, urinary tract infection
- Neurologic disorders
  - Arnold-Chiari malformation
  - Hydrocephalus with shunt dysfunction (or before surgery)
  - Intracranial hemorrhage or subdural hematoma
  - Subdural hematoma
- Psychosocial disorders (cyclic vomiting, psychogenic vomiting, bulimia)
- Renal disorders (obstructive uropathy, renal insufficiency)
- Cardiac disorders or congestive heart failure

WORKUP

- Infants and children presenting with uncomplicated regurgitation or heartburn may not need a confirmatory diagnostic test.
  - The positive predictive value of these symptoms is high.
  - Symptom resolution is often used as a clinical end point.
- Patients with atypical or extraesophageal symptoms, individuals not responding to empirical medical therapy, those with frequently recurring symptoms, and those with progressive symptoms should undergo diagnostic evaluation and may require referral to a gastroenterologist.
- The choice of diagnostic test depends on the clinical question.
- The 24-hour pH probe is the most sensitive method for diagnosing GER.
  - An episode of reflux is defined as a decrease in the intraluminal pH to <4.
  - The frequency of reflux, the overall time of esophageal exposure to acid, and the longest reflux episodes are recorded.
  - In infants, reflux more than 9% of the time and, in older children and adults, reflux more than 4% of the time is considered significant.
  - Prolonged alkaline reflux (pH > 7), which is usually caused by bile reflux, can cause symptoms and create significant tissue damage.
  - A pH probe is useful in determining the temporal relationship between episodes of reflux and symptoms.
- Endoscopy with biopsy is the most appropriate test to assess mucosal damage.
  - It is useful in the detection of esophagitis, Barrett's esophagus, hiatal hernia, strictures, and antral or duodenal webs.
  - It allows the opportunity for therapeutic intervention (i.e., stricture dilation).
- Multiple luminal electrical impedance measurements are rarely used in the diagnosis of GERD; however, it may be used to

evaluate peristalsis and to assess the function of the LES when an underlying motility disorder is suspected.
- Bravo, a small capsule containing a radio transmitter that is inserted endoscopically into the distal esophagus, is a new technology that can monitor pH for up to 48 hours, obviating the need for nasal catheter placement.

LABORATORY TESTS
- In general, laboratory tests are of little value in differentiating gastroesophageal reflux from other gastric conditions.
- Guaiac-positive stools are common.
- A complete blood cell count with a differential cell count may be useful to quantify the percentage of eosinophils (i.e., elevated in eosinophilic gastroenteritis and esophagitis).
- *H. pylori* serology or a breath test may exclude *H. pylori* infection as a contributing factor to symptoms

IMAGING STUDIES
- A contrast study of the upper gastrointestinal tract should be performed in all patients who have chronic regurgitation to eliminate the possibility of anatomic causes of delayed gastric emptying. (See Gastritis and Peptic Ulcer Disease in Diseases and Disorders [Section I].)
  - It is effective in detecting esophageal strictures.
  - It is useful in evaluating motor function and detecting hiatal hernia.
  - It is not useful for including or excluding the diagnosis of GER.
- Gastroesophageal scintiscan (i.e., radionuclide gastric emptying study) is the best method for calculating the rate of emptying.
  - It can also detect aspiration with greater sensitivity than a barium swallow.
  - Approximately 50% of children with GERD have delayed gastric emptying.
  - The scan is especially important when fundoplication is being considered to determine the need for pyloromyotomy.

TREATMENT (Rx)

NONPHARMACOLOGIC THERAPY
- Uncomplicated GER in infants is usually a self-limiting problem that resolves by 12 to 18 months of age, and only a thorough physical examination and parental reassurance and education are necessary.
- The infant should be kept upright as much as possible in the postprandial period.
- High-osmolality formulas should be avoided (osmolality: soy-based < lactose-based < elemental formulas), but hypoallergenic formulas may be useful. Whey-based formulas may empty more rapidly from the stomach, but they have not been shown to significantly decrease GER.
- Smaller and more frequent feedings.
- Thickened feeds may diminish the number of regurgitation episodes. However, this may lead to occult reflux episodes of long duration, possibly increasing the risk of esophageal and pulmonary complications.
- In older children, the following behavioral modifications should be recommended:
  - Prohibit eating 1 to 3 hours before bed.
  - Elevate the head of the bed.
  - Avoid known LES relaxants (e.g., tobacco, caffeine, chocolate, peppermint, garlic) and acidic foods (e.g., citrus, tomatoes).
  - Promote weight loss in obese patients.

ACUTE GENERAL Rx
- Medical intervention is indicated in patients with GERD who have recurrent symptoms or suspected complications.
- In adults, H_2-receptor antagonists (H_2RAs) lead to partial or complete resolution of symptoms in 50% to 70% of patients.
  - All H_2RAs are equally effective when used in equivalent doses.
  - Two randomized, controlled clinical trials enrolling children support the use of cimetidine and nizatidine in healing esophagitis and improving symptoms.
- Because of the greater antisecretory effect of proton pump inhibitors (PPIs), the success of this class of agent is superior to H_2RAs in terms of symptom relief and healing.
  - Between 70% and 90% of adult patients report partial or complete resolution of symptoms.
  - The various PPIs appear equally effective at equivalent doses.
  - Safety and dosing in young children are not well established although they are generally well tolerated.
  - Common side effects include headache, diarrhea, and constipation.
- Prokinetic agents (e.g., metoclopramide, bethanechol, low-dose erythromycin, cisapride) are no longer recommended as first-line therapy in children with delayed gastric emptying and GERD because of a lack of convincing data regarding efficacy and their considerable side effects.
  - Cisapride is no longer recommended because of its association with a prolonged QT interval and cardiac arrhythmias.
  - Therapy with erythromycin in very young infants may increase the risk of pyloric stenosis.
  - Metoclopramide rarely causes tardive dyskinesia and should not be used in patients with underlying seizure disorders.

CHRONIC Rx
- Therapy with a PPI is usually continued for 8 to 12 weeks if clinical improvement occurs. The patient is then often switched to an H_2RA. If no improvement occurs, further evaluation is necessary.
- The cause of reflux is often not correctable (e.g., motility disturbance, neurologic disease), and multiple courses of treatment are necessary.
- Surgery (i.e., laparoscopic or open Nissen fundoplication) may be considered in:
  - Cases refractory to medical therapy
  - Patients with severe complications (i.e. recurrent pneumonia or persistent asthma)
  - Children who face a lifetime of therapy because of recurrent relapses when medications are withdrawn

REFERRAL
- Patients with recurrent, complicated, or refractory disease should be referred to a gastroenterologist.
- A surgeon may be consulted when complications are severe, medications are ineffective, or the patient does not tolerate or desire long-term medical treatment.
- Neurologists, geneticists, psychiatrists, or toxicologists may be consulted if other causes for recurrent vomiting are being considered.

PEARLS & CONSIDERATIONS

COMMENTS
- Suspect reflux in patients with refractory asthma or recurrent pneumonia.
- Patients often have a family history of allergy or atopic disease.
- Children with GER often avoid spicy tomato sauces and acidic juices
- Some patients with reflux complain of a burning sensation in the throat and not in the chest.
- Reflux and constipation often coincide

PREVENTION
- Avoid tobacco, caffeine, and spicy and acidic foods.
- Eat frequent, small meals, and avoid eating for several hours before bedtime.

PATIENT/FAMILY EDUCATION
- Possible complications include esophagitis, esophageal stricture, Barrett's esophagus, recurrent pneumonia, asthma, nocturnal cough, apnea, and ALTEs.
- Infants commonly outgrow the illness, but in older children, the disease typically is one of dysmotility, possibly necessitating long-term or frequent courses of therapy.
- Dietary and behavioral changes may improve the course.

SUGGESTED READINGS

Boyle JT et al: Do children with gastroesophageal reflux become adults with gastroesophageal reflux? What is the role of acid suppression in children? *J Pediatr Gastroenterol Nutr* 37(Suppl 1): S65, 2003.

Dahms BB: Reflux esophagitis: sequelae and differential diagnosis in infants and children including eosinophilic esophagitis. *Pediatr Dev Pathol* 7:5, 2004.

Gold BD et al: What outcome measures are needed to assess gastroesophageal reflux disease in children? What study design is appropriate? What new knowledge is needed? *J Pediatr Gastroenterol Nutr* 37(Suppl 1):S72, 2003.

Rudolph CD: Are proton pump inhibitors indicated for the treatment of gastroesophageal reflux in infants and children? *J Pediatr Gastroenterol Nutr* 37(Suppl 1):S60, 2003.

AUTHOR: **ELIZABETH MANNICK, MD**

BASIC INFORMATION

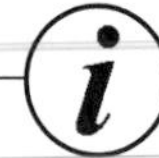

DEFINITION

Giardiasis is the infection of small intestines with the protozoan parasite *Giardia lamblia intestinalis.*

SYNONYMS

Giardia duodenalis
Giardia intestinalis

ICD-9-CM CODE
007.1 Giardiasis

EPIDEMIOLOGY & DEMOGRAPHICS

- *Giardia lamblia* is the most common human protozoal enteropathogen. It is seen in 4% of stool specimens submitted for examination to the clinical laboratories.
- Prevalence rates vary from 2% to 5% in the industrialized world to 20% to 30% in the developing world.
- The incubation period is 7 to 28 days.
- It can cause clinical infection with as few as 10 to 25 cysts.
- The infection is usually transmitted by contaminated water or food. Person-to-person transmission can occur in day-care settings or sexually among homosexual men.
- Untreated surface water from streams or lakes is the most common risk factor for acquiring this infection.
- Filtration of water is the most important step in water purification to prevent the infection. The cysts are not completely inactivated by chlorination, sedimentation, or flocculation methods that are commonly used for water purification.
- High-risk groups for giardiasis include the following:
  - Infants and young children, especially those attending day-care centers
  - Travelers
    - High attack rates (30% to 40%) with travel: certain parts of Russia and other developing countries
    - High prevalence areas within the United States: Colorado ski resorts, mountainous regions, and national parks
  - Immunocompromised patients
  - Sexually active male homosexuals
  - Inpatients in psychiatric institutions

CLINICAL PRESENTATION

History

- The patient may present as an asymptomatic carrier or may have acute or chronic diarrhea.
- Asymptomatic infection is the most common form.
- Host factors such as immune and nonimmune defense mechanisms, as well as variation in parasite virulence, may play a role in preventing disease expression.
- Acute giardiasis has an incubation period of 1 to 2 weeks, and 95% of patients have an acute onset with diarrhea.
  - Stools are typically profuse and watery.
  - There is usually no associated blood or mucus.
  - Other findings include the following:
    - Malaise (85%)
    - Cramping, abdominal pains (75%)
    - Bloating (70%)
    - Weight loss (65%)
    - Nausea (60%)
    - Marked flatulence (35%)
    - Vomiting (25%)
    - Fever (13%)
  - Untreated, some infections resolve in 1 to 2 weeks, up to 50% of patients develop chronic giardiasis.
- Chronic giardiasis has more profound constitutional symptoms.
  - Headache and malaise
  - Weight loss
  - Abdominal bloating
  - Persistent diarrhea, which can be intermittent in nature
  - Steatorrhea

Physical Examination

- May have signs of dehydration
- Failure to thrive or weight loss
- Abdominal distention
- Abdominal tenderness
- Stool usually heme negative
- Edema (i.e., protein-losing enteropathy occasionally seen in chronic giardiasis)

ETIOLOGY

- Infection is usually caused by ingestion of as few as 5 to 10 encysted forms of *G. lamblia.*
- After ingestion, excystation occurs, probably on contact with stomach acid.
- One or two trophozoites per cyst are released, and they are responsible for the disease.
- The cysts are 10 to 12 μm in diameter, whereas the trophozoites are tear shaped and 15 μm long. They have two nuclei and four flagella. They cause infection in the duodenum and upper intestines, probably due to the favorable alkaline pH.
- The trophozoites attach to the enterocytes by a ventral disk.
- A number of pathogenetic mechanisms have been proposed, including direct damage to the intestinal brush border, induction of an inflammatory response, and alterations in bile contents or duodenal flora.

DIAGNOSIS

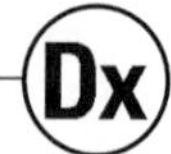

DIFFERENTIAL DIAGNOSIS

- Other forms of acute diarrhea
  - Infectious enteritis: viral, bacterial, or other protozoal agents
  - Traveler's diarrhea
  - Allergic reactions
  - Food poisoning
- Chronic diarrhea
  - Malabsorption syndromes, including celiac disease
  - Toddler's diarrhea
  - Cystic fibrosis
  - Lactase and other disaccharidase deficiency
  - Chronic constipation with overflow incontinence (i.e., encopresis)
  - Allergic enterocolitis
  - Irritable bowel syndrome
  - Inflammatory bowel disease
  - Motility disorders
  - Tuberculosis
  - Acquired immunodeficiency syndrome (AIDS)

LABORATORY TESTS

- Fecal specimen is assessed, with direct visualization of the parasite as a cyst or a trophozoite under a microscope.
  - Single stool specimen detect 70%
  - Three specimens increase sensitivity to 88%
- Fecal antigen detection tests have become more popular because of the ease of detection and higher sensitivity.
  - Direct fluorescence antibody test detects intact organisms. The sensitivity and specificity are 96% to 100%.
  - Enzyme immunoassays detect soluble stool antigens. The sensitivity is 94% to 97%, and specificity is 99% to 100%.
- Duodenal fluid aspirate or endoscopic biopsy specimens can sometimes be used to detect the trophozoite forms.

TREATMENT

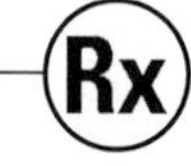

NONPHARMACOLOGIC THERAPY

Supportive care is needed for replacing fluid losses and correcting malnutrition.

ACUTE GENERAL Rx

- Nitroimidazoles (drugs of choice)
  - Dosage
    - Metronidazole: 5 mg/kg/dose (maximum dose of 250 mg), taken orally three times daily for 5 to 7 days
    - Tinidazole (for children > 3 years old: 50 mg/kg (maximum dose of 2 g), taken orally once
  - Efficacy (metronidazole and tinidazole): 90%
  - Side effects (metronidazole and tinidazole): nausea, vomiting, dizziness, headache, metallic taste, rash, neutropenia, disulfiram-like reaction with alcohol, peripheral neuropathy
  - Contraindications (metronidazole and tinidazole): pregnancy, interactions with alcohol and warfarin
- Nitazoxanide
  - Dosage
    - 100 mg, taken orally twice daily for 3 days (children 1 to 3 years old)

 - 200 mg, taken orally two times daily for 3 days (children 4 to 11 years old)
 - 500 mg, taken orally two times daily for 3 days (children older than 12 years); available in liquid and tablet formulations
 - Efficacy: About 90%
 - Side effects: dyspepsia, nausea, dizziness
 - Contraindications: not studied yet in pregnancy, renal or hepatic failure; may increase INR if taken with warfarin; may increase phenytoin levels
- Furazolidone
 - Dosage: 2 mg/kg/dose (maximum dose of 100 mg), taken three times daily for 7 to 10 days
 - Efficacy: 80%
 - Side effects: nausea and vomiting
 - Contraindications: Avoid in glucose-6-phosphate dehydrogenase deficiency because it can lead to hemolysis. Avoid using alcohol (i.e., disulfiram-like effect). Drug interactions occur with antidepressants and sympathomimetics.
- Mepacrine (Atabrine, Quinacrine)
 - Dosage: 2 mg/kg/dose (maximum dose of 100 mg), taken three times daily for 5 to 7 days
 - Efficacy: 90%
 - Side effects: nausea, vomiting, abdominal cramps, skin discoloration, toxic psychosis, hepatitis, anemia, psoriasis, and hepatic impairment (in elderly). Use only when conventional drug therapy fails, especially in immunocompromised individuals.
 - Contraindications: pregnancy. Avoid using with Primaquine, which can increase toxicity. Avoid using with alcohol, ritonavir, and aurothioglucose because they are associated with disulfiram-like effects.
- Paromomycin
 - Dosage: 30 mg/kg = dose (maximum dose of 500 mg), divided three times daily for 5 to 10 days
 - Efficacy: 55% to 90%
 - Side effects: diarrhea, vomiting, nausea, and abdominal cramps
 - Contraindications: pregnancy; no known drug interactions
- Albendazole
 - Dosage: 15 mg/kg/day (maximum dose of 400 mg), taken as a single oral dose daily for 5 days
 - Efficacy: 94% to 100%
 - Side effects: anorexia, abdominal pain, hypersensitivity, and rarely, alopecia
 - Contraindications: pregnancy; drug interactions with carbamazepine and phenytoin

DISPOSITION

Patients usually respond to treatment. Proper measures should be taken to avoid reinfection (see "Prevention").

REFERRAL

For confusing cases or those with negative results for stool ova and parasites, consider a pediatric gastroenterology consultation for a small bowel biopsy.

PEARLS & CONSIDERATIONS

PREVENTION

- Public health interventions are required to ensure that water supplies are free of *G. lamblia* and that methods are available to monitor the presence of the parasite in drinking water.
- Personal hygiene education is important.
- Most filtration devices provide satisfactory decontamination.
- Neither chlorine nor iodine-based chemical disinfection results in 100% cyst inactivation, although the latter is superior.
- Heating to 70°C for 10 minutes is also a practical alternative.

PATIENT/FAMILY EDUCATION

- Encourage good hand washing technique.
- Provide information on the proper methods of drinking water purification, especially to travelers.
- Identify people who belong to a high-risk group, and provide appropriate and specific guidelines (e.g., travelers, day-care attendees).

SUGGESTED READINGS

Ali SA, Hill DR: Giardia intestinalis. *Curr Opin Infect Dis* 16:453, 2003.

Centers for Disease Control and Prevention. Available at www.cdc.gov/ncidod/dpd/parasites/giardiasis/default.htm

Farthing MJG: Giardiasis. *Gastroenterol Clin* 25:493, 1996.

Gardner T, Hill DR: Treatment of giardiasis. *Clin Microbiol Rev* 14:114, 2001.

Goka AKJ et al: Diagnosis of giardiasis by specific IgM antibody enzyme-linked immunosorbent assay. *Lancet* 2:184, 1986.

Lewis DJM, Freedman AR: *Giardia lamblia* as an intestinal pathogen. *Dig Dis* 10:102, 1992.

Petri WA Jr: Treatment of giardiasis. *Curr Treat Options Gastroenterol* 8:13, 2005.

Zaat JOM et al: A systematic review on the treatment of giardiasis. *Trop Med Int Health* 2:63, 1997.

AUTHOR: **ALKA GOYAL, MD**

BASIC INFORMATION

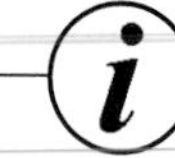

DEFINITION

Herpetic gingivostomatitis is a form of herpes simplex virus (HSV) infection. It is characterized by typical lesions of the mouth and gums.

SYNONYM

Herpetic gingivostomatitis

ICD-9-CM CODE

054.2 Herpetic gingivostomatitis

EPIDEMIOLOGY & DEMOGRAPHICS

- Humans are the sole reservoir for transmission to other humans.
- There is no seasonal variation.
- Distribution is worldwide.
- Transmission occurs by means of mucous membrane or skin contact.
- The typical age at onset is between 10 months and 4 years.
- Between 20% and 33% of children demonstrate serologic evidence of infection by 5 years of age.
- Acquisition and transfer is frequently asymptomatic.

CLINICAL PRESENTATION

- Symptoms include the following:
    - Fever (85% of patients) lasts a mean of 4 days (range, 0 to 8 days).
    - Painful oral lesions occur within the first 1 or 2 days of illness and last an average of 12 days (range, 7 to 18 days).
    - Poor oral intake occurs on average for 4 to 10 days.
    - Drooling (85%) typically lasts 6 to 7 days.
    - Extraoral lesions occur in 60% to 70% of individuals.
    - Coryza or otalgia may occur.
- Oral exanthema manifests with vesicular or ulcerated lesions on an erythematous base located largely on the gingivae (70%) and in the anterior mouth. Gums may be swollen, erythematous, ulcerated, and friable.
- Extraoral vesicular lesions may extend to the perioral area (e.g., lips, cheeks, chin), nares, and neck or, in the event of nail biting or thumb sucking, to the fingers ("herpetic whitlow"). They typically rupture and crust.
- Cervical, submental, submandibular, and preauricular lymph nodes are often swollen and tender.

ETIOLOGY

- Herpes simplex virus type 1 (HSV-1) and, rarely, herpes simplex virus type 2 (HSV-2) are the causative organisms.
- The incubation period is 2 to 20 days (mean, 4 days).
- Oral shedding during the primary infection occurs for up to 23 days (mean, 7 to 12 days).
- The immune response consists of antibody-dependent cellular cytotoxicity (ADCC) and interferon.
- After entry into sensory nerve endings at or near the site of inoculation, viral particles may travel by retrograde axonal transport to the trigeminal ganglion, where a permanent copy of viral genetic material is inserted into the host's genome. These features of latency allow recurrence of symptomatic disease and intermittent, asymptomatic shedding.

DIAGNOSIS

Dx

DIFFERENTIAL DIAGNOSIS

- Herpangina: Oral lesions are located in the posterior pharynx with little or no gingival or buccal involvement. Perioral lesions do not occur. Herpangina is often associated with a more acute onset, shorter duration, and milder oral discomfort.
- Hand, foot, and mouth (HFM) disease: Although oral lesions may be anterior, the gums and lips are typically spared. Cutaneous lesions on hands and feet are often bilateral (in contrast to herpetic whitlow, which is typically unilateral) and do not crust.
- Aphthous stomatitis: Oral lesions are not preceded by vesicle formation. Extraoral lesions do not occur. Fever and systemic illness are uncommon.
- Impetigo: Intraoral lesions do not occur. Although extraoral lesions in HSV infections often demonstrate a honey-colored crust, they rarely undergo secondary bacterial infection.
- Chemotherapy-associated mucositis: The most recognizable form is characterized by periapical erythema, swelling, and tenderness, with "punched-out" craters in the interdental papillae that may become covered with a pseudomembrane. Differentiation from HSV infection may require laboratory identification.

WORKUP

The diagnosis is usually based on clinical findings, without needing ancillary testing.

LABORATORY TESTS

- Rapid and specific tests
    - Fluorescent antibody (FA): Scraping with a cotton swab from the base of an unroofed vesicle provides the best material for analysis. Despite the significantly lower viral count, a swab from the crater of an ulcer may still be sufficient in the absence of intact lesions. FA alone is not HSV type specific. Placement of the specimen in 1 to 2 mL of liquid viral transport media kept on ice allows performance of a back-up culture and subsequent type-specific monoclonal antibody staining.
    - Polymerase chain reaction (PCR) is generally impractical for mucosal lesions due to the presence of inhibitors.
- Rapid but nonspecific tests
    - Tzanck smear
    - Giemsa or other tissue stains
    - Electron microscopy
- Less rapid but specific tests
    - Culture is still the gold standard and most specific method for diagnosing HSV outside of the cerebrospinal fluid (CSF). As with FA testing, recovery of virus is greatest in the vesicular stage. Samples should be obtained as for FA. Calcium alginate swabs inhibit HSV viral isolation. High-titer samples show evidence of growth by 24 hours, and low-titer samples show growth by 5 to 7 days (mean, 2 to 3 days).
- Serology is problematic and rarely useful in diagnosing primary gingivostomatitis.

TREATMENT

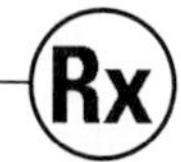

NONPHARMACOLOGIC THERAPY

- Therapy is usually supportive and provided on an outpatient basis.
- Adequate hydration is essential and may be the sole reason for hospitalization of children requiring inpatient care.
- Cold, nonacidic fluids; shakes; ice cream; yogurt; slush; or Popsicles may provide hydration, nutritive support, and symptomatic relief.

ACUTE GENERAL Rx

- Symptomatic relief of oral lesions
    - Diphenhydramine and aluminium magnesium hydroxide (Benadryl and Maalox) in a 1:1 solution as a swish and swallow or spit (maximum dose of 5 mg/kg/day of diphenhydramine).
    - Radiacare (an oral rinse derived from *Aloe vera L.*, often used for radiation-induced oral mucositis) is good tasting and safe if swallowed. The dose is 5 mL (younger child) to 15 mL (older child or adolescent) as a swish and spit four times per day. Increased oral contact time enhances effectiveness.
    - Viscous lidocaine is no longer recommended in young children.
    - Analgesia is also indicated.
        - Ibuprofen: 7 to 8 mg/kg/dose every 6 to 8 hours
        - Acetaminophen: 12 to 15 mg/kg/dose every 4 hours
- Antiviral therapy
    - Limited evidence suggests milder severity, a briefer course of illness, and shorter duration of viral shedding if oral acyclovir is begun within 72 hours of the onset of illness. However, the cost of therapy and limited data regarding disease recurrence and drug resistance prevent routine

recommendation for use of acyclovir in patients with herpetic gingivostomatitis.
  - For individuals with moderate to severe disease or who participate in large day-care programs, some experts recommend the use of oral acyclovir, even if initiated more than 72 hours after the onset of oral lesions. This may prevent or diminish length of hospital stay for intravenous hydration and pain management or decrease the likelihood of disease transmission. The dose is 70 to 80 mg/kg/day, divided in three or four doses (maximum of 1 g/day) for 5 days or until new lesion formation has ceased and sustained clinical improvement is evident.
  - Older children (>12 years) may use valacyclovir (2000 mg every 12 hours for 1 day).
  - HSV infection in neonates or immunocompromised patients or in extraoral lesions in contact with altered integument (e.g., eczema, burns, diaper dermatitis) may result in severe, disseminated disease, requiring hospitalization and intravenous therapy (see Herpes Simplex Virus Infections in Diseases and Disorders [Section I]).

CHRONIC Rx

- The most common manifestation of recurrent oral HSV infection is herpes labialis (i.e., fever blisters or cold sores), for which topical antiviral therapy is of little clinical benefit.
- Individuals with frequent herpes labialis recurrences may benefit from continuous, preventative therapy with 6 to 12 months of oral acyclovir (80 mg/kg/day in three divided doses, with a maximum of 1g/day).

DISPOSITION

- Outpatient follow-up is required to ensure adequate hydration.
- For return to day care or school, the patient or parent should understand that viral shedding with primary oral infection typically persists for 7 days (range, 2 to 12 days). Children who do not have control of oral secretions, are biters, or are too ill to comfortably participate in activities should be excluded from group child care.

REFERRAL

Referral is based on the occurrence of rare but potential complications, including dissemination of HSV infections; central nervous system infection; acute disseminated encephalomyelitis (ADEM); Bell's palsy; atypical, prolonged croup; herpetic epiglottis; Ludwig's angina; upper airway obstruction; lymphangitis; otitis media; recurrent gingivostomatitis; recurrent erythema multiforme or Stevens-Johnson syndrome; and secondary bacterial infection (particularly with *Kingella kingae* or group A streptococci).

PEARLS & CONSIDERATIONS

COMMENTS

- HSV-1 is an important cause of acute pharyngitis in the college-age population, accounting for 5% to 24% of cases (double to triple that caused by group A streptococci in this age group). HSV pharyngitis is usually clinically indistinguishable from other forms of viral or bacterial pharyngitis. Oral lesions accompany only 10% to 35% of cases
- Interpersonal skin-to-skin or oral-to-skin transmission may result in herpes gladiatorum among wrestlers or herpes rugbiaforum ("scrum pox") among rugby players.
- Bacterial cultures of HSV lesions growing *Staphylococcus aureus* are more likely to represent colonization than infection.
- Recurrent impetigo, especially in the same location with each recurrence, should prompt consideration of HSV.
- Recurrent HSV is the most common trigger of recurrent erythema multiforme minor.

PREVENTION

- Symptomatic and asymptomatic shedding occur, but it is particularly prudent to avoid direct contact with lesions during symptomatic periods.
- Avoidance of direct contact of lesions with neonates or individuals with eczema, burns, or immunodeficiency is imperative.

PATIENT/FAMILY EDUCATION

- Progression of lesions occurs over 4 to 6 days, followed by an additional week of resolution, for an approximate 2-week duration of symptoms.
- Because the epidermis (rather than the dermis) is typically involved, healing without scarring is the norm.
- Recurrence
  - Between 50% and 75% of individuals have no episodes of recurrence.
  - The most common manifestation of recurrent oral HSV infection is fever blisters or cold sores.
  - Recurrences may be triggered by intercurrent infection, local trauma, sun exposure, stress, the administration of immunosuppressive agents, and hormonal changes.
  - Recurrences are typically milder, of shorter duration, and more localized than primary disease.
  - A local prodrome (e.g., pain, burning, tingling, pruritus) often occurs, lasting from 6 hours to several days. Vesicles erupt at the site of initial inoculation (typically along the outer edge of the vermilion border), evolve into pustules or ulcers by 1 or 2 days, and subsequently crust.

SUGGESTED READINGS

Arvin AM: Herpes simplex viruses 1 and 2. *In* Feign R et al (eds): *The Textbook of Pediatric Infectious Diseases,* 5th ed. Philadelphia, WB Saunders, 2004, pp 1884–1907.

Herpes simplex. *In* Pickering LK et al (eds): *Red Book: 2003 Report of the Committee on Infectious Diseases,* 26th ed. Elk Grove Village, IL, American Academy of Pediatrics 2003.

Prober CG: Herpes simplex virus. *In* Long S et al (eds): *Principles and Practice of Pediatric Infectious Diseases,* 2nd ed. New York, Churchill Livingstone, 2003, pp 1032–1041.

Whitley RJ et al: Herpes simplex viruses. *Clin Infect Dis* 26:541, 1998.

AUTHOR: **C. ELIZABETH TREFTS, MD**

BASIC INFORMATION

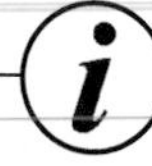

DEFINITION

Infantile (congenital) glaucoma results from high intraocular pressure that damages the optic nerve and other ocular structures.

SYNONYMS

Buphthalmos
Congenital glaucoma
Developmental glaucoma
Trabeculodysgenesis

ICD-9-CM CODES

365.4 Glaucoma associated with congenital anomalies, dystrophies, and systemic syndromes
365.14 Glaucoma of childhood

EPIDEMIOLOGY & DEMOGRAPHICS

- One case per 10,000 live births
- Sixty percent diagnosed by 6 months, 80% by 1 year
- Sixty-five percent males
- Seventy percent bilateral
- Ten percent familial

CLINICAL PRESENTATION

- Clinical triad: blepharospasm, epiphora, and photophobia
- Large eye (normal corneal diameter is 9 to 10 mm in the newborn)
- Cloudy cornea
- High intraocular pressure
- Increased optic nerve cupping
- Decreased visual acuity

ETIOLOGY

Dysgenesis of aqueous drainage pathways leads to decreased aqueous outflow, with a resultant increase in intraocular pressure that damages the eye.

DIAGNOSIS

DIFFERENTIAL DIAGNOSIS

- Tearing: nasolacrimal duct obstruction, foreign body, corneal abrasion
- Corneal clouding: corneal dystrophies, storage diseases (e.g., Hurler's syndrome)
- Prominent globe: craniofacial syndrome, orbital tumors

WORKUP

Refer the patient to an ophthalmologist to determine intraocular pressure under anesthesia, if necessary.

TREATMENT

NONPHARMACOLOGIC THERAPY

- Goniotomy is an incision that creates communication for the aqueous to access Schlemm's canal.
- Trabeculectomy or glaucoma drainage device creates a hole in sclera to let aqueous percolate into a subconjunctival bleb.
- Cycloablation damages the ciliary body to decrease aqueous production.

ACUTE GENERAL Rx

Aqueous suppressants (e.g., Diamox, Timoptic, Trusopt) are not as helpful in the pediatric population as in adults.

DISPOSITION

Lifelong follow-up is needed by an ophthalmologist to monitor intraocular pressure and follow for ocular damage.

REFERRAL

- Immediate referral is needed to an ophthalmologist familiar with the surgical treatment of childhood glaucoma.
- Consider a genetic workup.

PEARLS & CONSIDERATIONS

COMMENTS

Glaucoma is associated with Sturge-Weber syndrome, neurofibromatosis, Lowe syndrome, congenital rubella, and aniridia.

PATIENT/FAMILY EDUCATION

More information can be obtained from the Children's Glaucoma Foundation (www.childrensglaucoma.com).

SUGGESTED READINGS

Freedman SF, Walton DS: Approach to infants and children with glaucoma. *In* Epstein DL et al (eds): *Chandler and Grant's Glaucoma,* 4th ed. Baltimore, Williams & Wilkins, 1997, pp 586–597.

Kipp MA: Childhood glaucoma. *Pediatr Clin North Am* 50:89, 2003.

AUTHOR: **MATTHEW D. GEARINGER, MD**

BASIC INFORMATION

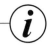

DEFINITION

Acute glomerulonephritis (AGN) is kidney disease characterized by proliferation and inflammation of the glomeruli. Clinically, there is sudden onset of hypertension, edema, hematuria, proteinuria, oliguria, and azotemia. The process generally is self-limited.

SYNONYMS

Acute postinfectious glomerulonephritis
Acute poststreptococcal glomerulonephritis

ICD-9-CM CODES
580.0 Poststreptococcal glomerulonephritis
580.9 Acute glomerulonephritis

EPIDEMIOLOGY & DEMOGRAPHICS

- Many cases are subclinical.
- Acute poststreptococcal glomerulonephritis (APSGN) occurs sporadically or in epidemics.
- It is mainly a disease of children between 2 and 12 years.
  - Fewer than 5% of patients are younger than 2 years old.
- Male:female ratio is approximately 2:1.
- Higher incidence is noted in siblings of affected patients.

CLINICAL PRESENTATION

- Most common presenting features are hematuria, proteinuria, edema, and hypertension.
  - Hematuria and proteinuria develop abruptly.
- Gross hematuria is present in 25% to 40%.
- Proteinuria is typically mild to moderate but may be in nephrotic range.
  - Acute onset of edema and weight gain occurs over several days.
  - Hypertension may be mild and asymptomatic or severe and associated with headaches or seizures.
- Oliguria occurs transiently in approximately 50% of patients.
- Pallor is present.
- History of pharyngitis (7 to 10 days) or impetigo (14 to 21 days) noted prior to onset of symptoms.
- Nonspecific symptoms include headache, malaise, lethargy, anorexia, fever, abdominal pain, weakness.
- Historical features suggesting possible alternative diagnosis:
  - Poor growth suggests possible underlying chronic illness, which could be presentation of chronic glomerulonephritis.
  - Concomitant pharyngitis or upper respiratory infection suggest possible immunoglobulin A nephropathy (IgAN).
  - Preceding illness symptoms suggest alternative infectious agent.
  - Purpuric rash, abdominal pain, and arthritis suggest Henoch-Schönlein purpura (HSP).
  - Malar rash, arthritis, fever, and malaise suggest systemic lupus erythematosus (SLE).
  - Persistent fever suggests glomerulonephritis associated with subacute bacterial endocarditis.
  - Persistent fever in patients with ventriculoatrial shunts suggests possible shunt nephritis.
- Family history of renal disease suggests hereditary nephritis such as Alport's nephritis and may be associated with hearing loss in affected individuals.

Physical Examination

- Head, eyes, ears, nose, and throat (HEENT)
  - Funduscopic examination with atrioventricular nicking or arteriolar narrowing indicates hypertensive changes.
  - Periorbital edema suggests volume overload.
  - Erythema or exudate of pharynx suggests concomitant infection.
- Cardiac
  - Hypertension, jugular venous distention, gallop, and tachycardia all indicate volume overload.
  - New murmur may be secondary to volume overload or suggestive of nephritis associated with subacute bacterial endocarditis.
- Pulmonary
  - Rales or cough may indicate pulmonary edema.
- Abdomen
  - Distention and ascites suggest fluid overload and significant proteinuria.
- Extremities
  - Edema
  - Joint swelling or erythema
- Skin
  - Pallor.
  - Healed skin lesions may suggest recent impetigo.
  - Purpura suggests HSP/vasculitis.
  - Malar rash suggests lupus.
- Neurologic
  - Seizures, encephalopathy, or coma may occur secondary to hypertensive crisis.
- Growth parameters
  - Weight and height, if decreased, suggest a chronic illness.

ETIOLOGY

- Most cases are postinfectious, with poststreptococcal glomerulonephritis being the most common. Other infectious agents include the following:
  - Bacteria (*Streptococcus viridans, Staphylococcus aureus, Klebsiella pneumoniae, Treponema pallidum*)
  - Viruses (hepatitis B, cytomegalovirus, Epstein-Barr, Coxsackie, mumps)
  - Rickettsiae
  - Fungi
  - Parasites
- APSGN is the most studied.
  - The exact pathogenetic mechanism remains controversial but is believed to be an immune complex-mediated process.
  - Not all strains of streptococci lead to nephritis, suggesting the importance of organism characteristics.
    - Nephritogenic strains of group A β-hemolytic streptococcal infection causing pharyngitis include strains M types 1, 3, 4 12, 25, and 49, while those causing skin infections include strains 2, 49, 55, 57, and 60.
- Histologically, AGN is characterized by a diffuse exudative and proliferative glomerulonephritis.
  - Immunofluorescence reveals granular immunoglobulin G (IgG) and C3 deposits along the capillary walls.
  - Electron microscopy reveals subepithelial deposits.

DIAGNOSIS

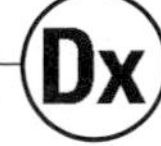

DIFFERENTIAL DIAGNOSIS

- Other postinfectious glomerulonephritides
- HSP
- Nephritis associated with subacute bacterial endocarditis
- Shunt nephritis
- Acute presentation of chronic glomerulonephritis
  - IgAN
  - Membranoproliferative glomerulonephritis (MPGN)
  - SLE
- Rapidly progressive glomerulonephritis

WORKUP

Diagnosis is generally made on clinical grounds with typical history, physical examination, and evidence of previous streptococcal infection either by culture done at time of infection or by serology in the setting of an acute nephritis picture.

LABORATORY TESTS

- Urinalysis with microscopic examination
  - Hematuria with or without red blood cell (RBC) casts
  - Proteinuria: generally trace to 2+; unusual to be in nephrotic range
- Chemistries
  - Blood urea nitrogen and creatinine may be increased.
  - Electrolyte disturbances may include:
    - Hyperkalemia
    - Acidosis
    - Hyperphosphatemia
- Hematology
  - Anemia
- Serologies
  - Hypocomplementemia (C3 and CH50) during the acute phase occurs in 90% of patients with APSGN. C4 may be normal or mildly depressed.
    - C3 typically normalizes within 6 to 8 weeks.
    - Failure of C3 to normalize after 6 to 8 weeks raises concern that the underlying disease is MPGN or SLE.

- Evidence of recent streptococcal infection or concomitant streptococcal infection will be present.
  - Elevated ASO titer occurs in 80% of patients with pharyngitis but only 30% of those with pyoderma.
    - Rise in titers starts approximately 2 weeks after infection and peaks at approximately 3 to 5 weeks.
    - Antibiotic therapy blunts the rise in antibody titer.
  - Anti-DNAse B titer is the most sensitive indicator of prior streptococcal infection.
  - Previous documented positive culture.
  - Positive throat culture at time of presentation.
- Definitive diagnosis requires renal biopsy, but biopsy is generally not necessary. Consider renal biopsy if atypical presentation:
  - Age younger than 2 years or older than 12 years
  - Presence of nephrotic syndrome
  - Normal serum complement levels
  - Deteriorating renal function
  - Significant systemic symptoms
  - Abnormal growth curve
  - Atypical course: delay in resolution of glomerulonephritis including prolonged period of hypocomplementemia (see "Patient/Family Education" for typical course description)

TREATMENT

NONPHARMACOLOGIC THERAPY

- Salt restriction
- Fluid restriction
  - If significantly volume overloaded, fluid restriction should equal insensible water losses plus urine output.
- Potassium and phosphate restriction: as indicated by laboratory values

ACUTE GENERAL Rx

- Antibiotics if concomitant pharyngitis, pyoderma, or other infection is documented.
- Diuretics:
  - For treatment of hypertension which occurs secondary to fluid and salt retention
  - To decrease edema
  - To improve urine output in oliguric states
- Additional antihypertensive agents administered as needed based on blood pressure elevation.
- Phosphate binders (e.g., calcium carbonate with meals) should be used in addition to dietary restriction of phosphorus if hyperphosphatemia present.
- Avoid nephrotoxic medications.
- Medications may require dose adjustment if significant renal impairment is present.
- If the patient has impaired renal function, severe electrolyte abnormalities, or uremia, consult pediatric nephrology.
  - Dialysis sometimes required
- Consider hospital admission if:
  - Oliguria, hypertension, renal insufficiency, electrolyte disorders (e.g., hyperkalemia)

CHRONIC Rx

- APSGN is generally self-limited with an excellent prognosis for recovery.
- Less than 2% of patients do not have a complete recovery and have residual renal abnormalities (hematuria, proteinuria, or impaired renal function). A pediatric nephrologist should be consulted.

DISPOSITION

- See "Patient/Family Education" for description of typical course for the disease.
- Monitor blood pressure, renal function, and urinalysis for presence of blood and protein.
- Frequency of follow-up depends on severity of disease.
  - Monitoring may be at weekly to monthly intervals (depending on disease severity) for the first 6 months and then at 3- to 6-month intervals until hematuria and proteinuria are resolved for 1 year.
  - Once hematuria and proteinuria are resolved for 1 year, yearly urinalysis and blood pressure checks are recommended.

REFERRAL

- Refer to a pediatric nephrologist if the patient has hypertension, oliguria, renal insufficiency, significant systemic symptoms, atypical course, nephrotic-range proteinuria, severe electrolyte abnormalities, uremia, or persistently low C3.

PEARLS & CONSIDERATIONS

COMMENTS

- Presence of RBC casts signifies glomerulonephritis, but its absence does not rule it out.
- The ideal time to examine urine is immediately after the patient voids.
- If gross hematuria is present, it may be easier to detect casts by examining one drop of unspun urine instead of spun urine.

PATIENT/FAMILY EDUCATION

- The typical course is as follows:
  - Oliguria and azotemia generally resolve within a few weeks.
  - Hypertension resolves within several weeks.
  - Gross hematuria resolves within several weeks.
  - C3 normalizes by 6 to 8 weeks.
  - Proteinuria generally resolves by 6 months.
  - Hematuria generally resolves by 12 months but may persist for several years.
- Recovery is generally complete for APSGN; however, 1% to 2% may have residual urinalysis abnormalities or hypertension.
- APSGN generally does not occur more than once but has been reported to recur in a small percentage of patients.

SUGGESTED READINGS

Brenner RM, Petersen J: Postinfectious glomerulonephritis. *Nephrol Rounds* 3, 2000.

Sulyuk E: Acute proliferative glomerulonephritis. *In* Avner ED et al (eds): *Pediatric Nephrology.* Philadelphia, Lippincott Williams & Wilkins, 2004, pp 601–613.

AUTHOR: **AYESA N. MIAN, MD**

BASIC INFORMATION

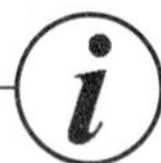

DEFINITION

The nephritic syndrome is characterized by hematuria, proteinuria, oliguria, and volume overload. Acute glomerulonephritis generally has an abrupt onset and is self-limited. Chronic glomerulonephritis may present with an abrupt or insidious onset and does not generally resolve on its own; indeed it may progress to chronic renal failure. The chronic glomerulonephritides of childhood discussed in this section include Henoch-Schönlein purpura (HSP), immunoglobulin A nephropathy (IgAN), systemic lupus erythematosus (SLE), Alport's nephritis, and membranoproliferative glomerulonephritis (MPGN).

SYNONYMS

Hereditary nephritis: Alport's nephritis
HSP: Henoch-Schönlein purpura, anaphylactoid purpura
IgAN: Berger's disease
MPGN: membranoproliferative glomerulonephritis, mesangiocapillary glomerulonephritis

ICD-9-CM CODES
287.0 Henoch-Schönlein purpura (HSP)
583.0 Immunoglobulin A nephritis (IgAN)
583.9 Membranoproliferative glomerulonephritis (MPGN)
710.0 Systemic lupus erythematosus (SLE) nephritis
759.89 Alport's nephritis

EPIDEMIOLOGY & DEMOGRAPHICS

- HSP
  - Predominantly affects children, though can occur rarely in adults
  - Rare in children younger than 2 years
  - Peak incidence age 4 to 5 years
  - Often follows an upper respiratory tract infection (URI)
  - Renal disease more likely to be severe in older children
- IgAN
  - Most common type of glomerulonephritis
  - Male:female ratio 2 to 6:1
  - Lower prevalence in African Americans
  - Occurs at all ages but most common in second and third decades of life
- SLE nephritis
  - Incidence and prevalence not well established in children
  - Increased frequency in Hispanic, Asian, and African Americans
  - Female predominance with F:M ratio as:
    - 2:1 prepubertal children
    - 4.5:1 adolescents
    - 8 to 12:1 adults
- Alport's hereditary nephritis
  - Prevalence 1:50,000 live births
  - Cases reported in all ethnic groups
  - Genetically heterogeneous
- X-linked Alport's syndrome (XLAS): approximately 80% of cases
  - Autosomal recessive: approximately 15% of cases
  - Autosomal dominant: 5% of cases
- MPGN
  - Occurs in older children and young adolescents (ages 8 to 16 years)
  - Incidence estimated to be 1 to 2 per 10^6 children

CLINICAL PRESENTATION

HSP (see chapter on Henoch-Schönlein purpura [HSP] in Diseases and Disorders [Section I])

- Symptoms may occur in any order
- Skin
  - Almost all children will exhibit skin lesions at some point in the course of disease.
  - Skin lesions start as erythematous macules; some develop into urticarial papules and then become purpuric.
  - In younger children, rash may be more urticarial and associated with localized edema.
  - Rash generally involves extensor surfaces of extremities and buttocks with symmetric distribution and sparing of trunk.
  - Recurrent crops of the purpuric rash may occur for several months.
- Joints
  - Joint involvement in approximately 70%
  - Consists of arthralgias and periarticular edema
  - Major joints affected: knees, ankles, elbows, wrists
  - Symptoms transient and leave no permanent damage
- Gastrointestinal disease
  - Gastrointestinal involvement in approximately 50% to 70%
  - Symptoms include colicky abdominal pain, vomiting, melena, and hematochezia
  - Intussusception is a potential complication
- Renal disease
  - Affects 20% to 100% of patients, depending on diagnostic criteria
  - Gross hematuria
  - Microscopic hematuria, isolated
  - Microscopic hematuria with proteinuria
  - Hypertension
- Involvement of other organs
  - See chapter on HSP
- IgAN
  - Variable presentations
    - Gross hematuria
      - May be asymptomatic
      - May be associated with loin pain
      - Often associated with URI and typically occurs after 1 to 2 days as compared to 1 to 2 weeks with poststreptococcal glomerulonephritis
      - Less frequently associated with other infections (e.g., diarrhea)
      - Variable intervals between episodes
    - Microscopic hematuria persists in between episodes of gross hematuria
      - More common presentation in children compared to adults
    - Asymptomatic hematuria with or without proteinuria
    - Acute nephritic syndrome with hematuria, hypertension, renal insufficiency, and edema
    - Nephrotic syndrome
    - Mixed nephritic-nephrotic syndrome
- SLE (see chapter on Systemic Lupus Erythematosus [SLE] in Diseases and Disorders [Section I])
  - Constitutional symptoms—common initial symptoms
    - Fever
    - Weight loss
    - Malaise
    - Fatigue
  - Oral mucosa
    - Ulcers
  - Skin
    - Malar rash: present in approximately one third of children
    - Photosensitivity
    - Discoid rash
  - Joint
    - Swelling
    - Arthritis
    - Pain
  - Central nervous system (CNS)
    - Seizures
    - Altered mental status or behavior
  - Cardiovascular
    - Hypertension (headaches, visual disturbances)
    - Pericarditis (chest pain)
  - Respiratory
    - Pleurisy
  - Gastrointestinal
    - Vasculitis (abdominal pain)
  - Renal manifestations when SLE nephritis present
    - Proteinuria: ~100%
    - Nephrosis: 45% to 65%
    - Granular casts: 30%
    - Red blood cell (RBC) casts: 10%
    - Microhematuria: 80%
    - Gross hematuria: 1% to 2%
    - Impaired renal function: 40% to 80%
    - Rapid decline in renal function: 30%
    - Acute renal failure: 1% to 2%
    - Hypertension: 15% to 50%
    - Hyperkalemia: 15%
    - Tubular abnormalities: 60% to 80%
- Alport's hereditary nephritis
  - Family history of renal failure and deafness
  - XLAS–affected males
    - Primary finding is hematuria which generally develops within the first decade.
      - Intermittent gross hematuria may follow a URI
    - Proteinuria eventually develops in affected males and the amount progressively increases with increasing age and may reach nephrotic range.
    - Affected males eventually progress to end-stage renal disease but rate of progression can be variable.

- XLAS–heterozygous females
  - Hematuria
    - Almost all have some degree of hematuria
  - Proteinuria may or may not be present
  - Course generally more benign than for affected males; may maintain reasonably good renal function even when elderly
  - Presence of gross hematuria in childhood, nephrotic syndrome, and diffuse glomerular basement thickening suggests progressive nephritis in affected women
- XLAS–associated findings
  - Hypertension also occurs with increasing age.
  - Sensorineural hearing loss is not congenital and generally is detectable by late childhood/early adolescence.
    - Hearing loss begins with high tones and progresses with time.
    - Deafness occurs in 30% to 50% of patients.
    - There is no relationship between severity of hearing loss and severity of renal disease.
  - Ocular anomalies occur in approximately 15% to 30% and include anterior lenticonus.
  - Presence of anterior lenticonus is virtually pathognomonic for Alport's syndrome.
- Autosomal recessive
  - Clinical symptoms similar to XLAS
  - Females affected as severely as males
- Autosomal dominant
  - Clinical features similar to XLAS but rate of deterioration of renal function is slower

- MPGN
  - Presentations
    - Asymptomatic hematuria and proteinuria detected on routine urinalysis
    - Acute nephritic picture
    - Acute nephrotic picture
    - Rapidly progressive glomerulonephritis—accounts for small percentage of patients
  - Symptoms/signs
    - Preceding respiratory infection: approximately 50% cases
    - Gross hematuria: approximately 20%
    - Nephrotic syndrome: approximately 70%; may have history of edema and weight gain (see chapter on Nephrotic Syndrome in Diseases and Disorders [Section I])
    - Hypertension: approximately 30%
      - May have headaches, blurry vision
    - Asymptomatic hematuria and proteinuria: approximately 20% to 40%
    - Azotemia: approximately 30%
    - Secondary forms may be suggested by:
      - History of malar rash, purpura, weight loss, arthritis, recurrent infections, cardiac disease, ventriculoatrial shunt, blood transfusion, jaundice

ETIOLOGY

- HSP
  - Immune complex disease is associated with IgA deposition in mesangial area of glomerulus and within vessel walls resulting in leukocytoclastic vasculitis.
- IgAN
  - Pathogenesis remains incompletely understood.
  - Presence of mesangial IgA deposition suggests immune complex-mediated disease.
- SLE
  - Characterized by production of autoantibodies
  - Etiology remains unclear
- Alport's nephritis
  - Mutations in genes encoding for the α-3, α-4, or α-5 chains of type IV collagen result in abnormal structure of glomerular basement membrane.
  - X-linked Alport's nephritis: genetic defect in COL4A5 (gene coding for α-5 chain of type IV collagen)
  - Autosomal recessive form involves mutations in COL4A3 or COL4A4.
  - Autosomal dominant form involves mutations in COL4A3 or COL4A4.
- MPGN
  - Immune complex disease with unknown antigen (type I, III)
  - May be associated with other chronic immune complex disorders or systemic diseases includes SLE, hepatitis B and C, and subacute bacterial endocarditis
  - Pathogenesis remains incompletely understood.

DIAGNOSIS Dx

DIFFERENTIAL DIAGNOSIS

The differential diagnosis for chronic glomerulonephritis in childhood includes:

- HSP
  - Histologically similar to IgA; clinical presentation differs
  - Other vasculitides such as SLE
  - See chapter on HSP
- IgAN
  - Histologically similar to HSP; clinical presentation differs
  - MPGN
  - Alport's nephritis
  - Other diseases associated with diffuse mesangial IgA deposits
    - SLE, cystic fibrosis, celiac disease, Crohn's disease, non-Hodgkin's lymphoma
- SLE
  - Other vasculitides (see chapter on SLE)
- Alport's nephritis
  - IgAN
  - MPGN
  - Thin basement membrane disease
    - Characterized by isolated hematuria which may be familial
    - Not associated with proteinuria, hypertension, renal insufficiency, deafness, or family history of renal failure
- MPGN
  - Low C3, when present, persists unlike with acute poststreptococcal glomerulonephritis (APSGN), which is associated with normalization of C3 within 6 to 8 weeks.
  - IgAN
  - Alport's nephritis—family history significant for renal failure and deafness
  - Can be associated with other conditions such as SLE, subacute bacterial endocarditis, human immunodeficiency virus (HIV), hepatitis B and C, sickle cell disease

WORKUP

- Renal biopsy
  - Early in course of Alport's syndrome, biopsy may be nondiagnostic
- Diagnosis of Alport's syndrome may be suspected based on family history of renal failure and deafness.
- Skin biopsy may be helpful in some cases but may also be inconclusive.

LABORATORY TESTS

- Complete blood cell count (CBC) with platelets
- Chemistries, renal function (blood urea nitrogen, creatinine), total protein, and albumin
- Complement levels—C3 and C4
  - Low C3 level suggests acute poststreptococcal glomerulonephritis, MPGN, or SLE.
- ASO titer—with initial episode to evaluate for possible APSGN
- Antinuclear antibodies—if suspect vasculitis
- IgA levels—may be elevated with HSP or IgA but not diagnostically helpful
- Prothrombin time/partial thromboplastin time—if petechiae or purpura noted
- Other serologies such as anti–double-stranded DNA or ANCA, if vasculitis suspected
- Urinalysis
- Random urine protein:creatinine ratio or 24-hour urine for protein and creatinine—to quantitate proteinuria
- Audiology and ophthalmology exam if suspect Alport's nephritis

TREATMENT Rx

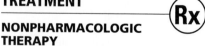

NONPHARMACOLOGIC THERAPY

- SLE (see chapter on SLE)
- Alport's nephritis
  - Hearing aids, if significant hearing impairment

ACUTE GENERAL Rx

Specific therapy for nephritis will be determined by the pediatric nephrologist or rheumatologist.

- HSP
  - Mild cases do not require therapy.
  - For moderate to severe cases of HSP nephritis (crescentic glomerulonephritis, nephrotic syndrome, or rapidly progressive disease), the nephrologist may treat with steroids, cyclophosphamide, azathioprine, and perhaps plasma exchange.
  - For management of extrarenal manifestations, see chapter on HSP.
- IgAN
  - Ideal therapy is not well established.
  - Possible treatments with steroids, fish oil, and angiotensin-converting enzyme (ACE) inhibitors should be considered by pediatric nephrologist.
- SLE
  - Treatment of lupus nephritis is guided by renal biopsy results and may include steroids, cyclophosphamide, cyclosporine, or mycophenolate mofetil.
  - For management of extrarenal symptoms, see chapter on SLE.
- Alport's nephritis
  - Supportive care for renal disease
    - ACE inhibitors may be beneficial for management of hypertension and proteinuria.
- MPGN (idiopathic)
  - Though still controversial, treatment with steroids appears to improve outcome.
  - Prescribe antihypertensive therapy as needed.
    - ACE inhibitors may be beneficial for management of both hypertension and proteinuria associated with any of the glomerulonephritides previously discussed.

CHRONIC Rx

- Outlined earlier under "Acute Rx"

DISPOSITION

All children with a chronic glomerulonephritis require regular follow-up with a pediatric nephrologist.

- HSP
  - Long-term morbidity from the disease is related to renal involvement.
    - Renal disease may not be present at onset but may develop within a few months.
      - All patients should have periodic urinalyses and blood pressure checks during the first 3 to 4 months after diagnosis of HSP.
    - The majority of patients recover well from acute illness, but an estimated 2% to 5% progress to chronic renal failure.
    - Poor prognostic indicators include nephrotic syndrome, renal insufficiency, and crescentic involvement.
  - Long-term studies show that up to 25% may have a late deterioration even if initial renal recovery was good.
- IgAN
  - Can be a slowly progressive disease
  - In adults, approximately one third develop chronic renal failure within 20 years.
- SLE
  - Natural history of renal involvement includes flares and remissions and therefore regular follow-up, even during quiescent periods, is important.
    - Complement levels (C3 and C4) may fall prior to development of clinical relapse.
    - Repeat renal biopsy may be necessary.
  - May be influenced by use of other therapies (e.g., nonsteroidal anti-inflammatory drugs)
  - See SLE chapter for additional information.
- Alport's nephritis
  - X-linked
    - Progressive renal disease with males developing renal failure
    - Course in females generally more benign
- MPGN
  - If untreated, 50% will lose renal function by 10 years.
  - Markers of poor outcome include nephrotic syndrome, renal insufficiency at diagnosis, and crescent formation.

REFERRAL

- Patients with suspected chronic glomerulonephritis (e.g., hematuria or proteinuria, RBC casts on urinalysis, renal insufficiency, hypertension) should be referred to a pediatric nephrologist.
- Patients with suspected lupus or other vasculitis should also be referred to a pediatric rheumatologist.

PEARLS & CONSIDERATIONS

COMMENTS

- Any chronic glomerulonephritis may have an acute presentation.
  - Patients with MPGN and low C3 may initially be diagnosed with APSGN and the diagnosis subsequently questioned when the C3 levels remain low 8 weeks after the initial illness.

PATIENT/FAMILY EDUCATION

- Educate the family about the chronic nature of the kidney disease and the importance of regular follow-up.
  - Monitor urine for worsening proteinuria, hematuria.
  - Monitor renal function and for the potential development of chronic renal failure and its sequelae (e.g., anemia, secondary hyperparathyroidism, poor growth).
  - Monitor blood pressure for the potential development of hypertension.
- In association with the nephrologist, educate the family regarding the natural history of the specific kidney disease, the therapeutic options, and the side effects of therapy.
- See chapters on HSP and SLE for additional information.

Web Sites and Support Groups

- National Kidney Foundation
- Lupus Foundation of America
- NephKids—Email support group for parents of children with chronic kidney disease. Available at http://www.mailman.srv.ualberta.ca/mailman/listinfo/nephkids

SUGGESTED READINGS

Andreoli SP: Chronic glomerulonephritis in childhood. *Pediatr Clin North Am* 42:1487, 1995.

Delos Santos NM et al: Pediatric IgA nephropathies: clinical aspects and therapeutic approaches. *Semin Nephrol* 24:269, 2004.

Hunley TE et al: IgA nephropathy. *Curr Opin Pediatr* 11:152, 1999.

Lau KK et al: Glomerulonephritis. *Adolesc Med* 16:67, 2005.

AUTHOR: **AYESA N. MIAN, MD**

BASIC INFORMATION

DEFINITION

Gonorrhea generally is referred to as an infection of the genital tract, but it may also include infection of the eye, skin, joint, pharynx, or blood by the gram-negative diplococcus *Neisseria gonorrhoeae.*

SYNONYMS

Pelvic inflammatory disease (PID)
Sexually transmitted disease (STD)
Sexually transmitted infection (STI)

ICD-9-CM CODES
098.0 Gonococcal infection
098.15 Cervical infection
098.19 Pelvic infection
098.40 Gonococcal conjunctivitis

EPIDEMIOLOGY & DEMOGRAPHICS

- In 2002, 351,852 cases of gonorrhea were reported in the United States to the Centers for Disease Control and Prevention (CDC).
- Those 15 to 29 years old represented 75% of the reported cases.
- Adolescent girls 15 to 19 years old and men 20 to 24 years old have the highest rates of infection.
- Ophthalmia neonatorum occurs in 2% to 4% of live births in the developed world, and in 0.5% of live births in the U.S.
- The most common complication of untreated gonorrhea is PID, an ascending infection of the upper genital tract.
- Gonorrhea is responsible for 50% of cases of PID.
- Up to one third of untreated cases of gonorrhea infection result in PID.
- Coinfection with *Chlamydia trachomatis* is common.

CLINICAL PRESENTATION

History

- Newborns
  - Ophthalmia neonatorum occurs after an incubation of less than 3 days.
  - No history of ocular prophylaxis in the newborn period.
  - Transmission is the result of exposure to infected cervical exudate during delivery.
  - Discharge is initially watery, becoming thick and mucopurulent.
  - Discharge occurs after the incubation period and, if not treated, progresses to corneal involvement leading to visual impairment.
  - Some cases do have a benign, limited course.
  - Disease is often bilateral.
  - Scalp abscesses can occur after in utero fetal monitoring.
  - Disseminated infections are rare.
- Prepubertal children
  - Disease manifests as vaginitis with discharge.
  - Dysuria, frequency, and urgency occur.
  - Suspect sexual abuse unless proved otherwise.
- Adolescents
  - One third of genital tract infections are asymptomatic.
  - Urethritis occurs approximately 1 week after exposure.
  - Dysuria is common.
  - Mucoid discharge becomes purulent.
  - In females, abdominal pain, pelvic pain or fullness, dysuria, and discharge are the common complaints.
  - Fever, vomiting, and anorexia also occur, especially with more extensive disease.
  - Extension from genital mucosal infections can lead to less common presentations.
    - Scrotal pain (epididymitis) may occur.
    - Right upper quadrant pain, vomiting, and anorexia occur with perihepatitis or Fitzhugh-Curtis syndrome.
    - Painful and enlarged lesions (bartholinitis) can be present.
    - PID manifests with mild to severe anorexia, abdominal or pelvic pain, and fever.
  - Pharyngitis is often asymptomatic but may manifest with an exudative sore throat.
  - Between 1% and 3% of adolescents who are untreated develop disseminated gonococcal infection.
    - Presents with septic arthritis or with systemic signs (i.e., fever, chills, and polyarthralgias).
    - A rash with tender skin lesions may be present.

Physical Examination

- Neonates
  - Mucopurulent eye discharge
  - Scalp abscesses
  - Sepsis (with lethargy, apnea, bradycardia, tachypnea, color changes, blood pressure instability, or hypotension)
- Prepubertal children: vaginal discharge
- Adolescents
  - Vaginitis occurs with a thick, white-green-yellow discharge.
  - Cervical tenderness can occur with motion.
  - Urethritis (i.e., penile discharge and dysuria) is the most common finding in infected males.
  - Pustules are seen on erythematous bases; petechiae, papules, and macules occur on extremities and often overlie septic joints in cases of disseminated disease.
  - Tenosynovitis and arthritis occur, especially of the knee.

ETIOLOGY

N. gonorrhoeae, a gram-negative diplococcus, may infect the mucosal surfaces of urogenital sites (e.g., cervix, urethra, rectum) and the oropharynx and nasopharynx (i.e., throat), causing symptomatic or asymptomatic infections.

DIAGNOSIS

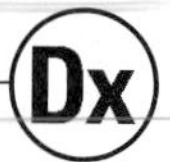

DIFFERENTIAL DIAGNOSIS

- Newborn conjunctivitis
  - Chemical conjunctivitis (i.e., silver nitrate prophylaxis)
  - *Chlamydia* conjunctivitis
  - Lacrimal duct obstruction
  - Viral conjunctivitis
  - Other bacterial conjunctivitis
- Vaginitis or PID
  - Coinfection with *Chlamydia trachomatis*
  - *Trichomonas*
  - Herpes simplex virus
  - Polymicrobial infections
- Septic arthritis
  - Other bacterial causes
  - Tumor
  - Osteomyelitis
  - Rheumatologic
  - Trauma

LABORATORY TESTS

- Gram stain of the exudate from the eyes, endocervix, vagina, male urethra, and skin lesions provides identification of gram-negative intracellular diplococci.
- Positive culture on selective media (i.e., Thayer-Martin-chocolate agar supplemented with antibiotics) is the gold standard.
- In newborns, cultures of blood and cerebrospinal fluid should be obtained to evaluate the possibility of dissemination.
- Culture should be the basis for diagnosis in the prepubertal child due to forensic concerns in the evaluation of sexual abuse.
- Nonculture methods include the following:
  - DNA probes (i.e., polymerase chain reaction and ligase chain reaction)
    - Urine-based tests (i.e., DNA probes) are used to screen for asymptomatic infections.
    - Urine-based tests are less invasive and increase compliance (i.e., acceptance of testing) in obtaining data.
  - Enzyme immunoassay tests
- It is important to test for coinfections (e.g., *Chlamydia,* syphilis, human immunodeficiency virus, *Trichomonas*) with any STI.

TREATMENT

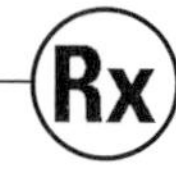

NONPHARMACOLOGIC THERAPY

Nonpharmacologic treatment is inappropriate even for an asymptomatic infection.

ACUTE GENERAL Rx

- Any one of the following may be used for uncomplicated infections:
  - Cefixime: 400 mg orally, taken once (unavailable in the United States)
  - Ceftriaxone: 125 mg, administered once intramuscularly
  - Ciprofloxacin: 500 mg, taken orally once
  - Ofloxacin: 400 mg, taken orally once

- Levofloxacin: 250 mg, taken orally once
- Azithromycin: 2 g, taken orally once

- Either of the following therapies may be provided for coinfection with *Chlamydia*:
  - Azithromycin: 1 g, taken orally once
  - Doxycycline: 100 mg, taken orally twice daily for 7 days
- Therapy should be provided for newborn conjunctivitis.
  - Ceftriaxone: 25 to 50 mg/kg, administered once intramuscularly or intravenously (maximum of 125 mg)
  - Saline irrigation of the affected eye

COMPLEMENTARY & ALTERNATIVE MEDICINE

Practice safe sex.

DISPOSITION

Anticipatory guidance regarding sexual behavior and risk taking needs to be addressed at health care visits.

REFERRAL

Positive gonorrhea culture results need to be reported to the appropriate public health authorities according to individual state laws.

PEARLS & CONSIDERATIONS

COMMENTS

In general, antibiotics are used to cover gonorrhea and *Chlamydia* because coinfection is common.

PREVENTION

- Primary prevention
  - Abstinence
  - Postponement of sexual involvement
  - Sexual risk reduction
  - Condom use
- Secondary prevention
  - Access to medical care
  - Partner notification

PATIENT/FAMILY EDUCATION

- Gonorrhea is a sexually transmitted disease. Abstinence or condom use can decrease or eliminate the risk of infection.
- Infection should be treated with antibiotics urgently to decrease the risk to sexual partners and to decrease the risk to unborn children of pregnant women.

SUGGESTED READINGS

Centers for Disease Control and Prevention. Available at www.cdc.gov

AUTHOR: **MAUREEN NOVAK, MD**

BASIC INFORMATION

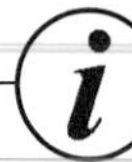

DEFINITION

Granuloma inguinale is a granulomatous ulcerative disease of the skin and subcutaneous tissues of the genital area. It is rare in the United States.

SYNONYM

Donovanosis

ICD-9-CM CODE

099.2 Granuloma inguinale

EPIDEMIOLOGY & DEMOGRAPHICS

- Granuloma inguinale is the major cause of genital ulcers in many tropical regions of the world, including Papua, New Guinea; southeast India; eastern South Africa; and the Caribbean.
- The highest incidence occurs in tropical and subtropical areas.
- The incubation period is 8 to 80 days.
- It is transmitted through sexual intercourse with a person with an active infection.
- Young children can become infected by contact with infected secretions.

CLINICAL PRESENTATION

History

- Any travel to endemic countries
- Any sexual contact with a person with genital ulcer disease

Physical Examination

- Subcutaneous genital nodules progress to painless ulcers that may bleed.
- There may be single or multiple nodules.
- Involvement of the anal area occurs in 5% to 10% of cases.
- Extragenital lesions of face, mouth, or liver occur in approximately 6% of cases.
- Pseudobubo is an inguinal mass that represents subcutaneous extension to the inguinal area and mimics inguinal lymphadenopathy.

ETIOLOGY

An intracellular gram-negative bacterium called *Calymmatobacterium granulomatosis* related most closely to the *Klebsiella* species

DIAGNOSIS

DIFFERENTIAL DIAGNOSIS

- In the United States, most young, sexually active patients with genital ulcers have genital herpes, syphilis, or chancroid (other possibilities include tuberculosis and carcinoma).
- Lymphogranuloma venereum, blastomycosis, and other granulomatous diseases are also part of the differential diagnosis.

WORKUP

Most cases are diagnosed on the basis of characteristic clinical findings.

LABORATORY TESTS

- Confirmation of the diagnosis can be made by the following methods:
  - Histologic examination is performed on punch biopsy specimens taken from the edge of active lesions.
  - Scrapings are obtained from the edges of active lesions.
  - A crush preparation is made from granulation tissue obtained with a thin scalpel. The preparation is made by taking a piece of granulation tissue from a lesion and crushing it between slides. The smear then should be air dried and stained with Wright or Giemsa stain. Donovan bodies are dark-staining, intracellular inclusions seen in large mononuclear cells.
- Polymerase chain reaction (PCR) and serologic testing are available only on a research basis.

TREATMENT

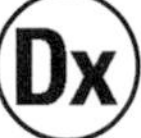

ACUTE GENERAL Rx

- Administer trimethoprim-sulfamethoxazole or doxycycline for children 8 years or older. Treat for a minimum of 3 weeks or until lesions heal.
- Alternative regimens include the following:
  - Ciprofloxacin for at least 3 weeks
  - Erythromycin (used in pregnant and lactating women) for at least 3 weeks
  - Azithromycin for at least 3 weeks
- Healing begins within 7 days of starting therapy.
- Evaluate the patient for other sexually transmitted diseases such as gonorrhea, syphilis, *Chlamydia trachomatis*, human immunodeficiency virus (HIV), and hepatitis B virus.

DISPOSITION

- Patients should be clinically followed weekly until signs and symptoms have resolved.
- Healing occurs in 3 to 5 weeks, except in severe cases.

PEARLS & CONSIDERATIONS

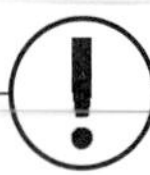

COMMENTS

- Most genital ulcer disease in the United States is caused by herpes, syphilis, or chancroid.
- A secondary bacterial infection may develop in the lesions, or coinfection with another sexually transmitted pathogen can occur.

PREVENTION

Safe sex practices should be used.

PATIENT/FAMILY EDUCATION

- Safe sex recommendations should be reviewed.
- Sexual contacts should be examined and treated prophylactically in the following cases:
  - If they had sexual contact with the patient during the 60 days preceding the onset of symptoms.
  - If they have clinical signs and symptoms of the disease.
- Relapse occurs frequently. It can occur 6 to 18 months later despite effective initial therapy.

SUGGESTED READINGS

American Academy of Pediatrics: Granuloma inguinale. *In* Pickering LK (ed): *2003 Red Book: Report of the Committee on Infectious Diseases,* 26th ed. Elk Grove Village, IL, American Academy of Pediatrics, 2003, pp 292–293.

Centers for Disease Control and Prevention: Granuloma inguinale (donovanosis). *In 2002 Guidelines for Treatment of Sexually Transmitted Diseases.* Atlanta, Centers for Disease Control and Prevention, 2002.

Centers for Disease Control and Prevention: www.cdc.gov/nchstp/dstd/STD98T06.htm

Hart GL: Donovanosis. *Clin Infect Dis* 25:24, 1997.

Paterson DL: Disseminated donovanosis (granuloma inguinale) causing spinal cord compression: case report and review of donovanosis involving bone. *Clin Infect Dis* 26:379, 1998.

AUTHOR: **CYNTHIA CHRISTY, MD**

BASIC INFORMATION

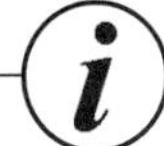

DEFINITION

Guillain-Barré syndrome is an acute polyradiculoneuropathy that classically manifests with ascending paresthesias, weakness, areflexia, and autonomic dysfunction.

SYNONYMS

Acute idiopathic demyelinating polyneuritis (AIDP)
Acute idiopathic polyneuritis
Acute motor axonal neuropathy (AMAN)
Postinfective polyneuritis

ICD-9-CM CODE
357.0 Guillain-Barré syndrome

EPIDEMIOLOGY & DEMOGRAPHICS

- The incidence is 1 to 2 cases per 100,000 people in the general population per year in the developed world.
- The male-to-female ratio is 1.25:1.
- Guillain-Barré syndrome affects all ages, but bimodal peaks occur, representing young adults and the elderly.

CLINICAL PRESENTATION

History

- Between 50% and 70% of patients have a nonspecific viral illness in the preceding month.
- Guillain-Barré syndrome most commonly manifests with symmetric weakness of the legs, low back and leg pain, paresthesias, and areflexia.
  - It begins in the lower extremities.
  - It progresses cephalad to the trunk, upper extremities, and bulbar muscles.
  - Weakness may begin in the upper extremities and progress caudad.
  - Weakness may progress to flaccid paralysis.
- It is a monophasic illness with three stages.
  - Progression phase: worsening symptoms for days to weeks (average, 5 to 10 days)
  - Plateau phase: static symptoms for days to weeks (usually less than 3 weeks)
  - Recovery: usually begins 2 to 4 weeks after halt of progression; recovery continues for weeks to months, up to 12 months in some cases
- Approximately 40% of patients have sensory complaints.
- Fifty percent of patients have bulbar involvement that may result in oculomotor weakness, dysphagia, facial weakness, and respiratory insufficiency.
- Miller-Fisher variant is characterized by acute external ophthalmoplegia, ataxia, and areflexia.
- Between 10% and 20% of patients progress to respiratory failure requiring mechanical ventilation.

Physical Examination

- The patient is usually afebrile.
- Examine the skin for ticks (to rule out tick paralysis).
- Examine the spine for tenderness (in consideration for diskitis, transverse myelitis, epidural abscess, other spinal cord or vertebral abnormalities).
- Meningismus and papilledema are rare and more compatible with other diagnoses.
- Symmetric motor weakness usually occurs with distal to proximal progression. Between 5% and 10% of patients may have initial involvement of upper extremities.
- Deep tendon reflexes are absent in areas of weakness. Very early in the disease course, there may be deep tendon reflexes in proximal areas, but they are absent in distal regions.
- Typically, patients complain of some nonspecific leg pain. Although some patients may have some mild distal sensory loss, a sensory level suggests another diagnosis.
- Patients have an ataxic gait out of proportion to weakness.
- Patients may have cranial nerve involvement with facial weakness, oculomotor palsy, and diminished swallowing.
- Between 10% and 20% of patients progress to respiratory failure, which is best monitored by forced vital capacity.
- Patients may have associated severe autonomic dysfunction, including tachyarrhythmias, bradyarrhythmias, and labile blood pressure.
- Bowel and bladder dysfunction are rare, and when they occur, they should prompt a thorough evaluation for spinal cord pathology.

ETIOLOGY

Infectious organisms probably share epitopes with components of peripheral nerve myelin (in AIDP) or peripheral nerve axons (in AMAN), causing the immune responses to cross-react with these nerve components (i.e., molecular mimicry).

DIAGNOSIS

Dx

DIFFERENTIAL DIAGNOSIS

- Acute cerebellar ataxia: deep tendon reflexes intact, cerebrospinal fluid (CSF) protein in the normal range
- Spinal cord diseases (e.g., compression myelopathy, transverse myelitis)
  - Patients usually have a distinct spinal level of sensory loss and paresthesias.
  - Transverse myelitis often manifests with back pain and a distinct sensory level with paraparesis.
  - Epidural abscess often manifests with fever, back pain, and lower extremity weakness.
- Poliomyelitis: symmetric paralysis, with no sensory deficits
- Diphtheria: early signs of palatal paralysis, difficulty swallowing, blurred vision followed by cranial nerve involvement, loss of reflexes, and neuropathy
- Tick paralysis
  - Irritability and anorexia are followed by ascending weakness.
  - Weakness is usually rapidly progressive.
  - Ticks are commonly located in nuchal or occipital area.
  - Removal of a tick is diagnostic.
- Porphyria: abdominal pain, disturbed consciousness, apparent psychosis, seizures, and rapidly progressive peripheral neuropathy
- Botulism
  - In children younger than 1 year with acute weakness, botulism is most likely.
  - In infants, constipation may be the first symptom, followed by decreased feeding and ptosis.
  - In older children, it commonly manifests with diplopia, photophobia, and blurred vision, followed by difficulty swallowing and increasing weakness.
- Myasthenia gravis
  - There is a history of slow progression and episodic weakness with ptosis or ophthalmoplegia.
  - Reflexes and sensation are normal.
- Heavy metal intoxication (e.g., lead, arsenic, mercury, thallium)
  - Encephalopathy almost always precedes peripheral nerve disease.
  - With lead intoxication, footdrop may precede encephalopathy.
  - Often, erythema and tremors are seen with mercury poisoning.
- Glue sniffing
- Drug-induced toxic neuropathy: reported with amitriptyline, dapsone, glutethimide, hydralazine, isoniazid, nitrofurantoin, and vincristine
- Organophosphate poisoning: usually includes pupillary changes, salivation, and gastrointestinal disturbance
- Lyme disease
  - In stage 2, patients may have neuropathy, encephalopathy, cranial neuropathy, or peripheral radiculoneuropathy.
  - A history of erythema chronicum migrans is helpful.
- Polymyositis
  - Onset can be sudden or chronic, with proximal muscle weakness, especially of the pelvic and shoulder girdles.
  - Dysphagia and neck weakness are common.
  - Levels of muscle enzymes are elevated.
- Black widow spider bite

WORKUP

- CSF examination (the following findings are typical during the second week of disease)
  - The opening pressure is normal.
  - CSF protein elevation: About 50% have elevations in first week of illness, with increasing CSF protein over the ensuing weeks.
  - Peak protein level is between 80 and 200 mg/dL.
  - The CSF cell count rarely exceeds 10 lymphocytes/mm^3.

    - A cell count greater than 50 suggests an alternative diagnosis.
    - The glucose level is normal.
    - Cultures show no growth.
- Electrodiagnostic studies are helpful.
    - Nerve conduction studies may show evidence of multifocal demyelination, with possible superimposed axonal degeneration.
    - Typically, conduction block, marked slowing of conduction velocity, prolonged distal latency, and temporal dispersion are seen.
    - Typical electrophysiologic features may not be apparent until clinical weakness is well established.
    - Electromyography may show abnormal recruitment of motor units. In AMAN, there is no evidence of demyelination. Electromyography is important for showing small CMAPs and dispersion.

LABORATORY TESTS

- Urine for porphyrins
- Complete blood cell count and erythrocyte sedimentation rate usually normal
- Lyme titer
- Human immunodeficiency virus (HIV) serology
- Urine screen for heavy metals

IMAGING STUDIES

Magnetic resonance imaging is useful if the presentation is consistent with a cord process rather than Guillain-Barré syndrome.

TREATMENT

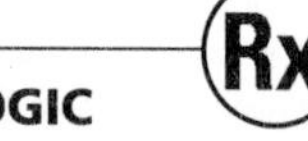

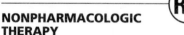

NONPHARMACOLOGIC THERAPY

- Admit the patient to the hospital to monitor respiratory status and autonomic instability and to provide supportive care.
- Provide nutritional support.
- Consult neurology and obtain electrodiagnostic studies.
- Monitor forced vital capacity every 6 hours for signs of impending respiratory failure.
- Monitor the patient's ability to protect the airway (intubation may be necessary if the gag reflex is absent or diminished gag reflex).
- Monitor the skin for decubiti.
- Indications of impending respiratory failure include the following:
    - Rapidly decreasing vital capacity
    - Breathlessness or fatigue
    - Deteriorating values of arterial blood gases
    - Dysphagia and shoulder weakness
    - Rapidly progressive paralysis
- Use respiratory support, intubation, and ventilation if indicated.
- Perform a tracheostomy if long-term ventilator support is anticipated.

ACUTE GENERAL Rx

- For patients with rapidly progressive disease, bulbar paralysis, or impending respiratory distress or for those unable to walk, plasmapheresis or intravenous immune globulin (IVIG) have been effective.
- Manage symptomatic pain.

CHRONIC Rx

- For relapses, refer the patient to a neurologist, who may suggest a repeat course of IVIG.
- Physical therapy may be useful.

DISPOSITION

- The recovery phase may continue for up to 1 year.
- Most rapid recovery occurs within the first 6 months, and approximately 85% of patients have full recovery in 12 months.
- Patients may need symptomatic support and physical therapy.
- Between 3% and 5% of patients have relapsing disease and may need repeated immunomodulatory treatment.

REFERRAL

Refer the patient to a neurologist.

PEARLS & CONSIDERATIONS

COMMENTS

- Fever is not typical.
- Bowel and bladder involvement is rare.
- Preceding *Campylobacter jejuni* infection is often associated with AMAN.
- Dysphagia and facial weakness should increase concern about respiratory failure.
- In an infant with sudden or rapidly progressive weakness, think first of botulism.
- Search the skin carefully for ticks.

PATIENT/FAMILY EDUCATION

- The National Institute of Neurological Disorders and Stroke web site (http://www.ninds.nih.gov/disorders/gbs/gbs.htm) has information on Guillain-Barré syndrome and other neurologic diseases.
- The Guillain-Barré Syndrome Support Group (http://www.gbs.org.uk/) provides information for patients and parents.

SUGGESTED READINGS

Neuromuscular home page. Available at http://www.neuro.wustl.edu/neuromuscular/antibody/gbs.htm

Newswanger DL, Warren CR: Guillain-Barré syndrome. *Am Fam Physician* 69:2405, 2004.

AUTHOR: **JENNIFER M. KWON, MD**

BASIC INFORMATION

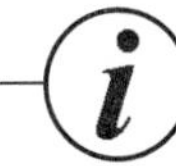

DEFINITION

Gynecomastia is benign glandular development of the male breast.

ICD-9-CM CODE
611.1 Gynecomastia

EPIDEMIOLOGY & DEMOGRAPHICS

- Between 60% and 90% of infants have transient gynecomastia.
- Between 30% and 50% of adolescent males have transient gynecomastia.
- Onset usually occurs at age 10 to 12 years (i.e., begins 6 months after puberty starts).
- The occurrence peaks at age 13 to 14 years (i.e., Tanner stage III).
- Regression usually occurs spontaneously in 6 months, affecting approximately 75% within 2 years and 90% within 3 years.

CLINICAL PRESENTATION

- Gynecomastia developing before puberty (excluding neonatal period) or later than 6 months after puberty requires further workup.
- Physical examination includes palpation of breast tissue by moving the thumb and forefinger on each side of the breast and moving them inward toward the nipple. Optimally, the patient should be positioned with hands behind his head.
  - Gynecomastia should be symmetric around the nipple.
  - Tissue should feel rubbery or firm.
  - Typically, a growth more than 0.5 cm in diameter is detectable; most studies consider gynecomastia as more than 2 cm of glandular tissue.
  - Adipose tissue (causing pseudogynecomastia) produces little resistance with palpation.
- Other relevant items on the physical examination include:
  - Testicular size (<3 cm may indicate hypogonadism)
  - Testicular masses (neoplasms)
  - Evidence of feminization (e.g., eunuchoid body habitus, female hair pattern, small testicles)

ETIOLOGY

- The cause is an imbalance of stimulatory estrogens and inhibitory androgens.
  - During puberty, most patients with gynecomastia have no significant differences in one-time measurements of testosterone, estradiol, estrone, or gonadotropins from those of pubescent boys without gynecomastia.
  - Some studies have shown transient rises in estradiol (preceding testosterone) as a contributing factor to adolescent gynecomastia.
  - Boys can have abnormal hormone production (i.e., adrenal or testicular tumor).
  - There may be an abnormal tissue response to hormones (i.e., androgen insensitivity syndromes).
  - Hormone binding by sex hormone-binding globulin (SHBG) may be altered.
  - Peripheral conversion of androgens to estrogens may occur (i.e., by adipose tissue).
  - Hormonal profiles may be altered by exogenous hormones (i.e., placenta in the neonate) or ingestion or injection of hormones directly.

DIAGNOSIS

Dx

DIFFERENTIAL DIAGNOSIS

- Pseudogynecomastia: adipose tissue
- Conditions causing acentric or asymmetric breast tissue:
  - Lipomas
  - Neurofibromas
  - Dermoid cysts
  - Lymphangiomas

WORKUP

- In the setting of adolescence with normal physical and genitourinary examination results, follow-up every 6 months is all that is indicated.
- Worsening or failure to improve may indicate a need for further workup.
- Investigate intentional or unintentional drug exposures, including drugs of abuse (e.g., marijuana, anabolic steroids) and prescription drugs (e.g., H_2-blockers, antibiotics, antifungals) (see Box 1-2).
- Targeted endocrinologic workup of gynecomastia included the following indications:
  - If severe (>5 cm)
  - Painful (not merely tender)
  - Develops before puberty
  - Associated with small testicular volume
  - Others signs of endocrine disease, such as weight loss or tachycardia related to thyroid disease
- Evaluation may be targeted toward physical findings.
  - Evaluation of possible neoplasm: testicular mass or abdominal mass
  - Evaluation of hard, nodular, or eccentric breast tissue

LABORATORY TESTS

- Follicle-stimulating hormone (FSH), luteinizing hormone (LH), estradiol, and testosterone (i.e., free testosterone is most useful because of variation in SHBG)
- Thyroid-stimulating hormone (TSH) (e.g., altered thyroid function alters SHBG, alters aromatization of androgens)
- Human chorionic gonadotropin (hCG) (i.e., elevated in germ cell testicular tumors, which account for 95% of testicular neoplasms)
- Serum creatinine to evaluate renal insufficiency (i.e., Leydig cell insufficiency with renal failure)
- Hepatic function tests (i.e., liver dysfunction and cirrhosis are associated with enhanced accumulation of androgens and elevation of SHBG)
- Karyotype if Klinefelter syndrome suspected (gynecomastia occurs in 80% of patients with klinefelter syndrome)

IMAGING STUDIES

- Mammography is good for evaluating gynecomastia to rule cut with pseudogynecomastia.
- Mammography or ultrasound can be used to evaluate other breast masses that may be confused with gynecomastia.
- Testicular ultrasound if mass is palpable and to evaluate testicular architecture or size.
- Computed tomography of the abdomen or pelvis if an adrenal tumor is suspected or an abdominal mass is palpable.

TREATMENT

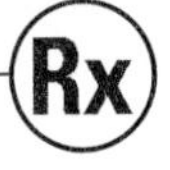

NONPHARMACOLOGIC THERAPY

Breast reduction surgery should be considered if the enlargement is severe or persistent.

ACUTE GENERAL Rx

- Withdraw precipitating drugs or medicines, including illicit substances (e.g., marijuana, anabolic steroids) and drugs that may alter the androgen-estrogen balance.
- Treat the underlying disorder, such as a testicular or adrenal neoplasm or hyperthyroidism.
- Treat severe or persistent pubertal gynecomastia with androgens such as dihydrotestosterone (DHT), antiestrogens (i.e., tamoxifen and raloxifene), or the aromatase inhibitor, testolactone.

DISPOSITION

Most neonatal and pubertal gynecomastia resolves without intervention.

REFERRAL

- Refer the patient to a plastic surgeon or breast surgical specialist in the following situations.
  - An abnormal breast mass on imaging is not consistent with gynecomastia, and biopsy may be indicated.
  - If the gynecomastia causes significant emotional distress, has failed to respond to watchful waiting, or has failed endocrine (drug) therapy (i.e., probable reduction mammoplasty candidate).
- Refer the patient to an endocrinologist for the following indications:
  - Breast tissue is more than 3 cm in diameter and enlarging or failing to decrease in size over repeated 6-month follow-up visits.
  - There is evidence of an abnormal hormonal profile (e.g., androgen insensitivity, primary hypogonadism, adrenal hormone source, hyperthyroidism).

- ○ The patient has Klinefelter syndrome.
- Refer the patient to a specialist in urology and/or oncology for the following indications:
  - ○ Testicular mass or elevated hCG level
  - ○ Adrenal mass

PEARLS & CONSIDERATIONS

COMMENTS

- Significant gynecomastia that is present for more than 1 year may not be reversible, and patients therefore need prompt evaluation or referral.
- Significant fibrosis may be detected histologically in 1 year.
- Breast cancer is extremely uncommon in the pediatric population.

PREVENTION

- Patients should avoid illicit substances, especially marijuana, heroin, or amphetamines.
- Caution should be exercised for certain prescription drugs (see Box 1-2).

BOX 1-2 **Drugs Associated with Gynecomastia**

Hormones
Estrogens
Aromatizable androgens
Gonadotropins

Psychoactive Drugs
Tricyclic antidepressants
Phenothaizines
Benzodiazepine

Cardiovascular Drugs
Calcium channel blockers
Angiotensin-converting enzyme Inhibitors
Digoxin

Diuretics
Spironolactone
Thiazides

Gastric Acid Inhibitor
Cimetidine
Omeprazole

Antibiotics
Isoniazid
Ketoconazole
Metronidazole

Cytotoxic Drugs
Cyclophosphamide
Methotrexate
Vincristine

Other
Aurafin
Ergotamine
Etretinate
Metoclopramide
Minoxidil
Penicillamine
Sulindac
Theophylline

Drugs of Abuse
Alcohol
Marijuana
Heroin
Methadone
Amphetamines

From Davis AJ, Kulig JW: Adolescent breast disorders. *Adolescent Health Update* 1996;9:7.

PATIENT/FAMILY EDUCATION

- Reassurance can safely be given to most adolescents and their parents when breast tissue development is consistent with their Tanner stage and age.
- Reassurance can be given to most parents of neonates.
- More information is available for parents and patients on the Internet (http://www.nlm.nih.gov/medlineplus/, http://www.keepkidshealthy.com/).

SUGGESTED READINGS

Braunstein GD: Gynecomastia. *N Engl J Med* 328:490, 1993.

Lawrence SE et al: Beneficial effects of raloxifene and tamoxifen in the treatment of pubertal gynecomastia. *J Pediatr* 145:71, 2004.

AUTHOR: **GUS GIBBONS EMMICK, MD**

BASIC INFORMATION

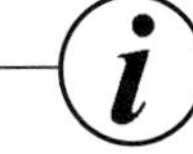

DEFINITION

Hand, foot, and mouth (HFM) disease is a viral infection characterized by a particular pattern of exanthem (rash) and enanthem (oral eruption).

SYNONYMS

Anterior stomatitis with exanthem
"Hoof and mouth disease" (popular misconstruction)

ICD-9-CM CODE

079.2 Hand, foot, and mouth disease

EPIDEMIOLOGY & DEMOGRAPHICS

- Information is extrapolated from data on enteroviral infection.
- While other animals may acquire infection from contact with people, humans are the only natural hosts.
- Distribution is worldwide.
- Disease may be endemic, epidemic, or pandemic.
- Seasonal variation: Attack rates peak in summer and fall, although sporadic cases may occur throughout the year in temperate climates. Occurrence is yearlong in tropical climates.
- Route of transmission is largely fecal-oral, and less commonly, via respiratory droplets. Indirect transmission via contaminated food, water, or fomites has been described.
- Enteroviral infection is frequently asymptomatic. In the case of Coxsackie A16, the most frequent cause of HFM disease, the rate of clinical expression is particularly high. Children less than 5 years of age demonstrate the highest clinical expression rates (up to 100%), followed by school-age children (38%), and adults (11%).
- Severity of infection varies inversely with age.
- Clinical manifestations of illness often differ markedly among household members.
- Spread within a community is typically from child-to-child, then within family groups.

CLINICAL PRESENTATION

History

- Sudden onset of fever (38.3°C to 41°C lasting 1 to 7 days) frequently accompanied by anorexia, malaise, and sore throat. Vomiting, diarrhea, or abdominal pain (3% to 33%), and rarely, conjunctivitis (0% to 18%) may occur.
- Enanthem occurs concomitantly with, or shortly after, the onset of fever and lasts up to 1 week.
- Exanthem follows 1 to 2 days after the onset of fever and oral eruption, and also persists for up to 1 week. Adults frequently experience symptomatic disease without the associated rash.

Physical Examination

- Enanthem:
  - Oral lesions chiefly involve the tongue and buccal mucosa but may also include the palate.
  - They begin as small, 3 to 8 mm erythematous macules, which rapidly progress to vesicles and may coalesce into bullae.
  - Most typically, they ulcerate before resolution.
- Exanthem:
  - Peripherally distributed, involving the extremities. Hands are more frequently involved than feet.
  - Lesions are more common on the dorsal and interdigital surfaces, but may often be found on the palms, soles, and buttocks.
  - They are small (3 to 7 mm), tender, and consist of mixed papules and vesicles with surrounding erythema.

ETIOLOGY

HFM is caused by several Enteroviruses, predominantly Coxsackie A16. Other agents include: Coxsackie types A5, A7, A9, A10, B1, B2 and B3; *Echovirus* 33; and *Enterovirus* 71.

- Incubation period: probably 2 to 10 days.
- Viremia potentially occurs twice.
  - The initial ("minor") viremia occurs on approximately the third post-exposure day, often coinciding with the onset of early symptoms. During this initial viremia, viral particles travel to secondary sites of replication (skin and mucous membranes, distant lymph nodes, and potentially, the respiratory tract, heart, central nervous system, pancreas, adrenals, liver, spleen). If by this point, host immune mechanisms are able to sufficiently limit viral replication, subclinical infection may occur.
  - A second ("major") viremia follows (approximately day 3 to 7 post-exposure), at which time an additional opportunity for distal seeding occurs.
- Immune response: not fully understood, but serotype-specific antibody probably plays the major role, followed by macrophage function.
- Shedding: occurs from the upper respiratory tract for 1 to 3 weeks and in the stool for up to 8 to 12 weeks following primary infection.
  - Asymptomatic shedding occurs frequently.
  - Following re-infection, fecal (but not oral) shedding may also occur, although this is usually at a lower titer and of shorter duration.

DIAGNOSIS

Dx

DIFFERENTIAL DIAGNOSIS

- *Varicella:* Patients with varicella are generally more ill appearing and demonstrate more extensive and centrally distributed skin lesions, but less oral involvement.
  - Unlike varicella, the lesions of HFM disease heal by absorption and thus do not form pustules or crusts.
- *Herpetic gingivostomatitis* (HGS): Lesions in HGS are both larger and more anteriorly located. Involvement of the gingivae, common in HGS, is not typically seen in HFM.
- *Herpangina:* The enanthem is also caused by enteroviral infection and resembles HFM, but is distributed more posteriorly. There are no cutaneous lesions.
- *Aphthous stomatitis:* Oral lesions are often larger, more anterior, and usually unaccompanied by fever or systemic symptoms.

WORKUP

For uncomplicated HFM, diagnosis is clinical.

LABORATORY TESTS

- Direct culture of nasopharynx, throat, rectum, or any body fluid may be obtained.
  - Specimens should be kept cool and protected from light.
  - Evidence of enteroviral growth is typically apparent within 3 to 6 days. Group A Coxsackieviruses are not grown as readily on standard viral culture media as other enteroviruses.
  - Rectal specimens must be interpreted with care. Due to the prolonged period of shedding in stool, enterovirus detected there may reflect prior infection rather than current disease.
- Polymerase chain reaction (PCR) testing of pharynx, cerebrospinal fluid (CSF), blood, or urine is available. In infants or individuals with suspected enteroviral meningitis, PCR on CSF has been shown to be a more rapid and sensitive technique than standard culture, depending upon lab availability.

TREATMENT

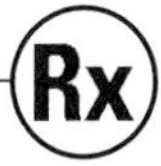

NONPHARMACOLOGIC THERAPY

- Treatment is typically supportive, including adequate oral hydration.
- Cold, nonacidic fluids (e.g., popsicles or slushes) may provide symptomatic relief.

ACUTE GENERAL Rx

- Analgesics (acetaminophen 12 to 15 mg/kg/dose every 4 hours or ibuprofen 7 to 8 mg/kg/dose every 6 to 8 hours) may be used for pain and fever control.
- Neonates or patients with humoral immune deficiency may experience severe, disseminated disease for which intravenous immune globulin may prove beneficial. (High titers of neutralizing antibody to several enteroviruses may be found in immunoglobulin.)
- Pleconaril, a novel antiviral agent which prevents viral attachment to host cell receptors, has been used on a limited basis in

complicated enteroviral infection. It has no role in typical HFM disease therapy.

DISPOSITION

- Outpatient management is the rule, as illness is typically mild and self-limited.
- Because other, more severe, manifestations of enteroviral illness may ensue (meningitis, encephalitis, myocarditis, pulmonary edema, etc.), clear guidelines for parent observation for signs and symptoms indicative of progression to more severe enteroviral illness or dehydration are warranted, with reevaluation as necessary.
- Vomiting (though present in up to 3% to 15% of individuals with uncomplicated HFM disease) and absence of oral lesions have each been associated with more severe disease and warrant close observation or additional evaluation for secondary sites of involvement (central nervous system, heart, liver, etc.).
- Children may return to day care and school when oral lesions are unaccompanied by drooling, and illness has resolved enough to allow comfortable resumption of activities.

REFERRAL

- As indicated for evidence of neurologic, cardiac, or hepatic disease.

PEARLS & CONSIDERATIONS

COMMENTS

- Enteroviruses are inactivated quickly by heat (>56°C), chlorination, formaldehyde, and ultraviolet light.
- *Enterovirus 71* has been identified as the etiologic agent in several fatal outbreaks of HFM disease characterized by progression, within 2 to 7 days, to refractory shock, cardiac dysfunction, pulmonary edema, and encephalomyelitis.

PREVENTION

- Control measures include personal hygiene, particularly hand washing around diaper changes and avoidance of oral secretions.
- Perinatal acquisition of an enterovirus can occur, including vertical transmission and postnatal infection. Special caution should be exercised to limit exposure to pregnant women, particularly in the third trimester.

PATIENT/FAMILY EDUCATION

- Typical HFM disease is self-limited, lasting approximately 3 to 7 days. Course may be biphasic, consistent with the minor and major viremias of enteroviral infection.

SUGGESTED READINGS

Cherry JD: Enteroviruses Parechoviruses. *In* Feigin RD et al (eds): *Textbook of Pediatric Infectious Diseases,* 5th ed. Philadelphia, WB Saunders, 2004, pp 1984–2025.

Chong CY et al: Hand, foot and mouth disease in Singapore: a comparison of fatal and non-fatal cases. *Acta Pediatr* 92:1163, 2003.

Modlin JF: Enteroviruses: Coxsackieviruses, echoviruses, newer enteroviruses. *In* Long S et al (eds): *Principles and Practice of Pediatric Infectious Diseases,* 2nd ed. New York, Churchill Livingstone, 2003, pp 1179–1187.

AUTHOR: **C. ELIZABETH TREFTS, MD**

BASIC INFORMATION

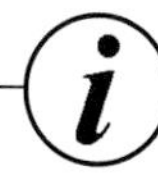

DEFINITION

Acute brain injury is accidental or inflicted trauma to the head resulting in the following:

- Mild head injury: Glasgow Coma Scale (GCS) (See GCS in Emergency Medicine, [Section IV]) score of 13 or 14 or a traumatically induced physiologic disruption of brain function, as manifested by one of the following:
  - Any period of loss of consciousness (LOC)
  - Any loss of memory for events surrounding the accident
  - Any alteration in mental state at the time of the accident
  - Focal neurologic deficits, which may or may not be transient
- Moderate head injury: GCS score of 9 to 12
- Severe head injury: GCS score of 8 or less and coma lasting 6 hours or more

SYNONYMS

Brain injury
Closed head injury
Head trauma
Intracranial injury
Traumatic brain injury

ICD-9-CM CODES
851-854 Intracranial hemorrhage
854 Brain injury
959.01 Head injury

EPIDEMIOLOGY & DEMOGRAPHICS

- Approximately 100,000 to 200,000 new head injuries occur in children each year.
- The population incidence is 193 to 367 per 100,000.
- The two peak periods are early childhood (younger than 5 years of age) and middle to late adolescence.
- Up to the age of 5 years, males and females are affected equally; after the age of 5 years, male predominance ranges from 2:1 to 4:1.
- In infants, toddlers, and young children, assaults/child abuse and falls account for 50% of injuries; 20% are related to motor vehicle accidents in infants and children to 4 years of age.
  - Younger children more commonly sustain pedestrian or bicycle-related injuries.
- Most injuries in older children and adolescents are related to motor vehicle accidents.
  - Falls and assaults/abuse account for less than 20% of injuries in older children.
  - Adolescents are more typically injured as passengers in motor vehicles.
  - Older children and adolescents also sustain sports or recreational injuries, as well as penetrating injuries.
- The highest rate of injuries is reported among those in the lower socioeconomic classes.
- Focal injuries, such as subdural, epidural, and intracerebral hematomas, occur in 15% to 20% of children, with a higher incidence in children younger than 4 years of age.
- Skull fractures occur in 5% to 25% of children and are associated with epidural hematomas 40% of the time.
- 10% to 15% of children hospitalized with head trauma have a severe head injury; of these, the mortality rate is approximately 33% to 50%, with most survivors having permanent deficits.
- Children are more susceptible to diffuse axonal injury (DAI) caused by rotational acceleration and deceleration because of their relatively higher head to body ratio, weak neck musculature, and lack of myelination.
- Children more frequently present with diffuse brain injury and cerebral swelling with resultant intracranial hypertension (up to 44%) when compared to adults.

CLINICAL PRESENTATION

History

- The source is usually clear; it is more important to define the extent of injury.
- Accidental: someone witnessed involvement in motor vehicle accident, high fall, or sports injury.
- Nonaccidental or abuse:
  - Suspicious "falls" or injuries not explained by proposed history
  - Penetrating injuries caused by gunshot wound or stabbing
- Alteration in mental status, such as behavior changes, irritability, or lethargy
- Neurologic abnormalities, such as headache, visual abnormalities, gait abnormalities, or weakness
- Emesis
- LOC

Physical Examination

- Altered GCS score (see Box 1-3)
- Abnormal cranial nerve examination; abnormal pupillary light reflex, eye position, or eye movements
- Abnormal motor, sensory, or reflex examination
- Lacerations, abrasions, or hematomas about head and scalp
- Depressed skull fracture by palpation
- Otorrhea, rhinorrhea, Battle's sign, or raccoon eyes
- Retinal hemorrhages with suspected abuse

ETIOLOGY

- Approximately 95% of traumatic brain injuries in children are closed head injuries.
- Penetrating brain injuries
- Shaken baby syndrome or shaken impact syndrome
- Primary injury: focal, diffuse, closed head injury or penetrating injury that occurs at the time of impact
- Secondary injury: cascade of biochemical and physiologic events within the brain that contribute to diffuse brain swelling, anoxia, or ischemia with further tissue loss or damage

DIAGNOSIS

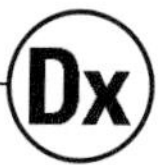

DIFFERENTIAL DIAGNOSIS

- Especially in the infant and toddler, differentiate between accidental and inflicted injury
- Anoxic or hypoxic encephalopathy
- Ruptured arteriovenous malformation or aneurysm
- Postictal phase
- Meningoencephalitis

WORKUP

- Adequately resuscitate (ABCs [airway, breathing, and circulation]), with particular attention directed toward assessing and securing an airway and ensuring adequate ventilation and circulation.
- Stabilize the cervical spine.
- Conduct a brief neurologic examination, including assigning a GCS score.
- Once the patient is stabilized, perform a thorough neurologic examination.
- If a cervical spine injury is possible based on the mechanism of injury, evaluate the cervical spine with anteroposterior, lateral, and open-mouth radiographic views.
  - Maintain cervical spine immobilization until cleared radiographically and no tenderness to palpation is present over cervical spine.
  - Additional flexion/extension views may need to be obtained to evaluate for ligamentous injury.
- For mild head injury:
  - No additional evaluation is necessary if the patient did not experience LOC or amnesia, has a GCS score of 15, has no focal deficits, and has no palpable skull fracture. Discharge home with written instructions for the parents about how to evaluate the child.
  - With brief LOC (shorter than 5 minutes), amnesia, a GCS score of 13 or 14, impaired alertness or memory, or palpable depressed skull fracture, evaluate with computed tomography (CT) scan. If no intracranial disease is present, may discharge home with written instructions for parents about how to evaluate the child.
  - If the child experiences LOC for more than 5 minutes, posttraumatic seizures, or focal neurologic deficits or an intracranial lesion is seen on CT scan, the child should be admitted for observation.
- For moderate head injury:
  - Children with GCS scores of 9 to 12, focal neurologic deficits, or intracranial disease on CT scan have the potential for deterioration and should be observed

closely in an intensive care unit (ICU) setting; obtain neurosurgical evaluation.

- For severe head injury:
  - CT scan of head and immediate neurosurgical evaluation should be obtained, with close observation in an ICU setting.
- In cases of child abuse:
  - Initial evaluation of head with CT should be performed to rule out immediate surgical hematomas, but then magnetic resonance imaging (MRI) scan of head, which is superior in determining traumatic hematomas of varying ages, should be performed.
  - Conduct a skeletal survey to evaluate for fractures of varying ages, posterior rib fractures, or metaphyseal fractures of long bones.
  - Perform an ophthalmologic evaluation of the retina.
  - Thoroughly examine the skin for bruises, burns, and other traumatic lesions.

LABORATORY TESTS

- Follow serum electrolytes and serum osmolarity, especially if using osmotic diuretics.

IMAGING STUDIES

- Head CT or MRI: see "Workup" for specific workup based on severity of clinical findings

TREATMENT

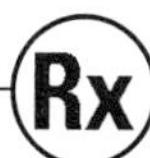

NONPHARMACOLOGIC THERAPY

- Mild or moderate head injury:
  - Closely observe the patient, with frequent neurologic evaluations.
- Severe head injury:
  - Place intracranial monitor if GCS score is less than 8 and monitor intracranial pressure (ICP).
  - Maintain cerebral perfusion pressure (CPP = mean arterial pressure − ICP) at 50 mm Hg or more in infants and young children and 70 mm Hg in older children and adolescents.
  - Keep head midline.
  - Elevate the head of bed 30 to 45 degrees.
  - Initiate controlled ventilation to maintain a $Paco_2$ of 32 to 35 mm Hg.
  - Maintain adequate oxygenation (Pao_2 between 90 and 100 mm Hg); avoid hypoxia.
  - Maintain normal blood pressure; avoid hypotension.
  - Intermittently drain cerebrospinal fluid to lower ICP and maintain adequate CPP.
  - Avoid noxious stimuli.
  - Prevent hyperthermia (consider adding a cooling blanket if antipyretics are ineffective, but must administer sedation and possibly muscle relaxants to prevent shivering).
  - In some centers, global jugular venous oxygen saturations are monitored continuously with a fiberoptic catheter to detect possible brain ischemia. Xenon-enhanced CT scans have been advocated as a means of discriminating between diffuse and local ischemia.
  - Studies are underway to evaluate the benefits of mild hypothermia (32° to 34°C) to limit cerebral oxygen demand.

ACUTE GENERAL Rx

- Mild or moderate head injury:
  - No medical therapy is available, except possible use of an anticonvulsant if a focal lesion is present.
- Severe head injury:
  - Sedatives, including propofol, benzodiazepines, narcotics, may be given.
  - Nondepolarizing muscle relaxants can be used for intubation and occasionally as needed if sedatives alone are unable to blunt the effects of noxious stimuli.
  - Osmotic diuretics (mannitol) can be used to reduce brain edema if the patient is hemodynamically stable (0.25 to 0.5 g/kg given every 2 to 6 hours to increase serum osmolarity to between 290 and 305 mOsm).
  - Loop diuretics (furosemide 1 mg/kg) may be effective to reduce transient intravascular volume increase that follows mannitol infusion.
  - Isotonic fluids can be used to restore and maintain adequate perfusion and blood pressure.
  - Infusion of hypertonic saline has been shown to be beneficial by having an osmotic effect on edematous cerebral tissue as well as exerting hemodynamic, vasoregulatory, immunologic, and neurochemical effects. Its use has replaced osmotic diuretic therapy in many centers.
  - Pressor support (e.g., dopamine, norepinephrine) can be initiated if unable to maintain adequate CPP with augmentation of intravascular volume.
  - Anticonvulsants (e.g., Dilantin, phenobarbital) can be used for antiseizure prophylaxis, but this remains controversial, especially beyond 7 days.
  - Antipyretics may be administered.
  - Lidocaine (1 mg/kg; maximum, 6 mg/kg/24 hours) given intravenously or intratracheally, or thiopental or pentobarbital (1 mg/kg intravenously) may be given to blunt the increase in ICP associated with tracheal suctioning.
  - High-dose barbiturates have been used to decrease brain metabolism when the ICP cannot be controlled and thus CPP cannot be maintained by other means.
  - Surgical evacuation of large epidural or subdural hematomas.
  - Decompressive craniectomy for severe elevated ICP remains controversial.

DISPOSITION

- Mild to moderate head injuries:
  - If discharged home, specific written instructions should be given to the caregiver.
- Severe head injuries:
  - Transfer the patient to a specialized, multidisciplinary rehabilitation program as soon as the patient is medically stable.
- For children with neurologic or psychiatric deficits, enroll in specialized school or early childhood development/stimulation programs.
- Sports injuries:
  - Grade 1 concussion: no LOC; amnesia lasting less than 30 minutes
    - First concussion: return to play if asymptomatic at rest and on exertion for 1 week
    - Second concussion: return to play in 2 weeks after asymptomatic for 1 week
    - Third concussion: terminate season; may return to play next season if asymptomatic
  - Grade 2 concussion: LOC less than 5 minutes; amnesia longer than 30 minutes but less than 24 hours
    - First concussion: return to play after asymptomatic at rest and on exertion for 1 week
    - Second concussion: no play for a minimum of 1 month; may return to play then if asymptomatic for 1 week; consider terminating the season
    - Third concussion: terminate season; may return to play next season if asymptomatic
  - Grade 3 concussion: LOC for 5 minutes or longer or amnesia longer than 24 hours
    - Transport to hospital for evaluation
    - First concussion: no play for a minimum of 1 month; may then return to play if asymptomatic for 1 week
    - Second concussion: terminate season; may return to play next season if asymptomatic
  - If neurosurgery needed, no contact or collision sports
- Abuse/assault:
  - Notify appropriate authorities

REFERRAL

- Refer to neurosurgeons and intensivists for acute management of symptomatic head trauma.
- Children with head injuries and residual cognitive, motor, speech, or behavioral deficits should be referred to a neurologist or neuropsychologist.

PEARLS & CONSIDERATIONS

COMMENTS

- Preventive measures are the only way to eliminate primary brain injuries. All therapies are focused only on preventing secondary brain injuries.

- Postinjury cerebral edema usually peaks at 24 to 48 hours and gradually resolves over 3 to 4 days.
- Seventy percent of all pediatric trauma deaths occurring within 48 hours of hospital admissions are the result of head injuries.
- Isolated, brief, immediate posttraumatic seizures occurring within seconds of impact require no therapy.
- The severity of head injury outcome is related directly to the duration and degree of coma.
- Children as a group have a better outcome than adults; however, children younger than 7 years of age fare worse, partly because of a higher incidence of child abuse and the functions of the developing brain. Disruption or damage to the centers for acquiring or interpreting new stimuli may adversely affect the child's ability to acquire new and higher functions.
- Children younger than 4 years of age at the time of severe head injury are unlikely to be able to work independently outside of a structured environment.

PREVENTION

- Use child-restraint devices appropriately in motor vehicles; place children in the back seat
- Obey speed limits
- Use sports equipment, especially helmets, appropriately
- Enforce and follow all sports rules
- Provide adequate adult supervision
- Provide information about parenting classes and support services for those at risk for child abuse
- Advocate for firearm legislation to decrease availability of guns

PATIENT/FAMILY EDUCATION

National Head Injury Foundation

Brain Injury Association of America (www.biausa.org)

SUGGESTED READINGS

Adelson PD, Kochanek PM: Head injury in children. *J Child Neurol* 13:2, 1998.

Adelson PD et al: Guidelines for Acute Medical Management of Severe Traumatic Brain Injury in Infants, Children, and Adolescents. *Ped Crit Care Med* 4(3):S1, 2003.

Alderson P et al: Therapeutic hypothermia for head injury. [Update of Cochrane Database Syst Rev (1):CD001048, 2002: Meta-Analysis.] *Cochrane Database Syst Rev* (4):CD001048, 2004.

Alderson P, Roberts I: Corticosteroids for acute traumatic brain injury. [Update of Cochrane Database Syst Rev (2):CD000196, 2000] *Cochrane Database Syst Rev* (1):CD000196, 2005.

Brain Injury Association, Inc. Available at www.biausa.org/

Brain Trauma Foundation, American Association of Neurological Surgeons, Joint Section on Neurotrauma and Critical Care: Guidelines for the management of severe traumatic brain injury. *J Neurotrauma* 17:451, 2000.

Dutton RP, McCunn M: Traumatic brain injury. *Curr Opin Crit Care* 9:503, 2003.

Guskiewicz KM et al: National Athletic Trainers' Association. Recommendations on management of sport-related concussion: summary of the National Athletic Trainers' Association position statement. *Neurosurgery* 55(4):891, 2004[discussion 896].

National Safe Kids Campaign. Available at www.safekids.org/

The Pediatric Critical Care Medicine. Available at http://anes01.wustl.edu/

Roberts I et al: Mannitol for acute traumatic brain injury. [Update of Cochrane Database Syst Rev (2):CD001049, 2000] *Cochrane Database Syst Rev* (2):CD001049, 2003.

Society of Critical Care Medicine: Guidelines for the acute medical management of severe traumatic brain injury in infants, children, and adolescents [see comment]. *Crit Care Med* 31(6 Suppl): S407, 2003.

AUTHOR: **KAREN S. POWERS, MD**

BASIC INFORMATION

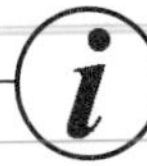

DEFINITION

Headache is a symptom. Three clinically defined symptom patterns (migraine, cluster, and tension) include most pediatric recurrent headaches.

SYNONYMS

Cephalgia
Chronic headache
Migraine
Migraine headache
Tension headache

ICD-9-CM CODES
307.81 Tension headache
346.2 Cluster headache
346.9 Migraine headache, idiopathic
784.0 Headache, NOS

EPIDEMIOLOGY & DEMOGRAPHICS

- Headaches are very common.
  - Nonmigraine, occasional headaches are seen in as many as 35% of 7-year-olds and 54% of 15-year-olds.
- Approximately 1% to 3% of 3- to 7-year-olds, 4% to 11% of 7- to 11-year-olds, and 8% to 23% of children older than 11 years have migraine headaches.
- In children 3 to 7 years: girls affected less than boys; 7 to 11 years: girls and boys affected equally; 11 to 15 years: girls affected more than boys.
- Family history is a significant risk factor for migraine headaches which are inherited by a heterogeneous autosomal dominant pattern with incomplete penetrance.
- Children who experience migraines have a 34% chance of going into remission, a 45% chance of having their headaches improve, and a 21% chance of having long-term problems with migraine headaches.

CLINICAL PRESENTATION

Three main chronic headache types include:

- Migraine headache
  - Age of presentation is usually 7 to 14 years of age.
  - Triggers of migraines include the following:
    - Foods and chemicals: monosodium glutamate (MSG), cheeses containing tyramine, caffeine, nitrites, sulfites, histamine, and phenolic flavonoids in red wine
    - Drugs
    - Environmental factors, such as bright lights or noise
    - Psychosocial factors, such as emotional stress
  - International Headache Society (ICHD-II) criteria for pediatric migraine *without aura* require five or more attacks with:
    - Headache of 1 to 72 hours duration
    - At least two of the following: bilateral or unilateral frontal/temporal location; pulsating, moderate to severe pain, aggravated by routine activities (bilateral presentation more common in children)
    - Nausea/vomiting or photophobia and phonophobia
    - History and physical exam not suggestive of another etiology
  - ICHD-II criteria for pediatric migraine *with typical aura* require at least two attacks with one of the following fully reversible auras with:
    - Visual symptoms such as loss of vision, or seeing things like spots or lines
    - Sensory symptoms such as numbness or feelings of pins and needles
    - Dysphasic speech
      - At least two of the following symptoms: homonymous visual symptoms or unilateral sensory symptoms, or one or more aura symptoms developing over 5 or more minutes
    - Each symptom should last at least 5 minutes and not longer than 60 minutes
  - Other migraine types exist including familial hemiplegic migraine, sporadic hemiplegic migraine, and basilar-type migraine.
  - Common precursors of migraines include: cyclical vomiting, abdominal migraine, and benign paroxysmal vertigo of childhood.
- Cluster headache based on ICHD-II criteria
  - Presents as severe, boring, unilateral orbital, supraorbital, or temporal pain
  - Lasts approximately 15 to 180 minutes each and occur in clusters
  - Cluster episodes may last for days or weeks
  - Headache accompanied by one of the following ipsilateral signs: conjunctival injection or lacrimation, nasal congestion or rhinorrhea, eyelid edema, forehead or facial swelling, miosis or ptosis, or agitation
  - Unusual in children younger than 10 years of age
- Tension headache based on ICHD-II criteria
  - Also known as *muscle contraction* or *stress* headache
  - Involves all locations in the head and is usually bilateral
  - No aura associated with this type of headache
  - Nausea and vomiting absent
  - Pain is nonpulsating and not aggravated by normal activity.
  - Pain is reported as mild to moderate in intensity.
  - Headache may last 30 minutes to 7 days.
  - Photophobia may be prominent and therefore hard to distinguish from migraines in children. Phonophobia may be present. Migraine more likely if both photophobia and phonophobia are present.
- In order to illicit a good history of the headache symptoms, ask patient to draw a picture of headache.
  - Show where it hurts
  - Demonstrate what it feels like
  - List/draw associated symptoms that precede the headache
- A complete physical, including thorough neurologic examination and blood pressure, is generally unremarkable in children with recurrent headaches but must be performed.
- Findings that are suspicious for another cause, include the following:
  - Seizure
  - Trauma
  - Pain in a single, specific location that can be pointed at with one finger or headache that stays in the one spot and is getting worse
  - A change in gait
  - Change in personality
  - Sudden and severe onset with the first episode
  - Pain with waking up that gets better after arising from bed or that is relieved with vomiting
  - Pain that is set off by coughing
  - Presence of an ill contact with meningitis/encephalitis or similar infection
  - Altered development or mental status
  - A constant headache that is worse with lying down or with Valsalva maneuver
  - Fever
  - Nuchal rigidity
  - Petechiae
  - Bulging fontanel or altered head circumference
  - Cushing's triad: increased blood pressure, increased respiratory rate, decreased heart rate
  - Severe hypertension
  - Papilledema
  - Any abnormality on complete neurologic exam

ETIOLOGY

- Migraines are believed to be caused by cortical neurons being stimulated by the brain stem which then sensitize the trigeminal nerve ganglion.
- Sterile inflammation of the vasculature mediated by neurotransmitters such as serotonin causes vasoconstriction and dilation of cerebral vessels.

DIAGNOSIS

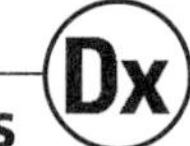

DIFFERENTIAL DIAGNOSIS

- Increased intracranial pressure (ICP)
  - Pseudotumor cerebri
  - Mass (benign or malignant tumor)
  - Hydrocephalus

- Intracranial bleeding (subdural, epidural, or intracerebral)
- Central nervous system (CNS) infection
  - Meningitis
  - Encephalitis
  - Brain abscess
- Vasculitis
- Arteriovenous malformation
- Aneurysm
- Analgesic abuse (use)
  - "Analgesic abuse headache" can occur with regular, frequent use of analgesics.
- Depression

WORKUP

If the patient has a normal physical exam including complete neurologic exam and funduscopic exam and no red flags on history, no laboratory and imaging studies are indicated.

IMAGING STUDIES

Computed tomography (CT) should be done if there are signs of increased ICP.

TREATMENT

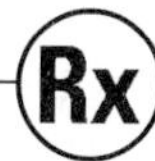

NONPHARMACOLOGIC THERAPY

- Sleep
- Trial of food elimination based on triggers identified in headache diary
- Physical therapy
- Biofeedback

ACUTE GENERAL Rx

- Acetaminophen (12 to 15 mg/kg/dose at 4-hour intervals, max. 325 to 500 mg) or ibuprofen (7 to 10 mg/kg/dose at 6- to 8-hour intervals, max. 600 mg) should be given early in the course of a migraine.
  - Acetaminophen has faster onset but ibuprofen has performed better in trials.
  - Ibuprofen may be more effective in boys than girls.
  - Both drugs are also effective for tension headaches.
- For children more than 12 years old, sumatriptan nasal spray has been proven effective at 5- mg and 20-mg spray doses.
  - Subcutaneous sumatriptan may be effective but currently there is not enough evidence to support this.
- Other medications for acute migraines not responding to home management include the following:
  - Promethazine: initial dose 0.25 to 1.0 mg/kg IV/PO/IM/PR every 4 to 6 hours; maximum 25 mg/dose
  - Prochlorperazine: 0.11 to 0.13 mg/kg IV/PO/PR every 6 hours; maximum 7.5 to 10.0 mg/day
  - Ketorolac: 0.5 mg/kg IV/IM every 6 hours; maximum 30 mg/dose
  - Dihydroergotamine (DHE):
    - 6 to 9 years: 0.1 mg/dose
    - 9 to 12 years: 0.15 to 0.2 mg/dose
    - 12 to 16 years: 0.25 to 0.5 mg/dose every 6 hours, max. 12 doses
  - Should be used with an antiemetic.
  - Only used when other treatments are not successful.
- Cluster headaches can be treated with 100% O_2, sumatriptan as dosed for migraines, and DHE as dosed for migraines.

CHRONIC Rx

- If a patient requires therapy for migraine headaches three or more times a week a preventive therapy should be considered. However, there is not enough data to currently recommend a specific therapy as effective. Some medications currently being used include:
  - Cyproheptadine:
    - less than 6 years: 0.125 mg/kg two to three times daily (max. 12 mg/day)
    - 6 to 14 years: 4 mg two to three times per day (max. 16 mg/day)
  - Propranolol: 1 to 4 mg/kg/day
  - Amitriptyline:
    - 6 to 12 years: 10 to 30 mg/day divided twice daily
    - More than 12 years: 10 to 50 mg/day divided into three doses
  - Divalproex sodium, topiramate, and levetiracetam are also being used but adequate data do not exist to prove effectiveness for any of these medications.
- Medicines used in prevention of cluster headache include the following:
  - Methysergide
  - Lithium
  - Corticosteroids
- Management of chronic tension headaches should focus on identifying and avoiding predisposing factors.

DISPOSITION

- Patient should be followed until resolution or significant improvement is achieved and as needed for acute recurrences and evaluation of medication side effects.

REFERRAL

- Difficult to manage headaches should prompt referral to neurologist or mental health specialist.

PEARLS & CONSIDERATIONS

COMMENTS

- Mnemonic for features of migraines:
  Mother (family history)
  Intermittent
  Grinding/throbbing
  Relief with rest
  Aura
  Idiopathic (rule out other causes of headache)
  Nausea/vomiting
  Eyes and ears (photophobia and phonophobia)
  Search for triggers
- All (oral) medications for migraines work best if given early in course. Thus, it is important for patients and caregivers to try to recognize sensations that precede an attack.

PREVENTION

- Limit use of analgesics to less than three times weekly
- Encourage adequate sleep
- Never skip meals
- Regular exercise
- Avoid triggers (e.g., caffeine, MSG, chemical fumes)

PATIENT/FAMILY EDUCATION

- See "Prevention"

SUGGESTED READINGS

Lewis D et al: Practice parameter: pharmacological treatment of migraine headache in children and adolescents. *Neurology* 63(12):2215, 2004.

Lewis D et al: Practice parameter: evaluation of children and adolescents with recurrent headache. *Neurology* 59:490, 2002.

Linder S, Winner P: Pediatric headache. *Med Clin North Am* 85(4):1037, 2001.

Millichap G, Yee M: The diet factor in pediatric and adolescent migraine. *Pediatr Neurol* 28:9, 2003.

Olesen J: The International Classification of Headache Disorders, 2nd ed. *Cephalgia* 24(Suppl 1):9, 2004.

Qureshi F, Lew D: Managing headache in pediatric emergency department. *Clin Pediatr Emerg Med* 4:149, 2003.

Stafstrom C, Rostasy K: The usefulness of children's drawings in the diagnosis of headache. *Pediatrics* 109:460, 2002.

AUTHOR: **DIANA BARNETT KUDES, MD**

BASIC INFORMATION

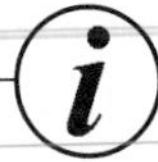

DEFINITION

Complete heart block (CHB) is a bradycardic rhythm caused by failure of impulse conduction from the atria to the ventricles with complete atrioventricular dissociation. The atrial rate is usually higher than the ventricular rate.

SYNONYMS

Complete atrioventricular block
Third-degree atrioventricular block
Unless bradycardia is concurrent, atrioventricular dissociation is not an acceptable synonym because this entity may exist with normal rates of at least one pacemaker (e.g., sinus bradycardia with an appropriate junctional rate) and with ventricular tachycardias.

ICD-9-CM CODE
746.86 Congenital heart block

EPIDEMIOLOGY & DEMOGRAPHICS

- Congenital CHB occurs in 1 in 15,000 to 1 in 25,000 births.
- The mortality of congenital CHB in utero is high if hydrops is present and in premature infants.
- The incidence of surgically induced CHB has progressively decreased and is currently quite low (less than 5%), seen most commonly in the setting of complex cardiac malformation repairs.
- The incidence of CHB in systemic disease and infection is very low.
- Atrioventricular nodal mesotheliomas, extremely rare cardiac tumors, may cause CHB.
- Congenital CHB caused by fetal exposure to anti-Ro (SSA/Ro) and anti-La (SSB/La) occurs in only 1% to 5% of mothers with collagen vascular disease, but the recurrence rate for subsequent pregnancies is 20%.
- No gender predilection is seen with congenital or acquired CHB.

CLINICAL PRESENTATION

History
- Fetal bradycardia
- Fetal hydrops/intrauterine death
- Congestive heart failure
- Fatigue
- Diminished exercise capacity
- Syncope
- Sudden death
- History of associated malformations or history of systemic illnesses (listed under "Etiology")

Physical Examination
- Bradycardia but usually regular rhythm
- Wide pulse pressure
- Low cardiac output
- Manifestations of associated malformations or systemic illnesses (see "Etiology")
- Late mitral regurgitation in non-paced patients

ETIOLOGY

- Congenital caused by transplacental immunoglobulin G (IgG-anti-Ro/SSA or anti-La/SSB) antibody transfer in occult or overt maternal connective tissue disease (lupus, primarily)
- Congenital in the setting of left atrial isomerism (polysplenia) with an atrioventricular septal defect or in patients with levotransposition of the great vessels
- Congenital with a late presentation (second decade) caused by SCN5A and NK×2.5 mutations (Gene mutations associated with congenital heart block.)
- Acquired as a result of damage to the atrioventricular node and His bundle during surgical repair of congenital and acquired cardiac defects
- Acquired as a result of infections: endocarditis, myocarditis, diphtheria, Lyme disease
- Acquired in systemic diseases: acute rheumatic fever, myotonic and muscular dystrophies, Kearns-Sayre syndrome
- Acquired as a result of tumor infiltration: mesothelioma and unknown degenerative processes

DIAGNOSIS

DIFFERENTIAL DIAGNOSIS

- Sinus bradycardia
- Blocked atrial bigeminy
- Type II second-degree atrioventricular block

LABORATORY TESTS

- Electrocardiogram/cardiac monitoring to determine atrial and ventricular rates
- Holter (ambulatory) monitor to assess
  - Lowest rate (e.g., during sleep)
  - Stability of escape pacemakers
  - Escape ventricular or higher-grade ventricular ectopy
  - Intermittent atrial capture of the ventricles
- Anti-Ro and anti-La antibodies
  - Congenital CHB in the absence of structural heart disease likely represents maternal collagen vascular disease.
- Exercise test in older patients

IMAGING STUDIES

- Echocardiogram to look for structural abnormalities, tumor, and myocardial dysfunction

TREATMENT

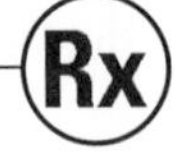

NONPHARMACOLOGIC THERAPY

- Temporary ventricular or, preferably, permanent cardiac pacemaker implantation

ACUTE GENERAL Rx

- In general, patients with CHB need to be paced if symptoms, structural heart disease, or rate-related low cardiac output is present.
- Isoproterenol infusion (0.05 to 0.4 μg/kg/minute) used to increase the ventricular rate as a bridge to more definitive therapy, but observe for ventricular ectopy.

CHRONIC Rx

- See "Disposition"

DISPOSITION

- All patients with CHB require follow-up by a pediatric cardiologist.
- All patients with pacemakers require enrollment in a pacemaker clinic with regularly scheduled transtelephonic assessment and office appointments.

REFERRAL

- All patients with CHB should be referred to a pediatric cardiologist.

PEARLS & CONSIDERATIONS

COMMENTS

- Surgically induced or myocarditis-related CHB may be transient. If reversion to sinus rhythm does not occur in 7 to 14 days, switch from temporary to permanent pacemaker implantation.
- Immune-mediated congenital CHB is permanent.
- Despite satisfactory pacing, the infant with immune-mediated CHB may succumb to the development of a congestive or dilated immune-related cardiomyopathy during the first 2 years of life.

SUGGESTED READINGS

Buyon JP et al: Autoimmune-associated congenital heart block: demographics, mortality, and recurrence rates obtained from a national neonatal lupus registry. *J Am Coll Cardiol* 31:1658, 1998.
Friedman RA: Congenital A-V block: pace me now or pace me later? *Circulation* 92:283, 1995.
Schmidt KL et al: Perinatal outcome of fetal complete atrioventricular block: a multicenter experience. *J Am Coll Cardiol* 17:1360, 1991.
Weindling SN et al: Duration of complete atrioventricular block after congenital heart disease surgery. *Am J Cardiol* 82:525, 1998.

AUTHORS: **J. PETER HARRIS, MD** and **SVETLANA TISMA-DUPANOVIC, MD**

BASIC INFORMATION

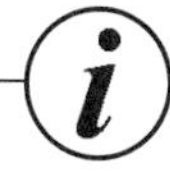

DEFINITION

Heat-related illness (HRI) represents a spectrum of clinical disorders characterized by temperature elevation, dehydration, and electrolyte disturbance.

- HRIs typically affect athletes surrounding participation in warm weather sports. Nonathletes (often the very young and the very old) become susceptible to HRI during seasonal heat waves, particularly in poor urban areas.
- *Heat cramps* result from painful, sustained contractions of leg muscles after prolonged exercise. Patients with this mildest form of exertional HRI have a normal core body temperature.
- *Heat exhaustion* represents a more serious level of exposure and dehydration resulting from excessive sweat production. Patients with heat exhaustion will have an elevated core temperature (typically 38°C to 40°C) and may exhibit a number of associated signs and symptoms including nausea, vomiting, orthostasis, and syncope.
- The diagnosis of *heat stroke* reflects the most extreme, life-threatening degree of environmental heat exposure. Patients with heat stroke demonstrate extreme core temperature elevations (higher than 40.5°C) accompanied by severe water and sodium losses. Heat stroke is classified as *exertional* when it occurs in otherwise healthy athletes, and *classic* when described in infants or the elderly.

SYNONYM

Sunstroke

ICD-9-CM CODES
992.0 Heat stroke
992.2 Heat cramps
992.5 Heat exhaustion

EPIDEMIOLOGY & DEMOGRAPHICS

- Highly at-risk individuals include infants, victims of diarrheal illness, and elderly persons with underlying medical conditions.
- Events increase during seasonal heat waves.
  - Those particularly at risk inhabit poor areas of northern U.S. cities.
  - Tenants in older buildings lacking air conditioning are highly susceptible to HRI.
- Global warming may increase the incidence in the future.
- Infants and child athletes are more prone to climatic heat stress than are adults because of their higher rate of heat transfer from the environment, higher baseline metabolic rates, and lesser ability to sweat.
- Child and adolescent athletes may exercise poor judgment and ignore, or be unaware of, the warning signs of HRI.
- Accidental deaths occur with infants and children locked in automobiles.
  - In summer climates, the interior and trunk temperature of automobiles can reach higher than 65°C (150°F) in just 15 minutes.
  - Cracking open the window does *not* prevent rapid overheating.

CLINICAL PRESENTATION

History

- Histories should include the type and the duration of exercise and environmental conditions to which the patient has been exposed.
- Inquire about chronic illness (i.e., cystic fibrosis) or recent activity (attempted weight loss) that may increase the risk of fluid and electrolyte imbalance.
- Symptoms may include:
  - Shaking chills
  - Headache
  - Nausea
  - Excessive sweating
  - Dry skin (anhydrosis)
  - Extreme fatigue
  - Leg cramps
  - Light-headedness or dizziness
  - Confusion
  - Syncope

Physical Examination

Findings may include:

- Tachycardia
- Elevated temperature (typically 38°C to 40°C with heat exhaustion, more than 40.5°C with heat stroke)
- Piloerection on chest and arms
- Either excessive perspiration or anhydrosis
- Combativeness, aggressiveness
- Mental status may degrade to obtundation with loss of consciousness

ETIOLOGY

- *Heat cramps* are thought to result from inadequate muscle perfusion secondary to dehydration and sodium depletion.
  - Both reactions accentuate calcium activity in skeletal muscle.
  - Cramps occur mainly in hamstring and calf muscles.
- *Heat exhaustion* represents a more severe level of dehydration.
  - Sustained exercise leads to massive sweat production with resultant water and electrolyte loses.
  - Plasma volume and sweat production decrease as dehydration progresses. Sweat production falls and cooling ability is greatly impaired.
  - Elevated core temperature (higher than 40°C) increases metabolic demand, further stressing the already compromised cardiovascular system.
- The diagnosis of *heat stroke* implies a life-threatening degree of hyperthermia with profound hemodynamic and metabolic abnormalities.
  - Dangerously elevated core temperature (may be higher than 42°C [107.6°F]).
  - Diffuse cellular injury occurs from shock (oxygen debt) and hyperpyrexia. Severe heat stroke can lead to neuronal injury, rhabdomyolysis, mitochondrial dysfunction, lactic acidosis, and death.
  - A generalized inflammatory response may develop, leading to disseminated intravascular coagulation (DIC) and multiorgan dysfunction, similar to that seen in the sepsis syndrome.
- Historically, mortality from heat stroke has been reported to be as high as 50% to 80%. More recent data in patients treated with aggressive intensive care strategies suggest a lower mortality of 15% to 20%.

DIAGNOSIS

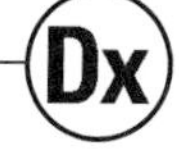

DIFFERENTIAL DIAGNOSIS

- In the presence of an appropriate history, the diagnosis of HRI is often straightforward.
- HRI should be expected during seasonal heat waves and may be clear in athletes with appropriate environmental exposure.
- The differential diagnosis includes many illnesses that induce fever and mental status changes, including, but not limited to, the following:
  - Generalized viral illnesses, bacterial sepsis
  - Encephalitis, meningitis
  - Head trauma

WORKUP

- Assess the ABCs (airway, breathing, and circulation).
- Airway control (endotracheal intubation) may be necessary for the most severely affected heat stroke patients.
- Volume status is presumably depleted, assess for signs of decompensated shock and end-organ compromise.
- Initial evaluation of core (rectal temperature) is indicated. If severely elevated, urgent external cooling measures are indicated.

LABORATORY TESTS

- Many electrolyte abnormalities can be found in HRI.
  - Disturbances of sodium and potassium balance (increased or decreased)
  - Hypocalcemia
  - Hyperphosphatemia
- Rhabdomyolysis can be detected by myoglobinuria or elevated serum creatine kinase (CK).
- In severe heat stroke, an arterial blood gas, liver function studies, coagulation assays, CK, and urinary myoglobin should be obtained.

IMAGING STUDIES

Imaging studies are generally not indicated for the child with a clear history and classic physical exam findings. Imaging, if required, should not be pursued prior to cooling the patient and assuring a stable cardiorespiratory status.

TREATMENT

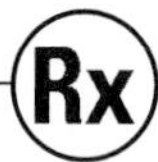

NONPHARMACOLOGIC THERAPY

- Heat cramps are treated nonpharmacologically with the following methods:
  - Rest
  - Oral rehydration
  - Local massage
    - If symptoms resolve, then further evaluation is not indicated.
    - Parents and coaches should reduce the child's activity level and begin a more gradual conditioning regimen.
- Heat exhaustion requires more aggressive interventions:
  - Rehydration: The typical adolescent or adult requires 1 to 2 L of fluid over the first several hours. Oral rehydration is appropriate for a fully conscious patient. Parental rehydration is indicated for the patient who demonstrates hemodynamic or mental status instability.
  - Immediate cooling measures should be initiated.
    - Move the patient into the shade.
    - Dry sweat and moisture from the skin (to increase evaporative heat loss).
    - Further cooling can be achieved by applying ice to sites of superficial great vessels (i.e., neck, axillae, and groin).
  - Monitor body temperature closely. An increasing core temperature despite initial therapy and cooling measures indicates the presence of heat stroke, which is a medical emergency.

ACUTE GENERAL Rx

- Heat stroke is a medical emergency necessitating care in an acute care facility. Core temperatures may rise above 42°C, putting the patient at risk for generalized cellular necrosis, imminent cardiovascular collapse, and death.
  - Begin external cooling with ice application to neck, axillae, and groin.
  - Remove the patient's clothing, cover the patient with a wet sheet, and focus a fan or air conditioning directly on the patient.
- Initiate rapid intravenous fluid administration.
  - Generally administer 0.9% normal saline, at least 20 mL/kg or 800 mL/m^2) over the first hour.
  - Give a normal saline bolus (10 mL/kg) as necessary for blood pressure support.
- Inotropic support may be necessary.
- Urine output should be monitored to assess the ongoing fluid resuscitation (urinary catheter should be placed).
- Monitor electrolytes and treat any imbalances accordingly.
- Continually reassess ABCs.
  - Assure an adequate airway. Endotracheal intubation is indicated for the comatose or seizing patient.
- Treat seizures if they occur.
  - Benzodiazepines are the first-line antiseizure therapy.
  - Lorazepam 0.1 to 0.2 mg/kg for children, 2.0 mg for adults.
- Consider treating rigors/shivering with similar benzodiazepine dosing.

DISPOSITION

- Children with heat cramps or mild heat exhaustion should be removed from play, hydrated, and cooled as previously described.
  - Body temperature should be monitored, and, if it remains or returns to normal, hospitalization is not required.
  - Preventive measures should be instituted (see "Prevention").
- Patients with heat stroke should be transferred immediately to an emergency medical center.
  - Children with this life-threatening condition should be cared for in pediatric intensive care units.
- Vital signs and metabolic parameters are generally monitored for 24 to 48 hours after reaching normothermia, in order to look for signs of secondary cellular damage.

PEARLS & CONSIDERATIONS

COMMENTS

Remember that environmentally induced hyperthermia is not relieved by antipyretic (e.g., acetaminophen, ibuprofen) administration. Manual cooling measures are necessary.

PREVENTION

- HRI is preventable.
- Children, parents, and coaches need to be familiar with the risks associated with HRI and focus on maintaining hydration, limiting participation in extreme heat and humidity, and recognizing early signs of over-exertion.
  - During exercise, a child should consume fluids at least every 15 to 20 minutes. Weight monitoring can be a useful means to identify excessive fluid loss (>5% of body weight).
  - Outdoor activity should be limited during periods of high heat and humidity.
- Morning or evening practice times may be beneficial.
- Water breaks and cool down periods are essential for safety.

SUGGESTED READINGS

American Academy of Pediatrics, Committee on Sports Medicine and Fitness: Climatic heat stress and the exercising child and adolescent. *Pediatrics* 106(1):158, 2000.

Center for Disease Control: Tips for preventing heat related illness. Available at http://www.bt.cdc.gov/disasters/extremeheat/heattips.asp

Naughton MP et al: Heat-related mortality during a 1999 heat wave in Chicago. *Am J Prev Med* 22(4):221, 2002.

AUTHOR: **WILLIAM G. HARMON, MD**

BASIC INFORMATION

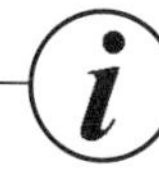

DEFINITION

The classification of Mulliken and Glowacki in 1982 separates hemangioma and vascular malfomation. *Hemangiomas* are benign vascular tumors in which a growth phase, marked by endothelial cell proliferation, is followed by involution and fibrosis. Hemangiomas are differentiated from *vascular malformations,* which are hamartomas. Vascular malformations do *not* proliferate or involute; are composed of aberrant but mature endothelial cells, which may be capillary (e.g., port-wine stain), lymphatic (e.g., cystic hygroma), venous, arterial, or combined channel anomalies; are always present; and grow with the child.

SYNONYMS

Strawberry birthmark
Strawberry hemangioma
Strawberry mark

ICD-9-CM CODE
228.00 Hemangioma

EPIDEMIOLOGY & DEMOGRAPHICS

- Hemangiomas are the most common soft tissue tumor of infancy.
- 1% to 12% of 1-year-olds have hemangiomas.
  - White (10% to 12%) greater than black (1% to 2%) greater than Asian (<1%)
- They are uncommonly (<10%) familial.
- The female:male ratio is 3:1; vascular malformations occur in equal female:male ratios.
- The incidence is increased in very-low-birth-weight premature infants (20% to 30% in < 1.0 kg preterm infant births).
- About one third of hemangiomas are present at birth; most (80%) of the rest develop within the first few weeks of life.
- Approximately 75% to 80% of patients have one, 15% to 20% have two, and less than 5% have three or more hemangiomas; rarely, disseminated neonatal hemangiomatosis is seen.
- Approximately 60% occur in the head and neck area, 25% on the trunk, and 15% on an extremity.
- 60% to 65% are superficial, 15% are deep, and 20% to 25% are combined superficial and deep.
- Neither site, size, depth, presence at birth, diameter of proliferative phase, sex, nor race predicts which hemangiomas will involute completely.
- Approximately 50% resolve by 5 years of age, and 90% resolve by 9 years of age.

CLINICAL PRESENTATION

History

- The history typically is of little help.
- The typical course is of an erythematous growth which may have been noted at or slighly after birth and is grown.
- Hemangioma associated with multiple anomalies is referred to as PHACES syndrome (female:male ratio is 8:1):
  Posterior fossa abnormality (Arnold-Chiari or Dandy-Walker malformation)
  Hemangiomas (facial and laryngeal)
  Arterial anomalies (carotid and vertebral arteries)
  Coarctation of the aorta (and other cardiac)
  Eye abnormalities (cataract, microphthalmia, abnormal retinal vessels)
  Sternal or abdominal cleft
- Hemangioma of the lumbosacral region is a potential marker for occult spinal malformations.
- Hemangioma of the face or neck may be associated with tracheal hemangioma.

Physical Examination

- A pale macule with threadlike telangiectasia may be present in newborns.
- Hemangiomas are bright red, elevated, and slightly compressible as they enlarge, especially if superficial.
- Deep hemangiomas are blue in color and have a soft fullness to palpation with poorly defined borders.
- Size can range from a few millimeters to centimeters.
- A rapid increase in size occurs over the first 1 to 6 months.
  - The maximum size is reached at approximately 6 to 8 months in superficial hemangiomas.
  - Maximum size may not be reached until 12 to 14 months in deep hemangiomas.
- Slower involution occurs after 6 to 9 months.
  - Involution begins with central pallor and fading of bright red color.
  - 10% to 40% of lesions have some residual skin changes.
    - Lesions may leave atrophic, wrinkled skin or fibrofatty residual at the site.
    - Telangiectases, superficial dilated veins, and hypopigmentation also seen residually.

Complications

- Ulceration
  - Most common complication
  - May be quite painful
  - Risk of infection, hemorrhage, and scar formation
- Kasabach-Merritt phenomenon (KMP)
  - Associated with consumptive coagulopathy, anemia, and thrombocytopenia
  - Most common within the first 4 to 5 months of life
  - Usually occurs in massive, deep hemangioma, which may be a different lesion than a simple hemangioma
  - The lesions in KMP may grow for 2 to 5 years.
- There can be vital structure compromise.
  - Periorbital lesions may lead to amblyopia, astigmatism, or myopia.
  - Periauricular lesions may obstruct the external auditory canal.
  - Airway lesions may present with hoarseness, stridor, or "noisy" breathing.
    - Hemangiomas involving the chin, lips, and mandibular region of the face increase the risk of airway hemangioma.
- Visceral hemangiomas
  - High morbidity occurs because of high flow with high-output cardiac failure and anemia.
  - If multiple (especially facial) hemangiomas are present, consider visceral lesions (especially liver).
- Lumbosacral hemangiomas
  - These are associated with lumbosacral spine abnormalities, in particular tethered cord.
- Large facial hemangiomas
  - These may be associated with Dandy-Walker syndrome or other posterior fossa abnormalities, such as PHACES syndrome.

ETIOLOGY

- Hemangiomas are generally caused by angiogenesis—new vessels arising from existing vasculature.
- Vasculogenesis, in which new blood vessels are made from endothelial cells, may play a role.
- The rapid increase in size with proliferation of cells followed by cessation of growth and eventual involution is not well understood.

DIAGNOSIS

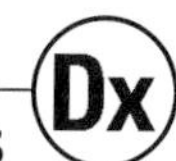

DIFFERENTIAL DIAGNOSIS

- Tumors (angiosarcoma, fibrosarcoma)
- Vascular malformations, lymphatic malformations
- Pyogenic granuloma
- Kaposiform hemangioendothelioma
- Spindle cell hemangioendothelioma
- Infantile hemangiopericytoma
- Maffucci syndrome (enchondromas with multiple angiomas)

WORKUP

- The diagnosis is usually clinical.
- Larger lesions, especially hepatic or other large congenital lesions, are more difficult to diagnose.

IMAGING STUDIES

- For large, difficult diagnoses:
  - Doppler ultrasonography is useful.
    - Differentiates from solid tumors
    - Differentiates from arteriovenous malformations and lymph vessel and capillary anomalies
  - Magnetic resonance imaging also differentiates hemangiomas from other vascular malformations and soft tissue tumors.

TREATMENT

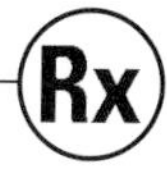

NONPHARMACOLOGIC THERAPY

- Wait and watch approach
- Significant parental emotional support

- More chance of scar with intervention than with waiting for natural involution
- Surgery rarely required
  - The patient may need tracheostomy for subglottic hemangioma.
  - Embolization is used for large cutaneous lesions that have not responded to medical therapy.
  - Surgical excision may be useful for pedunculated lesions and those that are life-threatening and unresponsive to medical management.
- Surgery may be needed to repair residual abnormalities after regression of hemangioma.
- Laser systems: flash lamp-pumped pulsed dye and others.
  - Less effective for hemangiomas compared with success in port-wine stains
  - Best used in thin superficial malformations and ulcerating lesions (penetrates only 1 mm)
  - Finger tip, nose tip, ear
  - Laser-trained physician should treat

ACUTE GENERAL Rx

- If large or life-threatening:
  - Systemic steroids
    - Administer 2 to 3 mg/kg/day for weeks to months.
      - Ideal length of therapy is controversial.
      - Rapid taper of steroid during proliferative phase may lead to rebound.
  - Intralesional steroid
    - 1 to 3 doses
    - Less than 3 to 5 mg/kg triamcinolone per lesion
  - Potent topical steroids
    - Improvement in one series only
    - Contraindicated in periocular area because of skin atrophy and necrosis with potential occlusion of central retinal artery
  - Recombinant interferon-alfa-2a
    - Angiogenesis inhibitor
    - Some success in patients with life-threatening lesions who failed corticosteroid therapy
    - Side effects: irritability, neutropenia, liver function test abnormalities, and spastic diplegia
  - Bleomycin
    - When injected into hemangiomas, bleomycin is reported to decrease size, but general use has not been evaluated.
  - Imiquimod: immune modifier
    - Case reports of success

DISPOSITION

- Follow patients for complete regression.
- Cosmetic surgical repair can be attempted late, if residual skin changes persist.

REFERRAL

- Dermatologic or surgical referral is warranted if specific therapy is needed.
- Also may consult (pediatric) ophthalmologist, (pediatric) otolaryngologist, (pediatric) plastic surgeon, or neurosurgeon depending on site of lesion.

PEARLS & CONSIDERATIONS

COMMENTS

- The course of hemangiomas is quite typical; an atypical course suggests a different diagnosis.
- Parents need significant emotional support, especially with hemangiomas that are on the head and neck (since noticed by others).

PATIENT/FAMILY EDUCATION

- Stress the benign nature and natural course of involution of these lesions.
- If the lesion ulcerates, bleeds, or suddenly increases in size, parents should seek medical attention.
- If the lesion obstructs a vital structure with its growth, parents should seek medical attention.

SUGGESTED READINGS

Antaya R: Infantile hemangioma. Available at www.emedicine.com=Derm=topiczol.html.

Dohil MA et al: Vascular and pigmented birthmarks. *Pediatr Clin North Am* 47:801, 2000.

Drolet BA et al: Hemangiomas in children. *N Engl J Med* 341:173, 1999.

Garzon MC, Frieden IJ: Hemangiomas: when to worry. *Pediatr Ann* 29:58, 2000.

HealthLink: Comprehensive review sheds new light on birthmarks. Available at www.healthlink.mcw.edu/article/936041445.html

Wahrman J, Honig P: Hemangiomas. *Pediatr Rev* 15:266, 1994.

Welsh O et al: Treatment of infantile hemangiomas with short-term application of imiquimod 5% cream. *J Am Acad Derm* 51:639, 2004.

AUTHOR: **LYNN C. GARFUNKEL, MD**

BASIC INFORMATION

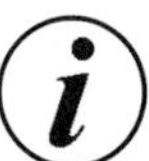

DEFINITION

Hemolytic disease with ABO incompatibility is hemolysis of neonatal red blood cells (RBCs) secondary to incompatibility between a type O mother and a type A or B newborn.

SYNONYM

ABO isoimmunization

ICD-9-CM CODE

773.1 Hemolytic disease caused by ABO isoimmunization

EPIDEMIOLOGY & DEMOGRAPHICS

- In one large series, 28% of ABO-incompatible babies had a weakly positive direct Coombs test and only 2% of these required an exchange transfusion.
- The severity of hemolysis does not increase with subsequent pregnancies as it does in RhD hemolytic disease

CLINICAL PRESENTATION

History

- Hydrops is very rare.
- Early neonatal jaundice, usually observed during the first 24 hours, may be reported.

Physical Examination

- Jaundice
- Liver and spleen usually normal in size

ETIOLOGY

In a type O mother, the naturally occurring maternal immunoglobulin G (IgG) anti-A or anti-B antibodies cross the placenta and attach to fetal and neonatal type A or type B RBCs. The degree of fetal and neonatal hemolysis is usually much milder than that which occurs with RhD hemolytic disease because of the following factors:

- Most anti-A and anti-B antibodies are immunoglobulin M (IgM) and do not cross the placenta.
- Anti-A and anti-B do not bind complement on the fetal RBC membrane.
- A and B antigens are present on many tissues other than RBCs, thus diluting the pool of anti-A and anti-B antibodies available to attach to RBC membranes.
- There are relatively few A and B antigen sites on fetal and neonatal RBCs.

DIAGNOSIS

DIFFERENTIAL DIAGNOSIS

- Hemolytic disease caused by other RBC antigen-antibody systems, including Rh disease, Kell, Duffy, Kidd, and so on
- Sepsis
- RBC membrane enzyme defects, such as glucose-6-phosphate dehydrogenase (G6PD) deficiency and pyruvate kinase deficiency

LABORATORY TEST(S)

- Anti-A or anti-B antibodies in cord and neonatal blood
- Positive direct Coombs test on cord and neonatal blood
- Anemia
- Spherocytes seen on peripheral blood smear

TREATMENT

ACUTE GENERAL Rx

- Intensive phototherapy is administered to control hyperbilirubinemia.
- An exchange transfusion is occasionally required to prevent the bilirubin level from reaching a degree that would put the infant at risk for acute bilirubin encephalopathy (kernicterus on neuropathology).

DISPOSITION

Neonates with significant hemolysis should have serial follow-up hematocrits at 1- to 2-week intervals to identify those infants with a continued slow hemolysis who may require a "top-up" transfusion with packed RBCs.

REFERRAL

Infants requiring an exchange transfusion should be referred to a level 3 neonatal intensive care unit.

PEARLS & CONSIDERATIONS

COMMENTS

The rapidity and degree of hemolysis are difficult to predict. Bilirubin levels must be monitored carefully.

SUGGESTED READINGS

American Academy of Pediatrics: Management of hyperbilirubinemia in the newborn infant 35 or more weeks of gestation. *Pediatrics* 114:297, 2004.

Bowman JM: Immune hemolytic disease. *In* Nathan DG, Orkin SH (eds): *Nathan Oski's Hematology of Infancy and Childhood,* 5th ed. Vol. 2. Philadelphia, WB Saunders, 1998, p 62.

AUTHOR: **JAMES W. KENDIG, MD**

BASIC INFORMATION

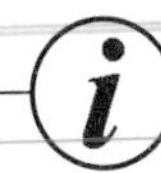

DEFINITION

Hemolysis of fetal and neonatal RhD-antigen-positive red blood cells (RBCs) caused by RhD antibodies acquired transplacentally from a sensitized RhD-negative mother.

SYNONYM

Erythroblastosis fetalis caused by RhD

ICD-9-CM CODE

773.0 Hemolytic disease caused by Rh isoimmunization

EPIDEMIOLOGY & DEMOGRAPHICS

- The prevalence of RhD-negative individuals varies by racial and geographic origin.
  - 15% to 20% in northern Europe
  - 5% in sub-Saharan Africa
  - Less than 1% in Asia
- With the introduction in 1968 of RhD immune globulin to prevent the sensitization of RhD-negative mothers, the incidence of this disease has declined exponentially.

CLINICAL PRESENTATION

- History of RhD mother with sensitization
- Fetal anemia and hydrops fetalis
- Neonatal anemia and hepatosplenomegaly
- Neonatal hyperbilirubinemia

ETIOLOGY

- Fetal RhD-positive RBCs (inherited from the father) cross the placenta of an RhD-negative mother and stimulate the maternal immune system to produce anti-RhD antibodies.
- These maternal immunoglobulin G (IgG) antibodies, in turn, cross the placenta of the current or future pregnancy to cause hemolysis of the fetal and neonatal RhD-positive RBCs.

DIAGNOSIS

DIFFERENTIAL DIAGNOSIS

- The differential diagnosis includes maternal sensitization with fetal and neonatal hemolysis secondary to other RBC antigen-antibody systems such as: ABO, Kidd, Kell, Duffy, and C/c and E/e alleles of the Rh system.

LABORATORY TESTS

Prenatal Diagnostic Workup

- The RhD-sensitized pregnancy is followed with serial RhD antibody titers and with serial ultrasound examinations (to look for hydrops).
- With climbing antibody titers, amniocentesis should be done to evaluate delta OD 450 values of the amniotic fluid.
- With increasing delta OD 450 values, cordocentesis should be performed to measure the fetal hematocrit.

Postnatal Diagnostic Workup

- Samples of umbilical cord blood and neonatal blood are positive for anti-D antibodies.
- Direct antiglobulin test (Coombs test) is positive.
- The reticulocyte count is elevated.
- Erythroblasts are seen on the blood smear.
- Progressive anemia and hyperbilirubinemia develop.

IMAGING STUDIES

- Serial prenatal ultrasound exams are employed to monitor for the development of hydrops.

TREATMENT

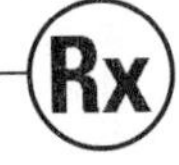

NONPHARMACOLOGIC THERAPY

Prenatal Therapy

- With recent technological developments in the field of fetal-maternal medicine, intravascular fetal transfusions (via cordocentesis) with packed RBCs may be administered to the fetus with severe anemia and early hydrops.

Delivery Room Therapy

- The infant delivered with severe hydrops requires aggressive resuscitation.
  - Intubation
  - Assisted ventilation
  - Administration of packed RBCs
  - Prompt thoracentesis and paracentesis if necessary

Neonatal Intensive Care Unit Therapy

- The infant may require one or more double-volume exchange transfusions to prevent the bilirubin from climbing into the toxic range.
- Phototherapy assists in controlling the rate of rise of the bilirubin.
- Intensive phototherapy using multiple banks of special blue fluorescent phototherapy lights may be employed.

ACUTE GENERAL Rx

The administration of intravenous immune globulin at 0.5 g/kg over 2 hours may help to avoid an exchange transfusion if the bilirubin is rising in spite of intensive phototherapy.

CHRONIC Rx

- Late anemia may develop because of continued slow hemolysis.
  - Serial hematocrits should be checked at 1- to 2-week intervals during the first 6 to 8 weeks.
- Transfusion with packed RBCs may be needed if symptomatic anemia develops.

DISPOSITION

- Late sequelae of neonatal bilirubin toxicity include choreoathetoid cerebral palsy, hearing impairment, and dental dysplasia.
- Follow-up hearing screens and neurodevelopmental evaluations are required.

REFERRAL

- Pregnant RhD-sensitized women should be referred to a regional center staffed with specialists in high-risk obstetrics and neonatology.

PEARLS & CONSIDERATIONS

COMMENTS

- ABO incompatibility between an RhD-negative mother and an RhD-positive fetus (i.e., mother O negative and fetus A or B positive) helps to protect the RhD-negative mother against RhD sensitization.

PREVENTION

Antepartum

- At 28 weeks' gestation, all RhD-negative mothers should have an RhD antibody screen.
- If negative, RhD immunoglobulin (300 μg) is administered intramuscularly.

Postpartum

- If the newborn infant is RhD positive, the mother should receive at least 300 μg of RhD immunoglobulin.
- The hospital blood bank should perform a Kleihauer-Betke stain of the maternal blood to evaluate the degree of fetal-to-maternal hemorrhage.
- In the case of a large fetal-to-maternal bleed, additional doses of RhD immunoglobulin may be required to prevent maternal sensitization.

SUGGESTED READINGS

American Academy of Pediatrics: Management of hyperbilirubinemia in the newborn infant 35 or more weeks of gestation. *Pediatrics* 114:297, 2004.

Gottstein R, Cooke RWI: Systematic review of intravenous immunoglobulin in hemolytic disease of the newborn. *Arch Dis Child Fetal Neonatal Ed* 88:F6, 2003.

Maisels MJ: Why use homeopathic doses of phototherapy? *Pediatrics* 98:283, 1996.

Prevention of RhD alloimmunization. *ACOG Pract Bull* 4, May 1999.

AUTHOR: **JAMES W. KENDIG, MD**

BASIC INFORMATION

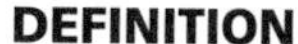
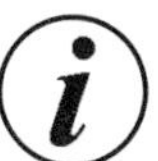

DEFINITION

Hemolytic uremic syndrome (HUS) is a syndrome of acute renal failure, microangiopathic hemolytic anemia, and thrombocytopenia.

ICD-9-CM CODES
283.11 Hemolytic uremic syndrome
584.9 Acute renal failure

EPIDEMIOLOGY & DEMOGRAPHICS

Most cases of HUS are secondary to infection with *Escherichia coli* O157:H7.

- D+ (diarrhea in prodrome) HUS is caused by *E. coli* O157:H7:
  - D+ HUS is the most common cause of acute renal failure in children in North America.
  - Peak incidence occurs in children younger than 5 years of age.
  - It occurs sporadically (most cases) and in epidemics.
  - The disease peaks between June and September.
  - Most cases result from contaminated beef products, but can also result from person-to-person contact, contaminated fruit, unpasteurized cider and milk, vegetables, and water.

CLINICAL PRESENTATION

- Typical (D+) HUS
  - Diarrheal prodrome in 90%; bloody in 75%
  - Abrupt onset of pallor, prostration, hematuria, oliguria, and edema, often as gastrointestinal symptoms are resolving
  - Signs and symptoms of renal failure predominate; may have involvement of any organ system
- History of offending drugs or affected family members and lack of diarrheal prodrome in atypical (D−) forms

ETIOLOGY

There are many causes of HUS. All involve endothelial cell injury of some kind.

- Infectious
  - *E. coli* O157:H7
    - *E. coli* O157:H7 is the most common cause of HUS in children, followed by other enterohemorrhagic *E. coli* strains and *Shigella dysenteriae* type 1.
    - These bacteria cause diarrhea-positive (D+) cases of HUS through the production of shigatoxins (verotoxins).
    - The secreted toxin is absorbed and binds to a cell surface glycolipid receptor. The complex is internalized and disrupts cellular protein synthesis. In the gastrointestinal tract, this leads to bloody diarrhea.
    - Systemically absorbed toxin affects many organs, especially the kidneys, in which there is a very high concentration of the glycolipid receptor on the glomerular endothelium in young children. Damaged endothelium induces thrombus formation.
  - *Streptococcus pneumoniae*
    - Neuraminidase exposes the Thomsen-Friedenreich antigen on cells leading to immune damage.
  - Human immunodeficiency virus (HIV)
  - Other infectious agents
- Noninfectious (These are known as atypical or diarrhea-negative [D−] HUS.)
  - Idiopathic
  - Hereditary
    - Autosomal dominant and autosomal recessive forms
    - Complement factor H deficiency
    - von Willebrand factor cleaving protease (ADAMTS 13) deficiency
    - Defects in vitamin B_{12} metabolism
  - Drugs: cyclosporine, tacrolimus, mitomycin C, oral contraceptives
  - Pregnancy
  - Malignant hypertension

DIAGNOSIS

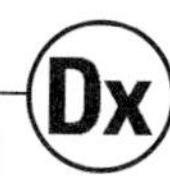

DIFFERENTIAL DIAGNOSIS

- Typical (D+) versus atypical (D−) HUS
- Thrombotic thrombocytopenic purpura
- Disseminated intravascular coagulation
- Henoch-Schönlein purpura

LABORATORY TESTS

- Blood urea nitrogen, creatinine, electrolytes for abnormalities
- Complete blood count, blood smear, platelet count, prothrombin time (PT), partial thromboplastin time (PTT), Coombs test, reticulocyte count, bilirubin level
  - Anemia, fragmented red blood cells (RBCs), thrombocytopenia, elevated white blood cell (WBC) count, reticulocytes elevated, bilirubin elevated
  - PT, PTT usually normal
  - Coombs test negative (except in pneumococcal-related HUS)
- Urinalysis: macroscopic hematuria, proteinuria, pyuria, cellular, granular, and hyaline casts
- Stool culture for bacteria (notify laboratory specifically that *E. coli* O157:H7 is being considered); approximately 30% of cultures are positive
- Free fecal Shigalike toxin (approximately 50% yield)
- Serologic testing for antibodies to verotoxin-producing *E. coli* (VTEC)
- Stool guaiac
- Amylase and lipase if pancreatitis suspected
- Kidney biopsy if atypical or a prolonged course

IMAGING STUDIES

- Imaging studies of gastrointestinal tract, central nervous system, chest, and kidneys as indicated by course and examination

TREATMENT

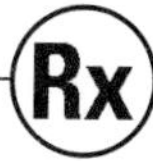

ACUTE GENERAL Rx

- Therapy of typical (D+) HUS is supportive, with correction of fluid, electrolyte, and acid-base abnormalities. Up to 90% of patients require dialysis.
- Judicious use of packed RBC and platelet transfusions (symptomatic anemia; bleeding) should be exercised.
- Plasmapheresis and plasma exchange are needed for atypical cases, but not for typical (D+) HUS.
- Corticosteroids and intravenous immunoglobulin do not appear to be effective.
- The role of antibiotics in the progression from *E. coli* hemorrhagic colitis to typical (D+) HUS is controversial. They do not appear to help and may lead to more severe disease.
- Antimotility medications are a known risk factor for progression from hemorrhagic colitis to HUS and should be avoided.

CHRONIC Rx

- According to sequelae

DISPOSITION

- Mortality is now less than 5% for typical (D+) HUS but is significantly higher for atypical forms.
- Long-term sequelae include the following:
  - As many as 40% of patients with typical (D+) HUS have some chronic renal abnormalities after 10 years (proteinuria [18%], hypertension [6%], decreased creatinine clearance [16%], end-stage renal disease [3%]).
  - Up to 48% of children with atypical forms of HUS progress to end-stage renal disease.
  - Proteinuria persisting longer than 1 year from HUS portends a poorer renal prognosis.
  - Approximately 8% of children with typical (D+) HUS have long-term neurologic sequelae (e.g., retardation, seizures, motor deficit, learning and behavioral problems, blindness).
  - Recurrence in a kidney transplant is uncommon with typical (D+) HUS.
  - There is a high risk of recurrence in atypical (D−) HUS.

REFERRAL

- Input of a pediatric nephrologist should be obtained.

PEARLS & CONSIDERATIONS

COMMENTS

- HUS often occurs abruptly just as the child appears to be improving from a bout of colitis.
- Siblings who develop HUS more than 1 year apart probably have a familial form of HUS.

PREVENTION

- Practice good hand-washing technique.
- Cook meats, particularly ground beef, thoroughly (to internal temperature of 155°F [68.3°C]).
- Avoid unpasteurized milk and cider.
- Wash fruits and vegetables thoroughly.
- Children with hemorrhagic colitis should not return to day care until two stool cultures for *E. coli* O157:H7 have been negative.

PATIENT/FAMILY EDUCATION

NEPHKIDS website has information on various kidney diseases with links to an email discussion group for parents of children with kidney disease. Available at http://cnserver0.nkf.med.ualberta.ca/nephkids/

Local chapters of the National Kidney Foundation (www.kidney.org) can provide information and support.

SUGGESTED READINGS

Kaplan BS et al: The pathogenesis and treatment of hemolytic uremic syndrome. *J Am Soc Nephrol* 9:1126, 1998.

Tarr PI et al: Shiga-toxin-producing *Escherichia coli* and haemolytic uremic syndrome. *Lancet* 365:1073, 2005.

Wong CS et al: The risk of the hemolytic-uremic syndrome after antibiotic treatment of *Escherichia coli* O157:H7 infections. *N Engl J Med* 342:1930, 2000.

Zipfel PF et al: Genetic screening in haemolytic uremic syndrome. *Curr Opin Nephrol Hypertens* 12:653, 2003.

AUTHOR: **WILLIAM S. VARADE, MD**

BASIC INFORMATION

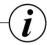

DEFINITION

Hemophilia is a hereditary bleeding disorder that is caused by a deficiency or defect in a blood clotting factor. Rare cases are acquired.

SYNONYMS

Hemophilia "A": "Classic hemophilia" caused by a factor VIII deficiency/defect
Hemophilia "B": "Christmas disease" caused by a factor IX deficiency/defect

ICD-9-CM CODES
286.0 Hemophilia A
286.1 Hemophilia B

EPIDEMIOLOGY & DEMOGRAPHICS

- Hemophilia A and B are X-linked recessive disorders.
- Hemophilia A is the most common, although it is rare in the population (1 in 10,000 live male births)
  - Hemophilia A is found in all ethnic groups throughout the world.
  - All sons of affected males are normal.
  - All daughters of affected males are obligate carriers.
  - Sons of carriers have a 50:50 risk of disease (daughters have a 50:50 carrier risk).
- Hemophilia B is clinically identical to hemophilia A.
  - Hemophilia B occurs in 1 in 30,000 male births; 4:1 ratio of hemophilia A:B.
  - Factor VIIIa is a cofactor for factor IXa; therefore deficiency of either factor causes decreased factor IX activity. It may be qualitative or quantitative.
  - Severity patterns, genetic patterns, laboratory features, and differential diagnosis are similar to those of hemophilia A.
  - Course and prognosis are similar to those seen with hemophilia A (although less likely to develop inhibitors).
- Other hemophilias include, in order of frequency, deficiencies of factors XI, X, VII, V, and II.
  - The degree of severity is important in management.
  - Specific products are available for some deficiencies; plasma is used for many.

CLINICAL PRESENTATION

Clinically, patients may have mild, moderate, or severe disease. The clinical features usually correlate with the severity of the factor deficiency. Clinical features are similar in hemophilia A and B.

- Hematomas
  - These are characteristic of hemophilia (unusual in patients with platelet disorders).
  - Patients with severe hematomas can have dissection (retropharyngeal/retroperitoneal).
  - Muscle bleeding can lead to compartment syndromes.
- Hemarthrosis
  - Approximately 75% of hemophilia bleeding is joint-related.
  - Joints are most commonly affected in the following order: knees, elbows, ankles, shoulders, wrists, and hips.
  - Patients often have a target joint, resulting in a cycle of inflammation and rebleeding.
  - If not treated quickly, hemarthrosis can result in chronic pain/joint destruction, and ultimately osteoporosis, bone cysts, and joint space narrowing.
- Pseudotumors
  - These tumors usually occur within the tendons or bones.
- Hematuria
  - Hematuria is often seen during the lifetime of a hemophiliac.
  - Hematuria is usually from the renal pelvis.
  - Treat with factor replacement.
    - Prednisone is sometimes used.
    - Avoid Amicar.
- Neurologic complications
  - Intracranial bleeding is usually seen with trauma.
  - Spinal bleeding is rare.
  - Peripheral nerve compression can be seen secondary to muscle bleeding.
- Mucous membrane bleeding
  - Epistaxis is common (hemoptysis often structural).
  - Ulcer disease is common secondary to nonsteroidal anti-inflammatory drugs used for arthritis.
    - Cyclooxygenase-2 (COX-2) inhibitors have been used but safety of these medications remains a concern.
- Surgery and procedures
  - It is common for patients to bleed with surgery. Prevention is key.
  - Mild bleeding in patients often is discovered postoperatively.
  - Dental extractions are a common cause of morbidity.
  - Bleeding may be delayed for hours or days.
  - Infected wound hematomas may occur.
  - Perioperative hemophilia needs are based on the type of surgery and the severity of the hemophilia.

ETIOLOGY

- Factor VIII or IX deficiency may be qualitative, quantitative, or both.
- Delayed clot formation secondary to reduced thrombin generation.
- Factor VIII is a very large gene (186 kb).
  - Multiple deletions, mutations, and insertions are described.
  - Intron 22 mutation (homologous recombination) is a common genetic defect in severe hemophilia A.

DIAGNOSIS

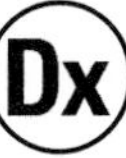

DIFFERENTIAL DIAGNOSIS

- von Willebrand disease (severe)
  - Usually has a prolonged bleeding time
  - Different inheritance pattern and different clinical manifestations
- Other hereditary bleeding disorders
  - Clinically similar with deficiency of factor IX and factor XI
  - Similar laboratory features: factor XII deficiency (prolonged activated partial thromboplastin time [aPTT] but no bleeding)

LABORATORY TESTS

- Prolongation of the aPTT is seen, with normal prothrombin time (PT) and normal bleeding time.
- Patients with mild hemophilia may have a normal aPTT.
- The aPTT corrects with normal plasma (unless inhibitor present).
- Functional factor VIII can be measured with a clotting assay.
  - Factor VIII: C measures coagulant activity.
- Immunologic factor VIII can be measured with an immunoassay.
  - Factor VIII: Ag can measure normal and abnormal factor VIII.
- Factor levels expressed in units: 1 unit in 1 mL of plasma—if normal (~100%).
  - Severe: less than 1% factor activity; spontaneous bleeding is recognized during infancy.
  - Moderate: 2% to 5% factor activity; may have spontaneous bleeding, trauma-related bleeding is common.
  - Mild: 6% to 30% factor activity; trauma-related bleeding, surgical bleeding; may go unrecognized until adult years.
  - Carriers may be symptomatic but if so are usually mild clinically.

TREATMENT

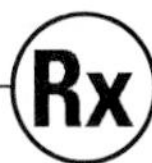

NONPHARMACOLOGIC THERAPY

General Principles

- Have a sense of urgency.
- Avoid acetylsalicylic acid (ASA, aspirin) and antiplatelet drugs (if possible).
- Avoid intramuscular injections.
- Follow patients in a specialized center.
- Trust the patients because they know the disease.
- Local measures include pressure, rest, ice, topical thrombin, fibrin glue, and sutures with caution.

Surgical Procedures

- Surgical intervention may be needed to evacuate a hematoma.
- Patients occasionally undergo synovectomy.
- Orthopedic procedures are fairly common.

- Venous access devices (ports) are common in children.

ACUTE GENERAL Rx

General Principles

- Have clotting factor concentrates available.
- Time procedures appropriately for factor coverage (not weekends).

Hemophilia A Treatment

- Factor replacement
  - Plasma-derived factor concentrates are still available (treated to increase purity and viral safety using solvent detergent, pasteurization, or monoclonal antibodies).
  - Recombinant factor is mainly used; in the future, gene therapy will likely be available.
- Dosing
  - Based on the following criteria:
    - Severity of the hemophilia
    - Severity and site of the bleeding
    - Size of the patient
  - Issues to consider include the dosing interval, the desired factor level, and the planned treatment duration. (Consultation with hematologist is recommended for dosing.)
- Other agents/modalities
  - DDAVP: In patients with mild to moderate hemophilia, factor VIII levels are transiently raised (peak at 30 to 60 minutes), often to a safe level, to control bleeding or prevent procedure-related bleeding. If use of this therapy is anticipated, a DDAVP trial should be performed to assess the patient's response (dose: 0.3 μg/kg intravenously).
  - Intranasal DDAVP (Stimate) is available.
    - Different formulation than DDAVP is used for enuresis and diabetes insipidus.
  - Amicar is an antifibrinolytic drug that is useful with dental work and mucosal bleeding.
    - Hematuria is a contraindication.
  - Corticosteroids are sometimes useful for hematuria and hemarthrosis.

Hemophilia B Treatment

- Basic principles are the same as those for hemophilia A.
- Until recently, the only available products were prothrombin complex concentrates, which have potential thrombotic risk with repeat dosing. More highly purified products are now available with minimal contamination of other proteins (monoclonal products). Recombinant factor IX (BeneFix) is available and widely used.
- Dosing is a *major difference with factor VIII;* only 50% plasma recovery. There is extravascular binding and a longer half-life. Therefore, dosing can be less frequent.

Medical Complications

- Factor VIII inhibitors
  - Antibodies to factor VIII develop in approximately 15% of patients with hemophilia A.
  - Usually seen in patients with severe disease and frequent exposure to factor. Exposure at an early age likely increases risk.
  - Inhibitors tend to run in families and are seen in blacks more than whites.
  - Patients with inhibitors may be low-responders or high-responders.
  - Treatment of inhibitors includes the following:
    - Factor VIII (high-dose or continuous infusion)—may saturate the antibody
    - Prothrombin complex concentrates (PCCs)/activated PCCs
    - Porcine factor VIII (may be cross-reactive)
    - Recombinant VIIa (NovoSeven)—commonly used currently
    - Immune tolerance regimens—to decrease the inhibitor level/activity
- Hepatitis
  - Almost all multitransfused patients (pre-1985) have evidence of hepatitis.
    - Approximately 90% are hepatitis B surface antibody (HBsAb) positive, and 10% are hepatitis B surface antigen (HBsAg) positive.
    - Fortunately, this is no longer an issue for pediatric patients with hemophilia.
    - The prevalence of hepatitis C is extremely high.
    - Approximately 50% of patients develop chronic active hepatitis or cirrhosis.
    - Some success has been achieved with α-interferon/ribavirin.
    - Human immunodeficiency virus (HIV) worsens the natural history of hepatitis C.
- HIV infection
  - Many early pediatric HIV cases were in people with hemophilia.
  - Most received contaminated factor and seroconverted between 1978 and 1985.
  - Approximately 80% to 90% of severe older hemophiliacs are HIV-positive.
    - Many have died in the last 10 to 15 years.
  - Essentially no treatment-related conversions have occurred since 1985.
- Other infections
  - Hepatitis A is associated with rare transfusion-related cases (can vaccinate now).
  - Parvovirus is also associated with rare transfusion-related cases.
  - Creutzfeldt-Jakob disease (CJD) is a theoretical concern.
    - Rare reports of CJD possibly linked with blood transfusion.
    - No cases have been reported in hemophiliacs.

CHRONIC Rx

Prophylaxis

- Commonly used in Europe
  - Increased use recently in the United States
  - Decreases chronic joint damage
  - Encouraged in those with frequent bleeds
- Overall may not increase cost/use
- Aim for factor level trough of more than 1%
- Can be timed with activities (e.g., Little League)

DISPOSITION

- Infants are usually treated at hemophilia centers.
- Parents of young children learn to infuse factor at home.
- Preteens often learn self-infusion.

REFERRAL

A multidisciplinary team should be involved in the care of patients with hemophilia. The team includes medical, nursing, social services, dental, orthopedic, physical therapy, infectious disease, and gastrointestinal personnel, as well as support groups.

PEARLS & CONSIDERATIONS

PATIENT/FAMILY EDUCATION

- By the late 1970s, life expectancy approached that of nonhemophiliacs.
  - Life expectancy for HIV-positive hemophiliacs is shortened.
  - Older uninfected patients and those patients born after 1985 have an excellent life expectancy.
- Cause of death was historically bleeding.
  - Other causes of death and related comorbidities include the following:
    - The development of inhibitors
    - Chronic liver disease secondary to hepatitis B or C
    - HIV-related complications

SUGGESTED READINGS

Manco-Johnson MJ et al: Advances in care of children with hemophilia. *Semin Thromb Hemost* 29(6):585, 2003.

Mannucci PM: Hemophilia: treatment options in the twenty-first century. *J Thromb Haemost* 1(7):1349, 2003.

The Mary M. Gooley Hemophilia Center, Inc. Available at www.hemocenter.org

The National Hemophilia Foundation. Available at www.hemophilia.org

The World Federation of Hemophilia. Available at www.wfh.org

AUTHOR: **RONALD L. SHAM, MD**

BASIC INFORMATION

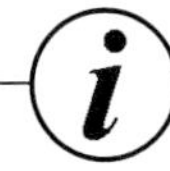

DEFINITION

Hemoptysis is expectoration of blood from sputum arising from the oral cavity, larynx, trachea, bronchi, or lungs.

SYNONYM

Expectoration of blood

ICD-9-CM CODE
786.3 Hemoptysis

EPIDEMIOLOGY & DEMOGRAPHICS

- In young children, the incidence of hemoptysis is difficult to gauge, as they often swallow their secretions rather than expectorate them.
- Older children are more likely to expectorate their secretions, yet reliable data are not found regarding epidemiology and demographics.
- Acute lower respiratory infection is the most common cause (approximately 40% of cases).
- Bronchiectasis, resulting from cystic fibrosis (CF) or other chronic pulmonary infections, is also common, especially in a referral population.
- Approximately 1% to 15% of patients with bronchiectasis develop hemoptysis.
- Congenital heart disease, once a common cause of hemoptysis in pediatric patients, is uncommon now because of the availability of early corrective surgery.

CLINICAL PRESENTATION

History

- One must first elucidate that the bleeding is actually coming from the tracheobronchial tree.
- Sputum is usually bright red, rust-colored, or frothy.
- Inquire about constitutional symptoms (e.g., fever, weight loss), choking spells, recent infections or trauma, calf pain, or hematuria.
- Hemoptysis may be preceded by dyspnea, pleuritic pain, or a gurgling noise in the airway.
  - With *hematemesis,* the vomited blood may be of coffee-ground consistency, clotted, darkened color, or mixed with food, or it may be preceded by epigastric discomfort or nausea.
  - With *epistaxis,* the differentiation may be more difficult, but blood is often spit or vomited, increased in production with the head tilted back, or associated with anterior nasal bleeding.

Physical Examination

- First examine the material, checking for food particles, acidity, or clots, all of which are more common in *hematemesis.*
- Pallor may indicate anemia from chronic disease.
- Digital clubbing may indicate chronic suppurative lung disease, pulmonary arteriovenous malformation (AVM), or congenital heart disease.
- Other bruises or signs of trauma may support concomitant pulmonary contusion.
- Check for telangiectasias elsewhere on the body.
- A missing tooth may support a foreign body aspiration.
- Localized pulmonary examination findings include consolidation, wheezes (foreign body, endobronchial lesions), unequal breath sounds, pleural rubs (pneumonia, collagen vascular disease, pulmonary embolism), and bruits (AVM).

ETIOLOGY

- Loss of integrity between pulmonary vasculature and bronchial tree, as in infection, bronchiectasis, or foreign body erosion
- Alveolar hemorrhage syndromes such as hereditary hemorrhagic telangiectasia or AVMs
- Pulmonary infarction (e.g., cocaine, pulmonary thromboembolism)
- Vasculitis
- Coagulopathy

DIAGNOSIS

DIFFERENTIAL DIAGNOSIS

- Diagnosis made primarily from history, with supportive features from physical examination
- Acute infection of the lower respiratory tract
  - Pneumonia: bacterial, viral, tuberculosis, fungal (especially aspergillosis), or parasitic
  - Tracheobronchitis
- Bronchiectasis, especially in patients with CF and ciliary dyskinesia
- Foreign body aspiration
- Lung abscess
- Pulmonary AVM
- Hereditary hemorrhagic telangiectasia (Osler-Weber-Rendu syndrome)
- Trauma (iatrogenic, penetrating, blunt)
- Alveolar hemorrhage syndrome (may be idiopathic or associated with systemic lupus erythematosus, Goodpasture's syndrome, Henoch-Schönlein purpura, or Wegener's granulomatosis)
- Congenital heart disease
- Primary pulmonary hemosiderosis: may be associated with cow's milk protein allergy (Heiner syndrome)
- Pulmonary thromboembolism
- Tracheostomy-related
- Tumor (uncommon as a cause overall, but a common feature in bronchial carcinoid syndrome)
- Coagulopathy
- Drugs (aspirin [acetylsalicylic acid, ASA], propylthiouracil, cocaine)
- Unexplained hemoptysis: following workup imperative

LABORATORY TESTS

- The pH of expectorated material is alkaline; in hematemesis, the pH is acidic.
- Laboratory tests include the following:
  - Complete blood count assessment for anemia with chronic disease or elevated white blood cell counts with acute infectious process
  - Erythrocyte sedimentation rate to look for collagen vascular disease
  - Prothrombin time (PT)/partial thromboplastin time (PTT) for vitamin K deficiency or liver disease
  - Sputum Gram stain and culture for bacteria, fungi, and mycobacteria
  - Urine analysis to assess hematuria
  - Blood urea nitrogen and creatinine
- Specialized testing should be performed as needed.
  - Tuberculosis or aspergillus skin testing
  - Immunoglobulin E
  - Sweat chloride test for CF
  - Milk precipitins (Heiner syndrome)
  - Antiglomerular basement membrane antibodies (Goodpasture's syndrome)
  - Antinuclear antibodies (systemic lupus erythematosus)
  - Antineutrophil cytoplasmic antibody (Wegener's granulomatosis)
  - Consideration of renal biopsy if signs of renal involvement

IMAGING STUDIES

- Chest radiograph (one third are normal)
  - AVM
  - Bronchiectasis
  - Infiltrates
  - Adenopathy
- Most foreign bodies are radiolucent; therefore consider expiratory-inspiratory films to check for ball-valve obstruction.
  - Technetium 99-tagged red blood cell scan can identify the site of bleeding in approximately 50% of cases.
  - Chest computed tomography (CT) scan is the procedure of choice to further define pulmonary parenchymal disease.
    - Magnetic resonance imaging (MRI) is more useful for vascular structures.
    - Ventilation-perfusion (V/Q) scan or spiral chest CT scan should be obtained to evaluate for pulmonary embolus.
- Selective bronchoscopy may be needed in the following cases:
  - Laboratory workup complete and cause not defined
  - Continued bleeding
- Bronchioalveolar lavage with or without biopsy may be needed.
- Removal of foreign bodies may be necessary.

TREATMENT

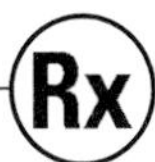

NONPHARMACOLOGIC THERAPY

In most cases, hemoptysis is self-limited and not a sign of more serious disease.

ACUTE GENERAL Rx

- In massive hemoptysis, remember airway, breathing, and circulation (ABCs of resuscitation).
  - Mechanical ventilation with frequent suctioning may be necessary to maintain airway patency.
- Once the airway is protected, a diagnostic/therapeutic rigid bronchoscopy (for concomitant mechanical ventilation) can be performed.
  - Clotted material is removed.
  - Iced saline or topical vasoconstrictors such as oxymetazoline or epinephrine can be instilled to control bleeding.
- If this does not control the bleeding, balloon tamponade may be attempted.
- If this fails, the patient should be sent for selective bronchial arteriography followed by embolization of the suspected vessel(s).
  - Gelfoam, Ivalon, bucrylate, metallic coils, or polyvinyl alcohol particles may be used.
  - Bronchial artery embolization is contraindicated if a spinal artery arises from the suspected bronchial artery.
    - In this case, the bronchial artery is cannulated.
    - Embolization material is injected.
- Up to 90% of bleeding can be controlled with the previous measures.
- Surgical intervention is necessary only for failed medical treatment.
  - Laser therapy may be an option in the future.
  - Approximately 70% of patients have minor and 20% have major recurrences.
  - Surgical therapy with resection of the affected segment is indicated for severe recurrences.

CHRONIC Rx

Usually, no chronic therapy is needed.

DISPOSITION

- As hemoptysis is usually a self-limited problem, specific diagnostic and therapeutic modalities are usually not needed.
- The prognosis is uniformly good for those with self-limited hemoptysis.
- For those with specific disease entities responsible for hemoptysis, their disposition is dependent upon the specific diagnosis.

REFERRAL

- Any patient with persistent, severe, or recurrent hemoptysis should be considered for referral to a pulmonologist or otolaryngologist.

PEARLS & CONSIDERATIONS

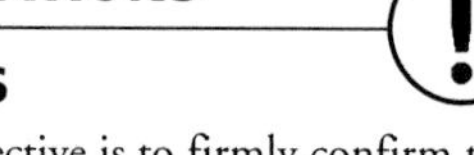

COMMENTS

- The first objective is to firmly confirm that one is dealing with hemoptysis rather than epistaxis or hematemesis.
- Infections of the respiratory tree account for nearly half of the cases overall, whereas foreign body aspiration is a common cause in toddlers.
- Malignancy is a rare cause.

PATIENT/FAMILY EDUCATION

- Most cases of hemoptysis are self-limited.
- For most cases, safe and effective therapeutic options are available.
- In more complex cases, a pulmonologist can often dictate the most effective strategy for the workup.

SUGGESTED READINGS

Batra PS, Holinger LD: Etiology management of pediatric hemoptysis. *Arch Otolaryngol Head Neck Surg* 127:377, 2001.

Fabian MC, Smitheringale A: Hemoptysis in children: the hospital for sick children experience. *J Otolaryngol* 25:44, 1996.

Nelson WE et al: *Nelson Textbook of Pediatrics,* 15th ed. Philadelphia, WB Saunders, 1999.

Pianosi P, Al-sadoon H: Hemoptysis in children. *Pediatr Rev* 17:344, 1996.

Quintero DR, Fan LL: Hemoptysis in children. *In* Rose BD (ed): *UpToDate.* Wellesley, MA, UpToDate, 2004.

AUTHOR: **STEVEN JOYCE, MD**

BASIC INFORMATION

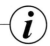

DEFINITION

Intracranial hemorrhage refers to bleeding that occurs inside the skull but not necessarily within the brain (intracerebral). It is classified by location. Epidural blood is situated between the skull and the dura, subdural blood is situated between the dura and the underlying brain, and subarachnoid blood is beneath the arachnoid and separated from the brain by the pia. Subdural bleeding is further classified by the time interval between injury and the onset of symptoms as acute (up to 24 hours), subacute (1 to 10 days), or chronic (more than 10 days).

SYNONYMS

Epidural hematoma, epidural hemorrhage, or epidural bleed
Head bleed
Intracranial hemorrhage, intracranial hematoma, or intracranial bleed
Subdural hematoma, subdural hemorrhage, or subdural bleed

ICD-9-CM CODES
431 Intracerebral hemorrhage
432 Nontraumatic extradural hemorrhage
432.1 Nontraumatic subdural hemorrhage
432.9 Nonspecified, nontraumatic intracranial hemorrhage
767 Subdural and cerebral hemorrhage due to birth trauma
852 Subarachnoid, subdural, and extradural hemorrhage following injury
853 Other and unspecified intracranial hemorrhage following injury

EPIDEMIOLOGY & DEMOGRAPHICS

- Trauma is the leading cause of death and disability among children in the United States, and brain injury is the leading cause of death from trauma. The major causes of pediatric brain injury (and traumatic intracranial bleeding) are falls, motor vehicle crashes, and recreational activities.
- As with all types of trauma, males have approximately twice the rate of brain injuries compared with females.
- Rates of injury are stable throughout childhood but increase dramatically at age 15 years.
- The more severe the head injury, the more likely there is to be intracranial bleeding.
  - Seventy percent of epidural hemorrhages are associated with skull fracture.
  - About 30% of subdural hemorrhages are associated with skull fracture.
- Among children younger than 2 years of age:
  - Approximately 25% of head injuries requiring hospital admission are caused by abuse.
  - Subdural hemorrhages more commonly result from child abuse than from unintentional injury.
  - Intracranial bleeding is caused by blunt trauma and shaking injury with secondary damage to the bridging cortical veins.
- Approximately 20% of subdural hemorrhages are bilateral.
- Epidural hematomas are usually unilateral, occur in older children with blunt unintentional trauma to the temporal lateral aspect of the skull, and are less common than subdural hematomas.
- Most falls resulting in intracranial bleeding are falls from heights of more than 10 feet.
  - Epidural hematomas can occur in infants from falls of less than 4 feet (especially with a skull fracture), because of their high center of gravity and tendency to land head first.
- The risk of bleeding complications in patients with coagulopathy is directly related to the severity of the condition (e.g., critically low factor level or platelet count $<5000/mm^3$).
  - The location of such bleeding is consistent with the mechanism of injury.
  - Rarely, such bleeding occurs as a spontaneous event.

CLINICAL PRESENTATION

History

- History of trauma should always be sought.
- Precise details should be elicited, including:
  - Time, location, and description of how the injury occurred
  - Whether there was loss of consciousness and the duration of the loss
  - Whether there were any posttraumatic neurologic changes or a lucent period before the onset of confusion or coma
- Explanations that are not consistent with the severity of the injury or the developmental level of the child should be investigated further.
- Intracranial bleeding can be associated with birth trauma.
  - Newborns may present with seizures after 48 hours of age.
  - Subarachnoid and subdural hemorrhages are the most commonly seen types of bleeding.
  - A history of cephalopelvic disproportion, abnormal presentation, precipitous delivery, or the use of mechanical devices may be elicited.
  - Significant intracranial bleeding may be found in the absence of external signs of trauma.

Physical Examination

- Physical assessment should begin with the familiar "ABCDE" mnemonic—airway, breathing, circulation, disability, and exposure.
  - Airway instability can be both a cause and an effect of head injury.
  - Recognition and control of shock is important for adequate central nervous system (CNS) perfusion.
  - Hypovolemic shock is rare in isolated head injury even with intracranial hemorrhage.
- Initial neurologic examination should focus on the level of consciousness, the presence of abnormal neurologic signs, and size and reactivity of the pupils.
  - The best indicator of insufficient perfusion and oxygenation of the brain is alteration of consciousness.
- Carefully examine the fundi for papilledema and retinal hemorrhages.
  - Retinal hemorrhages rarely occur in unintentional brain injury. Their presence usually implies that the child is the victim of shaken-impact syndrome.
- Abnormalities of ocular gaze suggest orbital fracture or impending herniation.
- The head should be examined carefully, looking for the following:
  - Lacerations and contusions of the scalp
  - Tenderness to palpation or indentations of the skull
  - Tension of the anterior fontanel in the infant
  - Signs of basilar skull fracture
    - Periorbital hemorrhage (raccoon eyes)
    - Ecchymosis behind the ears (Battle's sign)
    - Bleeding from the nose or ears
    - Cerebrospinal fluid (CSF) rhinorrhea or otorrhea (glucose-positive)
- The most important feature of the examination of children with a head injury is serial and frequent reassessment using a reliable, easily reproducible system with good interrater reliability, such as the Glasgow Coma Scale with its pediatric modification (see Emergency Medicine in Charts, Formulas, Laboratory Tests and Values [Section IV]). Deteriorations demand reevaluation and may require therapeutic intervention.

ETIOLOGY

- Most cases of intracranial bleeding in newborn and pediatric populations result from trauma.
- Subdural hematomas in newborns result from birth trauma caused by cephalopelvic disproportion, abnormal presentation, precipitant deliveries, and the use of mechanical devices during delivery.
- Trauma resulting from automobile accidents is the usual mechanism of injury resulting in intracranial bleeding.
- Inflicted injury caused by abuse or assault may also cause intracranial bleeding.
- Primary hematologic conditions (e.g., hemophilia, idiopathic thrombocytopenic purpura) can be associated with spontaneous intracranial bleeding. Most cases of bleeding in these patients also occur as a result of trauma.

DIAGNOSIS

DIFFERENTIAL DIAGNOSIS

- Newborns with intracranial bleeding associated with birth trauma may present with seizures, apnea, vomiting, or irritability. External signs of trauma may or may not be present.
- Differential diagnosis in infants with altered mental status includes:
  - Apparent life-threatening event (ALTE) (see Apparent Life-Threatening Event and Sudden Infant Death Syndrome in Diseases and Disorders [Section I])
  - Shaken baby syndrome
  - CNS infection
  - Seizure
  - Poisoning
  - Inborn error of metabolism
  - Hypoglycemia
  - Hyponatremia
  - Stroke
- Differential diagnosis in older children with altered mental status if trauma or history for trauma not obvious includes:
  - Meningitis
  - Encephalitis
  - Encephalopathy
  - Seizure disorder
  - Ingestion
  - Intoxication
  - Drug exposure
  - Overdose
  - Metabolic abnormality (inborn error of metabolism, hypoglycemia, hyponatremia)
  - Stroke
  - Tumor
  - Vitamin A intoxication

WORKUP

- With a known history of significant trauma or minor trauma in a patient at high risk for intracranial bleeding, diagnostic evaluation is done to determine the extent and nature of the injuries and to determine the potential need for emergent neurosurgical intervention.
- Children who present with physical findings that are inconsistent with the history given should be evaluated for other sites of traumatic injury. Abuse should be considered.

LABORATORY TEST

Evaluation and monitoring of hematologic parameters and the coagulation system is often indicated in the assessment of patients with intracranial bleeding.

IMAGING STUDIES

- Computed tomography (CT) scan is the test of choice for patients with a head injury who are suspected of having intracranial bleeding.
- CT scan of the head should be performed for patients with any of the following:
  - A history of or findings on examination that suggest an underlying bleeding problem
  - Posttraumatic loss of consciousness, seizures, amnesia, disorientation, mental status change
  - Hemiparesis, anisocoria, ocular palsy, or other focal neurologic signs
  - Severe head injury with a pediatric Glasgow Coma Score (PGCS) of 8 or less or a decline in the PGCS of ≥ 2 points
  - Presence of a penetrating skull injury or a palpably depressed skull fracture
  - Signs or symptoms of elevated intracranial pressure (ICP)
  - Retinal hemorrhages
  - Unconscious patients in need of emergent chest or abdominal surgery
- Contrast is not required; significant intracranial blood is quite evident without contrast.
- CT images of the head may miss some linear, stellate, and basilar skull fractures.
- Significant findings on CT scan may include:
  - Fresh blood—seen as an area of more increased density (whiter) than surrounding tissue.
  - Epidural hemorrhages—lens-shaped areas of increased signal located in the temporal-parietal regions.
  - Acute subdural hematomas—crescent-shaped areas of increased density, usually frontal in location, that spread diffusely along the inner table of the skull.
- Magnetic resonance imaging (MRI) is usually not needed in the acute situation.
  - MRI is more sensitive in detecting hypothalamic and brainstem infarcts and nonhemorrhagic intracranial lesions and in distinguishing acute on top of more chronic bleeding. It can also be used in subsequent evaluations of the child with persistent signs or symptoms.
  - Availability of MRI and the challenge of sedation and monitoring make MRI less practical than CT scan for the acutely injured patient.
- Ultrasonography can be helpful in newborns and young infants with open fontanelles.
- Radiologic evaluation should not be undertaken until the patient is stabilized.
- Because epidural hematomas result from arterial bleeding that can progress rapidly, some patients with hemiparesis, signs of herniation, and respiratory failure may require neurosurgical intervention before the diagnosis can be confirmed with CT.
- Although most cases of epidural bleeding and some cases of subdural bleeding are associated with a skull fracture, normal skull films do not exclude the possibility of intracranial bleeding.
- Subdural hemorrhages are a classic feature of the shaken baby syndrome. In these injuries, subdural hemorrhages occasionally may be bilateral and located posteriorly in the interhemispheric fissure.

TREATMENT

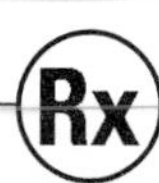

NONPHARMACOLOGIC THERAPY

- Initial management should be directed at correcting life-threatening problems and preventing secondary brain injury. Remember to elevate the head of the bed of all patients with head injuries.
- The frequency of pupil examination, level of consciousness checks, and repeated neurologic examination should be dictated by the patient's acuity in conjunction with neurosurgical consultation.
- Attention to the airway, respirations, and circulation take immediate precedence over the management of the head injury. If needed, orotracheal (not nasal) intubation using a rapid-sequence intubation technique to minimize elevations of ICP.
- If herniation is imminent, hyperventilation is indicated.
- Neurosurgical consultation is indicated for patients with severe head injury with loss of consciousness, depressed skull fractures, linear skull fractures that cross the middle meningeal artery groove, or basal skull fractures, and is indicated if imaging studies reveal acute bleeding that has a mass effect or the potential for one.
- Epidural and acute subdural hemorrhages are managed with emergent surgical drainage.
- In the young infant with open sutures, subdural taps can be performed for diagnostic and therapeutic purposes, but they generally are not used to evacuate acute bleeds.
- A burr hole approach to the hematoma may be required emergently.
- Depressed skull fractures are often associated with brain laceration and may require intraoperative hemostasis and elevation of the depressed fragment. In the absence of an intracerebral bleed, many pediatric depressed fractures are managed conservatively.
- Most subarachnoid and small intracerebral hemorrhages do not require surgical drainage and are managed conservatively.

ACUTE GENERAL Rx

- Pharmacologic agents have limited usefulness in the emergent management of head trauma.
  - Lidocaine can be given to suppress the cough reflex before intubation.
  - Rapid-sequence induction with Pavulon, atropine, succinylcholine, and thiopental is needed for intubation to protect the airway and minimize elevations of ICP.
  - Osmotic agents such as mannitol may rarely be necessary to decrease ICP but are never used prophylactically and are begun only if fluid resuscitation has been ensured. Furosemide is often used as an adjunct to mannitol therapy.

- Hypotonic fluids should be avoided and fluid status reevaluated frequently given the potential for inappropriate antidiuretic hormone release.
- Prophylactic use of anticonvulsants is unwarranted. Phenytoin is the most commonly used anticonvulsant for the treatment of acute, traumatic seizures.

CHRONIC Rx

Involvement of social services and rehabilitative services is almost always needed for children and families who have experienced severe head injury.

DISPOSITION

Children with serious head trauma associated with intracranial bleeding require hospitalization and monitoring in an intensive care setting.

REFERRAL

- Neurosurgical consultation and operative intervention are indicated for children with epidural and acute subdural hemorrhages and for children with depressed skull fractures associated with cerebral laceration.
- Consultation with a neurologist may be needed for the child with seizures or CNS disability resulting from the head injury.

PEARLS & CONSIDERATIONS

COMMENTS

- Most intracranial hemorrhages in pediatric patients are caused by moderate or severe head injury resulting from accidental or intentional injury.
- Epidural hematomas are seen with a history of a direct traumatic blow, usually across the middle meningeal artery groove.
  - There is generally a lucid period followed by headache with a change in mental status associated with pupillary changes and hemiparesis.
  - CT demonstrates a lens-shaped epidural collection of blood with mass effect.
  - Treatment consists of emergent surgical drainage and supportive care.
- Subdural hematomas are more common than epidural hematomas. They result from venous bleeding of the bridging veins that cross the dura and are a classic feature of shaken baby syndrome.
  - These are usually associated with a slower time course than epidural bleeding.
  - Generally, they present with symptoms of elevated ICP, and retinal hemorrhages may be found on physical examination.
  - CT shows a crescent-shaped collection of blood spreading along the inner table of the skull.
  - Acute subdurals usually require emergent surgical drainage and have a poorer prognosis than epidural bleeding because of the underlying brain injury. Most chronic subdurals are managed conservatively without surgery.
- A high index of suspicion for the possibility of intentional injury should be considered if the history contains discrepancies or is inconsistent with the extent of the observed trauma.

PREVENTION

- Most significant pediatric head trauma is caused by accidental injuries related to accidents involving motor vehicles or recreational vehicles and falls.
- Primary prevention of such accidental injuries through education and the use of restraints and safety equipment is strongly encouraged.
- Early recognition of infants and children at risk for or being victimized as a result of child abuse is crucial. Many children who subsequently become victims of serious abuse with significant head trauma have been previously identified as being at risk. Vigilant follow-up of such families is required.

PATIENT/FAMILY EDUCATION

- The prognosis for head injury is worse with associated intracranial bleeding.
- Many individuals have significantly reduced scores on neuropsychologic tests.
- About 15% of these children will subsequently develop epilepsy.
- The outcome for children with severe head injury is in general better than that for adults with the same severity score. Note, however, that children with epidural and subdural hemorrhage are a special subgroup with a poorer prognosis.
- All families whose children sustain major head injury experience major stress and require early intervention with social and rehabilitation services.

SUGGESTED READINGS

Dolan M: Head trauma. *In* Barkin RM (ed): *Pediatric Emergency Medicine: Concepts and Clinical Practice.* St. Louis, Mosby, 1992, pp 184–198.

Gedeit R: Head injury. *Pediatr Rev* 22:118, 2001.

Kaufman BA, Dacey RG: Acute care management of closed head injury in childhood. *Pediatr Ann* 23:18, 1994.

National Resource Center for Traumatic Brain Injury. Available at www.neuro.pmr.vcu.edu

Raphaely RC et al: Management of severe pediatric head trauma. *Pediatr Clin North Am* 27:715, 1980.

Rivara FP: Epidemiology and prevention of pediatric traumatic brain injury. *Pediatr Ann* 23:12, 1994.

Rossman NP et al: Acute head trauma in infancy and childhood: clinical and radiologic aspects. *Pediatr Clin North Am* 26:707, 1979.

Virtual Hospital. Available at www.vh.org/Patients/IHB/Neuro/BrainInjury/00TableOfContents.html

AUTHOR: **LYNN R. CAMPBELL, MD**

BASIC INFORMATION

DEFINITION

Henoch-Schönlein purpura (HSP) is a systemic vasculitis with palpable purpura, colicky abdominal pain, arthritis, and nephritis.

SYNONYMS

Anaphylactoid purpura
Purpura rheumatica
HSP
Hypersensitivity vasculitis

ICD-9-CM CODES
287.0 Henoch-Schönlein purpura

EPIDEMIOLOGY & DEMOGRAPHICS

- Peak age is 4 to 5 years but HSP can occur at any age.
- Males and females are affected equally.
- More common in winter and spring.
- HSP is often preceded by upper respiratory infection; rarely associated with drug or food ingestion.

CLINICAL PRESENTATION

- Symmetric, palpable, red petechial rash on buttocks and extensor surfaces of lower extremities occurring in crops; less extensive on upper extremities; becomes purpuric; macular, papular, urticarial, or bullous
- Edema of scalp, periorbital area, hands, and feet seen in infants in absence of renal disease
- Colicky abdominal pain (more than 50%)
- Abdominal tenderness
- Gastrointestinal bleeding (bloody stools, hematemesis)
- Arthralgias and arthritis (in up to 75%; ankles and knees more often than elbows and hands)
- Macroscopic hematuria
- Hemoptysis (rare; although 95% have subclinical lung involvement)
- Neurologic involvement (rare; headache, mental status changes, seizures, focal neurologic deficits, mononeuropathies, polyradiculoneuropathies)
- Hypertension
- Testicular swelling (~10% of males)

ETIOLOGY

Deposition of immunoglobulin A (IgA)-containing immune complexes in small blood vessel walls leading to leukocytoclastic vasculitis

DIAGNOSIS

DIFFERENTIAL DIAGNOSIS

- Typical rash in absence of clotting abnormality; arthralgias; acute hemorrhagic edema of childhood; systemic lupus erythematosus; drug reaction; erythema multiforme; urticaria; cryoglobulinemia; testicular torsion; juvenile rheumatoid arthritis; intussusception; acute surgical abdomen

WORKUP

- Skin biopsy (in questionable cases) shows leukocytoclastic vasculitis with IgA and C3 deposition.
- Kidney biopsy is indicated if renal insufficiency or nephrotic range proteinuria present. May show a proliferative, crescentic, necrotizing glomerulonephritis with IgA and C3 deposition

LABORATORY TESTS

- Blood urea nitrogen (BUN), creatinine, electrolytes, and albumin may be abnormal if there is significant renal involvement.
- Urinalysis may show hematuria (up to 90% of patients), proteinuria, leukocytes, and casts with renal involvement.
- Serum IgA level is elevated in 50% of cases.
- Prothrombin time, partial thromboplastin time, and platelet count usually normal.
- Stool guaiac is often positive.

IMAGING STUDIES

- Abdominal ultrasound may show intussusception (most are ileoileal in HSP, with average age 6 years).
- Kidneys may show "medical renal disease," a descriptive term that indicates abnormal appearance of the kidneys on ultrasound but is nonspecific regarding cause.

TREATMENT

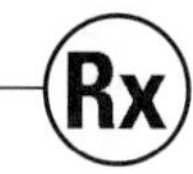

NONPHARMACOLOGIC THERAPY

If severe gastrointestinal involvement exists, intussusception, bowel infarction, or bowel ulceration with gastrointestinal bleeding can be present and should be treated.

ACUTE GENERAL Rx

- Nonsteroidal anti-inflammatory agents for arthritis; use with caution in presence of renal disease or gastrointestinal bleeding.
- Corticosteroids may hasten recovery of abdominal pain, arthralgias, and painful edema. Corticosteroids are *not* indicated for established mild renal involvement.
- Antihypertensives for elevated blood pressure.
- High dosages of pulse steroids or cytotoxic agents, and perhaps plasmapheresis, are used for rapidly progressive glomerulonephritis, crescentic glomerulonephritis, and nephrotic syndrome.

CHRONIC Rx

Dependent on sequelae

DISPOSITION

- The patient may have a relapsing course with recurrent bouts of rash and arthritis. Generally becomes milder over time with eventual resolution.
- Renal involvement generally occurs within 3 months of the onset of rash. Need to follow serial urinalyses even if rash, arthralgias, and abdominal pain are improving. Incidence of renal involvement in HSP has been reported to be 20% to 100% depending on the definition used. A true estimate is difficult to determine.
- Renal disease is the most significant complication, with 2% to 5% progressing to chronic renal failure. Renal insufficiency, heavy proteinuria with or without nephrotic syndrome, and significant hypertension are poor prognostic indicators.
- Deterioration of renal function has occurred even with apparent resolution of renal involvement up to 20 years after onset.
  - Patients must be monitored long term with blood pressure and urinalyses.
  - If these are abnormal, BUN and creatinine should also be evaluated.

REFERRAL

- Patients with significant renal involvement should be referred to a nephrologist.
- Gastroenterology or surgery referral may be indicated for severe findings.
- In questionable cases, referral to a dermatologist for skin biopsy may be indicated.

PEARLS & CONSIDERATIONS

COMMENTS

Patients who are older at presentation are more likely to have severe renal involvement and a poorer prognosis.

PREVENTION

Corticosteroids have been suggested to prevent renal involvement in early HSP, but this is controversial.

PATIENT/FAMILY EDUCATION

- The patient may have recurrent bouts of rash and arthralgias, but these generally become less frequent and milder with time.
- Most cases resolve without sequelae.
- Renal involvement is the most serious complication and may occur even as other symptoms are resolving. Even so, most renal findings resolve without sequelae, but long-term monitoring is important.
- NEPHKIDS website has information on kidney diseases with links to an email discussion group for parents. Available at http://cnserver0.nkf.med.ualberta.ca/nephkids/
- Local chapters of the National Kidney Foundation can provide information and support. (www.kidney.org)

SUGGESTED READINGS

Ballinger S: Henoch-Schönlein purpura. *Curr Opin Rheum* 15:591, 2003.
Choong CK, Beasley SW: Intra-abdominal manifestations of Henoch-Schönlein purpura. *J Paediatr Child Health* 34:405, 1998.
Davin JC, Weening JJ: Henoch-Schönlein purpura nephritis: an update. *Eur J Pediatr* 160:689, 2001.
Delos Santos NM, Wyatt RJ: Pediatric IgA nephropathies: clinical aspects and therapeutic approaches. *Semin Nephrol* 24:269, 2004.
Goldstein AR et al: Long-term follow-up of childhood Henoch-Schönlein nephritis. *Lancet* 39:280, 1992.

AUTHOR: **WILLIAM S. VARADE, MD**

BASIC INFORMATION

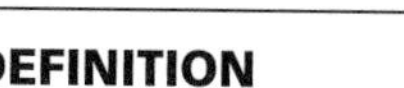

DEFINITION

Hepatitis A virus (HAV) infects hepatocytes and produces a clinical spectrum of disease ranging from asymptomatic infection to acute, fulminant hepatitis.

SYNONYM

Infectious hepatitis

ICD-9-CM CODE
070.1 Hepatitis A without coma

EPIDEMIOLOGY & DEMOGRAPHICS

- Overall seroprevalence of HAV in the United States is approximately 38%, with 11% by the age of 5.
- A historically low number of cases of HAV, approximately 7500, were reported in 2002, but due to the frequency of mild or asymptomatic illness, the true incidence is likely more than 10 times this number.
- In underdeveloped countries, HAV antibody can be found in virtually 100% of adults.
- Risk factors in U.S. are (1) contact with an infected individual (26%), (2) exposure to a day-care facility (14%), (3) intravenous drug use (11%), (4) recent travel (4%), and (5) as part of suspected water or food outbreak (3%).
- Forty-two percent of cases are without known risk factors, but half of these cases are in children younger than 6 years of age.
- Transmission is most likely to occur 2 weeks prior to the onset of symptoms. Children shed the virus longer than adults.

CLINICAL PRESENTATION

- The average incubation period is 28 days, with a range of 15 to 50 days.
- Greater than 80% of the infections are silent in infants and toddlers, whereas more than 75% of adolescents and adults experience symptoms.
- Abrupt onset of symptoms includes fever, malaise, nausea, vomiting, abdominal pain, and jaundice lasting for 1 to 3 months.
- Only a small percentage of symptomatic children are hospitalized, with a case fatality of approximately 0.1% compared with 1.8% in adults older than age 50.
- Fulminant liver failure is extremely rare. Chronic carrier state does not occur with HAV.
- Of symptomatic patients 85% have mild hepatomegaly and liver tenderness.
- Posterior cervical lymphadenopathy and splenomegaly occur in 15% of cases.
- Less than 5% of symptomatic children are icteric. Jaundice resolves in 2 weeks.

ETIOLOGY

- HAV is a 27-nm, icosahedral, non-enveloped, single-stranded RNA virus belonging to the Herpetovirus genus.
- HAV infects human and primate hepatocytes.
- Transmission is primarily by a fecal-oral route, with an attack rate as high as 90%.
- Infection is either by person-to-person contact or ingestion of contaminated water or food (e.g., undercooked shellfish).
- HAV exists at the highest concentrations in stool and bile. It can rarely be transmitted by blood transfusion but is not transmissible by saliva, urine, or semen.
- Infection can occur perinatally, but the outcome is usually benign.

DIAGNOSIS (Dx)

DIFFERENTIAL DIAGNOSIS

- See Jaundice/Hyperbilirubinemia in "Differential Diagnosis" and "Diagnostic Algorithms" sections.
- Hepatitis E, which is virtually nonexistent in the U.S., resembles HAV in transmission, course, and prognosis, with the exception of its greater association with complications during pregnancy and fetal loss.

LABORATORY TESTS

- In week 2 through the initial week of jaundice, HAV can be cultured in stool; however, this is impractical for standard workup.
- In week 2, serum aminotransferases (aspartate aminotransferase [AST] and alanine aminotransferase [ALT]) begin to rise, peak in weeks 3 to 6 at levels higher than 500, and normalize by week 8.
- Increase in AST and ALT is closely followed by a rise in serum bilirubin.
- Serum IgM-specific antibody is detectable 25 to 30 days after infection and persists for 2 to 3 months. This is the gold standard for detection of acute illness.
- IgG-specific antibody is detectable within 40 days of infection and persists indefinitely.
- Liver biopsy is seldom warranted.

TREATMENT (Rx)

NONPHARMACOLOGIC THERAPY

- HAV is generally self-limited, and recovery within 4 to 8 weeks is typical.
- Therapy is supportive; good nutrition and avoidance of further liver trauma (i.e., hepatotoxic drugs).

ACUTE GENERAL Rx

- For the rare patient with dramatic cholestasis, a short course of prednisolone can mitigate the disease process and symptoms.

DISPOSITION

- Infection confers lifelong immunity.
- Fulminant HAV, a rare event, most often strikes patients younger than 10 or older than 40. When acute liver failure does occur, transplant options should be promptly considered.

REFERRAL

- Consider referral to a gastroenterologist or hepatologist if patient presents with an extended or fulminant course of HAV.

PEARLS & CONSIDERATIONS

COMMENTS

Rare extrahepatic symptoms in HAV include evanescent rash, arthralgias, vasculitis, and glomerulonephritis.

PREVENTION

- Prevention includes attention to good hygiene and avoidance of contaminated water and food sources.
  - Strict handwashing especially in day-care and institutional settings.
  - Special precautions with regard to water sources and food preparation when visiting endemic areas; 84% of U.S. travel-related cases involve excursions to Mexico.
- Pooled human immune serum immunoglobulin (ISIG) has existed for more than half a century and can be used prophylactically before an exposure (i.e., travel) or within 2 weeks of exposure (i.e., HAV-positive household contact).
  - Serious adverse events associated with ISIG are extremely rare.
  - When administered within 2 weeks of HAV exposure, ISIG is more than 85% effective in preventing HAV infection.
  - When administered before exposure, ISIG prevents HAV infection in up to 95% and confers immunity for 3 to 5 months.
- Two inactivated HAV vaccines are available: HAVRIX and VAQTA.
  - A first dose of HAV vaccine is effective within 1 month but should be followed by a second dose in 6 to 12 months.
  - Vaccination efficacy is 95% or greater, confering immunity for at least 20 years.
  - HAV vaccine is now recommended at 1 year of age and for people traveling to endemic areas, intravenous drug users, male homosexuals, people with occupational exposures, and people with chronic liver disease.

PATIENT/FAMILY EDUCATION

- Sexual and household contacts of patients with acute HAV infection should receive 0.02 mL/kg immunoglobulin within 2 weeks of exposure.

SUGGESTED READINGS

Centers for Disease Control: Viral hepatitis. Available at www.cdc.gov/ncidod/diseases/hepatitis/

Jenson HB: The changing picture of hepatitis A in the United States. *Curr Opin Pediatr* 16: 2004.

Kane M: Hepatitis viruses and the neonate. *Clin Perinatol* 24:181, 1997.

Leach CT: Hepatitis A in the United States. *Pediatr Infect Dis J* 23:6, 2004.

Sokal E: Viral hepatitis throughout infancy to adulthood. *Acta Gastroenterol Belg* LXI:170, 1998.

AUTHOR: **JASON G. EMMICK, MD, FAAP**

BASIC INFORMATION

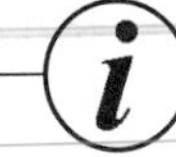

DEFINITIONS

Hepatitis B virus (HBV) is a highly infectious DNA virus. It primarily causes acute liver disease but also leads to chronic liver disease in many patients. Hepatitis D virus (HDV) is a passenger virus requiring the presence of HBV and may occur as a simultaneous coinfection or as a superinfection in an HBV carrier.

ICD-9-CM CODES
070.30 HBV, acute
070.32 HBV, chronic
070.33 HBV with HDV
070.52 HDV
V02.61 HBV carrier

EPIDEMIOLOGY & DEMOGRAPHICS

- Worldwide, HBV ranks as the ninth cause of mortality, with an estimated 350 million carriers.
- In the United States 1.25 million people have chronic HBV infection, resulting in 17,000 hospitalizations and 5000 deaths from its various complications annually.
- Each year in the United States, 20,000 children are born to mothers who are positive for HBsAg (hepatitis B surface antigen).
- Because of immunization programs, acute HBV reports have fallen from 0.66 to 0.16 cases per 100,000 in children less than 15 years of age between 1990 and 1998.
- Superinfection with HDV in a patient who is seropositive for hepatitis B e-antigen (HBeAg) is a major risk factor for chronic liver disease.
- Of those with chronic HBV, 15% to 30% develop cirrhosis. A small subset of this group develops hepatocellular carcinoma (HCC).

CLINICAL PRESENTATION

- Neonatal and early childhood HBV infections are often asymptomatic.
- Up to 90% of children younger than 1 year of age infected with HBV develop chronic infection, but only 5% to 15% of older children and adults develop chronic HBV infection.
- Early childhood carriers of HBV generally spend 10 to 20 years in an immunotolerant state during which silent and active replication of HBV occurs.
- Most older children and adults acquire protective levels of antibody, experience complete resolution of symptoms, and go on to have lifelong immunity.
- Symptomatic children develop malaise, nausea, anorexia, and low-grade fevers about 6 to 18 weeks after exposure.
- Liver tenderness, hepatomegaly, splenomegaly, and lymphadenopathy are common.
- Jaundice develops in one fourth of all infected children and peaks in weeks 8 to 12.
- More often than in hepatitis A virus (HAV) or hepatitis C virus (HCV) infections, there is skin or joint involvement including: arthritis of interphalangeal-metacarpal joints; urticaria/angioedema; Gianotti-Crosti syndrome (papular acrodermatitis with lymphadenopathy).
- A small subset of patients develop polyarteritis nodosa, glomerulonephritis, leukocytoclastic vasculitis, Raynaud's phenomenon, or Guillain-Barré syndrome.
- Only a few percent of children with elevated alanine aminotransferases (ALTs) present with cirrhosis or progress to cirrhosis in the childhood years.
- Acute HBV results in fulminant hepatitis and death in less than 1% of patients.

ETIOLOGY

- HBV is a double-stranded DNA virus from the family of Hepadnaviridae.
- HBV contains three primary structural antigens: surface (HBsAg), core (HBcAg), and e-antigen (HBeAg).
- HBV can be transmitted via infected blood, semen, vaginal secretions, and saliva.
- Although breastmilk contains HBV particles, breastfeeding does not seem to lead to increased rates of infection.
- In industrialized countries, infection most often results from sexual activity (26%), intravenous drug use (23%), occupational exposure (3%), and more rarely from perinatal transmission, household contact, or blood transfusion (risk now less than 1 in 60,000 units of blood transfused).
- No clear risk factor is identified in one fourth of HBV infections.
- Perinatal transmission occurs in as little as 10% of cases when the mother has only HBsAg, but it occurs as often as 90% when she is also seropositive for HBeAg.
- HDV is a small passenger virus that uses excess HBsAg to coat an inner core of single-stranded, circular RNA.

DIAGNOSIS

Dx

DIFFERENTIAL DIAGNOSIS

- See Jaundice/Hyperbilirubinemia in Differential Diagnosis (Section II) and Hyperbilirubinemia in Clinical Algorithms (Section III).

LABORATORY TESTS

- In acute HBV, aminotransferases begin to rise by 8 weeks after exposure, peak at 10 to 12 weeks, and normalize around months 5 to 6.
  - ALT tends to rise higher than aspartate aminotransferase (AST), and both generally peak at more than 500 IU/L.
  - Both rise soon after the presence of HBeAg, HBsAg, and HBV DNA.
- Elevations in bilirubin (5 to 10 mg/dL) are more modest and follow ALT/AST elevations.
- Acute HBV is demonstrated by detection of HBsAg and immunoglobulin M (IgM) antibody to the core antigen.
- HBV DNA by polymerase chain reaction is highly sensitive and a direct measure of infectivity.
- The presence of HBeAg is indicative of high HBV levels of inoculum or viral replication.
- Antibody to HBsAg confers protective immunity and is found in those immunized for HBV or who have cleared the infection.
- Patients with chronic HBV maintain HBsAg along with immunoglobulin G (IgG) antibody to the core antigen.
- In chronic HBV, AST/ALT often remain modestly elevated (50 to 200 IU/L).
- HDV can be detected by IgM to HDV, and its presence should be sought in flares of chronic HBV, and in particularly fulminant cases of HBV.
- In children with HBV, it is recommended that clinicians check the full battery of liver function tests along with a complete blood count and consider assessment for concurrent hepatitis C and human immunodeficiency virus infection.

IMAGING STUDIES

- Age and frequency of checking liver ultrasounds to monitor for HCC has not been fully established.

TREATMENT

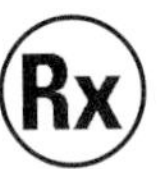

NONPHARMACOLOGIC THERAPY

- For both acute HBV and HDV, treatment is limited to supportive care and avoidance of further liver trauma (i.e., hepatotoxic drugs and alcohol).
- Hepatitis A vaccine should be provided to all children with HBV.
- Transplantation should be considered early in the course of impending liver failure.

ACUTE GENERAL Rx

- Only interferon-α and lamivudine are licensed in the United States for treatment of children with chronic HBV.
- Treatment is indicated for children older than 2 years of age who have: active viral replication; elevated liver function tests (especially an ALT greater than twice normal limits); serologic evidence of HBV that persists for more than 6 months; and a liver biopsy showing chronic inflammation.
- As in adults, pooled data from trials in children have demonstrated that treatment with interferon-α results in loss of HBV DNA and HBeAg 20% to 58% of the time, compared with 8% to 17% in controls.
- Successful interferon treatment results in histologic and clinical improvements.
- There appears to be no role for "steroid priming" for either children or adults.

- Lamivudine as both monotherapy and in combination with interferon-α has shown promise in increasing rates of HBV clearance with a relatively better side-effect profile than interferon-α alone.
- Pegylated interferon and other nucleoside analogues likely represent the next generation of HBV treatment.

DISPOSITION

- ALT monitoring and physical exams looking for signs of chronic liver disease are recommended at least yearly.
- HBeAg and anti-HBeAg values should be checked yearly to watch for spontaneous resolution.
- HCC risk is up to 390-fold greater in patients with chronic HBV and has been reported in childhood. Although there are no formal guidelines for children, many pediatric gastroenterologists recommend screening for HCC (hepatic ultrasound and α-fetoprotein) on at least an annual basis.

REFERRAL

- Consider referral to a gastroenterologist or hepatologist for all patients with chronic or complicated courses of HBV/HDV.

PEARLS & CONSIDERATIONS

COMMENTS

- Vaccine effectiveness is not altered by simultaneous administration of hepatitis B immunoglobulin (HBIG) but is compromised by gluteal rather than deltoid injection.
- Cesarean section delivery does not reduce the transmission rate of HBV to neonates.
- A small percentage of patients in the United States have viral mutations with no detectable HBeAg (but can be picked up by HBV DNA) and tend to have more virulent disease.

PREVENTION

- Most industrialized nations now routinely screen all pregnant mothers for HBV and vaccinate all children in early life.
- Transmission of HBV to newborns of HBV-positive mothers is preventable 95% of the time if HBIG is given within 12 hours of life along with starting the HBV vaccine series.
- There are now two thimerosal-free HBV vaccines available.
    - Both contain an inactivated portion of surface antigen in a yeast vector.
    - The vaccine series consists of three doses generally given in infancy with the first dose to be given shortly after birth or prior to hospital discharge.
    - Vaccines for HBV also exist in combination with other childhood immunizations and can be used for subsequent vaccinations. (Four doses of HBV may be administered if a birth dose was given.)
    - The vaccine confers protection in 95% of healthy recipients and likely lasts a lifetime.
    - Vaccination carries no risk of transmission and there are no absolute contraindications except severe hypersensitivity to yeast or other vaccine components.
    - Severe reactions are extremely rare with anaphylaxis occurring about once in 600,000 doses administered.
- HBIG should be given to seronegative patients who have been exposed to HBV. It is approximately 90% effective in preventing HBV in exposed patients.
- There is no cure for HDV, and strategies rely on treatment and prevention of HBV.

PATIENT/FAMILY EDUCATION

- The American Academy of Pediatrics still recommends breastfeeding in addition to immunoprophylaxis for infants born to mothers who have chronic HBV infection.
- Condoms reduce, but do not prevent, the spread of HBV to sexual partners.
- Seronegative household members or sexual partners of HBV-infected individuals should receive immunoprophylaxis with HBV HBIG, followed by the HBV immunization series.

SUGGESTED READINGS

Arnot R: The evolving efforts to control HBV. *Pediatr Infect Dis J* 17:S26, 1998.

Bortolotti F: Treatment of chronic hepatitis B in children. *J Hepatol* 39:1455, 2003.

Broderick AL et al: Hepatitis B in children. *Semin Liver Dis* 23:1, 2003.

Broderick AL et al: Management of hepatitis B in children. *Clin Liver Dis* 8:2, 2004.

Bunyamin D et al: Current therapeutic approaches in childhood chronic hepatitis B infection: a multicenter study. *J Gastroenterol Hepatol* 19:174, 2004.

Duff P: Hepatitis in pregnancy. *Semin Perinatol* 22:277, 1998.

Hochman JA et al: Chronic viral hepatitis: always be current! *Pediatr Rev* 24:12, 2003.

Kane M: Hepatitis viruses and the neonate. *Clin Perinatol* 24:181, 1997.

Lee W: Hepatitis B virus infection. *N Engl J Med* 337:1733, 1997.

Schwarz KB: Pediatric issues in new therapies for hepatitis B and C. *Curr Gastroenterol Rep* 5, 2003.

Sokal E: Viral hepatitis throughout infancy to adulthood. *Acta Gastroenterol Belg* LXI:170, 1998.

Zimmerman RK: Recommended childhood adolescent immunization schedule, United States, 2003 and update on childhood immunization. *Am Fam Physicians* 67:1, 2003.

AUTHOR: **JASON G. EMMICK, MD, FAAP**

BASIC INFORMATION

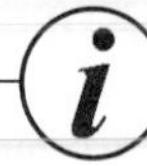

DEFINITION

Hepatitis C virus (HCV) infection is generally asymptomatic in its first 20 years but most often leads to chronic liver disease.

SYNONYM

Non-A/non-B hepatitis

ICD-9-CM CODES
070.51 HCV, acute
070.54 HCV, chronic
070.71 HCV without coma
V02.62 HCV carrier

EPIDEMIOLOGY & DEMOGRAPHICS

- Worldwide, it is estimated that 170 million people have chronic HCV.
- In the United States, 4 million people have HCV, with the full peak of known infection not expected to crest for 10 to 20 years.
- In children, the prevalence increases over the age spectrum with approximately 0.4% of 12- to 19-year-olds infected.
- Males and people ages 20 to 39 years are at highest risk for HCV infection.
- 1% to 3% of the present obstetric population is seropositive for HCV.
- Approximately 80% of infected children progress to chronic HCV insidiously over 20 to 40 years before their disease is recognized.

CLINICAL PRESENTATION

- 15% of patients report initial vague symptoms of fatigue, anorexia, nausea, malaise, and abdominal discomfort; only 4% have jaundice.
- The incubation time average is 6 to 7 weeks (range of 2 to 26 weeks).
- Jaundice is occasionally seen in acute infection but, when seen with chronic HCV, generally represents hepatic decompensation.
- HCV, well known for extrahepatic disease, may manifest in many ways including necrotizing skin lesions, arthritis, and purpura.

ETIOLOGY

- HCV is a single-stranded, enveloped RNA virus from the Flavirus family with six main genotypes that have clinical relevance.
- Major risk sources of acquisition of HCV are intravenous drug use, high-risk sexual behavior, tattooing, and maternal-fetal transmission.
- In one study, two thirds of intravenous drug users tested seropositive for HCV.
- Although HCV accounts for up to 90% of hepatitis resulting from transfusion, the blood supply has been relatively free of this virus since July 1992.
  - Risk of HCV from a single transfusion is now less than 1 in 100,000.
- Vertical transmission rates are about 5% to 10%, with an increased risk in mothers coinfected with human immunodeficiency virus (HIV) or who have high HCV viral loads.
- Sexual transmission appears to be rare among monogamous partners.
- Although low levels of HCV are found in breastmilk of HCV-infected mothers, this has not yet been proven to be a route of transmission.
- About 10% of HCV-infected individuals have no clear risk factor.

DIAGNOSIS

Dx

DIFFERENTIAL DIAGNOSIS

- See Jaundice/Hyperbilirubinemia in Differential Diagnosis (Section II) and Hyperbilirubinemia in Clinical Algorithms (Sections III).

LABORATORY TESTS

- Initially, enzyme immunoassay (EIA) is used, with positive results confirmed by recombinant immunoblot assay (RIBA) or HCV RNA by polymerase chain reaction (PCR).
  - EIA has a sensitivity and specificity that approaches 99%, but it may not be accurate in the first 6 weeks after exposure.
  - EIA cannot distinguish among acute, chronic, and resolved HCV infections.
  - There are RIBA assays for four HCV antigens.
  - A RIBA that is positive for two or more antigens is confirmatory for HCV infection.
  - A RIBA with only one antigen detected is considered indeterminant.
- The alanine aminotransferase (ALT) is most often used to follow liver disease but may often fluctuate or be normal despite ongoing hepatic damage.
- HCV RNA uses PCR amplification and exists in qualitative and quantitative forms.
  - Qualitative HCV RNA is a more sensitive test and can detect the virus as soon as 2 weeks after exposure.
  - Quantitative HCV RNA can be used to judge prognosis and treatment response.
- Genotype testing exists in several versions and can help predict prognosis and treatment response (i.e., the common U.S. genotype 1 is the least responsive).
- Liver biopsy is a valuable tool in determining patients who are likely to progress to cirrhosis: those with marked necroinflammation, septal fibrosis, or partial nodularity.

TREATMENT

Rx

NONPHARMACOLOGIC THERAPY

- Strict emphasis is placed on avoiding additional liver insults (i.e., alcohol and hepatotoxic drugs) as well as preventing or immunizing against other types of viral hepatitis.

ACUTE GENERAL Rx

- In general, treatment criteria for adults and children older than 2 years of age are elevated transaminases, abnormal liver histology, and positive HCV RNA viral load.
- Trials of treatment for HCV in children are limited and generally uncontrolled, but a sustained response of around 36% has been seen with interferon monotherapy.
- Positive prognostic factors include young age, HCV genotypes other than type 1, short duration of disease, low HCV RNA levels, and absence of cirrhosis.
- Interferon generally results in flulike symptoms shortly after administration.
- Complications associated with therapy include bone marrow suppression, severe depression, alopecia, thyroid dysfunction, and interstitial pulmonary fibrosis.
- Pegylated interferon in combination with ribavirin has become the standard treatment for adults, but the data in children are still limited.

DISPOSITION

- HCV-related liver disease is the single most common reason for liver transplantation in the U.S., but rarely in childhood.
- Recurrence of HCV occurs in as many as 95% of the transplant cases.
- Periodic measurement of ALT as a rough marker of disease activity is recommended.
- Periodic ultrasound and α-fetoprotein levels should be performed as a screening test for hepatocellular carcinoma (HCC) in long-standing HCV infection.
- Hepatitis C patients are at high risk for developing extrahepatic manifestations: essential mixed cryoglobulinemia, porphyria cutanea tarda, leukocytoclastic vasculitis, keratoconjunctivitis, arthritis, glomerulonephritis, thyroiditis, and pulmonary fibrosis.
- Risk factors for progression to end-stage chronic disease include alcohol intake, age older than 40, male gender, and necroinflammatory findings on liver biopsy.
- Of those with chronic HCV, 20% progress to cirrhosis after 20 to 50 years, with as many as 1% to 4% of these patients developing HCC per year.

REFERRAL

- Consider referral to a gastroenterologist or hepatologist for all pediatric patients with acute or chronic infections with HCV.

PEARLS & CONSIDERATIONS

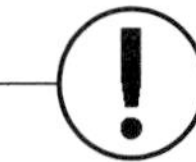

COMMENTS

- A single HCV DNA can be negative despite HCV infection, and ALT can be normal despite ongoing necroinflammation.

PREVENTION

- Prevention mainly relies on avoidance of previously mentioned risk factors.

- Immune globulins are ineffective, and the promise of an HCV vaccine is distant.

PATIENT/FAMILY EDUCATION

- While there is no clear increased risk of HCV with breastfeeding, HCV does exist in breastmilk and the decision to breastfeed must be individualized.
- HCV-infected individuals should be cautioned against sharing razors and toothbrushes with household members or having unprotected sexual activity.
- Strict avoidance of alcohol should be adamantly encouraged because its use is the single strongest risk factor for progression to end-stage liver disease.

SUGGESTED READINGS

Di Ciommo V et al: Interferon alpha treatment of chronic hepatitis C in children: a meta-analysis. *J Viral Hepatitis* 10:210, 2003.

Duff P: Hepatitis in pregnancy. *Semin Perinatol* 22:277, 1998.

Emerick K: Treatment of hepatitis C in children. *Pediatr Infect Dis J* 23:257, 2004.

Hochman JA et al: Chronic viral hepatitis: always be current. *Pediatr Rev* 24:12, 2003.

Kane M: Hepatitis viruses and the neonate. *Clin Perinatol* 24:181, 1997.

Kesson A: Diagnosis and management of paediatric hepatitis C virus infection. *J Paediatr Child Health* 38:213, 2002.

Moyer M: HCV infection. *Adv Pediatr Infect Dis* 14:109, 1999.

Schwarz KB: Pediatric issues in new therapies for hepatitis B and C. *Curr Gastroenterol Rep* 5:233, 2003.

Zignego A: Extrahepatic manifestations of HCV infection: facts and controversies. *J Hepatol* 31:369, 1999.

AUTHOR: **JASON G. EMMICK, MD, FAAP**

BASIC INFORMATION

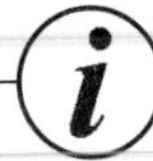

DEFINITIONS

Hernia is a protrusion of a loop or knuckle of an organ or tissue through an abnormal opening.

- Umbilical hernia—type of abdominal hernia in which part of the intestine protrudes at the umbilicus and is covered by skin and subcutaneous tissue
- Epigastric hernia—an abdominal hernia through the linea alba above the level of the umbilicus
- Spigelian hernia—an abdominal hernia through the linea semilunaris
- Lumbar hernia—herniation of omentum or intestine in the lumbar region of the back
- Parastomal hernia—herniation of omentum or intestine adjacent to the fascial exit of an enterostomy
- Incisional hernia—an abdominal hernia at the site of a previously made incision

SYNONYMS

Bulge
Mass
Rupture

ICD-9-CM CODES
533.1 Umbilical
553.8 Lumbar
553.21 Incisional
553.29 Epigastric, Spigelian
569.69 Parastomal

EPIDEMIOLOGY & DEMOGRAPHICS

- Umbilical hernias are seen in 1 of every 6 children.
  - They are 6 to 10 times more common in black children than in white children.
  - These hernias are often associated with low birth weight and occur with higher incidence among premature infants.
  - They are more common with trisomy 13, 18, and 21.
  - They are more common with hypothyroidism, mucopolysaccharidoses, and Beckwith-Wiedemann syndrome.
- Epigastric hernias are common hernias in children and are small and may be multiple.
  - Preperitoneal fat protrudes through small defects in the linea alba.
  - If located immediately above the umbilicus, they are called *supraumbilical hernias* and may contain bowel, or omentum.
- Spigelian hernias are rarely seen in childhood.
- Lumbar hernias are among the rarest of abdominal wall hernias and may be congenital, posttraumatic, or postoperative. Congenital lumbar hernias are associated with rib and vertebral anomalies, leading to the designation of lumbocostovertebral syndrome.
- Parastomal and incisional hernias occur with incidences below 5%. Symptomatic hernias require repair.

CLINICAL PRESENTATION

- Umbilical hernias protrude when the child strains or cries and spontaneously reduce when the child is supine and at rest.
  - Fascial rings smaller than 1 cm in toddlers usually close spontaneously.
  - Proboscoid hernias may be referred for surgical repair early for social, cosmetic, or skin integrity concerns.
- Epigastric hernias present as palpable protrusions in the midline from the xiphoid to the umbilicus.
  - They are readily apparent when the child holds his or her arms above the head and performs a Valsalva maneuver.
  - Most are irreducible and produce discomfort out of proportion to their size.
- Spigelian hernias are difficult to diagnose because they are interparietal and are contained by the aponeurosis of the external oblique.
  - They may appear as intermittent masses in the lower abdomen, lateral to the edge of the rectus abdominus muscle.
  - They are accentuated by crying or straining.
- Lumbar hernias present as flank swellings that protrude with crying.
  - Most are easily reducible on examination.
- Parastomal hernias are more common with colostomies than with ileostomies.
- Incisional hernias underlie visible scars. Often, there is a palpable defect in the fascia. Abdominal content protrudes with increased intra-abdominal pressure.
  - Overlying skin is atrophic and devoid of subcutaneous fat.

ETIOLOGY

- Umbilical hernias result from a failure of obliteration of the site in the abdominal wall through which the umbilical vessels exited the fetus to join the placenta.
  - In teens and adults, obesity, multiple pregnancies, and ascites may be precursors.
- Epigastric hernias, which are located between the xiphoid process and the umbilicus, result from fascial defects arising at the site of penetration of the fascia by blood vessels or from tears in the linea alba induced by coughing, straining, or abdominal distension.
  - Epigastric hernias are differentiated from diastasis recti, which is an attenuation, but not a defect, in the linea alba.
- Spigelian hernias occur along the subumbilical portion of Spieghel's semilunar line and through Spieghel's fascia, which is an intrinsically weak area of the abdominal wall. The defect is located at the intersection of the internal oblique and transversus abdominis muscles at the lateral border of the rectus sheath.
- Lumbar hernias of congenital origin result from a diffuse muscle deficiency of the musculofascial layers and occur in the following areas:
  - The inferior lumbar triangle of Petit is bounded by the latissimus dorsi, the external oblique muscle, and the iliac crest.
  - The superior lumbar triangle of Grynfeltt-Lesshaft is bounded by the 12th rib, the internal oblique muscle, and the sacrospinalis muscle.
- Parastomal hernias occur adjacent to a stoma. The hernia is usually composed of bowel and results in ischemia or obstruction.
- Incisional hernias are caused by wound infection, obesity, or errors in surgical technique.
  - Primary repair should be performed with nonabsorbable suture material. Often, prosthetic material is needed to help close the defect without tension.

DIAGNOSIS

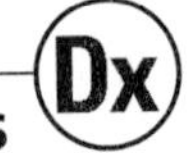

DIFFERENTIAL DIAGNOSIS

- Lipoma
- Hematoma
- Soft tissue neoplasm

WORKUP

- Umbilical hernias are recognized on physical examination.
  - The diameter of the fascial defect and not the length of protrusion is prognostically significant.
  - The incarceration rate is 1 per 1500 hernias in childhood.
- Epigastric hernias are accentuated on physical examination by the Valsalva maneuver and by having the child raise his or her arms above the head.
  - Protuberance is seen midline, above the level of the umbilicus.
- Spigelian hernias, unless large, are difficult to diagnose on physical examination.
  - Ultrasound and computed tomography (CT) may reveal hernias that are too small to detect clinically.
- Lumbar hernias may be apparent on physical examination, but CT may define the precise anatomy of the defect.
- Parastomal and incisional hernias after surgery are accentuated on physical examination by maneuvers that increase intra-abdominal pressure.

IMAGING STUDIES

- Ultrasound or CT can provide radiologic guidance for marking the site of a spigelian hernia.
- CT or ultrasound may be necessary to identify the exact location of a lumbar hernia defect.

TREATMENT

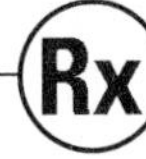

NONPHARMACOLOGIC THERAPY

- Surgical repair of hernial defects is generally warranted.
- Umbilical hernias that persist as a child approaches school age should be repaired.
  - Earlier repair is warranted if symptoms of incarceration or recurring pain develop or if the fascial defect is in excess of 1.5 cm diameter.
- Epigastric hernias do not spontaneously resolve and therefore should be surgically repaired.
  - Their small size makes identification problematic in the anesthetized child.
  - The exact location of the hernia should be marked in relation to the umbilicus with the child awake.
- Spigelian hernias are more frequently associated with incarceration and strangulation (20%) and hence necessitate repair.
- Lumbar hernias usually bulge with retroperitoneal fat and rarely incarcerate or strangulate.
  - The tension-free closure of a lumbar hernia may require placement of a prosthetic mesh or use of a muscle flap.
- Parastomal hernias may be repaired at the time of reversal of an ileostomy or colostomy in a child or if pain, incarceration, or maintenance of the integrity of a stomal appliance become problematic.

DISPOSITION

In the absence of wound infection, chronic disease states, connective tissue disorders, or malnutrition, recurrence rates after operative repair of abdominal wall hernias in children are negligible.

REFERRAL

Children with abdominal wall hernias should be referred to a pediatric surgeon. Operative repair is generally an outpatient procedure requiring general anesthesia.

SUGGESTED READINGS

Hernia information. Available at www.hernia.org

Kapur P et al: Pediatric hernias and hydroceles. *Pediatr Clin North Am* 45:773, 1998.

Oldham KT et al: *In* Oldham KT (ed) *Principles and Practice of Pediatric Surgery.* Philadelphia, Lippincott Williams & Wilkins, 2005, pp 1087–1101.

Wantz G (moderator): Incisional hernia: the problem and the cure: Symposium. *J Am Coll Surg* 188:429, 1999.

YourHealth.com. Available at www.yourhealth.com

AUTHORS: **WALTER PEGOLI, JR., MD** and **GEORGE T. DRUGAS, MD**

BASIC INFORMATION

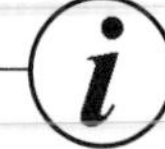

DEFINITIONS

Hernias arising above the femoral skin crease are *inguinal,* and those arising below the crease are *femoral.* Indirect inguinal hernias pass obliquely through the groin. If the sac extends down toward the scrotum, they are called *scrotal hernias.* Direct inguinal hernias protrude directly through the floor of the inguinal canal and rarely descend into the scrotum. Femoral hernias extend through a defect medial to the femoral vein.

SYNONYM

Inguinal bulge or rupture

ICD-9-CM CODES
550.10 Incarcerated hernia
550.90 Inguinal hernia
553.00 Femoral hernia
603.9 Hydrocele

EPIDEMIOLOGY & DEMOGRAPHICS

- Inguinal hernia
  - The incidence of inguinal hernias in children ranges from 0.8% to 4.4%. It is highest in infancy.
  - Approximately one third of children with hernias are younger than 6 months at operation.
  - The incidence of inguinal hernia is highest in premature infants, ranging from 16% to 25% of all premature infants.
  - Males are affected approximately six times more often than females.
  - Right-sided hernias are predominant.
    - Sixty percent occur on the right
    - Thirty percent occur on the left
    - Ten percent bilateral
  - Approximately 11.5% of patients have a positive family history of inguinal hernia.
- Femoral hernia
  - Femoral hernias account for less than 1% of all groin hernias in children.

CLINICAL PRESENTATION

- Inguinal or scrotal bulge, which may come and go:
  - Accentuated with increased intra-abdominal pressure (cough, strain, Valsalva)
- Perinatal factors that increase risk of hernias:
  - Prematurity
  - Mechanical ventilation
  - Bronchopulmonary dysplasia
  - Asthma
- A mass that is visible above the inguinal ligament, which may extend to the ipsilateral scrotum, is a classic physical finding in patients with an indirect inguinal hernia.
- "Silk glove sign" (thickening "smoothness" of the spermatic cord) is a useful finding in patients in whom an inguinal hernia is suspected clinically, but is not evident.
- Inguinal hernias may be associated with undescended testis.
- Noncommunicating hydroceles (peritesticular fluid collections) do not change in size or decompress with manual compression.
  - They have a high incidence of spontaneous resolution by 1 year of age.
- Femoral hernias are located medial to the femoral vessels and do not extend into the scrotum.
  - From 15% to 20% are incarcerated at initial presentation.

ETIOLOGY

- Failure of the processus vaginalis to close accounts for nearly all inguinal and scrotal abnormalities seen in infancy and childhood.
- Direct hernias result from congenital or acquired muscular defect in the floor of the inguinal canal.
- For women, the increased diameter of the true pelvis, as compared with that of men, widens the femoral canal, and predisposes women to femoral hernias.
- Femoral hernias are extremely rare, with a 2:1 female:male ratio.

DIAGNOSIS

Dx

DIFFERENTIAL DIAGNOSIS

- Made on physical examination
- Testicular torsion
- Inguinal or femoral lymphadenitis
- Torsion of appendix testis
- Lipoma of the spermatic cord
- Hydrocele of the spermatic cord

IMAGING STUDIES

- Ultrasound (duplex) if differential includes torsion of testis or appendix testis
- Nuclear medicine study if differential includes torsion of testis

TREATMENT

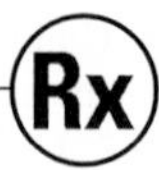

NONPHARMACOLOGIC THERAPY

- Femoral and inguinal hernias do not spontaneously resolve. They should be repaired due to the risk of incarceration.
- In patients younger than 1 year with a unilateral inguinal hernia, contralateral exploration is indicated because of the high risk of bilaterality.
- Most patients can undergo elective ambulatory hernia repair. Symptomatic hernias should be repaired semi-urgently. Incarcerated hernias should be reduced. Irreducible hernias or strangulated hernias require emergent surgical intervention to prevent intestinal or testicular ischemia.
- Femoral hernias should be repaired to prevent incarceration and strangulation.

DISPOSITION

- Several complications that are associated with herniorrhaphy require long-term follow-up.
  - Iatrogenic undescended testis (trapped testicle)
  - Injury to vas deferens (sterility if bilateral)
  - Testicular atrophy
- Repeated evaluation of the scrotal content over time is necessary to evaluate for possible postoperative complications. This is especially true for patients with a history of incarcerated/strangulated inguinal hernias.

REFERRAL

Children with inguinal and femoral hernias should be referred to a pediatric surgeon for definitive surgical correction.

SUGGESTED READINGS

Rescorla F: Hernias umbilicus. *In* Oldham KT et al (eds): *Principles and Practice of Pediatric Surgery.* Philadelphia, Lippincott Williams & Wilkins, 2005, pp 1087–1101.

AUTHOR: **WALTER PEGOLI, JR., MD**

BASIC INFORMATION

DEFINITION

Herpangina, a viral illness with a distinct clinical course, is characterized by fever and oral lesions. The enanthem found in herpangina can be found in other enteroviral illnesses.

SYNONYMS

Enteroviral stomatitis
Mouth ulcer

ICD-9-CM CODE
074.0 Herpangina

EPIDEMIOLOGY & DEMOGRAPHICS

- Information is extrapolated from data on enteroviral infection in general.
- Humans are the only natural hosts for enteroviruses.
- Distribution is worldwide.
- Disease may be endemic, epidemic, or pandemic.
- In temperate climates, attack rates peak in summer and fall, although sporadic cases may occur throughout the year. Shellfish may allow enteroviral storage during cold weather intervals. Prevalence is the same all year in tropical climates.
- Fecal-oral transmission is predominant, and less commonly, by respiratory droplets. Indirect transmission occurs through contaminated food, water, or fomites. Viral particles can survive the acidic pH of the stomach and persist at room temperature for several days.
- Spread within a community is likely child-to-child and then within families.
- Infection is frequently asymptomatic, although when apparent, clinical manifestations of illness often differ markedly among household members.
- Children are the primary susceptible cohort, and the severity of infection varies inversely with age.

CLINICAL PRESENTATION

History

- Onset is abrupt, with a short (few hours) prodrome of listlessness or anorexia followed by: fever (not universal, but common and may exceed 41°C), drooling, sore throat, oral lesions as well as headache, backache, coryza, vomiting, diarrhea

Physical Examination

- Enanthem lesions begin as moderately painful, discrete, punctate macules, which rapidly progress through papular, vesicular, and then ulcerative stages; the latter form has an erythematous base.
- Lesions are initially small (1 to 2 mm), but they may enlarge to 3 to 5 mm. The size of the erythematous base varies in diameter, but may reach 10 mm.
- Number of lesions ranges from 2 to 14.
- Lesions are located in the posterior pharynx, including the tonsillar pillars, soft palate, uvula, tonsils, posterior buccal mucosa, and rarely, the dorsum or tip of the tongue.
- Aside from the lesions, the remainder of the pharynx may be erythematous but is often unremarkable.
- The remainder of the physical examination is nonspecific.

ETIOLOGY

- Most commonly group A coxsackieviruses (typically serotype A16, but also 1 through 10 and 22); less commonly, group B coxsackieviruses 1 through 5, and echoviruses 6, 9, 11, 16, 17, 22, 25, and 32.
- Incubation period: 3 to 12 days
- Site of inoculation: nasopharynx
- Viremia: potentially occurs twice
  - The initial (minor) viremia occurs on the third postexposure day, coinciding with the onset of symptoms. Viral particles travel to secondary sites of replication (i.e., skin and mucous membranes, distant lymph nodes, and potentially, the respiratory tract, heart, central nervous system, pancreas, adrenals, liver, and spleen). If host immune mechanisms are able to sufficiently limit viral replication, subclinical infection occurs.
  - A second (major) viremia follows 3 to 7 days after exposure, with an additional opportunity for distal seeding.
- Immune response is not fully understood, but serotype-specific antibody probably plays the major role, followed by macrophage function.
- Shedding, occurs from the upper respiratory tract for 1 to 3 weeks and in the stool for up to 12 weeks after primary infection. Asymptomatic shedding occurs frequently. After repeat infection, fecal shedding may occur.

DIAGNOSIS

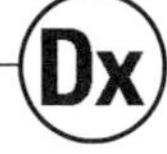

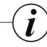

DIFFERENTIAL DIAGNOSIS

- Herpetic gingivostomatitis (HGS): Lesions are larger and more anteriorly located; lymphadenopathy and involvement of the gingivae, is more common and patients typically appear more ill in HGS.
- Hand, foot, and mouth disease: Oral lesions may be more anterior and occur with a typical exanthem.
- Aphthous stomatitis: Oral lesions are often larger, more anterior, and usually unaccompanied by fever or systemic symptoms.

WORKUP

The diagnosis is based on clinical findings.

LABORATORY TESTS

Confirmation, if necessary, may be obtained by culture or by pharyngeal polymerase chain reaction (PCR) methods.

TREATMENT

NONPHARMACOLOGIC THERAPY

- Treatment is usually outpatient and supportive, including adequate oral hydration.
- Cold, nonacidic fluids, Popsicles, or slush may provide symptomatic relief.

ACUTE GENERAL Rx

- Analgesics may be used for pain.
  - Ibuprofen, 7 to 8 mg/kg/dose every 6 to 8 hours *or*
  - Acetaminophen, 12 to 15 mg/kg/dose every 4 hours
- Follow-up visits are scheduled as required to ensure adequate hydration and reassess in the event of complications.
- Children may return to day care and school when lesions are unaccompanied by drooling and child has normal resumed activities.

REFERRAL

The enanthem found in herpangina can be found in other clinical enteroviral entities associated with more serious illness, including meningitis, encephalitis, acute flaccid paralysis, myocarditis. Referral may be required in these cases.

PEARLS & CONSIDERATIONS

COMMENTS

- Enteroviruses are inactivated quickly by heat (>56°C), chlorination, formaldehyde, and ultraviolet light.
- Acute lymphonodular pharyngitis is a variant of herpangina associated with coxsackievirus A10 infection. Found in the same distribution as herpangina, lesions are small, firm, white nodules packed with lymphocytes, that do not progress to vesicles or ulcerate, but simply recede.

PREVENTION

- Hand washing, especially after diaper changes.
- Limit exposure to pregnant women, particularly in the third trimester, because perinatal enterovirus can occur.
  - Vertical transmission manifests as neonatal sepsis within the first week of life.
  - Postnatal infection during the first 10 days of life may result from limited macrophage function.

PATIENT/FAMILY EDUCATION

- Typical illness is self-limited and lasts 3 to 7 days, but it may be biphasic.
- Give clear instructions for observation for signs and symptoms indicative of progression to more severe illness or dehydration.

SUGGESTED READINGS

Cherry JD: Enteroviruses and parechoviruses. *In* Feigin RD et al (eds): *Textbook of Pediatric Infectious Diseases,* 5th ed. Philadelphia, WB Saunders, 2004, pp 1984–2025.

Cherry JD, Nielsen K: Herpangina. *In* Feigin RD et al (eds): *Textbook of Pediatric Infectious Diseases,* 5th ed. Philadelphia, WB Saunders, 2004, pp 170–172.

Modlin JF: Enteroviruses: coxsackieviruses, echoviruses, and newer enteroviruses. *In* Long S et al (eds): *Principles and Practice of Pediatric Infectious Diseases,* 2nd ed. New York, Churchill Livingstone, 2003, pp 1179–1187.

AUTHOR: **C. ELIZABETH TREFTS, MD**

BASIC INFORMATION

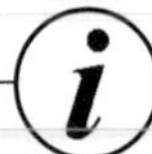

DEFINITION

Herpes simplex type 1 (HSV1) and herpes simplex type 2 (HSV2) cause a range of cutaneous, mucocutaneous, central nervous system (CNS), and disseminated infections. Primary infections are defined as the initial infection in individuals who have not previously been infected with either HSV1 or HSV2. Once infected, HSV1 and HSV2 can reactivate from latent infection in regional sensory nerves. Herpetic infections usually are described by their locations.

SYNONYMS

Cold sores (recurrent oral herpes lesions)
Fever blisters (recurrent oral herpes lesions)
Genital herpes
Herpes meningoencephalitis
Herpetic conjunctivitis
Herpetic gingivostomatitis
Herpetic keratoconjunctivitis
Herpetic pharyngitis
Herpetic whitlow
Neonatal herpes infection
Oral herpes or herpes labialis

ICD-9-CM CODES

054.2 Herpetic gingivostomatitis
054.3 Herpes meningoencephalitis
054.6 Herpetic whitlow
054.9 Herpes simplex, herpes labialis
054.10 Genital herpes
054.43 Herpetic conjunctivitis
054.43 Herpetic keratoconjunctivitis
054.79 Herpetic pharyngitis
771.2 Congenital (neonatal) HSV infection

EPIDEMIOLOGY & DEMOGRAPHICS

- HSV1 and HSV2 infections are extremely common; the seroprevalence depends on the population studied.
- In many parts of the world, most individuals acquire HSV1 infection during childhood.
- In the United States, HSV1 infection has become less common in childhood.
- The prevalence of HSV2 infection has increased in the United States. Overall, 22% of the adult U.S. population is infected with HSV2, with higher prevalence rates in general for women.

CLINICAL PRESENTATION

- In most cases of HSV infections, there are no symptoms, and the individual is unaware of the infection.
- Individuals with primary mucocutaneous or cutaneous herpes infections may complain of a painful rash at the site and manifest other constitutional symptoms, such as fever and malaise.
- Children with herpetic gingivostomatitis have painful oral ulcers accompanied by
  - Fever and malaise
  - Decreased oral intake
  - Drooling
  - Cervical lymphadenopathy
- Distribution of gingivostomatitis typically includes the lips, anterior oral cavity, gingiva, buccal mucosa, and tongue, and it may involve the posterior palate, pharynx, and face.
- Those with symptomatic recurrent infections may recognize a prodrome of pain, itching, or diatheses in the area before the appearance of the rash.
- Localized vesicular rash on an erythematous base is characteristic of symptomatic infections but often is absent in cases of disseminated or CNS herpes infections.
- Vesicles may rupture, drain, and crust, giving the impression of purulence.
- Mucous membrane lesions may evolve into ulcers.
- HSV infection of the pharynx typically causes an exudative pharyngitis.
- Infants with neonatal herpes infections may have a history of delivery after prolonged rupture of membranes.
  - Rarely is there a history of maternal genital herpes or oral herpes contact.
  - Infants may develop meningoencephalitis, disseminated disease, or disease localized to the skin, eyes, and mouth.
  - Infants may have symptoms attributable to pneumonitis or sepsis syndrome.
- Beyond the newborn period, disseminated HSV infection is rare but may occur in immunocompromised patients.
- Patients with disseminated HSV infections may have tachypnea, respiratory distress, or hemodynamic instability.
- Patients with HSV meningoencephalitis usually have fever and altered mental status and may have nuchal rigidity or focal neurologic signs, including seizures.

ETIOLOGY

- HSV1 and HSV2 enter the host by direct skin or mucous membrane contact with the virus.
- HSV1 usually causes infections above the waist.
- HSV2 usually causes infections below the waist.
- In individuals beyond the newborn age, HSV typically causes an asymptomatic or localized initial infection at the site of inoculation and then enters regional sensory nerves, where it establishes latent infection.
- When HSV subsequently reactivates, it may cause asymptomatic shedding or recurrent lesions. Known triggers of reactivation of HSV include ultraviolet light, trauma to the skin or sensory nerve ganglia, and immunosuppression.

DIAGNOSIS

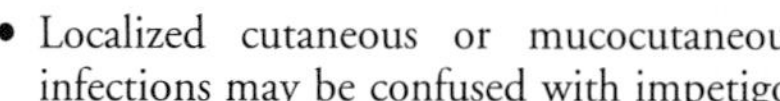

DIFFERENTIAL DIAGNOSIS

- Localized cutaneous or mucocutaneous infections may be confused with impetigo, varicella-zoster virus infections, candidiasis, or noninfectious dermatitis.
- Genital HSV infections may be confused with other sexually transmitted infections, including chancroid and syphilis.
- Gingivostomatitis may be confused with enterovirus infections (i.e., herpangina) or aphthous stomatitis.
- Neonatal herpes infection may be confused with bacterial sepsis, cutaneous staphylococcal infection, enterovirus infection, or congenital cytomegalovirus infection.
- Herpetic meningoencephalitis or meningitis may be confused with aseptic meningitis or meningoencephalitis of other causes, bacterial meningitis, or subarachnoid hemorrhage.

LABORATORY TESTS

- HSV can be identified in skin or mucous membrane lesions by virus isolation in tissue culture or fluorescent antigen detection.
- Except in cases of HSV2 meningitis associated with primary genital infections, HSV is generally not isolated from cerebrospinal fluid (CSF) in tissue culture.
  - Polymerase chain reaction is a sensitive method to detect HSV in CSF.
  - HSV meningoencephalitis causes CSF pleocytosis, often predominantly lymphocytes, red blood cells, and elevated CSF protein.
  - Electroencephalogram typically shows focal spike and wave abnormalities. A characteristic finding of paroxysmal lateralizing epileptiform discharges (PLEDs) is described.
- Disseminated infections, including neonatal infections, may be associated with the following:
  - Pneumonitis apparent on a chest radiograph
  - Hepatitis detected by liver function tests
  - Disseminated intravascular coagulation detected by clotting studies
- Serology can detect individuals who are at risk for primary disease.

IMAGING STUDIES

- Magnetic resonance imaging (MRI) can help in the diagnosis of HSV meningoencephalitis.
- MRI can detect lesions in the limbic system before computed tomography (CT).

TREATMENT

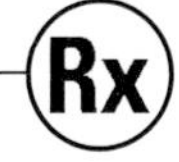

ACUTE GENERAL Rx

- Administer the following treatment for primary or first episode of genital HSV infection in normal hosts (similar doses have been used for primary or moderately severe cutaneous or mucocutaneous infections):
  - Oral acyclovir, 40 to 80 mg/kg/day divided every 6 to 8 hours or 400 mg three times daily for 5 to10 days, *or*

- Oral valacyclovir, 1000 mg twice daily for 5 days, *or*
- Oral famciclovir, 250 mg every 8 hours for 5 days
- Topical acyclovir: limited benefit for cutaneous lesions

- Administer the following treatment for severe infections, including neonatal HSV infection and HSV meningoencephalitis:
  - Intravenous acyclovir, 10 to 20 mg/kg/dose every 8 hours, with the higher dose recommended for neonatal disease
- Resistance to acyclovir occurs in some immunocompromised patients. These infections may respond to foscarnet.
- Ophthalmologic HSV infections can be treated with systemic and topical antivirals, usually in consultation with an ophthalmologist.

CHRONIC Rx

- Recurrent episodes are usually treated with the following:
  - Oral acyclovir, 40 to 80 mg/kg/day divided every 6 to 8 hours *or* 800 to 1200 mg divided three times daily, *or*
  - Oral valacyclovir, 500 mg twice daily, *or*
  - Oral famciclovir, 125 mg twice daily for 5 days
- Suppression of frequent HSV recurrences is maintained with oral acyclovir (80 mg/kg/day in three divided doses, 1000 mg/day maximum) for up to 12 continuous months.

DISPOSITION

- Patients with uncomplicated cutaneous or mucocutaneous herpes infections do not require additional follow-up.
- Patients who experience frequent recurrences require regular follow-up to assess the need for and the effectiveness of suppressive therapy.
- Patients with severe herpes infections, including neonatal HSV infections, meningoencephalitis, and keratoconjunctivitis, require close monitoring to assess the effectiveness of therapy and to evaluate for the development of complications or side effects from antiviral therapy.
- Patients with CNS or ophthalmologic infection require subsequent evaluation for long-term morbidity.

REFERRAL

- Neonates and other individuals with severe HSV infection should be referred to a specialist in infectious diseases.
- Patients with ophthalmic HSV infection or facial lesions in the area of the eye should be referred to an ophthalmologist.
- Patients with HSV meningoencephalitis or radiculomyelopathy should be referred to a neurologist.

PEARLS & CONSIDERATIONS

COMMENTS

- HSV should be considered in the differential diagnosis of infections that fail to respond to antibiotics and are associated with negative bacterial cultures.
- Although HSV lesions often appear somewhat purulent, they rarely become superinfected.
- A young child with suspicious genital lesions requires a thorough evaluation and a high index of suspicion for child sexual abuse.

PREVENTION

- Frequent recurrences and virus shedding may be suppressed with antiviral therapy. After suppressive therapy is withdrawn, recurrences will continue at the previous rate.
- Regular and correct condom use can decrease, but not prevent completely, the transmission of genital herpes.
- Individuals such as intensive care unit nurses and respiratory therapists, who have occupational exposures to oral or genital secretions, should wear gloves to prevent herpetic whitlow.
  - Gloves should be worn for contact with herpetic lesions.
  - Transmission of HSV to infants of mothers with active genital lesions during labor may be decreased by delivering the infant by cesarean section before or as soon as possible after rupture of membranes ($\leq$4 hours).

PATIENT/FAMILY EDUCATION

- Neonates are particularly vulnerable to severe HSV infection.
  - Limit contact with people with oral lesions.
  - When contact between a neonate and an individual with active HSV lesions is unavoidable, the person should cover the lesion and wash his or her hands carefully before handling the infant.
  - Infants at risk for neonatal HSV infection or who have had neonatal infection should be evaluated if rash, fever, or lethargy occurs.
- Patients with HSV infection may feel stigmatized and require reassurance to alleviate feelings of guilt and embarrassment.
  - HSV is transmitted by physical contact with infected skin or mucous membranes.
  - Asymptomatic infections and asymptomatic shedding are common, and people may transmit the virus without realizing that they are infected.
- Immunocompromised patients and neonates should not come in contact with children with gingivostomatitis because they transmit HSV in their oral secretions.
- Individuals with genital HSV infections should always use condoms because the virus may be transmitted when no symptoms are apparent.

SUGGESTED READINGS

Brown ZA et al: The acquisition of herpes simplex during pregnancy: its frequency and impact on pregnancy outcome. *N Engl J Med* 337:509, 1997.

Fleming DT et al: Herpes simplex virus type 2 in the United States, 1976 to 1994. *N Engl J Med* 337:1105, 1997.

Kimberlin DW et al: Natural history of neonatal herpes simplex virus infections in the acyclovir era. *Pediatrics* 108:223, 2001.

Kimberlin DW et al: Safety and efficacy of high-dose intravenous acyclovir in the management of neonatal herpes simplex virus infections. *Pediatrics* 108:230, 2001.

Kimberlin DW Whitley, RJ: Neonatal herpes: what have we learned. *Semin Pediatr Infect Dis* 16:7, 2005.

Prober CG et al: The management of pregnancies complicated by genital infections with herpes simplex virus. *Clin Infect Dis* 15:1031, 1992.

AUTHOR: **MARY T. CASERTA, MD**

BASIC INFORMATION

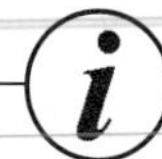

DEFINITION

The primary infection caused by the varicella-zoster virus is chickenpox. Reactivation of the latent varicella-zoster virus results in herpes zoster or shingles.

SYNONYMS

Herpes zoster: shingles
Varicella: chickenpox

ICD-9-CM CODES
052.9 Chickenpox
053.9 Zoster

EPIDEMIOLOGY & DEMOGRAPHICS

- Varicella is highly contagious.
- It is generally spread by direct contact of virus with the upper respiratory tract or conjunctiva.
- Patients are contagious from 1 to 2 days before the onset of rash until lesions have crusted. The incubation period is 10 to 21 days or up to 28 days if varicella zoster immune globulin (VZIG) is given.
- In temperate climates, varicella has been a disease of childhood with a peak in late winter and early spring. The epidemiologic pattern is expected to change with immunization.
- Some cases go unrecognized.
- Maternal varicella infection can result in fetal infection.
- Zoster is more common after 50 years of age. It is also seen in children who had varicella at a young age and in immunocompromised children.
- More severe varicella and zoster infections are seen in individuals with T-cell deficiencies and those receiving steroids.

CLINICAL PRESENTATION

Varicella

- Varicella is a systemic infection characterized by fever and a generalized vesicular, pruritic rash.
- There may be a history of exposure to varicella 10 to 21 days earlier.
- The rash typically develops in crops over 2 to 4 days, changing from papule to vesicle to crusted lesion over about 5 days.
- Children usually develop hundreds of skin lesions.
- Varicella is often more severe in adolescents and adults.
- Infants born to mothers who develop varicella 5 days before to 2 days after delivery are at increased risk for severe disease.
- Bacterial superinfection with *Streptococcus pyogenes* or *Staphylococcus aureus* is the most frequent complication. These infections may be life threatening.
- Other complications include encephalitis, cerebellar ataxia, hepatitis, pneumonia, thrombocytopenia, and glomerulonephritis.

Herpes Zoster

- Herpes zoster results from reactivation of the varicella-zoster virus.
- Typically, vesicular lesions are unilateral in the distribution of one to three dermatomes.
- Eye involvement may be significant.
- The lesions may be difficult to distinguish from herpes simplex.
- Lesions may become widespread, particularly in the immunocompromised patient.
- There is usually pain before the appearance of skin lesions.
- Pain may persist after the rash has resolved; this occurs more commonly in adults.

ETIOLOGY

- Chickenpox and herpes zoster are caused by the varicella-zoster virus, which is an alphaherpesvirus.
- Chickenpox is the primary infection. During this infection, a latent infection is established in sensory nerve ganglia.
- Zoster occurs when there is reactivation of the latent virus in the sensory nerve ganglia.

DIAGNOSIS

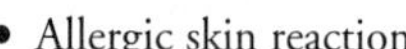

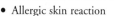

DIFFERENTIAL DIAGNOSIS

- Allergic skin reaction
- Herpes simplex virus infection
- Insect bites
- Smallpox
- Staphylococcal or streptococcal skin infection

WORKUP

The diagnosis of varicella-zoster infections is often determined by the history and results of the physical examination.

LABORATORY TESTS

- Viral culture of vesicular lesion may be helpful particularly if the rash is atypical or if herpes simplex virus infection is a consideration.
- Lesion may be aspirated with a fine needle and fluid placed immediately in viral culture medium.
- The base of the lesion may be swabbed for fluorescent antigen testing or Tzanck smear. Tzanck smear is not specific for varicella infections.
- Additional testing, such as a complete blood cell count, liver function tests, blood culture, or chest radiograph, may be indicated for patients with complications.
- Antibody testing is not helpful in the acute setting for making the diagnosis of varicella infections.
- Antibody testing may later contain a varicella diagnosis or test immunity to varicella.
- Standard commercial testing for varicella may not detect vaccine-induced immunity.

TREATMENT

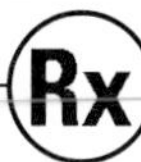

NONPHARMACOLOGIC THERAPY

Oatmeal baths may be soothing for varicella infections.

ACUTE GENERAL Rx

Varicella

- Acetaminophen may be used for fever or discomfort.
- Aspirin should not be used with varicella infection.
- Acyclovir is not routinely recommended for healthy children.
- Acyclovir should be considered for healthy patients who are at risk for more severe disease.
- Oral acyclovir is given for 5 days or until crusting of all lesions.
- Intravenous acyclovir is recommended for seriously ill or immunocompromised patients.
- Acyclovir is most effective when started at onset of disease.

Herpes Zoster

- Oral acyclovir may be used to treat healthy patients, but it is usually not recommended for children.
- Intravenous acyclovir is recommended for seriously ill or immunocompromised patients.

DISPOSITION

- Most healthy children with varicella or herpes zoster may be managed as outpatients.
- Immunocompromised patients with these infections are usually hospitalized for intravenous acyclovir and close monitoring.
- Patients at risk for complications should be followed closely.

REFERRAL

- Referral to an infectious disease specialist is recommended for severe or complicated cases of varicella.
- Refer to other specialists, such as an ophthalmologist or neurologist, as indicated.

PEARLS & CONSIDERATIONS

COMMENTS

- Many adults without an apparent history of varicella have detectable antibodies to varicella and are immune.
- Children who acquire varicella in utero or during the first years of life are at increased risk for herpes zoster at a young age.

PREVENTION

- The varicella vaccine is recommended for healthy individuals 1 year old or older who have not had a prior varicella infection.

- The varicella vaccine is a live attenuated vaccine. One dose is recommended for children 12 years of age or younger.
- For individuals older than 12 years, two doses are used.
- Individuals with varicella should stay home, out of public areas (i.e., school, day care, work, or stores) until lesions are crusted.
- Patients with zoster that cannot be covered should be excluded from public areas until the lesions are crusted.
- In the hospital, airborne and contact precautions are used for patients with varicella or disseminated zoster and for immunocompromised persons with zoster.
- Varicella-exposed susceptible patients should be on airborne and contact precautions during the incubation period for varicella.
- For varicella-susceptible individuals at high risk for severe disease, VZIG should be given within 96 hours of an exposure.
- VZIG is recommended for hospitalized premature infants ($\leq$28 weeks' gestation or birth weight $\leq$ 1000 g), hospitalized premature infants whose mother has not had varicella, newborn whose mother develops varicella 5 days before or 2 days after delivery, immunocompromised susceptible individuals, and pregnant susceptible women.

PATIENT/FAMILY EDUCATION

- Parents should be encouraged to have eligible children vaccinated against varicella to protect them and others against varicella and its potential complications.
- Patients with varicella infections should be evaluated if they have concerning symptoms such as lethargy, high fever, cellulitis, or respiratory distress.

SUGGESTED READINGS

American Academy of Pediatrics: Varicella-zoster infections. *In* Pickering LK (ed): *Red Book: 2003 Report of the Committee on Infectious Diseases,* 26th ed. Elk Grove Village, IL, American Academy of Pediatrics, 2003, pp 672–686.

Centers for Disease Control and Prevention. Available at www.cdc.gov

Feder HM, Hoss DM: Herpes zoster in otherwise healthy children. *Pediatr Infect Dis J* 23:451, 2004.

Gershon AA: Varicella-zoster virus. *In* Feigin RD et al (eds): *Textbook of Pediatric Infectious Diseases.* Philadelphia, WB Saunders, 2004, pp 1962–1971.

Whitley RJ: Varicella-zoster virus. *In* Mandell GL, et al (eds): *Mandell, Douglas, and Bennett's Principles and Practice of Infectious Diseases.* Philadelphia, Elsevier, 2005, pp 1780–1786.

AUTHOR: **CAROL A. MCCARTHY, MD**

BASIC INFORMATION

DEFINITION

Hirschsprung's disease is a genetic disorder characterized by congenital absence of ganglion cells in the colon extending proximally to a variable distance from the internal anal sphincter (i.e., rectum).

SYNONYMS

Colonic aganglionosis
Congenital megacolon

ICD-9-CM CODE
751.3 Hirschsprung's disease

EPIDEMIOLOGY & DEMOGRAPHICS

- The incidence is 1 case per 5000 live births.
- No racial predilection is seen.
- The male-to-female ratio is as follows:
  - Rectosigmoid disease: 4:1
  - Total colonic aganglionosis: 2:1
- Family history may be positive.
  - Approximately 6% to 8% of patients have a positive family history.
  - About 21% in patients with total colonic aganglionosis have a positive family history.
  - The risk of Hirschsprung's disease in siblings of an affected child is 4%, and the risk increases as the length of affected bowel increases.
- Increased prevalence of other disorders is seen.
  - Multiple endocrine neoplasia types IIa and IIb
  - Trisomy 21 (4% to 13%)
  - Waardenburg's syndrome
  - Smith-Lemli-Opitz syndrome
  - Ondine's curse
  - Von Recklinghausen's syndrome
  - Type D brachydactyly
- Only 4% to 8% of patients with Hirschsprung's disease are premature.
- Age at diagnosis varies, but most children are diagnosed in the first month of life.
  - Younger than 1 month: 41% to 64%
  - From 1 month to 1 year: 21% to 35%
  - Older than 1 year: 15% to 26%
- Various lengths of the colon can be involved.
  - Rectosigmoid (75%)
  - Variable lengths beyond the rectosigmoid (10% to 15%)
  - Entire colon (8%)
  - Short-segment and ultrashort-segment (<5 cm) Hirschsprung's disease also described
  - Small and large bowel (<1%)
- Mortality rate is 2.4% to 6%.
  - Mortality may be related to other underlying disorders.
  - Mortality is higher in the presence of enterocolitis.

CLINICAL PRESENTATION

History

- Presentation in the newborn period
  - Vomiting (most common clinical feature)
  - Abdominal distention
  - Constipation (since birth)
  - Failure to pass meconium within 48 hours of birth
  - General symptoms of bowel obstruction
  - Evidence of sepsis in the presence of enterocolitis
- Presentation in older infants and children
  - Constipation (most common clinical feature)
  - Abdominal distention
  - Vomiting
  - History of problems with stooling since birth
  - Absence of significant encopresis
  - Poor weight gain

Physical Examination

- Rectal examination
  - Increased rectal tone on digital examination
  - Explosive bowel movement after digital examination
  - No stool in rectal vault
- Abdominal distension
- Signs of enterocolitis: fever, explosive stools (with or without gross blood), significant abdominal distention, and in severe cases, hypovolemic shock
- Failure to thrive (older children with underlying chronic enterocolitis)

ETIOLOGY

- Approximately 80% of cases are caused by genetic mutations that are autosomal dominant with incomplete penetrance. Mutations in the *RET* proto-oncogene and the endothelin 3 genes have been identified.
- Genetic defect or mutation causes failure of neural crest cells to migrate caudad along the vagus and enter the bowel wall, with a resulting absence of ganglion cells for variable distances in the colon, starting at the internal anal sphincter in the rectum.
- The ganglion cells in the myenteric plexus of Auerbach and the submucosal plexus of Meissner are part of the enteric nervous system. Their absence interrupts the expression of the parasympathetic nerves, inhibiting relaxation of the affected muscles.
  - Affected bowel remains contracted.
  - There is loss of peristalsis.
  - There is loss of the rectosphincteric reflex. A bolus of stool in the rectum does not result in relaxation of the internal anal sphincter.

DIAGNOSIS

DIFFERENTIAL DIAGNOSIS

- Infants
  - Atresia (anal, colonic, jejunoileal)
  - Meconium plug syndrome or ileus, small left colon syndrome
  - Microcolon
  - Hypothyroidism
  - Anal stenosis
  - Congenital pseudo-obstruction
  - Neuronal dysplasia
  - Incarcerated hernia (inguinal or internal)
  - Gastrointestinal tract duplications
  - External obstruction (ovarian or mesenteric cysts)
  - Sepsis with ileus (in severely ill infants)
- Older children
  - Functional constipation
  - Pseudo-obstruction, primary or secondary
  - Anterior displacement of the anus

WORKUP

- Early diagnosis is important to avoid complications associated with the development of enterocolitis.
  - Although an unprepped barium enema can be diagnostic of Hirschsprung's disease (see "Imaging Studies"), the diagnosis is confirmed with a rectal biopsy.
  - Anorectal manometry may also be helpful in cases of short-segment disease
- Diagnosis requires a rectal biopsy.
  - Rectal biopsy is required for definitive diagnosis (performed by pediatric gastroenterologists and surgeons).
  - Suction rectal biopsy is the initial procedure of choice and can be done at the bedside without sedation.
  - Findings on the biopsy that support the diagnosis include an absence of ganglion cells and a positive acetylcholinesterase stain (i.e., allows identification of hypertrophied nerves).
  - Complications of the suction rectal biopsy are rare but include perforation (<1%) and an inadequate specimen (i.e., biopsy with insufficient submucosa or taken too low in the rectum).
  - It may be difficult to diagnose short-segment Hirschsprung's disease.
  - If an adequate specimen cannot be obtained by suction rectal biopsy, a full-thickness surgical biopsy is required to make the diagnosis.
- Anorectal manometry is used to assess disease.
  - Anorectal manometry measures the reaction of the internal anal sphincter (aganglionic in all cases of Hirschsprung's disease) to balloon distention in the rectum.
    - Normal: the sphincter relaxes when the balloon is inflated.
    - Hirschsprung's disease: The sphincter does not relax, or the tone increases.
  - The positive predictive value is approximately 90%, and there are few false-negative test results.
  - This is a more reliable screening test than barium enema but requires expertise in anorectal manometry.

- This test is particularly reliable for short-segment Hirschsprung's disease.
- Diagnostic tests are selected as follows:
  - Highly suspicious: rectal biopsy (if surgeon or gastroenterologist readily available)
  - Suspicious: barium enema before rectal biopsy
  - Suspicious but barium enema is nondiagnostic: manometry or rectal biopsy
  - Suspected short-segment disease and barium enema and rectal biopsy are nondiagnostic: manometry

IMAGING STUDIES

- Plain abdominal radiograph (kidney, ureter, and bladder) may suggest the diagnosis of Hirschsprung's disease.
  - Distended bowel loops with an abrupt cutoff below the pelvic brim
  - Relatively airless rectum (unless a digital rectal examination has been performed or the infant has received an enema or suppository)
  - In infants with enterocolitis, grossly distended loops of bowel with bowel wall thickening and, in some cases, evidence of perforation
- Barium enema (unprepped) may be used to confirm the diagnosis:
  - There is no bowel preparation before the study because it could modify the findings.
  - Findings suggesting Hirschsprung's disease include the following:
    - Transition zone between the narrow aganglionic bowel and the dilated unaffected bowel
    - Rectal diameter narrower than the sigmoid colon
    - Delayed evacuation of barium at 24 hours (least reliable finding)
  - Barium enema is diagnostic in approximately 80% of patients with Hirschsprung's disease.
    - No transition zone in total colonic aganglionosis
    - Less diagnostic in patients with short- or ultrashort-segment disease

TREATMENT

Rx

NONPHARMACOLOGIC THERAPY

- Operative intervention is the definitive treatment.
- Remove affected bowel, and place normally innervated bowel at the anus. There are three established surgical procedures:
  - Duhamel (side-to-side rectal colonic anastomosis)
  - Soave (endorectal pull-through)
  - Swenson (coloanal anastomosis)
- Traditionally, a diverting colostomy was created at a level in which the presence of ganglion cells was verified histologically. The definitive procedure was performed at a later time.
- All three procedures can now be performed as a single stage, and even newer techniques include the laparoscopically assisted approach.
- Staged repairs are still recommended for some patients:
  - Ill patients and those who require emergent fecal diversion
  - Those with massive gastrointestinal dilation who require defunctionalization to shrink the bowel before the definitive procedure
- A more limited procedure may be used for patients with ultrashort-segment Hirschsprung's disease.
  - Anorectal myectomy: A full-thickness, 2- to 3-cm-long strip is cut through the internal anal sphincter.

ACUTE GENERAL Rx

- Medical management is reserved for stabilizing the infant before surgery.
  - Restore fluid and electrolyte balance.
  - Perform adequate evacuation of the colon with saline enemas.
  - Provide broad-spectrum antibiotics if enterocolitis is expected.
- Treatment of enterocolitis includes the following:
  - Intravenous hydration (hypovolemic shock)
  - Frequent rectal irrigation with warm saline enemas
  - Intravenous antibiotics, including metronidazole

DISPOSITION

- Enterocolitis is the most significant complication.
  - Overall incidence varies from 20% to 60%.
  - Until recently, enterocolitis was the major cause of mortality.
  - Enterocolitis usually manifests with the clinical triad of explosive watery diarrhea, abdominal distention, and fever.
- Surgical results vary.
  - Approximately 65% to 85% of patients eventually achieve good results with normal bowel habits, no soiling, and infrequent constipation.
  - About 5% to 10% have severe constipation or incontinence.
  - Approximately 25% of patients require reoperation for stenosis, prolapse, obstruction, abscess drainage, sphincterotomy, or surgical revision.
  - Children with neurologic compromise and those with trisomy 21 tend to have more problems with constipation and incontinence.
  - Postoperative enterocolitis may occur in up to 25% of patients. Postoperatively, mechanical factors (anastomotic stricture or leak, intestinal obstruction) contribute to an increased risk of developing enterocolitis.

REFERRAL

- Refer to a gastroenterologist or pediatric surgeon for definitive diagnosis (rectal biopsy) if Hirschsprung's disease is suspected by the history and physical examination results.
- If the clinical diagnosis is equivocal, a barium enema can be performed before referral.
- If the barium enema results support the diagnosis, the patient should be referred directly to the surgeon.
- An infant or child who develops clinical symptoms of enterocolitis postoperatively should be stabilized if necessary (e.g., fluid resuscitation, intravenous antibiotics) and immediately referred to the surgeon.

PEARLS & CONSIDERATIONS

!

COMMENTS

- Consider Hirschsprung's disease in any infant or child who does not pass meconium in the first 48 hours of life or who is constipated from birth.
- Consider Hirschsprung's disease in an older child who has a history of long-standing constipation not associated with encopresis and who cannot have a bowel movement without a laxative.
- Consider Hirschsprung's disease with increased tone, empty rectal vault, and explosive evacuation of stool after a digital rectal examination.
- The clinical triad of explosive watery stools, abdominal distention, and fever in a child with Hirschsprung's disease requires immediate intervention with intravenous fluids, antibiotics, and rectal irrigation.

PATIENT/FAMILY EDUCATION

- American Pseudo-obstruction and Hirschsprung's Disease Society (APHS): phone: 978-685-4477; email: aphs@mail.tiac.net
- Pull-thru Network: www.pullthrough.org

SUGGESTED READINGS

Amiel J, Lyonnet S: Hirschsprung's disease, associated syndromes, and genetics: a review. *J Med Genet* 38:729, 2001.

Baker SS et al: Constipation in infants and children: evaluation and treatment. *J Pediatr Gastroenterol Nutr* 29:612, 1999.

Swenson O: Hirschsprung's disease: a review. *Pediatrics* 5:224, 2002.

AUTHOR: **M. SUSAN MOYER, MD**

BASIC INFORMATION

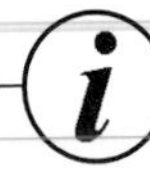

DEFINITION

The histiocytoses are a group of disorders characterized by infiltration and proliferation of cells of monocyte-macrophage or dendritic cell lineage. The major forms of childhood histiocytoses can be grouped into three classes (see "Synonyms") based on the involvement of normal monocytic or dendritic cell types and the histopathologic findings of the lesion.

SYNONYMS

- Class I histiocytoses
  - Langerhans' cell histiocytosis (LCH). This term replaces the histiocytosis X and the syndromes:
    - Eosinophilic granuloma (bone lesions alone)
    - Hand-Schüller-Christian disease (bone lesions, diabetes insipidus, exophthalmos)
    - Letterer-Siwe disease (disseminated disease)
- Class II histiocytoses
  - Familial erythrophagocytic lymphohistiocytosis (FEL)
  - Histiocytic necrotizing lymphadenitis (Kikuchi's disease)
  - Infection-associated hemophagocytic syndrome (IAHS)
  - Juvenile xanthogranuloma
  - Primary hemophagocytic lymphohistiocytosis (HLH)
  - Self-healing reticulohistiocytosis
  - Sinus histiocytosis with massive lymphadenopathy (SHML), Rosai-Dorfman disease
  - Sporadic hemophagocytic lymphohistiocytosis
  - Virus-associated hemophagocytic syndrome (VAHS)
- Class III histiocytoses
  - Acute monocytic leukemia (M5 AML)
  - Malignant histiocytosis, histiocytic medullary reticulosis
  - True histiocytic lymphoma, histiocytic sarcoma

ICD-9-CM CODES
202.3 Malignant histiocytosis
202.5 Histiocytosis X, acute
206.0 Acute monocytic leukemia
277.8 Histiocytosis X, chronic

EPIDEMIOLOGY & DEMOGRAPHICS

- Class I histiocytoses
  - Incidence is estimated at 2 to 5 cases per million children per year.
  - Peak age is between 1 and 4 years.
  - Male-to-female ratio is 2:1.
  - Disseminated LCH is more common in children younger than 2 years.
- Class II histiocytoses
  - Most children with FEL present before 3 months of age.
  - The familial form of the disorder has an autosomal recessive pattern of inheritance.
  - IAHS is most common among individuals with underlying immune suppression.
  - SHML occurs primarily during the first 2 decades. The male-to-female ratio is 1:1, and it is more common among blacks than whites.
- Class III histiocytoses
  - Malignant histiocytosis (MH) is reported in all decades of life.
  - Most previously reported cases of MH in children were actually anaplastic large cell lymphomas.
  - True MH is rare and accounts for less than 1% of non-Hodgkin's lymphoma (NHL).

CLINICAL PRESENTATION

- Class I histiocytoses
  - Symptoms reflect the extent and location of disease because LCH can be localized or generalized. Common signs and symptoms are detailed below in order of decreasing frequency.
  - Lytic bone lesions are present in 80% of cases.
    - Lesions may be associated with pain and swelling at affected sites.
    - The most common sites are the skull, pelvis, femur, orbit, ribs, humerus, mandible, tibia, vertebrae, and clavicle.
    - Exophthalmos, otitis media, and dental anomalies, including early loss of deciduous teeth, may be observed.
  - A rash resembling seborrheic dermatitis with crops of scaling, crusted, yellow-brown macules and papules may be present. The rash often occurs on the scalp, and in young children, it may be mistaken for cradle cap.
  - Lymphadenopathy and hepatosplenomegaly are present in about one third of cases.
  - Pancytopenia arising from bone marrow infiltration or splenomegaly may result in petechiae, signs of anemia, and mucositis.
  - With central nervous system (CNS) involvement, signs and symptoms include the following:
    - Diabetes insipidus (i.e., polydipsia and polyuria) from pituitary involvement is seen at diagnosis in 15% of cases but may develop years after the initial presentation of LCH
    - Subtle neurologic findings, ataxia, tremor
    - Seizures
  - Pulmonary involvement may manifest as acute respiratory illness with tachypnea, shortness of breath, and cough.
  - Signs of multisystem disease include the following:
    - Fever and recurrent fever (common with disseminated disease)
    - Irritability
    - Weight loss, failure to thrive
- Class II histiocytoses
  - The clinical presentations of the HLH syndromes, including FEL, IAHS and VAHS, are generalized, nonspecific, and typically follow a fulminant course. Signs include fever, anorexia, irritability, disorientation, failure to thrive, hepatosplenomegaly, lymphadenopathy, jaundice, edema, pallor, petechiae, and hemorrhagic rash.
  - The diagnosis of FEL requires a family history of HLH.
  - Patients with SHML generally present with systemic symptoms.
    - Fever
    - Massive lymph node enlargement, typically cervical, that may be locally destructive
    - Other sites of involvement, including the skin, orbit, bone, salivary glands, and upper respiratory tract
- Class III histiocytoses
  - Symptoms are nonspecific but suggest generalized disease, including fever, wasting, weight loss, lymphadenopathy, hepatosplenomegaly, abdominal pain, and jaundice.
  - Raised skin lesions and subcutaneous nodular infiltrates may be seen. In monocytic leukemia, the gingiva may be involved.

ETIOLOGY

- Class I histiocytoses
  - This reactive disorder is characterized by a proliferation of Langerhans' cells, perhaps caused by a defect in immunoregulation.
  - Although generally not considered a neoplasm, studies demonstrate that lesional cells are clonal in origin.
- Class II histiocytoses
  - This is a nonmalignant accumulation of mononuclear phagocytic cells (non-Langerhans' cells) throughout the reticuloendothelial system.
  - HLH is characterized by hemophagocytosis in the lymphoreticular system, marrow or central nervous system, and it may result from an inappropriate response to various infectious or noninfectious stimuli. A defect in humoral or cellular immunity is postulated.
  - A wide range of viral, bacterial, fungal, mycobacterial, rickettsial, and parasitic diseases have been associated with hemophagocytic syndromes.
  - SHML is a nonmalignant, locally invasive disorder of unknown origin.
- Class III histiocytoses
  - Each of these disorders arises from the clonal proliferation of malignant cells of monocyte-macrophage lineage.

DIAGNOSIS

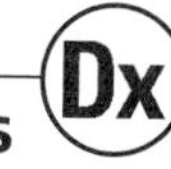

DIFFERENTIAL DIAGNOSIS

- The forms of childhood histiocytoses have overlapping symptoms and signs, making them difficult to differentiate based on the clinical picture alone. A correct pathologic diagnosis is imperative, however, because they have different treatment strategies.
- The differential diagnosis for the skin lesions includes:
  - Diaper rash
  - Atopic dermatitis
  - Scabies
  - Seborrhea
- Because benign and malignant disorders may manifest as lytic bone lesions, the following diagnoses should be considered:
  - Bone cysts
  - Osteosarcoma or Ewing's sarcoma
  - Metastatic neuroblastoma
  - Primary lymphoma of the bone
  - Giant cell tumor
  - Malignant fibrous histiocytoma
- Cytopenias or bone marrow involvement should raise the possibility of leukemia. The differential diagnosis of leukemia includes the following:
  - Juvenile rheumatoid arthritis
  - Infectious mononucleosis
  - Immune thrombocytopenic purpura
  - Leukemoid reactions
  - Common pediatric malignancies known to metastasize to the bone marrow: neuroblastoma, Ewing's sarcoma, Hodgkin's or non-Hodgkin's lymphoma, and rhabdomyosarcoma
- When generalized symptoms of fever, adenopathy, or organomegaly are present, the differential diagnosis should include the following:
  - Sepsis or systemic infection
  - Lymphoid malignancies
  - Underlying immune deficiency
- When MH is suspected, care must be taken to distinguish it from advanced-stage Hodgkin's disease or the non-Hodgkin's lymphomas, particularly anaplastic large cell subtypes.

WORKUP

Tissue from involved lesions is required to confirm any of these diagnoses.

- Class I histiocytoses
  - The presumptive diagnosis of LCH may be based on light microscopy identification of granulomatous lesions and cells consistent with Langerhans' cells in a biopsy specimen from involved tissues.
  - Definitive diagnosis requires immunohistochemical staining positive for CD1a, S-100, or Birbeck granules by electron microscopy.
- Class II histiocytoses
  - Diagnostic criteria for HLH include the following:
    - Fever >38.5°C for 7 days *and*
    - Splenomegaly (>3 cm) *and*
    - Cytopenias affecting at least two cell lines (hemoglobin less than 9 g/dL, platelet count <100,000/µL, or absolute neutrophil count <1000/µL) *and*
    - Laboratory evidence of hypertriglyceridemia (>2.0 nmol/L) or hypofibrinogenemia (<150 mg/dL) *and*
    - Histopathologic evidence of hemophagocytosis in the bone marrow, spleen, or lymph nodes
    - Additional findings in HLH not required for diagnosis may include increased transaminases, prolonged prothrombin time (PT) or activated partial thromboplastin time (aPTT), hyponatremia, hyperferritinemia, and cerebrospinal fluid pleocytosis
  - A detailed family history looking for HLH, death in infant of unknown cause, and parental consanguinity is important. A family history of HLH is required to make the diagnosis of FEL.
  - SHML and the other class II histiocytoses usually are diagnosed by lymph node biopsy. The characteristic findings include a reactive infiltration of morphologically normal macrophages within the nodes without effacement of architecture or cellular atypia. Immunostains for CD1a and S-100 are negative. Other findings may include elevated sedimentation rate, polyclonal hypergammaglobulinemia, and neutrophilic leukocytosis; however, these are not diagnostic.
- Class III histiocytoses
  - MH is diagnosed by biopsy of involved tissue, usually a lymph node or bone marrow, that shows sheets of atypical mononuclear cells with histiocytic differentiation, with effacement of normal architecture of the lymph node, and a high mitotic rate. Immunophenotype and special stains are crucial to confirm the histiocytic or monocytic nature of the malignant cells.
  - Acute monocytic leukemia (M5 AML) is typically diagnosed by bone marrow biopsy that shows replacement with monoblasts. Hyperleukocytosis and involvement of the skin and gingiva are highly suggestive of this subtype of leukemia.
  - True histiocytic lymphoma is a localized neoplasm. Biopsy shows tissue macrophages with malignant morphology and staining pattern of the monocyte lineage.

LABORATORY TESTS

- Initial evaluation should include the following:
  - Complete blood cell count, differential and platelet counts
  - Comprehensive chemistry panel, including transaminases and uric acid
  - Coagulation tests (PT, aPTT, fibrinogen at a minimum)
- Consider additional testing:
  - Titers and cultures as appropriate for underlying infections such as Epstein-Barr virus, cytomegalovirus, or adenovirus for suspected HLH
  - Triglyceride level and ferritin for suspected HLH
  - Urine osmolality to look for diabetes insipidus for suspected LCH
- Diagnostic and staging evaluation may include bone marrow aspirate and biopsy and examination of the cerebrospinal fluid.

IMAGING STUDIES

- Chest radiograph is used to look for adenopathy or pulmonary involvement.
- Skeletal survey is used to look for bone lesions, especially for LCH.
- Computed tomography of the chest, abdomen, pelvis, and head may be necessary to define the extent of disease.

TREATMENT

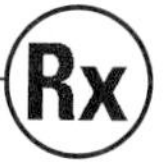

NONPHARMACOLOGIC THERAPY

- Class I histiocytoses
  - The treatment approach to LCH is not universally agreed on. Most experts advise the use of less intensive and toxic therapies directed at preventing the progression of lesions and controlling the disease symptoms while minimizing systemic toxicities.
  - Patients with localized disease of the skin, bone, or lymph node have an excellent prognosis and a high rate of spontaneous disease remission.
  - Treatment options may include the following:
    - Observation
    - Intralesional steroids
    - Surgical curettage
    - Low-dose radiation therapy (500 to 800 cGy)
- Class II histiocytoses
  - SHML has an excellent prognosis without specific therapy but may have a protracted course of 3 to 9 months.
  - Chemotherapy and radiation therapy have been successful.
- Class III histiocytoses are aggressive neoplasms, and multiagent chemotherapy is required.

ACUTE GENERAL Rx

- Class I histiocytoses
  - The clinical course of LCH depends on the extent of organ involvement and the age of the child, with mortality rates as high as 10% to 50% for children younger than 2 years.
  - For patients with multiple organ involvement, organ dysfunction, or progressive lesions after treatment with less intensive treatment, combination chemotherapy and systemic steroids may be indicated.

- The Histiocyte Society is conducting large international clinical trials to identify effective regimens to decrease the disease reactivation rate, morbidity, and mortality for high-risk patients.
- Class II histiocytoses
  - For patients with IAHS or VAHS, specific antibiotics or antiviral therapy may be of benefit, as may chemotherapy with etoposide.
  - FEL is rapidly fatal without aggressive supportive care.
    - Corticosteroids, chemotherapy, and cyclosporine may induce a short-term response.
    - Bone marrow transplantation is the only known curative therapy.
- Class III histiocytoses
  - The rate of prolonged disease-free survival with combination chemotherapy approaches 50%.
  - Bone marrow transplantation is a therapeutic option.

CHRONIC Rx

Occasionally, patients with aggressive LCH require lengthy courses or repeated pulses of corticosteroids.

DISPOSITION

- Physicians caring for patients with LCH must be aware that diabetes insipidus and subtle neurologic dysfunction can develop years after diagnosis.
- Children treated with chemotherapy or radiation therapy should be monitored for possible late effects of the treatment, including secondary malignancy.

REFERRAL

Although most histiocytic disorders of childhood are not true malignancies, a pediatric hematology-oncology specialist usually follows children with one of these disorders.

PEARLS & CONSIDERATIONS

COMMENTS

- The "punched-out" lytic bone lesion is the clinical hallmark of LCH.
- Seborrheic dermatitis is often present on the scalps of infants with LCH; biopsy and appropriate electron microscopy or histopathologic studies are diagnostic.
- The age of onset is the major clinical feature distinguishing HLH from malignant histiocytosis.
- The chemotherapeutic agent etoposide should be used with caution in patients with LCH or HLH because of concerns about an increased risk of secondary malignancy.
- Acute monocytic leukemia (M5 AML) may have an increased risk of fatal hemorrhage.

PATIENT/FAMILY EDUCATION

- The Histiocytosis Association of America: http://www.histio.org/association/index.shtml

SUGGESTED READINGS

Ladisch S, Jaffe ES: The histiocytoses. *In* Pizzo PA, Poplack DG (eds): *Principles and Practice of Pediatric Oncology,* 4th ed. Philadelphia, Lippincott Williams & Wilkins, 2002, pp 733–750.

Sullivan JL, Woda BA: Lymphohistiocytic disorders. *In* Nathan DG, Orkin SH (eds): *Nathan and Oski's Hematology of Infancy and Childhood,* 6th ed. Philadelphia, WB Saunders, 2003, pp 1375–1395.

Writing Group of the Histiocyte Society: Histiocytosis syndromes in children. *Lancet* 1:208, 1987.

AUTHOR: **BARBARA L. ASSELIN, MD**

BASIC INFORMATION

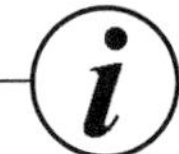

DEFINITION

Hydrocephalus is an increased volume of cerebrospinal fluid (CSF) within the cerebral ventricles that typically is associated with increased intracranial pressure (ICP).

SYNONYM

Water on the brain

ICD-9-CM CODES
331.3 Acquired communicating
331.4 Acquired obstructive
741.0 Spina bifida with hydrocephalus (fifth digit for level of lesion)
742.3 Congenital

EPIDEMIOLOGY & DEMOGRAPHICS

- Birth prevalence is 5 to 10 cases per 1000 in preterm infants and 0.5 to 1 case per 1000 term infants.
- X-linked hydrocephalus is caused by a mutation of the *L1CAM* gene at Xq28.
- In general, most congenital cases are multifactorial, with a recurrence risk of 4%.

CLINICAL PRESENTATION

History

- If congenital, a family history of hydrocephalus or neural tube defect may be found.
- Signs of acutely increased ICP include the following:
  - Headache, vomiting, lethargy, irritability, high-pitched cry
  - Change in vision
  - Seizures
- Signs of chronically increased ICP include the following:
  - Learning disabilities (i.e., difficulties with attention, information processing problems, or memory difficulties)
  - Discrepancy between verbal and performance scales on IQ score
  - Change in personality or performance in school
  - Precocious puberty

Physical Examination

- Progressive enlargement of head circumference
- Strabismus or paralysis of upward gaze (e.g., setting sun sign, Parinaud's syndrome)
- Spasticity of lower extremities
- Bulging fontanelle, spreading of sutures in infancy
- Papilledema; a late sign of increased ICP

ETIOLOGY

- Imbalance between the production and absorption of CSF
- Communicating form
  - Obstruction of the subarachnoid space (e.g., posthemorrhagic, postinfectious)
  - Developmental failure of arachnoid villi
  - Excessive CSF production (as seen with choroid plexus tumor)
  - Associated with Chiari malformation
- Obstructive form
  - Aqueductal stenosis
  - Mass lesions (e.g., neoplasm, cyst, hematoma, aneurysm)
  - Acquired obstruction from hemorrhage, infection, or scarring.
  - Obstruction of fourth ventricle (e.g., Dandy Walker malformation, arachnoiditis)
  - May develop with achondroplasia or Hurler's disease (i.e., mucopolysaccharidosis)

DIAGNOSIS

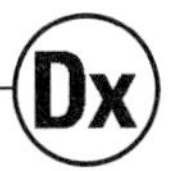

DIFFERENTIAL DIAGNOSIS

- Large head may be caused by the following:
  - Subdural hematoma
  - Degenerative diseases (e.g., Tay-Sachs disease, Canavan disease, metachromatic leukodystrophy, Alexander disease)
  - Skeletal disorders (e.g., achondroplasia, Russell-Silver syndrome, mucopolysaccharidosis)
  - Benign macrocephaly
  - Meningeal infiltration (e.g., neuroblastoma, histiocytosis)
- Cerebral atrophy may lead to large ventricles (i.e., hydrocephalus ex vacuo) but small head size.
- Hydranencephaly is characterized by complete absence of cerebrum supplied by the anterior and middle cerebral arteries.
- Pseudotumor cerebri may cause signs and symptoms of increased ICP without enlarged ventricles.

WORKUP

- Serial measurements of head circumference are obtained.
- ICP may be determined through a ventricular tap or lumbar puncture (if not contraindicated).

LABORATORY TESTS

Pathologic evaluation of tissue if hydrocephalus is caused by a brain tumor.

IMAGING STUDIES

- Cranial imaging (i.e., ultrasound, computed tomography [CT], or magnetic resonance imaging) can be done to evaluate ventricular size and detect structural abnormalities.
- Radionuclide studies can be used to determine ventricular and spinal perfusion.
- Neuroimaging and shunt series are used to evaluate for ventricular shunt dysfunction.

TREATMENT

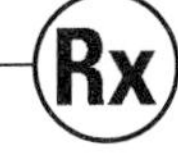

NONPHARMACOLOGIC THERAPY

- Ventricular shunt procedure
  - Ventriculoperitoneal (VP) shunt is most commonly used. Some newer valves have adjustable pressures.
  - Ventriculosubgaleal shunt may be used temporarily.
  - Ventriculoatrial (VA) or ventriculopleural shunts may be used as alternatives to VP shunts.
  - VA shunts have a high risk of pulmonary microemboli and shunt-related nephritis.
- Endoscopic third ventriculostomy is useful to treat obstructive hydrocephalus.
- Appropriate referral is needed for educational evaluation, stimulation, and therapies (e.g., early intervention program).
- Braces (e.g., ankle-foot orthosis) can be applied if the patient has spasticity.
- Repeated lumbar or ventricular punctures (i.e., taps) have been used to treat hydrocephalus caused by intracranial hemorrhage.

ACUTE GENERAL Rx

- The combination of acetazolamide (Diamox) plus furosemide (Lasix) has been used to transiently reduce ICP. However, even when it was effective, adverse effects were common, and it is no longer recommended.
- Serial spinal taps or ventricular taps may be useful to manage hydrocephalus with elevated ICP in neonates

CHRONIC Rx

Oral medications such as diazepam (Valium), baclofen (Lioresal), and tizanidine (Zanaflex); injections with botulinum toxin (Botox); intrathecal baclofen; and selective dorsal rhizotomy may help decrease spasticity.

DISPOSITION

- Routine clinical monitoring, including monitoring of pubertal development, is advised.
- Routine head CT scans should be obtained to evaluate ventricular size.
- Close communication should be maintained with the school or early intervention program.
- Children should have psychological and educational testing when they enter school.

REFERRAL

- All children should be referred to a neurosurgeon for treatment and follow-up.
- All children 0 to 3 years old, who have significant hydrocephalus, should be referred to an early intervention program.
- All children older than 3 years who have neural tube defects should be referred to their school district's committee on special education or committee on preschool special education.

PEARLS & CONSIDERATIONS

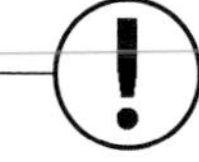

COMMENTS

- The signs and symptoms of ventricular shunt malfunction may be subtle. Consider CT of the head and a shunt series.
- Papilledema is a late sign of increased ICP. If it is present, it is useful, but lack of this sign is not meaningful.
- Determining how a ventricular shunt valve empties and fills is not reliable in deciding whether a shunt has failed.
- Tapping a malfunctioning shunt with a 25-gauge butterfly needle may save the life of a child whose shunt is obstructed.
- In a child who has meningomyelocele with hydrocephalus, ventricular shunt failure may cause signs of a Chiari malformation or tethered spinal cord.
- Precocious puberty is common in girls with hydrocephalus.

PREVENTION

- All women of child-bearing age should receive 1.0 mg of folic acid daily periconceptionally to decrease the occurrence of neural tube defects.
- Prenatal surgery to shunt hydrocephalus has not been successful; however, research continues in this area.

PATIENT/FAMILY EDUCATION

- Inform the family and child about signs and symptoms of increased ICP (i.e., ventricular shunt failure).
- Help families and educators develop realistic expectations for the child.

SUGGESTED READINGS

Garton HJ, Piatt JH Jr: Hydrocephalus. *Pediatr Clin North Am* 51:305–325, 2004.

Hydrocephalus Association. Available at http://www.hydroassoc.org/

Hydrocephalus Center. Available at www.patient-centers.com/hydrocephalus/

Liptak GS: Spina bifida hydrocephalus. *In* Coffey CE, Brumback RA (eds): *Essential Textbook of Pediatric Neuropsychiatry.* Baltimore, Lippincott Williams & Wilkins, 2005.

AUTHOR: **GREGORY S. LIPTAK, MD, MPH**

BASIC INFORMATION

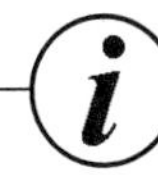

DEFINITION

Hydronephrosis is a descriptive term indicating dilation of the renal pelvis or calyces, or both. When the ureter is involved in this process, the term applied is hydroureteronephrosis.

SYNONYMS

Caliectasis
Pyelectasis
Pyelocaliectasis

ICD-9-CM CODE
753.29 Hydronephrosis

EPIDEMIOLOGY & DEMOGRAPHICS

- The prevalence in the general population is 0.15% to 0.67%.
- The frequency determined by antenatal ultrasound is 1 case per 100 to 200 fetuses.
- The male-to-female ratio is 2:1.
- The rate of bilateral cases is 10% to 20%.

CLINICAL PRESENTATION

History

- Most infants with antenatal hydronephrosis are asymptomatic at birth.
- Abdominal pain is associated with or relieved by emesis.
- Flank pain occurs with or without a radiating component to the gonads.
- Hematuria occurs after minor trauma.
- Urinary tract infection is a common complaint.
- Failure to thrive is associated with the condition.

Physical Examination

- Asymptomatic palpable mass in newborn
- Hypertension

ETIOLOGY

- Developmental form: Prenatal hydronephrosis may be transient and resolve as systems grow and mature.
- Obstruction
  - Bilateral hydronephrosis with hydroureter may point to posterior urethral valves, an anterior urethral valve, prune-belly syndrome, bilateral congenital megaureters, or a large ureterocele.
  - Unilateral hydronephrosis without hydroureter may indicate a ureteropelvic junction (UPJ) obstruction.
  - Unilateral hydronephrosis with hydroureter may indicate a ureterovesical junction obstruction by a ureterocele or congenital megaureter.
  - Unilateral hydronephrosis can also be caused by bladder outlet obstruction (do not be led astray by the unilateral finding).
- Vesicoureteral reflux is associated with hydronephrosis.
- High urine output is associated with renal concentrating defects.
- The condition is associated with syndromes such as prune-belly syndrome.

DIAGNOSIS

Dx

DIFFERENTIAL DIAGNOSIS

- Extrarenal pelvis (normal variant)
- Megacalycosis
- Multicystic dysplastic kidney (MCDK)
- Peripelvic cyst

LABORATORY TESTS

- For children with confirmed significant hydronephrosis:
  - Blood urea nitrogen (BUN), creatinine, and electrolyte levels.
  - BUN and creatinine provide an estimate of the glomerular filtration rate (GFR).
  - Abnormalities in potassium and bicarbonate may indicate subtle renal dysfunction.
- A urinalysis should be done on first-morning urine to evaluate concentrating ability (specific gravity of 1.020 or higher) and to assess for the presence of proteinuria, which can indicate renal parenchymal scarring.

IMAGING STUDIES

- Renal ultrasound to confirm the presence and laterality of hydronephrosis and to evaluate the renal parenchyma and bladder.
  - A grading system has been established by the Society for Fetal Urology.
    - Grade 0: intact central renal complex (renal pelvis)
    - Grade I: mild splitting of central renal complex
    - Grade II: pelviectasis (i.e., dilation of the pelvis) but no caliectasis (i.e., dilation of the calyx)
    - Grade III: markedly split central renal complex with uniformly dilated calyces, but normal renal parenchyma
    - Grade IV: characteristics of grade III with thinning of renal parenchyma
- Voiding cystourethrogram (VCUG) to identify vesicoureteral reflux, bladder appearance, and urethral anatomy.
- Diuretic renal scan to assess perfusion, function, and drainage of the kidneys.
  - Nuclear scintigraphy with technetium-labeled Mag-3 (^{99m}technetium Mertiatide, ^{99m}Tc-diethylenetriaminepentaacetic acid) is the study of choice.
  - Water-loading and a diuretic study help to assess obstruction.
  - These studies also provide information on the relative differential function of kidneys.
  - A standard intravenous urogram may not be adequate to detect obstruction.
  - MCDK is characterized by poor perfusion of and no function in the affected kidney.
- For infants with a history of antenatal hydronephrosis who are clinically well:
  - Renal ultrasound should be performed within 4 to 6 weeks after birth.
  - Corticomedullary differentiation and echogenicity may be sensitive indicators of renal integrity.
  - VCUG can be performed at any time, and results are abnormal (i.e., vesicoureteral reflux) in 25% of patients with normal postnatal ultrasound scans.
  - Diuretic renal scan should be done after 2 weeks of age because of physiologically low GFR in the immediate postnatal period precludes appropriate assessment if done too early.

TREATMENT

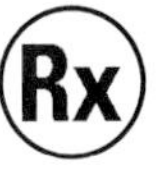

NONPHARMACOLOGIC THERAPY

- Surgical correction depends on the cause of hydronephrosis.
- Posterior urethral valves require surgical relief of the obstruction.
- Bladder catheterization may provide temporary drainage.
- Surgical repair of unilateral hydronephrosis caused by a UPJ obstruction may be deferred if no impairment of renal function is observed.
- Twenty-five percent of hydronephrosis is attributed to UPJ obstruction, but contributes 40% to overall renal function, ultimately necessitating surgical repair.

ACUTE GENERAL Rx

- Newborns with a history of antenatal hydronephrosis should receive antibiotics to reduce the incidence of urinary tract infection until the cause of hydronephrosis is determined.
  - Amoxicillin, 10 to 15 mg/kg/dose twice daily
  - Cephalexin, 20 to 30 mg/kg/day divided twice daily

DISPOSITION

- The immediate postoperative course of children with obstruction may be complicated by polyuria caused by postobstruction diuresis.
- Most obstructed kidneys improve or retain their level of preoperative function.
- Maximal return of function occurs within the first 12 to 24 months.
- Long-term follow-up of renal function is required for all children with obstruction because of the risk of delayed renal deterioration.
- Children with hydronephrosis resulting from vesicoureteral reflux require periodic VCUG and antibiotic prophylaxis until resolution of reflux. Endoscopic or operative correction may be offered, depending on the grade and clinical course.

REFERRAL

All children with hydronephrosis should be referred to a pediatric urologist for evaluation.

PEARLS & CONSIDERATIONS

PATIENT/FAMILY EDUCATION

- Although up to 1% of newborns have a prenatal diagnosis of hydronephrosis, those found to have significant urinary pathology postnatally are often managed non-emergently with close follow-up.
- Nephkids is an Internet-based support group for parents with children with kidney disease. It is moderated by a pediatric nephrologist and supported by the National Kidney Foundation. Information on enrolling is available at http://cnserver0.nkf.med.ualberta.ca/nephkids
- For parents and physicians, information on neonatal hydronephrosis can be found on the Internet: Digital Urology Journal: Neonatal Hydronephrosis (www.duj.com/); E-Medicine; Society for Pediatric Urology (spu.org); and Urology Health.org

SUGGESTED READINGS

Aksu N et al: Postnatal management of infants with antenatally detected hydronephrosis. *Pediatr Nephrol* 20:253–259, 2005.

Atug F et al: Robotic assisted laparoscopic pyeloplasty in children. *J Urol* 174:1440–1442, 2005.

Capello SA et al: Prenatal ultrasound has led to earlier detection and repair of ureteropelvic junction obstruction. *J Urol* 174:1425–1428, 2005.

Carr MC: Prenatal management of urogenital disorders. *Urol Clin North Am* 31:389–397, 2004.

Moorthy I et al: The presence of vesicoureteric reflux does not identify a population at risk for renal scarring following a first urinary tract infection. *Arch Dis Child* 90:733–736, 2005.

Rodriguez MM: Developmental renal pathology: its past, present future. *Fetal Pediatr Pathol* 23:211–229, 2004.

AUTHORS: **ROBERT A. MEVORACH, MD, WILLIAM C. HULBERT, MD,** and **RONALD RABINOWITZ, MD**

BASIC INFORMATION

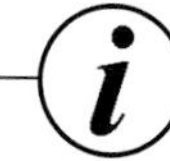

DEFINITION

Hypercholesterolemia is elevation above specified levels of total or low-density lipoprotein (LDL) cholesterol. This is important because it is one of several risk factors associated with atherosclerosis and coronary artery disease (CAD). Screening for elevated levels of lipids, although recommended by the American Academy of Pediatrics (AAP) for children in high-risk families, remains controversial.

SYNONYM

Hyperlipidemia

ICD-9-CM CODES
272.0 Pure hypercholesterolemia
272.1 Pure hypertriglyceridemia
272.2 Mixed hyperlipidemia

EPIDEMIOLOGY & DEMOGRAPHICS

- All people in the Bogalusa Heart Study between birth and 38 years old had fatty streaks in the aorta.
- For children between 2 and 15 years old, 50% had fatty streaks in the coronary arteries.
- For adults between 21 and 39 years old, 85% had fatty streaks in the coronary arteries.
- The presence of three or four cardiac risk factors increases the extent of fatty lesions in the coronary arteries 8.5 times.
- Risk factors for hypercholesterolemia include the following:
  - Parent with elevated cholesterol ($\geq$240 mg/dL)
  - Elevated body mass index (BMI), especially a truncal fat pattern
  - Persistently high intake of dietary cholesterol
  - Sedentary lifestyle
  - Cigarette smoking
  - Hypertension
  - Male gender (female cholesterol level increases after menopause)
  - Age (i.e., men > 45 years and women > 55 years)
  - Other medical diseases (e.g., renal disease, diabetes mellitus, hypothyroidism)
  - Medications (i.e., some diuretics, corticosteroids, and immunosuppressants)
- Additional risk factors for CAD include the following:
  - Family history of premature heart disease (parent or grandparent < 55 years)
  - Elevated total cholesterol or LDL cholesterol
  - High levels of lipoprotein a [Lp(a)]
  - Low levels of high-density lipoprotein (HDL) cholesterol
  - Elevated homocysteine level
  - Peripheral vascular disease
  - Cocaine or stimulant use or abuse

CLINICAL PRESENTATION

History

- Patients may have the following:
  - Family history of premature heart disease or high cholesterol
  - Obesity (BMI $\geq$ 95% for age and gender)
- Obtain diet details: milk and dairy, types of meats and fats.
- Obtain history of activity levels and cigarette smoking.
- Most patients with atherosclerosis are asymptomatic.
- Look for symptoms of diseases that secondarily cause hyperlipidemia.
  - Hypothyroidism, diabetes mellitus, Cushing's syndrome
  - Renal disease
  - Drug use and abuse (e.g., glucocorticosteroids, oral contraceptives, seizure medications, Retin-A, anabolic steroids, alcohol)

Physical Examination

- Growth (weight), especially truncal adipose deposition
- Blood pressure
- Evidence of lipid deposition
  - Xanthomas: yellow, orange, nonpainful, palpable lesions commonly found on the elbow, knee, or Achilles tendon
  - Corneal arcus
- Goiter
- Hepatomegaly
- Signs of nephrosis (e.g., hypertension, edema)
- Acanthosis nigricans

ETIOLOGY

- Defects in apolipoprotein or lipoprotein receptors lead to elevations in cholesterol or triglycerides (TGs), or both.
- Lipoproteins transport lipids in blood, and they consist of the following:
  - Chylomicrons and remnants are dietary triglycerides
  - Very-low-density lipoproteins (VLDLs) are endogenous triglycerides; practically, they are equivalent to TGs ÷ 5.
  - Intermediate-density lipoproteins (IDLs) are cholesteryl esters and TGs.
  - LDLs are cholesteryl esters. Elevated LDL levels increase the risk of CAD.
  - HDLs are cholesteryl esters and phospholipids. High HDL levels decrease risk of CAD.
  - Lp(a) is composed of cholesteryl esters.
- Apolipoproteins have a variety of functional and structural roles.
  - Defects in apolipoproteins have been associated with inherited disorders of lipid metabolisms.
    - Apo B-100 functions in the secretion of VLDLs from the liver and is a ligand for LDL receptors.
    - Apo E is a ligand for binding of IDL and remnants of LDL to receptors and LRP.
    - Apo C-II is an activator of lipoprotein lipase.

DIAGNOSIS

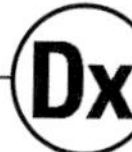

DIFFERENTIAL DIAGNOSIS

- Primarily high cholesterol
  - Familial hypercholesterolemia
    - LDL receptor defect or absence causes elevated LDL levels.
    - The disorder has an autosomal dominant inheritance pattern.
    - Approximately 10% also have mildly elevated TGs.
    - Aortic valve disease, tendon xanthomas, and premature arcus cornea are common.
    - Homozygote status is associated with an incidence of 1 case per 1,000,000 births, LDL elevated to 6 to 10 times normal, and severe coronary atherosclerosis beginning at 10 years of age.
    - Heterozygote status is associated with an incidence of 1 case per 500 births, LDL elevated two to three times normal, and development of atherosclerotic heart disease by age 30.
  - Familial defective apolipoprotein B-100
    - A defect in the ligand-binding region of the LDL receptor causes elevated LDL levels.
    - The disorder has an autosomal dominant inheritance pattern.
    - The prevalence is 1 case per 700 persons in Europe and North America.
    - The condition may be associated with tendon xanthomas.
    - Patients have an increased risk of early CAD.
  - Familial hyperalphaproteinemia
    - The disorder has autosomal dominant and polygenic patterns of inheritance.
    - The conditions result in elevated HDL levels.
    - Patients have a decreased incidence of CAD.
- Mixed high cholesterol and TG levels
  - Familial combined hyperlipidemia
    - It probably is caused by increased hepatic production of LDLs or VLDLs, or both, and decreased clearance of TG-rich particles.
    - The disorder has an autosomal dominant pattern of inheritance and is the most common familial lipid abnormality.
    - The prevalence is approximately 1 case per 200 births.
    - Approximately 10% to 20% of the affected population has premature atherosclerosis.
    - The condition often is associated with abdominal obesity, glucose intolerance, hyperinsulinemia, and hypertension.
  - Familial hyperapobetalipoproteinemia
    - Patients have an increased risk of CAD.

- The condition is a variant of familial combined hyperlipidemia.
    - Familial dysbetalipoproteinemia
        - The condition is caused by mutations in the Apo E protein.
        - The disorder has an autosomal recessive pattern of inheritance.
        - Patients have elevated levels of LDL, cholesterol, and TGs and have normal levels of HDL.
        - It can occur in adulthood with palmar or tuberous xanthomas, high cholesterol levels, peripheral vascular disease, and premature CAD.
- Primarily high TG levels
    - Familial chylomicronemia syndrome
        - The TG levels are greater than 1000 mg/dL.
        - Lipoprotein lipase deficiency (LPL) is a rare autosomal recessive trait; clinically expressed as eruptive xanthomas, recurrent episodes of pancreatitis, failure to thrive, hepatomegaly, and splenomegaly; and possibly associated with Apo C-II deficiency.
        - The laboratory values and clinical appearance of familial chylomicronemia syndrome are similar to those of LPL deficiency.
    - Type V hyperlipoproteinemia
        - The condition can manifest with acute pancreatitis.
        - The TG levels usually are greater than 1000 mg/dL.
        - It is associated with medications such as estrogens, retinoids, and alcohol and with medical conditions such as diabetes mellitus and nephritic syndrome.
    - Familial hypertriglyceridemia
        - Clinical findings include elevated TGs, low HDL cholesterol, and normal to low LDL levels.
        - The condition has an autosomal dominant inheritance pattern and is not expressed until adulthood.
        - It is unknown whether it is associated with an increased risk of CAD.
- Secondary causes
    - Medications
        - Androgens
        - Anticonvulsants
        - Corticosteroids
        - Diuretics (thiazide and loop diuretics)
        - Immunosuppressants (cyclosporine, tacrolimus)
        - Oral contraceptives
        - Retinoids
    - Drugs of abuse: alcohol and anabolic steroids
    - Endocrine causes
        - Diabetes mellitus
        - Hyperaldosteronism or hyperreninemia
        - Hypopituitarism
        - Hypothyroidism
    - Renal causes
        - Nephrotic syndrome
        - Renal failure
    - Hepatic causes
        - Cholestasis (e.g., benign recurrent intrahepatic cholestasis, congenital biliary atresia, Alagille syndrome)
        - Hepatitis
    - Metabolic causes
        - Gaucher's disease
        - Niemann-Pick disease
        - Tay-Sachs disease
        - von Gierke's disease
    - Miscellaneous causes
        - Acute intermittent porphyria
        - Anorexia nervosa
        - Obesity
        - Systemic lupus erythematosus

LABORATORY TESTS

- Screening
    - Assessment of total cholesterol recommended for children with a parental history of total cholesterol greater than 240 mg/dL.
    - Total cholesterol assessment is at the discretion of the provider if the family history is incomplete or unavailable and if risk factors for CAD are present.
    - Full fasting lipid profile should be obtained if premature CAD occurred in parents or grandparents.
- Total cholesterol = LDL cholesterol + HDL cholesterol, when HDL cholesterol = TG ÷ 5 (for TG level less than 400 mg/dL)
    - Average total cholesterol in children 2 to 18 years old: <150 mg/dL
    - Total cholesterol <170 mg/dL: no intervention but reassess in 5 years
    - Total cholesterol 170 to 199 mg/dL (borderline, 75th to 95th percentile)
        - Recheck the total cholesterol level, and average the two numbers: for an average total cholesterol >170 mg/dL check a fasting lipid profile.
    - Total cholesterol >200 mg/dL: check fasting lipid profile
- Average LDL cholesterol in children 2 to 18 years old: <100 mg/dL
    - LDL <100 mg/dL
        - Reassess in 5 years.
        - Provide information on risk reduction.
    - LDL = 100 to 129 mg/dL (borderline, 75th to 95th percentile)
        - Recheck, and average the two numbers.
        - Provide a step 1 diet (see Step 1 and 2 Diets in Prevention [Section V]) and other risk reduction recommendations.
        - Reassess in 1 year.
    - LDL >130 mg/dL
        - Evaluate for underlying causes and start treatment.
        - Screen for symptoms of secondary causes of hyperlipidemia for all children with elevated cholesterol levels (see "Differential Diagnosis").
    - Laboratory workup as appropriate (e.g., thyroid-stimulating hormone, blood sugar, cortisol, renal function, liver function)

TREATMENT

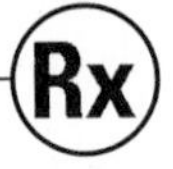

NONPHARMACOLOGIC THERAPY

- Lifestyle modifications: weight loss, increase exercise, decrease sedentary activities, and discontinue smoking
- Step 1 diet (for children ≥2 years old) (see Step 1 and 2 Diets in Prevention [Section V])
    - Diet must provide adequate calories for growth and development.
    - Calories are maintained by increasing carbohydrate:
        - Between 20% and 30% of total calories as fat, less than 10% saturated fat
        - Less than 300 mg/day of cholesterol
        - Generally does not lower LDL by more than 10% to 15%
- Step 2 diet (for children >2 years old) (see Step 1 and 2 Diets in Prevention [Section V])
    - Use if failure to reduce LDL to less than 130 mg/dL after 6 to 12 months of step 1 diet
    - Between 20% and 30% of calories as fat, but less than 7% saturated fats
    - Cholesterol limited to less than 200 mg/day

CHRONIC Rx

- Pharmacologic treatment is reserved for the following cases:
    - Children older than 10 years
    - Children who failed dietary manipulation for 6 to 12 months
- Drug therapy is indicated if the preceding two parameters are met along with one of the following:
    - Greater than 190 mg/dL of LDL cholesterol
    - Greater than 160 mg/dL of LDL cholesterol and family history of premature heart disease
    - Greater than 160 mg/dL of LDL cholesterol and multiple associated risk factors
- Goal is to lower total cholesterol and LDL cholesterol levels by 15%.
- Bile acid sequestrants (resins)
    - First-line medication for children
    - Primarily reduces LDL cholesterol (10% to 32%); can increase triglycerides
    - Usually need to supplement with vitamin D and folic acid
    - Cholestyramine
        - Familial hypercholesterolemia: 40mg/kg/day divided three times daily
        - Hypercholesterolemia: limited data for infants and children, but for ages 6 to 12 years, start at 80 mg/kg/day divided three times daily, not to exceed 8 g/day

- Unpalatable
- Side effects: nausea, bloating, constipation
- Hydroxymethylglutaryl coenzyme A (HMG-CoA) reductase inhibitors (i.e., statins)
  - Inhibit rate-limiting step in cholesterol synthesis and secondarily stimulate synthesis and activity of LDL cholesterol receptors, enhancing LDL cholesterol clearance
  - May also have modest effect on lowering TG and raising HDL cholesterol levels
  - Familial hypercholesterolemia (for children 10 to 17 years old):
    - Atorvastatin: recommended starting dose 10 mg, maximum of 20 mg/day
    - Lovastatin: recommended dose of 10 to 40 mg/day; start with 10 mg/day, 20 mg/day if greater than 20% reduction in LDL is needed
    - Simvastatin: recommended starting dose of 10 mg/day, 5 mg/day if also taking cyclosporin or manazol, maximum of 40 mg/day
    - Pravastatin: approved for ages 8 to 13 years; recommended dose of 20 mg/day and 40 mg/day for children 14 years or older, but start at 10 mg/day if patient is on immunosuppressants or other potentially myopathic medication and monitor LFTS frequently and before and after dose changes.
  - Limited data for dosing patients with nonfamilial hypercholesterolemia
  - Few long-term studies available that included children
  - Potential use in those with significantly elevated LDL levels or significant risks or premature heart disease in close family members and those who cannot tolerate or do not respond to bile acid sequestrants
  - Side effects: gastrointestinal upset, headaches, sleep disturbance, fatigue, muscle or joint pains, rhabdomyolysis, and severe myopathy
  - Risk of severe myopathy increased when combined with fibrates
  - Dosing must be adjusted with renal impairment
- Fibric acid derivatives (i.e., fibrates)
  - Reduces TG, increases HDL cholesterol, and has variable effects on LDL cholesterol
  - Few data on use in children; currently not recommended for children
- Nicotinic acid (i.e., niacin)
  - Reduces LDL cholesterol and TG levels; increases HDL cholesterol level
  - Limited use in children; not currently recommended for children younger than 12 years
  - Side effects: skin flushing, glucose intolerance, elevated liver enzymes, supraventricular arrhythmias, syncope, orthostasis, and hypotension

COMPLEMENTARY & ALTERNATIVE MEDICINE

- Fish oil (i.e., omega-3 fatty acids)
  - There is questionable evidence of generalizable effectiveness.
  - Short-term use in children with renal disease showed decreased TG levels.
- Other natural therapies for lowering cholesterol with adult data but few or no data on children include the following:
  - Probably effective: β-sitosterol, blond psyllium, flaxseed, oats, red yeast, sitosterol, soy protein
  - Possibly effective: alfalfa, artichokes, avocado, barley, β-glucans, black psyllium, calcium, English walnut, garlic, green tea, guar gum, macadamia nut, magnesium, olive, pectin, policosanol, rice bran, safflower, soybean oil, sweet orange, yogurt

DISPOSITION

Long-term lifestyle changes are needed.

REFERRAL

Help can be sought through local diet and weight-control groups.

PEARLS & CONSIDERATIONS

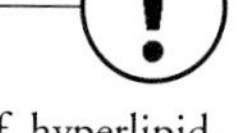

COMMENTS

- Never make the diagnosis of hyperlipidemia on the basis of total cholesterol alone.
- Address other risk factors for CAD.
  - Discourage cigarette smoking.
  - Identify and treat high blood pressure.
  - Instruct patients to avoid obesity, especially a high waist-to-hip ratio, by reducing weight and limiting fat intake.
  - Encourage exercise, and discourage a sedentary lifestyle.
  - Diagnose and treat diabetes mellitus.
  - Diagnose and treat renal disease.

PREVENTION

- Direct proof that intervention and treatment decrease the risk of CAD is not available.
- Evidence suggests early awareness and appropriate care can decrease risks later in life.

PATIENT/FAMILY EDUCATION

- It is unusual for atherosclerotic heart disease to be the result of one cause.
- Contributing factors include the following:
  - Age: increases with increasing age
  - Weight: increases with increasing weight
  - Sex: higher risk of CAD later in life for men
  - Family history of premature heart disease
  - Cigarette smoking
  - Diabetes mellitus
  - Low level of exercise
  - Dietary intake high in fat and total calories

SUGGESTED READINGS

American Academy of Pediatrics, Committee on Nutrition: Cholesterol in childhood. *Pediatrics* 101:141, 1998.

American Heart Association. Available at www.americanheart.org/Heart_and_stroke_A-Z_Guide/cholscr.html

Natural Medicines Comprehensive Database. Available at www.naturaldatabase.com

Newman TB, Garber AM: Cholesterol screening in children and adolescents. *Pediatrics* 105:637, 2000.

Tershakovec AM, Rader D: Disorders of lipoprotein metabolism transport. *In* Berhman R et al (eds): *Nelson Textbook of Pediatrics.* Philadelphia, Elsevier Science, 2004, pp 445–457.

Tonstad S: Role of lipid-lowering pharmacotherapy in children. *Paediatr Drugs* 2:12, 2000.

AUTHOR: **S. NICHOLE FEENEY, MD**

BASIC INFORMATION

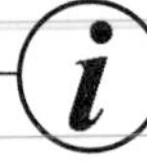

DEFINITION

Hyperkalemia is characterized by a serum potassium level greater than 5.5 mEq/L (normal = 3.5 to 5.5 mEq/L; mEq/L is equivalent to moles/L). Although there is some variability among laboratories in the definition of the normal range of values for potassium, all consider a value higher than 5.5 mEq/Lto indicate hyperkalemia. Urgent treatment is usually considered when the potassium level is higher than 6.0 mEq/L.

ICD-9-CM CODE
276.7 Hyperkalemia

EPIDEMIOLOGY & DEMOGRAPHICS

- Spurious values are common and are caused by blood sampling techniques (e.g., heelsticks, fingersticks, tourniquets).
- The epidemiologic and demographic features of true hyperkalemia correlate with the conditions causing it.
- Risk factors for hyperkalemia include exogenous administration of potassium and renal failure.

CLINICAL PRESENTATION

History

- Dietary history (e.g., potassium-rich foods such as bananas or potatoes)
- Medications (especially a combination of spironolactone, captopril or enalapril, other diuretics, and potassium chloride supplement)
- Urine output: evidence of oliguria (i.e., renal failure), polyuria (e.g., diabetes, renal failure)
- Pink, red, or dark urine (e.g., myoglobinuria, hemoglobinuria, glomerulonephritis)
- Fatigue or weakness (e.g., adrenal insufficiency, hyperkalemic familial periodic paralysis, renal failure)

Physical Examination

- Usually, no direct physical examination findings are apparent, except those related to the underlying disease process (e.g., tachypnea may suggest a compensatory respiratory alkalosis induced by an underlying metabolic acidosis).
- Cardiac arrhythmias may be identified.
- Muscle weakness or ascending paralysis may occur with high levels of potassium or with the syndrome of hyperkalemic periodic paralysis.

ETIOLOGY

- Spurious hyperkalemia
  - Caused by hemolysis during blood sampling
  - Caused by blood sampling distal to potassium infusion (e.g., blood drawn from a central line's distal port, when total parenteral nutrition solution is infusing into a proximal port)
  - Thrombocytosis (>500,000 platelets/mm^3), leukocytosis (>50,000/mm^3): potassium release during the clotting process (serum) but not in plasma (in vivo)
- Acidemia
- Hyperosmolality
- Diabetic ketoacidosis
- Renal failure (acute or chronic)
- Salt-losing congenital adrenal hyperplasia (i.e., 21-hydroxylase deficiency)
- Adrenal insufficiency
- Hypoaldosteronism or pseudohypoaldosteronism
- Rhabdomyolysis
- Crush injuries and burns
- Tumor lysis syndrome
- Intravascular hemolysis
- Rapid transfusion with old (hemolyzed) blood
- Excessive intake (e.g., salt substitutes, potassium-containing antibiotics, intravenous administration in maintenance fluids, total parenteral nutrition, acute replacement)
- Drug-induced
  - Succinylcholine (hyperkalemia peaks after 5 minutes)
  - Potassium-sparing diuretics (e.g., spironolactone, amiloride)
  - Angiotensin-converting enzyme (ACE) inhibitors (e.g., captopril, enalapril)
  - β-Blockers
  - Heparin
  - Digoxin toxicity
  - Propofol (likely related to severe induced metabolic acidosis after prolonged use of high-dose propofol; acidosis causes potassium to be extruded from red blood cells)
  - Malignant hyperthermia

DIAGNOSIS

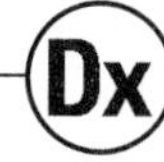

WORKUP

- The workup for hyperkalemia is determined by the possible causes.
- Serum potassium from a nonhemolyzed specimen: Obtain from free-flowing blood by venipuncture or arterial puncture to avoid hemolysis and falsely elevated values.
- Whole-blood potassium from a nonhemolyzed specimen: Values are always somewhat lower, but reference ranges (normal values) are also somewhat lower.

LABORATORY TESTS

Confirm serum and whole-blood potassium levels by repeating tests by sampling from free-flowing venous or arterial blood.

- Supportive tests
  - Electrocardiogram (ECG): Progression of findings often correlates with increasing potassium levels,
    - Peaked T waves (precordial leads)
    - Decreased amplitude of R wave
    - Widened QRS
    - Prolonged PR interval
    - Absent P wave
    - Sine wave (potassium > 8.0)
  - Ventricular arrhythmias may occur at any point, and progression of findings may occur extremely rapidly (i.e., in minutes).
  - A normal ECG does not rule out hyperkalemia. Only 20% of patients with hyperkalemia have a peaked T wave.

TREATMENT

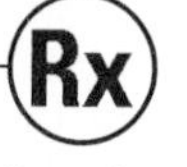

ACUTE GENERAL Rx

- If the potassium level is higher than 6.0 mEq/L:
  - Maintain continuous cardiac monitoring.
  - Discontinue all exogenous potassium (intravenous and oral).
  - Prepare for management of ventricular arrhythmias.
  - Monitor potassium at least every 2 hours until level is decreasing.
- If potassium is more than 6.0 mEq/L but less than 6.5 mEq/L:
  - Perform steps outlined previously.
  - Administer sodium polystyrene sulfonate (Kayexalate): 1 to 2 g/kg orally, nasogastrically, or rectally in 20% sorbitol every 6 hours (will drop potassium by 0.5 to 1 mEq/L in 1 to 2 hours) and monitor for sodium overload.
  - Consider furosemide (0.5 to 1.0 mg/kg intravenously).
  - Consider albuterol nebulization (2.5 mg in 3.0 mL of saline); its β-agonist effect drives potassium intracellularly.
  - Monitor potassium levels every 2 hours.
- If potassium is higher than 6.5 mEq/L or lower than 6.5 mEq/L and likely to rise rapidly (e.g., renal failure, tissue necrosis):
  - Place patient on a cardiac monitor, discontinue potassium, give Kayexalate, and consider furosemide.
  - Administer intravenous 10% calcium gluconate (100 mg/kg [1 ml/kg] up to 20 mL) over 10 minutes while monitoring for bradycardia and hypotension, or administer 10% calcium chloride (20 mg/kg [0.2 mL/kg] up to 5 mL [500 mg]) if a central line is available.
    - Myocardial cell membranes are stabilized immediately.
    - May repeat dose in 1 hour; follow calcium level.
    - Calcium infiltration causes severe tissue necrosis. For infiltrates, inject hyaluronidase into area as soon as possible to diminish the effect.
  - Sodium bicarbonate ($NaHCO_3$) (1 to 2 mEq/kg as an intravenous bolus over 5 to 15 minutes) can be used to shift potassium intracellularly by inducing alkalemia.
    - May repeat every 1 to 4 hours as necessary for persistent metabolic acidosis.
    - Follow pH levels.

- Administer a glucose and insulin infusion: 1 g/kg glucose with 0.3 unit of insulin/g glucose mixed together and administered over 2 hours.
- Monitor the potassium level hourly until it is lower than 6.0; if no response, prepare for dialysis to remove potassium from the body. Hemodialysis more effective than peritoneal dialysis.

DISPOSITION

- Determine the cause of hyperkalemia.
- Monitor potassium if the cause is not amenable to therapy or continued risks exist. If the underlying disease can be treated, hyperkalemia usually resolves.

REFERRAL

- Consider hospital admission and possible intensive care unit placement for the following conditions:
  - Potassium level greater than 6.0 mEq/L and risk factors present
  - Potassium level greater than 6.5 mEq/L and not responsive to initial treatments
- Referral to an endocrinologist, metabolic specialist, or nephrologist may be required.

PEARLS & CONSIDERATIONS

COMMENTS

- When hyperkalemia is suspected to be caused by the technique only, a repeat venous specimen should be drawn immediately without a tourniquet or an arterial puncture performed with free-flowing blood. Do not assume a spurious value until a clear reason is determined.
- Administration of potassium supplements to a patient with an intestinal ileus or poor intestinal motility may result in acute hyperkalemia when the ileus or dysmotility resolves because of the sudden absorption of the previously administered, unabsorbed, accumulated potassium.
- Combinations of potassium-sparing diuretics (e.g., spironolactone), ACE inhibitors (e.g., captopril), and oral potassium may result in acute hyperkalemia. Frequent monitoring is advised.

PREVENTION

- Careful calculation of potassium dosing, including intravenous potassium, particularly when given to correct hypokalemia
- Frequent blood level monitoring if on potassium supplements and potassium-sparing diuretics

PATIENT/FAMILY EDUCATION

- Risks of diuretics and potassium-containing solutions should be clearly explained.
- Methods for obtaining a rapid blood level at all times must be determined in conjunction with the family.

SUGGESTED READINGS

Brem AS: Disorders of potassium homeostasis. *Pediatr Clin North Am* 37:419, 1990.

Cronan KM, Norman ME: Renal and electrolyte emergencies. *In* Fleisher GR, Ludwig SL (eds): *Textbook of Pediatric Emergency Medicine,* 4th ed. Philadelphia, Lippincott Williams & Wilkins, 2000.

Kemper MJ et al: Hyperkalemia: therapeutic options in acute and chronic renal failure. *Clin Nephrol* 46:67, 1996.

Wood EG, Lynch RE: Fluids electrolyte balance. *In* Fuhrman BP, Zimmerman JJ (eds): *Pediatric Critical Care,* 2nd ed. St Louis, Mosby, 1998.

AUTHOR: **ELISE W. VAN DER JAGT, MD, MPH**

BASIC INFORMATION

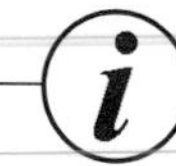

DEFINITION

Hypernatremia is characterized by a serum sodium concentration higher than 150 mEq/L; the normal level is approximately 135 to 145 mEq/L. Hypertonicity is a result of hypernatremia. Other substances besides sodium (e.g., mannitol, glucose) may cause hypertonicity, which is an increased amount of solute in the extracellular space compared with the intracellular space.

ICD-9-CM CODE
276.0 Hypernatremia

EPIDEMIOLOGY & DEMOGRAPHICS

- Hypernatremia is most commonly associated with dehydration from gastroenteritis. About 10% of infants with dehydration from gastroenteritis have hypernatremia.
- The mortality rate for acute hypernatremia is 8% to 45%, but estimates are based on older literature, and current practices may produce better results.
- The mortality rate for chronic hypernatremia is 10%, and morbidity is high among survivors.
- Hypernatremia is often associated with hypocalcemia and hyperglycemia.
- Hypernatremia has been associated with breastfed infants in the first several weeks of life.
- It is associated with the first infant, age (older women), middle and upper socioeconomic class, and higher levels of education.

CLINICAL PRESENTATION

History

- Diarrhea, nausea, or vomiting
- Thirst (unless gastritis)
- Type and quantity of fluid intake (high salt content?)
- Breastfed infant in first 2 to 3 weeks of life
- Amount of urine output
  - For high urine output, consider central or nephrogenic diabetes insipidus (DI), salt poisoning, excess diuresis from diuretics, hyperglycemia, or use of osmolar agents.
  - For low urine output, consider dehydration from poor intake or excess diarrheal or skin losses.
- Weight loss or gain
- Neurologic symptoms: irritability, high-pitched cry, seizures, coma
- Medications: furosemide, thiazides, mannitol, sorbitol, sodium bicarbonate, intravenous fluid sodium content

Physical Examination

- Weight (compare with a previous weight if known)
- Temperature: fever caused by infection or dehydration
  - Fever increases insensible water loss.
  - For every 1°C increase, fluid requirements increase by 10% to 12%.
- General and neurologic symptoms: obtunded, lethargic, irritable, high-pitched cry, seizures
- State of hydration: cardiovascular examination
  - Fluid deficit: tachycardia, decreased pulses, decreased capillary refill, decreased distal extremity temperature, decreased skin turgor, decreased blood pressure, dry mucous membranes
  - Fluid overload: edema, puffy eyelids, moist mucous membranes, hypertension
- Skin turgor: relatively well preserved compared with hyponatremic and isonatremic dehydration
  - Velvety skin
  - Doughy abdomen
- Anterior fontanelle: sunken, flat, or depressed; may be bulging if sagittal sinus thrombosis or bleed
- Respiratory rate: tachypnea (e.g., fever, acidosis, hyperventilation from increased intracranial pressure from intracranial bleeding)

ETIOLOGY

- Increased sodium intake
  - Oral route: improperly made-up formula, boiled skim milk, accidental poisoning, rarely elevated sodium in breast milk
  - Intravenous: intravenous fluids containing excess sodium or sodium bicarbonate
  - Salt water near-drowning (i.e., salt absorbed through stomach)
- Decreased fluid intake
  - Water
  - Formula or breast milk
- Increased water loss compared with sodium loss
  - Diarrhea: infectious, malabsorptive, sorbitol induced
  - DI: central or nephrogenic
  - Renal tubular dysfunction caused by obstructive uropathy or renal dysplasia
  - Drugs: diuretics, mannitol, glucose, lithium, cyclophosphamide, cisplatin
  - Increased respiratory or dermal water (insensible) losses

DIAGNOSIS

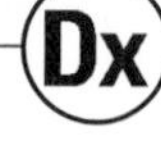

DIFFERENTIAL DIAGNOSIS

Causes discussed under "Etiology"

WORKUP

- Serum sodium should be obtained.
- Urine output should be determined.
  - Low urine output suggests dehydration.
  - Normal to high urine output suggests diabetes insipidus, renal tubular dysfunction, or salt poisoning.
- Additional laboratory tests aid in determining the cause of hypernatremia
  - Blood urea nitrogen (BUN), creatinine, chloride, potassium, bicarbonate, and glucose levels
  - Urine specific gravity; pH; osmolality; and sodium, potassium, and chloride levels
  - High urine sodium (>40 mEq/L)
    - Sodium and volume overloads
    - Renal tubular dysfunction or renal failure
    - Cerebral salt wasting
    - Diuretic use (e.g., furosemide, thiazides)
  - Low urine sodium (<10 to 20 mEq/L) with low urine osmolality (<100 mOsm/L) or low urine specific gravity (<1.003)
    - Diabetes insipidus
    - Primary hyperaldosteronism or use of spironolactone
    - Inadequate circulating blood volume with secondary aldosterone secretion (patients have low urine sodium, low urine output, high urine osmolality, and high urine specific gravity)
  - Fractional excretion of sodium: $(U_{Na} \div P_{Na}) \times (P_{Cr} \div U_{Cr}) \times 100\%$
    - Fractional excretion of sodium less than 1% suggests a prerenal cause, such as dehydration, or an absolute deficit sodium.
    - Fractional excretion of sodium more than 2% suggests renal disease (serum sodium is usually low or normal, however).

TREATMENT

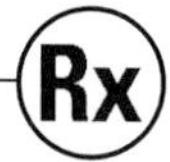

NONPHARMACOLOGIC THERAPY

- Observe for neurologic deterioration suggesting cerebral edema and increased intracranial pressure (e.g., anterior fontanelle, Glasgow Coma Scale score).
- Provide assistance with breastfeeding, including lactation aids.

ACUTE GENERAL Rx

- Hypernatremia caused by water loss
  - For signs of circulatory failure, restore intravascular volume rapidly with 20 mL/kg of intravenous normal saline.
  - Then slowly replace water deficit so that the serum sodium level falls 10 to 12 mEq/24 hours.
  - Use 5% dextrose (D_5) in ¼ (25%) normal saline with potassium chloride (as appropriate) at rates that result in replacement of deficit over the predicted number of days it takes to decrease sodium to normal while providing maintenance fluids.
    - This should take at least 48 hours and may require 4 to 5 days, depending how hypernatremic the child is.
    - Fluid should be given no faster than over 48 hours because the sodium level may drop too fast otherwise.
  - Although D_5 in ¼ (25%) normal saline with potassium chloride (combination of replacement and maintenance fluid) is hypotonic compared with serum, slow replacement results in a slow decrease in serum sodium with a decreased risk of cerebral edema.

- If caused by central DI, administer either of the following:
  - Desmopressin acetate (DDAVP) intranasally at 5 to 40 μg every 8 to 24 hours as needed or intravenously at 0.5 to 4 μg/dose every 8 to 24 hours as needed
  - Aqueous vasopressin (50 mU/kg/hr) by continuous intravenous drip and increase as necessary to 150 to 300 mU/kg/hr while monitoring urine output, urine specific gravity, and osmolality
  - Aim for urine output of 1 mL/kg/hr and urine specific gravity of 1.010 or higher.
- Hypernatremia caused by excess intake or decreased excretion
  - Discontinue all sodium intake and provide hyponatremic fluids for maintenance.
  - Furosemide helps promote natriuresis and may be considered.
  - Allow sodium level to decrease at a rate of 10 to 12 mEq/24 hours.
  - In the case of oliguric renal failure, dialysis should be considered.

DISPOSITION

- Monitor serum sodium every 4 hours initially to ensure slow (10 to 12 mEq/24 hours) decrease.
- Monitor by neurologic examinations every 2 hours until stable for 24 hours and then at longer intervals.
- Ongoing neurologic and developmental assessments by the primary care provider are necessary.

REFERRAL

Consider placing the patient in the intensive care unit for the following conditions:

- Sodium level higher than 160 mEq/L
- Ten percent dehydration or evidence of circulatory compromise
- Neurologic signs or symptoms, with the need for hourly neurologic monitoring
- Newly diagnosed central DI
- Need for multiple blood draws for laboratory tests; may require arterial line
- Other electrolyte abnormalities, along with significant hypernatremia

PEARLS & CONSIDERATIONS

COMMENTS

- Meticulous fluid calculations are essential, especially for deficits.
- If serum sodium is dropping too fast when correcting, decrease the rate of fluid administration (probably overestimated deficit) or increase sodium in the fluids.
- In DI, the degree of hypernatremia does not correlate well with the BUN; often, the BUN is minimally elevated, even though the patient is depleted of free water and the sodium level is high.
- Aqueous vasopressin is easier to regulate than intranasal or intravenous bolus desmopressin.

PREVENTION

- Proper intake of fluids, including formula and breast milk
- Proper use of medications
- Proper identification of signs of dehydration

PATIENT/FAMILY EDUCATION

- Instruct parents regarding the proper mixing of formulas.
- Provide instruction on the sodium content of various fluids (e.g., Gatorade).
- Explain normal urine output, the signs of dehydration, and the symptoms of DI (e.g., polyuria, polydipsia).
- Ensure that proper administration of intranasal DDAVP is given if the patient has central DI.

SUGGESTED READINGS

Conley SB: Hypernatremia. *Pediatr Clin North Am* 37:365, 1990.

Cronan KM, Norman ME: Renal and electrolyte emergencies. *In* Fleisher GR, Ludwig SL (eds): *Textbook of Pediatric Emergency Medicine,* 4th ed. Philadelphia, Lippincott Williams & Wilkins, 2000.

Wood EG, Lynch RE: Fluids electrolyte balance. *In* Fuhrman BP, Zimmerman JJ (eds): *Pediatric Critical Care,* 2nd ed. St Louis, Mosby, 1998.

AUTHOR: **ELISE W. VAN DER JAGT, MD, MPH**

BASIC INFORMATION

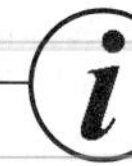

DEFINITIONS

Hypertension is defined as the average systolic blood pressure (SBP) or diastolic blood pressure (DBP) that is at or above the 95th percentile for gender, age, and height on three or more occasions. Stage I hypertension is more than 95% to 99% plus 5 mm Hg, and stage II hypertension is more than 99% plus 5 mm Hg. Prehypertension (formerly designated high normal BP) is defined as SBP or DBP levels that are more than the 90th percentile but less than the 95th percentile. White-coat hypertension refers to patients with BP levels at or above the 95th percentile in a physician's office or clinic but who are normotensive outside the clinical setting (see Table 1-9).

SYNONYM

High blood pressure

ICD-9-CM CODES
401 Essential hypertension
401.0 Malignant hypertension
401.1 Benign hypertension
402 Hypertensive heart disease
403 Hypertensive renal disease
404 Hypertensive heart and renal disease
405 Secondary hypertension

EPIDEMIOLOGY & DEMOGRAPHICS

- By definition, 5% of children and adolescents have BP high enough to be defined as hypertensive (refer to Blood Pressure in Charts, Formulas, Laboratory, Tests and Values [Section IV]).
- There appears to be a familial genetic influence on development because children from families with hypertension tend to have higher BP readings than children from normotensive families.
- Hypertension and prehypertension have become a significant health issue in the young because of the strong association of high BP with obesity and the marked increase in the prevalence of obesity in childhood.

CLINICAL PRESENTATION

History

- Neonatal history (especially umbilical artery catheterization)
- Medical history: renal disease (e.g., glomerulonephritis, polycystic kidneys, Henoch-Schönlein purpura), systemic lupus erythematosus, urinary tract infections, renal trauma, diabetes mellitus, cardiac surgery
- Family history: hypertension, atherosclerosis, preeclampsia, toxemia, renal disease, tumors (i.e., risk for essential hypertension and inherited renal or endocrine diseases)
- Review of systems: abdominal pain, dysuria, hematuria, frequency, nocturia, enuresis (may suggest underlying renal disease or infection); joint pains or swelling, facial or peripheral edema (nephrosis or nephritis); weight loss, failure to gain weight, flushing, sweating, fevers, palpitations (e.g., pheochromocytoma); muscle cramps, weakness, constipation (e.g., hypokalemia, hyperaldosteronism); age of menarche, sexual development (e.g., hydroxylase deficiency); ingestion of prescription, over-the-counter, or illicit drugs

Physical Examination

- General: pallor, facial or pretibial edema (i.e., renal disease)
- Café au lait spots, neurofibromas (i.e., von Recklinghausen's neurofibromatosis)
- Moon face, hirsutism, buffalo hump, truncal obesity, striae (i.e., Cushing's syndrome)
- Webbing of the neck, low hairline, wide-spaced nipples (i.e., Turner syndrome)
- Elfin facies, poor growth, retardation (i.e., Williams syndrome)
- Thyroid enlargement or nodules (i.e., hyperthyroid or hypothyroid)
- Cardiovascular conditions
  - Murmur, absent or delayed femoral pulses, low leg BP relative to arm BP (i.e., aortic coarctation)
  - Heart size, tachycardia, hepatomegaly, tachypnea (i.e., heart failure)
  - Bruits over great vessels (i.e., arteritis or arteriopathy)
- Abdomen
  - Epigastric bruit (i.e., renovascular disease or arteritis)
  - Unilateral or bilateral masses (i.e., Wilms' tumor, neuroblastoma, pheochromocytoma, polycystic kidneys)
- Neurologic conditions: hypertensive funduscopic changes, Bell's palsy, neurologic deficits (i.e., chronic or severe acute hypertension)

ETIOLOGY

The most common causes of hypertension vary by age group.

- Newborn: renal artery thrombosis, renal artery stenosis, renal vein thrombosis, congenital renal abnormalities, and coarctation of the aorta
- Infant: coarctation of the aorta, renovascular disease, and renal parenchymal disease
- Age 1 to 6 years: renal parenchymal disease, renovascular disease, and coarctation of the aorta
- Age 6 to 12 years: renal parenchymal disease, renovascular disease, essential hypertension, and coarctation of the aorta
- Age 12 to 18 years: essential hypertension, iatrogenic, and renal parenchymal disease

DIAGNOSIS

WORKUP

- Evaluation for identifiable causes (consider on all patients)
  - History: sleep history, family history, risk factors, diet and habits such as smoking and drinking alcohol
  - Levels of blood urea nitrogen, creatinine, and electrolytes; urinalysis and urine culture
  - Complete blood cell count
  - Renal ultrasound
- Evaluation for comorbidity (i.e., obesity, family history, or risk factors)
  - Fasting lipid panel
  - Fasting glucose
  - Drug screen
  - Polysomnography
- Evaluation for target-organ damage (i.e., all patients with hypertension and those patients with prehypertension plus comorbid risk factors)
  - Echocardiogram (i.e., left ventricular mass)
  - Retinal examination
- Additional evaluation as indicated
  - Ambulatory BP monitoring
  - Plasma renin determination
  - Renovascular imaging (i.e., renal ultrasound and renal artery flow studies)
  - Plasma and urine steroid levels
  - Plasma and urine catecholamines

TREATMENT

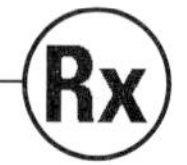

NONPHARMACOLOGIC THERAPY

The following therapies should be advocated for prehypertensive patients and as a complement to pharmacologic interventions in hypertensive patients:

- Weight reduction: This is the primary therapy for obesity-related hypertension. Prevention of excess or abnormal weight gain can limit future increases in BP.
- Exercise: Regular physical activity and restriction of sedentary activity can improve efforts at weight management and may prevent an excess increase in BP over time.
- Dietary interventions include sodium restriction and a heart-healthy diet to decrease fat intake. (See Dash Diet in Prevention [Section V])
- Encourage smoking cessation.
- Discourage alcohol and drug use.
- Family-based interventions improve success.

ACUTE GENERAL Rx

- Severe (BP > 1.3 to 1.5 times the 95th percentile) or symptomatic (i.e., heart failure, renal failure, funduscopic changes, or encephalopathy) hypertension should be treated emergently with intravenous antihypertensive drugs.

CHRONIC Rx

- Refer to Table 1-12.
- Indications for antihypertensive drug therapy in children include secondary hypertension and insufficient response to lifestyle modifications.
- Pharmacologic therapy, when indicated, should be initiated with a single drug. Acceptable drug classes for use in children include angiotensin-converting enzyme

TABLE 1-12 Antihypertensive Drugs for Outpatient Management of Hypertension in Children 1-17 Years Old

Class	Drug	Dose	Dosing Interval	Evidence	FDA Labeling	Comments
ACE inhibitor	Benazepril	Initial: 0.2 mg/kg per d up to 10 mg/d Maximum: 0.6 mg/kg per d up to 40 mg/d	qd	RCT	Yes	1. All ACE inhibitors are contraindicated in pregnancy; females of childbearing age should use reliable contraception. 2. Check serum potassium and creatinine periodically to monitor for hyperkalemia and azotemia. 3. Cough and angioedema are reportedly less common with newer members of this class than with captopril. 4. Benazepril, enalapril, and lisinopril labels contain information on the preparation of a suspension; captopril may also be compounded into a suspension. 5. FDA approval for ACE inhibitors with pediatric labeling is limited to children ≥6 years of age and to children with creatinine clearance ≥30 ml/min per 1.73 m^2.
	Captopril	Initial: 0.3–0.5 mg/kg/dose Maximum: 6 mg/kg per d	tid	RCT, CS	No	
	Enalapril	Initial: 0.08 mg/kg per d up to 5 mg/d Maximum: 0.6 mg/kg per d up to 40 mg/d	qd-bid	RCT	Yes	
	Fosinopril	Children >50 kg: Initial: 5–10 mg/d Maximum: 40 mg/d	qd	RCT	Yes	
	Lisinopril	Initial: 0.07 mg/kg per d up to 5 mg/d Maximum: 0.6 mg/kg per d up to 40 mg/d	qd	RCT	Yes	
	Quinapril	Initial: 5–10 mg/d Maximum: 80 mg/d	qd	RCT, EO	No	
Angiotensin-receptor blocker	Irbesartan	Children 6–12 years: 75–150 mg/d Children ≥13 years: 150–300 mg/d	qd	CS	Yes	1. All ARBs are contraindicated in pregnancy; females of childbearing age should use reliable contraception. 2. Check serum potassium, creatinine periodically to monitor for hyperkalemia and azotemia. 3. Losartan label contains information on the preparation of a suspension. 4. FDA approval for ARBs is limited to children ≥6 years of age and to children with creatinine clearance ≥30 ml/min per 1.73 m^2.
	Losartan	Initial: 0.7 mg/kg per d up to 50 mg/d Maximum: 1.4 mg/kg per d up to 100 mg/d	qd	RCT	Yes	
α- and β-Blocker	Labetalol	Initial: 1–3 mg/kg per d Maximum: 10–12 mg/kg per d up to 1200 mg/d	bid	CS, EO	No	1. Asthma and overt heart failure are contraindications. 2. Heart rate is dose-limiting. 3. May impair athletic performance. 4. Should not be used in insulin-dependent diabetics.
β-Blocker	Atenolol	Initial: 0.5–1 mg/kg per d Maximum: 2 mg/kg per d up to 100 mg/d	qd-bid	CS	No	1. Noncardioselective agents (propranolol) are contraindicated in asthma and heart failure. 2. Heart rate is dose-limiting. 3. May impair athletic performance. 4. Should not be used in insulin-dependent diabetics. 5. A sustained-release formulation of propranolol is available that is dosed once-daily.
	Bisoprolol/HCTZ	Initial: 2.5/6.25 mg/d Maximum: 10/6.25 mg/d	qd	RCT	No	
	Metoprolol	Initial: 1–2 mg/kg per d Maximum: 6 mg/kg per d up to 200 mg/d	bid	CS	No	
	Propranolol	Initial: 1–2 mg/kg per d Maximum: 4 mg/kg per d up to 640 mg/d	bid-tid	RCT, EO	Yes	
Calcium channel blocker	Amlodipine	Children 6–17 years: 2.5–5 mg once daily	qd	RCT	Yes	1. Amlodipine and isradipine can be compounded into stable extemporaneous suspensions. 2. Felodipine and extended-release nifedipine tablets must be swallowed whole. 3. Isradipine is available in both immediate-release and sustained-release formulations; sustained-release form is dosed qd or bid. 4. May cause tachycardia.
	Felodipine	Initial: 2.5 mg/d Maximum: 10 mg/d	qd	RCT, EO	No	
	Isradipine	Initial: 0.15–0.2 mg/kg per d Maximum: 0.8 mg/kg per d up to 20 mg/d	tid-qid	CS, EO	No	
	Extended-release nifedipine	Initial: 0.25–0.5 mg/kg per d Maximum: 3 mg/kg per d up to 120 mg/d	qd-bid	CS, EO	No	

National High Blood Pressure Education Program Working Group on High Blood Pressure in Children and Adolescents: The fourth report on the diagnosis, evaluation, and treatment of high blood pressure in children and adolescents. *Pediatrics* 114:555, 2004.

TABLE 1-13 Indications for Antihypertensive Drug Therapy in Children

Symptomatic hypertension
Secondary hypertension
Hypertensive target-organ damage
Diabetes (types 1 and 2)
Persistent hypertension despite nonpharmacologic measures

National High Blood Pressure Education Program Working Group on High Blood Pressure in Children and Adolescents: The fourth report on the diagnosis, evaluation, and treatment of high blood pressure in children and adolescents. *Pediatrics* 114:555, 2004.

TABLE 1-14 Classification of Hypertension in Children and Adolescents, with Measurement Frequency and Therapy Recommendations

	sbp or dbp Percentile*	Frequency of BP Measurement	Therapeutic Lifestyle Changes	Pharmacologic Therapy
Normal	<90th	Recheck at next scheduled physical examination	Encourage healthy diet, sleep, and physical activity	—
Prehypertension	90th to <95th or if BP exceeds 120/80 even if <90th percentile up to <95th percentile†	Recheck in 6 mo	Weight-management counseling if overweight; introduce physical activity and diet management‡	None unless compelling indications such as chronic kidney disease, diabetes mellitus, heart failure, or LVH exist
Stage I hypertension	95th-99th percentile plus 5 mm Hg	Recheck in 1-2 wks or sooner if the patient is symptomatic; if persistently elevated on 2 additional occasions, evaluate or refer to source of care within 1 mo	Weight-management counseling if overweight; introduce physical activity and diet management‡	Initiate therapy based on indications in Table 1-13 or if compelling indications (as shown above) exist
Stage II hypertension	>99th percentile plus 5 mm Hg	Evaluate or refer to source of care within 1 wk or immediately if the patient is symptomatic	Weight-management counseling if overweight; introduce physical activity and diet management‡	Initiate therapy§

*For gender, age, and height measured on at least 3 separate occasions; if systolic and diastolic categories are different, categorize by the higher value.
†This occurs typically at 12 years old for SBP and at 16 years old for DBP.
‡Parents and children trying to modify the eating plan to the Dietary Approaches to Stop Hypertension Study eating plan could benefit from consultation with a registered or licensed nutritionist to get them started.
§More than one drug may be required.
National High Blood Pressure Education Program Working Group on High Blood Pressure in Children and Adolescents: The fourth report on the diagnosis, evaluation, and treatment of high blood pressure in children and adolescents. *Pediatrics* 114:555, 2004.

(ACE) inhibitors, angiotensin-receptor blockers, β-blockers, calcium channel blockers, and diuretics.
- The goal for antihypertensive treatment in children should be reduction of BP to less than the 95th percentile unless concurrent conditions are present, in which case BP should be lowered to less than the 90th percentile.

DISPOSITION

See Table 1-14.

REFERRAL

- Referral to a cardiologist, nephrologist, or endocrinologist may be considered if a specific disorder is suspected or diagnosed.
- Patients with stage II hypertension may be referred to a provider with expertise in pediatric hypertension.

PEARLS & CONSIDERATIONS

COMMENTS

- Cuff size is important.
  - Cuff bladder width should be at least 40% of the circumference of the arm measured midway between the olecranon and acromion.
  - Cuff bladder length should encompass 80% to 100% of the arm.
- The preferred method of BP measurement is auscultation.
  - SBP is determined by the onset of the "tapping" Korotkoff sounds (K1).
  - DBP is established as the disappearance of Korotkoff sounds (K5).
- Secondary hypertension is more common in children than in adults.
- After hypertension is confirmed, BP should be measured in both arms and a leg (to assess for coarctation).
- Because left ventricular hypertrophy is the most prominent evidence of target-organ damage and is an indication to initiate or intensify therapy, patients with hypertension should have echocardiographic assessment of left ventricular mass at diagnosis and periodically thereafter.
- Because of the teratogenic risk with fetal exposure during second and third trimester, ACE inhibitors should be used with extreme caution in sexually active female adolescents.

PREVENTION

Hypertension screening in children should be initiated after age 3 years, but it may be started sooner in children with risk factors, including history of prematurity, congenital heart disease, or recurrent urinary tract infections.

PATIENT/FAMILY EDUCATION

More information can be found in Doctor's Guide articles on the Internet: http://www.docguide.com/news/content.nsf/PatientResAllCateg/Hypertension

SUGGESTED READINGS

Bartosh SM, Aronson AJ: Childhood hypertension: an update on etiology, diagnosis and treatment. *Pediatr Clin North Am* 46:235, 1999.
National High Blood Pressure Education Program Working Group on High Blood Pressure in Children and Adolescents: The fourth report on the diagnosis, evaluation, and treatment of high blood pressure in children and adolescents. *Pediatrics* 114:555, 2004.
Sinaiko AR: Hypertension in children. *N Engl J Med* 335:1968, 1996.

AUTHOR: **MARC A. RASLICH, MD**

BASIC INFORMATION

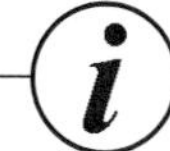

DEFINITION

Hyperthyroidism is a clinical condition typified by manifestations of elevated concentrations of circulating triiodothyronine (T_3) or thyroxine (T_4), or both. It usually is caused by Graves disease in children.

SYNONYM

Thyrotoxicosis

ICD-9-CM CODES

242.00 Graves disease without thyroid storm
242.90 Thyrotoxicosis without mention of goiter

EPIDEMIOLOGY & DEMOGRAPHICS

- Graves disease is six times more prevalent in females than in males.
- It is much less common in children than adults, with increased incidence at puberty and in families with autoimmune thyroid disease (i.e., Graves disease or Hashimoto's thyroiditis).

CLINICAL PRESENTATION

History

- General characteristics
  - Weight loss (less commonly, weight gain occurs early in the course)
  - Increased urination and thirst
  - Heat intolerance
- Endocrine features
  - Goiter commonly develops
  - Menstrual disturbances (i.e., decreased flow)
- Nervous system complaints
  - Sleep disturbance: difficulty falling asleep or difficulty staying asleep
  - Difficulty concentrating
  - Emotional lability
  - Decline in school performance
  - Fatigability
  - Tremor or worsening of handwriting
- Cardiovascular features
  - Palpitations or perception of tachycardia
- Gastrointestinal features
  - Increased appetite
  - Loose stools

Physical Examination

- General features
  - Markedly "fidgety"
  - Weight loss
- Endocrine features
  - Diffusely enlarged thyroid gland without palpable nodules
- Nervous system characteristics
  - Fine motor tremors
  - Tongue fasciculations
  - Proximal muscle weakness
  - Hyperreflexia
- Cardiovascular features
  - Increased pulse pressure
  - Tachycardia
  - Hyperactive precordium
  - High-output flow murmur
- Dermal features
  - Warm skin
  - Sweaty palms
  - Absence of acne in adolescents
- Ocular features
  - Exophthalmos (less common in children than adults; only one third of children)

ETIOLOGY

- Graves disease is an autoimmune condition caused by production of immunoglobulin G (IgG) thyroid-stimulating immunoglobulins (TSIs).
- The antibodies bind to the thyroid-stimulating hormone (TSH) receptors on the thyroid gland and stimulate production of thyroid hormones and stimulate thyroid growth.
- Hyperthyroidism occasionally is caused by a hyperfunctioning thyroid nodule (i.e., adenoma), McCune-Albright syndrome, exogenous thyroid ingestion, or a TSH-secreting adenoma (rare).
- "Hashitoxicosis" is transient hyperthyroidism associated with Hashimoto's thyroiditis, presumably caused by release of preformed thyroxine during autoimmune thyroid destruction.

DIAGNOSIS

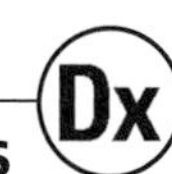

DIFFERENTIAL DIAGNOSIS

- Hyperthyroidism is often confused with nonthyroid conditions involving the central nervous system, including the following:
  - Attention deficit/hyperactivity disorder, behavioral problems
  - Psychiatric conditions
  - Stimulant use
- Hyperthyroidism may be confused with cardiovascular conditions.
  - Tachycardia (from anemia)
  - Arrhythmia
- The differential diagnosis for the hyperthyroid state includes the following:
  - Hyperfunctioning nodule
  - Exogenous thyroxine ingestion
  - Hashitoxicosis: hyperthyroid phase of Hashimoto's thyroiditis

WORKUP

The diagnosis often is obvious from the history and physical examination, especially if a diffusely enlarged thyroid is evident, obviating need for any further evaluation beyond simple thyroid function tests.

LABORATORY TESTS

- Thyroid function tests
  - TSH should be suppressed below the normal range in all forms of hyperthyroidism (except for rare cases of TSH-secreting adenoma).
  - The concentration of free T_4 should be elevated.
- Obtaining the total T_4 level is unnecessary if free T_4 is measured.
  - T_3 determination may be helpful in the diagnosis if TSH is suppressed and the free T_4 level is normal. Adenomas and some instances of Graves disease primarily result in elevated T_3.
- TSIs are present.
  - Levels are elevated but do not need to be measured if the diagnosis is evident from the history and physical examination.
  - Anti-thyroid antibodies are present in Graves disease and Hashimoto's thyroiditis

IMAGING STUDIES

- Radioiodine uptake and imaging usually are not needed if the diagnosis is evident from the history and physical examination.
  - Studies are helpful in identifying a hyperfunctioning nodule.
  - Studies are helpful in differentiating Hashitoxicosis (low uptake) from Graves disease (high uptake).

TREATMENT

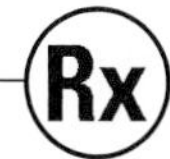

NONPHARMACOLOGIC THERAPY

- Partial thyroidectomy as treatment for Graves disease is less common than medical management and radioiodine therapy; there is a small risk of surgical complications, including hypoparathyroidism and recurrent laryngeal nerve damage.
- Surgery is the treatment of choice for pregnant patients; for those who require immediate, definitive therapy; and if radioiodine therapy is not possible (e.g., iodine allergy) after failure of medical management.
- Excision of a hyperfunctioning nodule is the treatment of choice, is curative, and is not associated with complications of thyroidectomy.

ACUTE GENERAL Rx

- Methimazole (Tapazole) or propylthiouracil (PTU) is the usual first-line therapy in children and adolescents.
  - Initial dosing in adolescents is typically 10 mg of methimazole three times daily or 100 mg of PTU three times daily (one half of this amount for preadolescent children).
  - A repeat free T_4 level should be obtained in 4 to 6 weeks; if the free T_4 concentration is dropping into the normal range, the medication dosage can be gradually reduced, often to once-daily dosing if using methimazole.
- Propranolol, starting at 10 mg three times daily and adjusted upward as needed, can be used in selected patients to help control symptoms while awaiting the therapeutic effects of medication or radioiodine.
- Radioiodine therapy with ^{131}I is usually considered second-line therapy in adolescents.

- It is used primarily in context of adverse reaction to medical therapy (e.g., neutropenia), for failure to control hyperthyroidism on medication, or because of patient preference for definitive therapy.
- It is associated with a high risk of permanent hypothyroidism requiring lifelong thyroid replacement.

DISPOSITION

- For patients treated with PTU or methimazole, the key to management is consistent, regular thyroid function testing with subsequent appropriate adjustments of medication.
- After thyroid values are stabilized, thyroid function tests performed every 3 to 4 months is usually adequate.
- A trial off medication can be considered after several years if the dosage of medication is low (i.e., 5 to 7.5 mg of methimazole daily), there have been no recent relapses of the free T_4 concentration into the hyperthyroid range, and the thyroid gland is small.

REFERRAL

- Many pediatricians refer all patients with hyperthyroidism to a pediatric endocrinologist for management and education.
- For children with hyperthyroidism that does not readily come under control with medical management, those with adverse effects to therapy, or those being considered for radioiodine or surgery, referral should be strongly considered.

PEARLS & CONSIDERATIONS

COMMENTS

- TSH may not be a reliable indicator of the hyperthyroid state early after beginning therapy because of the lag in pituitary recovery.
- The duration of Graves disease in children is much longer than in adults and may take years to remit. If the euthyroid state is maintained for 1 year or longer off medications, there is a good chance that long-term remission from Graves disease will be achieved.
- Neonatal Graves disease, caused by the transplacental passage of maternal stimulating antibodies, is rare but life threatening, and it should receive immediate attention.

PATIENT/FAMILY EDUCATION

- It is imperative that patients and family understand that neutropenia, a rare, reversible adverse effect of methimazole and PTU, can be life threatening if it goes unrecognized.
- Perioral lesions or fevers should be evaluated immediately with a complete blood cell count with a differential white cell count.
- Significant changes in clinical status between regular visits should be reported to the physician as soon as they are identified, and they should be followed with repeat thyroid function tests.

SUGGESTED READINGS

Lazar L et al: Thyrotoxicosis in prepubertal children compared with pubertal and postpubertal patients. *J Clin Endocrinol Metab* 85:3678, 2002.

Rivkees SA et al: Clinical review 99: the management of Graves' disease in children, with special emphasis on radioiodine treatment. *J Clin Endocrinol Metab* 83:3786, 1998.

Segni M et al: Special features of Graves' disease in early childhood. *Thyroid* 9:871, 1999.

Zimmerman D, Lteif AN: Thyrotoxicosis in children. *Endocrinol Metab Clin North Am* 27:109, 1998.

AUTHOR: **CRAIG ORLOWSKI, MD**

BASIC INFORMATION

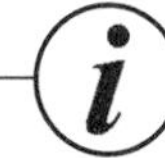

DEFINITION

Hypocalcemia occurs when the total serum calcium concentration is less than 7.0 mg/dL and the ionized calcium is less than 3.5 mg/dL (depending on the particular ion-selective electrode used).

ICD-9-CM CODE
275.41 Hypocalcemia

EPIDEMIOLOGY & DEMOGRAPHICS

- Thirty percent to 90% of preterm infants develop hypocalcemia. Less mature infants have a greater probability of developing hypocalcemia; the incidence of hypocalcemia is inversely proportional to gestational age and birth weight.
- About 20% to 50% of infants of diabetic mothers develop hypocalcemia.
- About 30% of newborns who have an Apgar score below 7 at 1 minute of age may develop hypocalcemia.
- The incidence of "late" hypocalcemia decreased dramatically when the phosphorus content of infant formula was reduced. It does not occur in breastfed infants.

CLINICAL PRESENTATION

- Generalized neuromuscular irritability can manifest as paresthesias, muscle cramps, laryngospasm, or tetany.
- Nonspecific signs include apnea, seizures, jitteriness, increased extensor tone, clonus, hyperreflexia, and stridor (laryngospasm). Jitteriness and generalized convulsions are the main clinical signs.
- Asymptomatic or clinically mild signs occur in preterm infants with early-onset hypocalcemia.
- High-pitched cry, Chvostek's sign (i.e., tapping on face just anterior to the ear at the zygomatic bone elicits facial muscle twitching on that side), and Trousseau's sign (i.e., carpopedal spasm, a painful flexion of wrist and metacarpal phalangeal joints with hyperextension of fingers) after brief occlusion of brachial artery (i.e., blood pressure cuff inflated to systolic blood pressure for longer than 3 minutes) are useful in older infants but are of little diagnostic value in the first few days of life.

ETIOLOGY

- Early-onset neonatal hypocalcemia (during the first 3 days of life)
  - Maternal illness: diabetes mellitus, toxemia of pregnancy, hyperparathyroidism, gestational exposure to anticonvulsants
  - Low birth weight, prematurity
  - Birth asphyxia
  - Respiratory distress, sepsis
  - Hypomagnesemia
- Late-onset neonatal hypocalcemia (most commonly during the first 5 to 10 days of life but occasionally as late as 6 weeks of age)
  - High phosphate load: term infants fed a cow's milk–derived formula or other high-phosphate diet (e.g., cereals) with immaturity of renal tubular phosphate excretion
  - Hypoparathyroidism: transient or permanent
  - Hypomagnesemia
  - Intestinal calcium malabsorption (usually accompanies other malabsorption syndromes)
  - Phototherapy: may relate to melatonin disturbance
  - Maternal factors: decreased vitamin D intake or sunlight exposure
  - Exchange transfusion with citrate-containing blood

DIAGNOSIS

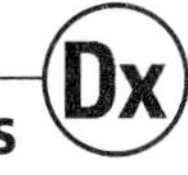

DIFFERENTIAL DIAGNOSIS

- Diagnosis is based on the serum calcium level.
  - Rickets
  - DiGeorge syndrome
  - Renal tubular acidosis
  - Hypercalciuria
  - Hyperphosphaturia
  - Hyperphosphatemia
- Metabolic or respiratory alkalosis
- Differential diagnosis for jittery infants includes
  - Seizure
  - Central nervous system malformation or injury
  - Sepsis
  - Hypoglycemia
  - Hypomagnesemia
  - Narcotic withdrawal or maternal drug ingestion (e.g., cocaine)

WORKUP

- A history of maternal hypercalcemia is helpful. When an infant is the product of an uncomplicated term pregnancy, delivery, and postpartum course, the maternal calcium concentration should be measured to identify asymptomatic hyperparathyroidism or familial hypocalciuric hypercalcemia (FHH).
- Most infants with early hypocalcemia do not require an extensive workup for unusual causes of hypocalcemia, unless the hypocalcemia is refractory to usual therapy or is prolonged.
- Most children with hypocalcemia and no clear cause require a comprehensive evaluation.
- Late hypocalcemia is so unusual with current infant formulas that a workup for other causes is necessary unless the history reveals excessive phosphorus intake.

LABORATORY TESTS

- The diagnosis is based on the serum total or ionized calcium level.
- Monitor serum calcium levels in infants at risk for developing hypocalcemia.
  - Preterm infants weighing less than 1500 g: at 12, 24, 48 hours of life
  - Sick or stressed infants: at 12, 24, 48 hours of life and then as indicated
- Measure serum calcium, ionized calcium, phosphorus, and magnesium levels.
  - Elevated serum phosphorus concentration suggests phosphorus loading, renal insufficiency, or hypoparathyroidism.
  - Magnesium level of 1 mg/dL or less strongly suggests primary hypomagnesemia.
- Assess albumin and parathyroid hormone (PTH) as needed; rarely assess 25-hydroxyvitamin D, 1,25-dihydroxyvitamin D, and renal function; measurement of calcium-regulating hormones is not routinely recommended unless hypocalcemia is prolonged, refractory, or recurrent.
- An electrocardiographic QTc interval longer than 0.4 second (because of prolonged systole) is an indicator of hypocalcemia and may help in monitoring therapy.

IMAGING STUDIES

Examine the chest radiograph for the thymic silhouette if DiGeorge syndrome is suspected.

TREATMENT

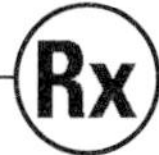

NONPHARMACOLOGIC THERAPY

- Early-onset neonatal hypocalcemia
  - Hypocalcemic preterm infants who have no clinical signs and are not ill from any other cause may not require specific treatment.
  - This condition often resolves spontaneously by day 3.

ACUTE GENERAL Rx

- Calcium preparations: Use a 10% solution of calcium gluconate (elemental calcium content of 9 mg/mL) for intravenous use or oral use; provide calcium supplementation at dosages of 30 to 75 mg of elemental calcium/kg/day (in four to six divided doses), titrated to the response of patient.
- Early-onset neonatal hypocalcemia
  - Ill infants or infants with severe hypocalcemia (serum calcium < 6 mg/dL, ionized calcium < 3 mg/dL) are usually treated.
- Late-onset neonatal hypocalcemia
  - In phosphorus-induced hypocalcemia, use a low-phosphorus formula (or human milk) and oral calcium supplementation to increase calcium and decrease phosphorus absorption.
  - Hypoparathyroidism requires therapy with vitamin D or one of its metabolites: 1,25-dihydroxyvitamin D (or 1α-hydroxyvitamin D_3, a synthetic analog).
- Treat hypocalcemic seizures, apnea, or tetany (serum calcium level is usually less than 5.0 to 6.0 mg/dL).

- Emergency calcium therapy
  - Use 1 to 2 mL of 10% calcium gluconate per kilogram of body weight, given by intravenous infusion over 10 minutes.
  - Monitor heart rate to avoid cardiac arrhythmia; calcium infusion should be temporally stopped if bradycardia occurs.
  - Monitor the infusion site to avoid skin necrosis. Repeat the dose in 10 minutes if no clinical response occurs.
- Maintenance calcium therapy
  - After the initial dose, maintenance calcium should be given parenterally or orally: 75 mg/kg/day for the first day, one half of the dose on the next day, one half again, and discontinue.
  - The duration of supplemental calcium therapy varies with the cause of hypocalcemia: 2 to 3 days for early hypocalcemia and possibly for lifetime for hypocalcemia caused by hypoparathyroidism or malabsorption.

- Symptomatic hypocalcemia unresponsive to calcium therapy may be caused by hypomagnesemia.
  - Use a 50% solution of magnesium sulfate (500 mg or 4 mEq/mL); administer 0.1 to 0.2 mL (50 to 100 mg)/kg intravenously (infuse slowly over 10 minutes) or intramuscularly (may cause local tissue necrosis).
  - Repeat the dose every 6 to 12 hours. Obtain a serum magnesium concentration before each dose.

CHRONIC Rx

Supplemental calcium and vitamin D metabolites may be required for a lifetime for hypocalcemia caused by hypoparathyroidism.

DISPOSITION

- In most cases, early neonatal hypocalcemia resolves within the first week of life.
- Prolonged hypocalcemia should prompt the physician to investigate other, more permanent causes.
- Regular follow-up monitoring of the serum calcium concentration and appropriate monitoring of underlying disease (e.g., PTH concentration) are necessary to watch for recurrence of hypocalcemia.

REFERRAL

A neonatologist, endocrinologist, or nephrologist may be consulted if the course is unusual or to manage differential considerations.

PEARLS & CONSIDERATIONS

COMMENTS

If neonatal hypocalcemia accompanies hypomagnesemia, hypocalcemia may not be corrected unless hypomagnesemia is first rectified.

PREVENTION

- Early neonatal hypocalcemia can be prevented in neonates at risk by oral and parenteral calcium supplementation (75 mg of elemental calcium/kg/day).
- Maintenance of normal maternal vitamin D status may secondarily prevent late hypocalcemia in some infants.
- Treatment should be used to prevent hypocalcemia for high-risk newborns who exhibit cardiovascular compromise and require cardiotonic drugs or blood pressure support.
  - Use a continuous calcium infusion by a central catheter to maintain a total calcium level higher than 8.0 mg/dL and an ionized calcium level higher than 4.0 mg/dL.
  - Commonly used dosages range from 20 to 75 mg/kg/day.
- The most effective prevention of neonatal hypocalcemia includes prevention of prematurity and birth asphyxia, judicious use of bicarbonate therapy, and minimization of the occurrence of respiratory alkalosis from excessive mechanical ventilation.

SUGGESTED READINGS

Demarini S et al: Disorders of calcium, phosphorus and magnesium metabolism. *In* Fanaroff AA, Martin RJ (eds): *Neonatal Perinatal Medicine: Diseases of the Fetus and Infant,* 7th ed. St. Louis, Mosby, 2001, pp 1376–1386.

Itani O, Tsang RC: Calcium, phosphorus, and magnesium in the newborn: pathophysiology and management. *In* Hay WW (eds): *Neonatal Nutrition and Metabolism.* St. Louis, Mosby, 1991, pp 171–202.

AUTHORS: **RAN NAMGUNG, MD, PHD** and **REGINALD TSANG, MBBS**

BASIC INFORMATION

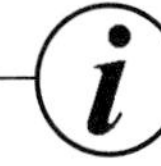

DEFINITION

Hypokalemia occurs when the serum potassium level is less than 3.5 mEq/L (normal is approximately 3.5 to 5.5 mEq/L).

ICD-9-CM CODE
276.8 Hypokalemia

EPIDEMIOLOGY & DEMOGRAPHICS

- The most common cause of hypokalemia is diuretic use.
- The epidemiologic and demographic features of hypokalemia correlate with the conditions causing it.

CLINICAL PRESENTATION

History

- Medication
- Dietary history and eating habits
- Fatigue or weakness (e.g., hypokalemic familial periodic paralysis, hypomagnesemia)
- Diarrhea
- Vomiting or ileus
- Nasogastric suction

Physical Examination

- Weight and height
- Cardiac arrhythmias: premature ventricular or atrial contractions, heart block ventricular tachycardia, ventricular fibrillation
- Decreased cardiac output and perfusion: severe hypokalemia
- Decreased bowel sounds from intestinal ileus
- Mental apathy
- Muscle weakness
- Ascending paralysis: associated with the syndrome of hypokalemic periodic paralysis

ETIOLOGY

- Decreased intake: anorexia nervosa, high-carbohydrate diet
- Increased renal or urinary losses
  - Diuretics (e.g., furosemide, thiazides), gentamicin, amphotericin, carbenicillin, corticosteroids
  - Hyperaldosteronism, adrenal adenomas, renin-producing tumors, Cushing's syndrome, licorice ingestion
  - Renovascular disease
  - Renal tubular disease: renal tubular acidosis, Fanconi's syndrome, chronic cystic renal disease, Bartter's syndrome, Gitelman's syndrome
  - Osmotic diuresis from glycosuria
  - Hypomagnesemia, hypochloremia
- Increased gastrointestinal losses
  - Diarrhea, malabsorption
  - Vomiting or nasogastric suction, including bulimia
  - Laxative abuse
  - Ileostomy
- Redistribution of potassium from extracellular or intravascular space to intracellular space
  - Endogenous catecholamines, exogenous β-agonists, including inhaled medications (e.g., albuterol)
  - Alkalemia
  - Increased insulin levels
- Malaria (severe)
- Trauma; brain injury

DIAGNOSIS

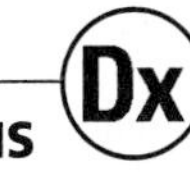

DIFFERENTIAL DIAGNOSIS

- Muscle weakness (see Hypotonia in Clinical Algorithms [Section III])
- Congestive heart failure and arrhythmia (see Congestive Heart Failure in Diseases and Disorders [Section I])
- Hypokalemia (see "Etiology")

WORKUP

- The whole-blood potassium level is somewhat lower than the serum potassium level.
- Electrocardiogram shows flattened or inverted T wave, U wave, ST-segment depression, and atrial and ventricular arrhythmias.
- Urine potassium analysis
  - Low level suggests total-body potassium depletion.
  - High level suggests renal potassium wasting.

TREATMENT

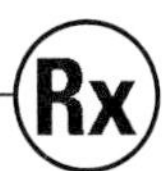

ACUTE GENERAL Rx

- Urgency of treatment depends on the level of serum potassium, the rate of potassium loss, the number of risk factors present for cardiac arrhythmias or neurologic abnormalities, and the physical signs and symptoms caused by hypokalemia.
- The presence of signs or symptoms suggests that immediate and aggressive treatment is necessary.
  - Cardiac arrhythmias
  - Muscle weakness (lower extremities, then upper extremities and respiratory muscles)
- The absence of symptoms but a high number of risk factors suggests that rapid treatment is required:
  - With use of potassium-depleting diuretics, especially furosemide, because even one dose can cause significant kaliuresis within 1 hour of administration
  - Ongoing significant gastrointestinal losses
  - Association with other electrolyte abnormalities, such as hypomagnesemia, hypophosphatemia, hypocalcemia, or hypochloremia
  - Intrinsic cardiac conduction abnormalities, such as prolonged QT syndrome
  - Myocarditis or cardiomyopathy (especially dilated)
  - Low potassium levels within the first few days after cardiac surgery, especially after cardiopulmonary bypass or ventriculotomy
  - Digoxin
  - Known history of hypokalemic periodic paralysis
- The absence of symptoms and risk factors suggests that correction may be done less emergently.
- If risk factors (especially cardiac) are present and the serum potassium level is less than 3.0 mEq/L (<3.5 if immediately preoperative or postoperative for cardiac surgery), do the following:
  - Place patient on a cardiac monitor.
  - Increase the concentration of potassium in maintenance fluids to 40 mEq/L (peripherally) and up to 100 mEq/L centrally.
  - Immediately administer 1 mEq/kg of potassium chloride enterally.
    - Administer 40 mEq per dose maximum.
    - The enteral route preferable because fewer potential arrhythmogenic side effects occur and absorption is almost as rapid (within 1 hour) as giving potassium intravenously over 1 hour.
  - If the enteral route is not possible (e.g., ileus, emesis), administer 0.5 mEq/kg up to a maximum of 20 mEq of potassium chloride intravenously over 1 hour.
    - Peripherally, use a concentration of less than 40 mEq/L to avoid the potential for serious infiltration and injury.
    - When risk factors are present and in the absence of a central line but with an extremely well-functioning intravenous line, higher concentrations may be needed because of volume considerations.
    - Centrally, up to a concentration of 100 mEq/L (0.1 mEq/mL) of potassium chloride may be used.
  - Check the potassium level 1 hour after infusion is complete or 2 hours after enteral administration, and repeat as necessary until the potassium level is within 3.0 to 3.5 mEq/L.
  - Hold diuretics until the potassium concentration is corrected to greater than 3.0 mEq/L.
  - Avoid alkalemia.
  - Correct other electrolyte abnormalities, especially magnesium and chloride levels.
- If no risk factors or signs and symptoms are present and the serum potassium level is higher than 3.0 mEq/L, use oral medications and a high-potassium diet.
  - Medications: Various preparations are available in liquid, tablet, or capsule formulations.
    - The starting dose in a low-risk situation is 1 to 2 mEq/kg/24 hours divided twice daily.
    - Use up to 10 to 20 mEq twice daily.
  - Consider potassium-sparing diuretics (e.g., spironolactone, amiloride) if required.
  - Dietary intake should include potassium-rich foods (e.g., prune juice, tomato juice, orange juice, grape juice, bananas [1 mEq of potassium/inch]).

DISPOSITION

Follow-up with frequent serum potassium determinations is imperative until the patient is stable, especially if the underlying cause has not been resolved.

REFERRAL

Consider endocrinologic, metabolic, and renal consultations based on the underlying cause.

PEARLS & CONSIDERATIONS

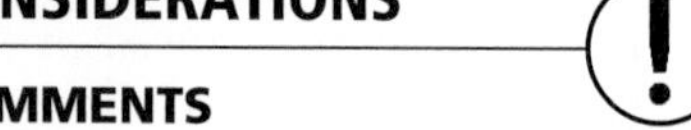

COMMENTS

- Administration of potassium supplements in a patient with intestinal ileus or poor intestinal motility may result in acute hyperkalemia (caused by sudden absorption of the previously administered, accumulated potassium) when the ileus or dysmotility is resolved.
- If potassium chloride infiltrates a peripheral vein, hyaluronidase should be infiltrated into the area to minimize tissue injury.
- Because a significant risk of arrhythmias exists, a cardiac monitor should always be used while infusing a potassium bolus into a central vein or catheter. Serial boluses should not be administered in rapid succession without measuring the serum potassium level between doses.
- If the serum chloride level is low, the potassium concentration will be difficult to replete. Replete chloride aggressively along with potassium supplementation. Arginine chloride may be needed.

PATIENT/FAMILY EDUCATION

- Educate the patient and family about the importance of compliance with oral potassium preparations, especially if taking multiple diuretics.
- Educate the patient and family about potassium-rich foods. This may require a nutrition consultation.

SUGGESTED READINGS

Brem AS: Disorders of potassium homeostasis. *Pediatr Clin North Am* 37:419, 1990.

Cronan KM, Norman ME: Renal and electrolyte emergencies. *In* Fleisher GR, Ludwig SL (eds): *Textbook of Pediatric Emergency Medicine,* 4th ed. Philadelphia, Lippincott Williams & Wilkins, 2000.

Wood EG, Lynch RE: Fluids and electrolyte balance. *In* Fuhrman BP, Zimmerman JJ (eds): *Pediatric Critical Care,* 2nd ed. St Louis, Mosby, 1998.

AUTHOR: **ELISE W. VAN DER JAGT, MD, MPH**

BASIC INFORMATION

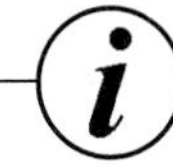

DEFINITION

Hyponatremia is present when the serum sodium concentration is less than 130 mEq/L (130 mmol/L), although some would consider a value less than 135 to be hyponatremic. Normal range generally falls between 133 to 146 mEq/L, with some variability dependent on individual laboratories.

SYNONYMS

Hyponatremia is not synonymous with *hypotonic* or *hyposmolar.* Patients with hyponatremia may be isotonic, hypotonic, or hypertonic depending on other solutes in the extracellular space that cannot traverse the cell membrane.

ICD-9-CM CODE
276.1 Hyponatremia

EPIDEMIOLOGY & DEMOGRAPHICS

- Hyponatremia is most commonly associated with dehydration secondary to gastroenteritis, especially from rotavirus.
- In hospitalized patients, it is the most common electrolyte disturbance (3% to 6%). It is often related to the following conditions:
  - Excess antidiuretic hormone (ADH) secretion secondary to surgery, pain, and mechanical ventilation
  - Excess use of relatively hypotonic intravenous fluid administration
  - Diuretic therapy
  - Third-space losses (e.g., peritonitis, pancreatitis, ascites)

CLINICAL PRESENTATION

History

- Diarrhea
- Nausea and vomiting
  - Central nervous system disease
  - Gastroenteritis
  - Adrenal disease/insufficiency
  - Renal disease
- Type and quantity of fluid intake (low salt content?)
- Amount of urine output
  - High urine output in the face of hyponatremia suggests physiologic correcting of fluid overload with associated:
    - Dilutional hyponatremia
    - Salt wasting from renal, adrenal, or cerebral disease
    - Diuretic therapy
  - Low urine output in the face of hyponatremia suggests an excess of ADH resulting in a dilutional hyponatremia or hyponatremic dehydration with an attempt to preserve intravascular volume
- Weight loss/gain
- Neurologic symptoms
  - Headache
  - Altered sensorium
  - Lethargy or coma
  - Seizures
- Muscle weakness and cramps
- Medications (e.g., furosemide, thiazides)
- Hyperlipidemia

Physical Examination

- State of hydration
  - Fluid deficit: tachycardia, decreased pulses, decreased capillary refill, decreased distal extremity temperature, decreased skin turgor, decreased blood pressure, dry mucous membranes
  - Fluid overload: edema, puffy eyelids, moist mucous membranes, hypertension
- Weight (compare with a previous weight if known)
- Anterior fontanelle: sunken, flat, or bulging
- Respiratory rate: tachypnea (seen with fever, acidosis, congestive heart failure, fluid overload, respiratory disease)
- Fever: infection
- Neurologic: obtunded, lethargic, hyperreflexia or hyporeflexia, muscle weakness, seizures

ETIOLOGY

- Sodium losses
  - Gastrointestinal
    - Secretory and nonsecretory diarrhea
    - Ileostomy
  - Renal disease
    - Tubular dysfunction
    - Postobstructive uropathy
    - Polyuric renal failure, chronic renal disease
    - Heavy metal poisoning
  - Hypoadrenalism with salt wasting
    - Congenital adrenal hyperplasia
    - Addison's disease
    - Hypoaldosteronism
  - Cerebral salt wasting
  - Diabetic ketoacidosis, hyperglycemia with secondary urinary sodium losses
  - Excessive skin losses
    - Cystic fibrosis
    - Heat exhaustion
  - Third-space losses
    - Peritonitis
    - Burn edema
    - Postsurgery
  - Diuretics
    - Furosemide
    - Thiazides
    - Potassium-sparing (e.g., spironolactone)
    - Mannitol
- Increased intravascular or total body water
  - Excessive oral or intravenous administration of hyponatremic fluids
    - Inappropriate formula mixing
    - Psychogenic
    - Forced water intoxication
    - Medical error/miscalculation
  - Syndrome of inappropriate antidiuretic hormone secretion (SIADH)
  - Hyperglycemia
    - Intravascular osmolar substance attracts water and thus results in hyponatremia (dilutional effect) with sodium decreasing by 1 to 2 mEq/L for every 100 mg/dL glucose.
    - Once the hyperglycemia overrides the renal threshold, glycosuria with water loss and eventual total body water depletion occurs.
  - Severe pulmonary disease
    - Asthma
    - Pneumonia
    - Bronchiolitis
  - Congestive heart failure
  - Oliguric renal failure
  - Liver failure
  - Medications (DDAVP [1-deamino-8-D-arginine-vasopressin])
  - Hypothyroidism
- Inadequate intake (dietary salt restriction)
- Artificially low
  - High blood lipid content
  - High blood protein content

DIAGNOSIS

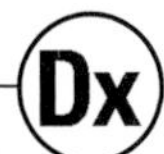

DIFFERENTIAL DIAGNOSIS

See "Etiology"

WORKUP

- Obtain serum sodium
- Obtain blood urea nitrogen (BUN), creatinine, chloride, potassium, bicarbonate, and glucose
- Obtain urine specific gravity, pH, sodium, potassium, and creatinine
  - High urine sodium (>40 mEq/L) suggests the following:
    - Volume overload
    - Adrenal insufficiency
    - Renal tubular dysfunction
    - Renal failure
    - Cerebral salt wasting
    - Increased ADH, SIADH
    - Diuretic use (e.g., furosemide, thiazides)
  - Low urine sodium (<20 mEq/L) suggests the following:
    - Inadequate circulating blood volume with secondary aldosterone secretion
    - Absolute sodium deficit from lack of intake or excess gastrointestinal or skin losses
    - Primary hyperaldosteronism
    - Spironolactone use
- Fractional excretion of sodium:

$$\frac{(U_{Na} \times P_{Cr})}{(P_{Na} \times U_{Cr})} \times 100$$

  - Fractional excretion of sodium less than 1% suggests a prerenal cause or absolute deficit of sodium.
  - Fractional excretion of sodium more than 2% suggests renal or adrenal disease.

TREATMENT

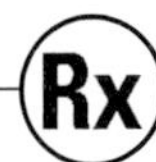

ACUTE GENERAL Rx

- If seizures or coma are present and sodium is less than 125 mEq/L, give 3% saline.
  - Calculate mEq sodium to give (125 − serum sodium) × (weight in kg) × 0.6.

  - Give over 4 hours and preferably in a central line or large peripheral intravenous administration (3% saline has very high osmolarity and may cause tissue necrosis if it infiltrates).
- If patient is hyponatremic from water overload, restrict water and give furosemide (water greater than sodium loss).
- If renal failure, may require dialysis or oral sorbitol administration to induce diarrhea with sodium losses.
- If dehydrated and sodium is 120 to 130 mEq/L without neurologic deficits, make up deficit fluids in 24 hours (one half in first 8 hours and remainder in next 16 hours) using normal saline to replace the sodium deficit and maintenance sodium requirements.
- If sodium is less than 120 mEq/L and has decreased over longer than 48 hours, correct sodium no faster than 10 to 12 mEq/24 hours.
- If sodium is less than 120 mEq/L and has decreased over less than 48 hours, may correct more rapidly.
- Monitor for neurologic deterioration if sodium is less than 125 mEq/L and has occurred acutely over 48 hours.

DISPOSITION

- Neurologic intensive monitoring is not required when sodium is higher than 125 mEq/L.
- The cause must be determined so that hyponatremia does not recur.

REFERRAL

Hospitalization and potential intensive care setting should be considered for the following:

- Serum sodium less than 125 mEq/L
- Hyponatremia associated with any neurologic symptoms
- Hyponatremia and renal failure
- Hyponatremia and more than 10% dehydration
- Hyponatremia and any disease that requires frequent monitoring of cardiovascular, neurologic, renal, or respiratory systems

PEARLS & CONSIDERATIONS

COMMENTS

- Urine sodium, specific gravity, osmolality, and serum BUN and osmolality provide the critical information for making an etiologic diagnosis of hyponatremia.
- Strict attention to type and exact amount of input and output of fluids in hospitalized patients is critical for preventing iatrogenic hyponatremia, especially in very young patients.

PREVENTION

- Careful evaluation of fluid balance—intake and output.
- Careful monitoring of urine output for patients at risk for SIADH.
- Proper intravenous and oral fluid administration (containing sufficient sodium). Some have recommended increasing the sodium content of maintenance fluids as a preventive measure in hospitalized patients
- Avoidance of the administration of large volumes of low sodium fluids rapidly. If rapid fluid resuscitation is necessary, isotonic saline or lactated Ringer's solution should be used.

PATIENT/FAMILY EDUCATION

- Proper formula mixing
- Side effects of diuretics
- Information about underlying illness or disease process

SUGGESTED READINGS

Berry PL, Belsha CW: Hyponatremia. *Pediatr Clin North Am* 37:35, 1990.

Cronan K, Norman ME: Renal and electrolyte emergencies. *In* Fleisher GR, Ludwig G (eds): *Textbook of Pediatric Emergency Medicine,* 4th ed. Philadelphia, Lippincott Williams & Wilkins, 2000.

Gruskin AB, Sarnaik A: Hyponatremia: pathophysiology and treatment—a pediatric perspective. *Pediatr Nephrol* 6:280, 1992.

Hoorn EJ et al: Acute hyponatremia related to intravenous fluid administration in hospitalized children: an observational study. *Pediatrics* 113:1279, 2004.

Subramanian S, Ziedalski T: Oliguria, volume overload, Na balance and diuretics. *Crit Care Clin* 21:291, 2005.

Wood EG, Lynch RE: Fluids and electrolyte balance. *In* Fuhrman BP, Zimmerman JJ (eds): *Pediatric Critical Care,* 2nd ed. St. Louis, Mosby, 1998.

AUTHOR: **ELISE W. VAN DER JAGT, MD, MPH**

BASIC INFORMATION

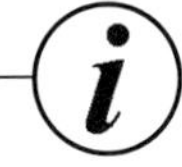

DEFINITIONS

- Hypothermia is a reduction of core body temperature to 35°C (89°F) or lower. Hypothermia may be divided into mild (core temperature 32°C to 35°C), moderate (28°C to 32°C), and severe (<28°C).
- Frostbite is the actual freezing of tissue, and may be divided into superficial and deep forms.

SYNONYMS

Cold injury is a general term encompassing hypothermia, frostbite, frostnip, immersion foot (trench foot), and chilblains (pernio).

ICD-9-CM CODES

Frostbite of the: Face (991.0), Hand (991.1), Foot (991.2), Other/unspecified (991.3)
991.4 Immersion foot
991.5 Chilblains
991.6 Hypothermia
991.8 Other specified effects of reduced temperature
991.9 Other unspecified effects of reduced temperature

EPIDEMIOLOGY & DEMOGRAPHICS

- Often associated with outdoor activities.
- May complicate injury, especially multiple trauma and near-drowning.
- The homeless are at increased risk, as are those with mental illness or intoxication.
- Frostbite is more common in males, probably reflecting behavioral rather than biological differences.
- Incidence varies by geographic location and season.

CLINICAL PRESENTATION

History

- Usually obvious—exposure to cold environment.

Hypothermia

- May be missed, especially in association with other injury, such as multiple trauma.
- More subtle complaints include dizziness, confusion/poor judgment, mood changes, or irritability seen in very young or old.
- May present with unresponsiveness, coma, or cardiac arrest of unknown etiology.

Frostbite

- Initial complaints include a feeling of cold and thickness, usually in an extremity, which then becomes associated with numbness. At this point, the injury is termed *frostnip*; rewarming will cause tingling in the affected area, and will prevent permanent injury.
- Without rewarming, numbness and cold may become associated with a stinging or burning sensation, which diminishes as a feeling of clumsiness or absence of the limb develops, and frostbite occurs.

Physical Examination

Hypothermia

- Accurate temperature recording may be problematic because many thermometers do not accurately record low body temperatures.
  - Ideally, use a rectal thermometer designed for a wide range of temperatures, the end of which should not be buried in cold stool.
  - Bladder or esophageal temperature probes may also be used.
- Bradycardia or other dysrhythmias are common in moderate to severe hypothermia.
- Bradypnea may be appropriate because metabolic demands are diminished.
- Coma and apparent lifelessness, including absent cardiac activity and respiratory effort, may be present in severe hypothermia.
- At 34°C to 35°C, vigorous shivering is seen. Shivering ceases below 30°C to 32°C, as glycogen stores are depleted (may occur earlier in small children).
- Central nervous system changes, such as amnesia and dysarthria, develop as core temperature falls below 33°C. These progress to ataxia, apathy, and stupor as temperature continues to fall.

Frostbite

- Superficial injury: waxy, edematous skin may be erythematous, with firm white plaques and decreased sensation. Clear blisters form, which reach the distal portion of the affected extremity.
- Deep injury: absent sensation and hemorrhagic blister formation occur.

ETIOLOGY

Hypothermia and frostbite are the result of exposure to conditions resulting in excessive heat loss.

- This may be a body of water, such as with near drowning.
  - Hypothermia may also be the result of abnormal control of body temperature, seen in such conditions as sepsis, hypothyroidism, hypopituitarism, and hypoadrenalism. Infants are at relatively higher risk for hypothermia, as are those with immature or inappropriate behavioral response to the cold.
  - Hypothermia and frostbite may be the result of inflicted injury (child abuse), such as punishment by cold exposure, or neglect.

DIAGNOSIS

Dx

DIFFERENTIAL DIAGNOSIS

- Immersion foot (trench foot) is the result of prolonged exposure to cold, wet conditions. Its course and treatment are generally similar to those of frostbite.
- Chilblains (pernio) is localized skin changes, such as erythema, cyanosis, plaques, and nodules, as a result of chronic cold exposure. Treatment is supportive.
- Stroke or toxic ingestions (barbiturate, benzodiazepine, or cocaine) can mimic the altered mental status of severe hypothermia.

WORKUP

Frostbite and mild hypothermia do not require diagnostic testing.

LABORATORY TESTS

Moderate to severe hypothermia may need laboratory testing for monitoring treatment.

- Arterial blood gas: reflects overall acid-base and respiratory status.
- Glucose: hypoglycemia may precipitate or complicate hypothermia.
- Complete blood cell count/platelet count, prothrombin time/partial thromboplastin time, fibrinogen level: may reveal hemoconcentration and disseminated intravascular coagulation; low fibrinogen is associated with poorer outcomes. Hematocrit increases 2% for every 1°C drop in temperature.
- Urinalysis: for myoglobinuria.
- Electrolyte panel: serum potassium greater than 10 mEq/L predicts poor outcome.
- Electrocardiogram (ECG), continuous cardiorespiratory monitoring
  - ECG may show a characteristic "J" or "Osborne" wave, a positive deflection immediately following the R wave.
  - Dysrhythmias are commonly seen in severely hypothermic patients.
    - Atrial dysrhythmias are often benign.
    - Asystole or ventricular fibrillation can also occur.
- Consider toxicology screen.

IMAGING STUDIES

- Consider cervical spine imaging.
- Consider chest radiograph.

TREATMENT

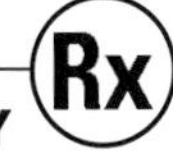

ACUTE GENERAL THERAPY

- Treatment of hypothermia takes priority over treatment of frostbite!
  - Carefully remove cold, wet clothing.
  - Wet skin should be carefully dried.

Hypothermia

- Although the patient may appear lifeless, resuscitative efforts, including cardiopulmonary resuscitation (CPR) , should generally be continued until the temperature is at least 30°C to 32°C.
- Severely hypothermic patients should be handled gently, as even minor jostling may precipitate dysrhythmias.
- Obtunded or unresponsive patients should undergo gentle endotracheal intubation.
- Asystole or ventricular fibrillation (seen at core temperatures below 25°C) should be

treated with CPR. Intravenous drugs are generally ineffective at temperatures below 30°C; bretylium (10 mg/kg) is probably the most effective drug for treatment of ventricular fibrillation in hypothermia. Defibrillation of the hypothermic patient is often ineffective, but may be attempted.

- Mild hypothermia: passive external rewarming (warm environment, insulated blankets) or active external rewarming (truncal application of warm packs or warmed blankets); avoid thermal injury to damaged skin.
- Moderate hypothermia: core rewarming is needed: warmed intravenous fluids (normal saline not lactated Ringer's solution) (replaces old-induced diuresis and third-spacing); warm, humidified oxygen (40°C to 42°C); consider warm peritoneal, gastric, bladder, rectal, or thoracic lavage.
- Severe hypothermia: cardiopulmonary bypass with extracorporeal rewarming, as well as warmed oxygen and IV fluids.
- Hypoglycemia should be treated with IV glucose.
- If sepsis is suspected, broad-spectrum antibiotics should be administered.
- Endocrine insufficiency may require hormonal supplementation.

Frostbite

- Rubbing or application of snow should be avoided. Do not use hair dryers or heaters.
- Rapidly rewarm by immersion of extremity in warm (38°C to 43°C) water bath, usually for 20 to 30 minutes, longer if fully frozen. This should wait until core body temperature is at least 32°C. Thawing takes 20 to 40 minutes for superficial frostbite and up to 1 hour for deep injuries.
- Clear blisters should be debrided, but hemorrhagic blisters should be left intact.
- Tetanus immunization status should be updated if necessary.
- Wound infection is common; consider administration of broad-spectrum antibiotics.
- Intense pain on rewarming is common; analgesia will be needed.
- Amputation should be delayed until devitalized tissue is clearly demarcated.
- Involve a surgeon (for fasciotomy) if compartment syndrome is suspected.

CHRONIC Rx

- Frostbite may affect growth plates, leading to bone growth abnormalities, requiring orthopedic referral.
- Sensory changes, including increased sensitivity to cold, may be lifelong.

COMPLEMENTARY & ALTERNATIVE MEDICINE

- Apply aloe vera cream every 6 hours to affected areas.

DISPOSITION

- Discharge home. Survival is usually complete in healthy patients (mortality rate < 5 %).

REFERRAL

- Patients with moderate to severe hypothermia or deep frostbite may be best managed at a pediatric referral center with critical care, burn unit, and surgical support.

PEARLS & CONSIDERATIONS

COMMENTS

- "No one is dead until they are warm and dead." Clinical evidence has shown excellent full neurologic recovery even after cardiac arrest.
- External active rewarming should be applied to the trunk only, avoiding extremities.
- External rewarming of the moderately to severely hypothermic patient may make matters *worse.*
- *Avoid* gradual rewarming of frostbitten extremities; further tissue damage may result. Partial thawing followed by refreezing is even worse.
- When giving warmed (42°C to 44°C) intravenous fluids, avoid lactated Ringer's solution, which is poorly metabolized by the hypothermic liver. Normal saline or dextrose 5% normal saline is preferred. To warm, place 1 L bag in microwave for 1 to 2 minutes on "high" setting; mix thoroughly.

PREVENTION

- Appropriate clothing, along with avoidance of drugs/alcohol, when encountering cold conditions.
- Eyes, testicles, and nipples should be protected to prevent frostbite of these sensitive areas.
- Awareness of signs and symptoms and survival packs for those involved in winter sports (i.e., hiking, skiing, camping).

PATIENT/FAMILY EDUCATION

- Information for parents. Available at http://www.kidshealth.org/parent/firstaid/frostbite.html
- Hypothermia. Available at http://mayoclinic.com/health/hypothermia/DS00333

SUGGESTED READINGS

Cheng D: Frostbite. *In* Simon HK (ed): *Emedicine: Emergency Medicine.* Boston, Boston Medical Publishing, 2004. Available at http://www.emedicine.com/ped/topic803.htm

Decker W: Hypothermia. *In* Adler J (ed): *Emedicine: Emergency Medicine.* Boston, Boston Medical Publishing, 1998. Available at http://www.emedicine.com/emerg/topic279.htm

Decker W: Hypothermia. *In* Danzl D (ed): *Emedicine: Emergency Medicine.* Boston, Boston Medical Publishing, 2001. Available at http://www.emedicine.com/emerg/topic279.htm

Hofstrand HJ: Accidental hypothermia and frostbite. *In* Barkin RM (ed): *Pediatric Emergency Medicine: Concepts and Clinical Practice,* 2nd ed. St. Louis, Mosby, 1997, pp 500–510.

Mechem CC: Frostbite. *In* Adler J (ed): *Emedicine: Emergency Medicine.* Boston, Boston Medical Publishing, 1998. Available at http://www.emedicine.com/emerg/topic209.htm

AUTHORS: **GREGORY P. CONNERS, MD, MPH, MBA, FAAP** and **MADELYN GARCIA, MD**

BASIC INFORMATION

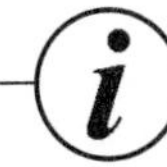

DEFINITION

Hypothyroidism is an abnormally low level of circulating thyroid hormones (i.e., thyroxine [T_4] and triiodothyronine [T_3]) resulting in various clinical manifestations.

SYNONYMS

Acquired hypothyroidism (immune mediated)
Autoimmune thyroiditis
Chronic lymphocytic thyroiditis
Hashimoto thyroiditis
Congenital hypothyroidism
Cretinism (archaic term used to describe clinical constellation of mental and physical developmental delays resulting from untreated congenital hypothyroidism)

ICD-9-CM CODES
243.00 Congenital hypothyroidism
245.2 Hashimoto's thyroiditis

EPIDEMIOLOGY & DEMOGRAPHICS

- Congenital form: 1 case in 3000 to 4000 births
- Usually sporadic, except in dyshormonogenesis
- Autoimmune form: about 2% prevalence among U.S. teenagers, with peak incidence in early to middle puberty
- Female-to-male ratio is 2:1 in adolescence (10:1 in adults); higher in patients with Turner and Down syndrome and those with type 1 diabetes mellitus

CLINICAL PRESENTATION

History

- Symptoms of clinical hypothyroidism include the following:
  - Poor energy level
  - Constipation
  - Cold intolerance
  - Weight gain
  - Reduced appetite
  - Paleness
  - Change in school performance
- Thyroid enlargement may occur, especially in Hashimoto's thyroiditis.
- In infants, symptoms of clinical hypothyroidism include the following:
  - Delayed development and poor growth if untreated
  - Prolonged hyperbilirubinemia, feeding difficulties, delayed stooling

Physical Examination

- Signs of clinical hypothyroidism in newborns and infants (may be subtle or absent)
  - Poor linear growth
  - Poor weight gain
  - Relative bradycardia
  - Large anterior and posterior fontanelles
  - Large tongue
  - Hoarse cry
  - Umbilical hernia
  - Facial puffiness
  - Jaundice (unconjugated hyperbilirubinemia)
- Signs of clinical hypothyroidism in children and adolescents
  - Poor linear growth
  - Bradycardia
  - Excessive weight gain (rarely extreme)
  - Dry skin
  - Paleness
  - Lethargy
  - Slow relaxation phase of deep tendon reflexes (test at Achilles tendon)
- Thyroid examination in congenital cases
  - Usually, no thyroid tissue palpable with dysgenesis
  - Goiter with dyshormonogenesis (may not be present at birth)
  - Lingual thyroid may be present (ectopic)
- Thyroid examination in cases of Hashimoto's thyroiditis
  - Goiter with cobblestone surface (bosselation)
  - May have no palpable tissue if late in process
  - Initially, gland may be smooth and soft but later becomes firm or hard

ETIOLOGY

- Congenital disease
  - About 85% of cases are associated with dysgenesis (i.e., abnormal gland formation) or with an ectopic gland (i.e., lack of normal migration). Thyroid gland dysgenesis occurs mostly sporadically, with only 2% caused by known specific gene defects.
  - Between 10% and 15% have a hormonogenesis defect inherited in an autosomal recessive pattern.
  - Five percent are central (pituitary or hypothalamic).
- Acquired disease
  - Hashimoto's thyroiditis is T-cell autoimmune-mediated destruction of the thyroid gland.
  - Other non-autoimmune forms of hypothyroidism include the following:
    - Exposure to neck irradiation
    - Neck surgery
    - Low dietary intake of iodine
    - Excessive intake of goitrogens (e.g., Brassica family of vegetables)
    - Antithyroid medications (e.g., propylthiouracil [PTU], methimazole)

DIAGNOSIS Dx

DIFFERENTIAL DIAGNOSIS

- Primary (i.e., thyroid underactivity) acquired forms
  - Hashimoto's thyroiditis (chronic lymphocytic thyroiditis)
  - Iodine deficiency
  - Iatrogenic radiation-induced hypothyroidism
  - Surgical removal of thyroid
- Primary (i.e., thyroid underactivity) congenital forms
  - Transient hypothyroidism from transplacental passage of maternal blocking antibodies (i.e., maternal autoimmune thyroid disease)
  - Transient from maternal use of antithyroid medications (i.e., PTU or methimazole)
- Rarely, secondary or tertiary hypothyroidism (i.e., pituitary or hypothalamic, respectively) from pituitary or central nervous system tumors or from pituitary or hypothalamic malformation or destruction

LABORATORY TESTS

- Thyroid function tests for congenital and acquired forms include the following:
  - Thyroid-stimulating hormone (TSH) determination alone is generally sufficient for screening for primary hypothyroidism, and the level should be elevated, often markedly.
  - The level of free (or total) T_4 should be measured if a secondary (pituitary) or tertiary (hypothalamic) pathologic condition is suspected or possible.
- The TSH level may be low in secondary hypothyroid states or low, normal, or slightly elevated in tertiary (hypothalamic) states. It is therefore not useful as the sole test in this situation.
- Anti-thyroid antibodies (anti-thyroglobulin and anti-peroxidase) are helpful in confirming the autoimmune nature of thyroiditis in acquired hypothyroidism.
- Newborn screening programs using dried blood spots collected at 24 to 48 hours of age are routine in almost all industrialized countries.
  - In the United States, the primary screen most commonly measures TSH values in all infants or selected infants with total T_4 values below a certain threshold.
  - These programs, initiated in the 1970s, have dramatically reduced the incidence of mental retardation associated with unrecognized congenital hypothyroidism because hypothyroid infants were rarely diagnosed clinically before several months of age.

IMAGING STUDIES

- Thyroid scan (i.e., technetium 99m or iodine 123) or Doppler ultrasound in cases of congenital hypothyroidism is used to detect an ectopic gland. This is not needed in all babies because treatment is instituted based on thyroid function test results.
- Ultrasound usually is not needed in cases of acquired hypothyroidism from Hashimoto's thyroiditis, but scans are often obtained for patients presenting with goiter. In this case, ultrasound reveals a heterogeneous thyroid corresponding to intrathyroidal lymphoid follicles.

TREATMENT

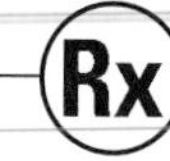

NONPHARMACOLOGIC THERAPY

Therapy consists of dietary iodine supplementation in areas where endemic goiters occur as a result of nutritional iodine deficiency.

ACUTE GENERAL Rx

- The dose of synthetic L-thyroxine or T_4 (e.g., Synthroid, Levoxyl) is 75 to 100 μg/m^2/day for children and adolescents. The initial dose of L-thyroxine for congenital hypothyroidism is 10 to 15 μg/kg/day. T_4 levels should be normalized as rapidly as possible.
- T_3 (e.g., Cytomel) is used only in special circumstances.
- Desiccated thyroid preparations are antiquated and are not recommended. There is no good clinical evidence that combinations of T_4 and T_3, as found in desiccated preparations, are superior to T_4 alone when used in the treatment of children.

DISPOSITION

- Congenital hypothyroidism requires very close follow-up with frequent thyroid function testing.
- The American Academy of Pediatrics and the American Thyroid Association recommend repeat testing of T_4 and TSH levels on the following schedule:
  - Between 2 and 4 weeks after initiation of therapy
  - Every 1 to 2 months during the first year of life
  - Every 2 to 3 months from age 1 to 3 years
  - Then every 3 to 12 months until growth is completed
  - After 2 to 3 years of age, a trial off therapy for infants believed to have had transient hypothyroidism
- Acquired hypothyroidism can usually be managed adequately by again measuring TSH and free T_4 levels at 4 to 6 weeks after initiation of therapy (and after dose changes) and then every 6 months during the growing years or every 6 to 12 months in older adolescents.

REFERRAL

- All patients with severe congenital hypothyroidism should be managed, if possible, by a pediatric endocrinologist in the first several years of life because of the possibility of developmental problems if they are not treated optimally.
- Uncomplicated cases of Hashimoto's thyroiditis can be treated in the primary care setting by physicians familiar with thyroid replacement therapy.
- Premature infants may have thyroid function test results that are more difficult to interpret, and they preferably should be managed by those with experience in this area.

PEARLS & CONSIDERATIONS

COMMENTS

- Soy formula can significantly impede thyroid hormone absorption and should be avoided.
- Newborn infants should not have thyroid function tests during the first 24 hours of life because the postnatal surge in TSH immediately after birth complicates interpretation of thyroid function results.
- Because of the wide range of normal free or total T_4 values and the sensitivity of TSH to small changes in thyroid hormone levels, an individual with an elevated TSH level can be hypothyroid despite normal population range of thyroid hormone levels.

PREVENTION

- Iodine supplementation (usually in salt) effectively prevents hypothyroidism resulting from iodine deficiency in persons living in iodine-deficient areas.
- In families with multiple first-degree relatives with autoimmune thyroid disease, screening with TSH and anti-thyroid antibodies may identify affected children early in course of disease.

PATIENT/FAMILY EDUCATION

- Thyroid replacement should ideally be taken on an empty stomach and should not be taken with iron or soy products.
- Missed doses can be made up by doubling the dose the next day.
- Any change in clinical status in a patient receiving replacement therapy suggestive of hypothyroidism or hyperthyroidism should prompt communication with the physician, and thyroid function tests should be repeated.

SUGGESTED READINGS

Brown R, Larsen PR: Thyroid gland development and disease in infancy and childhood. *In* DeGroot LJ, Hennemann G (eds): *The Thyroid and Its Diseases,* 1999. Online text available at www.thyroidmanager.org/Chapter15/15-frame.htm

Fisher DA: Thyroid disorders in childhood and adolescence. *In* Sperling MA (ed): *Pediatric Endocrinology.* Philadelphia, WB Saunders, 2002, pp 187–209.

Ogilvy-Stuart AL: Neonatal thyroid disorders: a review. *Arch Dis Child* 87:F165, 2002.

AUTHOR: **CRAIG ORLOWSKI, MD**

BASIC INFORMATION

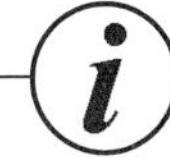

DEFINITION

Thrombocytopenia is caused by an antibody-mediated destruction of platelets. Children typically present with signs and symptoms of mucocutaneous bleeding. Idiopathic thrombocytopenic purpura (ITP) can be acute (resolves within 6 months) or chronic (persists longer than 6 months).

SYNONYMS

Autoimmune thrombocytopenic purpura
Immune thrombocytopenic purpura
Werlhof's disease

ICD-9-CM CODE
287.3 Immune thrombocytopenic purpura

EPIDEMIOLOGY & DEMOGRAPHICS

- The peak age of acute ITP is 2 to 4 years, but it can occur at any age.
- The annual incidence is 4 to 8 per 100,000 population.
- The male-to-female ratio is 1:1 in childhood and 1:3 in adolescence.
- A slight increase occurs in winter and spring.
- Most cases in children (80% to 90%) resolve within 6 to 12 months.
- Chronic ITP is more common in children older than 10 years (especially girls) or younger than 1 year of age.

CLINICAL PRESENTATION

History

- A relatively short history (days to weeks) of easy bruising or petechiae is reported in a child who is otherwise healthy.
- Minimal or no trauma is associated with bruises.
- Less commonly, children present with epistaxis, prolonged menses, hematuria, or gastrointestinal bleeding.
- Two thirds of children have a history of an antecedent viral illness in the month before presentation.
- No other systemic or constitutional illnesses are present.

Physical Examination

- General: well-appearing child, normal vital signs
- Skin
  - Bruises (large and small)
  - Sometimes palpable hematomas
  - Petechiae
- Mucus membranes ("wet" purpura): palatal/buccal petechiae, subconjunctival or retinal hemorrhage
- No lymphadenopathy or hepatosplenomegaly

ETIOLOGY

- Antibody-mediated destruction of platelets occurs.
- Antibody-coated platelets are removed by the reticuloendothelial system, especially the spleen.
- Acute ITP is associated with a recent viral illness in two thirds of cases.
  - Acute ITP can be caused by specific viral infections, such as Epstein-Barr virus (EBV), human immunodeficiency virus (HIV), or varicella.
- Many children with chronic ITP have autoantibody to platelet antigens, such as glycoprotein (GP) IIbIIIa or GP IbIX, and thus have true autoimmune disease.
- ITP may be associated with other autoimmune disorders, such as lupus, Evans syndrome, and antiphospholipid antibody syndrome.
- ITP may be caused by certain medications: carbamazepine, valproate, quinidine, heparin.
- ITP is also associated with recent vaccinations (e.g., measles-mumps-rubella, tetanus)

DIAGNOSIS

DIFFERENTIAL DIAGNOSIS

- Differential causes of ITP:
  - Autoimmune: systemic lupus erythematosus (SLE), antiphospholipid antibody syndrome, Evans syndrome
  - Infection: HIV, EBV, varicella
  - Medications: carbamazepine, quinidine, valproate, heparin
- Other causes of thrombocytopenia:
  - Bone marrow disorders: thrombocytopenia-absent radii syndrome, aplastic anemias, leukemias, Wiskott-Aldrich disease
  - Platelet disorders: type IIB von Willebrand disease, Bernard-Soulier syndrome, giant platelet syndromes
  - Neonatal thrombocytopenia, alloimmune thrombocytopenia
  - Medications: sulfonamides
  - Other: hemolytic uremic syndrome, disseminated intravascular coagulation, thrombotic thrombocytopenic purpura, Kasabach-Merritt syndrome (cavernous hemangioma)
- Other causes of bleeding:
  - von Willebrand disease
  - Nonsteroidal anti-inflammatory drugs (NSAIDs)
  - Trauma
  - Abuse
  - Hemophilia
  - Liver disease

WORKUP

- Made on the basis of the history, physical examination, and limited laboratory studies.
  - A well-appearing child with a brief history of bruising, petechiae, or bleeding
  - Isolated profound thrombocytopenia
  - No other hematologic or other laboratory abnormalities

LABORATORY TESTS

- Complete blood count, differential, platelet count, reticulocyte count, type and screen
- Prothrombin time, activated partial thromboplastin time should be normal
- Peripheral blood smear to look at platelet size and number, red blood cell and white blood cell morphology
- Optional: Coombs test, antinuclear antibodies, immunoglobulin G, immunoglobulin A, immunoglobulin M
- Bone marrow aspirate (optional): recommended in the thrombocytopenic child who has anemia or leukopenia, the child who has hepatosplenomegaly, or a child with presumed ITP who will be treated with glucocorticoids

TREATMENT

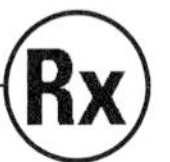

NONPHARMACOLOGIC THERAPY

- The decision to treat and what to treat with is based primarily on the extent of bleeding and the platelet count.
- The child's desired level of activity and family concerns and wishes should be considered.
- Observation: Because there is a high rate of spontaneous recovery (50% to 75% within 1 month of diagnosis), selected children with minimal signs of bleeding and platelet counts higher than $20,000/mm^3$ can be observed.
  - Children should not be given NSAIDs or aspirin.
  - They should not participate in contact sports or activities that put them at risk of head trauma.
- Splenectomy is reserved for children older than 5 years of age with severe ITP refractory to, or only transiently responsive to, medical therapies beyond 12 months.
  - ITP permanently resolves in 70% to 80% of children after splenectomy.
  - The risks of splenectomy include surgical and anesthesia complications and postsplenectomy sepsis.

ACUTE GENERAL Rx

- Treatment is indicated for any patient with active bleeding, extensive bruising or petechiae, or a very low platelet count (e.g., $<10,000/mm^3$).
- Treatment of asymptomatic patients with low ($<20,000/mm^3$) platelet counts is controversial.
- Prednisone is given at 2 mg/kg/day divided twice a day orally.
- In general, a bone marrow aspirate is done first.
  - This is done to ensure that no leukemia is present.
  - Prednisone partially treats and could mask an early diagnosis of leukemia.
  - Taper over 1 to 4 weeks to maintain the platelet count in a safe range (20,000 to 50,000) with no evidence of bleeding.

- Toxicity for short-term use includes mood changes, increased appetite, weight gain, hypertension, and diabetes.
- Anti-D antibody (WinRho) is dosed at 50 to 75 μg/kg and is given intravenously over 3 to 5 minutes.
  - This treatment is effective only in Rh-positive children.
  - The platelet count rises in a few days and drops again in 2 to 3 weeks.
  - Toxicity includes anemia, chills, and headache.
- Intravenous gamma globulin (IVIG) is dosed at 1 g/kg and given intravenously over 6 to 12 hours.
  - This treatment is most effective in quickly raising the platelet count (24 to 72 hours).
  - Treatment usually requires admission to the hospital.
  - The platelet count remains elevated for 3 to 4 weeks.
  - More than 50% of children develop headaches, vomiting, and fever.
  - Allergic reaction and blood product-associated infections are two risks.
- Platelet transfusions are usually not helpful in ITP.
- Platelet transfusions are reserved for life-threatening bleeding (e.g., intracranial bleed).

CHRONIC Rx

- Many options for chronic ITP
- Intermittent treatment with agents that were effective for the patient previously (e.g., Anti-D immunoglobulin every few months)
- Immunomodulation with rituximab
- Immunosuppression with chemotherapeutic agents
- Splenectomy (see "Nonpharmacologic Therapy")

DISPOSITION

- The aforementioned therapies do not cure ITP, but they are effective in temporary control.
- ITP resolves within 1 month of diagnosis in 50% of children, within 6 months in 75%, and within 12 months in 90%.
- The likelihood of life-threatening hemorrhage, such as a central nervous system hemorrhage, is less than 1%.
- Patients should be followed closely by their pediatrician and pediatric hematologist/oncologist until the platelet count is consistently within the normal range.
  - Decisions regarding ongoing therapy depend on the extent of bleeding, the platelet count, and the child's desired level of activity.
  - Children with ongoing thrombocytopenia should be periodically reevaluated for autoimmune diseases such as SLE, Evans syndrome, immunodeficiency, or the antiphospholipid antibody syndrome.

REFERRAL

Children with thrombocytopenia should be referred to a pediatric hematologist/oncologist.

PEARLS & CONSIDERATIONS

COMMENTS

- Platelets are often large on the peripheral blood film of children with ITP.
- Children with ITP may have bruises in unusual places (e.g., inner thighs, axillae).
- Splenomegaly and lymphadenopathy are *not* seen in ITP and suggest another illness.

PATIENT/FAMILY EDUCATION

- ITP is a self-limited disease with a low likelihood of recurrence.
- ITP is not cancer or leukemia and is not associated with and does not lead to cancer.
- Children with ITP must avoid activities that put them at risk of head trauma and should not take medications that increase their risk of bleeding, especially NSAIDs.
- The ITP Society, Contact a Family program at www.cafamily.org.uk

SUGGESTED READINGS

Beardsley DS, Nathan DG: Platelet abnormalities in infancy and childhood. *In* Nathan DG, Orkin SH (eds): *Nathan and Oski's Hematology of Infancy and Childhood,* 5th ed. Philadelphia, WB Saunders, 1998.

George J et al: Idiopathic thrombocytopenic purpura: a practice guideline developed by explicit methods for the American Society of Hematology. *J Am Soc Hematol* 88:3, 1996.

Medeiros D, Buchanan G: Current controversies in the management of idiopathic thrombocytopenic purpura during childhood. *Pediatr Clin North Am* 43:757, 1996.

Murphy S et al: Thrombocytopenia. *Pediatr Rev* 20:64, 1999.

National Institute of Diabetes and Digestive and Kidney Diseases. Available at www.niddk.nih.gov/health/hematol/pubs/itp/itp.htm

UltraNet Communications, Inc. Available at www.ultranet.com/itpsoc/

AUTHOR: **MATTHEW RICHARDSON, MD**

material in the stomach that has already dissolved may not be apparent.

TREATMENT

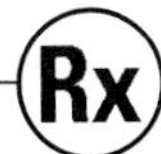

NONPHARMACOLOGIC THERAPY

- It is important to emphasize that serum iron concentrations correlate best with clinical symptoms when they are obtained 3 to 5 hours following ingestion.
- Asymptomatic patients who are known to have ingested less than 20 mg/kg of elemental iron require no intervention.
- Patients with serum iron levels less than 300 μg/dL who remain asymptomatic may be discharged home after 6 hours of observation.
- Patients with serum iron levels greater than 500 μg/dL or evidence of toxicity require treatment.

ACUTE GENERAL Rx

- In symptomatic patients, maintain the airway, assist with ventilation if necessary, and support intravascular volume.
- In patients with evidence of shock, intravascular volume should be aggressively repleted with intravenous crystalloid or blood, as appropriate.
- Serial reevaluation of intravascular volume status is critical, especially if there is ongoing metabolic acidosis.
- Because of iron-induced myocardial dysfunction and loss of vasomotor tone, some patients require inotropes or vasopressors.
- Gastrointestinal decontamination is best achieved by whole bowel irrigation with a polyethylene glycol solution (GoLYTELY) administered by nasogastric tube at a rate of 250 to 500 mL/hour, with attention to airway security in the patient with altered consciousness. Whole bowel irrigation is contraindicated in the presence of obstruction, perforation, ileus, or significant gastrointestinal bleeding. Its use should be guided by advice from a qualified toxicologist or regional poison control center.
  - If a sizable tablet mass is suspected or identified radiographically, endoscopy or surgical gastrotomy may be indicated to remove it.
- Gastric lavage (with appropriate airway protection) using room-temperature normal saline may also be considered, especially for intentional ingestions, when imaging studies reveal evidence of pill fragments in the stomach, and when the amount of elemental iron ingested is greater than 20 mg/kg.
  - Large tablet size and viscous consistency of iron preparations makes recovery of gastric contents difficult.
  - Do not lavage with bicarbonate or phosphate-containing solution, or with enterally administered deferoxamine.
  - Syrup of ipecac is no longer recommended for routine use.
- Activated charcoal does not adsorb iron.
- Chelation therapy should be administered to symptomatic patients with 4- to 6-hour serum iron levels greater than 300 μg/dL and in all patients with 4- to 6-hour levels in excess of 500 μg/dL. The agent of choice for chelation in acute iron toxicity is deferoxamine.
  - Give by continuous intravenous infusion at 10 to 15 mg/kg/hour.
    - The intramuscular route of administration is not recommended.
    - Rapid infusion of deferoxamine may be associated with shock.
      - Reduce the rate of administration
      - Support the intravascular volume
  - The duration of chelation therapy is guided by the patient's clinical status.
  - Chelation should continue until physiologic disturbances, laboratory values and imaging studies are normal.
  - Deferoxamine can be given safely to pregnant women.
- Throughout the clinical course of the iron-intoxicated patient, assess for signs of electrolyte derangement and shock so that fluid resuscitation can proceed if needed.
  - Renal failure may ensue as a result of shock and hypoperfusion or from nephrotoxicity of deferoxamine-iron complex.
  - Hemodialysis may be useful to assist clearance of the chelated iron complex.

DISPOSITION

- All patients with intentional ingestions should receive an evaluation by psychiatry once they are clinically stable.
- In cases of accidental ingestion, social work consultation is often helpful to assess the degree of supervision in the home.

REFERRAL

- Patients suspected of having a potentially toxic exposure should be stabilized and referred to the nearest tertiary care center with experience in managing critically ill children.
- Consult the nearest regional poison center in all cases of toxic ingestion.

PEARLS & CONSIDERATIONS

COMMENTS

- Clinicians should not base therapeutic decisions solely on serum iron levels, as their value in predicting systemic toxicity depends in large part on the timing of the serum level relative to the time of ingestion.
- Deferoxamine interferes with serum iron estimation. Therefore, levels should be drawn prior to the initiation of treatment.
- Infusion of deferoxamine is typically associated with a change of urine color to orange-red or pink, "vin-rose," but efficacy of chelation therapy should not be judged according to whether or not the color change has occurred.
  - Even in patients with markedly toxic serum iron levels, urine color change may not be observed, especially if the patient is in some degree of hypovolemic or distributive shock.

PREVENTION

- The danger of accidental poisoning in the home should be discussed routinely at pediatric health supervision visits, beginning at the 6-month visit.
  - Parents should be instructed to "childproof" the home, including locking vitamin preparations and all other medicines out of the reach of children.
  - Parents should be provided with the phone number of the regional poison center. They should be instructed to call immediately when they suspect that an inappropriate ingestion may have occurred.

PATIENT/FAMILY EDUCATION

- Parents should be educated about the potential toxicity of iron-containing compounds in the home, including multivitamin preparations. These and other medications should be kept locked and out of the reach of children, even if they are packaged with childproof caps.
- Families should be provided with the phone number of the nearest regional poison center (1-800-222-1222).

SUGGESTED READINGS

AAP, Committee on Injury, Violence, and Poison Prevention: Poison treatment in the home. *Pediatrics* 112:1182, 2003.

Baranwal AK et al: Acute iron poisoning: management guidelines. *Indian Pediatr* 40:534, 2003.

Kronfol R: Acute iron intoxication in children and adolescents. Available at Up to Date On Line 12.2. http://www.utdol.com/ Accessed February 2, 2005.

Riordan M et al: Poisoning in children: 3 common medicines. *Arch Dis Child* 87:400, 2002.

Shannon M: Ingestion of toxic substances by children. *N Engl J Med* 342(3):186, 2000.

Shannon M: The demise of ipecac. *Pediatrics* 112(5):1180, 2003.

Watson WA et al: 2003 annual report of the American Association of Poison Control Centers Toxic Exposure Surveillance System. *Am J Emerg Med* 22(5):335, 2004.

AUTHORS: **MEREDITH E. REYNOLDS, MD** and **KATHLEEN M. VENTRE, MD**

Irritable Bowel Syndrome

BASIC INFORMATION

DEFINITION

Irritable bowel syndrome (IBS) is defined by the presence of recurrent abdominal pain (RAP) associated with disordered defecation in the absence of demonstrable organic disease. Rome II criteria for IBS include at least 12 weeks (which need not be consecutive) in the preceding 12 months of abdominal discomfort or pain that has two of the three following features: relieved with defecation, onset associated with a change in frequency of stool, and onset associated with a change in form (appearance) of stool. There also are no structural or metabolic abnormalities to explain the symptoms.

SYNONYMS

Functional gastrointestinal disorders
IBS
Irritable colon
Spastic colon

ICD-9-CM CODES
536.9 Unspecified functional disorder of the stomach
564.1 Irritable colon

EPIDEMIOLOGY & DEMOGRAPHICS

- IBS is a common cause of school absenteeism and use of medical care resources by children and adolescents.
- It is the most common digestive disease encountered by gastroenterologists treating adults.
- In community-based studies, abdominal pain occurred weekly in 13% to 30% of middle and high school students.
    - Six percent of middle school students and 14% of high school students could be classified as having IBS.
    - A community-based study performed in New England revealed that 32% to 37% of eighth and tenth graders had abdominal pain in the previous 6 months.
    - In referral specialty clinics, two thirds of children with chronic abdominal pain have symptoms compatible with IBS.
- The relation between RAP and IBS has not been clearly defined.
    - Approximately 30% to 50% of patients with RAP continue with pain and may develop IBS that persists into adulthood.
    - Females with RAP seemed to be at greater risk for IBS.
- The number of adults seeking medical advice may be only a small portion of those with IBS.
    - Other factors are likely to influence the decision to obtain medical advice.
    - The same is probably true for children.

CLINICAL PRESENTATION

History

- Different symptoms may predominate.
- Abdominal pain (e.g., recurrent, colicky, periumbilical), particularly in children 5 years and older, should be assessed.
    - Abdominal pain varies in intensity.
    - Pain may be periumbilical, epigastric, or in the right or left side.
    - Pain may be severe enough to interfere with daily activities.
    - A bowel movement may relieve pain.
    - Food ingestion may worsen pain.
- Bowel movements may be abnormal.
    - In older children, IBS follows a pattern similar to that seen in adults, including constipation, diarrhea, or diarrhea alternating with constipation.
    - There may be a sensation of difficult or incomplete evacuation.
- Symptoms of upper gastrointestinal dysfunction include heartburn, nausea, vomiting, bloating.
- Autonomic symptoms include the following: pallor, fatigue, headache, dizziness, palpitations, low-grade fever, nausea, vomiting.
- Anxiety and depression scores are higher for patients with IBS.

Physical Examination

- Normal growth and development
- Normal abdominal examination results
    - Occasionally, mild abdominal distention
    - Occasionally, periumbilical or generalized tenderness
- Normal physical examination results otherwise
- Malnutrition, mass lesions, organomegaly, jaundice, ascites, perianal disease, costovertebral pain, skin problems, joint swelling, neuropathy, guaiac-positive stool: *not* compatible with a IBS diagnosis

ETIOLOGY

- The cause is unknown.
    - May result from visceral hypersensitivity after a host of potential initiating events (e.g., infection or inflammation, allergy, trauma, stress, abnormal motility)
    - Gastrointestinal dysmotility: inconsistent abnormal small bowel and colonic motility patterns
    - Genetic predisposition, familial clustering
    - Stress and psychological disturbances: possible additive and modulating effects
- IBS is frequently associated with comorbid psychopathology.

DIAGNOSIS

Dx

- In the absence of structural or biochemical markers, the diagnostic criteria are symptom based.
- The diagnosis is made on clinical grounds using the Rome II criteria, outlined earlier.

DIFFERENTIAL DIAGNOSIS

- Gastrointestinal infections (particularly giardiasis)
- Celiac disease
- Inflammatory bowel disease (IBD)
- Lactose intolerance
- *Helicobacter pylori* infection
- Food intolerances or allergies
- Malabsorption
- Gallstones
- Pancreatitis
- Urinary tract infection
- Gynecologic abnormalities (e.g., PID)
- Toxin (e.g., lead)
- Constipation
- Lymphocytic colitis
- Unlikely in child who appears ill or has progressive symptoms, weight loss, symptoms at night, bleeding, evidence of malabsorption, fever, bilious vomiting, an abnormal physical examination, or a positive family history (e.g., peptic ulcer disease, IBD, gallstones)

WORKUP

The diagnosis is made based on the symptoms and the fulfillment of Rome II criteria.

LABORATORY TESTS

- Screening tests that may be considered for
    - Complete blood cell count with differential and reticulocyte counts
    - Erythrocyte sedimentation rate
    - Total protein and albumin
    - Liver function tests, including albumin and total protein
    - Pancreatic amylase and lipase
    - Serum electrolytes
    - Blood urea nitrogen and creatinine
    - Celiac screening (IgA and tissue transglutaminase or anti-endomysial antibody)
    - Urinalysis and urine culture
    - Stool guaiac test
    - Stool examination for ova and parasites
- Additional tests should be performed only if indicated by the history, findings on physical examination, or screening laboratory tests:
    - Lactose breath test
    - Breath testing for bacterial overgrowth
    - Blood screening for inflammatory bowel disease (i.e., perinuclear antineutrophil cytoplasmic antibodies [p-ANCA] and anti-*Saccharomyces cerevisia* antibodies [ASCA])
    - Tests to exclude infection with *H. pylori* (i.e., stool antigen test and breath tests)
    - Esophagogastroduodenoscopy
    - Colonoscopy
    - Electroencephalography
    - Laparoscopy
    - Other assays (e.g., porphyrins, lead)

IMAGING STUDIES

- Frequently needed studies:
    - Abdominal ultrasound (if possible during acute attack)
    - Rarely and depending on the presentation and results of the screening tests, the following imaging studies may be indicated:
        - Upper gastrointestinal series with small bowel follow-through

- Barium enema
- Intravenous pyelogram
- Abdominal computed tomography scan
- Functional gallbladder imaging (nuclear medicine study with gallbladder emptying)

TREATMENT

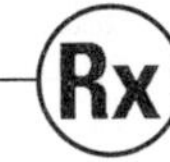

NONPHARMACOLOGIC THERAPY

- Reassurance, education, and emotional support are critical.
- Nutrition:
  - Dietary fiber (age + 5 g of fiber/day)
  - Elimination of potentially exacerbating foods (consider lactose-free diet)

ACUTE GENERAL Rx

- Supportive care
- Antispasmodics and anticholinergics (e.g., dicyclomine, hyoscyamine)

CHRONIC Rx

- Initial therapy consists of suppression of gastric acid and treatment of other gastrointestinal symptoms.
  - Use H_2-blockers (e.g., ranitidine, cimetidine, famotidine).
  - Proton pump inhibitors (e.g., omeprazole, lansoprazole) may be beneficial, particularly if there is a component of dyspepsia.
  - Laxatives can be used by patients with constipation.
  - Prokinetics may be useful in patients with dyspepsia and constipation.
  - Antibiotics can be used for bacterial overgrowth in selected patients with severe bloating.
  - Loperamide is effective in patients with diarrhea.
- If the previous nonpharmacologic and medical interventions mentioned fail, try others:
  - Antispasmodics and anticholinergics (e.g., dicyclomine, hyoscyamine) or calcium channel blockers (e.g., diltiazem, pinaverium).
    - Peppermint oil has properties similar to calcium channel blockers.
    - Although placebo-controlled studies in adults have had mixed results, these agents may be effective in children with severe and debilitating symptoms.
  - Antidepressants and anxiolytics have central and peripheral effects. They may be used at low doses and have been shown in randomized studies in adults and open-label studies in children to be effective
    - They are effective in patients with visceral hyperalgesia.
    - Most of the experience has been with tricyclic antidepressants (e.g., amitriptyline, desipramine) benzodiazepines and selective serotonin reuptake inhibitors (SSRIs) (e.g., citalopram).
  - Newer medications that manipulate serotonin receptors are available.
    - Tegaserod is a $5HT_4$ agonist that has been shown in placebo-controlled trials to be effective in women with constipation-predominant IBS. It has been successful in uncontrolled studies in children, although there is no pediatric dose.
    - Alosetron, a $5HT_3$ antagonist was proved to be effective in the treatment of diarrhea-predominant IBS in adult women, but its use was associated with ischemic colitis. It was removed from the market and can be obtained only under a special program and only for adult patients.

COMPLEMENTARY & ALTERNATIVE MEDICINE

- Psychotherapy, biofeedback, and cognitive behavioral therapy are useful.
- A multidisciplinary approach is necessary.

DISPOSITION

- Close follow-up should be maintained, with frequent physician contact.
- Avoid school absence.

REFERRAL

- Patients with a poor response to nonpharmacologic and initial medical interventions may need to be evaluated by a gastroenterologist.
- If patients with IBS have a high degree of disability, they may require a multidisciplinary approach.

PEARLS & CONSIDERATIONS

COMMENTS

- Abdominal pain in children younger than 4 years should be investigated thoroughly.
- Even though the symptoms of IBS are functional in nature, they are real.
- The diagnosis of IBS needs to be a positive diagnosis, not one of exclusion.
- Reassurance is important.
  - There is a low likelihood of finding an organic cause.
  - There is no physical danger to the child.
- Establish specific goals of therapy.
- Unnecessary diagnostic tests and referrals may only reinforce an already problematic symptom.
- Do not let the symptoms become the disease.
- IBS symptoms are associated with high levels of disability and health service use.
- Visits to a physician are related to parental perceptions of the severity of the symptoms.

PREVENTION

- Early intervention is important in children.
- Treat triggers.

PATIENT/FAMILY EDUCATION

- American Academy of Family Physicians: www.aafp.org/patientinfo/bowel.html
- International Foundation for Functional Gastrointestinal Disorders: www.iffgd.org
- National Institute of Diabetes & Digestive & Kidney Diseases: www.niddk.nih.gov/health/digest/summary/ibskids/index.htm
- National Institute of Diabetes & Digestive & Kidney Diseases: www.niddk.nih.gov/health/digest/pubs/irrbowel/irrbo

SUGGESTED READINGS

Campo J et al: Citalopram treatment of pediatric recurrent abdominal pain and comorbid internalizing disorders: an exploratory study. *J Am Acad Child Adolesc Psychiatry* 43:1234, 2004.

Di Lorenzo C et al: Visceral hyperalgesia in children with functional abdominal pain. *J Pediatr* 139:838, 2001.

Drossman DA et al: AGA technical review on irritable bowel syndrome. *Gastroenterology* 123:2108, 2002.

Drossman DA et al: Cognitive-behavioral therapy vs. education and desipramine versus placebo for moderate to severe functional bowel disorders. *Gastroenterology* 125:19, 2003.

Hyams JS: Irritable bowel syndrome, functional dyspepsia, and functional abdominal pain syndrome. *Adolesc Med Clin* 15:1, 2004.

Walker LS et al: Recurrent abdominal pain: symptom subtypes based on the Rome II criteria for pediatric functional gastrointestinal disorders. *J Pediatr Gastroenterol Nutr* 38:187–191, 2004.

Weydert J et al: Systematic review of treatments for recurrent abdominal pain. *Pediatrics* 111:e1–e10, 2003.

AUTHOR: **SAMUEL NURKO, MD, MPH**

BASIC INFORMATION

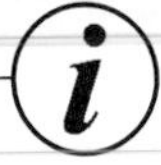

DEFINITION

Kawasaki disease (KD) is an acute, self-limited, multisystemic vasculitis of unknown origin. It is the leading cause of acquired heart disease in children.

SYNONYMS

Kawasaki syndrome
Mucocutaneous lymph node syndrome

ICD-9-CM CODE
446.1 Kawasaki disease

EPIDEMIOLOGY & DEMOGRAPHICS

- KD usually occurs in children 6 months to 5 years old.
- It is unusual in patients younger than 3 months or older than 8 years.
- The U.S. annual attack rate is 9 cases per 100,000 children younger than 5 years.
- The male-to-female ratio is 1.5:1.
- KD occurs all year but is more common in the winter and early spring.
- Geographic and temporal clustering does occur.
- Person-to-person transmission is not documented; it is rare in siblings.
- Recurrence is reported in less than 2% of patients.
- Coronary artery ectasia (i.e., dilation) or aneurysms develop in 15% to 25% of untreated children.
- Risk factors for coronary artery abnormalities include the following:
  - No treatment with intravenous gamma globulin (IVIG)
  - Male gender
  - Age younger than 1 year
  - Long duration of fever (>10 days) or biphasic febrile course
  - Persistent high elevation of acute-phase reactants
  - High absolute band count
  - Hemoglobin lower than 10 mg/dL, low platelet count, low albumin level
- Coronary dilation occurs as early as 7 days after onset and peaks at 3 to 4 weeks.
- Previously, there were 2 to 3 deaths per 1000 untreated patients as a result of an acute myocardial infarction.
- The highest risk of death, persistence of aneurysms, and late sequelae are most common in patients with giant coronary aneurysms (>8 mm internal diameter).
- Fifty percent of aneurysms regress in 1 to 2 years; the remainder persist or develop stenosis at the mouth or outlet of the aneurysm.

CLINICAL PRESENTATION

- Diagnostic criteria are as follows:
  - Fever, usually high and spiking, of at least 5 days' duration and four or more of the five principal clinical features:
    - Bilateral nonexudative bulbar conjunctivitis
    - Red, edematous cracked lips; strawberry tongue; pharyngeal erythema
    - Polymorphous exanthem with perineal accentuation
    - Palmar and solar erythema with tender induration of the hands and feet and subsequent desquamation 1 to 3 weeks after onset, beginning in the periungual areas
    - Anterior cervical adenopathy (one or more nodes with a diameter larger than 1.5 cm), usually unilateral, the least common finding, and present in 50%
  - Other diseases with similar findings must be excluded.
- Other findings include extreme irritability, headache, vomiting, abdominal pain, diarrhea, urethritis, and arthralgia or arthritis.
- Rarely, hearing loss, or testicular swelling occurs.
- Tachycardia greater than expected from fever, gallop rhythm, cardiogenic shock from acute myocarditis, or later myocardial infarction may occur.
- Nuchal rigidity caused by aseptic meningitis may be found.
- Audible mitral regurgitation is present in 1% of patients.

ETIOLOGY

The cause is unknown but likely to be infectious with immunoregulatory derangements.

DIAGNOSIS

Dx

DIFFERENTIAL DIAGNOSIS

- Measles
- Scarlet fever
- Drug reactions
- Stevens-Johnson syndrome
- Other febrile viral exanthemas
- Rocky Mountain spotted fever
- Staphylococcal scalded skin syndrome or toxic shock syndrome
- Bacterial cervical lymphadenitis
- Juvenile rheumatoid arthritis
- Leptospirosis
- Mercury hypersensitivity reaction (i.e., acrodynia)

LABORATORY TESTS

- Elevated levels of acute-phase reactants are seen: erythrocyte sedimentation rate (ESR), C-reactive protein (CRP), α_1-antitrypsin, platelet count.
- The following are common:
  - Neutrophilia with immature forms
  - Anemia
- The following may be seen:
  - Hypoalbuminemia
  - Proteinuria
  - Sterile pyuria
  - Cerebrospinal fluid mononuclear pleocytosis
  - Elevated levels of serum transaminases
- Thrombocytosis peaks at 10 to 14 days.
- Abnormal lipid metabolism (e.g., low levels of high-density lipoprotein, high levels of triglycerides) may persist for years.

IMAGING STUDIES

- Subclinical pericardial effusions are seen in 30% of patients on echocardiography.
- Gallbladder hydrops may be identified on abdominal ultrasound.
- These laboratory findings may be helpful if some of the principal findings are not present (i.e., incomplete or atypical KD).

TREATMENT

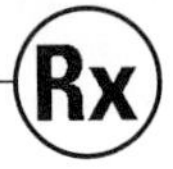

NONPHARMACOLOGIC THERAPY

- Consider coronary artery bypass grafts (i.e., revascularization) for reversible ischemia caused by coronary artery stenosis if
  - The myocardium is viable.
  - No distal stenoses are present.
- Coronary angioplasty has not been effective for stenotic lesions, but stent placement may be effective.

ACUTE GENERAL Rx

- IVIG is administered at a dose of 2 g/kg over 12 hours.
- IVIG may be repeated for recrudescent or persistent fever (10% of patients).
- Intravenous methylprednisolone has been used in patients who are resistant to IVIG.
- Aspirin is administered at 80 to 100 mg/kg/day orally until the patient is afebrile.

CHRONIC Rx

- Aspirin is then administered at 3 to 5 mg/kg/day for at least 8 weeks.
- A cardiology evaluation, including echocardiograms 2 and 8 weeks after the onset of KD, is necessary.
- If no coronary artery abnormalities are seen at 2 and 8 weeks, aspirin can be discontinued; otherwise, aspirin should continue indefinitely.
- Add clopidogrel (Plavix) if stable small to moderate aneurysms are seen.
- If giant coronary artery aneurysms (>8 mm in diameter) are present, heparin given immediately followed by warfarin is usually added for anticoagulation.
- Tissue plasminogen activator (tPA) is used for acute coronary occlusion.
- Administer varicella and influenza vaccines to patients taking aspirin long term.

DISPOSITION

- All patients with KD should initially be evaluated by a pediatric cardiologist, with repeat echocardiography at 2 and 8 weeks after onset to detect coronary artery abnormalities.
- Patients with coronary abnormalities require long-term follow-up, with anticoagulation, activity restrictions, and serial diagnostic testing based on the severity of their coronary lesions.

- Patients with aortic or mitral regurgitation require infective endocarditis prophylaxis.

REFERRAL

- All patients with suspected acute KD should be seen by a pediatric cardiologist and have a baseline echocardiogram.
- Patients with a history suggesting KD but no cardiovascular evaluation should be seen by a pediatric cardiologist.

PEARLS & CONSIDERATIONS

COMMENTS

- The constellation of marked persistent irritability, refusal to bear weight, and confluent perineal erythema may be helpful if KD is in an early stage or is incompletely expressed.
- Approximately 90% of patients treated with IVIG are afebrile within 48 hours.
- Despite appropriate therapy, up to 4% of patients with KD develop coronary aneurysms (giant aneurysms in 1%).
- Consider obtaining an echocardiogram for an infant, child, or adolescent with unexplained fever lasting 1 week or more, especially with any of the principal clinical features and with elevated acute phase reactants (ESR > 40 mm/hr, CRP > 3.0 mg/dL).

PATIENT/FAMILY EDUCATION

- If coronary artery abnormalities are identified, parents should learn basic cardiopulmonary resuscitation.
- The patient's cardiologist should be notified immediately if syncope or acute exercise intolerance develops.
- Whether KD is a risk factor for premature atherosclerotic coronary disease is unknown; nevertheless, a cardiac-healthy lifestyle should be emphasized for patients who have had KD.

SUGGESTED READINGS

Akagi T et al: Outcome of coronary artery aneurysms after Kawasaki disease. *J Pediatr* 121:689, 1992.

Newburger JW et al: Diagnosis, treatment, and long-term management of Kawasaki disease: a statement for health professionals from the committee on rheumatic fever, endocarditis, and Kawasaki disease, Council on Cardiovascular Disease in the Young, American Heart Association. *Pediatrics* 114:1708, 2004.

AUTHOR: **J. PETER HARRIS, MD**

BASIC INFORMATION

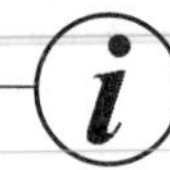

DEFINITION

A characteristic phenotype in the presence of a 47,XXY chromosome pattern.

ICD-9-CM CODE
758.7 Klinefelter syndrome

EPIDEMIOLOGY & DEMOGRAPHICS

- The incidence of 47,XXY karyotype is 1 case in 500 to 1000 male live births.
- Approximately one half of 47,XXY conceptions are lost prenatally.

CLINICAL PRESENTATION

History

- Early literature describes an increased incidence of childhood behavior problems, learning difficulties, and intelligence quotients 10 to 15 points below siblings in boys with Klinefelter syndrome. The typical presentation was a boy who came to medical attention in the school years because of behavior or learning problems in conjunction with the characteristic body habitus.
- The most commonly reported developmental abnormality is verbal fluency or delayed expressive speech.
- Older reports appear to demonstrate an ascertainment bias in that only boys who manifested the behavior or learning problems were likely to come to medical attention before puberty. An undefined percentage of boys with a 47,XXY genotype actually demonstrate the phenotype of Klinefelter syndrome as defined by Dr. Klinefelter's original report.
  - Most males diagnosed prenatally with a 47,XXY karyotype appear to perform relatively normally in childhood.
  - Diagnosis of a 47,XXY karyotype is not unusual in infertility clinics or during an evaluation for small testicles in otherwise apparently normal postpubertal males.
- Postpubertally, boys with a 47,XXY karyotype generally have some degree of decreased testosterone production, although they may produce adequate testosterone for virilization at puberty.
- Most affected males appear to have normal sexual function.
- Most affected males are infertile; however, a few men with a 47,XXY karyotype have successfully fathered normal children by intracytoplasmic sperm injection (ICSI). (In this procedure, sperm are harvested from the testis or ejaculate and injected directly into the oocyte in vitro.) There does appear to be a slightly increased risk of sex or autosomal chromosome abnormalities in children conceived through ICSI.

Physical Examination

- Normal to tall stature
- Thin body habitus with relatively long legs
- Normal male external genitalia, with small testicles (especially postpubertally)
- Significant incidence of the following: gynecomastia, elbow dysplasia, intention tremor.
- Occasional incidence of the following: cryptorchidism or hypospadias, scoliosis, diabetes mellitus, bronchitis, ataxia, skin breakdown over lower legs, germ cell tumors.
- Mental deficiency, growth deficiency, and more severe elbow abnormalities in males with more than two X chromosomes (e.g., 48,XXXY)

ETIOLOGY

- Eighty percent of males with two or more X chromosomes have a 47,XXY genotype.
- In general, the higher the number of X chromosomes (e.g., 48,XXXY), the higher the number of abnormalities.
- Usually results from aberrant segregation of sex chromosomes in meiosis; maternal or paternal errors appear equally likely.
- The phenotype appears to be associated with genes mapping to the long arm of the X chromosome. It appears that males with a smaller number of CAG repeats in the X-linked androgen receptor gene may have less inactivation of the androgen receptor and therefore few symptoms.
- Males who are mosaic for a 47,XXY cell line with a normal 46,XY cell line may have a variable phenotype (from normal to Klinefelter syndrome) and a higher likelihood of fertility.

DIAGNOSIS

Dx

DIFFERENTIAL DIAGNOSIS

- Other chromosome abnormalities
- Fragile X syndrome
- Primary endocrine abnormalities
- Marfan's syndrome
- Homocystinuria

LABORATORY TESTS

- Chromosome karyotype is 47,XXY.
- Buccal smears no longer recommended as they are unlikely to detect mosaicism, structurally abnormal X chromosomes, or autosomal karyotypic abnormalities.

TREATMENT

Rx

NONPHARMACOLOGIC THERAPY

- The patient may be referred to a developmental or behavioral specialist.
- Referral for special educational services is helpful if the child has learning problems.

CHRONIC Rx

- Testosterone therapy is typically needed at adolescence.
- Many adult men report enhanced well-being on testosterone supplementation.
  - Traditionally, the recommendation for testosterone supplementation in adulthood was controversial.
  - An increasing number of physicians are recommending supplementation to prevent long-term complications of androgen deficiency, such as obesity, diabetes mellitus, osteoporosis, and thromboembolic disease.

DISPOSITION

- Routine pediatric follow-up is needed, with special attention to developmental and behavioral issues in early childhood and virilization, sexual function, and self-esteem in adolescence.
- Slightly increased risk for germinal tumors.

REFERRAL

- The patient and family should be referred for genetic counseling.
- Affected boys should undergo endocrine evaluation at adolescence.
- Psychological therapy referral may be necessary for poor self-esteem or depression.

PEARLS & CONSIDERATIONS

COMMENTS

- Some individuals recommend that the eponym *Klinefelter syndrome* be reserved only for males who exhibit the characteristic phenotype.
- Those diagnosed prenatally or for other reasons who do not experience difficulties with growth or performance should be referred to as having a 47,XXY karyotype, not Klinefelter syndrome.

PATIENT/FAMILY EDUCATION

- A relatively normal childhood can be expected if the child is diagnosed prenatally.
- Any behavior or learning issues may require special evaluation and school placement.
- Sexual intercourse is normal, although some men receive testosterone supplementation.
- Infertility may be amenable to sperm manipulation (i.e., ICSI) in some men.
- Support group information can be obtained through the Klinefelter Syndrome Support Group: http://klinefeltersyndrome.org/
- *The Even Exchange,* a newsletter of Klinefelter Syndrome and Associates, provides useful information for parents and adult patients (P.O. Box 119, Roseville, CA 95678-0119).
- *Klinefelter Syndrome, The X-tra Special Boy,* and *For Boys Only* are publications available from the Genetics Clinic, Crippled Children's Division, Oregon Health Sciences University.

SUGGESTED READINGS

Jones K-L: 47,XXY. *In Smith's Recognizable Patterns of Human Malformations.* Philadelphia, WB Saunders, 1997.

Klinefelter HF et al: Syndrome characterized by gynecomastia, aspermatogenesis, without aleydigism and increased excretion of follicle stimulating hormone. *J Clin Endocrinol* 2:615, 1942.

Lanfranco F et al: Klinefelter's syndrome. *Lancet* 364:273, 2004.

Robinson A et al: Sex chromosome aneuploidy: the Denver prospective study [original article series]. *Birth Defects* 26:59, 1990.

Willard HF: The sex chromosomes and X chromosome inactivation. *In* Scriver CR et al (eds): *The metabolic and molecular bases of inherited disease.* New York, McGraw-Hill, 1995, pp 1202–1203.

AUTHOR: **GEORGIANNE ARNOLD, MD**

BASIC INFORMATION

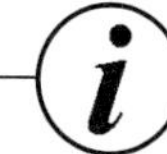

DEFINITION

- Knee extensor tendonitis includes three entities:
  - Patellar tendonitis (jumper's knee) affects the patellar tendon along its course from the inferior pole of the patella to, but not including, the tibial tuberosity.
  - Quadriceps tendonitis affects the quadriceps tendon and its attachment on the superior pole of the patella.
  - Sinding-Larsen-Johansson syndrome (SLJ) is a traction apophysitis (or [multiple] stress fracture[s]) at the inferior pole of patella and generally affects active and growing younger children (pre- and early puberty).

SYNONYMS

Patella tendonitis—jumper's knee
Quadriceps tendonitis
SLJ syndrome
Stress fracture of patella
Traction apophysitis of knee (patella)

ICD-9-CM CODES
726.64 Patellar tendinitis
727.2 Jumper's knee
732.4 Sinding-Larsen-Johansson syndrome (SLJ), patella fracture

EPIDEMIOLOGY & DEMOGRAPHICS

- Generally seen in association with repetitive microtrauma to the knee such as jumping and kicking sports—especially volleyball, soccer, basketball, and dance.
- SLJ is most common in younger children usually between 10 and 13 years.
- May be more common in those with decreased quadriceps and hamstring flexibility.

CLINICAL PRESENTATION

- Pain noted with kicking, jumping (push off and landing), and weight bearing on a flexed knee.
- General examination to assess stance and posture, evaluate range of motion, test ligament stability.
- In patellar tendonitis, the pain is along the patellar tendon (between the inferior pole of patella and tibial tuberosity). (See Knee Maneuvers in Charts, Formulas, Laboratory Tests and Values [Section IV].)
- Pain at distal attachment of quadriceps on superior pole of patella while straightening knee seen with quadriceps tendonitis.
- Pain localized specifically over the lower patella in SLJ.
  - No point tenderness on tibial tuberosity (Osgood-Schlatter disease)
- Tight and weak quadriceps may be appreciated.

ETIOLOGY

- These three entities all believed to be overuse syndromes.
- Rapid acceleration, deceleration, jumping, and landing may result in significant trauma to extensor knee mechanism.
- Trauma with ensuing inflammation of patella tendon or quadriceps tendon at or near insertion to patella, or microfracture of patella in cases of SLJ.

DIAGNOSIS

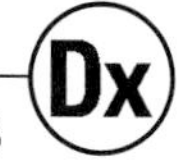

DIFFERENTIAL DIAGNOSIS

- Other anterior knee pain syndromes (PFPS, patellar dislocation)
- Osgood-Schlatter disease, also a traction apophysitis but at distal patellar tendon attachment onto tibial tuberosity
- Meniscal tears
- Ligament tears or ruptures within knee joint (anterior cruciate ligament, medial collateral ligament, etc.)
- Bursitis (prepatellar)
- Arthritis, synovitis
  - Inflammatory (e.g., juvenile arthritis, rheumatic fever)
  - Infectious (e.g., staphylococcal, salmonellal infections)
- Any hip pathology can radiate to knee
  - Slipped capital femoral epiphysis (SCFE)
  - Legg-Calvé-Perthes
  - Transient synovitis hip

IMAGING STUDIES

- Ultrasound may be considered, specifically to localize area for steroid injection if significant pain persists after appropriate therapy (done by orthopedic or sports medicine physicians).
- Hypoechoic area may be visualized within patellar tendon at or near attachment to inferior pole of patella.

TREATMENT

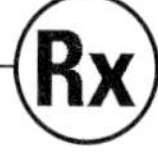

NONPHARMACOLOGIC THERAPY

- Restricted activity may be necessary temporarily.
- Ice
- Quadriceps stretching and strengthening
- Cross-training
- Immobilization is not usually necessary.
- Rarely, athletes require surgical intervention for persistent pain or limitation of movement.

ACUTE GENERAL Rx

- Nonsteroidal anti-inflammatory agents (NSAIDs) for pain and inflammation

CHRONIC Rx

- Ongoing strengthening and stretching of knee joint (leg and thigh) muscles
- Rarely, intralesional steroids

DISPOSITION

- Athletes may be unable to return to sports for 6 or more months if significant extensor tendonitis exists.

REFERRAL

- Referral to sports medicine or physical therapy for rehabilitation or exercise training
- Referral to an orthopedic surgeon if the diagnosis is unclear, for acute trauma necessitating surgery, and for unresolving pain or weakness

PEARLS & CONSIDERATIONS

COMMENTS

All children presenting with knee pain should also be evaluated for ipsilateral hip disorders, which can present with knee pain.

PREVENTION

For many pediatric knee problems, adequate stretch and strengthening with a decrease in repetitive trauma (overuse) will allay problems.

PATIENT/FAMILY EDUCATION

SLJ, like OSGD, is usually self-limited.

SUGGESTED READINGS

Cook JL et al: Reproducibility and clinical utility of tendon palpation to detect patellar tendinopathy in young basketball players. *Br J Sports Med* 35:65, 2001.

Ferretti A et al: Patellar tendonitis: a follow-up study of surgical treatment. *J Bone Joint Surg* 84A:2179, 2002.

Fredberg U et al: Ultrasonography as a tool for diagnosis, guidance of local steroid injection and, together with pressure algometry, monitoring of the treatment of athletes with chronic jumper's knee and Achilles tendonitis: a randomised, double-blind, placebo-controlled study. *Scand J Rheum* 33:94, 2004.

Hergenroeder AC: Approach to the young athlete with acute knee pain or injury. UpToDate online 13.3 Sept. 3, 2006.

AUTHOR: **LYNN C. GARFUNKEL, MD**

BASIC INFORMATION

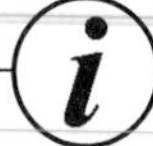

DEFINITIONS

- Anterior cruciate ligament (ACL): strain or rupture of the ligament that goes from the medial aspect of the lateral femoral condyle to the central anteromedial tibial plateau.
- Posterior cruciate ligament (PCL): injury of the ligament that extends from the lateral portion of the medial femoral condyle to the posterior lateral central tibial plateau.
- Lateral collateral ligament (LCL): injury of the ligament that extends from the lateral distal femoral epiphysis to the proximal tibial epiphysis.
- Medial collateral ligament (MCL): injury of the ligament that extends medially from the medial femoral epicondyle to the proximal (medial) tibial epiphysis.
- Anterior and posterior crucial ligaments (ACL, PCL) stabilize tibia and femur in frontal plane.
- The lateral and medial collateral ligaments (LCL, MCL) protect from varus and valgus forces.
- See Knee Maneuvers in Charts, Formulas, Laboratory Tests and Values (Section IV).

ICD-9-CM CODES

717.83 Old tear anterior cruciate ligament (ACL)
717.84 Old tear posterior cruciate ligament (PCL)
844.0 Lateral collateral ligament (LCL) sprain
844.1 Medial collateral ligament (MCL) sprain
844.2 Acute anterior cruciate ligament (ACL) sprain

EPIDEMIOLOGY & DEMOGRAPHICS

- Avulsion fracture of the tibial eminence is more common in child than ACL disruption.
  - Growth plate is weaker than ligament before puberty (epiphyseal closure); therefore fractures are more common.
- ACL and MCL are most commonly injured knee ligaments, but rare before puberty.
- ACL injuries are two to four times more common in girls.
- ACL tears are commonly associated with meniscal tears.
- Basketball and soccer are the most commonly associated sports, but football, hockey, lacrosse, skiing, gymnastics, wrestling, and volleyball also increase risk for ACL tears.
- Graded for severity:
  - Minor fiber dysfunction (stretching, grade I)
  - Moderate, partial fiber disruption (partial tear, grade II)
  - Severe injury, complete ligament disruption (grade III)

CLINICAL PRESENTATION

ACL Tears

- Acute pop (appreciated in one third of patients)
- Fall to ground and unable to walk without assistance
- Large effusion within hours (hemarthrosis) indicates intra-articular injury which may preclude positive Lachman or anterior drawer tests (see Knee Maneuvers in Charts, Formulas, Laboratory Tests and Values [Section IV]).
- Lachman test
  - With patient supine, the hip and knee are flexed 20 to 30 degrees.
  - Stabilize the femur and move the tibia anteriorly from the femur.
  - The test is positive, indicating an ACL tear, if the anterior translation of the tibia on the femur occurs with a soft end point.
- Anterior drawer test
  - With the patient sitting with the knee flexed 90 degrees, anteriorly displace the tibia from the femur.
  - Patient may be supine with the hip flexed 45 degrees and the knee flexed 90 degrees.
    - The examiner may stabilize the foot by sitting on it.
    - The examiner wraps his or her fingers around the calf near the hamstring insertion with the thumbs on either side of the patella along the tibial plateau.
    - Significant anterior translation occurs after an ACL tear.

MCL Tears

- Maintenance of stability for walking is usual.
- Erythema may occur along medial knee.
- Pain and stiffness of gait can occur.
- Laxity of knee with valgus stress with knee partially flexed.
- Swelling is common.
- Tenderness along medial knee may be present.

LCL Tear

- Pain and stiffness along lateral joint line may be present.
- Swelling within hours if complete rupture.
- Instability is uncommon with isolated LCL sprains.
- Tenderness along lateral knee may be present.
- Effusion is common.
- Limited range of motion but tenderness and laxity laterally with varus stress on partially flexed knee.

ETIOLOGY

ACL

- Hyperextension (especially on landing from a jump), sudden deceleration (or stopping), or a valgus stress with rotational force on planted or pronated foot

MCL

- Valgus force to partially flexed knee with foot planted
- "Clipping" injury in football

LCL

- Tear occurs with varus force to the knee or hyperextension injury

PCL

- Extreme (hyper) flexion and fall on shin with toe pointed
- Bent knee with sudden force on proximal tibia (dashboard injury)

DIAGNOSIS

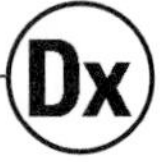

DIFFERENTIAL DIAGNOSIS

- Patella dislocation (mechanism of noncontact injury identical to ACL tear)
- Patellar fracture
- Proximal tibia/tibial spine avulsion fracture
- Meniscal injury
- Femoral condyle fracture
- Chondral avulsion patella
- Bursitis
- Arthritis, synovitis
- Slipped capital femoral epiphysis (SCFE)
- Legg-Calvé-Perthes disease
- Other hip pathology

WORKUP

- Definitive diagnosis is made at arthroscopy.
- Acute knee effusion is associated with trauma.
  - May be indication for arthroscopy and orthopedic workup
  - Usually indicates hemarthrosis (ligament tear, meniscal tear, fracture, or combination)

IMAGING STUDIES

- With ligament injuries, consider radiographic studies
  - Rule out fractures (anteroposterior, lateral, tunnel, and skyline views of knee)—physeal and tibial eminence, osteochondral lesions, and loose bodies
  - May need stress radiographic study under fluoroscopy to visualize nonossified disruptions
- Magnetic resonance imaging
  - Discouraged as screening tool (75% false-positive and false-negative readings in skeletally immature in one study)
  - Evaluation of soft tissues not visualized on plain radiography
  - Used by surgeon involved with definitive therapy

TREATMENT

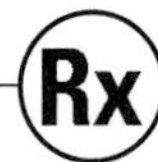

NONPHARMACOLOGIC THERAPY

- Compression
- Ice
- Elevation
- Immobilization with partial weight bearing

- Protected motion in brace begins as soon as possible
- Weight bearing and strengthening follow
- Surgical repair usually necessary, but not emergently, in grade III tears

ACUTE GENERAL Rx

- Nonsteroidal anti-inflammatory drugs (NSAIDs) for pain

CHRONIC Rx

- Rehabilitation for significant tears may take months before return to full activity is advised.

DISPOSITION

- Return to sports when the following have occurred:
  - Full range of motion
  - Normal strength
  - Nontender
  - No complaints (of pain, weakness, agility, endurance) with sport/activity
- Both nonoperative and operative care of significant knee injuries are wrought with complications and long-term disabilities.
- Methods of repair may vary based on skeletal maturation.

REFERRAL

Referral should be made to an orthopedic surgeon for suspected full or partial rupture, if the diagnosis is unclear, for surgery, for persistent pain, or for instability.

PEARLS & CONSIDERATIONS

COMMENTS

In prepubertal child, avulsion fractures are more common than ligamentous injuries.

PREVENTION

- Sports guidelines that prevent clipping

SUGGESTED READINGS

Bales CP et al: Anterior cruciate ligament injuries in children with open physes. *Am J Sports Med* 32:1978, 2004.

Davids JR: Pediatric knee: clinical assessment of common disorders. *Pediatr Clin North Am* 43:1067, 1996.

Dorizas JA, Stanitski CL: Anterior cruciate ligament injury in the skeletally immature. *Orthop Clin N Am* 34:355, 2003.

Shea KG et al: Anterior cruciate ligament injury in paediatric and adolescent patients. *Sports Med* 33:455, 2003.

Vaquero J et al: Intra-articular traumatic disorders of the knee in children and adolescents. *Clin Orthop Rel Res* 432:97, 2005.

AUTHOR: **LYNN C. GARFUNKEL, MD**

BASIC INFORMATION

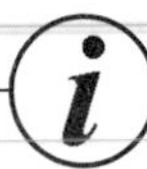

DEFINITION

Meniscal tears and injuries involve the disk-shaped medial or lateral fibrocartilage pads that lie between the femoral condyles and the tibial plateau (see Orthopedics and Sports Medicine in Charts, Formulas, Laboratory Tests and Values [Section IV]).

SYNONYMS

Locked knee
Torn cartilage

ICD-9-CM CODE

836.2 Meniscal tear

EPIDEMIOLOGY & DEMOGRAPHICS

- Rare among prepubertal children
- More common with high-impact sports
- Medial meniscal tears more common than lateral tears (young and old alike)
- Commonly seen with concurrent ligament (especially anterior cruciate ligament) ruptures

CLINICAL PRESENTATION

- Specific event often recalled by teen, but one sixth to one third of patients with meniscal tears will report no history of antecedent injury.
- Pain
- Mechanical symptoms—clicking, popping, catching, locking, or giving way
  - May especially occur if there is a loose fragment of cartilage in joint space
- Weight bearing may be preserved, especially in small injuries, or limited by pain
- Joint (femoral-tibial) line tenderness
- Decreased range of motion
- Pain with duck-walking
- Effusion of knee usually occurs within 24 hours of acute tears; chronic effusion may also be seen.
- Positive McMurray test (see Knee Maneuvers in Charts, Formulas, Laboratory Tests and Values [Section IV])
  - Nonspecific
  - Place fingers along the joint line on a flexed (greater than 120 degrees) knee, then internally (or externally) rotate the tibia, while bringing the knee joint to full extension.
  - A painful pop in the lateral or medial joint line will be elicited.

ETIOLOGY

- These tears result from a twisting motion with the knee flexed and foot planted (landing from jump).
- The meniscus splits because of firm attachments to the rotating femur on the fixed tibia.

DIAGNOSIS

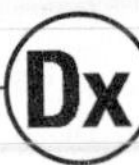

DIFFERENTIAL DIAGNOSIS

- Discoid meniscus
- Popliteus tendonitis
- Osteochondritis dissecans
- Patellofemoral instability
- PFPS
- Iliotibial band syndrome
- Anterior cruciate ligament (ACL), medial collateral ligament (MCL) tears (which may also accompany meniscal injuries)
- Osteochondral or avulsion fractures of femur, tibia, or patella
- Other knee sprain/strain
- Tumor, bone cyst
- Bursitis
- Arthritis, synovitis
- Osteomyelitis
- Slipped capital femoral epiphysis (SCFE)
- Legg-Calvé-Perthes disease
- Other hip disorders with referred pain

WORKUP

- Acute effusions associated with trauma are usually caused by hemarthrosis and generally indicate meniscal tear, ACL or other ligament rupture, or osteochondral fracture.
- Chronic effusions may be associated with tumor, infection, rheumatologic, or metabolic abnormalities as well as overuse.
- Arthroscopy may be indicated for diagnosis and treatment especially if persistent pain with mechanical symptoms.

IMAGING STUDIES

- Clinical diagnosis is 92% to 93% sensitive and specific, respectively, compared with magnetic resonance imaging (MRI) sensitivity and specificity of 50% and 38%, respectively, in one study.
- MRI high false-positive rate may be because of increased hydration of pediatric meniscus.
  - However, evaluation of soft tissues is not visualized on plain radiography.
  - Improved sensitivity and specifically when used by experienced physicians, but cost is very high compared with examination (and arthroscopy).

TREATMENT

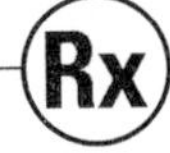

NONPHARMACOLOGIC THERAPY

- Avoid positions and activity that are painful and place extra forces on knees—squatting, kneeling, kicking, cycling, repetitive bending/straightening (stair climbing), twisting, and pivoting.
- Small, peripheral tears often heal without specific therapy.
- Surgical therapy may be needed for:
  - Repair of unstable tears
  - Removal of fragments, especially medial central, because avascular and poor healing
  - Meniscectomy; not preferred because poor long-term results
- Begin quadriceps contractions as soon as they can be done without pain (including day of injury) to avoid losing muscle bulk and strength.

ACUTE GENERAL Rx

- Nonsteroidal anti-inflammatory drugs (NSAIDs) for acute pain
- Ice for 10 to 20 minutes several times per day

CHRONIC Rx

- Gradual quadriceps and hamstring strengthening with increasing weights and eventual weight bearing
- Begin with straight leg, advance starting with 30-degree flexion then 45 degrees, then 75 degrees, then 90 degrees
- Increase weight at each degree of flexion, advance slowly
- Training for endurance and flexibility ongoing and overlapping with strength rehabilitation

DISPOSITION

Return to activity and eventually sports after rehabilitation complete (pain-free with normal strength and normal range of motion).

REFERRAL

- Referral to an orthopedic surgeon or sports medicine specialist
- Referral to physical therapist for strengthening and stretching education and oversight

PEARLS & CONSIDERATIONS

PREVENTION

For many pediatric knee problems, adequate stretching and strengthening will help in preventing injury (and reinjury).

PATIENT/FAMILY EDUCATION

- Familydoc.com. Available online at www.familydoc.com

SUGGESTED READINGS

Anderson B: *Meniscal injury of the knee.* UpToDate online, May 12, 2005.

Hergenroeder AK: *Approach to young athlete with acute knee pain or injury; Cases of knee pain or injury in young athlete.* UpToDate online, 2004.

Kocher MS et al: Meniscal disorders: normal, discoid, and cysts. *Orthop Clin North Am* 34:329, 2003.

Moti AW, Micheli LJ: Meniscal and articular cartilage injury in the skeletally immature knee. *AAOS Instr Course Lectures* 52:683, 2003.

AUTHOR: **LYNN C. GARFUNKEL, MD**

BASIC INFORMATION

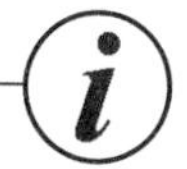

DEFINITION

Labyrinthitis is a viral or bacterial infection of the inner ear that causes dizziness and reduced or distorted hearing. Closely related is vestibular neuritis, which is caused by a viral infection of one of the two vestibular nerves. The imbalance of information about head positioning is interpreted by the brain to be movement, resulting in the sensation of vertigo. Symptoms include dizziness, vertigo, disequilibrium or imbalance, and nausea.

SYNONYMS

Inner ear infection
Vertigo

ICD-9-CM CODE
386.30 Labyrinthitis

EPIDEMIOLOGY & DEMOGRAPHICS

- Five percent of all dizziness is caused by labyrinthitis or vestibular neuritis.
- It occurs in all age groups but is more common in 30 to 50 year olds.
- Females are slightly more susceptible than males, at a ratio of 1.5:1.

CLINICAL PRESENTATION

History

- The early stages may be mild.
- Disequilibrium and hearing loss occur.
- Nausea is common.
- Symptoms are often precipitated by sudden movements or a sudden turn of the head.

Physical Examination

- The middle ear may show signs of infection or serous fluid.
- Nystagmus (usually horizontal) may be present at rest or when provoked by head turning.
- Meningeal signs should be evaluated carefully to distinguish it from meningitis.
- Careful neurologic examination is important to detect other conditions.

ETIOLOGY

- An upper respiratory infection precedes the onset of symptoms in 50% of cases.
- Viruses (or occasionally bacteria) can enter the inner ear and cause inflammation of the labyrinth system or directly affect the vestibular nerve. Viruses causing labyrinthitis include adenovirus, coxsackievirus, respiratory syncytial virus (RSV), influenza, herpesvirus, hepatitis, polio, cytomegalovirus (CMV), Epstein-Barr virus, measles, rubella, and mumps.
- Chronic, untreated middle ear infections can create a serous labyrinthitis resulting from inflammation or cholesteatoma formation.
- Bacteria from the middle ear can spread locally, leading to suppurative labyrinthitis.

DIAGNOSIS (Dx)

DIFFERENTIAL DIAGNOSIS

- Closed head injury
- Hypertension
- Ear trauma
- Allergies
- Anxiety
- Neurologic disease (i.e., central nervous system tumor or infection)
- Headache or migraine
- Ménière's disease
- Many drugs can cause dizziness:
  - Alcohol
  - Tobacco
  - Caffeine
  - β-Blockers or antihypertensives
  - Illicit drugs: cocaine, amphetamines, glue sniffing
  - Antiepileptics

WORKUP

- Initially, only a history and physical examination are necessary.
- No specific laboratory studies are available for labyrinthitis. To rule out other associated conditions, a lumbar puncture, complete blood cell count, or tympanocentesis may be indicated.

LABORATORY TESTS

- If symptoms persist beyond 1 month, recur, or become debilitating, an audiogram and electronystagmography (ENG) may help distinguish labyrinthitis from Ménière's disease and migraine.
  - An audiogram shows reduced hearing (especially high frequency) in labyrinthitis.
  - ENG characteristically shows reduced responses to motion of one ear.

IMAGING STUDIES

- Magnetic resonance imaging (MRI) can detect evidence of stroke, tumor, or vestibular nerve impingement.
- The cochlea, vestibule, and semicircular canals enhance on T1-weighted, postcontrast images of persons with acute and subacute labyrinthitis. This finding is highly specific and correlates with objective and subjective patient assessment.
- Improvements in MRI techniques may make this the study of choice for suspected labyrinthitis.

TREATMENT (Rx)

NONPHARMACOLOGIC THERAPY

- Lying still with the eyes closed may help reduce the severity of vertigo.
- If complicated by otitis media, mastoiditis, or cholesteatoma, a surgical procedure (e.g., myringotomy, mastoidectomy) may be needed.

ACUTE GENERAL Rx

- The initial treatment for viral labyrinthitis consists of bed rest and hydration.
- Patients with severe nausea and vomiting may benefit from intravenous fluid and antiemetic medications (promethazine, 0.25 to 1 mg/kg/dose PO every 6 hours; ondansetron (Zofran) for 4 to 11 year olds, 4 mg every 8 hours and for 12 years to adult, 8 mg every 8 hours).
- Diazepam is occasionally helpful as a vestibular suppressant (oral dose of 0.1 to 0.2 mg/kg/dose every 6 to 8 hours).
- A short course of oral corticosteroids may be helpful (1 to 2 mg/kg/day).
- The role of antiviral therapy is not established.
- Antibiotics should be used only in suppurative conditions (e.g., otitis media, mastoiditis).

DISPOSITION

- Patients should be monitored to ensure adequate hydration.
- It may take 3 weeks to recover from labyrinthitis. Recovery involves a combination of resolution of acute infection and compensation by the brain for persistent vestibular imbalance.
- Some patients experience intermittent symptoms for months, especially associated with sudden head movements.
- Minor sensitivity to head motion can persist for years and may reduce the ability to perform certain activities and sports, such as racquetball, volleyball, or aerobics.

REFERRAL

- Formal hearing testing should be performed at the end of symptoms to detect subtle hearing deficits that may persist.
- For those whose symptoms persist or who exhibit concerning neurologic findings, referral should be made to a specialist who is familiar with vestibular disorders.

PEARLS & CONSIDERATIONS

COMMENTS

- About 5% of all dizziness is caused by vestibular neuritis or labyrinthitis.
- Children as young as 1 year of age can experience vertigo, which may mimic seizure activity.
- Any neurologic finding besides nystagmus suggests conditions other than labyrinthitis.

PATIENT/FAMILY EDUCATION

- The Vestibular Disorders Association (VEDA) offers information on support groups, children's educational sites, and reference books: www.vestibular.org

SUGGESTED READINGS

Boston ME: Labyrinthitis. *In* Adler J et al (eds): *E-medicine.com,* May 2005.

Curtis JA: Dizziness and vertigo. *In* Hoekelman RA et al (eds): *Primary Pediatric Care,* 4th ed. Mosby, St Louis, 2001, pp 1034–1035.

AUTHOR: **NEIL E. HERENDEEN, MD**

BASIC INFORMATION

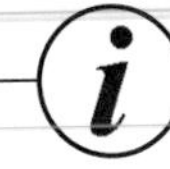

DEFINITION

Lacrimal duct obstruction is blockage of the nasolacrimal duct drainage system leading to increased eye tearing and potential infection.

SYNONYMS

Blocked tear duct
Dacryocystitis (infection of obstructed duct)
Dacryostenosis
Nasolacrimal duct obstruction

ICD-9-CM CODES
375.32 Dacryocystitis, acute and subacute
375.42 Chronic dacryocystitis
375.55 Neonatal tear duct occlusion
375.56 Dacryostenosis
743.65 Congenital dacryostenosis

EPIDEMIOLOGY & DEMOGRAPHICS

- The nasolacrimal duct system is not fully patent in as many as 73% of term infants.
- More than 90% of cases of lacrimal duct obstruction resolve spontaneously in the first 9 to 12 months of life.
- Obstruction resolves spontaneously or remains asymptomatic in all but approximately 4% of patients.

CLINICAL PRESENTATION

History

- Intermittent and recurrent tearing and mucoid discharge is produced from one or both eyes, usually without conjunctival injection.
- Symptoms usually begin within days to weeks after birth and are often variable and cyclical.
- Associated conjunctival injection and infection may occur and, in rare cases, progress to dacryocystitis.
  - Mucopurulent discharge with tender swelling of the nasolacrimal sac
  - Swelling noted along the medial canthus and lower lid

Physical Examination

- Assess for conjunctival injection.
- Assess for erythema or swelling of lacrimal sac and surrounding periorbital tissues.
- Digital pressure of the nasolacrimal sac can be diagnostic as well as therapeutic.
  - If obstructed, pressure may cause tears and mucus to be released from the puncta.
  - This may help relieve the distal obstruction.

ETIOLOGY

- Congenital
  - Obstruction of the nasolacrimal duct (the bony canal that carries tears into the nose) prevents drainage of tears produced by the lacrimal gland and promotes mucus buildup within the lacrimal sac.
  - Obstruction occurs during development of the lacrimal system and typically involves the distal portion of the duct.
  - Obstruction may represent failure of canalization of the epithelial cells that form the duct, resulting in a thin membrane that occludes the lumen.
- Acquired
  - Far less common in children and adolescents than in adults
  - May result from trauma, infection, sinus disease, nasal polyps, tumor, sarcoid, Wegener's granulomatosis, or other granulomatous disease

DIAGNOSIS (Dx)

DIFFERENTIAL DIAGNOSIS

- In a newborn with obstruction and associated infection, other causes of conjunctivitis (*Neisseria gonorrhoeae, Chlamydia,* nonspecific, or allergic) or keratitis need to be considered.
- Congenital glaucoma can present with excessive tearing and light sensitivity, but associated signs include increased intraocular pressure; an enlarged, hazy cornea; and occasionally, lid spasm.
- In an older infant with tearing, consider a foreign body or corneal abrasion.
- Other disorders of the lacrimal drainage system can present with similar symptoms.
  - Atresia of the lacrimal puncta: increased tearing but milder and without mucoid discharge
  - Congenital mucocele (dacryocystocele) of the lacrimal sac
    - Rare; bluish subcutaneous swelling in the medial canthal area
    - Results from a nonpatent lacrimal sac with both proximal and distal obstruction
    - Prone to infection and may progress to cellulitis
- In cases of dacryocystitis, assess closely for signs of periorbital or orbital cellulitis.

WORKUP

Consider culture of the eye discharge in cases with associated conjunctivitis or dacryocystitis.

TREATMENT (Rx)

NONPHARMACOLOGIC THERAPY

- Directed toward avoiding infection and minimizing additional obstruction of the sac with discharge and debris
- Application of warm compresses to the eye to cleanse away discharge and debris
- Massage of nasolacrimal sac
  - Digital compressing of the nasolacrimal sac results in increased hydrostatic pressure within the canal.
  - This pressure may force the duct to open (see "Patient/Family Education").
- For cases that do not resolve spontaneously by 1 year of age, referral to a pediatric ophthalmologist is indicated for probing and irrigation of the nasolacrimal duct.
- Additional surgical options include nasolacrimal duct intubation with silastic tubing and pediatric balloon dacryoplasty.

ACUTE GENERAL Rx

- For mild or low-grade infection accompanying obstruction, use topical antibiotics (ointment preferred over drops) combined with nasolacrimal sac massage.
- If infection is more severe or with accompanying dacryocystitis, take a culture of the discharge and begin treatment with systemic antistaphylococcal antibiotics (oral or intravenous).
  - Close monitoring is critical.
  - Orbital cellulitis is a possible complication.

DISPOSITION

See "Nonpharmacologic Therapy."

REFERRAL

Infants who do not experience spontaneous resolution by 1 year of age should be referred to a pediatric ophthalmologist.

PEARLS & CONSIDERATIONS

COMMENTS

- Congenital nasolacrimal duct obstruction is the most common abnormality of the entire lacrimal system in children.
- It presents with recurrent tearing and eye discharge in the early newborn period without conjunctival injection or photophobia.
- Digital massage can be therapeutic in relieving the distal congenital duct obstruction.

PREVENTION

See "Nonpharmacologic Therapy" described previously to minimize secondary infection.

PATIENT/FAMILY EDUCATION

- Parents should be instructed to massage the nasolacrimal sac three to four times daily.
  - Appropriate massage technique should be performed in the medial canthal area and not down the nasal bone, where the duct is interosseous and not affected by compression.
  - The initial motion should milk any discharge from the sac upward, followed by firm downward pressure on the nasolacrimal sac.
- Parents should call their child's physician to report signs of infection such as conjunctival infection or periorbital erythema and swelling.

SUGGESTED READINGS

Lavrich JB, Nelson LB: Disorders of the lacrimal system apparatus. *Pediatr Clin North Am* 40:767, 1993.

Robb RM: Congenital nasolacrimal duct obstruction. *Ophthalmol Clin North Am* 14(3):443, 2001.

AUTHOR: **LAURA JEAN SHIPLEY, MD**

BASIC INFORMATION

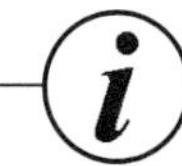

DEFINITION

Lactose intolerance is the inability to digest the milk sugar lactose, resulting in a constellation of clinical symptoms after the ingestion of milk products.

SYNONYMS

Hypolactasia
Lactase deficiency
Lactose malabsorption

ICD-9-CM CODE
271.3 Intestinal lactase deficiency and lactose malabsorption

EPIDEMIOLOGY & DEMOGRAPHICS

- Primary acquired lactase deficiency is more common in some populations.
  - Up to 70% to 100% prevalence in Asians, Africans, Eskimos, and Native Americans
  - Less than 20% prevalence in Scandinavians and Anglo-Saxons
- Primary lactose intolerance develops after lactase levels decrease, usually between 3 and 5 years of age. Symptoms may manifest at any age.
- Secondary lactose intolerance occurs during and often after its causal illness.

CLINICAL PRESENTATION

History
- Flatulence
- Abdominal pain
- Bloating
- Loose stools (develop within hours after milk ingestion)
- Symptom severity, timing after milk ingestion, and amount of lactose required to elicit them vary depending on the following:
  - Intestinal lactase levels
  - Lactose dose and presenting vehicle
  - Gastric emptying and intestinal transit time
  - Intestinal secretion in response to osmotic challenge
  - Bacterial flora

Physical Examination
- Tympanitic or distended abdomen
- Hyperactive bowel sounds
- Weight loss or poor weight gain (rare)

ETIOLOGY

- Lactose malabsorption is caused by a deficiency of the intestinal brush border enzyme lactase.
  - Lactase breaks down lactose into the monosaccharides glucose and galactose.
  - Unlike disaccharides, monosaccharides are absorbed by the small intestine.
- Undigested, and therefore unabsorbable, lactose passes through the intestine, drawing water into the lumen.
- Colonic bacteria ferment lactose, producing gas and volatile fatty acids.
- Congenital alactasia is rare.
- Primary acquired deficiency results from decreasing enzyme activity in the small intestine with age or maturity (i.e., postweaning).
- Secondary lactase deficiency results from disease processes or treatments that injure the small bowel lining (e.g., celiac disease, Crohn's disease, giardiasis, rotavirus infection, cow's milk or soy protein sensitivity, irradiation).
- Transient lactase deficiency occurs in premature infants.
- Developmental lactose intolerance is defined by the following:
  - At 26 to 34 weeks' gestation, lactase levels are 30% of term infants' levels.
  - At 35 to 38 weeks' gestation, lactase levels are 70% of term infants' levels.

DIAGNOSIS

Dx

DIFFERENTIAL DIAGNOSIS

- Cow's milk protein sensitivity
- Giardiasis
- Constipation with encopresis
- Irritable bowel syndrome or functional abdominal pain
- Other diseases causing small bowel mucosal injury

WORKUP

- The breath hydrogen test measures exhaled hydrogen gas produced in the colon by bacterial fermentation of undigested lactose.
- Serial measurements are obtained after ingestion of a 2 g/kg lactose load.
  - Abnormal peak demonstrated within 1 to 2 hours indicates lactose malabsorption.
  - Associated symptoms indicate lactose intolerance.
  - In the absence of bacteria that produce hydrogen, symptoms may occur without an abnormal peak in breath hydrogen (i.e., false negative).

LABORATORY TESTS

- Serum lactose tolerance test
  - Serial blood glucose levels are drawn after oral lactose ingestion.
  - Patients with lactase deficiency do not have a normal elevation of blood glucose levels after oral ingestion of lactose.
- Direct assay of enzyme activity (can be obtained from intestinal biopsy)
- Stool pH
  - Acid stool (pH < 5) indicative of carbohydrate malabsorption
  - Not specific for lactose malabsorption
  - May be helpful in infants and toddlers

TREATMENT

Rx

NONPHARMACOLOGIC THERAPY

- A lactose-free or low-lactose diet should be initiated.
  - Strict elimination may be instituted for 2 to 3 weeks to demonstrate complete resolution of symptoms.
  - Liberalize slowly, depending on the symptoms.
- Some patients tolerate digested or fermented milk products such as yogurt, cultured buttermilk, and curds.
- Hidden sources of lactose may be found in baked goods, margarine, lunch meats, salad dressings, candy, and medications.

ACUTE GENERAL Rx

- Lactase supplements may be taken with milk products.
- Milk containing hydrolyzed lactose is available (i.e., Lactaid).
- Calcium supplements are necessary if few dairy products are tolerated.

CHRONIC Rx

Patients may need lifelong lactase supplementation.

DISPOSITION

With avoidance of lactose, patients do well.

REFERRAL

- Patients should be referred to a pediatric gastroenterologist if an underlying intestinal illness is suspected (e.g., associated weight loss) or if symptoms do not resolve with strict elimination of lactose.
- Consider referral to nutritionist for parental education and advice about diet, especially if caloric or calcium intake is a concern.

PEARLS & CONSIDERATIONS

PATIENT/FAMILY EDUCATION

- National Digestive Diseases Information Clearinghouse (NIDDIC): http://digestive.niddk.nih.gov/ddiseases/pubs/lactoseintolerance
- North American Society for Pediatric Gastroenterology, Hepatology and Nutrition: www.naspghan.org (click on "public information," then "disease information," then "lactose intolerance in children")
- American Gastroenterological Association: www.gastro.org (click on "patient center," then "digestive conditions," then lactose intolerance)

SUGGESTED READINGS

Bahna SL: Cow's milk allergy versus cow milk intolerance. *Ann Allergy Asthma Immunol* 89(Suppl):56, 2002.
Shaw AD, Davies GJ: Lactose intolerance: problems in diagnosis and treatment. *J Clin Gastroenterol* 28:208, 1999.
Vesa TH et al: Lactose intolerance. *J Am Coll Nutr* 19(Suppl):165S, 2000.

AUTHOR: **M. SUSAN MOYER, MD**

BASIC INFORMATION

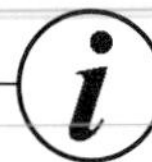

DEFINITION

Lead poisoning is the potential impairment caused by lead ingestion, and it affects almost every organ in the body. Lead poisoning usually has no overt symptoms. The developing central nervous system of the young child is particularly likely to be affected. Common manifestations are an irreversible reduction in neurocognitive potential, decreased attention span, and increased aggressiveness. These effects may occur at blood lead levels currently designated as being below the Centers for Disease Control and Prevention (CDC) lead level of concern (10 μg/dL). Very high blood lead levels (≥70 μg/dL) are rare and can result in encephalopathy, coma, and death.

SYNONYM

Lead toxicity

ICD-9-CM CODE
984.9 Lead poisoning

EPIDEMIOLOGY & DEMOGRAPHICS

- Children are primarily susceptible to the toxic effects of lead.
- Lead poisoning occurs in all populations.
- The highest prevalence is found among poor, black children 5 years or younger who live in older inner-city housing.

CLINICAL PRESENTATION

- Pica
- Exposure to lead-containing dust, old peeling paint, contaminated soil, or other lead sources (i.e., paint used before 1950 had a high lead content)
- Low dietary intake of iron or calcium
- Physical exam usually noncontributory

ETIOLOGY

- Lead-contaminated dust and soil; deteriorated lead-based paint; cosmetics, ceramics, home remedies, lead pipes, and solder
- Occupational exposure (e.g., pottery making, glass production, battery manufacture or recycling, work in lead smelters or incinerators, iron working, pipe fitting, plumbing, demolition work, remodeling, chemical manufacturing, work on firing ranges)
- Airborne exposure near industrial point sources
- Associated with iron deficiency anemia

DIAGNOSIS

DIFFERENTIAL DIAGNOSIS

The diagnosis is based on laboratory testing, with nothing else in the differential diagnosis.

LABORATORY TESTS

- The diagnosis depends on the result of a venous lead assay.
- Erythrocyte protoporphyrin levels can help differentiate children with acute and chronic lead exposure.
- Iron studies should be obtained for child with venous lead levels ≥ 15 μg/dL.

IMAGING STUDIES

- Long-bone radiographs may show "lead lines" in cases of chronic lead exposure.
- Abdominal radiographs to look for lead chips or other ingested sources of lead should be considered before starting chelation for children with a venous lead level of 45 μg/dL or higher.

TREATMENT

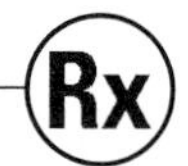

NONPHARMACOLOGIC THERAPY

- Ensure adequate iron and calcium intake.
- Environmental home inspection should occur expeditiously for any child whose venous lead level is 20 μg/dL or higher.
- Child should be removed from environment in which lead source is found.

ACUTE GENERAL Rx

- Children with a venous lead level of 45 μg/dL or higher should undergo chelation with a 5-day parenteral course of 1000 mg/m^2/day of $CaNa_2EDTA$ or a 19-day oral course of 2,3-DMSA (Succimer, Chemet). Home chelation should never be performed in a hazardous home environment.
- A venous lead level of 70 μg/dL or higher is considered a medical emergency. These children should receive a 5-day parenteral course of 1500 mg/m^2/day of $CaNa_2EDTA$ and 75 mg/m^2 of intramuscular dimercaprol (BAL) every 4 hours for 3 days.
- Good hydration should be ensured during the administration of $CaNa_2EDTA$ because of the possibility of nephrotoxicity associated with this chelating agent.
- Chelation does not reverse the neurocognitive effects.

DISPOSITION

- Children completing chelation should not return to a home environment until lead hazards are remediated.
- Children with moderately elevated venous lead levels (10 to 19 μg/dL) should undergo follow-up blood lead testing every 3 to 4 months. Children with higher blood lead levels should be tested more frequently.
- Children who are iron deficient at the time of chelation should begin receiving iron supplements 1 to 2 weeks after chelation is completed.
- Developmental follow-up is important for children with significantly elevated blood lead levels.

REFERRAL

Referral to the city or county health department should be undertaken when a child is found to have with a venous lead level of 20 μg/dL or higher.

PEARLS & CONSIDERATIONS

COMMENTS

- Lead is toxic wherever it is found, and it is found everywhere.
- Lead poisoning rarely has obvious clinical manifestations. Screening is required.

PREVENTION

- Risk assessment should be performed at every health supervision visit between 6 months and 6 years of age.
- Children who are at risk for significant lead exposure by history or who live in areas where 12% or more of children have blood lead levels of 10 μg/dL or higher or where 27% or more of housing was built before 1950 should have a blood lead assay at 12 and 24 months of age and whenever a specific risk factor is identified.

PATIENT/FAMILY EDUCATION

- Minimize environmental exposures to lead through the following steps: wet-mop uncarpeted floors, and wet-wipe window sills often; do not allow children to play with soil; wash children's hands often; limit children's exposure to peeling or chipping paint; avoid children's presence in homes being renovated.
- Maintain an adequate dietary intake of iron and calcium for affected children.
- More information can be obtained from:
  - Alliance for Healthy Homes (202-543-1147; http://www.afhh.org)
  - Housing and Urban Development Office of Hazard Control (www.hud.gov/offices/lead/)
  - Lead Poisoning Prevention Outreach Program, National Safety Council, Environmental Health Center (202-974-2476; http://www.nsc.org/issues/lead/)
  - National Lead Information Center (part of the National Safety Council), Environmental Protection Agency, Office of Pollution Prevention and Toxics (800-424-LEAD; www.epa.gov/lead/nlic.htm)
  - The National Center for Healthy Housing (410-992-0712; www.centerforhealthyhousing.org)

SUGGESTED READINGS

American Academy of Pediatrics Committee on Environmental Health: Screening for elevated blood lead levels. *Pediatrics* 101:1072, 1998.

Canfield RL et al: Intellectual impairment in children with blood lead concentrations below 10 μg per deciliter. *N Engl J Med* 348:1517, 2003.

Centers for Disease Control and Prevention: Preventing lead poisoning in young children: a statement by the Centers for Disease Control. Atlanta, Department of Health and Human Services, 1991.

Centers for Disease Control and Prevention: Screening young children for lead poisoning: guidance for state and local public health officials. Atlanta, Department of Health and Human Services, 1997.

National Academy of Sciences: Measuring lead exposure in infants, children, and other sensitive populations. Washington, DC, National Academy Press, 1993.

Rogan WJ et al: The effect of chelation therapy with succimer on neuropsychological development in children exposed to lead. *N Engl J Med* 344:1421, 2001.

AUTHORS: **STANLEY J. SCHAFFER, MD, MS** and **JAMES R. CAMPBELL, MD, MPH**

BASIC INFORMATION

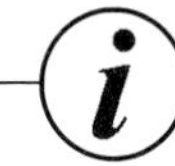

DEFINITION

Legg-Calvé-Perthes disease (LCPD) is an idiopathic avascular necrosis of the femoral head that may be partial or total.

SYNONYMS

Legg-Perthes disease
Osteochondrosis, hip
Perthes disease

ICD-9-CM CODE
732.1 Legg-Calvé-Perthes disease

EPIDEMIOLOGY & DEMOGRAPHICS

- The incidence varies from 1 case in 1200 to 12,500 children.
- The male-to-female ratio is 4:1.
- Bilateral involvement occurs in approximately 10%.
- LCPD generally occurs at 4 to 8 years of age (range, 2 to 13 years).
- LCPD is more common in whites and Asians; it is rare in blacks and Native Americans.
- LCPD may be associated with low birth weight, abnormal birth position, increased parental age, urban setting, psychological profiles suggesting attention deficit/hyperactivity disorder, and exposure to passive smoke.
- A delayed bone age may be seen.
- Short stature for age may be identified.

CLINICAL PRESENTATION

History

- A painless limp that is exacerbated by activity is reported.
- Pain, if present, is located in the groin, anterior thigh, or knee.
- Pain in the knee of any growing child should prompt a thorough examination of the hip because hip pathology often presents as pain in the knee.

Physical Examination

- Antalgic limp
- Limitation of abduction and internal rotation
- Disuse thigh atrophy (may also have atrophy of the buttock and calf)
- Leg length discrepancy
- Hip flexion contracture

ETIOLOGY

- The cause is unknown.
- Theories have focused on a compromise of blood flow to the femoral head.
  - Intraosseous venous hypertension and venous congestion
  - Arterial occlusion
  - Disorders of coagulation (i.e., thrombophilia and hyperfibrinolysis, caused by factor V Leiden or anticardiolipin antibodies)
  - Probably multifactorial

DIAGNOSIS

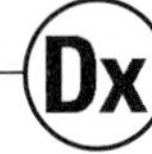

DIFFERENTIAL DIAGNOSIS

- Before radiologic evaluation:
  - Transient synovitis
  - Synovitis of any cause (e.g., juvenile arthritis, early septic arthritis)
- After radiologic evaluation, usually obvious:
  - For bilateral symmetric involvement; consider the following:
    - Hypothyroidism
    - Skeletal dysplasia (e.g., multiple epiphyseal dysplasia)
  - Bilateral involvement also may occur in other systemic disorders:
    - Renal disease
    - Steroid medication use
    - Sickle cell disease
  - Follow-up should continue until skeletal maturity to monitor the hip and the limb length.
  - Long-term follow-up suggests that osteoarthritis will develop in the fourth or fifth decade.

LABORATORY TESTS

- Laboratory results:
  - Generally normal complete blood cell count and erythrocyte sedimentation rate
  - May show thrombophilia or hyperfibrinolysis

IMAGING STUDIES

- Plain radiographs reveal various stages of the disease.
  - Normal
  - Cessation of growth (i.e., decreased size of ossific center)
  - Subchondral fracture or lucency (i.e., crescent sign)
  - Fragmentation (e.g., epiphysis appears fragmented, areas of increased radiodensity and radiolucency)
  - Re-ossification (i.e., uniform density of the epiphysis)
  - Healed (i.e., residual deformity)
- A bone scan may be helpful early, before bony changes occur. Decreased uptake may be seen in the involved femoral head.
- Magnetic resonance imaging may be useful before radiographic changes or during the course of the disease.
  - Ascertain shape of the femoral head.
  - Image for congruency of joint.
  - Look for presence of osteochondritis dissecans.

TREATMENT

Rx

NONPHARMACOLOGIC THERAPY

- The prognosis depends primarily on the age of the child and the extent of femoral head involvement.
- Children younger than 6 years of age tend to have less severe disease.
- The presence of subluxation or extrusion, the duration of the disease process, premature closure of the growth plate, and limited range of motion also may affect outcome.
- No treatment has been reported to speed healing of the femoral head.
- Treatment is indicated for pain, limitation of motion, and those with severe disease and poor prognosis.
- Nonpharmacologic treatment measures include the following:
  - Limitation of activities
  - Crutches
  - Physical therapy
  - Traction
  - Petrie casts
  - Abduction bracing: shown to be ineffective treatment
- Surgical approaches include the following:
  - Adductor tenotomy or medial release, or both, to help restore motion
  - Innominate osteotomy
  - Proximal femoral osteotomy
  - Arthroscopy or arthrotomy to remove symptomatic osteochondritis dissecans of the femoral head
  - Treatment goals: restoring a normal range of motion and obtaining as round a femoral head as possible by containing the femoral head within the acetabulum

ACUTE GENERAL Rx

Nonsteroidal medication can be used for hip joint irritability and pain.

DISPOSITION

- Follow-up should take place until skeletal maturity to monitor the hip and limb length.
- Long-term follow-up suggests that osteoarthritis will develop in the fourth or fifth decade.

REFERRAL

- Pediatric orthopedic surgeons should be involved in the assessment and care of children with persistent, unexplained limp or pain in the hip, thigh, or knee.
- An abnormal radiograph should prompt referral to a pediatric orthopedist.

SUGGESTED READINGS

Gruppo R et al: Legg-Calvé-Perthes disease in three siblings, 2 heterozygous and one homozygous for the factor V Leiden mutation. *J Pediatr* 132:885, 1998.

Herring JA et al: Legg-Calve-Perthes disease. Part 1. Classification of radiographs with use of the modified lateral Pillar and Stulberg classification. *J Bone Joint Surg Am* 86:2103, 2004.

Herring JA et al: Legg-Calve-Perthes disease. Part II. Prospective multicenter study of the effect of treatment on outcome. *J Bone Joint Surg Am* 86:2121, 2004.

Pediatric Orthopaedic Society of North America. Available at www.posna.org

Roy DR: Current concepts in Perthes disease. *Pediatr Ann* 28:748, 1999.

Thompson GH: Legg-Calvé-Perthes disease. *In* Pizzutillo PD (ed): *Pediatric Orthopaedics in Primary Practice.* New York, McGraw-Hill, 1997.

AUTHOR: **DENNIS ROY, MD**

BASIC INFORMATION

DEFINITION

Acute lymphoblastic leukemia (ALL) is the malignant transformation and proliferation of a lymphoid progenitor cell.

SYNONYMS

Acute lymphatic leukemia
Acute lymphocytic leukemia
ALL

ICD-9-CM CODE
204.00 Acute lymphoblastic leukemia

EPIDEMIOLOGY & DEMOGRAPHICS

- ALL is the most common cancer in the pediatric age group; it comprises 25% to 30% of all pediatric cancers and 75% of all acute leukemias.
- The incidence is 3 to 4 cases per 100,000 children.
- The peak incidence occurs between 2 and 5 years of age.
- A higher incidence occurs in boys and whites.

CLINICAL PRESENTATION

History
- Symptom duration of days to weeks
- Unexplained fever (intermittent or persistent)
- Easy or excessive bruising, other unusual bleeding
- Bone pain, limp, refusal to walk
- Anorexia, fatigue

Physical Examination
- Ill appearance
- Weight loss, usually not significant
- Pallor (often not appreciated by family members)
- Lymphadenopathy: nontender, firm nodes; usually disseminated
- Splenomegaly or hepatomegaly
- Petechiae, purpura; mucosal bleeding

ETIOLOGY

- The cause is unknown, although certain genetic and environmental factors, viral infections, and immunodeficiency syndromes have been indicated.
- Most patients have a chromosomal abnormality in the leukemic blast; it is unclear how the genetic change occurs, although most are somatic changes and therefore are not inherited.
- Other genetic factors play a role, and increased incidence is associated with certain constitutional abnormalities such as trisomy 21 (Down syndrome) or neurofibromatosis, identical twins (20% risk if one twin develops disease during the first 5 years of life), and familial cases (siblings have a fourfold increased risk over the general population).
- Environmental exposures to ionizing radiation and alkylating agents may play a role in the pathogenesis.

DIAGNOSIS (Dx)

DIFFERENTIAL DIAGNOSIS

- Infections: infectious mononucleosis (Epstein-Barr virus), cytomegalovirus, pertussis (associated with reactive lymphocytosis), osteomyelitis
- Hematologic disorders: idiopathic thrombocytopenic purpura, aplastic anemia
- Other malignant disorders: neuroblastoma, non-Hodgkin's lymphoma, other leukemias
- Nonmalignant disorders: juvenile rheumatoid arthritis

LABORATORY TESTS

- Complete blood cell count (CBC)
  - More than one half of pediatric patients present with a white blood cell (WBC) count less than 10,000/mm^3.
  - It is important to demonstrate evidence of more than one cell line affected: neutropenia (absolute neutrophil count < 1000), anemia (e.g., normocytic, normochromic), or thrombocytopenia.
- Review the blood smear for blasts (i.e., large cells with a small amount of basophilic cytoplasm surrounding a large nucleus).
- Definitive diagnosis can be made only by bone marrow aspiration.
  - More than 25% blasts in the marrow are required for a diagnosis of leukemia.
  - Most patients have complete replacement by blasts (80% to 100% blasts).
- Multiple biologic studies are performed on marrow blasts for confirmation of the diagnosis and stratification for treatment purposes and prognosis.
  - Immunophenotype surface antigens by flow cytometry
  - Chromosome analysis (i.e., cytogenetics)
  - Other research tools (i.e., cytochemistry, molecular genetics)
- Chemistries: electrolytes, blood urea nitrogen, creatinine, uric acid, liver function tests
- Tumor lysis laboratory tests include levels of uric acid, potassium, phosphorus, and calcium
- Spinal tap to evaluate cerebrospinal fluid for presence of blasts
- Other tests: coagulation profile, electrocardiogram and echocardiogram, immunologic survey (necessary before many treatment regimens)

IMAGING STUDIES

Chest radiographs are used to assess for significant mediastinal lymphadenopathy.

TREATMENT (Rx)

NONPHARMACOLOGIC THERAPY

Because of the intensity of current treatment regimens, most pediatric patients have a central venous access catheter placed at diagnosis to facilitate treatment.

ACUTE GENERAL Rx

- Aggressive intravenous hydration and allopurinol should be started as soon as possible in all cases to reduce the effects of tumor lysis.
- Plasmapheresis may be necessary if white cell counts are greater than 100,000.
- Combined-modality treatment (divided into various phases) should be initiated as soon as possible:
  - Induction
    - Goal: produce remission during the initial 4 to 5 weeks of therapy.
    - Drugs: vincristine (VCR), prednisone or dexamethasone (DEX), asparaginase (ASP) with or without an anthracycline (DOXO), intrathecal methotrexate (IT-MTX)
  - Consolidation
    - Therapy: directed at the central nervous system (CNS)
    - Weekly IT-MTX (for prophylaxis) or cranial irradiation: CNS leukemia at diagnosis and if patient is 3 years or older
    - Continued systemic chemotherapy: mercaptopurine (6MP), VCR
  - Interim maintenance (IM) and delayed intensification (DI)
    - Multiple drugs administered in an intensive schedule to intensify remission (DI) but allow for normal cell recovery (IM)
    - IM-VCR, MTX, 6MP, DEX, and IT-MTX
    - DI-VCR, DEX, ASP, doxorubicin, Cytoxan, 6-thioguanine, cytarabine, and IT-MTX
  - Maintenance
    - Primarily consists of outpatient therapy (oral 6MP and MTX)
    - Monthly visits for pulses of vincristine, corticosteroids
    - IT-MTX every 12 weeks
- The duration of treatment is approximately 2 years for girls and 3 years for boys after consolidation.
- Most children are (and should be) treated on national cooperative group study protocols (e.g., Children's Oncology Group).
  - Evidence suggests that the outcome is improved when patients are treated on pediatric protocols.
  - A large proportion of adolescents is not included in studies because of poor accrual rates.

CHRONIC Rx

- Maintenance therapy for ALL is described in "Acute General Rx."
- Prophylaxis for *Pneumocystis pneumoniae* is trimethoprim-sulfamethoxazole or pentamidine.
- Prompt evaluation for fever or other signs of infection (varicella) is required,

especially for patients with a low absolute neutrophil count (ANC).
- Use transfusions and nutritional support as needed.

DISPOSITION

- On completion of therapy, patients should be followed intermittently for relapse (e.g., bone marrow, CNS, and testicular) and late effects of treatment.
- Seventy percent of patients with ALL are cured.
- Good-risk patients (i.e., initial WBC count < 50,000/mm^3, age 1 to 10 years) have an 85% to 90% cure rate.
- High-risk patients (i.e., >10 years; WBC count > 50,000/mm^3) have a 65% to 70% cure rate.
- Other factors also determine risk categories: immunophenotype, DNA index, cytogenetics, presence of CNS disease, and rate of response to induction therapy.
- Most relapses occur while on therapy. A 20% risk of relapse exists after treatment is complete.

REFERRAL

All children and adolescents (0 to 21 years old) should be referred to a tertiary care center for care managed by a pediatric hematologist-oncologist, ideally one participating in cooperative group trials.

PEARLS & CONSIDERATIONS

COMMENTS

- Leukemia should always be considered in the differential diagnosis of unexplained fever, bruising, or bone pain.
- When a CBC is obtained, look for abnormalities of more than one cell line (increasing the suspicion that the bone marrow is affected).
- Abnormality of more than one lymphoid organ (e.g., nodes, spleen, liver) on examination should raise the suspicion of ALL.

PREVENTION

Because the cause of ALL is unknown, prevention is not applicable. Early diagnosis, however, can greatly affect outcome.

PATIENT/FAMILY EDUCATION

- Parents need to understand that childhood cancer is different from adult cancer and that most patients with ALL are cured.
- Parents should be educated about the side effects of chemotherapy and the signs and symptoms for which they need to contact the medical team.
- School-related issues include repeated absences and learning difficulties after CNS therapy (especially in patients < 6 years old).
- Support groups are available through the Leukemia Society of America, 600 Third Avenue, New York, NY 10016 (212-573-8484).
- Support groups are available through the Candlelighters Childhood Cancer Foundation, Inc., 7910 Woodmont Avenue, Suite 460, Bethesda, MD 20814 (800-366-2223 or 301-657-8401).

SUGGESTED READINGS

American Cancer Society. Available at www.cancer.org

Friebert SE, Shurin SB: ALL: diagnosis and outlook. *Contemp Pediatr* 15:118, 1998.

Friends Network (interactive site for kids). Available at www.cancerfunletter.com

Greaves M: A natural history for pediatric acute leukemia. *Blood* 82:1043, 1993.

Lanzkowsky P: Leukemias. *In Manual of Pediatric Hematology and Oncology,* 3rd ed. California, Academic Press, 2000, pp 359–411.

Margolin JF, Poplack DG: Acute lymphoblastic leukemia. *In Principles and Practice of Pediatric Oncology,* 4th ed. Philadelphia, Lippincott williams & wilkins, 2001.

National Childhood Cancer Foundation (Children's Oncology Group). Available at www.nccf.org

Pui CH et al: Acute lymphoblastic leukemia [review article]. *N Engl J Med* 350:1535, 2004.

AUTHOR: **SHERRY L. BAYLIFF, MD, MPH**

BASIC INFORMATION

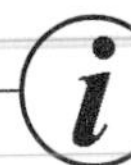

DEFINITION

Acute myelogenous leukemia (AML) is the malignant transformation and proliferation of any myeloid progenitor cell.

SYNONYMS

Acute nonlymphocytic leukemia
AML

ICD-9-CM CODE

205.00 Acute myelogenous leukemia

EPIDEMIOLOGY & DEMOGRAPHICS

- There are approximately 500 new cases of AML per year, accounting for 20% of cases of pediatric leukemia.
- No sex or ethnic predisposition exists for AML. There is a slight increase in case numbers during the teenage years.
- Most cases of congenital leukemia (i.e., within the first 4 weeks of life) are AML.

CLINICAL PRESENTATION

History

- Unexplained fever, serious infection or sepsis; pallor, fatigue, weight loss; bruising or bleeding; bone pain; persistent respiratory or gastrointestinal symptoms; "blueberry muffin" rash in neonates.

Physical Examination

- Cutaneous or mucosal hemorrhage, menorrhagia; hepatosplenomegaly, lymphadenopathy; gingival hypertrophy; leukemia cutis (i.e., bluish skin nodules), especially in the neonate; retinal hemorrhage or cotton-wool spots on funduscopic examination.

ETIOLOGY

- The cause is unknown.
- Specific genetic abnormalities are present in the leukemia cell, but it is unknown how they arise; myelodysplasia often converts to AML.
- Children with genetic conditions such as trisomy 21 (i.e., Down syndrome) or Fanconi's anemia are at increased risk.
- Environmental exposures, such as ionizing radiation, benzene, epipodophyllotoxins (i.e., etoposide), and alkylating agents, are associated with AML.

DIAGNOSIS

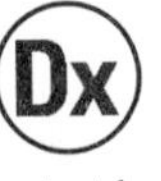

DIFFERENTIAL DIAGNOSIS

- Hematologic disorders: aplastic anemia, idiopathic thrombocytopenic purpura
- Infection or sepsis: disseminated intravascular coagulation (DIC), osteomyelitis

LABORATORY TESTS

- Complete blood cell count is required; most patients have significant anemia and thrombocytopenia.
  - Immature white blood cells (WBCs) (e.g., promyelocytes, myelocytes) are seen on the differential count.
  - Twenty-five percent of patients present with hyperleukocytosis with a WBC count greater than 100,000/mm^3.
- Review the blood smear for blasts and nucleated red blood cells.
- Bone marrow aspiration is necessary to make the diagnosis of AML. A concentration of more than 25% myeloblasts in the sample is diagnostic.
- Multiple biologic tests are performed on leukemic cells for confirmation of the diagnosis and stratification for treatment and prognosis.
  - Seven subtypes of AML exist: myeloblastic (M0, M1), promyelocytic (M3), myelomonocytic (M4), monocytic (M5), erythroblastic (M6), and megakaryocytic (M7). All subtypes are treated similarly, except for promyelocytic leukemia.
  - Immunophenotype surface antigens are determined by flow cytometry.
  - Chromosome analysis (i.e., cytogenetics) is necessary.
  - Other research tools include cytochemistry and molecular genetics.
    - Coagulation tests include prothrombin time (PT), partial thromboplastin time (PTT), fibrinogen, and D-dimer to screen for DIC.
    - Blood chemistry determinations include electrolytes, blood urea nitrogen, creatinine, transaminases, and bilirubin.
    - Spinal tap is done to evaluate cerebrospinal fluid for involvement by leukemia.

TREATMENT

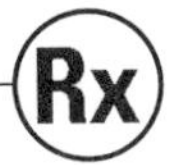

NONPHARMACOLOGIC THERAPY

Because of the intensity of current treatment regimens, most pediatric patients have a central venous access device placed at diagnosis to facilitate treatment.

ACUTE GENERAL Rx

- Stabilization of any life-threatening complications (i.e., bleeding, infection, tumor lysis syndrome, and leukostasis) must precede disease-directed therapy.
- Treatment entails intensive chemotherapy.
  - Marrow must be put into a state of severe hypoplasia to induce remission, resulting in prolonged periods of pancytopenia and hospitalization.
  - Common side effects include severe mucositis, liver damage, bleeding complications, and bacterial and fungal infections. These patients require aggressive supportive care.
- The main chemotherapeutic agents for treatment of AML are cytosine arabinoside and anthracyclines; central nervous system (CNS) prophylaxis is also used.
  - Several courses of intensive chemotherapy are given to prevent relapse.
  - Overall cure rate for AML is about 40%.
- Allogeneic bone marrow transplantation is performed in first remission for all patients with AML who have a matched donor in the family. The cure rate after transplantation is 50% to 70%.

DISPOSITION

- The risk of relapse is about 50%.
- Patients need to be monitored closely for signs and symptoms of recurrent leukemia.
- Survivors need to be followed for late-occurring side effects such as cardiac dysfunction from anthracyclines, secondary cancers, and fertility problems.

REFERRAL

All children and adolescents (0 to 21 years old) should be referred to a tertiary care center for treatment managed by a pediatric hematologist-oncologist, ideally one participating in cooperative group trials.

PEARLS & CONSIDERATIONS

COMMENTS

- Persistent fever of unknown origin, persistent infections, or other chronic signs and symptoms should raise suspicion of AML.
- Patients presenting with AML can be seriously ill because of infection or a very high WBC count, and they should be referred promptly for care.
- Patients with trisomy 21 have a 15-fold to 20-fold increased risk of leukemia, especially after transient myeloproliferative syndrome as a neonate.

PREVENTION

Because the cause of AML is unknown, prevention is not applicable. Early diagnosis, however, can significantly affect outcome.

PATIENT/FAMILY EDUCATION

- AML requires aggressive treatment, with many serious side effects and prolonged hospitalizations.
- Family members are tested at diagnosis to identify compatible bone marrow donors.
- Even with successful completion of treatment, a significant risk of relapse exists.
- Support groups are available: Leukemia Society of America (212-573-8484); Candlelighters Childhood Cancer Foundation, Inc., (800-366-2223 or 301-657-8401)

SUGGESTED READINGS

American Cancer Society. Available at www.cancer.org

Friends Network (interactive site for kids). Available at www.cancerfunletter.com

Golub TR et al: Acute myelogenous leukemia. *In Principles and Practices of Pediatric Oncology,* 3rd ed. Philadelphia, Lippincott-Raven, 1997.

Greaves M: A natural history for pediatric acute leukemia. *Blood* 82:1043, 1993.

Lanzkowsky P: Leukemias. *In Manual of Pediatric Hematology and Oncology,* 3rd ed. California, Academic Press, 2000, pp 359–411.

National Childhood Cancer Foundation (Children's Oncology Group). Available at www.nccf.org

Pui CH et al: Childhood leukemias [review]. *N Engl J Med* 332:1618, 1995.

AUTHOR: **SHERRY L. BAYLIFF, MD, MPH**

BASIC INFORMATION

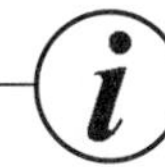

DEFINITION

Head lice is an arthropod infestation by the head louse of the scalp and neck, and it most commonly occurs in children.

SYNONYMS

Head lice
Pediculosis capitis

ICD-9-CM CODE
132.0 Head lice

EPIDEMIOLOGY & DEMOGRAPHICS

- Infection occurs worldwide, with 6 to 12 million persons infected each year in the United States.
- The highest incidence occurs among school-aged children between 4 and 11 years old.
- No significant differences exist by sex or socioeconomic status, but head lice in the United States are rarely found among blacks, likely due to difficulty in grasping the oval hair shaft.
- The prevalence ranges from 1% to 3%, but it occasionally exceeds 25% in elementary schools.
- It is estimated that children in the United States lost 12 to 24 million days of school in 1998 due to "no nit" policies in schools.
- The annual cost of head lice is estimated at $367 million, including the cost of over-the-counter pediculicides and costs to school systems.

CLINICAL PRESENTATION

- Most children with lice are asymptomatic, although there may be a history of pruritus if the infestation has been present for a longer time.
- Children usually present for evaluation after an adult (e.g., caregiver, teacher, school nurse, camp counselor) identifies presumed lice or nits on the scalp or in the case of an outbreak in daycare or at school.
- Physical examination is important to verify active infection; misdiagnosis is common.
- Active infestation is characterized by seeing crawling lice.
  - Some sources consider the presence of viable nits as indicative of active infestation, but this is difficult to determine.
  - In one study, 77 patients had "nits" present, but only 4 had live lice.
  - Diagnosis based on nits alone seen within 0.25 inch of the scalp will result in many unnecessary treatments.
- Adult lice are difficult to locate because they are sensitive to light and hide in hair strands.
- The adult head louse is grayish white to red or brown, is 3 to 4 mm long, and favors the front of the scalp.
- Unhatched eggs are small, oval, whitish, and transparent, and they are attached firmly to one side of the hair shaft 1 to 3 mm from the scalp, often at the nape of the neck and behind the ears.
- Artifacts, such as dandruff, hair gel, hair spray residue, dirt, or other insects, may be mistaken for lice or nits.

ETIOLOGY

- *Pediculosis humanus capitis* is a six-legged, wingless, bloodsucking insect that infests only the human head.
- The parasite requires the vascular environment of the scalp for a blood meal every 4 to 6 hours.
- The insect has a 30-day, three-stage life cycle: egg, nymph, and adult.
- Once the egg has hatched (in 6 to 9 days), it takes 7 to 10 days to reach the adult stage.
- Adult lice are the size of a sesame seed, and females can lay up to 10 eggs per day.
- Most people in the United States are infested with fewer than 10 lice.
- Transmission occurs by direct contact with an infected person's hair and possibly by sharing combs, hats, and other accessories.
- The adult louse may remain on bedding or upholstery for a brief time, but viability after being removed from the scalp is less than 2 days.
- Nits require an ambient temperature similar to that near the human scalp to hatch.

DIAGNOSIS

Dx

DIFFERENTIAL DIAGNOSIS

Ensure the appropriate diagnosis and eliminate confusion with benign particles; there is no other differential diagnosis for scalp infection of this type.

WORKUP

- Perform the examination in a well-lighted room or in natural sunlight for 3 to 5 minutes, carefully parting the hair and looking for lice.
- Visual inspection of the hair and scalp may miss 75% of infections identifiable by the use of a fine toothed nit comb. Examination may be made easier by wet combing and looking for live lice, but this is less practical in the clinical office.
- Detecting live lice on the head secures the diagnosis.
- Nits detected farther out on the hair shaft are not an indication of active infection.

LABORATORY TESTS

Samples of presumed lice or eggs may be collected and sent to the Harvard School of Public Health for analysis (see website below for more information).

TREATMENT

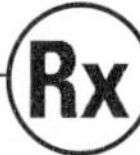

NONPHARMACOLOGIC THERAPY

- Treatment should be considered when active lice or viable eggs are observed.
- Mechanical removal of lice with the use of wet combing is recommended as an alternative to the use of insecticides, particularly in the case of children younger than 2 years old (only permethrin is labeled for use on children younger than 2 years).
- "Bug busting," or combing wet hair lubricated with hair conditioner or oil for 15 to 30 minutes per session every 3 to 4 days for several weeks using a nit comb, cures between 38% and 58% of cases.
  - Successful therapy requires patience and perseverance and, ideally, the removal of viable eggs from the hair shafts.
  - Some advocate a prerinse of 50% water and 50% vinegar to aid in the removal of the eggs or use of over-the-counter preparations that claim to loosen the egg from the shaft for easy removal. No scientific evidence supports this approach, and these products may influence the efficacy or residual activity of pediculicides.
- Environmental controls have centered on careful cleaning of the clothing, bedding, hats, stuffed animals, and upholstery, but this is probably unnecessary because viability of the louse once removed from the host is less than 48 hours, and nits require a very warm environment to hatch.
- Cleaning of combs and brushes, changing and laundering bedding and clothing, and simple vacuuming are likely sufficient environmental measures.
- No scientific data indicate that fomite control has any effect on re-infestation.
- Pediculide spray is unnecessary. It is of little benefit, so avoid exposure.

ACUTE GENERAL Rx

- Medical therapies can best be divided into topical pediculicides (i.e., insecticides) and oral agents.
- The safety of the child is the overriding concern, because the infestation presents no risk to the host.
- For topical medications, treatments should be used as directed on the package labeling (i.e., on dry hair or recently shampooed hair). The product should be applied to wet the entire scalp, but it need not be applied to the ends of long hair below the level of the shirt collar.
- Permethrin is a synthetic pyrethroid that is the treatment of choice for head lice due to its excellent safety profile and labeling for children down to 2 months old.
  - It is an insecticide that acts on the nerve cell membrane of the parasite, disrupting the sodium channel transport, delaying

repolarization, and paralyzing the insects. All pediculicides potentially affect mammalian nervous systems.
  - Permethrin has extremely low toxicity to humans.
  - Insecticidal activity approaches 100%, and ovicidal activity is approximately 70% to 80%.
  - There is residual activity for up to 2 weeks after the initial application to kill emerging nymphs from unkilled eggs.
  - A second treatment 7 to 10 days later is recommended if crawling lice are still seen.
  - Permethrin is available as an over-the-counter 1% crème rinse (Nix), which is applied to hair that is first shampooed with a nonconditioning shampoo and towel dried. After 10 minutes, it should be rinsed off over a sink with cool water to minimize skin contact and absorption.
  - A 5% permethrin compound (Elimite) is available by prescription and can be used with a shower cap overnight when resistance is suspected.
- Synergized pyrethrins are natural insecticidal compounds derived from the chrysanthemum flower that are neurotoxic to adult lice, but they have very low mammalian toxicity.
  - Given the derivation from ragweed or chrysanthemums, there is a possibility of allergic reaction in sensitized patients, and it is labeled for use only for children older than 2 years.
  - Insecticidal activity approaches 100%, and ovicidal activity is approximately 70% to 80%, necessitating a second treatment 7 to 10 days later to kill newly hatched eggs that may have survived. There is no residual activity.
  - Products are mostly shampoos applied to dry hair. They should be rinsed over a sink with cool water to minimize skin contact and absorption.
  - Over-the-counter preparations include RID, Pronto, A-200, R & C shampoo, and others.
- Malathion (Ovide) is an irreversible cholinesterase inhibitor that has been reintroduced to the U.S. market after having been pulled from the market twice due to prolonged application times, flammability, and odor concerns.
  - Malathion is a fast-acting insecticide and the most effective ovicide (<5% of eggs hatch after a 10-minute treatment). It binds to sulfur atoms in the hair, providing residual activity against lice.
  - It is available as a lotion that is applied to the hair, allowed to dry naturally, and washed off after 8 to 12 hours over a sink with cool water.
  - Safety has not been established for children younger than 2 years.
    - The alcohol base is highly flammable.
    - Patients should avoid the use of hair dryers, curling irons, or any flame (including smoking cigarettes) during use.
    - There is a risk of severe respiratory depression if ingested.
    - Use with caution when resistance is strongly suspected.
- Lindane (Kwell) is an organochloride that exhibits central nervous system toxicity and has been associated with seizures in some patients who used it incorrectly.
  - The insecticidal and ovicidal activity is less than that seen with permethrin or pyrethrin.
  - Resistance has been reported worldwide; there are better choices for therapy.
- Trimethoprim-sulfamethoxazole is an antibiotic that has been shown in two studies to eradicate lice infestations when given at otitis media doses.
  - Rare but severe allergic reactions make this a less desirable treatment option if alternatives are effective.
- Ivermectin is an anthelmintic agent that has been shown in one study to be effective against head lice. However, the drug is not approved by the U.S. Food and Drug Administration as a pediculicide.
  - The oral dose is 200 μg/kg, repeated once 10 days later.
  - Use with caution in young children or those weighing less than 15 kg because of possible neurologic effects.

COMPLEMENTARY & ALTERNATIVE MEDICINE

- Occlusive agents, such as petroleum jelly, olive oil, pork fat, or mayonnaise, have been recommended.
- These agents can be placed on the scalp in large quantities and covered overnight with a shower cap.
- Presumably, these products occlude the respiratory systems of the lice.
- Removal of eggs is critical because unhatched eggs are likely unaffected by the occlusive treatment and will ultimately mature into adult lice.
- Only anecdotal information is available concerning efficacy, which may result from intensive grooming and removal of lice and nits. Diligent shampooing is often required to remove the residue from these treatments.

DISPOSITION

- Careful reexamination of the scalp for lice or eggs is necessary, even after a pediculicide application, in conjunction with manual removal techniques.
- Suspected treatment failures have been reported in increasing frequency and may be the result of the following factors:
  - Misdiagnosis (i.e., misidentification or lack of active infection)
  - Noncompliance
  - New infestation
  - Lack of ovicidal or residual properties of the product
  - Resistance by lice to the insecticide
- Examination by a member of the health care team should be performed before labeling the child as a treatment failure.
- Patients should not repeatedly treat with over-the-counter medications if lice persist; they should seek medical advice.

PEARLS & CONSIDERATIONS

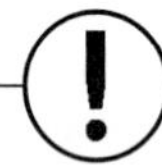

COMMENTS

- Because generics may be provided if a prescription is written, package labeling may not include detailed instructions; therefore, provide written or printed instructions to parents.
  - When applying topical pediculicides, follow directions carefully.
  - When using the permethrin (Nix) product, do not use conditioning shampoos or conditioners for 2 to 3 weeks after application, because they may interfere with the residual action of the medication.
- Prophylactic treatment of all household members is not routinely advised.
- Extensive environmental measures are not needed; laundering and vacuuming suffice.
- Only those with active infection should be treated to help prevent true lice resistance.

PREVENTION

- It is likely impossible to totally prevent head lice infestation because of the close head-to-head contact between young children at play.
- Children should be taught not to share combs, brushes, or hats, which are possible vehicles for live lice.
- Parents should be aware of the signs of lice so that prompt treatment can minimize further spread.

SUGGESTED READINGS

Frankowski BL, Weiner LB: Head Lice. *Pediatrics* 110:638, 2002.

Jones KN, English JC: Review of common therapeutic options in the United States for the treatment of pediculosis capitus. *Clin Infect Dis* 36:1355, 2003.

National Pediculosis Association. Available at www.headlice.org

AUTHOR: **SUSANNE E. TANSKI, MD**

BASIC INFORMATION

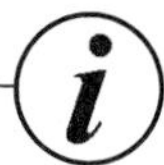

DEFINITION

Infection caused by *Listeria monocytogenes* is an important zoonosis that is uncommon in the general population. Although transmitted by food, it is an unusual cause of food poisoning and gastroenteritis. More often, systemic infection, such as life-threatening meningoencephalitis or bacteremia, results in patients of certain risk groups (e.g., neonates, pregnant women, and immunocompromised hosts).

SYNONYMS

Granulomatosis infantiseptica
Listeriosis

ICD-9-CM CODES
005.8 Other bacterial food poisoning
027.0 *L. monocytogenes*
771.2 Granulomatosis infantiseptica, fetal, or congenital listeriosis

EPIDEMIOLOGY & DEMOGRAPHICS

- *L. monocytogenes* is widespread in nature.
  - Found commonly in soil, decaying vegetation, and sewage
  - Also found in the fecal flora of many mammals, including 5% of healthy adults
- Modes of transmission include the following:
  - Foodborne mode is predominant, although gastroenteritis itself is not the predominant disease seen. The most common foods associated with transmission are ready-to-eat foods such as milk, soft cheeses, pâté, delicatessen meats, raw meat, and raw vegetables. Also commonly associated with listeriosis are unreheated hot dogs and turkey franks and undercooked poultry.
  - Vertical transmission is most often responsible for neonatal disease.
- Incidence and prevalence
  - *L. monocytogenes* is the sixth most common enteric bacterial cause of foodborne illness in the United States (following *Salmonella, Campylobacter, Shigella, Escherichia coli* O157:H7, and *Yersinia*). About 600 to 700 cases of *L. monocytogenes* disease are reported yearly in the United States.
  - The annual incidence in the United States has decreased in recent years because of stricter food-handling practices. The average overall annual incidence in 1989 was 0.8 case per 100,000 population; in 2003, it was approximately 0.3 per 100,000. However, the incidence rates of perinatal *Listeria* disease are more than 10-fold higher than the general population rates of roughly 12 per 100,000 in 2003. About 1.5% of U.S. early-onset neonatal sepsis is caused by *Listeria.*
- Risk factors and affected groups
  - Pregnant women
  - Infants younger than 1 month old
  - Patients with malignancy, organ transplantation, or human immunodeficiency virus-induced immunosuppression
  - Iron overload (e.g., chronic transfusion, hemochromatosis)
  - Adults older than 50 years

CLINICAL PRESENTATION

- History and physical examination
  - Patients often have ingested foods associated with transmission in the preceding month, and many patients presenting with bacteremia, central nervous system (CNS) infection, or infection during pregnancy have experienced symptomatic gastroenteritis in the preceding month.
  - The incubation period is about 21 days for all forms of listeriosis, except for acute gastroenteritis (discussed later).
- Infection in pregnancy
  - Febrile bacteremia with flulike illness (sometimes accompanied by lower back pain and gastrointestinal symptoms) is most commonly observed in the third trimester.
  - The condition may be self-limited, but it can persist or cause chorioamnionitis; premature labor is common.
  - The risk of stillbirth and neonatal death after maternal listeriosis is about 25%.
- Neonatal infection
  - *Granulomatosis infantiseptica* is a disseminated form of neonatal disease resulting from in utero infection.
  - It is uncommon but usually fatal. Widespread granulomatous microabscesses occur, especially in the liver, spleen, and skin; cutaneous lesions are papular or pustular, 1 to 3 mm in diameter with an erythematous base.
  - Early-onset neonatal sepsis and bacteremia: mimics group B streptococcal disease. It occurs shortly after birth, especially in premature infants.
  - Late-onset meningitis occurs at about 2 weeks of age. It is notably less common than early-onset disease.
- Systemic infection in immunocompromised children and adults
  - It most commonly manifests as pyogenic meningitis with somewhat atypical features; nuchal rigidity is less common, and fluctuating mental status is more common. Blood cultures are more likely positive than cerebrospinal fluid (CSF) cultures, and CSF Gram stains may not show organisms.
  - It less commonly manifests as brainstem encephalitis (i.e., rhombencephalitis), which has been described in adults with systemic listeriosis but not in infants.
  - Brain abscesses and cerebritis may occur at all ages.
  - Other focal sites of infection are rare.
  - Systemic infection occurs in nonimmunocompromised older adults (>50 years).
- Acute gastroenteritis is an unusual manifestation of listeriosis, despite its transmission by food, but it has been reported in point-source outbreaks. It is accompanied by fever and abdominal pain, and it has an incubation period of about 1 day.

ETIOLOGY

- *L. monocytogenes:* gram-positive, rod-shaped, facultative anaerobic bacterium
- The only one of six *Listeria* species pathogenic for humans

DIAGNOSIS

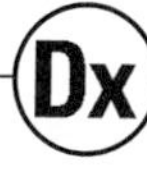

DIFFERENTIAL DIAGNOSIS

- Neonatal sepsis or meningitis
- Atypical meningitis
- Parenchymal brain infection, especially in immunosuppressed patients
- Febrile illnesses in third-trimester pregnant women
- Foodborne outbreaks of febrile gastroenteritis that are not found to have a more common cause

LABORATORY TESTS

Bacterial cultures should be obtained for samples of blood, CSF, and stool.

IMAGING STUDIES

For CNS disease, magnetic resonance imaging is superior to computed tomography in the demonstration of early cerebritis or brainstem involvement (e.g., rhombencephalitis).

TREATMENT

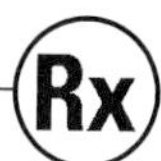

ACUTE GENERAL Rx

- Although no controlled clinical trials are available, in vitro data, animal model data, and clinical experience suggest that the therapy of choice is a combination of ampicillin plus gentamicin.
- For penicillin-allergic patients, trimethoprim-sulfamethoxazole may be given.
- Cephalosporins are not active against *L. monocytogenes.*

PEARLS & CONSIDERATIONS

COMMENTS

- Unlike group B streptococcal infections, recurrent maternal disease in humans is not documented, and antibiotics are not indicated for future pregnancies.
- Isolation of "diphtheroids" from blood or CSF should alert the clinician to consider misdiagnosed *L. monocytogenes.*
- *L. monocytogenes* received its name by causing monocytosis in the blood of laboratory

rabbits, not humans. The CSF pleocytosis in *Listeria* meningitis in adults and children is most often polymorphonuclear.

PREVENTION

The Centers for Disease Control and Prevention (CDC) provide recommendations for consumer prevention of listeriosis.

- For all persons:
  - Thoroughly cook raw food from animal sources (e.g., beef, pork, poultry).
  - Thoroughly wash raw vegetables.
  - Keep uncooked meats separate from other foods.
  - Avoid raw or unpasteurized milk.
  - Wash hands, knives, and cutting boards after handling uncooked meat.
- Additional recommendations for persons at high risk (i.e., immunocompromised hosts, pregnant women, elderly persons):
  - Avoid soft cheeses (e.g., Mexican-style, Feta, Brie, Camembert, blue-veined cheese) but not hard cheeses, cream cheese, cottage cheese, or yogurt; pasteurization may not be fully effective against intracellular *Listeria.*
  - Reheat leftover foods and ready-to-eat preprocessed meats (e.g., hot dogs) until steaming hot before eating.
  - Consider avoiding cold cuts and delicatessen foods, although the risk is relatively low.

PATIENT/FAMILY EDUCATION

More information can be found at the CDC web site (disease information topic "A to Z" list, www.cdc.gov/az.do).

SUGGESTED READINGS

Bortolussi R, Mailman T: Listeriosis. *In* Feigin RD et al (eds): *Textbook of pediatric infectious diseases,* 5th ed. Philadelphia, WB Saunders, 2004.

Lorber B: *Listeria monocytogenes. In* Mandell GL et al (eds): *Mandell, Douglas, and Bennett's Principles and Practice of Infectious Diseases,* 6th ed. Philadelphia, Elsevier, 2005.

Mylonakis E et al: Listeriosis during pregnancy: a case series and review of 222 cases. *Medicine (Baltimore)* 81:260, 2002.

Posfay-Barbe KM, Wald ER: Listeriosis. *Pediatr Rev* 25:151, 2004.

Tappero JW et al: Reduction in the incidence of human listeriosis in the United States: effectiveness of prevention efforts? *JAMA* 273:1118, 1995.

AUTHOR: **GEOFFREY A. WEINBERG, MD**

BASIC INFORMATION

DEFINITION

Lyme disease is the most common tick-borne illness in the United States. It is caused by *Borrelia burgdorferi.*

ICD-9-CM CODE
088.81 Lyme disease

EPIDEMIOLOGY & DEMOGRAPHICS

- The Lyme disease bacterium, *B. burgdorferi,* normally lives in mice, squirrels, and other small animals. It is transmitted among these animals and to humans through bites of certain kinds of ticks.
- In the Northeast and upper north-central regions of the United States, *Ixodes scapularis* (the black-legged tick, previously known as *Ixodes dammini*) is the main vector for *B. burgdorferi.*
- *Ixodes pacificus* (the Western black-legged tick) is the primary vector in the Pacific coast states.
- Infestation occurs in rural, heavily wooded areas near the vector.
- Cases peak in summer and fall.
- More than 95% of cases are concentrated in the Northeast, Eastern Seaboard, and the upper Midwest.
- Children and adolescents account for 33% to 50% of reported cases.
- Lyme disease is most common among boys between 5 and 19 years old and persons age 30 or older.
- Seventy-five percent of reported children presented with their initial symptoms in the summer months (i.e., June, July, and August).

CLINICAL PRESENTATION

History

- Tick bite
- Travel to endemic area
- Arthritis, neurologic disorder, cardiac problems, typical rash of erythema migrans (EM)

Physical Examination

- Stage 1 occurs within days to weeks after an infected tick inoculates the human host with *B. burgdorferi,* and between 60% and 80% of children develop the characteristic cutaneous finding of EM.
  - EM begins as a red papule or macule, usually in the groin, axilla, or thigh, and steadily and rapidly (over 24 to 48 hours) expands to a round or oval lesion (at least 5 cm in diameter) with an erythematous periphery and central clearing.
  - Symptoms associated with the rash are reminiscent of a viral syndrome and can include fever, arthralgia, myalgia, chills, headache, malaise, and fatigue, as well as physical signs such as lymphadenopathy, hepatosplenomegaly, and less commonly, nonexudative pharyngitis, nonproductive cough, and orchitis.
- Stage 2 occurs 3 to 4 weeks after infection. Dissemination of the spirochete occurs, and one half of patients manifest secondary skin lesions, which are also annular with central clearing but removed from the original point of inoculation and usually smaller than the primary lesion.
  - This second stage of the illness is similar to other spirochetal infections (e.g., syphilis), in which these early disease manifestations resolve even without antibiotic therapy.
  - Other complications seen in the early disseminated stage of the illness involve multiple organs systems, including the following:
    - Ophthalmologic: optic neuritis, keratitis, conjunctivitis, uveitis, choroiditis
    - Cardiac (4% to 8% of patients): most commonly see complete heart block and can include myopericarditis
    - Neurologic (15% to 20% of patients): meningitis, subtle signs of encephalitis (including somnolence, poor memory, and mood change); peripheral neuritis: asymmetric with motor, sensory or mixed manifestations; commonly presenting as paralysis of the seventh or facial nerve (Bell's palsy)
    - Other: pancreatitis
  - Serum antibody to *B. burgdorferi* develops during this phase.
- The late phase of Lyme disease is characterized by more persistent findings and occurs within months to years after the initial infection.
  - Two thirds of untreated patients have episodic oligoarthritis lasting approximately 1 week, especially involving the knee but also reported in the elbow, wrist, hip, shoulder, and ankle.
  - Late-stage neurologic disease is less common than arthritis but can persist much longer.
  - Transplacental passage of *B. burgdorferi* does occur, and case reports of prematurity, syndactyly, rash, cortical blindness, developmental delay, and intrauterine fetal death are found in the literature.

ETIOLOGY

Lyme disease is caused by infection with the spirochete *B. burgdorferi.*

DIAGNOSIS

Dx

DIFFERENTIAL DIAGNOSIS

- Pauciarticular juvenile arthritis
- Aseptic meningitis
- Multiple sclerosis
- Septic arthritis
- Acute rheumatic fever
- Fibromyalgia syndrome
- Bell's palsy
- Peripheral neuropathy

WORKUP

- The diagnosis of Lyme disease is made primarily by clinical criteria and secondarily supported by serologic data.
  - Isolation of *B. burgdorferi* from a clinical specimen
  - Diagnostic levels of immunoglobulin M (IgM) or immunoglobulin G (IgG) antibody response to the spirochete in serum or cerebrospinal fluid (CSF)
  - Significant change in IgM or IgG antibody response to *B. burgdorferi* in paired acute and convalescent serum samples
- IgM antibody becomes detectable in 2 to 4 weeks and peaks between 3 and 6 weeks after the onset of infection.
- The secondary IgG response corresponds to the development of early arthritic symptoms, occurs at 4 to 6 weeks after the onset (later than the IgM response), and can be detectable for years afterward.

LABORATORY TESTS

- Serologic testing for Lyme disease focuses on these antibody responses using three assays:
  - Indirect immunofluorescence assay
  - Enzyme-linked immunosorbent assay
  - Immunoblotting or the Western blot assay
- Ongoing work toward a standardized methodology for identification of *B. burgdorferi* antigen using polymerase chain reaction technology for amplification of minute quantities of DNA in serum or urine specimens has resulted in increasing test availability.
- None of these antibody assays is appropriate for screening patients who do not demonstrate a consistent clinical picture, even in hyperendemic areas.

TREATMENT

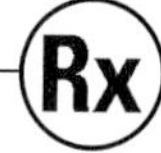

NONPHARMACOLOGIC THERAPY

- Antibiotics are effective in most cases of Lyme disease, although few controlled trials have been done enrolling children or adults.
- Oral therapy with amoxicillin (500 mg three times daily; 50 mg/kg/d divided in three doses for children) or doxycycline (100 mg twice daily for those 8 years or older) for 14 to 21 days is indicated for the early manifestations of Lyme disease such as EM. A 28-day course is recommended for arthritis.
- Equivalent efficacy for the treatment of early Lyme disease has been demonstrated for other oral agents such as cefuroxime, amoxicillin/probenecid, and azithromycin in adults.
- Parenteral regimens for 2 to 3 weeks are preferred therapy for late manifestations such as persistent or recurrent arthritis, severe carditis, meningitis, or encephalitis.

- Ceftriaxone (2 g IV once daily for 14 to 28 days) is probably the therapy of choice because of its long half-life and penetration into the CSF in concentrations consistently higher than the MIC_{90} of *B. burgdorferi.*
- Treatment failure can occur with any of the recommended regimens, and repeat treatment may (rarely) be necessary.

PEARLS & CONSIDERATIONS

COMMENTS

- Lyme disease is a multisystem spirochetal disease with numerous clinical presentations.
- Think of it in a case of rash and arthritis in a child from an endemic area with a history of tick bite.

PREVENTION

- Prevention of Lyme disease involves avoidance of tick exposure in endemic areas.
- Tick repellents, such as DEET (*N,N*-diethylmetatoluamide) for the exposed skin of adults or permethrins for clothing, should be used sparingly.
- Appropriate light-colored clothing with long sleeves and long pants is recommended.
- Tick "patrols" or intense scrutiny of the body after potential exposures should be conducted.
  - Embedded ticks must be removed with tweezers, being careful not to squeeze the body and promote mixing of the tick and human blood.
  - Studies of antibiotic prophylaxis after a tick bite have shown no definite advantage.
  - Antibiotic prophylaxis after a tick bite even in an endemic area is not indicated.
- The ultimate strategy in Lyme disease prevention is effective vaccination for humans.
  - On December 22, 1998, the U.S. Food and Drug Administration approved a Lyme disease vaccine for individuals 15 to 70 years old. It was subsequently withdrawn in 2002 because of low demand and is not available.

SUGGESTED READINGS

American Academy of Pediatrics: Lyme disease *(Borrelia burgdorferi). In* Pickering LK (ed): *Red Book 2003: Report of the Committee on Infectious Diseases,* 26th ed. Elk Grove Village, IL, American Academy of Pediatrics, 2003, pp 407–411.

Centers for Disease Control and Prevention. Available at www.cdc.gov

Steere AC: Lyme disease. *N Engl J Med* 345:115, 2001.

Worsmer GP et al: Guidelines from the Infectious Diseases Society of America. Practice guidelines for the treatment of Lyme disease. *Clin Infect Dis* 31:S1–S14, 2000.

AUTHOR: **CYNTHIA CHRISTY, MD**

BASIC INFORMATION

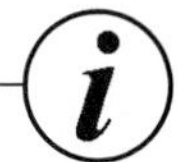

DEFINITIONS

Lymphangitis is inflammation or an infection of the lymphatic system. Lymphedema is an excess amount of lymph in soft tissue resulting from primary or secondary lymphatic insufficiency. Cystic hygroma is a congenital malformation of the lymphatic system, resulting in multiloculated, cystic masses.

SYNONYMS

Cystic hygroma
Lymphangioma
Lymphedema, primary
  Milroy's disease
  Meige's disease (i.e., lymphedema praecox)
  Lymphedema tarda

ICD-9-CM CODES
228.1 Cystic hygroma
457.1 Lymphedema
457.2 Lymphangitis
759.89 and 759.90 Congenital anomaly

EPIDEMIOLOGY & DEMOGRAPHICS

- Lymphangitis
  - The most common cause of lymphangitis worldwide is *Filaria* infection, but bacterial infection (e.g., streptococci) is more common in North America.
  - Infections are often seen as a result of chronic obstruction or malformation.
  - May occur with cellulitis.
- Lymphedema, primary
  - The incidence is 1 case per 10,000 people younger than 20 years.
  - A female preponderance exists.
  - One third of cases are caused by agenesis, hypoplasia, or obstruction of the distal system.
  - One half of cases are caused by proximal obstruction.
  - A few patients have a positive family history.
  - Primary lymphedema is associated with Turner syndrome, Noonan syndrome, yellow nail syndrome, intestinal lymphangiectasia, lymphangiomyomatosis, and arteriovenous malformation.
- Lymphedema, secondary
  - This form is more common than primary lymphedema.
  - Increased incidence exists in India and Southeast Asia.
  - Tumor is an uncommon cause in children.
- Cystic hygroma
  - The incidence is 1 case per 12,000.
  - There is a predilection for the head and neck, but it may involve the axilla, limbs, trunk, and mediastinum.
  - Approximately 50% to 65% of cystic hygromas are present at birth.

CLINICAL PRESENTATION

- Lymphangitis
  - Redness and pain of an extremity
  - Occasionally, fever and systemic symptoms
  - May have history of break of integument (abrasion, insect bite, etc.)
  - History of lymphedema
  - Travel history
  - Painful, tender erythematous extremity (often lower) with red "streaking".
  - The extremity may be diffusely swollen, especially when associated with lymphedema.
  - Fever and local adenopathy may develop
- Lymphedema, primary
  - Unilateral or bilateral swelling of an extremity
  - May present at birth/infancy, adolescence, or after age 35
  - May have family history
  4. Diffuse swelling and pitting of the extremity (often lower).
  - Occasionally, lymphedema is associated with infection.
- Lymphedema, secondary
  - Unilateral or bilateral swelling of an extremity
  - Medical history of recurrent infections, cancer, radiation
  - Clinical findings are similar to primary lymphedema however surgical or radiation changes in the area or extremity may be noted.
- Cystic hygroma
  - Painless mass involving the neck, axilla, head
  - Stridor and/or cough secondary to airway compression
  - Dysphagia because of tongue or neck involvement
  - Sometimes history of fever, redness, pain
  - Small or large cystic mass involving the neck, axilla, and tongue is seen.
  - Masses are usually non tender, soft, mobile, and not erythematous (although can get infected).
  - The mass may transilluminate.
  - Stridor and respiratory compromise may be noted.
  - When Cystic hygroma is infected may present as lymphangitis, cellulitis, or abscess

ETIOLOGY

- Lymphangitis
  - Infection
  - Radiation therapy
  - Tumor
  - Obstruction
- Lymphedema, primary
  - Different forms are based on age of presentation: congenital lymphedema in infancy, lymphedema praecox in childhood and adolescence, lymphedema tarda in later life.
  - A few cases have a positive family history with autosomal dominant inheritance: Milroy's and Meige's disease.
  - Several different pathologic forms exist, including agenesis, hypoplasia, and obstructive.
  - Obstruction can be proximal or distal.
  - A less common hyperplastic type can be seen and occasionally is associated with megalymphatics.
- Lymphedema, secondary
  - Acquired from a variety of causes: bacterial lymphangitis (usually streptococci), tumor, filariasis, irradiation, surgery, trauma, tuberculosis, dermatitis, parenteral drug use, and rheumatoid arthritis.
  - Edema associated with abnormalities of the heart, liver, and kidney is not true lymphedema because the lymphatic system is normal in those conditions.
- Cystic hygroma
  - Congenital failure of the embryologic lymphatic system to establish drainage into the venous system
  - Results in the formation of multiloculated, cystic lymphatic malformations

DIAGNOSIS

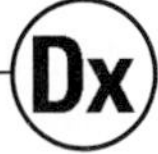

DIFFERENTIAL DIAGNOSIS

- Lymphangitis
  - Superficial thrombophlebitis
  - Reflex sympathetic dystrophy
  - Cellulitis
- Lymphedema
  - Congestive heart failure
  - Nephrotic syndrome
  - Deep vein thrombosis (DVT)
  - Cirrhosis
  - Hypoalbuminemic states
  - Myxedema
  - Reflex sympathetic dystrophy
  - Pelvic mass or tumor
- Cystic hygroma
  - Hemangioma
  - Branchial cleft cyst
  - Thyroglossal duct cyst
  - Dermoid or epidermoid cyst
  - Ranula
  - Cervical lymphadenitis
  - Mediastinal mass

WORKUP

- The history and physical examination (fever, adenopathy, swelling) may be enough to make a diagnosis of lymphangitis.
  - Leukocytosis may be found on a complete blood cell count.
  - An ultrasound or phlebogram is sometimes necessary to rule out DVT.
- Lymphedema
  - The diagnosis is generally based on history and physical examination to rule out nonlymphatic causes of edema.
  - Occasionally, an ultrasound or phlebogram can help differentiate lymphedema from DVT.

- Computed tomography (CT) may be needed to assess a focal (pelvic) mass.
- Rarely, a lymphangiogram, lymphoscintigram, or CT scan can be used to define abnormal lymphatics.
- Consider genetic testing or workup for Turner or Noonan syndrome.

- Cystic hygroma
  - History and physical examination are important.
  - Ultrasound can help in the assessment.
  - CT can be used to evaluate the extent of complicated masses.
  - Occasionally, needle aspiration is used for culture or pathology to ensure that no infection or tumor is present.
  - Genetic testing/workup for Turner or Noonan syndrome.

TREATMENT

NONPHARMACOLOGIC THERAPY

- Lymphangitis
  - Elevation and local compresses
  - Occasionally, surgical intervention (i.e., incision and drainage of abscess)
- Lymphedema
  - Elevation; compression stockings or devices
  - Exercise; skin and foot hygiene
  - Salt restriction
  - Surgery (e.g., drainage procedures, limb reduction, grafting): mostly palliative
- Cystic hygroma
  - Repeated aspiration and radiation treatment in an attempt to shrink or involute and injection with sclerosing agents have been tried with little success.
  - Surgical removal of abnormal lymphatic structures can be attempted.

ACUTE GENERAL Rx

- Lymphangitis
  - Antibiotics, especially antistreptococcal antibiotics, can be used.
  - Antiparasitic medications can be tried.
- Lymphedema
  - Diuretics
  - Antibiotics, antifungals, or antiparasitics if infection coexistent
  - Treatment of cause in secondary cases (e.g., malignancy)
- Cystic hygroma
  - No known medical therapies are available.
  - Occasionally, immediate aspiration to relieve an airway obstruction is necessary.

CHRONIC Rx

- Lymphangitis and lymphedema
  - Often a chronic, recurring problem requiring repeated treatment with antibiotics.
  - Emphasis should be placed on vigorous foot and skin care to try to reduce episodes of bacterial superinfection.
- Cystic hygroma
  - Regression is rare, and most should be removed at the time of diagnosis.

DISPOSITION

- Lymphangitis
  - This is a recurrent problem for many individuals, especially if an underlying lymphatic vessel obstruction or abnormality is present.
  - Antibiotic treatment is effective.
  - A recurring problem can lead to secondary obstruction or increased obstruction.
- Lymphedema
  - This is a chronic problem with progressive increase within the first year of diagnosis, but progression is rare after that.
  - Approximately 15% of patients require surgical intervention.
- Cystic hygroma
  - Close follow-up and removal are necessary.
  - Regression is rare.

REFERRAL

- Lymphangitis
  - Referral is rarely necessary for an initial episode.
  - Consultation with an infectious disease specialist is indicated for resistant infections or if a parasitic cause is suspected.
  - Occasionally, surgical consultation for drainage of abscess or wound care is needed.
- Lymphedema
  - A genetics consultation may be helpful for families if a hereditary cause is suspected.
  - Consultation with a vascular surgeon may be indicated if other measures have not been helpful, but surgical intervention may only be palliative.
- Cystic hygroma
  - All cases should be referred to a surgeon with expertise (usually pediatric surgeons and otolaryngologists).
  - Consider refferral to pediatric genetics for Turner or Noonan syndrome.

PEARLS & CONSIDERATIONS

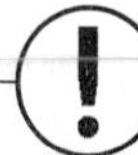

COMMENTS

- Cystic hygroma often involves the left side of the neck and is usually not subtle or confused with other items in the differential diagnosis.
- Nonlymphatic causes of edema are far more common than lymphedema and should always be ruled out.

PATIENT/FAMILY EDUCATION

- Lymphangitis
  - Good skin hygiene
  - Prompt attention to infection
- Lymphedema
  - Dietary education
  - Exercise and compression stockings
  - Prompt attention to infection
- Cystic hygroma
  - Parents should be educated about the complications (i.e., acute change in size, hemorrhage, infection, and respiratory compromise).
- Web sites, support groups, and resources are available:
  - Cystic Hygroma Online Support Group: members.tripod.com/SCchsupport
  - Cystic Hygroma-Parent's Place Message Board: rainforest.parentsplace.com/dialog/get
  - Lymphedema Foundation: www.lymphedemafoundation.org
  - Lymphedema International Network: www.lymphedema.com
  - Lymphedema Products: home.earthlink.net
  - Lymphedema Support Group: super.sonic.net/LSG/
  - National Lymphedema Network: www.lymphnet.org

SUGGESTED READINGS

Brown R, Azizkhan R: Pediatric head and neck lesions. *Pediatr Clin North Am* 45:889, 1998.

Cooke JP, Rooke TW: Lymphedema. In Loscalzo J et al (eds): *Vascular Medicine.* Boston, Little, Brown, 1992.

Harel L et al: Lymphedema praecox seen as isolated unilateral arm involvement: case report and review of the literature. *J Pediatr* 130:492, 1997.

Lewis JM, Wald ER: Lymphedema praecox. *J Pediatr* 104:641, 1984.

Ninh T, Ninh T: Cystic hygroma in children: a report of 126 cases. *J Pediatr Surg* 9:191, 1974.

AUTHOR: **STEVEN SCOFIELD, MD**

BASIC INFORMATION

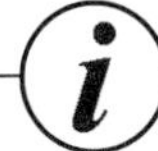

DEFINITION

Hodgkin's disease (HD) or lymphoma is a malignancy characterized by the presence of Reed-Sternberg (RS) cells or variants with a background of a non-neoplastic, reactive cellular infiltrate in involved tissue, usually lymph nodes.

SYNONYM

Hodgkin's lymphoma

ICD-9-CM CODE

201.9 Hodgkin's disease

EPIDEMIOLOGY & DEMOGRAPHICS

- HD accounts for 6% of pediatric cancers.
- In developed countries, two age peaks occur, one in early adulthood (middle to late 20s) and the second in late adulthood (after age 50). Approximately 18% of pediatric patients with HD are younger than 10 years.
- The male-to-female ratio is 3:1 to 4:1 for children younger than 10 years and 1.3:1 for older children.
- Increased incidence is seen in family members: twofold to fivefold increase in siblings, ninefold increase in same-sex siblings, and 99-fold increase in monozygotic twins.

CLINICAL PRESENTATION

History

- Enlarged lymph nodes are usually painless and most commonly located in the cervical or supraclavicular region.
- Mediastinal disease is present in 76% of adolescents and 33% of 1- to 10-year-old children.
- Symptoms include the following:
  - Coughing or shortness of breath
  - About 30% of patients with "B" symptoms (fever > 38°F, drenching night sweats, unexplained weight loss > 10% of body weight in preceding 6 months)
  - Fatigue
  - Abdominal pain, occurring in older patients, especially after consuming alcohol
  - Pruritus

Physical Examination

- Enlarged lymph nodes are generally firm and immobile. Ninety percent of patients present with a pattern that suggests contiguous lymphatic spread.
- Decreased breath sounds can be heard if a large mediastinal mass is present.
- Superior vena cava syndrome is observed if a large mediastinal mass is present.

ETIOLOGY

- There is increased incidence among patients with evidence of Epstein-Barr virus (EBV) infection, although approximately one half of patients with HD have no evidence of EBV. Anti-EBV titers are elevated before the diagnosis of HD. Presence of EBV tumor genomes is age related, occurring in 75% of affected children younger than 10 years of age and only 20% of older children; it also varies by ethnicity.
- EBV-associated antigens are found to a variable degree in HD subtypes as follows:
  - Mixed cellularity: up to 96%
  - Nodular sclerosing: 34%
  - Lymphocyte predominant: 10%
- A complex deficiency of cellular immunity exists in HD patients.
- There may be an increased incidence in immunocompromised patients, including patients with human immunodeficiency virus (HIV), infection or acquired immunodeficiency syndrome (AIDS), organ transplant recipients, and patients with congenital immunodeficiency syndromes.
- HD is rarely seen as a secondary malignancy, unlike non-Hodgkin's lymphoma.

DIAGNOSIS

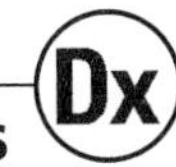

DIFFERENTIAL DIAGNOSIS

- Non-Hodgkin's lymphoma
- Leukemia, particularly T-cell acute lymphoblastic leukemia
- Metastatic disease from another tumor (e.g., neuroblastoma, rhabdomyosarcoma)
- Infection, including viral (e.g., EBV, cytomegalovirus), atypical mycobacterium, cat-scratch disease
- Normal thymus

WORKUP

- Biopsy of enlarged node (i.e., excisional or open biopsy recommended)
- Bone marrow aspirates and biopsies in patients with high-risk disease to evaluate for metastatic disease
- Frequency of RS cell in pathologic specimen is variable. Reactive infiltrate likely results from cytokine release by RS cell. RS cells are large cells with abundant cytoplasm and multiple nuclei or multilobed nuclei. They are not pathognomonic, however, and can be found in other disorders. A clone of B lymphocyte origin may be most common, but there is evidence for multilineage origin.
- Four subtypes exist (first three are considered classic Hodgkin's disease):
  - Nodular sclerosing
    - Distinctive because of collagenous bands that divide the lymph node into nodules.
    - Approximately 77% of adolescents and 44% of children younger than 10 years are diagnosed with this subtype.
  - Mixed cellularity
    - Approximately 11% of adolescents and 33% of children younger than 10 years have this subtype.
    - This subtype is associated with advanced disease, extranodal extension, and B symptoms.
  - Lymphocyte depleted
    - This form is rare in children.
    - This type of disease often is advanced at diagnosis.
    - The prognosis is poor.
  - Lymphocyte predominant
    - This type is more common in males and young children than in adults (33% of cases are in children younger than 15 years).
    - Clinically localized disease commonly involves one lymph node region and spares the mediastinum.
- Ann Arbor Staging System
  - Involvement of single lymph node region or extralymphatic region
  - Involvement of two or more lymph node regions or one extranodal region and contiguous lymph node region on same side of diaphragm
  - Involvement of lymph node regions on both sides of diaphragm; may include spleen involvement or contiguous involvement of one extranodal site
  - Diffuse or disseminated involvement of one or more extranodal sites, with or without lymphatic involvement. Potential sites of involvement include liver, bone marrow, and lungs.
- Additional designations:
  - Asymptomatic, no B symptoms
  - Presence of one or more of the following symptoms: fever higher than 38°F, drenching night sweats, or unexplained weight loss of more than 10% of body weight in preceding 6 months
- Approximately 65% of children are stage I/II; stage IV is less common in children younger than 10 years.
- Pathologic staging:
  - It is rarely performed because of use of combined-modality therapy (i.e., chemotherapy and radiation therapy).
  - Laparotomy is performed to examine organs, biopsy liver and lymph nodes, and remove the spleen.
  - Indications for pathologic staging vary, depending on risk of abdominal disease, radiologic imaging, and potential use of combined-modality therapy versus radiation therapy alone.

LABORATORY TESTS

- Complete blood cell count and renal and liver function tests are obtained at baseline. Elevated liver enzymes may indicate liver involvement.
- The erythrocyte sedimentation rate (ESR) values are often elevated and may be followed to monitor disease response and recurrence.
- C-reactive protein (CRP) is being investigated for a role in disease risk and response monitoring.

IMAGING STUDIES

- Chest radiograph
- Computed tomography (CT) of the neck, chest, abdomen, and pelvis; approximately 50% of patients with normal chest radiographs have chest CT abnormalities.
- Gallium scan to identify extent of gallium avid disease.
- Positron emission tomography (PET) replacing gallium scan
- Lymphangiography rarely used, especially in children

TREATMENT

NONPHARMACOLOGIC THERAPY

- Hodgkin's disease is sensitive to radiation therapy, and patients may be cured with irradiation alone. Risk of relapse and effects of radiation, particularly in doses required as single modality, on growing children and adolescents led to development of and emphasis on combined-modality therapy.
- Role of radiation therapy and appropriate radiation field continue to be investigated in high-risk patients with complete response to chemotherapy and low- and intermediate-risk patients with rapid early response to chemotherapy. Patients with incomplete response or without rapid early response to chemotherapy should receive radiation therapy.

ACUTE GENERAL Rx

- Therapy decisions are based on age, stage, pathology, and risk stratification (including B symptoms), number of disease sites, and presence of bulky disease. Protocols include low-, intermediate-, and advanced-stage or high-risk designations and treatment pathways based on response to therapy.
- There are multiple active chemotherapy regimens. The mechlorethamine (nitrogen mustard), Oncovin (vincristine), prednisone, and procarbazine (MOPP) regimen has been replaced because of a high incidence of infertility, especially in males, and the risk of secondary leukemia. Regimens may include doxorubicin, bleomycin, vinblastine, and dacarbazine (ABVD) or doxorubicin, vincristine, cyclophosphamide, and prednisone with or without bleomycin and etoposide. Other agents are being investigated for treating resistant or recurrent disease.
- Survival is excellent for all stages of disease, with most recent studies demonstrating 85% to 95% 10-year survival for early-stage disease and 70% to 90% 10-year survival for advanced-stage disease.
- High stage (i.e., more than four sites of involvement), large mediastinal adenopathy (LMA, defined as mass exceeding one third the transverse diameter of the chest on a posteroanterior chest radiograph), and B symptoms, particularly fever and weight loss, are poor prognostic factors.
- Unlike many other malignancies, salvage rates or cures after relapse are significant. Intensive therapy, such as autologous hematopoietic stem cell transplant, may be required.
- Overall survival has been compromised by death from causes other than HD, including second malignancies and cardiovascular deaths. Current therapy and investigations include efforts to minimize late toxicities without compromising disease-free survival.

DISPOSITION

- The schedule of radiologic monitoring depends on the site and stage of disease. CT of initial disease sites and chest radiography may be followed every 3 to 6 months for 3 to 5 years and then yearly until 10 years from therapy. CT scans of the chest, abdomen, and pelvis may be periodically performed.
- ESR may be repeated on the same schedule if the value was abnormal at diagnosis.
- Gallium scan or PET scan is used to assess response and may be used to monitor patients off therapy for disease recurrence.
- Long-term toxicities of chemotherapy may include cardiomyopathy, pulmonary fibrosis, infertility or early menopause, and secondary malignancies, especially leukemia.
- Long-term toxicities of radiation therapy may include hypothyroidism, musculoskeletal hypoplasia, coronary artery and valvular disease, and salivary dysfunction, and secondary malignancies include breast, thyroid, gastrointestinal, and skin cancers. The risk of breast cancer is particularly significant for girls receiving irradiation during early adolescence. Annual screening mammograms starting 8 years from diagnosis are recommended.

REFERRAL

- Patients should be referred to pediatric oncologists and radiation therapists with experience in treating pediatric patients.
- Although medical oncologists have experience treating patients with HD, the medical, psychosocial, and long-term needs of children and adolescents are best met by a team of pediatric specialists.

PEARLS & CONSIDERATIONS

COMMENTS

- Chest radiographs should be obtained before the surgical procedure because patients may have significant mediastinal adenopathy that may compromise the airway.
- Thymic rebound after therapy may be misinterpreted as relapse, and repeat evaluations may be necessary.
- Children and adolescents who have had splenectomies should take prophylactic penicillin and have booster immunizations as appropriate.

PREVENTION

No preventive interventions are available.

PATIENT/FAMILY EDUCATION

- HD is curable using a variety of chemotherapy and radiation therapy regimens. Parents and patients should ask to be fully informed about treatment options and potential risks and benefits.
- Pediatric oncologists can refer patients and parents to local or national support organizations for children with cancer and their families. National organizations include the American Cancer Society and CureSearch, a component of the Children's Oncology Group.

SUGGESTED READINGS

Diehl V et al: Hodgkin's lymphoma—diagnosis and treatment. *Lancet Oncol* 5:19, 2004.

Hudson MM, Constine LS: Hodgkin's disease. *In* Halperin EC et al (eds): *Pediatric Radiation Oncology,* 4th ed. Philadelphia, Lippincott Williams & Wilkins, 2005, pp 223–259.

Hudson MM, Donaldson SS: Hodgkin's disease. *In* Pizzo PA et al (eds): *Principles and Practice of Pediatric Oncology,* 4th ed. Philadelphia, Lippincott Williams & Wilkins, 2002, pp 637–660.

www.curesearch.org

www.cancer.org

AUTHOR: **ANDREA S. HINKLE, MD**

BASIC INFORMATION

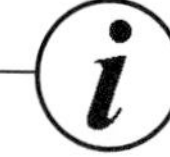

DEFINITION

Non-Hodgkin's lymphoma (NHL) represents a heterogeneous group of malignant neoplasms arising from the transformation of cells of lymphocytic or histiocytic origin, which most often appear in lymph nodes or other lymphoid tissue (i.e., tonsils, thymus, or Peyer's patches). Heterogeneous by histology, site of origin, and clinical manifestations, NHL often involves the bone marrow and the central nervous system. Childhood NHL bears little resemblance to adult NHL or Hodgkin's disease in terms of biology, clinical behavior, or therapy.

SYNONYMS

Malignant lymphoma
Reticuloendothelial neoplasm
Specific subtypes
- Anaplastic large cell lymphoma (ALCL)
- Burkitt's or small, noncleaved cell (non-Burkitt's) lymphoma
- Diffuse large cell lymphoma (DLCL)
- Lymphoblastic lymphoma
- True histiocytic lymphoma (rare)

Former terms
- Giant follicular lymphoma
- Lymphoreticular neoplasm
- Lymphosarcoma
- Reticulum cell sarcoma

ICD-9-CM CODES
200.1-200.8 Specific subtypes
202.8 Non-Hodgkin's lymphoma

EPIDEMIOLOGY & DEMOGRAPHICS

- In the United States, approximately 800 children and adolescents younger than 20 years are diagnosed with NHL each year.
- A higher incidence is seen among males and whites compared with blacks.
- Peak age is 5 to 15 years.
  - Burkitt's and non-Burkitt's small, noncleaved cell tumors predominate among 5- to 14-year-old patients.
  - DLCLs are most common among 15- to 19-year-old patients.
- Most tumors are in extranodal sites. The prevalence of primary site varies:
  - Abdominal: 35%
  - Mediastinal: 26%
  - Peripheral nodal outside of head and neck: 14%
  - Head and neck region, including tonsils, Waldeyer's ring, and cervical nodes: 13%
  - Skin, orbit, thyroid, bone, kidney, breast, or gonads: 11%
- Childhood NHLs are among the most rapidly growing tumors, and the duration of symptoms is therefore short. The average time from onset of symptoms to diagnosis is 2 to 6 weeks.
- The 5-year survival rate is 72% for those younger than 20 years, although this varies from 60% to 90%, depending on the specific subtype, stage, and treatment regimen.

CLINICAL PRESENTATION

- The history depends on the anatomic sites and extent of involvement.
- Systemic symptoms are not common but may include fever, malaise, anorexia, and mild weight loss, particularly in ALCL.
- Evaluate for potential urgent medical situations:
  - Cord compression can occur abruptly with early warning signs of paresthesias or extremity weakness.
  - Mediastinal mass with respiratory distress can manifest with airway compression, causing shortness of breath, cough, wheezing, increased work of breathing, or stridor.
  - Superior vena cava (SVC) syndrome as a result of mediastinal mass compression of the SVC occurs with facial edema, plethora, headache, and altered mental status.
  - Hyperuricemia or renal failure can be present at diagnosis as a result of tumor lysis syndrome.
  - With signs of cranial nerve palsy must look for other signs of increased intracranial pressure to rule out brain tumor or cerebrovascular accident.
    - Double vision: usually associated with asymmetric extraocular movements on physical examination
    - Facial droop: facial asymmetry that may be indistinguishable from a Bell's palsy
  - Intussusception, intestinal obstruction, or hydronephrosis is associated with an abdominal mass.
- Abdominal pain and a change in bowel habits may be the primary presenting complaints.
- Painless masses (i.e., lymph node enlargement) may be identified. Involved lymph nodes are enlarged, firm, rubbery, nontender, and nonmobile.
- Organomegaly should be assessed by careful examination for an enlarged liver or spleen during the initial evaluation.
- A primary mass may occur in the head or neck.
  - Jaw mass or swelling
  - Unilateral tonsillar enlargement
  - Congestion, nasal obstruction
  - Eye bulging, proptosis

ETIOLOGY

- The cause is unknown in most cases; rare cases of familial NHL have been reported.
- A small proportion of cases are associated with the inherited and acquired immunodeficiency syndromes that are known to carry an increased risk.
- Associated congenital immunodeficiency syndromes include the following:
  - Wiskott-Aldrich syndrome
  - Ataxia-telangiectasia
  - X-linked lymphoproliferative syndrome
  - Severe combined immunodeficiency syndrome, x-linked agammaglobulinemia, and common variable agammaglobulinemia
  - Chédiak-Higashi syndrome
- Associated acquired immunodeficiency states include the following:
  - Acquired immunodeficiency syndrome (AIDS)
  - Immunosuppressive therapy: after organ or marrow transplantation, high-dose glucocorticosteroids, or androgen steroid abuse
- Epstein-Barr virus (EBV) infection is associated with African-type Burkitt's lymphoma or NHL occurring in patients with an underlying immunodeficiency.
- Specific biologic subtypes are associated with distinctive gene translocations, but their role in the pathogenesis of the disease is not known.

DIAGNOSIS

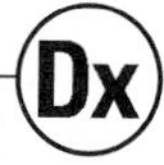

DIFFERENTIAL DIAGNOSIS

- Benign
  - EBV or cytomegalovirus mononucleosis
  - Cat-scratch disease
  - Histiocytosis
  - Teratoma
- Malignant
  - Hodgkin's disease
  - Leukemia
  - Rhabdomyosarcoma
  - Neuroblastoma
  - Ewing's sarcoma
  - Germ cell tumor

WORKUP

- Confirm the diagnosis and subtype and stage the disease.
  - The urgent medical situations detailed previously (i.e., cord compression, mediastinal mass with respiratory distress, SVC syndrome, or tumor lysis syndrome) may require minimal investigations to be performed based on the presenting history and physical examination results so that emergent treatment such as radiation therapy or steroids can be instituted without delay. Whenever possible this should be done in consultation with the pediatric oncologist to avoid interfering with the documentation of the diagnosis.
  - The final diagnosis is based on histology, cytochemistry, cytogenetics, immunophenotype, and molecular studies of biopsy of the primary lesion, lymph node, or marrow biopsy when positive.
  - Biopsy should be done at a center with the capacity to perform all necessary analyses on the tissue sample.

LABORATORY TESTS

- Obtain a complete blood cell count and differential count. If counts are abnormal, suspect marrow involvement and do a marrow aspirate.
- Obtain blood chemistry tests. Abnormal levels of urate, calcium, phosphate, or creatinine suggest tumor lysis syndrome. Lactate dehydrogenase is usually elevated.
- Use a bone marrow aspirate and biopsy.
  - When positive, this test can be used to establish the diagnosis without performing a lymph node biopsy.
  - Marrow involvement (i.e., stage IV lymphoma) is defined as marrow with less than 25% blasts.
  - If more than 25% blasts are found or blasts are circulating in the peripheral blood, the diagnosis is leukemia.
- Analyze spinal fluid.
- Obtain pleural or peritoneal fluid analysis when applicable may be diagnostic.

IMAGING STUDIES

- Obtain a chest radiograph to look for a mediastinal mass, adenopathy, effusions, and degree of airway compression.
- Obtain computed tomography (CT) of the involved areas (i.e., neck, chest, abdomen, and pelvis) as indicated.
- Gallium scan or positron emission tomography (PET) scan can be used.
  - The scans may be useful in detecting occult metastatic disease.
  - The scans can identify areas of high metabolic activity and can be very useful in follow-up evaluation of disease response to therapy. Although there may be residual mass on plain CT scans, if the mass no longer shows uptake of the radionuclear contrast, it suggests there is no longer viable tumor in the area.
  - PET scan has virtually replaced the use of gallium scan for adult lymphomas, but its role in pediatric lymphomas is under investigation.
- Magnetic resonance imaging may be helpful if bony or paraspinal involvement is suspected.

TREATMENT

NONPHARMACOLOGIC THERAPY

- Surgery has no role except for biopsy. Aggressive tumor resection is not indicated and may result in excessive morbidity.
- Radiation may be used emergently to treat complications arising from space-occupying lesions (i.e., mediastinal mass, hydronephrosis, or spinal cord compression). Otherwise, its role is limited to central nervous system (CNS) treatment and local therapy of chemotherapy-refractory disease.

ACUTE GENERAL Rx

- Initial management often requires treatment of complications arising from the following:
  - Space-occupying nature of the tumor
  - Tumor lysis syndrome
    - The metabolic complications of onset of chemotherapy or the tumor itself.
    - Characterized by hyperuricemia, hypocalcemia, hyperphosphatemia, and renal insufficiency.
- Multiagent chemotherapy is the mainstay of treatment.
  - Specific treatment recommendations are based on the stage of disease, the histologic features, and immunologic subtype.
  - Commonly used chemotherapy agents include vincristine, corticosteroids, methotrexate, and mercaptopurine. Intrathecal chemotherapy may be used.
  - Other agents may include anthracycline, cyclophosphamide, and cytosine arabinoside.
  - Length of treatment varies with the stage and subtype of NHL, and it continues for 6 weeks (i.e., localized except lymphoblastic) to 2 years (i.e., lymphoblastic and any advanced-stage disease).
  - CNS prophylaxis is an essential part of treatment of patients with advanced-stage disease. The risk for CNS disease recurrence is especially high in patients with lymphoblastic or Burkitt's lymphomas. Common strategies for CNS-directed therapy include high-dose systemic therapy (i.e., methotrexate or cytarabine), intrathecal chemotherapy, and cranial irradiation in high-risk cases.
- Stem cell transplantation has been effective as part of salvage therapy for recurrent disease.

CHRONIC Rx

- Continued follow-up with the oncologist is important to monitor for late side effects of therapy, recurrence, and development of a second malignancy.
- Many pediatric cancer centers have specific clinical programs for long-term follow-up.

COMPLEMENTARY & ALTERNATIVE MEDICINE

There is no evidence for the role of complementary and alternative medical approaches. They usually are not recommended because of concern that they may interfere with the anticancer effects of traditional chemotherapy regimens.

DISPOSITION

- Periodic imaging of affected organs is performed during therapy and at regular intervals for 3 to 4 years from the diagnosis to monitor for evidence of recurrence.
- Regular medical evaluation with a history, examination, and laboratory tests, as appropriate, should continue yearly for 20 years or longer.
  - Monitor for late effects of chemotherapy.
  - Monitor for secondary malignancies.

REFERRAL

All patients should be referred to a pediatric cancer center for diagnosis, management, and follow-up as soon as the diagnosis of NHL or other malignancy is suspected.

PEARLS & CONSIDERATIONS

COMMENTS

- The presence of a mediastinal mass with respiratory symptoms is an emergency.
  - The patient should be kept in a sitting position.
  - Use of general anesthesia is avoided. After an airway is stabilized, immediately refer the patient to a pediatric cancer center.
- An abdominal primary lesion is the most common cause of intussusception in children older than 6 years.
- Acute lymphoblastic leukemia (ALL) and lymphoblastic or Burkitt's NHL are virtually indistinguishable cytologically. Blast cells are identical, and the clinical features are similar. Clinical distinction between NHL and ALL is based on the degree of bone marrow infiltration.

PATIENT/FAMILY EDUCATION

- National Candlelighters Childhood Cancer Foundation can be reached at 800-366-2223 or through their web site (www.candlelighters.org).
- National Children's Cancer Society can be reached at 800-5-FAMILY.
- Many cities and state regions have support groups and summer camp programs for patients, parents, siblings, and friends.
- Local cancer centers are aware of local support groups and resources available for each stage of treatment.
- Physicians and families can access several web sites: National Cancer Institute CancerNet (www.cancer.gov), OncoLink (www.oncolink.upenn.edu), and Children's Oncology Group (www.childrensoncologygroup.org).

SUGGESTED READINGS

Link MP, Donaldson SS: The lymphomas and lymphadenopathy. *In* Nathan DG et al (eds): *Hematology of Infancy and Childhood.* Philadelphia, Elsevier, 2003, pp 1333–1374.

Magrath IT: Malignant non-Hodgkin's lymphomas in children. *In* Pizzo PA, Poplack DG (eds): *Principles and Practice of Pediatric Oncology.* Philadelphia, Lippincott Williams & Wilkins, 2002, pp 661–705.

Percy CL, et al: Lymphomas and reticuloendothelial neoplasms. *In* Ries LAG et al (eds): *Cancer incidence and survival among children and adolescents.* US SEER Program 1975–1995, NIH publication no. 99-4649. Bethesda, MD, National Cancer Institute, 1999.

AUTHOR: **BARBARA L. ASSELIN, MD**

BASIC INFORMATION

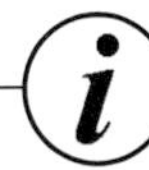

DEFINITION

Malaria is a febrile disease caused by intracellular protozoa of the genus *Plasmodium.*

SYNONYM

Foul air

ICD-9-CM CODE
084.6 Malaria

EPIDEMIOLOGY & DEMOGRAPHICS

- Malaria is endemic in tropical areas; most U.S. cases are imported.
- *Plasmodium falciparum* and *Plasmodium vivax* are the most common species.
- Because of persistent hepatic infection, relapses occur with *P. vivax* and *Plasmodium ovale* infection.
- Widespread drug resistance has important implications for prevention and treatment.

CLINICAL PRESENTATION

- Cyclical febrile paroxysms are typical.
- Fevers may be irregular (*P. falciparum*) or occur at periodic intervals (every 48 hours for *P. vivax* or *P. ovale*) or every 72 hours (*Plasmodium malariae*).
- Paroxysm begins with chill, followed by high fever. There may be systemic symptoms, including malaise, headache, seizures, vomiting, and diarrhea. The sweating stage is characterized by fatigue and resolution of fever.
- Patients often appear well between paroxysms.
- In addition to fever, tachycardia and hypotension may occur.
- Hepatosplenomegaly is common.
- Central nervous system findings (e.g., confusion, seizures, coma) are common in children.

ETIOLOGY

- Four species cause disease in humans: *P. falciparum, P. malariae, P. ovale,* and *P. vivax.*
- Malaria is most commonly acquired from the bite of infected female *Anopheles* mosquito.
- Sporozoites travel from the blood to the liver, where infection is amplified and from which merozoites are released into the blood.
- Rupture of infected red blood cells is responsible for periodic fever.
- Some parasites develop gametes taken up by mosquitoes to produce sporozoites.
- Infection also results from inoculation of infected blood through transfusion, contaminated needles, or across the placenta.

DIAGNOSIS

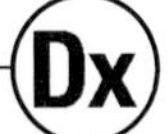

DIFFERENTIAL DIAGNOSIS

- Bacteremia
- Endocarditis
- Influenza
- Meningoencephalitis
- Tuberculosis
- Typhoid fever

LABORATORY TESTS

- A microscopic examination of the blood should be done for detection of parasites. In hyperendemic areas, a low-level parasitemia may not be the cause of presenting illness.
- Thick blood smears concentrate red blood cells. Multiple smears may be necessary to find the parasite.
- Thin blood smears are needed for species identification and determination of the parasite load.
- Determining whether *P. falciparum* is present is critical because of the potential severity of the disease.
- *P. falciparum* is suggested by parasitemia in more than 2% of red blood cells, multiple parasites in a single erythrocyte, and banana-shaped gametocyte.
- Antigen assays and polymerase chain reaction (PCR) are used in selected settings.

TREATMENT

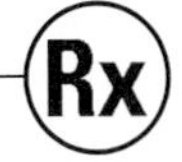

ACUTE GENERAL Rx

- Drug choice depends on the *Plasmodium* species, drug resistance patterns, and severity of the illness.
- Chloroquine is used for all *Plasmodium* infections except *P. falciparum* and *P. vivax* resistant to chloroquine.
- Drugs used for parenteral therapy include quinidine gluconate, quinine dihydrochloride, and artemether.
- Numerous drugs may be used alone or in combination for chloroquine-resistant *P. falciparum* and *P. vivax.*
- Primaquine phosphate is used to prevent relapses with *P. vivax* and *P. ovale.* Screening for glucose-6-phosphate dehydrogenase (G6PD) deficiency is necessary because of associated hemolytic anemia with this drug.
- Current drug recommendations and dosages can be found in the various editions of the *Red Book: Report of the Committee on Infectious Diseases and Centers for Disease Control.*
- Intravenous therapy may be necessary in very ill patients.
- Exchange transfusion has been used for parasitemia greater than 10%.

DISPOSITION

Follow-up blood smears should be evaluated for patients with *P. falciparum.*

REFERRAL

- Patients should be seen by an infectious disease specialist or a health care provider experienced with travel preparation 6 to 8 weeks before travel.
- Referral to an infectious disease specialist is recommended for children who have acquired malaria.

PEARLS & CONSIDERATIONS

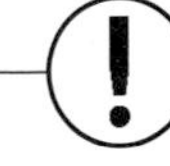

COMMENTS

- Think of malaria in patients with fever and an appropriate travel history.
- Patients infected with species of *Plasmodium* other than *P. falciparum* may present years after travel.

PREVENTION

- No vaccine against malaria is available.
- Chloroquine is used in chloroquine-sensitive areas.
- In chloroquine-resistant areas, the main drugs used are atovaquone or proguanil, mefloquine, and doxycycline.
- Medications should be in childproof containers and out of children's reach.
- For small children, special drug formulations are necessary and can be prepared at a full-service pharmacy.

PATIENT/FAMILY EDUCATION

- Travelers to endemic areas should obtain advice from health care providers familiar with travel medicine.
- In some situations (e.g., pregnancy, very young children, drug sensitivities), standard chemoprophylaxis cannot be used, and travel should be avoided.
- Patients should limit the amount of exposed skin and use a DEET (*N,N*-diethylmetatoluamide)–containing repellent.
- Instructions for DEET repellents should be followed carefully.
- Patients should avoid outside activity from dusk until dawn and use protective measures when sleeping.
- Information can be obtained from the Centers for Disease Control and Prevention (CDC) (www.cdc.gov/travel); the CDC Fax Information Service (888-232-3299); and the CDC Malaria Hotline (770-488-7788; for emergency consultation after hours: 770-488-7100).

SUGGESTED READINGS

American Academy of Pediatrics: Malaria. *In* Pickering LK (ed): *Red Book: 2003 Report of the Committee on Infectious Diseases,* 26th ed. Elk Grove Village, IL, American Academy of Pediatrics, 2003.

Centers for Disease Control and Prevention: Health Information for International Travel. 2003–2004. Atlanta, GA U.S. Department of Health and Human Services, 2003.

Fairhurst RM, Wellens TE: *Plasmodium* species (malaria). *In* Mandel GL et al (eds): *Mandell, Douglas and Bennett's Principles and Practices of Infectious Diseases,* 6th ed. Philadelphia, Elsevier, 2005.

Strickland GT: Malaria. *In* Strickland GT (ed): *Hunter Tropical Medicine and Emerging Infectious Diseases,* 8th ed. Philadelphia, WB Saunders, 2000, pp 614–643.

AUTHOR: **CAROL A. MCCARTHY, MD**

Section I DISEASES AND DISORDERS

BASIC INFORMATION

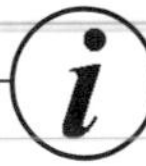

DEFINITION

Malrotation is any abnormal rotation or fixation of the intestines as they return from the umbilical cord to the abdomen during early fetal life. The abnormal position and lack of fixation within the abdomen predisposes the infant to volvulus, abnormal twisting of the intestine around the superior mesenteric vessels, and obstruction, often with secondary ischemia and infarction.

SYNONYMS

Midgut volvulus
Nonrotation

ICD-9-CM CODES

537.3 Volvulus of the duodenum
560.2 Volvulus of the bowel, colon, or intestine
751.4 Malrotation of the intestine
751.5 Volvulus, congenital

EPIDEMIOLOGY & DEMOGRAPHICS

- Malrotation occurs in 1 in 6000 live births.
- 55% present within the first week and 80% in the first month of life.
- The male-to-female ratio is approximately 2:1.
- There are no known ethnic, racial, or gender associations.
- Volvulus rarely predates delivery.

CLINICAL PRESENTATION

- Malrotation may manifest with volvulus, duodenal obstruction, or intermittent abdominal pain or as an incidental finding.
- The development of bilious emesis in a newborn is the classic presentation of volvulus and requires urgent evaluation.
- Lethargy or failure to thrive may be observed, especially in older children.
- Physical examination may reveal any of the following: irritability and lethargy, signs of dehydration, ill or toxic appearance, tachycardia, tachypnea, grunting, hypotension, distended abdomen or vague abdominal fullness.
- Signs and symptoms may be subtle early during volvulus, but observing an infant with bilious emesis for development of additional findings should be condemned.

ETIOLOGY

- Normal rotation and fixation of the intestine occurs in the first 3 months of fetal life.
  - The intestine lengthens and extends outside the abdominal cavity.
  - As the gut returns to the abdominal cavity, it rotates 270 degrees counterclockwise and becomes fixed in the retroperitoneum.
  - The duodenum falls behind the superior mesenteric vessels.
  - The ligament of Treitz attaches to the posterior wall of the abdominal cavity.
  - The cecum attaches in the right lower quadrant.
- Failure of the intestine to return to the abdominal cavity, rotate, or become correctly fixed in the retroperitoneum results in a variety of rotational anomalies.
- Abortive attempts to form the normal retroperitoneal fixation result in Ladd's bands, fibrous bands of connective tissue that can lead to obstruction.
- The most common and dangerous anomaly of rotation is "nonrotation."
  - Neither the duodenojejunal limb nor the cecocolic limb undergoes rotation, resulting in the duodenum descending along the right paravertebral gutter.
  - The proximal colon ascends parallel to the duodenum.
  - The normal broad-based mesentery does not exist.
  - This anatomic arrangement is particularly prone to twisting along the vascular axis, creating an intestinal volvulus.
  - Further twisting of the intestine results in venous obstruction followed by arterial obstruction, leading to intestinal ischemia and necrosis.
- Other rare rotational anomalies include:
  - Nonrotation of the duodenum with normal colonic rotation.
  - Reversed rotation of duodenum and colon, leads to transverse colon obstruction
  - Reversed rotation, paraduodenal hernias, and anomalies of attachment of the normally rotated intestine

DIAGNOSIS

DIFFERENTIAL DIAGNOSIS

- Necrotizing enterocolitis (NEC)
- Stenosis or stricture, especially after NEC
- Duplication
- Toxic megacolon
- Sepsis
- Bowel obstruction without volvulus (e.g., duodenal atresia)

IMAGING STUDIES

- Plain abdominal radiographs are not diagnostic and may be deceptively normal.
- An upper gastrointestinal series (UGI) is the study of choice and the gold standard.
  - With malrotation, the duodenojejunal junction is to the right of the spine and inferior to the duodenal bulb.
  - In volvulus, the obstruction is in the second or third portion of the duodenum and has the appearance of a bird's beak. If the duodenum is partially obstructed, a spiral or corkscrew appearance is seen.
- Barium enema may demonstrate malrotation with abnormal cecal position, but it cannot rule out duodenal obstruction caused by malrotation with a normally positioned cecum.
- Ultrasonography may identify orientation of the superior mesenteric vessels and suggest the diagnosis of malrotation.

TREATMENT

NONPHARMACOLOGIC THERAPY

- Malrotation with volvulus is a surgical emergency.
- Surgical correction is the only therapy.
- Operative treatment includes counterclockwise rotation of the volvulus to restore normal perfusion.
- Ladd's bands are divided to free duodenal lumen from extrinsic compression.
- The mesenteric base is broadened by placing the small bowel on the right side of the abdomen and the colon on the left side.
- Appendectomy is usually done to prevent later diagnostic confusion.
- If significant ischemic damage has occurred appropriate resection decisions may need to await a second-look 18 to 24 hours after correction of the volvulus.
- When significant irreversible ischemic damage has occurred, enterectomy is needed.
- When anomalies of intestinal rotation are recognized during the evaluation of recurrent abdominal pain or failure to thrive, operative correction is indicated.

ACUTE GENERAL Rx

The child with bilious emesis requires prompt surgical consultation and radiographic evaluation without delay.

DISPOSITION

Volvulus recurs in 3% of patients, most commonly in the early postoperative period, but it requires lifelong attention whenever bilious emesis or similar signs of obstruction occur.

REFERRAL

- Emergency pediatric surgical consultation is mandatory for an infant with bilious vomiting.
- Non-emergent consultation with a pediatric surgeon is appropriate for older infants or children with failure to thrive.

PEARLS & CONSIDERATIONS

COMMENTS

- Bilious vomiting in an infant is a surgical emergency until proved otherwise.
- Although there are many causes of bilious vomiting in infancy, no condition can result in irreversible damage in such a short time as malrotation with volvulus.
- Evaluation and treatment must proceed with haste.
- The physician evaluating a newborn with bilious emesis must expeditiously rule out volvulus to minimize the potentially devastating complications, including short gut and death.

SUGGESTED READINGS

Millar AJ et al: Malrotation and volvulus in infancy and childhood. *Semin Pediatr Surg* 12:229, 2003.
Torres AM et al: Malrotation of the intestine. *World J Surg* 17:326, 1993.

AUTHOR: **RICHARD A. FALCONE, JR., MD**

BASIC INFORMATION

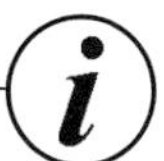

DEFINITION

Stinging marine animals constitute a large group of marine creatures that are capable of human envenomation. This group includes sponges, jellyfish, and corals. Most envenomations in the United States are relatively benign.

SYNONYMS

Marine envenomations
Marine scrapes
Sea bather's eruption
Sea envenomations

ICD-9-CM CODE
989.5 Marine sting

EPIDEMIOLOGY & DEMOGRAPHICS

- Marine stings typically occur in the warm waters of the south but can occur anywhere in the United States.
- In 2003, the American Association of Poison Control Centers received 2881 reports of marine envenomation with no reported deaths.
- Envenomations by exotic creatures not found in the coastal waters of the United States have occurred in tropical aquariums.

CLINICAL PRESENTATION

History

- Many victims of marine stings are beachgoers who are bathing along the shore.
- Victims also include divers who handle these creatures.
- Stings typically seen in the United States cause painful skin lesions usually in a linear pattern.

Physical Examination

- Toxicity is dose related.
- Urticaria and vesicles in a linear pattern.
- Systemic symptoms occasionally occur and include respiratory distress.
- Envenomations with the Portuguese man-of-war jellyfish may result in severe anaphylaxis.

ETIOLOGY

- The stings of marine animals are medically significant in the United States because of their common rate of occurrence.
- Stinging marine animals are members of the phylum Cnidaria and include the following:
  - Jellyfish
  - Atlantic Portuguese man-of-war
  - Sea nettles
  - Coral species
- All stinging marine animals use the nematocyst, an injection device for venom, to envenomate their victims.
  - Nematocysts are located along the length of tentacles.
  - Even after detachment from the body of the animal, nematocysts may remain active in water for weeks.

DIAGNOSIS

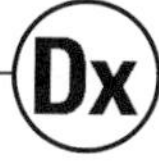

DIFFERENTIAL DIAGNOSIS

- Contact dermatitis
- Marine puncture wounds
- Sea snake envenomation

WORKUP

Laboratory tests and imaging studies are not appropriate for most marine stings in the United States.

TREATMENT

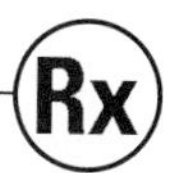

NONPHARMACOLOGIC THERAPY

- Initial management of airway, breathing, and circulation (ABCs), if necessary, should begin.
- Therapy is aimed at deactivating any remaining nematocysts and venom.
  - Immediately rinse the wound with saltwater, not with fresh water.
  - Remove remaining tentacles with forceps or a well-gloved hand.
  - Apply 5% acetic acid (i.e., vinegar) topically for 30 minutes, which inactivates the toxin.
  - Apply shaving cream and shave the affected area with a razor to remove any remaining nematocysts.

ACUTE GENERAL Rx

- Topical anesthesia such as a eutectic mixture of lidocaine anesthetics (EMLA) or Lidocaine Multilamellar X/fer (LMX4) may be applied. Apply topical anesthetic cream to small areas under occlusive dressing for 30 to 60 minutes.
- Systemic analgesia with narcotics is sometimes necessary.
  - Morphine sulfate: 0.05 to 0.2 mg/kg/dose intravenously, intramuscularly, or subcutaneously (maximum dose of 15 mg) or 0.2 to 0.5 mg/kg/dose orally (maximum dose of 30 mg), every 4 hours as needed
  - Codeine: 0.5 to 1 mg/kg/dose orally (maximum dose of 60 mg), every 4 hours as needed
  - Acetaminophen: 15 mg/kg/dose orally or rectally, every 4 hours as needed
- Systemic antihistamines may be used.
  - Diphenhydramine: 1 to 1.25 mg/kg/dose intravenously, intramuscularly, or orally (maximum dose of 50 mg), every 6 hours as needed
- Topical steroids may be used. Apply 1% or 2% hydrocortisone cream for itching.
- Systemic steroid therapy remains controversial.
- Antivenin administration is species specific.
  - An antivenin for the box-jellyfish (*Chironex fleckeri*) is available.
  - An antivenin for stonefish stings is available.

CHRONIC Rx

Long-term effects from marine stings in the United States are rare.

DISPOSITION

- Most patients can continue symptomatic therapy at home.
- Local discomfort and rash should resolve within 1 to 2 weeks.

REFERRAL

- Envenomation by the box jellyfish (*C. fleckeri*), which is found in the waters of Northern Australia, and severe envenomation by the Portuguese man-of-war (*Physalia physalis*) can be life threatening.
- These stings require immediate care in a facility that is capable of airway and cardiac management.
- Assistance from the regional poison control center can be helpful in management.

PEARLS & CONSIDERATIONS

COMMENTS

- Household vinegar and isopropyl alcohol can be used to inactivate the toxin.
- Perfume and high-proof liquor may be less efficacious and may be harmful.

PREVENTION

- All swimmers should be aware of the risks posed by marine stings. Bathers should avoid waters infested by jellyfish.
- Swimmers should obey all posted warnings, and children should be watched carefully along the beach.
- Divers should avoid handling corals and sponges unless proper protective clothing is worn.
- Normal clothing and petrolatum jelly applied to the skin do not reliably prevent stings.

SUGGESTED READINGS

Auerbach PS: Marine envenomation. *In* Auerbach PS (ed): *Wilderness Medicine. Management of Wilderness and Environmental Emergencies,* 3rd ed. Mosby–Year Book, St. Louis, 1995, pp 1327–1374.

Watson WA et al: 2003 Annual Report of the American Association of Poison Control Centers Toxic Exposure Surveillance System. *Am J Emerg Med* 22:335, 2004.

Women's and Children's Hospital: CSL Antivenom Handbook. Available at www.wch.sa.gov.au/paedm/clintox/cslavh_marine.html (for physicians).

AUTHORS: **WILLIAM T. TSAI, MD** and **ROBERT J. FREISHTAT, MD, MPH**

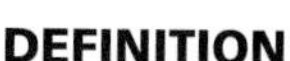

BASIC INFORMATION

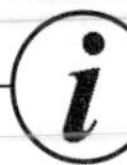

DEFINITION

Infant mastitis or breast abscess is breast inflammation, often occurring with abscess formation in the first 2 months of life.

ICD-9-CM CODES
771.5 Neonatal infective mastitis
778.7 Neonatal noninfective mastitis

EPIDEMIOLOGY & DEMOGRAPHICS

- The overall incidence is low. The highest incidence was seen in the 1940s and 1950s, during the staphylococcal epidemics in hospital nurseries.
- This condition occurs only in term infants because premature infants lack full mammary development.
- Mastitis occurs at age 2 to 8 weeks of life and usually peaks in the third week.
- The female-to-male ratio is 2:1.
- Bilateral breast involvement is rare.

CLINICAL PRESENTATION

History

- Increased swelling and redness of the breast.
- Discharge from the affected nipple may be reported.
- Signs of systemic illness are absent.

Physical Examination

- Fever present in 25% of patients
- Variable irritability
- Breast tenderness on palpation
- Marked erythema and induration of affected breast
- Breast fluctuance and warmth variably present
- Other possible skin findings:
  - More extensive cellulitis beyond the mammary area
  - Pustular or bullous rash elsewhere

ETIOLOGY

- Physiologic breast enlargement is caused by in utero exposure to maternal estrogen.
- Potentially pathogenic bacteria occur on mucous membranes and skin.
- Virtually all cases are caused by *Staphylococcus aureus.*
- Rare cases are associated with gram-negative organisms (i.e., *Salmonella* and *Escherichia coli*), group B streptococci, and anaerobes.

DIAGNOSIS

DIFFERENTIAL DIAGNOSIS

The diagnosis is clinical and microbiologic, with the differential diagnosis focusing on the etiologic organism.

WORKUP

- Gram stain and culture (aerobic and anaerobic) of the purulent material must be obtained using one of the following methods:
  - Gentle manipulation of the nipple
  - Needle aspiration of the abscess
  - Surgical incision and drainage of the abscess
- Blood culture results are usually negative.
- Urine and cerebrospinal fluid cultures are not indicated unless there is clinical evidence of sepsis.

TREATMENT

NONPHARMACOLOGIC THERAPY

- Initial parenteral antimicrobial coverage should be directed at the organism observed on Gram stain.
  - Generally, a β-lactamase–resistant penicillin is used.
  - An aminoglycoside is an appropriate choice if gram-negative organisms are found on the Gram stain.
- After the organism and sensitivities are microbiologically determined, antibiotic coverage can be narrowed.
- The total length of therapy depends on the overall clinical response but usually need not extend beyond 10 to 14 days.
- Prompt incision and drainage is indicated for all abscesses that have not spontaneously drained.
- Use of incision and drainage is essentially curative.
- An experienced surgeon should perform the surgery to minimize mammary tissue destruction.

DISPOSITION

- Close clinical follow-up is necessary, especially when oral antimicrobial agents are being used.
- Long-term follow-up may reveal evidence of decreased breast tissue compared with the contralateral side after pubertal development is complete.

PEARLS & CONSIDERATIONS

COMMENTS

- More than two thirds of all breast abscesses in females are found in nursing mothers (2 to 8 weeks postpartum) and not in neonates.
- All infants with mastitis or abscess caused by *Salmonella* have signs and symptoms of gastroenteritis.

SUGGESTED READINGS

Rudoy RC, Nelson JD: Breast abscess during the neonatal period. *Am J Dis Child* 129:1031, 1975.
Walsh M, McIntosh K: Neonatal mastitis. *Clin Pediatr* 25:395, 1986.

AUTHOR: **CYNTHIA CHRISTY, MD**

BASIC INFORMATION

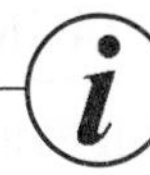

DEFINITION

Mastoiditis is an acute or subacute infection of the mastoid air cells. Mastoiditis is often a complication of otitis media.

ICD-9-CM CODES
383.00 Mastoiditis (acute or subacute)
383.1 Mastoiditis (chronic)

EPIDEMIOLOGY & DEMOGRAPHICS

- Children younger than 5 years are most commonly affected, mirroring the incidence of otitis media in this population.
- Mastoiditis is relatively uncommon, but an increasing frequency of mastoiditis is reported.
- Risk factors include acute otitis media and inadequate treatment of acute otitis media.

CLINICAL PRESENTATION

History

- Acute presentation
  - Fever
  - Otalgia
  - Retroauricular swelling, erythema, and pain with downward and outward deviation of the auricle
  - Otorrhea or a bulging, immobile, opaque tympanic membrane
  - With antibiotics, initial improvement and then relapse with fever, pain, and swelling or no response
  - Fluctuance if pus disrupts the bone and forms a subperiosteal abscess
    - In infants, fluctuance above the ear pushes the pinna inferiorly and out.
    - In children, fluctuance posterior to the ear pushes the pinna superiorly and out.
  - With or without postauricular swelling
  - Mucopurulent drainage from a perforated tympanic membrane
  - Hearing loss
- Chronic presentation
  - Chronic otitis media (months to years)
  - Possible fever
  - Persistent or intermittent otorrhea
  - Hearing loss
  - Persistent otalgia
- Complications
  - Subperiosteal abscess
  - Bezold abscess (i.e., dissection of pus into deep neck structures)
  - Cerebellar abscess
  - Epidural abscess
  - Subdural abscess
  - Empyema
  - Labyrinthitis
  - Venous sinus thrombosis
  - Bacteremia
  - Temporal bone osteomyelitis
  - Conductive hearing loss
  - Septic emboli
  - Facial nerve palsy
  - Meningitis
  - Otitic hydrocephalus (i.e., intracranial hypertension from lateral sinus obstruction)

ETIOLOGY

- Acute mastoiditis (i.e., symptoms for less than 1 month)
  - *Streptococcus pneumoniae*
  - *Streptococcus pyogenes*
  - *Staphylococcus aureus*
- Chronic mastoiditis (i.e., symptoms for 1 month or longer)
  - *S. aureus*
  - Gram-negative bacilli (e.g., *Pseudomonas aeruginosa*)
  - Anaerobes (i.e., *Peptococcus*, *Actinomyces*, and *Bacteroides melaninogenicus* most common)
  - Mycobacteria (uncommon in the US)

DIAGNOSIS

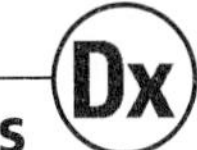

DIFFERENTIAL DIAGNOSIS

- Bone cysts
- Histiocytosis
- Leukemia
- Lymphoma
- Mastoid tumors
- Mumps
- Posterior auricular lymphadenopathy

WORKUP

Consider further workup in all cases of acute otitis media not responsive to antibiotics and in all cases of suppurative intracranial processes with no known focus.

LABORATORY TESTS

- Tympanocentesis for Gram stain and culture of fluid
- Lumbar puncture when meningeal signs are present
- Immunologic evaluation in cases in which other recurrent infections have occurred

IMAGING STUDIES

- Computed tomography (CT) scan of the temporal bone for confirmation of clinical impression
  - Nonspecific clouding of mastoid cells (serious otitis media can cause cloudy mastoids on CT scan)
  - Necrosis and coalescence of bony septa
  - Bony destruction
  - Hypoaeration

TREATMENT

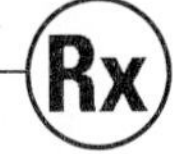

NONPHARMACOLOGIC THERAPY

- Tympanocentesis is done for diagnosis and treatment.
  - Tympanostomy tubes
  - Myringotomy
- Surgical intervention is indicated for therapeutic drainage or débridement if any of the following are present:
  - Fluctuance
  - CT scan indicative of bony involvement
  - Complications of mastoiditis (see Clinical Presentation)
  - Failure of medical therapy within 48 hours

ACUTE GENERAL Rx

- Antibiotics are tailored to Gram stain results and known etiologic agents.
- Acute mastoiditis: ceftriaxone, cefotaxime, or clindamycin (in penicillin-allergic patient)
- If central nervous system involvement is suspected: vancomycin to cover resistant pneumococci or staphylococci

CHRONIC Rx

- Chronic mastoiditis: no treatment until surgical cultures are obtained
- Examples of empirical therapeutic regimens for chronic mastoiditis: Ticarcillin and clavulanate, piperacillin and tazobactam, ceftazidime, or imipenem.
- Tailor therapy according to culture results.
- Intravenous therapy is given until a clinical response is achieved and then may be changed to oral therapy.
- If adequate oral absorption can be maintained, the etiologic organism has been identified, and an appropriate oral agent is available.
- Treat for a minimum of 3 weeks.

DISPOSITION

- Evaluate for hearing loss
- Careful follow-up for response to therapy and complications

REFERRAL

Consultation with otolaryngologists, surgeons, and neurosurgeons for specific complications. Consultation with pediatric infectious disease specialists may be warranted.

PEARLS & CONSIDERATIONS

COMMENTS

- Mastoiditis is uncommon.
- With increasing concerns about antibiotic use, the prevalence may increase.

PREVENTION

Early and complete treatment of acute otitis media reduces the risk of mastoiditis.

SUGGESTED READINGS

Ghaffar F et al: Acute mastoiditis in children: a seventeen-year experience in Dallas, Texas. *Pediatr Infect Dis J* 20:376, 2001.

Katz A et al: Acute mastoiditis in Southern Israel: a twelve year retrospective study (1990 through 2001). *Pediatr Infect Dis J* 22:878, 2003.

AUTHOR: **MAUREEN NOVAK, MD**

BASIC INFORMATION

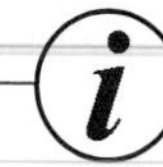

DEFINITION

Measles is an acute viral illness characterized by fever, cough, coryza, conjunctivitis, and a characteristic exanthem and enanthem.

SYNONYM

Rubeola

ICD-9-CM CODE
055.9 Measles

EPIDEMIOLOGY & DEMOGRAPHICS

- Although uncommon in the United States, measles is the leading vaccine-preventable cause of mortality in the world.
- The World Health Organization (WHO) estimated 30 to 40 million cases of measles worldwide in 2001, with 745,000 deaths attributed to the disease.
- Vaccination efforts have reduced the incidence of measles by 99% in developed countries.
- In the prevaccine era, 400,000 cases were reported in the United States each year. Measles was epidemic and occurred in biennial cycles in urban areas.
- Measles is transmitted by direct contact with infectious droplets and less commonly by airborne spread.
- Peak incidence in temperate areas is in the winter and spring.
- The highest attack rates were among children 5 to 9 years old.
- Encephalitis occurs in approximately 1 of 2000 reported cases.
- Mortality rates are highest for infants and adults with 1 death occurring for every 3000 cases.

CLINICAL PRESENTATION

History

- The incubation period is 10 ± 2 days.
- A 3-day prodrome of upper airway tract symptoms with fever is seen.
- Malaise, fever, coryza, conjunctivitis, and cough follow, with increasing severity over the next 2 to 4 days.
- Conjunctivitis is associated with tearing and photophobia.
- Exanthem appears 2 weeks after exposure.
  - At peak of fever and respiratory symptoms
  - Appears first on head, behind ears, and spreads centrifugally to the feet
  - Becomes confluent by the third day
  - Fades, following the reverse course of its appearance; desquamation possible
- Modified illness occurs in the partially immune individual.
  - Same sequence, but milder
  - Most commonly after immune globulin is given to an exposed, susceptible host
  - Also occurs in infected, unimmunized infants modified by transplacentally acquired maternal antibody
- Atypical illness occurs in some immunized patients exposed to wild-type virus.
  - Seen primarily in the 1970s in young adults who received killed measles vaccine
  - Similar incubation period
  - Sudden, high fever in prodrome, along with headache, abdominal pain, and myalgia
  - Rash occurs distally, with spread upward
  - Vesicular rash possible
  - Respiratory distress with pneumonia
  - Atypical measles: not contagious
- Complications of measles include pneumonia and secondary bacterial infection, which are the leading causes of death.
  - Diarrhea is the most common complication, occurring in 8% of cases.
  - Otitis media complicates measles in 7% of cases.
  - Clinically significant myocarditis and pericarditis occur rarely.
  - Encephalitis may occur during the rash.
  - Black measles (i.e., hemorrhagic measles) is a severe, often fatal complication, but it is rarely seen in the United States.
  - Subacute sclerosing panencephalitis (SSPE) is a rare, degenerative, central nervous system disease caused by persistent infection.
  - Measles is the leading cause of blindness in African children.

Physical Examination

- Prodrome lasts approximately 3 days.
  - Fever, coryza, rhinitis, and conjunctival infection predominate.
  - Koplik spots are the pathognomonic enanthem. White spots (about 1 mm) appear on a bright red background on the buccal mucosa and increase in number to coalesce on the buccal mucosa adjacent to the lower molars.
- The exanthem stage typically begins on the 14th day after exposure, at the peak of the respiratory symptoms.
  - Fever peaks then and begins to clear after the third or fourth day.
  - Koplik spots disappear over the next 3 days.
  - Exanthem starts behind the ears and along the hairline.
  - By the third day, the rash involves the face and spreads to the lower extremities sequentially from head to toe (centrifugally).
  - Maculopapular, erythematous, discrete lesions appear and progress to a confluent rash.
  - Appearance of lesions can be vesicular on an erythematous base.
  - On day 3 or 4, the rash fades to a copper color, and fine desquamation occurs.
  - Fever breaks on day 3 or 4, with resolution of respiratory symptoms.
  - Pharyngitis and generalized lymphadenopathy are often present.

ETIOLOGY

The measles pathogen is an RNA virus of one serotype, classified in the *Morbillivirus* genus in the Paramyxoviridae family.

DIAGNOSIS

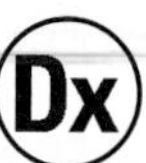

DIFFERENTIAL DIAGNOSIS

- Exclude illnesses whose main signs include an exanthematous rash.
  - Infectious mononucleosis, especially with amoxicillin
  - Drug eruptions, especially from penicillin, cefalospamos, and antiepileptic medications
  - Enteroviral coxsackievirus and other viral exanthems sometimes mimic measles
- Exposure and immunization history are helpful in limiting the differential diagnosis.

WORKUP

The presence of Koplik spots is pathognomonic.

LABORATORY TESTS

- Specific diagnosis is made by viral isolation.
- Serology is important in surveillance but not for routine diagnosis.
- Enzyme-linked immunosorbent assay (ELISA) for IgM, if positive, is diagnostic. Results are 20% negative at onset of rash; repeat within first month after onset of rash.
- IgG responses require paired sera (two specimens 10 to 30 days apart).

TREATMENT

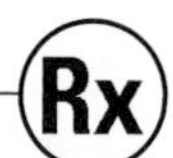

ACUTE GENERAL Rx

- No specific antiviral treatment is available.
- Symptomatic treatment of fever, maintenance of hydration, and antitussive therapy should be provided.
- Vitamin A (single dose of 200,000 IU orally; 100,000 IU for children 6 to 12 months old and 50,000 IU for infants 0–6 months) repeated the following day and at 4 weeks in clinically deficient children should be administered to all infected children who live in areas of known vitamin A deficiency.
- Any infected child with any of the following risk factors should be considered for vitamin A supplementation:
  - Hospitalized, 6-month-old to 2-year-old children with measles
  - Immunodeficiency (e.g., human immunodeficiency virus [HIV], immunosuppressive therapy, congenital immunodeficiencies)
  - Clinical evidence of vitamin A deficiency (i.e., by ophthalmologic criteria)
  - Impaired intestinal absorption (e.g., short gut syndrome, cystic fibrosis, biliary obstruction)
  - Moderate to severe malnutrition, including eating disorders
  - Recent immigration from areas where measles mortality rates are 1% or higher
- Postexposure prophylaxis
  - Vaccinate susceptible individuals within 72 hours of exposure.

- Immune globulin can be given to susceptible children within 6 days of exposure to prevent or modify infection.
  - The usual dose is 0.25 mL/kg administered intramuscularly.
  - Immunocompromised children should receive 0.5 mL/kg given intramuscularly.
  - Maximum total dose is 15 mL.
- Immune globulin is indicated for susceptible household contacts, infants younger than 12 months, pregnant women, immunocompromised hosts, and HIV-infected children regardless of immunization status, unless the patient is receiving intravenous immune globulin at regular intervals and the last dose was given within 3 weeks of exposure.

REFERRAL

Consultation with a pediatric infectious disease specialist may be warranted in complicated cases and exposures.

PEARLS & CONSIDERATIONS

PREVENTION

- Live measles virus vaccine
  - Attenuated
  - Monovalent or in combination (e.g., measles-rubella, measles-mumps-rubella [MMR], measles-mumps-rubella-varicella [MMRV] preferred)
  - Produces mild, noncommunicable infection
  - Development of antibodies in 95% of susceptible children
  - Lifelong protection
  - First dose on or after first birthday
  - Second dose preferably given between 4 and 6 years
  - Consider the patient susceptible if born after 1957 and without documentation of vaccination, physician-diagnosed illness, or titers confirming infection
  - In outbreaks: at least 1-month interval between vaccinations
- Adverse events
  - Fever occurs in 5% to 15% of recipients 7 to 12 days after receiving the vaccine.
  - Transient rashes appear in 5% of vaccine recipients.
  - Transient thrombocytopenia can occur.
  - Rare hypersensitivity reactions are usually minor and consist of urticaria or a wheal and flare reaction at the site of injection.
    - Children with egg allergies should be vaccinated without testing.
    - Reactions are attributed to small amounts of neomycin or gelatin in the vaccine.
- Precautions
  - Minor illnesses with fever are not a contraindication.
  - The risk of thrombocytopenia is increased in children with history of thrombocytopenia. The benefit versus risk of vaccine and illness need to be considered.
  - Recent administration of immune globulin may interfere with the serologic response to measles vaccine, and measles immunization should be delayed.
- Immunodeficient hosts
  - Live virus should not be given to severely immunodeficient children.
  - An interval of 3 months should be observed from cessation of any immunosuppressive therapy and vaccination.
  - High-dose corticosteroids (>2 mg/kg for 2 weeks or more) necessitate an interval of 1 month before immunization.
  - HIV infection is not a contraindication unless the child is severely immunocompromised (i.e., low CD4 T lymphocyte counts).
  - Pregnant women should not receive the vaccine.

PATIENT/FAMILY EDUCATION

Immunization results in serologic evidence of immunity in 99% of those receiving two doses at least 1 month apart starting after 12 months of age.

SUGGESTED READINGS

American Academy of Pediatrics: Measles. *In* Pickering LK (ed): *Red Book: 2003 Report of the Committee on Infectious Diseases,* 26th ed. Elk Grove Village, IL, American Academy of Pediatrics, 2003, pp 419–429.

AUTHOR: **MAUREEN NOVAK, MD**

BASIC INFORMATION

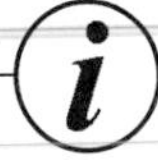

DEFINITION

Meckel's diverticulum is an ileal outpouching that occurs from the incomplete atresia of the vitelline duct (i.e., omphalomesenteric duct [OMD]) in the embryo. It may contain ileal mucosa or ectopic mucosa of gastric, pancreatic, or jejunal-colonic origin. Partial or incomplete attenuation of the OMD can lead to persistent fistula to the umbilicus, manifesting with umbilical drainage, umbilical sinus or cysts in which distal duct portions remain intact, or fibrous bands. These bands course from the Meckel's diverticulum to the base of the mesentery and may act as sites for internal herniation of the small intestine or intestinal obstruction. Meckel's diverticulitis is inflammation of the Meckel's diverticulum. This results from obstruction at the base leading to infection within the blind-ending diverticulum (similar to the mechanism of appendicitis).

SYNONYMS

Persistent omphalomesenteric duct (anomaly)
Persistent vitelline duct (anomaly)
Persistent yolk stalk (anomaly)

ICD-9-CM CODES
751.0 Meckel's diverticulum
751.0 Omphalomesenteric duct
759.89 Umbilical cyst

EPIDEMIOLOGY & DEMOGRAPHICS

- Generally follows the *rule of twos*:
  - Meckel's diverticulum occurs in approximately 2% of the population (prevalence of 0.2% to 4%).
  - The typical diverticulum is approximately 2 inches (3 cm) long and about 2 cm wide, and it arises within the terminal 2 feet (average of 60 cm proximal to the isocercal valve of the ileum).
  - There are two primary types of ectopic mucosa: gastric and pancreatic.
  - The two most common complications are bleeding and obstruction of the diverticulum or the small intestine.
- Males represent 75% of symptomatic patients.
- Approximately 60% of diverticula manifest in childhood, with 50% occurring by the third year of life.

CLINICAL PRESENTATION

- The type of presentation depends on the patient's age.
  - Hemorrhage is the most common complication (40%) and occurs more often in younger infants.
  - Older patients present more commonly with symptoms of inflammation.
- Meckel's diverticulum may be discovered incidentally.
  - A Meckel's diverticulum may be discovered at the time of operation for other reasons.
  - Selective indications must be used for resection, and consideration should be given to other simultaneous procedures to minimize the risk of complications.
  - Between 60% and 80% of patients have ectopic gastric or pancreatic tissue, increasing chance of future symptoms.
  - Most pediatric surgeons resect an incidental Meckel's diverticulum in the preadolescent child when the resection adds minimal additional risk to the procedure.
- A bleeding Meckel's diverticulum may be identified.
  - The lesion may result from mucosal ulceration in the diverticulum itself or in the ileum near the junction with the diverticulum.
  - Bleeding from a Meckel's is the most common cause of significant lower gastrointestinal hemorrhage in children.
  - Typically, the bleeding is painless, intermittent, and massive; it can occasionally be chronic or associated with pain or perforation.
- Bowel obstruction may result from Meckel's diverticulum.
  - It may manifest with emesis and abdominal distention.
  - It may have intermittent colicky pain caused by intussusception.
- Meckel's diverticulitis may develop.
  - It often manifests similar to acute appendicitis, and the diagnosis is often confused.
  - Meckel's diverticulitis may manifest with more "shifting" pain and more diffuse peritonitis than typical appendicitis.
- Umbilical lesions may be identified.
  - Fistulas to the umbilicus through an omphalomesenteric duct manifest with drainage at the base of the umbilicus.
  - Drainage may be of enteric secretions if the OMD is completely patent.
  - A periumbilical rash and inflammation surrounding the umbilicus may occur.
  - Incomplete patency (i.e., fibrosed at the intestinal end) may lead to mucoid drainage at the umbilicus.
  - Other umbilical anomalies (e.g., cysts) may manifest as a mass or an infection under the umbilicus.
  - Persistence of umbilical "granulation tissue" in the newborn should provoke further investigation.

ETIOLOGY

- The causes of persistence and incomplete atresia of the omphalomesenteric duct are unknown.
- Complications of a Meckel's diverticulum result from the presence of this diverticulum.
- Bleeding is precipitated by ulceration of the ileal mucosa at a site adjacent to the ectopic gastric mucosa. The ulcer may be within the main ileal lumen or within the diverticulum.
- Intussusception is caused by the Meckel's diverticulum acting as a lead point.
- Persistence of a portion of the embryonic fistula tract (e.g., intraumbilical fistula, umbilical cyst) may lead to mucoid or meconium drainage from the umbilicus.
- Residual omphalomesenteric duct bands may cause obstruction.

DIAGNOSIS

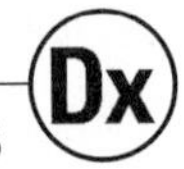

DIFFERENTIAL DIAGNOSIS

- The differential diagnosis depends on the anomaly and presentation.
- Intestinal obstruction and diverticulitis manifest as an acute abdomen.
- In most cases, the definitive diagnosis is made at the time of laparotomy.
- The differential diagnosis of mildly symptomatic or asymptomatic rectal bleeding includes the following:
  - Rectal fissure or trauma
  - Juvenile polyp or polyposis syndrome
  - Ulcerative colitis
  - Foreign body
  - Vascular malformation
  - Coagulopathy

WORKUP

Laparoscopy is diagnostic and therapeutic, and it has become the primary mode of diagnosis and treatment for suspected Meckel's bleeding when the diagnosis is not secured.

LABORATORY TESTS

For significant bleeding or syncope, consider a complete blood cell count, blood typing, and crossmatch.

IMAGING STUDIES

- ^{99m}Tc sodium pertechnetate scanning assists in the identification of a Meckel's diverticulum if there is ectopic gastric mucosa in the diverticulum.
  - When the lesion can be visualized, this is a helpful procedure.
  - Unfortunately, the rate of false-negative studies approaches 40%, even with enhancement using H_2-blockers or pentagastrin.
- Barium studies and computed tomography (CT) are rarely helpful.
- In patients with persistent drainage from the umbilicus, a direct sinogram with water-soluble contrast often discloses the tract and any communication with the intestinal tract.
- Ultrasound or CT helps to identify cysts and sinus tract remnants.

TREATMENT

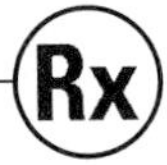

NONPHARMACOLOGIC THERAPY

- Patients with symptomatic Meckel's diverticulum should undergo operative removal of the diverticulum and correction of coincidental complications.

- When resection is undertaken for bleeding, care to excise all ectopic mucosa and the diverticulum is necessary.
- In the face of active bleeding, resection of the ulcer is curative.
- In the case of intussusception, the diverticulum is resected along a healthy margin after reduction.
- Inflamed diverticulum should be excised.
- Omphalomesenteric duct bands should be excised in all cases; any intestinal obstruction is also relieved.
- Laparoscopy has simplified the risk of exploration in the case of undiagnosed rectal bleeding in the young child. This procedure has replaced more complex imaging and angiography, simplifying and expediting management.

ACUTE GENERAL Rx

- Fluid resuscitation is provided for patients with bowel obstruction or bleeding as indicated.
- Appropriate blood products are given if needed for acute and massive bleeding.

DISPOSITION

After surgical treatment, normal postoperative follow-up is needed.

REFERRAL

Referral to a pediatric surgeon should occur if there is concern about symptoms that may indicate Meckel's diverticulum.

PEARLS & CONSIDERATIONS

COMMENTS

- The *rule of twos* indicates the following:
  - Two years old
  - Two feet from the terminal ileum
  - Two inches long
  - Two types of ectopic mucosa: gastric and pancreatic
  - Two major complications: bleeding and obstruction
  - Two primary routes for diagnosis: scan for Meckel's diverticulum and laparoscopy
- In cases of undiagnosed intractable abdominal pain, consider Meckel's diverticulum: intermittent intussusception, recurrent inflammation, and ectopic ulceration.
- Intractable granulation tissue at the umbilicus may represent ectopic tissue from an incompletely patent omphalomesenteric duct.

SUGGESTED READINGS

Brown RL, Azizkhan RG: Gastrointestinal bleeding in infants and children: Meckel's diverticulum and intestinal duplication. *Semin Pediatr Surg* 8:202, 1999.

Emil SG, Laberge JM: Meckel's diverticulum. *In* Mattei P (ed): *Surgical Directives: Pediatric Surgery.* Philadelphia, Lippincott Williams & Wilkins, 2003, pp 327–330.

AUTHOR: **RICHARD A. FALCONE, JR., MD**

BASIC INFORMATION

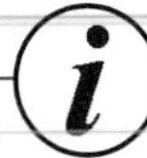

DEFINITION

Bacterial meningitis is inflammation of the meninges, the membranes covering the brain and spinal cord, as a result of bacterial infection.

SYNONYM

Leptomeningitis

ICD-9-CM CODE
320.9 Bacterial meningitis

EPIDEMIOLOGY & DEMOGRAPHICS

- The incidence of bacterial meningitis has varied between 0.7 and 7.3 cases per 100,000 people per year, depending on the period of time in which the study was conducted and the age group analyzed.
- The greatest risk for acquiring this infection is in infants between 6 and 12 months old. Most cases occur in children between 1 month and 5 years old.
- The epidemiology of bacterial meningitis depends on the etiologic agent.
- Characteristics of pneumococcal meningitis include the following:
  - There are 90 pneumococcal serotypes, but 7 cause most invasive disease in children younger than 6 years.
  - The highest rate for invasive pneumococcal infection is among children age 2 years or younger, with the highest incidence among children younger than 6 months. The pneumococcus is also the most common cause of bacterial meningitis in cerebrospinal fluid (CSF) leaks that develop after head trauma.
  - The risk of pneumococcal meningitis is significantly higher among blacks than whites.
  - The organism is a frequent inhabitant of the upper respiratory tract.
  - The incidence of antibiotic resistance to penicillin and the third-generation cephalosporins increased significantly in the 1980s and 1990s, although the incidence has declined recently in some locations.
- Characteristics of meningococcal meningitis include the following:
  - There are 13 serogroups, 5 of which (A, B, C, Y, W-135) are major.
  - There has been a shift in the distribution of serogroups causing invasive disease over the past 10 to 15 years, with an increasing percentage of cases caused by group Y. Most infections in children are caused by groups B (particularly in younger children), C, and Y.
  - Between 2% and 15% of healthy individuals (particularly adults) harbor the organism in the nasopharynx.
  - The endemic attack rate for invasive meningococcal disease is 1 to 3 cases per 100,000 people per year. The highest attack rates are among children younger than 1 year, with the peak occurring in infants 6 to 12 months old. The attack rate then falls until early adolescence, when it again rises.
  - The secondary attack rate among household and other close contacts (e.g., daycare contacts) of an index case is about 1000-fold greater than the endemic attack rate.
- Characteristics of group B streptococcal meningitis include the following:
  - Nine serotypes, but meningitis is usually caused by serotype III organisms.
  - Meningitis can be a manifestation of early-onset (<5 to 7 days old) or late-onset (>7 days old) infection, but it is more common as a manifestation of late-onset infection.
  - Early-onset infection results from vertical transmission from mother to infant shortly before or during delivery. The risk increases with premature labor, prolonged rupture of membranes, chorioamnionitis, intrapartum fever, and group B streptococcal bacteriuria. With the introduction of antibiotic prophylaxis administered during labor to colonized women, an almost 70% reduction in the incidence of early-onset disease to the current incidence of approximately 0.5 cases per 1000 live births has occured.
  - Late-onset infection usually occurs at 3 to 4 weeks of age (range, 1 week to 8 months). The incidence of 0.3 to 1.8 cases per 1000 live births has not changed significantly with the widespread use of chemoprophylaxis of maternal carriers of the organism at the time of delivery.
  - Although late-onset infection may result from vertical transmission of the organism from mother to infant at the time of delivery, with delayed hematogenous dissemination, it most likely results from horizontal transmission from nursery personnel, caregivers at home, or others close to the infant.

CLINICAL PRESENTATION

History

- Fever: variable degree; may or may not be present in neonates; almost always present in non-neonates
- Nausea and vomiting
- Headache
- Back pain
- Altered mental status (most helpful symptoms in infants are excessive irritability or lethargy; only 15% of patients are semicomatose or comatose)
- Poor feeding

Physical Examination

- Signs of meningeal irritation include nuchal rigidity; positive Kernig's sign (i.e., with leg flexed 90 degrees at the hip, knee cannot be straightened beyond 135 degrees); positive Brudzinski's sign (i.e., legs are flexed involuntarily when neck is flexed). These usually occur in older children and may not be present (or be present late in the course) in infants younger than 1 year.
- Bulging fontanelle may be found in infants.
- Apnea or respiratory distress may occur in neonates.
- Petechiae or purpura may occur with meningococcal infection.
- Shock is manifested by diminished peripheral perfusion, tachycardia, decreased urine output, depressed mental status, and late hypotension.
- Papilledema is rare; when present, look for brain abscess, venous sinus thrombosis, and subdural fluid collection.
- Seizures occur in approximately 20% to 30%; those occurring before or during the first 2 to 4 days of hospitalization and that are not difficult to control are not associated with a poor neurologic prognosis.
- Focal neurologic signs occur in 14% to 24% at the time of admission and are associated with an increased risk of poor neurologic outcome.
- Palsies of cranial nerves controlling extraocular movements (III, IV, VI) are usually transient; VIII nerve involvement (cochlear or vestibular) is often permanent.
- Signs of significantly increased intracranial pressure (ICP) include marked depression of consciousness; hypertension; bradycardia; irregular respirations; dilated, unreactive, or sluggishly reactive pupils; and decorticate or decerebrate posturing.
- Because most cases of bacterial meningitis arise hematogenously, there may be evidence of concomitant metastatic infection, such as cellulitis, pneumonia, or septic arthritis.

ETIOLOGY

- The microbiologic cause of bacterial meningitis depends on the patient's age.
- Younger than 1 to 2 months:
  - Group B streptococci: 52%
  - *Escherichia coli* and other gram-negative bacilli: 27%
  - *Listeria monocytogenes*: 6%
  - Anaerobes: 3%
  - Other gram-positive organisms: 7%
    - Enterococci
    - *Streptococcus pneumoniae*
    - Staphylococci
  - Other gram-negative organisms: 5%
    - *Haemophilus influenzae*
    - *Neisseria meningitidis*
    - *Pseudomonas* species
- Older than 2 months:
  - *S. pneumoniae* and *N. meningitidis* account for 90% to 95% of cases, although the frequency of pneumococcal infection has decreased in recent years as a result of the widespread use of the conjugate pneumococcal vaccine.
  - Other agents are occasionally observed: *H. influenzae*, *Salmonella* species, group

B streptococci, *L. monocytogenes*, and anaerobes.

DIAGNOSIS

Dx

DIFFERENTIAL DIAGNOSIS

- Other causes of meningitis: viral, tuberculous, fungal, parasitic, or protozoal agents
- Encephalitis
- Brain abscess
- Subdural empyema
- Spinal epidural abscess
- Ruptured intracranial or spinal cyst
- Head injury
- Intoxication
- Brain tumor

LABORATORY TESTS

- A lumbar puncture to collect CSF for analysis is the principal diagnostic test.
- Performance of a lumbar puncture is usually safe, although there is risk of cerebral herniation in patients with significantly elevated ICP, and it may not be tolerated in infants with significant hemodynamic instability.
- Lumbar puncture should be deferred in patients with significant depression of consciousness (i.e., no response to pain), hypertension, bradycardia, decorticate or decerebrate posturing, irregular respirations, fixed pupillary dilatation or sluggish pupillary response to light, or significant hemodynamic instability. In these situations, it is prudent to treat the patient presumptively for bacterial meningitis, lower the ICP, improve the patient's hemodynamic status, and perform the lumbar puncture at a later time when it is deemed safe to do so.
- CSF may be collected for the following tests:
  - Cell count: usually > 1000 white blood cells (WBCs)/mm^3; may be less early in infection or with fulminant disease
  - WBC differential count: usually a predominance of polymorphonuclear leukocytes
  - Glucose: usually moderately or severely depressed (<60% of the blood sugar level)
  - Protein: usually elevated
  - Gram stain: usually positive, unless the patient has very early infection, has received prior antibiotic therapy, or has *L. monocytogenes* infection (because *Listeria* meningitis often is a relatively low-inoculum infection)
  - Culture: CSF should be inoculated onto sheep's blood agar, chocolate agar, and into nutrient broth; the culture is usually positive, although if the patient has received prior antibiotic therapy, it may be negative.
  - Latex agglutination: commercial kits available for the detection of the capsular antigens of *S. pneumoniae, H. influenzae* type b, *N. meningitidis*, and group B streptococci in CSF
- The sensitivity of these tests in detecting bacterial antigen in CSF varies with the specific organism and the bacterial inoculum, although the specificity (when testing CSF) is excellent.
- Routine performance of these tests has fallen into disfavor because the results rarely alter the initial approach to antimicrobial therapy.
- There are two situations in which their performance may be useful:
  - When the patient has received prior antibiotic therapy and the Gram stain result is negative
  - In helping to differentiate pneumococcal from group B streptococcal infection in young infants with gram-positive cocci seen in CSF, because optimal empirical therapy for these two infections differs
- CSF analysis can be used to differentiate among the various types of meningitis.
- Viral meningitis can be determined by the following:
  - The CSF WBC count is usually 50 to 500/mm^3, although it can be lower or higher.
  - There is a predominance of polymorphonuclear leukocytes early, but the shift to a mononuclear WBC predominance usually occurs within 6 to 12 hours.
  - The CSF glucose level is usually normal or only mildly depressed, and the protein concentration is usually modestly elevated.
  - The Gram stain and bacterial cultures are negative, although viral cultures and polymerase chain reaction (PCR) testing may identify the etiologic agent.
- Tuberculous meningitis can be diagnosed by the following:
  - The CSF WBC count is usually 50–500/mm^3.
  - There is often polymorphonuclear WBC predominance early, and a shift to mononuclear WBC predominance occurs later.
  - The glucose level is moderately low (typically 15 to 35 mg/dL), lower than what is observed in viral meningitis but not as low as in many patients with bacterial meningitis.
- Blood cultures should be obtained for all patients suspected of having bacterial meningitis, because they are positive in 80% to 90% of patients who did not receive prior antibiotic therapy.
- Gram stain of the aspirate of purpuric lesions can assist in the diagnosis of meningococcal infection if the rash is present.

IMAGING STUDIES

Head computed tomography and magnetic resonance imaging may be useful in identifying complications of meningitis (e.g., hydrocephalus, subdural effusions, infarcts caused by vasculitis), but they are not used in establishing a diagnosis of bacterial meningitis.

TREATMENT

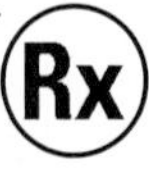

NONPHARMACOLOGIC THERAPY

- Patients should usually be admitted to a pediatric intensive care unit or neonatal intensive care unit initially for close observation.
- Monitor vital signs, peripheral perfusion, urine output, and mental status for evidence of shock.
- Monitor for evidence of the syndrome of inappropriate secretion of antidiuretic hormone (SIADH), manifested by hyponatremia, hypo-osmolality, possible oliguria, high urinary sodium concentration, and increasing body weight. Urine output and serum electrolytes should be monitored twice daily for at least the first 48 hours, the time when SIADH is most likely to develop. Restrict fluid intake if SIADH develops.
- Perform neurologic evaluation at the time of admission and every few hours for the first 2 to 3 days and at least daily thereafter.
- Monitor head circumference daily in infants.
- Occasionally, surgical intervention may be necessary to deal with complications of the infection. This may include drainage of significant, symptomatic subdural effusions or insertion of a ventriculoperitoneal shunt for hydrocephalus.

ACUTE GENERAL Rx

Antibiotic Therapy

- Antibiotic therapy should always be given parenterally and should be begun promptly at the hospital to which the patient first presents for care.
- Empirical therapy varies with age.
- For infants younger than 1 month old for empirical therapy or if gram-negative rods are seen on Gram stain, consider the following:
  - Use ampicillin plus cefotaxime.
  - If the Gram stain is negative but the other CSF analysis suggests bacterial meningitis, consider addition of gentamicin for synergy with ampicillin for *Listeria* treatment.
  - If evidence of group B streptococcal infection is shown by Gram stain or latex agglutination, use ampicillin or penicillin plus gentamicin.
  - If evidence of pneumococcal infection is shown by Gram stain or latex agglutination or if gram-positive cocci seen on Gram stain but latex agglutination testing is not available to help distinguish pneumococcal from group B streptococcal infection, use vancomycin plus cefotaxime.
- For children older than 1 month for empirical therapy or evidence of pneumococcal infection by Gram stain or latex agglutination, consider the following:

- Use vancomycin plus cefotaxime or ceftriaxone.
- If the Gram stain result is negative in an infant younger than 3 months, consider adding ampicillin for optimal coverage of a late-onset *Listeria* infection.
- If there is evidence of meningococcal infection (i.e., gram-negative kidney bean–shaped diplococci seen or positive latex agglutination testing), vancomycin is not essential; use penicillin, cefotaxime, or ceftriaxone.

- Therapy for specific pathogens include the following:
  - Group B streptococci: Use penicillin or ampicillin plus gentamicin. This combination is synergistic against most isolates of the organism and should be used initially. After a satisfactory clinical and microbiologic response has been achieved, penicillin or ampicillin alone can be given. Therapy is usually administered for a minimum of 14 days.
  - Gram-negative enteric bacilli or Enterobacteriaceae: Use cefotaxime with or without an aminoglycoside (usually gentamicin); if the patient is infected with a third-generation cephalosporin–resistant extended spectrum β-lactamase (ESBL)–producing organism, meropenem may be useful. Therapy is usually continued for a minimum of 21 days.
  - Pneumococcus: Vancomycin plus cefotaxime or ceftriaxone should be used initially pending susceptibility testing. If the organism is sensitive to penicillin by a reliable testing method (e.g., E test, quantitative microdilution methods), penicillin, cefotaxime, or ceftriaxone alone can be used. If the organism is not susceptible to penicillin (minimum inhibitory concentration [MIC] > 0.1 μg/mL) but sensitive to cefotaxime or ceftriaxone, either of these cephalosporins may be used. If the organism is resistant to penicillin and to the third-generation cephalosporins, use vancomycin plus either of these cephalosporins because the combination may demonstrate synergistic activity against the organism. Consider adding rifampin after 24 to 48 hours of therapy if the organism is susceptible to rifampin for the following reasons:
    - The patient's condition has not improved or worsened despite therapy with vancomycin plus cefotaxime or ceftriaxone.
    - A repeat lumbar puncture shows failure to substantially reduce or eradicate the number of organisms.
    - The organism has an unusually high cefotaxime or ceftriaxone MIC (≥ 4 μg/mL).
    - Occasionally, meropenem has been used in highly resistant pneumococcal meningitis. Consultation with an expert in pediatric infectious diseases should be considered in most of these situations. Therapy should be administered for a minimum of 10 to 14 days.
  - Meningococcus: Use penicillin, cefotaxime, or ceftriaxone. Therapy is administered for a minimum of 7 days.

Anti-Inflammatory Therapy

- Use dexamethasone.
  - Efficacy of this agent, when given shortly before or at the time of administration of the first dose of parenteral antibiotic therapy, was established to reduce the frequency of hearing loss and neurologic sequelae in patients with *H. influenzae* type b meningitis.
  - The drug reduces overall unfavorable outcomes and mortality in adults with pneumococcal meningitis.
  - Beneficial effects of dexamethasone have not conclusively been demonstrated in studies of pneumococcal or meningococcal meningitis in children, and there are no data pertaining to its use in children younger than 6 weeks old.
  - Based on the benefits seen in *H. influenzae* type b meningitis, the favorable experience in adults, and the probable lack of serious adverse effects, adjunctive therapy with this agent may be considered in children age 6 weeks or older.

Other Treatments

- Treat shock initially with isotonic fluids (usually crystalloids, occasionally colloids); inotropic agents may be necessary if myocardial depression is evident.
- Correct dehydration and shock, but do not overhydrate because it may aggravate cerebral edema.
- Observe for seizures. If they occur and are not caused by a metabolic disturbance (e.g., hypoglycemia, hyponatremia, hypocalcemia), treat with phenytoin or fosphenytoin (either is preferred in children older than 1 month because they do not depress mental or respiratory status) or phenobarbital, with or without a concomitant benzodiazepine (administered for rapid seizure control).
- Monitor for evidence of life-threatening increased ICP. Treat suspected marked increased ICP with transient hyperventilation (only for acute management of suspected impending cerebral herniation) and mannitol, with or without furosemide
- Monitor for evidence of disseminated intravascular coagulation (DIC). Treat DIC with fresh frozen plasma, cryoprecipitate, and platelets as needed.

DISPOSITION

- The mortality rate for bacterial meningitis is 1% to 5% (15% to 20% for neonates).
- Morbidity is influenced by many factors, including the age of the patient, duration of illness before initiating effective therapy, the specific pathogen, the bacterial inoculum, and host defenses. Overall, up to 50% of patients demonstrate neurologic sequelae with various degrees of severity.
- Follow-up is directed at monitoring for the rare (<1%) occurrence of relapse of infection after the course of antibiotic therapy and monitoring for neurologic sequelae, including hearing loss, seizures, motor abnormalities, language disorders or delay, hydrocephalus, and mental retardation.
  - Screening for hearing loss using audiometry or, in the young child, brainstem auditory-evoked potentials is usually done at the completion of the course of parenteral antibiotic therapy.
  - Careful assessment of the child's neurodevelopmental status is essential.

REFERRAL

- Children with bacterial meningitis should be admitted to a facility experienced in the management of this illness, where they can be closely observed and complications can be dealt with if they arise.
- Subspecialty consultation with a pediatric infectious diseases specialist, pediatric neurologist, neonatologist, or a pediatric neurosurgeon may be helpful in selected cases.

PEARLS & CONSIDERATIONS

COMMENTS

- Physicians caring for children must maintain a high level of vigilance to identify the child who has bacterial meningitis. The most common clinical manifestations are fever, vomiting, headache, and altered mental status.
- The diagnosis is established through performance of a lumbar puncture to collect CSF for analysis unless contraindications to lumbar puncture exist.
- Parenteral antibiotic therapy should be promptly administered.

PREVENTION

- The widespread use of the conjugate *H. influenzae* type b vaccines has largely eliminated this organism as a cause of bacterial meningitis.
- The heptavalent conjugate pneumococcal vaccine (containing purified capsular polysaccharides of serotypes 4, 6B, 9V, 14, 18C, 19F, 23F conjugated with a diphtheria protein) became available in 2000 and has significantly reduced the frequency of invasive pneumococcal disease, including meningitis.
- It is indicated for routine administration to all children younger than 24 months old (usually given at 2, 4, 6, and 12 to 15 months) and for immunization of children 24 to 59 months old at high risk for invasive pneumococcal infection.
- New conjugate pneumococcal vaccines containing a greater number of serotypes are under development.

- A quadrivalent meningococcal vaccine against serogroups A, C, Y, and W-135 is available but is not reliably immunogenic in children younger than 24 months. Routine immunization of children with this vaccine is not recommended.
- Its administration is recommended for children age 2 years or older in high-risk groups, including those with functional or anatomic asplenia and terminal complement component or properdin deficiencies.
- Because college students living in dormitories for the first time are at increased risk for invasive meningococcal infection, students and their parents should be educated about this risk, and vaccine should be administered if requested by them, if required by the educational institution the student will be attending, or if mandated by state law.
- A conjugate meningococcal vaccine that contains the aforementioned serogroups has been developed, appears to have immunological benefits over the existing licensed vaccine, and has been licensed by the U.S. Food and Drug Administration. This vaccine is recommended for routine administration in older children.
- Chemoprophylaxis of household and other close contacts of an index patient with invasive meningococcal disease is usually effective in preventing secondary cases.
- Prophylaxis is warranted for household, child care and nursery school contacts, others who frequently ate or slept in the same dwelling as the index case during the 7 days before onset of disease in the index case, or those who have had contact with the index patient's oral secretions through kissing or sharing of toothbrushes or eating utensils during this same period.
- Prophylaxis should also be administered to the index patient before hospital discharge, unless the patient was treated with ceftriaxone or cefotaxime.
- Available effective chemoprophylactic agents include rifampin, azithromycin, ceftriaxone, and ciprofloxacin.

PATIENT/FAMILY EDUCATION

- Educate parents about the mortality rate and the overall frequency and types of neurologic sequelae of bacterial meningitis.
- Inform parents that their child's hearing will be evaluated before hospital discharge and that close neurodevelopmental follow-up will be needed.
- Discuss the small (<1%) risk of relapse and what the parents would observe in the case of relapse.
- The Meningitis Foundation of America (www.musa.org) has information to assist patients who have had meningitis or families who have had a family member with meningitis.

SUGGESTED READINGS

American Academy of Pediatrics: Group B streptococcal infections. *In* Pickering LK (ed): *Red Book: 2003 Report of the Committee on Infectious Diseases,* 26th ed. Elk Grove Village, IL, American Academy of Pediatrics, 2003, pp 584–591.

American Academy of Pediatrics: Meningococcal infections. *In* Pickering LK (ed): *Red Book: 2003 Report of the Committee on Infectious Diseases,* 26th ed. Elk Grove Village, IL, American Academy of Pediatrics, 2003, pp 490–500.

American Academy of Pediatrics: Pneumococcal infections. *In* Pickering LK (ed): *Red Book: 2003 Report of the Committee on Infectious Diseases,* 26th ed. Elk Grove Village, IL, American Academy of Pediatrics, 2003, pp 430–436.

American Academy of Pediatrics, Committee on Infectious Diseases: Therapy for children with invasive pneumococcal infections. *Pediatrics* 99:289, 1997.

Bashir HE et al: Diagnosis and treatment of bacterial meningitis. *Arch Dis Child* 88:615, 2003.

Duke T et al: The management of bacterial meningitis in children. *Expert Opin Pharmacother* 4:1227, 2003.

Feigin RD: Use of corticosteroids in bacterial meningitis. *Pediatr Infect Dis J* 23:355, 2004.

Feigin RD, Pearlman E: Bacterial meningitis beyond the neonatal period. *In* Feigin RD et al (eds): *Textbook of Pediatric Infectious Diseases,* 5th ed. New York, WB Saunders, 2004, pp 443–474.

Kaplan SD: Management of pneumococcal meningitis. *Pediatr Infect Dis J* 21:589, 2002.

Saez-Llorens X, McCracken GH: Bacterial meningitis in children. *Lancet* 361:2139, 2003.

Tunkel AR et al: Practice guidelines for the management of bacterial meningitis. *Clin Infect Dis* 39:1267, 2004.

AUTHOR: **ROBERT A. BROUGHTON, MD**

BASIC INFORMATION

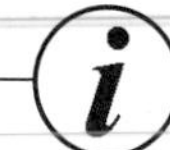

DEFINITION

Viral meningitis is inflammation of the meninges caused by many different viruses.

SYNONYM

Aseptic meningitis

ICD-9-CM CODE
047.9 Unspecified viral meningitis

EPIDEMIOLOGY & DEMOGRAPHICS

- Enteroviruses
  - Most common in infants younger than 1 year.
  - In temperate climates, most cases occur in summer and fall; cases occur year round in tropical and subtropical climates.
  - Spread is from person to person, by the fecal-oral route, and through respiratory droplets.
  - Incubation period is 4 to 6 days.
  - Meningitis develops in less than 1 per 1000 infected persons.
- Other agents
  - Arboviruses are usually accompanied by brain involvement (meningoencephalitis) unless caused by St. Louis and California viral infections (see Encephalitis, Acute Viral in Diseases and Disorders [Section I]).
  - Mumps are usually accompanied by brain involvement.
  - Most infections with measles, rubella, and variola viruses that involve the central nervous system (CNS) are encephalitic.

CLINICAL PRESENTATION

History

- Fever
- Headache (usually retro-orbital or frontal)
- Photophobia
- Anorexia, nausea, vomiting, abdominal pain, diarrhea
- Meticulous history for exposures in past 2 to 3 weeks
  - Travel
  - Insects
  - Pets (especially horses)
  - Medications
  - Injections
  - Other exposures
- Seizures: occur occasionally, may occur because of high fever alone

Physical Examination

- Meningeal signs
  - Nuchal rigidity
  - Positive Kernig's sign and Brudzinski's sign
    - Kernig's sign: When the leg is flexed 90 degrees at the hip, the knee cannot be extended beyond 135 degrees.
    - Brudzinski's sign: The legs are flexed involuntarily when the neck is flexed.
    - These signs may be present in older children. They are often not present in infants.
- Young infants: fever, irritability, and lethargy most commonly, bulging fontanelle
- Exanthem, enanthem
- Myalgia (occasionally)
- Muscle weakness (rare)

ETIOLOGY

- Enteroviruses account for 85% to 95% of cases for which an etiologic agent is identified. The most common enteroviruses are coxsackievirus B5 and echoviruses 4, 5, 9, and 11.
- Five percent of cases are caused by arboviruses (occur in summer and fall).
  - St. Louis encephalitis virus is the most common vector-transmitted cause of aseptic meningitis.
  - It is seen throughout the United States.
  - Aseptic meningitis accounts for 15% of all symptomatic cases of St. Louis encephalitis.
- Aseptic meningitis is the most common neurologic presentation of mumps infection.
  - It occurs in winter and spring.
  - Cerebrospinal fluid (CSF) pleocytosis occurs in more than 50% of patients with mumps.
  - Except for parotitis, the clinical manifestations differ little from enteroviral cases; encephalitis may also occur.
  - Neurologic involvement is three times more common in male than female patients.
- Many other viruses may cause meningitis, including the following:
  - Herpes simplex type 2 (see Herpes Simplex Virus Infections in Diseases and Disorders [Section I])
  - Human herpesvirus type 6
  - Human immunodeficiency virus type 1 (HIV-1)
  - Adenovirus
  - Varicella-zoster virus
  - Epstein-Barr virus
  - Lymphocytic choriomeningitis (transmitted by rodents, clinical manifestations in only 15% of those infected, remainder asymptomatic or mildly ill)
  - Encephalomyocarditis virus
  - Cytomegalovirus
  - Rhinoviruses
  - Measles
  - Rubella
  - Influenza types a and b
  - Parainfluenza
  - Parvovirus B19
  - Rotavirus
  - Coronavirus
  - Variola

DIAGNOSIS

DIFFERENTIAL DIAGNOSIS

- Manifestations of other forms of meningitis may be identical to those of cases caused by viruses.
  - Bacteria, including certain bacteria that do not readily stain or grow in standard culture systems (i.e., *Mycoplasma*)
  - Fungi
  - Tuberculosis
  - Parasites or protozoa
- Parameningeal infections (e.g., pneumonia, vertebral osteomyelitis)
- Malignancy
  - Leukemia
  - Brain tumor
- Immune diseases
  - Behçet's syndrome
  - Systemic lupus erythematosus
  - Sarcoidosis
- Miscellaneous causes
  - Kawasaki disease
  - Heavy metal poisoning
  - Intrathecal injections
  - Foreign bodies
  - Antimicrobial agents or other drugs
    - Trimethoprim-sulfamethoxazole
    - Nonsteroidal anti-inflammatory drugs
    - Chemotherapy
  - Epidermoid lesions (i.e., dermoid or other cysts)

WORKUP

- Perform lumbar puncture to collect CSF for the following:
  - Cell count: white blood cell (WBC) count of 50 to 500/mm^3; may be up to 1000/mm^3
  - Differential count: may be a polymorphonuclear WBC predominance early, but shift to mononuclear predominance usually occurs within 12 to 24 hours
  - CSF glucose level: usually normal or mildly depressed
  - CSF protein level: usually normal to mildly elevated
  - Gram stain: negative for bacteria
  - Cultures: negative for bacteria
- CSF, blood, rectal, and nasopharyngeal swabs should be collected for viral cultures.
- Paired serum specimens (day 0 and days 10 to 21) can be collected for antibody titer rises if cultures do not grow viruses or bacteria.
- History and clinical findings may require additional culture for mycobacteria, fungal, or protozoal infection.
- Atypical cells may require examination of cytopathology to exclude tumor.
- Enterovirus and herpes simplex virus infections can be confirmed by polymerase chain reaction (PCR). At least 65% to 70% of culture-negative CSF infections in patients with aseptic meningitis are enterovirus positive by PCR.
- Identification of specific viral pathogen is possible in as many as 55% to 70% of cases when consistent diagnostic methods are applied.

TREATMENT

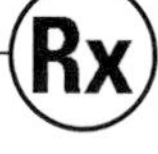

NONPHARMACOLOGIC THERAPY

- Supportive care
  - Fluids
  - Analgesics (avoid aspirin because of associated risk of Reye's syndrome)
  - Need for hospital admission based on possibility of treatable bacterial disease,

toxicity, and need for hydration and pain control
  - Observation for seizures (rare)

ACUTE GENERAL Rx

- No specific antibiotic therapy is available for enteroviral disease, but there is some efficacy of intravenous gamma-globulin in agammaglobulinemic patients.
- Acyclovir is available to treat meningitis caused by herpes simplex virus.
- Antibiotics may be started empirically while awaiting results of bacterial cultures (see Meningitis, Bacterial in Diseases and Disorders [Section I]) if diagnosis unclear.
  - Antibiotics should be given parenterally.
  - Antibiotics may be used in some cases such as: a toxic looking patients, a CSF with high WBC counts, a young patient with an atypical or severe clinical presentation.
- Pleconaril is available for compassionate release for selected patients with enteroviral disease (i.e., antibody-deficient patients with chronic enteroviral infection).

DISPOSITION

- Prognosis depends on the cause.
- Most children with enteroviral meningitis recover completely.
- Ten percent have CNS complications, including focal seizures, weakness, and obtundation or coma.
- Infants in first few months of life may have an increased risk for problems with language and development.
- These infants need formal developmental evaluation at age 3 to 6 years.

REFERRAL

- Most patients with viral meningitis can be treated by their primary care provider.
- Subspecialty consultation may be needed in complicated cases.
  - Pediatric infectious disease
  - Neurology

PEARLS & CONSIDERATIONS

COMMENTS

- The common presenting signs of fever, vomiting, headache, and irritability need careful assessment to exclude meningitis, especially in the young infant.
- The diagnosis is established by lumbar puncture CSF cell count and culture results.
- Parenteral antibiotics are not needed to treat viral meningitis but may be used empirically if bacterial meningitis cannot be reasonably excluded from the differential diagnosis.

PREVENTION

- Wash hands thoroughly and frequently.
- For child-care centers, wash objects and surfaces with which children have contact with a diluted bleach solution regularly. Use 1 cup of chlorine-containing household bleach in 1 gallon of water.

PATIENT/FAMILY EDUCATION

- Parents should be educated about the usually good prognosis (this is cause specific and most true for enteroviral infection).
- The low risk of neurologic sequelae can be discussed.
- Parents should be aware that the child's hearing and neurodevelopmental status should be monitored.
- The Meningitis Foundation of America has a large amount of information on its web site (www.musa.org) that can be of considerable assistance to patients who have had meningitis or families who have had a family member with meningitis.

SUGGESTED READINGS

AOL Government Guide. Available at www.governmentguide.com

Berlin LE et al: Aseptic meningitis in infants <2 years of age: diagnosis and etiology. *J Infect Dis* 168:888, 1993.

Centers for Disease Control and Prevention. Available at www.cdc.gov/viralmeningitis

Cherry JD: Aseptic meningitis and viral meningitis. *In* Feigin RD et al (eds): *Textbook of Pediatric Infectious Diseases,* 5th ed. Philadelphia, WB Saunders, 2004, pp 497–505.

Rorabaugh ML et al: Aseptic meningitis in infants younger than 2 years of age: acute illness and neurologic complications. *Pediatrics* 92:206, 1993.

Rotbart HA: Aseptic meningitis and viral meningitis. *In* Long SS et al (eds): *Principles and Practice of Pediatric Infectious Diseases.* New York, Churchill Livingstone, 2003, pp 284–291.

AUTHOR: **CYNTHIA CHRISTY, MD**

BASIC INFORMATION

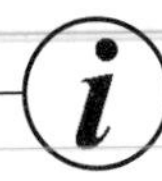

DEFINITION

Meningococcemia is a bacteremia and sepsis syndrome with fever, petechiae, purpura, and hemodynamic instability caused by the organism *Neisseria meningitidis,* a gram-negative intracellular diplococcus.

SYNONYMS

Meningococcal septicemia
Purpura fulminans
Waterhouse-Friderichsen syndrome

ICD-9-CM CODES
036.2 Meningococcemia
320 Bacterial meningitis
V03.89 Meningococcal vaccine

EPIDEMIOLOGY & DEMOGRAPHICS

- Transmission occurs from person to person by the respiratory route through pharyngeal secretions.
- Approximately 60% to 90% of cases occur in children.
- Overcrowding, such as in day-care centers, barracks, and households, is a risk factor for spread.
- Most people exposed become carriers and do not develop disease; however, they are the major source of organism spread because most patients with invasive disease have not had contact with another patient with invasive disease.
- The prevalence of asymptomatic carriage varies among populations; the average rate is 5% to 15% colonized in nonendemic areas.
- The incubation period is 2 to 10 days; patients are infectious up to 24 hours after treatment.
- The risk of household transmission is greatest in the first week after contact; 70% of secondary household cases occur in this period.
- The annual incidence of all meningococcal disease in the United States is 1.1 cases per 100,000 people, with the peak incidence occurring in late winter and early spring.
- It occurs in a worldwide distribution as endemic disease in certain countries or in epidemics; *meningitis belt* is a term used for increased prevalence and outbreaks in sub-Saharan Africa.
- Worldwide, group A strains are responsible for the largest epidemics, but in the United States, outbreaks have been increasingly related to serotype C disease.
- Serotype C represents 45% of isolates in the United States; serotype B accounts for another 45%.
- Attack rates are highest among children, with 46% of cases occurring in children 2 years old or younger.
- Other patients at high risk include splenectomized patients and those with congenital asplenia, terminal complement (C6, C7, C8), or properdin deficiency.
- Immunoglobulin and early complement deficiencies may also be associated with risk for meningococcemia.

CLINICAL PRESENTATION

History

- A prodrome of upper respiratory infection is common.
- Headache, fever, and nausea.
- A rash is noticed by the patient or caregiver. Rash may at first be faint maculopapular, with rapid change to petechiae with or without larger purpura.
- Rarely, a history of exposure to a known case in a cluster or outbreak setting is reported.
- Obtain histories of family members by the following criteria:
  - Age
  - Occupations
  - Day-care attendance
  - School attendance and other extracurricular activities, especially sports teams
  - Contacts who may need postexposure prophylaxis (discussed later)
- Obtain a history of medication use and prior antibiotic therapy, which may influence the outcome of culture results.

Physical Examination

- Vital signs usually include a high fever; blood pressure may be normal and then rapidly drop, or frank hypotension may be seen on presentation.
- Mental status may be normal, with rapid obtundation caused by shock with or without meningitis.
- Purpura and petechiae may be minimal or profound with massive skin necrosis and mucosal hemorrhage.
- Petechiae may appear first in areas of pressure (blood pressure monitoring, tourniquets).
- Patient may not have a stiff neck; meningococcemia is often seen with early subclinical meningitis or no meningitis.

ETIOLOGY

- Asymptomatic colonization of *N. meningitidis* is found in the nasopharynx.
- Bloodstream invasion occurs when complex interactions involving organism attachment factors, cofactors such as other infective agents, often respiratory viruses, and host immune status act in concert.
- Lipopolysaccharide endotoxin mediates cytokine release from activated monocytes, macrophages, and endothelial cells.
- Cytokines such as tumor necrosis factor, interleukins 1 and 6, and interferon-γ result in hypotension, myocardial depression, and increased vascular permeability.
- Direct capillary leakage, endothelial tissue damage, and end-organ damage result in necrosis of skin, digits, and mucosal surfaces, as well as adrenal hemorrhage (i.e., Waterhouse-Friderichsen syndrome).
- *N. meningitidis* has an outer polysaccharide capsule that serves to identify different serotypes; A, B, C, W-135, and Y account for invasive disease.
- Almost all isolates in the United States are still susceptible to penicillin; other parts of the world may have increasing penicillin resistance.
- U.S. isolates are often resistant to sulfonamides but rarely resistant to rifampin.
- *N. meningitidis* can also cause meningitis, septic arthritis, pericarditis, pneumonia, and conjunctivitis.
- Chronic meningococcemia is an uncommon presentation of periodic fever without shock or sepsis syndrome, often accompanied by recurrent petechiae and splenomegaly, and it may mimic Henoch-Schönlein purpura.

DIAGNOSIS

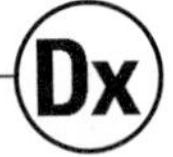

DIFFERENTIAL DIAGNOSIS

- Clinical presentation as described previously, with the presence of purpura and hypotension, is highly suggestive of meningococcemia.
- Many mild viral illnesses may manifest with fever and petechial exanthems—and commonly include enteroviruses and parvovirus B19.
- Other bacterial causes of sepsis and meningitis may manifest similarly.
  - Pneumococci
  - *Haemophilus influenzae* type b
  - *Neisseria gonorrhoeae*
- Hemorrhagic fever viruses should be excluded.
- Causes of similar fulminant shock syndromes include Dengue virus and hantaviruses.
- Rickettsial causes include Rocky Mountain spotted fever and others in the spotted fever group.
- Henoch-Schönlein purpura or anaphylactoid purpura is often preceded by an upper respiratory prodrome.
  - Palpable purpura
  - Abdominal pain (does not present with shock unless acute bowel process)
  - Arthritis
- Drug reaction or rashes can result from the following:
  - Sulfa drugs
  - Dilantin
  - Heparin
  - Thiazide diuretics
  - Rifampin
- Thrombocytopenias may be caused by blood disorders.
  - Immune thrombocytopenia
  - Aplastic anemia
  - Leukemias
  - Wiskott-Aldrich syndrome
- Other vasculitic diseases, such as polyarteritis and Kawasaki disease, may manifest with fever and petechiae.

WORKUP

- Confirmation of a case is by isolation of *N. meningitidis* from blood, cerebrospinal fluid (CSF), or another normally sterile site.
- All patients with suspected meningococcemia who can tolerate the procedure should have a lumbar puncture to confirm or exclude meningitis.
- Latex agglutination of CSF may be done if a patient received antibiotics before sampling.
- Petechial skin lesions can be scraped and then Gram stained and cultured.

LABORATORY TESTS

- Blood cultures
- Complete blood profile with differential and platelet count
- Parameters to assess for disseminated intravascular coagulation (DIC) includes clotting studies, such as D-dimer, fibrinogen, prothrombin time, and partial thromboplastin time

TREATMENT

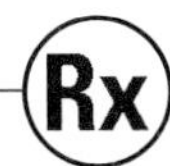

NONPHARMACOLOGIC THERAPY

- Cortisol may be considered if profound shock is present; it is given in replacement doses with hydrocortisone sodium phosphate or succinate.
- Pharmacologic doses of steroids have not been proved to be beneficial.
- Sympathetic blockade and topical nitroglycerin may be tried to improve perfusion locally.
- A hypercoagulable state may be treated with a heparin infusion.
- Experimental therapies, such as recombinant tissue plasminogen activator and concentrated antithrombin III, have been tried in DIC.
- Access to wound care units and hyperbaric oxygen therapy is beneficial for patients with extensive tissue necrosis.

ACUTE GENERAL Rx

- Rapid administration of antibiotics is important; obtaining blood cultures and performing a lumbar puncture should not delay treatment. Often, antibiotics can be given immediately after obtaining blood.
- The ability to give antibiotics in an outpatient office setting has been documented to decrease adverse outcomes.
- Appropriate antibiotics may be given by the intramuscular or intraosseous route if no intravenous access is available.
    - Penicillin G: 250,000 to 300,000 U/kg/day, divided every 4 to 6 hours (maximum, 24 million U/day)
    - Cefotaxime: 300 mg/kg/day, divided every 6 to 8 hours (maximum, 12 g/day)
    - Ceftriaxone: 100 mg/kg/day, divided every 12 to 24 hours (maximum, 4 g/day)
- Patients should be isolated in the hospital for 24 hours after the first dose of appropriate antibiotic therapy. The length of therapy is 7 days.
- Release of endotoxin after administering antibiotics may cause further symptoms of shock, and intensive care support is required for all cases initially for fluid resuscitation and often for respiratory support, management of blood products, and inotropic support.
- Central venous access is usually necessary.

DISPOSITION

- Poor prognosis is associated with the following:
    - Petechiae present for less than 12 hours
    - Hypotension (systolic blood pressure < 70 mm Hg)
    - Absence of meningitis (<20 white blood cells [WBCs] in CSF)
    - Low peripheral WBCs (<10,000) or erythrocyte sedimentation rate (<10)
    - Thrombocytopenia, coma, seizures, and extremes of age

REFERRAL

Plastic surgery and orthopedic surgery consultations may be needed to remove and replace necrotic areas of skin and limbs.

PEARLS & CONSIDERATIONS

COMMENTS

- Although patients with fever, hypotension, and shock with petechiae and purpura should be treated emergently, most children with fever and petechiae do not have meningococcemia; however, the diagnosis must *always* be considered because of the rapidity of deterioration that can occur.
- Most children with meningitis without fulminant meningococcemia fare well; younger infants without shock may present with occult bacteremia (5% to 8% of cases of occult bacteremias).
- Very high WBC count on presentation is usually a good prognostic factor but may be associated with development of postinfectious (immune-mediated) arthritis.
- Pediatric offices should have the ability to rapidly administer antibiotics.

PREVENTION

- Chemoprophylaxis for all family members of the index case is warranted.
- Close contacts of the index patient who sleep or eat together should be given prophylaxis. Close contact with oral secretions warrants prophylaxis.
- All day-care contacts in the same care room with close contact should receive prophylaxis.
- The drug of choice for prophylaxis is rifampin.
    - Penetrates secretions well
    - Eliminates carriage of the organism if it is not resistant
    - Rifampin: 10 mg/kg/dose (up to 600 mg/dose) every 12 hours for four doses
- Sulfonamides should be used only if resistance testing of the organism is done.
- Ceftriaxone and ciprofloxacin are effective in eradicating carriage and may be used.
    - Ceftriaxone: 250 mg intramuscularly as a single dose for adults, 125 mg intramuscularly as a single dose for children younger than 12 years
    - Ciprofloxacin: 500 to 750 mg as a single dose for adults
- The index patient who has received at least one dose of ceftriaxone does not need to receive other prophylaxis.
- Ceftriaxone is the drug of choice for prophylaxis of a pregnant contact.
- Tetravalent vaccine containing capsular polysaccharides of serogroups A, C, Y, and W-135 meningococci is licensed in the United States and approved for use in children older than 2 years.
- The serotype B capsule is poorly immunogenic, and no vaccine is available in the United States. A meningococcal vaccine specific for type B outer membrane protein is being tested in New Zealand.
- Meningococcal conjugate vaccines are available in Europe for constructs that contain serotypes C and A, with a promising reduction in serotype C disease reported from the United Kingdom with a serotype C conjugate vaccine.
- Tetravalent meningococcal conjugate vaccine (MCV4) has been approved by the U.S. Food and Drug Administration for persons 11 to 55 years old. It is administered intramuscularly as a single dose. These vaccines may provide longer lasting immunity than the polysaccharide vaccine.
- Tetravalent vaccine is indicated for patients at high risk for acquiring disease, such as splenectomized or functionally asplenic patients and patients with terminal complement component or properdin deficiency. The Advisory Committee on Immunization Practices (ACIP) has recommended vaccination for young adolescents (11 to 15 years old) with MCV4 vaccine.
- Immunization of incoming freshman college students living in dormitories is recommended.
- Discussion with students and their families should be provided regarding the moderately increased risk of meningococcal illness of first-year students living in dormitories and the potential benefit of the vaccine.
- Students should be immunized at the request of the student or if required by their institution.
- Travelers to areas with current outbreaks or high background rates of disease should receive vaccine.
- Vaccine may be considered for widespread administration in the setting of an outbreak. It should always be done in

conjunction with local and state public health recommendations.

- Meningococcemia is a reportable disease to public health authorities, who will assist in tracking cases and contacts and aid in making postexposure prophylaxis recommendations.
- Revaccination of high-risk patients may be considered.
  - If the patient was younger than 4 years of age at first vaccination
  - If exposure occurs 2 to 3 years after the first dose
  - If patient remains in a high-risk category, in which case a subsequent dose may be given 3 to 5 years after the first dose
  - Need for revaccination in older children and adults is not established

PATIENT/FAMILY EDUCATION

Information and support can be found through the Meningitis Foundation of America (www.musa.org).

SUGGESTED READINGS

Advisory Committee on Immunization Practices, U.S. Public Health Service: Prevention and control of meningococcal disease. *MMWR Morb Mortal Wkly Rep* 54:RR07, 2005.

American Academy of Pediatrics: Meningococcal infections. *In* Pickering LK (ed): *Red Book: Report of the Committee on Infectious Diseases,* 26th ed. Elk Grove, IL, American Academy of Pediatrics, 2003, pp 430–436.

American College Health Association. Available at www.acha.org

Centers for Disease Control and Prevention, ACIP Recommendations. Available at www.cdc.gov/epo/mmwr

Centers for Disease Control and Prevention for travel recommendations. Available at www.cdc.gov/travel

Harrison LH et al: Risk of meningococcal infection in college students. *JAMA* 281:1906, 1999.

Healy MA, Baker CJ: The future of meningococcal vaccines. *Pediatr Infect Dis J* 24:175, 2005.

Kirsch EA et al: Pathophysiology, treatment and outcome of meningococcemia: a review and recent experience. *Pediatr Infect Dis J* 15:967, 1996.

Rosenstein NE et al: Meningococcal disease. *N Engl J Med* 344:1378, 2001.

AUTHOR: **DONNA J. FISHER, MD**

BASIC INFORMATION

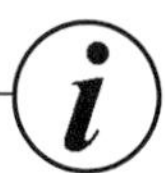

DEFINITION

Meningomyelocele, a neural tube defect, is the most complex malformation of the spinal cord. Anomalous nerve roots protrude through meninges, abnormal vertebral arches, and soft tissue. Associated abnormalities of the brain, such as the Chiari II malformation, occur commonly, as do learning disorders. Spinal lipomas or dermoid cysts may accompany the meningomyelocele. Syrinx is an accumulation of cerebrospinal fluid within the central spinal canal. Syringobulbia refers to accumulation of fluid in the central canal of the brainstem. Syringomyelia is the accumulation of fluid in the spinal cord. A tethered spinal cord is abnormally attached to surrounding tissue, usually in a more caudal (lower) position than normal. In children without meningomyelocele, tethering may be caused by a thickened filum terminale or a mass, such as a lipoma (see Occult Spinal Dysraphism in Diseases and Disorders [Section I]).

SYNONYMS

Meningomyelocele
- Myelomeningocele
- Spina bifida aperta
- Spina bifida cystica

Syrinx
- Syringobulbia, hydrosyringobulbia
- Syringomyelia, hydromyelia, hydrosyringomyelia

ICD-9-CM CODES

336.0	Syringomyelia and syringobulbia
741.0	Meningomyelocele with hydrocephalus
741.0	Use fifth digit classification with category, unspecified region; 1, cervical; 2, thoracic; 3, lumbar
741.9	Meningomyelocele without hydrocephalus
742.0	Encephalocele
742.53	Hydromyelia
742.59	Tethered spinal cord

EPIDEMIOLOGY & DEMOGRAPHICS

- The birth prevalence is approximately 4 to 6 per 10,000 live births in the United States.
- The birth prevalence has been decreasing because of improved maternal nutrition, use of folic acid supplementation, and enhanced prenatal detection, with elective termination of pregnancies.
- The risk for a second affected child from the same parents is 2 or 3 per 100 births; for a third, it is 10 per 100 births.
- Neural tube defects are more common in female children and in persons of British ancestry.

CLINICAL PRESENTATION

History

- Family history of neural tube defects or spontaneous abortions
- Maternal nutrition during gestation and prenatal exposures
- Family functioning (including social support and stress) and parental expectations and understanding of the problem
- Assessment of child's growth, development, mobility, and activities of daily living (e.g., personal hygiene, ability to feed self, self-help skills)
- Onset of new neurologic symptoms (e.g., weakness, changes in bowel and bladder function, tripping, clumsiness), usually indicating treatable conditions such as tethered spinal cord, diastematomyelia, syrinx, or ventricular shunt malfunction
- History of reactions to products made of latex (up to 50% of children who have meningomyelocele have allergies to latex)

Physical Examination

- The backs of *all* infants and children new to the practice should be examined for pigmented spots, hairy patches, and sinuses that extend into the spine.
  - Certain findings may be signs of occult spinal dysraphism (OSD), which predisposes to meningitis.
  - Neurologic deterioration may occur as a result of diastematomyelia, lipoma, syrinx, or tethering of the spinal cord.
  - Scoliosis is common in patients with myelomeningocele.
- Perform a neurologic examination.
  - Motor function, sensory level, and anal wink
  - Upper extremity strength, including grip (i.e., deterioration may indicate syrinx or malfunction of a ventricular shunt)
- Evaluate for shunt function.
  - Head circumference and palpation of the anterior fontanelle
  - Visualization of the eye grounds
  - Assessment of the cranial nerves (especially of extraocular movements)
  - Palpation of the shunt valve and tubing
- Perform an orthopedic examination.
  - Assessment of posture (e.g., scoliosis, lordosis, kyphosis)
  - Assessment of mobility
  - Joint mobility and stability
- Perform a dermatologic examination. Seek evidence of lesions (e.g., decubitus ulcers) in insensate areas.
- Developmental assessments are especially important before school entry to optimize learning.
  - Visual-spatial functioning
  - Verbal, performance, and educational measures
  - Fine motor, gross motor, language, and social-adaptive skills
  - Executive functions (e.g., planning future activities, organizing, inhibiting competing (inappropriate) responses, self-regulation, remembering rules, initiating tasks, remembering to remember an activity)

ETIOLOGY

- Failure of the neural tube to close 23 to 28 days after fertilization of the egg is believed to be caused by an interaction between multiple genes and the environment.
- Maternal exposure to any of the following increases the risk: valproic acid, malnutrition (especially folate deficiency), obesity, hyperthermia, alcohol, and maternal diabetes.
- Abnormalities in the gene that regulates methylenetetrahydrofolate reductase, an enzyme associated with folate metabolism, have been associated with neural tube defects.
- Chromosome anomalies, such as trisomy 18 or 13.

DIAGNOSIS

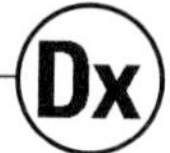

DIFFERENTIAL DIAGNOSIS

- Diagnosis is based on results of the physical examination, with little else in the differential diagnosis.
- Meningocele, with no peripheral nerve involvement, should be differentiated from meningomyelocele, which has sensory and motor loss below the level of the lesion.

WORKUP

- Renal structure and function
  - Urine culture
  - Renal ultrasound: hydronephrosis and structural anomalies such as a duplex collecting system
  - Serum levels of blood urea nitrogen and creatinine
  - Voiding cystourethrogram if vesicoureteral reflux is suspected
  - Urodynamics: bladder capacity, outlet pressure, and synergy between detrusor and sphincter

LABORATORY TESTS

Tests of serum blood urea nitrogen and creatinine levels should be obtained.

IMAGING STUDIES

- Ultrasound or computed tomography (CT) scan of the head: 75% to 85% have hydrocephalus
- Cranial and cervical spinal magnetic resonance imaging (MRI) if stridor and hoarseness, vocal cord paralysis, dysphagia, aspiration, apnea, central hypoventilation, breath-holding spells, opisthotonos, or weakness of the upper extremities develop—suggesting Chiari II malformation (i.e., downward displacement of hindbrain and cerebellum)
- MRI of spine if weakness in lower extremities, deterioration of gait, atrophy of muscles in lower extremities, sensory loss or change in lower extremities, change in deep tendon reflexes, change in bladder or bowel function, leg or back pain, new orthopedic contracture, foot or leg length discrepancy, progressive scoliosis in absence

of vertebral anomalies, trophic ulceration—suggesting tethered spinal cord
- Radiograms of the spine and hips
  - Abnormal vertebrae such as hemivertebrae, butterfly vertebrae
  - Scoliosis and kyphosis, especially in those with high spinal lesions
- Voiding cystourethrogram if vesicoureteral reflux suspected

TREATMENT

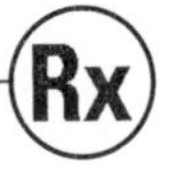

NONPHARMACOLOGIC THERAPY

- All operative procedures should be performed in a latex-free environment.
- Neurosurgical procedures
  - Closure of the lesion on the back within 72 hours after birth
  - Insertion of a shunt (usually ventriculoperitoneal) for progressive hydrocephalus
  - Revision of failed ventricular shunt
  - Untethering of tethered spinal cord
  - Posterior fossa decompression for symptomatic Chiari malformation
- Orthopedic procedures
  - Casting or surgery of fixed joint contractures or deformities
  - Surgery for severe or progressive kyphosis or scoliosis
- Urologic procedures
  - Urologic reconstruction, bladder augmentation, creation of continent vesicostomy (e.g., Mitrofanoff procedure) if conservative treatment fails
- General procedure: antegrade continence enema (ACE) surgery (i.e., cecostomy or Malone procedure) to enhance bowel management
- Access to interdisciplinary care: pediatrician, nurse, social worker, neurosurgeon, orthopedist, physical therapist, urologist, nutritionist, orthotist
- Referral to early intervention program: physical therapy, occupational therapy, special education services
- Clean intermittent catheterization is used to manage urinary tract. Contact to latex-containing products should be restricted from the first day of life.
- Sleep study for suspected apnea (associated with Chiari II malformation)
- Braces (e.g., ankle-foot-orthosis) and mobility devices (e.g., parapodium, wheelchair)
- High-fiber diet, regular toileting, and biofeedback to manage bowels
- Surgery, if necessary, for decubitus ulcers resistant to healing

ACUTE GENERAL Rx

- Antibiotic coverage in neonates with leaking lesions for gram-negative bacteria and staphylococci
- Intensive neurologic care for acute shunt dysfunction

CHRONIC Rx

- Antibiotic prophylaxis may be used for recurrent symptomatic urinary tract infection or ureteral reflux.
  - Cephalexin or amoxicillin in infants
  - Trimethoprim-sulfamethoxazole or nitrofurantoin in older children
- Medications to relax the detrusor muscle or increase sphincter tone to enhance continence include the following:
  - Imipramine
  - Oxybutynin
  - Pseudoephedrine
- Laxatives or enemas for constipation
- Sildenafil (Viagra) or tadalafil (Cialis) for erectile dysfunction

DISPOSITION

- Regular evaluation by a specialty team
- Routine renal ultrasound scans
- Routine head CT scans to evaluate ventricular size
- Routine radiograms if kyphosis or scoliosis progress
- Routine urine cultures for children who have ureteral reflux
- Close communication with the school or early intervention program
- Avoidance of all latex products

REFERRAL

- See Nonpharmacologic Therapy above
- All children 0 to 3 years old who have neural tube defects should be referred to an early intervention program.
- All children older than 3 years who have neural tube defects should be referred to their school district's committee on special education or committee on preschool special education. Children entering school should have formal psycho-educational evaluation.
- All children who have neural tube defects should be referred to an interdisciplinary specialty program for ongoing care.
- All adolescents who have neural tube defects should be referred to a transition program.

PEARLS & CONSIDERATIONS

COMMENTS

- Ventricular shunt failure in a child who has hydrocephalus may manifest with subtle or confusing signs and symptoms that can be mistaken for those of Chiari II malformation, syringomyelia, or tethered cord.
- Neural tube defects are static conditions. Any clinical deterioration should be evaluated for a treatable cause, such as ventricular shunt failure, tethered spinal cord, syrinx, or Chiari II malformation.
- Erythema and swelling of a joint or bone in an area that lacks sensation represent a fracture until proved otherwise.

PREVENTION

- All women of childbearing age should receive 0.4 mg of folic acid daily periconceptionally to decrease the occurrence of neural tube defects.
- Women who have a first-degree relative who has a neural tube defect should receive 4.0 mg of folic acid daily.
- Prenatal diagnosis can be made using maternal serum levels of alpha-fetoprotein at 14 to 16 weeks' gestation, combined with high-resolution ultrasonography with or without amniocentesis.
- Prenatal surgery to cover the open lesion on the back during the second trimester may diminish the severity of the Chiari II malformation.

PATIENT/FAMILY EDUCATION

- Prescribe folic acid (4.0 mg/day periconceptionally) for mothers and affected females to prevent recurrences.
- Help families and educators with their reactions to the child's condition and with developing realistic expectations for the child.
- Help patients understand their condition and develop increasing independence.
- Offer financial counseling.
- Avoid latex products, including in the hospital and operating suite.
- Discuss sexuality issues. Males have difficulty with erection and have retrograde ejaculation.
- Consider genetic counseling because affected individuals have a 3% chance of having an affected child.

SUGGESTED READINGS

American Academy of Pediatrics, Committee on Genetics: Folic acid for the prevention of neural tube defects. *Pediatrics* 104(Pt 1):325, 1999.

Children with Spina Bifida, A Resource Page for Parents. Available at http://www.waisman.wisc.edu/~rowley/sb-kids/index.htmlx

Liptak GS: Spina bifida and hydrocephalus. *In* Coffey CE, Brumback RA (eds): *Essential Textbook of Pediatric Neuropsychiatry.* Baltimore, Lippincott Williams & Wilkins, 2005.

Mitchell LE et al: Spina bifida. *Lancet* 364:1885, 2004.

Spina Bifida Association of America. Available at www.sbaa.org

Spina Bifida and Hydrocephalus Association of Canada. Available at www.sbhac.ca

AUTHOR: **GREGORY S. LIPTAK, MD, MPH**

BASIC INFORMATION

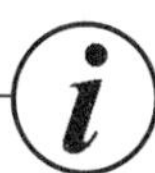

DEFINITION

Mental retardation is cognitive limitation as characterized by scores greater than 2 standard deviations below the mean on a valid intelligence quotient (IQ) measure, with limitation of adaptive function in communication, self-care, daily living skills at home or in the community, or social skills.

SYNONYMS

Cognitive limitation
Developmental delay (global)
Learning disability (in Europe, not in United States)
Slow learner

ICD-9-CM CODES
317 Mild mental retardation
318.0 Moderate mental retardation
318.1 Severe mental retardation
318 Profound mental retardation
319 Mental retardation, unspecified
783.4 Global delays

EPIDEMIOLOGY & DEMOGRAPHICS

- The incidence is 1% of the population, with a male preponderance.
- Most affected individuals have mild mental retardation (IQ of 50 to 70).
  - Moderate mental retardation is defined by a tested IQ of between 35 to 40 and 50 to 55.
  - Severe mental retardation is defined by a tested IQ of between 20 to 25 and 35 to 40.
  - Profound mental retardation is defined by a tested IQ of less than 20 to 25.
- Approximately 70% of cases of severe to profound mental retardation have a known cause.
- About 24% of cases with an IQ in the 50 to 70 range have a specific medical cause identified.

CLINICAL PRESENTATION

- Relative preservation of motor skills may delay diagnosis.
- Initial manifestation in early childhood may be language delay.
- Medical and family histories help guide the workup (see "Etiology").
- Careful physical examination with attention to the following:
  - Skin examination to rule out neurocutaneous syndromes
  - Hearing and vision assessment
  - Motor examination
  - Head circumference: evaluation for large or small heads
  - Syndrome stigmata: examination should include dysmorphic features to allow diagnosis of specific syndromes associated with mental retardation

ETIOLOGY

- A cause has been identified for 70% of individuals with severe or profound mental retardation and for 24% with mild mental retardation.
- Embryologic causes
- Microcephaly
  - Early decreased cell proliferation (e.g., genetic, embryologic origin)
  - Prenatal events with disruption of architecture (e.g., viral infections, vascular insults, migrational errors)
  - Early perinatal events (e.g., hypoxic encephalopathy, intracranial bleeding)
- Macrocephaly
  - Hydrocephalus
  - Sotos' syndrome
  - Fragile X syndrome
  - Autism
  - Chronic subdural bleeding
- Genetic causes
  - Fragile X syndrome, also called X-linked mental retardation, causes developmental delays in male maternal relatives and is the most common inherited form of mental retardation.
  - Trisomy 21, also known as Down syndrome, is the most common genetic cause of mental retardation.

DIAGNOSIS

Dx

DIFFERENTIAL DIAGNOSIS

- Autism
- Language disorders
- Learning disabilities
- Sensory impairment
- Epileptic aphasia
- Mental illness
- Profound environmental deprivation

WORKUP

- The workup is guided by the history and physical examination results.
- A hearing test should be performed.
- Karyotype and DNA analysis for fragile X syndrome should be considered if there is no other known cause.
- If anomalies of the head (e.g., increased or decreased head circumference) or abnormal neurologic examination results are found, consider neuroimaging.
- If history is compatible with seizures or if loss of speech or extreme behavioral variability is present, obtain an electroencephalogram (EEG).
- If loss of milestones, hypotonia, dietary avoidance of protein, suggestive examination results, or family history consistent with metabolic or neurodegenerative disease, consider metabolic or neurodegenerative work.
  - It may be prudent to refer patients to a tertiary care center at this point.
  - A preliminary workup may include, but is not limited to, fasting levels of plasma amino acids and urinary organic acids.
  - If hypotonic, determining lactate, pyruvate, and carnitine levels may be indicated.
- Formal psychologic testing using an appropriate instrument is critical for diagnosis. Functional abilities need to be formally assessed.

LABORATORY TESTS

- Family history of mental retardation or "slow learners," especially if it follows inheritance of fragile X, suggests that genetic evaluation is needed.
  - A sibling, parent, grandparent, aunt, or uncle is affected.
  - Mental retardation predominantly in males on the mother's side of the family support evaluation for the fragile X syndrome.
- Plateau or loss of skills, behavioral variability (related to dietary intake), refusal of protein foods (e.g., in urea cycle disorders), or specific findings such as smells consistent with organic acidurias (e.g., sweet smell of the urine in maple syrup urine disease) suggest the need for a metabolic workup.
- Pica and exposures may suggest the need to evaluate for lead and other toxins.

IMAGING STUDIES

Magnetic resonance imaging (MRI) of the head may be indicated if there is a loss of milestones, a distinct change in behavior, cutaneous markings consistent with a neurocutaneous syndrome (e.g., tuberous sclerosis), craniofacial abnormality, or abnormal result of a focal neurologic examination.

TREATMENT

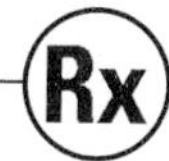

NONPHARMACOLOGIC THERAPY

- The primary therapies are educational and behavioral.
- It may be necessary to actively teach social and functional life skills.

CHRONIC Rx

- Psychiatric disorders can and do occur in people with mental retardation. Disorder-specific treatments depend on the proper diagnosis.
- Medication is often used for amelioration of specific symptoms such as hyperactivity. Stimulants may be useful in individual cases.
- Medication to treat aggression, self-injury, and stereotyped behaviors, among others, should be coordinated with a structured behavioral plan to teach appropriate behaviors.

COMPLEMENTARY & ALTERNATIVE MEDICINE

- Complementary treatments are specific to the disorder (e.g., megavitamin mixtures for trisomy 21).
- Use of complementary therapies is common

- Off-label use of medications as nosotropics (i.e., cognitive enhancers) remains unproved.

DISPOSITION

- Children 0 to 3 years old receive educational services through the early intervention programs.
- An appropriate public education is provided to students between the ages of 3 to 21 years by the home school district.
- School provides triennial formal testing or review and at least yearly program review.
- Families need to arrange legal guardianship (if appropriate) when the child is 18 years old and plan for adulthood.

REFERRAL

- Early intervention provides evaluation for children 0 to 3 years old.
- School districts provide testing and services for children 3 to 21 years old.
- Psychologists, developmental or behavioral pediatricians, child neurologists, child psychiatrists, and geneticists may be consulted for aspects of care.

PEARLS & CONSIDERATIONS

COMMENTS

- It is difficult to predict the ultimate cognitive outcome from testing in toddlers unless there is a known cause with an established course, such as trisomy 21.
- Children with mental retardation may be well served in inclusive classrooms with appropriate supports.
- Many adults with mental retardation work in competitive or supported employment in the community.
- Institutional care should be considered a thing of the past. Children with mental retardation should anticipate living and working in their communities.

PREVENTION

- Prenatal vitamins (e.g., folic acid) prevent spina bifida; prenatal care and good nutrition may prevent prematurity.
- Prenatal screening, such as alpha-fetoprotein and amniocentesis for chromosomal testing, is appropriate for older or high-risk mothers.
- Neonatal metabolic screening, such as for phenylketonuria, leads to instituting a preventive diet.
- Education, such as prenatal avoidance of alcohol, should be provided.
- Potential amelioration of some symptoms may occur with early intervention.

PATIENT/FAMILY EDUCATION

- The risk of recurrence depends on the underlying cause.
- Sexuality issues need to be addressed with education at the appropriate time.
- Families need to work with the agencies that coordinate young adult services well in advance of the anticipated need for them.

SUGGESTED READINGS

Association for Retarded Citizens. Available at www.thearc.org

Accardo P, Capute A: Mental retardation. *In* Capute A, Accardo P (eds): *Developmental Disabilities in Infancy and Childhood,* 2nd ed. Baltimore, Paul Brookes, 1996, pp 211–219.

AUTHOR: **SUSAN L. HYMAN, MD**

BASIC INFORMATION

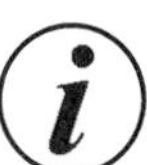

DEFINITION

Metabolic syndrome is a clustering of cardiovascular risk factors that leads to an increased risk for premature cardiovascular disease and increased susceptibility of developing type 2 diabetes mellitus. The syndrome represents a collection of multiple derangements that include elevated blood pressure, impaired glucose tolerance or insulin resistance, atherogenic dyslipidemia (i.e., high triglycerides, low high-density lipoprotein [HDL] cholesterol, and small low-density lipoprotein [LDL] particles), proinflammatory and prothrombotic properties, and obesity, with a particular contribution of abdominal obesity. There are two definitions for adults: World Health Organization, 1998 and the National Cholesterol Education Panel (NCEP), Third Adult Treatment Panel, 2001 .

SYNONYMS

Dysmetabolic syndrome X
Insulin resistance syndrome
Syndrome X

ICD-9-CM CODES

277.7 Metabolic syndrome
278.0 Obesity
278.01 Morbid obesity
577.8 Hyperinsulinemia
790.6 Abnormal blood glucose test
790.21 Impaired fasting glucose
790.22 Abnormal oral glucose tolerance test
790.29 Prediabetes

EPIDEMIOLOGY & DEMOGRAPHICS

- The metabolic syndrome affects 6% to 7% of adolescents in the United States. Among overweight adolescents with a body mass index (BMI) greater than the 95th percentile for age and gender, it affects about 40%.
- Obesity and insulin resistance appear relatively stable over time, but blood pressure and lipid abnormalities show variation over time.
- There are differences in prevalence rates among the components of the metabolic syndrome, with males being more affected than females.
- Racial differences exist. White and Hispanic youths have higher rates of lipid abnormalities than black youths, and blacks have higher rates of elevated blood pressure.
- Racial differences in central fat measurements are similar to racial differences in obesity, with Hispanics and blacks having higher rates than white youth.
- Hispanic males have the highest rates of the metabolic syndrome when using age-adjusted NCEP criteria.

CLINICAL PRESENTATION

History

- Asymptomatic disease is detected by screening for medical complications in overweight youths.
- The syndrome is rarely seen in children with normal weights and BMI values.
- Metabolic syndrome may coexist with type 2 diabetes mellitus in youths.
- It is more common among youths with a family history of type 2 diabetes.
- Children who were small for gestational age at birth, infants of diabetic mothers, and infants of mothers who smoked during pregnancy are at increased risk for developing the metabolic syndrome.

Physical Examination

- Excessive weight gain is demonstrated by the crossing of BMI percentiles, especially over relatively short periods.
- Excess abdominal adiposity, assessed by waist circumference, is particularly concerning and can be tracked over time.
- Acanthosis nigricans is common among overweight adolescents but is an insensitive finding for insulin resistance.

ETIOLOGY

- The metabolic syndrome is a manifestation of genetic predisposition to insulin resistance that is worsened by social and environmental factors that predispose to the development of excess weight, particularly central obesity.
- Genetic predisposition of insulin resistance can coexist with a family history of type 2 diabetes, premature coronary heart disease, or metabolic syndrome in parents and first- or second-degree relatives.
- Poor dietary behaviors predispose to obesity.
  - High consumption of saturated fats and trans fats
  - Low consumption of natural fibers (e.g., whole grains, fruits, vegetables)
  - Low consumption of dairy products
  - High consumption of sugar-sweetened beverages and foods with high glycemic index values may increase risk of insulin resistance.
- Physical inactivity and lack of exercise predispose to obesity.
- In adults, smoking increases insulin resistance; psychosocial and emotional stress are associated with insulin resistance.
- Visceral adipose tissue, even without being overweight, is a risk for metabolic syndrome.

DIAGNOSIS

Dx

DIFFERENTIAL DIAGNOSIS

- Type 2 diabetes mellitus
- Congenital or acquired lipodystrophy syndromes
- Medications that have weight gain as a side effect, particularly chronic use of oral corticosteroids, atypical antipsychotic medications, oral retinoic acid preparations, and antiretroviral therapy.

WORKUP

- Accurate measurements of weight and height to determine and track BMI.
- Measure waist circumference at annual visits for youths who are at risk for overweightness or are overweight by the BMI (see Growth Curves [Section IV]).
  - Waist circumferences greater than 102 cm for males and 88 cm for females are above the adult thresholds for central adiposity.
  - Waist circumference norms greater than the 90th percentile for age and gender have been created from the Third National Health and Nutrition Examination Survey from 1988 through 1994.
  - A patient is at risk if the BMI is consistently above the 95th percentile for age and gender without appearance of excess lean muscle mass, especially in the face of excess fat around the middle.
- Blood pressure values consistently greater than the 90th percentile for age, gender, and height on three or more occasions are in a range to consider the patient at risk factor for the metabolic syndrome, and they warrant closer monitoring for progress to primary or secondary hypertension.

LABORATORY TESTS

- Fasting lipid profile
  - Triglycerides above 110 mg/dL for adolescents and 90 mg/dL for preadolescent children are abnormal.
  - HDL cholesterol levels lower than 40 mg/dL are abnormal.
- Fasting insulin, glucose and hemoglobin A1C levels
  - A fasting glucose level greater than 100 mg/dL on two occasions or more is consistent with impaired fasting glucose.
  - A fasting insulin level greater than 20 mU/L is consistent with hyperinsulinemia, but fasting insulin levels are higher at baseline for black youths compared with white children.
  - HBA_{1C} values greater than 6%, which is greater than 2 standard deviations above the mean and raises concern for impaired glucose tolerance warranting evaluation (oral glucose tolerance test).
- Consider repeating laboratory tests annually or every other year, especially if the child gains excessive weight.
- Consider glucose tolerance testing because impaired glucose tolerance predicts individuals who will develop type 2 diabetes.
- Test for an elevated urine albumin-to-creatinine ratio (ACR).
  - This is one of the criteria for the metabolic syndrome using the WHO definition for adults.
  - Preliminary analyses have shown teens with the metabolic syndrome have lower mean urine ACR than teens without.
  - This may not represent a good marker for the metabolic syndrome in youths.

TABLE 1-15 **Waist Circumference (cm) Cutoffs for >90th and >95th Percentiles by Age and Sex; NHANES III, 1988-1994***

	>90% CUTOFFS		>95% CUTOFFS	
Age (years)	Males	Females	Males	Females
2	52.1	52.4	53.0	53.9
3	53.4	54.6	55.4	57.2
4	55.5	56.7	57.4	61.5
5	57.3	60.5	61.2	63.7
6	66.1	62.5	71.1	70.6
7	69.0	68.4	75.9	76.6
8	70.9	69.0	72.0	73.5
9	78.0	80.8	81.5	83.9
10	79.9	79.0	83.2	87.1
11	84.2	80.9	89.5	85.2
12	85.9	81.2	89.5	86.4
13	90.0	89.5	93.5	97.7
14	97.4	91.9	114.6	99.0
15	95.9	89.0	111.8	91.8
16	90.6	91.3	107.0	97.7
17	98.0	94.6	102.9	99.8
18	97.2	92.8	107.1	98.1
19	101.6	97.7	106.2	110.2

Values applied for national analysis in Cook, et al. 2003.
*Third National Health and Nutrition Examination Survey 1988-1994.

TREATMENT

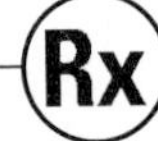

NONPHARMACOLOGIC THERAPY

- A 5% to 10% weight loss has been shown to reverse components of the metabolic syndrome and improve insulin resistance.
- Regular exercise and physical activity protect against the metabolic syndrome.
- Decrease in sedentary behavior (television watching) facilitates efforts to lose or maintain weight.

ACUTE GENERAL Rx

- There is not an acute treatment for the metabolic syndrome. Urgent medical treatment of hyperglycemia and possible ketoacidosis takes priority. (See DKA and Diabetes Type II in Section I)
- Medications that worsen insulin resistance or cause obesity may need to be adjusted.

CHRONIC Rx

- Lifestyle behaviors that include prevention of further weight gain.
- Persistent hypertension needs pharmacotherapy. Adult studies have indicated that angiotensin-converting enzyme inhibitors have protective affects against the development of diabetes and a protective effect for the kidneys.
- Insulin-sensitizing medications such as metformin may be considered for persistence of hyperglycemia in nondiabetic ranges. Consider only in conjunction with lifestyle and behavioral changes.
- Adolescents with type 2 diabetes who have elevated LDL cholesterol levels and other risk factors merit consideration for cholesterol-lowering therapy with HMG-CoA reductase inhibitors (i.e., statins).
  - Reserved for high-risk youth
  - Done in consultation with a specialist comfortable with pharmacotherapy for hyperlipidemia
- Smoking cessation and prevention reduce insulin resistance and decelerate premature atherosclerosis.
- Consider adjusting of medications that worsen insulin resistance or increase weight.

DISPOSITION

- Overweight children warrant frequent, regular follow-up for weight management. Include partnering with a parent or friend for appropriate lifestyle changes.
- Monitor weight and bp every 3 months.
- Education about signs or symptoms of hyperglycemia or diabetes.

REFERRAL

- Referral to an endocrinologist may be warranted, urgent referral for those with diabetes.
- Referral or management of persistent hypertension.
- Pharmacotherapy is rarely considered for lipid abnormalities, unless
  - Significant cardiac risk factors coexist
  - Type 2 diabetes exists
  - A strong family history for premature coronary heart disease exists

PEARLS & CONSIDERATIONS

COMMENTS

- Values used for children and adolescents are not yet well established.
- The adult definitions from the WHO or the NCEP are the most conservative approaches to apply for youths.
- Risk factors should be tracked annually.
- Metabolic syndrome factors change throughout adolescence and in association with lifestyle changes.

PREVENTION

- Maintenance of normal weight
- Prevent initiation of smoking
- Exclusive breast-feeding for at least 4 to 6 months
- Prevention of low-birth-weight infants
- Model healthy and appropriate eating and activity habits

PATIENT/FAMILY EDUCATION

- Lifestyle changes for the entire family: less television, more physical activity, better food choices, meal planning.
- If there is a parent who is overweight, partner with the child in weight loss. Parent changes in lifestyle behaviors is the best predictor of child's changes.

SUGGESTED READINGS

Cook S et al: Prevalence of the metabolic syndrome phenotype in adolescents: Findings from the third National Health and Nutrition Examination Survey, 1988-1994. *Arch Pediatr Adolesc Med* 187:821, 2003.

Cruz M et al: The metabolic syndrome in overweight Hispanic youth and the role of insulin sensitivity. *J Clin Endocrinol Metab* 89:108, 2004.

Fernandez J et al: Waist circumference percentiles in nationally representative samples of African-American, European-American and Mexican-American children and adolescents. *J Pediatr* 145:439, 2004.

Kahn R et al: Follow-up report on the diagnosis of diabetes mellitus: the expert committee on the diagnosis and classifications of diabetes mellitus. *Diabetes Care* 26:3160, 2003.

Knowler W et al: Reduction in the incidence of type 2 diabetes with lifestyle intervention or metformin. *N Engl J Med* 346:393, 2002.

Ten S et al: Insulin resistance syndrome in children. *J Clin Endocrinol Metab* 89:2526, 2004.

Williams C et al: Cardiovascular health in childhood: a statement for health professionals from the Committee on Atherosclerosis, Hypertension, and Obesity in the Young (AHOY) of the Council on Cardiovascular Disease in the Young, American Heart Association. *Circulation* 106:143, 2002.

AUTHOR: **STEPHEN COOK, MD**

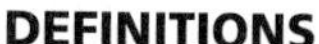

BASIC INFORMATION

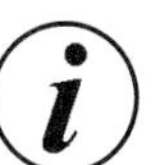

DEFINITIONS

Milia and miliaria are common neonatal dermatoses that result from the incomplete differentiation of the epidermis and its appendages at birth. Miliaria also can occur in older children. Milia are 1- to 2-mm, pearly white or yellow papules that result from retention of keratin and sebaceous material within the pilosebaceous apparatus of neonatal skin. Miliaria results from keratinous plugging of eccrine ducts, with subsequent escape of sweat into the skin below the level of obstruction. Miliaria crystallina (i.e., sudamina) are clear, pinpoint, superficial, thin-walled, noninflammatory vesicles created from sweat retention in the epidermis just below the stratum corneum. Miliaria rubra (i.e., prickly heat) are erythematous, grouped papules or vesicles that result from rupture of the intraepidermal portion of the sweat duct. The vesicle is at the level of the basal layer of the epidermis and may be surrounded by inflammatory cells. Miliaria pustulosa is rare and involves leukocytic infiltration of the vesicles. Miliaria profunda and miliaria pustulosa are rarely seen in temperate climates.

SYNONYMS

Milia
- Epidermal inclusion cyst
- Single lesion called *milium*

Miliaria
- Miliaria crystallina (i.e., sudamina)
- Miliaria rubra (i.e., prickly heat)

ICD-9-CM CODE
705.1 Miliaria
706.2 Inclusion (epidermal)

EPIDEMIOLOGY & DEMOGRAPHICS

- Milia
  - Present in 40% of all races of term infants
  - Less common in preterm infants
- Miliaria
  - More common before the advent of humidity and temperature control in nurseries
  - May affect febrile older children or occur with exercise in hot, humid climates
  - May occur in a neonate exposed to external sources of heat (e.g., phototherapy lights, radiant warmers)

CLINICAL PRESENTATION

History
- Milia
  - Well infant at birth
  - Full-term normal pregnancy
  - Lack of risk factors for bacterial or yeast infection (e.g., prolonged rupture of membranes, maternal fever, chorioamnionitis)
- Miliaria
  - Sometimes associated with maternal fever during labor
  - Exposure to hot, humid conditions
  - Fever, overdressing, ointment use, external sources of heat such as phototherapy or infant warmer, exercise in the older child
  - In older child, possible itching or a pins-and-needles sensation

Physical Examination
- Milia
  - Predilection for the cheeks, nasolabial folds, forehead, nose, ears, chin, and periorbital areas of the face; rarely found on arms and legs or penis
  - Cystic, white lesions 1 to 2 mm in diameter
  - Expressed contents of lesions resemble tiny white pearls
- Miliaria
  - Characteristic distribution is on the face, scalp, and intertriginous areas.
  - Miliaria crystallina (i.e., sudamina) are clear, pinpoint, superficial, thin-walled, noninflammatory vesicles.
  - Miliaria rubra (i.e., prickly heat) are erythematous, grouped papules or vesicles. If inflammation is prominent, the lesion may appear pustular.

ETIOLOGY

Causes include incomplete differentiation of the epidermis and its appendages at birth (milia and miliaria) in combination with hot, humid conditions (miliaria).

DIAGNOSIS

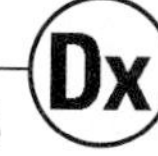

DIFFERENTIAL DIAGNOSIS

- Milia
  - Large milia (>2 mm) are found in the orofacial-digital syndrome (OFD).
  - Sebaceous gland hyperplasia is a result of exposure to maternal androgens. Lesions are pinpoint lesions, more yellow, and express sebaceous material.
  - Epstein's pearls are an oral mucosal variant of cutaneous milia.
- Miliaria
  - Erythema toxicum
  - Candidal infection
  - Early pyoderma
  - Herpes simplex

WORKUP

The diagnosis is based on the clinical features of milia or miliaria.

LABORATORY TESTS

- Milia: no tests needed
- Miliaria
  - Culture, Gram stain, Wright stain, and KOH preparation may be done.
  - On Wright stain, expect sparse squamous cells and lymphocytes.
  - Expect no bacteria or yeast.
  - Erythema toxicum vesicles have eosinophils but no bacteria.

TREATMENT

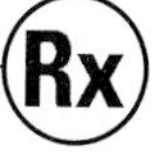

NONPHARMACOLOGIC THERAPY

- Milia
  - Conservative treatment is indicated because lesions are self-limited.
  - Lesions exfoliate within a few weeks without scarring. Even the large milia of the OFD syndrome exfoliate in 3 to 4 months, but they do leave pitted scars.
- Miliaria
  - Conservative treatment is indicated. The infant should be cared for in a cooler, less humid environment.
  - Give cool-water baths and avoid soap.

ACUTE GENERAL Rx

- Miliaria
  - Application of calamine lotion to body folds should result in resolution in several days.
  - Apply 1% hydrocortisone cream to itchy spots two to three times per day.

PEARLS & CONSIDERATIONS

PREVENTION

- Miliaria
  - Avoid hot, humid conditions.
  - Avoid the use of ointments on neonates.

SUGGESTED READINGS

Drolet BA, Esterly NB: The skin. *In* Fanaroff AA, Martin RJ (eds): *Neonatal-Perinatal Medicine,* 7th ed. St. Louis, Mosby, 2002.

Hurwitz S: *Clinical Pediatric Dermatology: A Textbook of Skin Disorders of Childhood and Adolescence.* Philadelphia, WB Saunders, 1993.

Hurwitz S: Skin lesions in the first year of life. *Contemp Pediatr* 15:110, 1998.

Pielop JA, Levy ML: Benign skin lesions in the newborn. UpToDate online (12.3), 2004. Available at www.uptodate.com/ Accessed January 7, 2005.

Van Praag et al: Diagnosis and treatment of pustular disorders in the neonate. *Pediatr Dermatol* 14:131, 1997.

Vasiloudes P et al: A guide to rashes in newborns. *Contemp Pediatr* 14:156, 1997.

AUTHOR: **CYNTHIA R. HOWARD, MD, MPH, FAAP**

BASIC INFORMATION

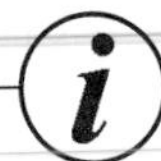

DEFINITION

Mitral valve prolapse (MVP) is focal or diffuse redundancy of mitral valve leaflets (predominantly the posterior cusp) with or without lengthening of subvalvar chordal structures, leading to abnormal coaptation (i.e., closure) of mitral leaflets in systole.

SYNONYMS

Barlow syndrome
Click-murmur syndrome
Floppy valve syndrome
Myxomatous degeneration of the mitral valve

ICD-9-CM CODE
424.0 Mitral valve disorders

EPIDEMIOLOGY & DEMOGRAPHICS

- First described in 1966 by Barlow and Bosman in the *American Heart Journal*
- Most common valvular disease in industrialized nations
- Prevalence in children and adolescents: 6% to 11%
  - Mean age of presentation: 9.9 years; rare presentation before adolescent growth spurt in children without connective tissue disorders
  - Before age 20, female-to-male ratio is 2:1, with significant genetic causes in females
  - After age 20, female-to-male ratio is equal; after age 50, higher rates for males
- May have a familial predisposition (i.e., developmental malformation) or result from maternal diabetes during pregnancy

CLINICAL PRESENTATION

History

- "Atypical" auscultatory findings first noticed after febrile illness (34% of patients)
- Abnormality on routine physical examination in asymptomatic child (33% of patients)
- Nonexertional, atypical chest pain (18% of patients); described as short and stabbing
- Arrhythmia and fatigue (each 3%); more common symptoms in adolescents and adults

Physical Examination

- Cardiac examination is best completed with the diaphragm of the stethoscope.
- Auscultatory findings may vary on multiple examinations of the patient.
- Midsystolic, "nonejection" click is heard at the left sternal border.
  - Can vary throughout systole
  - May have single or multiple clicks
- Second heart sound may be widely split.
- Variable late-systolic crescendo-decrescendo apical murmur (i.e., "honking" or "whooping" quality) is changed by postural maneuvers (see "Comments").
- Other findings include an early diastolic sound (similar to fixed second heart sound or opening snap of second heart sound).
- Abnormalities may be seen in other systems (e.g., high-arched palate, joint laxity, pectus excavatum, straight back syndrome).

ETIOLOGY

- MVP is called the silent form of congenital heart disease.
- Abnormalities include the myxomatous matrix of valve leaflets or collagenous structure of the chordae tendineae. Proteoglycan accumulates in elastic fibers of the valvar and extravalvar tissues, including the atrioventricular nodal arteries.
- MVP may reflect an abnormality of the chordal insertion rather than a leaflet abnormality.
- Redundancy of leaflet tissue is similar to Ebstein's anomaly of the tricuspid valve.
- Echocardiographic studies of neonates without connective tissue disorders reveal infrequent evidence of congenital MVP (i.e., MVP more developmental than congenital).
- MVP is associated with the following:
  - Atrial septal defects (15% to 41%)
  - Ebstein's anomaly
  - l-transposition of the great arteries
- Noncardiac associations include the following:
  - Connective tissue disorders (e.g., Marfan's syndrome, Ehlers-Danlos syndrome, osteogenesis imperfecta, pseudoxanthoma elasticum)
  - Fragile X syndrome
  - Turner syndrome
  - Mucopolysaccharidoses
  - Autosomal dominant polycystic kidney disease
  - Rheumatic fever
  - Kawasaki disease
- MVP is found in 46% of Down syndrome patients without other obvious congenital heart lesions.

DIAGNOSIS

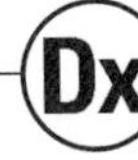

DIFFERENTIAL DIAGNOSIS

- Rheumatic mitral insufficiency (differentiated by responses to postural maneuvers and lack of click)
- Apical muscular ventricular septal defect (usually lacks clicks)

LABORATORY TESTS

- Electrocardiogram (ECG)
  - Repolarization abnormalities (prolonged QT interval, T-wave inversion in leads II, III, aVF) at rest or during exercise (49% to 63% of patients)
  - Uniform premature atrial or ventricular contractions and conduction disturbances (15% to 38% of patients); may also result in short bursts of paroxysmal atrial tachycardia
  - Exercise or ambulatory ECG of limited use because neither clinical features nor symptoms correlate with high-grade arrhythmias
  - Worsening arrhythmias may correlate with increasing mitral regurgitation (MR)

IMAGING STUDIES

- Chest radiograph: normal unless patient has other associated thoracoskeletal abnormalities (e.g., pectus excavatum, scoliosis, straight-back syndrome)
- Echocardiogram
  - "Prolapsing" systolic movement of mitral valve leaflets (more than 2 mm superior to annular ring); high rate of false-positive results
  - Identifies associated anomalies (e.g., atrioseptal defect, l-transposition of the great arteries)

TREATMENT

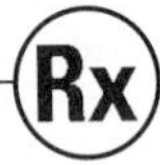

NONPHARMACOLOGIC THERAPY

- Family counseling is crucial to prevent cardiac "neurosis" caused by possible morbidity.
- Surgery is indicated based on the severity of MR.
- Surgery similar to that for congenital MR: resection of redundant leaflet tissue, annuloplasty ring, repair of chordal attachments (see Mitral Valve Regurgitation in Diseases and Disorders [Section I])

ACUTE GENERAL Rx

- Antiarrhythmics (e.g., β-blockers) are used for ventricular and atrial arrhythmias.
- β-Blockers may improve atypical chest pain.
- Oral antacids may be used because of a possible association between MVP and esophageal dysmotility.

CHRONIC Rx

When indicated, treatment is the same as found under "Acute General Rx."

DISPOSITION

- Asymptomatic: cardiac evaluation every 1 to 2 years to ascertain changes in examination results or appearance of symptoms
- MVP with MR: yearly evaluation

REFERRAL

Refer to a cardiologist for new-onset murmur, a click identified on physical examination, atypical chest pain, or arrhythmias.

PEARLS & CONSIDERATIONS

COMMENTS

- Timing of clicks varies with postural maneuvers.
  - Earlier in systole: Valsalva, squatting-to-standing positions

- Later in systole: standing-to-squatting, sitting-to-supine positions
- The murmur of MR also varies with position.
  - Louder, longer: supine-to-sitting, squatting-to-standing positions
  - Softer, shorter: sitting-to-supine, standing-to-squatting positions

PREVENTION

- Subacute bacterial endocarditis (SBE) prophylaxis is indicated for MR.
- For patients with isolated clicks, MVP, and no MR, the need for SBE prophylaxis is controversial.
- Systemic, chronic anticoagulation is not indicated for MVP.

PATIENT/FAMILY EDUCATION

- In childhood, MVP is a relatively benign condition. Malignant arrhythmias and near sudden death episodes are anecdotal.
- Pathological studies indicate that sudden death may occur more frequently in adolescent female patients with trivial MR, and there is limited evidence for ruptured chordae tendineae.
- Uncommon but major complications (i.e., endocarditis, chordal rupture or progressive MR, transient ischemic attacks, ventricular arrhythmias, sudden death) can occur in adulthood.
- Approximately 10% to 15% of patients with MVP have significant degenerative valvar changes over time.
- Morbidity of MVP is increased in patients with connective tissue disorder.

SUGGESTED READINGS

Alpert JS et al: Mitral valve disease. *In* Topol EJ (ed): *Textbook of Cardiovascular Medicine,* 2nd ed. Philadelphia, Lippincott-Raven, 2002, pp 483–509.

American Heart Association National Center. Available at www.americanheart.org

Baylen BG, Waldhausen JA: Diseases of the mitral valve. *In* Adams FH et al (eds): *Moss' Heart Disease in Infants, Children and Adolescents.* Baltimore, Williams & Wilkins, 1995, pp 647–664.

Bisset GS III et al: Clinical spectrum and long-term follow-up of isolated mitral valve prolapse in 119 children. *Circulation* 62:423, 1980.

Dollar AL, Roberts WC: Morphologic comparison of patients with mitral valve prolapse. *J Am Coll Cardiol* 17:921, 1990.

Shappell SD et al: Sudden death and the familial occurrence of mid-systolic click, late systolic murmur syndrome. *Circulation* 48:1128, 1973.

Society for Mitral Valve Prolapse Syndrome. Available at www.mitralvalveprolapse.com

AUTHOR: **ALAN M. MENDELSOHN, MD, FACC**

BASIC INFORMATION

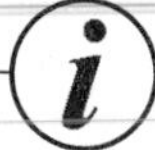

DEFINITION

Mitral valve regurgitation (MR) is incompetence of the mitral valve (lack of coaptation/closure of anterior and posterior mitral leaflets) and backward ejection of flow into the left atrium during left ventricular systole.

SYNONYM

Mitral insufficiency

ICD-9-CM CODE
746.6 Mitral regurgitation

EPIDEMIOLOGY & DEMOGRAPHICS

- Rare event in isolation (fewer than 1% of children with congenital heart defects)
- Most common manifestation of rheumatic heart disease

CLINICAL PRESENTATION

History

- Murmur in an otherwise asymptomatic patient.
- In absence of other etiologies, murmur may represent remnant of subclinical rheumatic carditis.
- Symptoms: dyspnea on exertion, orthopnea, and paroxysmal nocturnal dyspnea (more common in patients with chronic, severe MR).

Physical Examination

- Increased precordial activity, diffuse apical impulse
- Diminished first heart sound, increased pulmonary component of second heart sound
- Second heart sound may be narrowly split (with pulmonary hypertension)
- High-frequency, mid- to late blowing, or harsh holosystolic murmur at apex, with radiation to axilla and back

In moderate to severe MR:

- Third heart sound
- Low-frequency apical diastolic murmur
- Hepatosplenomegaly
- Peripheral edema

ETIOLOGY

- Usually associated with other forms of left ventricular outflow tract disease
  - Atrioventricular canal
  - Ventricular septal defect
  - Coarctation of the aorta
  - Patent ductus arteriosus
  - Anomalous left coronary artery from pulmonary artery
  - Isolated cardiac tumors
- May also be associated with tetralogy of Fallot, double outlet right ventricle or transposition of great arteries.
- Acquired: secondary effects of dilated cardiomyopathy, Kawasaki disease, rheumatic or viral myocarditis.
- Congenital abnormality of leaflets (e.g., leaflet cleft) or support structures (anomalies of papillary muscles or chordae tendineae).
- Common cardiac manifestation of connective tissue disorders:
  - Hurler's syndrome
  - Pseudoxanthoma elasticum
  - Marfan's syndrome
  - Ehlers-Danlos syndrome
  - Homocystinuria
- Can be associated with other rheumatoid diseases:
  - Systemic lupus erythematosus (SLE)
  - Ankylosing spondylitis
  - Systemic sclerosis
- MR may be associated with sickle cell disease.

DIAGNOSIS

DIFFERENTIAL DIAGNOSIS

- Ventricular septal defect (VSD)
  - Murmur of MR is mid- to late systolic unlike the early or holosystolic murmur of VSD
- Tricuspid insufficiency
- Aortic stenosis, hypertrophic (obstructive) cardiomyopathy (HOCM)
  - These murmurs tend to radiate more to the upper sternal border.
  - More ejection in quality.

LABORATORY TESTS

- Electrocardiogram
  - Left atrial and ventricular enlargement with severe MR; otherwise normal voltages.
  - Changes may be secondary to associated lesions (see "Etiology").
  - Up to 33% of cases may demonstrate left axis deviation (0 to −30 degrees).

IMAGING STUDIES

- Chest radiograph
  - Left atrial or ventricular enlargement
  - Increased pulmonary vascular markings
- Echocardiogram
  - Definitive test; confirms diagnosis
  - Delineates possible causes (i.e., abnormal mitral anatomy, leaflet clefts, cardiomyopathic changes, coronary abnormalities)
  - Defines left atrial and ventricular dimensions
- Cardiac catheterization
  - Primarily indicated for preoperative testing
  - Determines angiographic degree of MR
  - Defines pulmonary artery hemodynamics, left ventricular systolic and diastolic function

TREATMENT

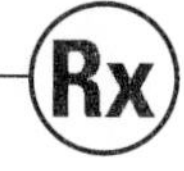

NONPHARMACOLOGIC THERAPY

- Intervention required in cases unresponsive to medical therapy.
- Type of surgery individualized by anatomic abnormality:
  - Suture closure of mitral leaflet cleft
  - Resection of redundant leaflet tissue
  - Annuloplasty ring to improve annular competence
  - Valve replacement with mechanical valve because of short (5- to 7-year) life span of bioprosthetic valve in mitral position
  - As techniques have advanced and materials have improved there is 75% 10-year freedom from reintervention
- Elective repair of hemodynamically significant MR in asymptomatic patients to prevent increasing complexity of later surgical repair is controversial.

ACUTE GENERAL Rx

- Moderate to severe MR:
  - Afterload-reducing agents: angiotensin-converting enzyme inhibitors (e.g., captopril, enalapril, or Monopril)
  - Positive inotropic agents (e.g., digoxin) or diuretic therapy for clinical congestive heart failure

CHRONIC Rx

Same as "Acute General Rx" when indicated.

DISPOSITION

- In most cases, mild MR from static causes (e.g., cleft mitral valve) does not progress.
- Trivial or mild MR (i.e., no electrocardiographic, radiographic, or echocardiographic evidence of atrial or ventricular dilation): conservative follow-up (every 1 to 2 years).
- Patients with an annuloplasty ring or mechanical mitral valve usually require anticoagulation therapy with warfarin.
  - Ring: anticoagulation for 3 to 6 months
  - Valve: lifelong anticoagulation
- Valve replacement before adolescence usually requires reoperation in adolescence or adulthood to implant a more appropriately sized valve.

REFERRAL

Refer to pediatric cardiologist for confirmation of diagnosis and grading of MR.

PEARLS & CONSIDERATIONS

COMMENTS

- Tricuspid insufficiency murmur: early systolic, ends before second heart sound
- Positional changes: see Mitral Valve Prolapse in Diseases and Disorders (Section I).

PREVENTION

- Subacute bacterial endocarditis (SBE) prophylaxis is necessary to prevent worsening of condition.
- Treatment of culture-proven group A β-hemolytic streptococcal pharyngitis is

needed to prevent (worsening) rheumatic carditis.

PATIENT/FAMILY EDUCATION

- Patients receiving chronic anticoagulation therapy should avoid contact sports and trauma.
- Appropriate group A β-hemolytic streptococcal prophylaxis (See Carditis Prophylaxis tables in Prevention [Section V]) should be administered if cause of MR was rheumatic fever.
- SBE prophylaxis is always indicated (see "Endocarditis Prophylaxis in Prevention [Section V]).
- The natural history varies according to the cause.
  - Rheumatic MR: progressive fibrosis and calcification, worsening MR or mitral stenosis.
  - Myxomatous MR (as with connective tissue disorders): higher incidence of spontaneous rupture of subvalvar structures, acute cardiac failure.
  - Patients with mechanical valves have a higher incidence of hemolysis and vegetations.

SUGGESTED READINGS

Alexson C et al: Mitral valve replacement with mechanical prostheses in children: improved operative risk and survival. *Eur J Cardiovasc Surg* 20:105, 2001.

Alpert JS: Mitral valve disease. *In* Topol EJ (ed): *Textbook of Cardiovascular Medicine,* 2nd ed. Philadelphia, Lippincott, 2002, pp 483–509.

American Heart Association. Available at www.americanheart.org

Baylen BG, Waldhausen JA: Diseases of the mitral valve. *In* Adams FH et al (eds): *Moss' Heart Disease in Infants, Children and Adolescents.* Baltimore, Williams & Wilkins, 1995, pp 647–664.

Davachi R et al: Diseases of the mitral valve in infancy: anatomic analysis of 55 cases. *Circulation* 43:565, 1971.

drkoop.com web site. Available at www.drkoop.com

Oregon Health Sciences University. Available at www.ohsu.edu/bicc-informatics/

AUTHOR: **ALAN M. MENDELSOHN, MD, FACC**

BASIC INFORMATION

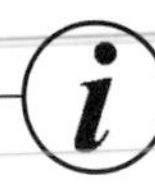

DEFINITION

Mitral value stenosis (MVS) indicates obstruction to left ventricular inflow at the valvar, subvalvar, or supravalvar level and is secondary to a single or to multiple etiologies.

SYNONYMS

Mitral stenosis
Mitral valve obstruction

ICD-9-CM CODE
746.5 Mitral stenosis

EPIDEMIOLOGY & DEMOGRAPHICS

- (See Endocarditis Prophylaxis in Prevention [Section V].) 0.4% to 0.5% of congenital cardiac anomalies; rarely an isolated lesion.
- Median survival (untreated): 35 months, mainly due to associated lesions.
- Progression of stenosis generally slow (e.g., mean period between acute rheumatic fever episode and symptomatic MVS is 20 years).
- Poor outcome: presentation in early infancy, evidence of low cardiac output or congestive heart failure (CHF).

CLINICAL PRESENTATION

History

- Mild disease: asymptomatic; approximately 50% of patients beyond infancy
- Moderate disease:
  - Forty-seven percent present beyond neonatal period; 36% of infants with moderate MVS are symptomatic and require intervention within first 2 years of life.
  - Symptoms include:
    - Multiple recurrent pulmonary infections
    - Failure to thrive
    - Irritability, dyspnea on exertion, diaphoresis with feeds
- Severe disease:
  - Symptoms in early postnatal period following ductus arteriosus closure; 86% within 13 days of life
  - Vascular collapse with dyspnea, tachypnea, hypotension, grunting, and ashen color

Physical Examination

- Soft first heart sound, absent mitral valve opening sound (findings usually reversed in patients with rheumatic mitral stenosis)
- Second heart sound
  - Variable splitting
    - Widely split in mild disease
    - Narrow split, accentuated pulmonary component secondary to pulmonary hypertension in severe disease
- Usually low-frequency, low-intensity mid-diastolic apical murmur; sometimes loud, high-frequency diastolic murmur
- Severe MVS:
  - Diminished peripheral perfusion and pulses
  - Jugular venous distention
  - Hyperdynamic right ventricular impulse
  - Third, fourth heart sounds: secondary to right ventricular diastolic dysfunction
  - Variable systolic ejection click, diastolic pulmonary insufficiency murmur (Graham-Steel murmur) in face of severe pulmonary hypertension

ETIOLOGY

- Congenital
  - Abnormal deposition of fibrous and myxomatous materials
  - Commissural fusion or hypoplasia—60% to 70% (hypoplastic mitral valve, double orifice mitral valve)
  - Excessive supravalvar connective tissue 20% (“ring”)
  - Abnormal insertion or fusion or quantity of chordae tendineae—8% to 11% (e.g., parachute mitral valve)
  - Predominantly associated with other forms of left ventricular (LV) and right ventricular (RV) disease: hypoplastic left heart syndrome, aortic coarctation, aortic stenosis (valvar, subvalvar), double-outlet right ventricle, atrial septal defect (primum, secundum)
- Inborn errors of metabolism (e.g., Fabry’s disease, Hunter’s syndrome, Hurler-Scheie syndrome)
- Rheumatoid disease (e.g., systemic lupus erythematosus, rheumatoid arthritis, rheumatic heart disease)

DIAGNOSIS

Dx

DIFFERENTIAL DIAGNOSIS

- Primary pulmonary artery hypertension; usually lacks apical diastolic murmur
- Pulmonary venous obstruction/pulmonary vaso-occlusive disease
- Cor triatriatum (obstructive membrane within left atrium limiting pulmonary venous drainage)
- Atrial myxoma
- Large atrial or ventricular septal defects

LABORATORY TESTS

- Electrocardiogram
  - Left atrial enlargement
  - Severe MVS: findings of right heart disease
    - Right ventricular enlargement
    - Right atrial enlargement
    - Right QRS axis deviation (+90 degrees to 150 degrees)
  - In adolescents and adults, paroxysmal (or chronic) atrial fibrillation

IMAGING STUDIES

- Chest radiograph
  - Left atrial enlargement
  - Increased pulmonary vascular markings
  - Increased right heart silhouette
- Echocardiogram
  - Definitive test confirms diagnosis
  - Provides diagnostic abnormal Doppler inflow patterns
  - Demonstrates chamber sizes
  - Defines all levels of involved mitral valve apparatus
- Cardiac catheterization
  - Valuable as diagnostic and therapeutic test
  - Defines degree of MVS, pulmonary hemodynamics, and cardiac index
  - Aids to rule out other pulmonary venous abnormalities
  - Defines associated LV outflow tract obstruction

TREATMENT

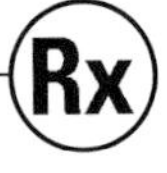

NONPHARMACOLOGIC THERAPY

- Surgical therapy: indicated for symptomatic relief or for inadequate improvement with medical intervention.
- Long-term outcomes impacted by pre- and postoperative LV function.
- Intervention depends on the etiology of MVS.
  - Simple commissurotomy (separation of leaflets)
  - Resection of excessive subvalvar/supravalvar tissue
  - Mitral valve replacement with mechanical prosthesis for multiple levels of MVS
- Optimal age for repair in asymptomatic patients with moderate to severe MVS is 3 years.
- Transcatheter balloon valvuloplasty: first proposed by Lock in 1985.
  - Procedure: limited use in infants, small children, patients with calcified valves
    - Two-year mortality approximately 40% regardless of treatment modality
  - Approximately 40% to 50% mid- (12 to 72 months) and long-term success when normal subvalvar anatomy and adequate annulus size present
  - Procedural complications: mitral regurgitation (rare), transient ischemic attacks, ventricular perforations (anecdotal), second- or third-degree atrioventricular block (in up to 22% of patients)

ACUTE GENERAL Rx

- Standard anticongestive therapy (e.g., diuretics, nitrates): mild to moderate symptomatic MVS.
- Surgical/transcatheter therapy is the treatment of choice in severe MVS.
- Digoxin may be useful in the face of right ventricular failure.
- Antiarrhythmics (e.g., digoxin, β-blockers, calcium channel blockers) as necessary.
- Chronic anticoagulation with warfarin as necessary.
- Aggressive treatment of pulmonary infections.

CHRONIC Rx

Same as "Acute General Rx" when indicated.

DISPOSITION

- Chronic anticoagulation (if necessary) requires close monitoring.
- Patients with chronic pulmonary vascular disease, concomitant pulmonary illnesses: follow-up every 6 to 12 months.
- Pulmonary vascular changes usually resolve within 2 years of treatment.
  - Most studies show no permanent vascular abnormalities (i.e., plexiform lesions) in patients even if treated late (i.e., 16 years of age).
- Acute pulmonary hypertensive crises may be responsive to inhaled nitric oxide.

REFERRAL

Refer to pediatric cardiologist for full evaluation and management if diagnosis is suspected by clinical history or physical examination.

PEARLS & CONSIDERATIONS

COMMENTS

Short periods of exercise or deep expiration may accentuate the murmur in larger patients.

PREVENTION

- Aggressive antibiotic therapy is indicated for rheumatic fever prophylaxis. (See Endocarditis Prophylaxis in Prevention [Section V].)
- Subacute bacterial endocarditis prophylaxis should be administered at times of appropriate risk. (See Endocarditis Prophylaxis in Prevention [Section V].)

PATIENT/FAMILY EDUCATION

- Patients with untreated MVS (regardless of degree) are at increased risk for cerebral embolic phenomena.
- Chronic atrial fibrillation: 40% of patients, even with effective gradient relief.
- Pulmonary vascular changes or pulmonary hypertension may be slow to resolve even after gradient resolution.

SUGGESTED READINGS

Alpert JS et al: Mitral valve disease. *In* Topol EJ (ed): *Textbook of Cardiovascular Medicine,* 2nd ed. Philadelphia, Lippincott-Raven, 2002, pp 483–509.

Baylen BG, Waldhausen JA: Diseases of the mitral valve. *In* Adams FH et al (eds): *Moss' Heart Disease in Infants, Children and Adolescents.* Baltimore, Williams & Wilkins, 1995, pp 647–664.

Mendelsohn AM, Beekman RH: Interventions in congenital heart disease. *In* Topol EJ (ed): *Comprehensive Cardiovascular Medicine.* Philadelphia, Lippincott-Raven, 1998, pp 2529–2553.

Moore P et al: Severe congenital mitral stenosis in infants. *Circulation* 89:2099, 1994.

AUTHOR: **ALAN M. MENDELSOHN, MD, FACC**

BASIC INFORMATION

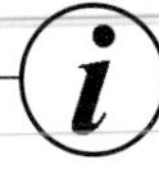

DEFINITION

Mixed connective tissue disease (MCTD) is an autoimmune, rheumatic disease with clinical features overlapping systemic lupus erythematosus (SLE), polymyositis, and systemic sclerosis, and associated with anti-U1 RNP (ribonucleoprotein) antibodies. Four classification criteria are published, but these are not validated in children.

SYNONYMS

MCTD
Overlap syndrome
Undifferentiated connective tissue disease (not all patients qualify by diagnostic serologies)

ICD-9-CM CODE
710.9 Connective tissue disease, diffuse (not specifically listed as MCTD)

EPIDEMIOLOGY & DEMOGRAPHICS

- No epidemiologic studies have been conducted in the United States.
- Estimated in 0.6% of all pediatric rheumatologic patients.
- The incidence is 0.10 per 100,000 children 0 to 15 years old in Finland and 0.05 per 100,000 children in Japan compared with 0.37 per 100,000 children with SLE in Finland and 0.47 per 100,000 children with SLE in Japan.
- Approximate female-to-male ratio is 6:1.
- Youngest reported patient was 4 years old.
- Increased association with HLA DR2/DR4 and anti-U1-70-kd RNP antibodies.

CLINICAL PRESENTATION

- Fever (occasional)
- Fatigue (ubiquitous symptom in connective tissue diseases)
- Arthralgia and arthritis (SLE-like or juvenile rheumatoid arthritis [JRA]-like in 90%) with associated joint swelling, large and small joints, symmetric distribution
- Raynaud's phenomenon (approximately 93% to 100%)
- Swollen hands (79% to 91%), diffuse induration or "sausage digits"
- Sclerodactyly (47% to 86%), rarely digital ulcers or pits
- Malar erythema, photosensitivity
- Esophageal dysmotility (dysphagia and reflux symptoms)
- Myositis with proximal muscle weakness
- Abnormal diffusion capacity for carbon monoxide (DL_{CO})—may be asymptomatic
- Signs of Sjögren's syndrome: swollen parotid glands, xerostomia, xerophthalmia
- Pericarditis, myocarditis
- Glomerulonephritis, proliferative or membranous (up to 36%, severe 15%)
- Rare central nervous system (CNS) complications, cerebrovascular accident
- Thrombocytopenia, leukopenia, direct Coombs-positive hemolytic anemia (uncommon)
- Thyroiditis
- Rheumatoid nodules (uncommon)

ETIOLOGY

Unknown, as are all autoimmune rheumatic diseases.

DIAGNOSIS

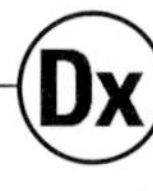

DIFFERENTIAL DIAGNOSIS

- Classification criteria provide systemic signs and symptoms and serologies to establish provisional diagnosis.
- Any autoimmune disease needs to be considered; however, MCTD manifests overlap components of SLE, SS, polymyositis (dermatomyositis), plus components of JRA and Sjögren's syndrome.
- Anecdotal reports of viral myocarditis and one case of malignancy confused with MCTD.

LABORATORY TESTS

- Antinuclear antibody test (ANA)—expect high titer, speckled pattern
- Positive RNP antibodies (U1–70 kd RNP)
- Much less commonly positive are ds DNA, Sm antibodies (Sharp criteria would exclude these patients.). These antibodies strongly suggest lupus.
- Complete blood cell count (CBC) with differential, platelet count
- Urine analysis, blood urea nitrogen (BUN), creatinine
- Muscle enzymes; creatine kinase (CK), aldolase, aspartate aminotransferase (AST), alanine aminotransferase (ALT), lactate dehydrogenase (LDH)
- Pulmonary function tests with routine flow loops and DL_{CO}; chest radiograph
- Quantitative immunoglobulins (likely elevated)—hypergammaglobulinemia
- C3, C4—occasionally low
- DAT/direct Coombs test
- Rheumatoid factor, positive in 50%

IMAGING STUDIES

- Esophageal studies, barium cine-esophagram
- Joint radiographs—cumulative may show erosive bone changes over time
- Electrocardiogram (ECG), echocardiogram

TREATMENT

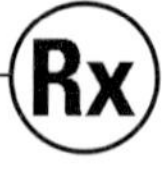

NONPHARMACOLOGIC THERAPY

Nonpharmacologic

- "Raynaud's prophylaxis"—mittens/gloves, avoidance of cold, no tobacco!
- Physical therapy—range of motion exercises, joint/hand protection
- Biofeedback; may be helpful for Raynaud's phenomenon
- Gastroesophageal reflux precautions

Surgical

- Usually none necessary; however, system-specific intervention may be necessary

ACUTE GENERAL Rx

- Nonsteroidal anti-inflammatory drugs (naproxen, tolmetin sodium, etc.) for arthritis and mild serositis
- Corticosteroids, usually oral administration for myositis, serositis, thrombocytopenia (clinically relevant), pulmonary manifestations
- Raynaud's phenomenon—calcium channel blockers, topical nitroglycerin products
- More intense immunosuppression may be used for serious renal, CNS, cardiac, or pulmonary involvement.
- Esophageal protection—H_2 blockers, proton pump inhibitors
- Intervention targeted at systems affected or symptoms (i.e., Raynaud's phenomenon) elicited.

CHRONIC Rx

- Intervention targeted at specific symptoms or organ systems affected.
- See also "Acute General Rx."

DISPOSITION

- Serial evaluation for evolution of disease (i.e., progressive arthropathy, sclerodactyly)
- Surveillance for hematologic, muscular, CNS, renal, or pulmonary involvement
- Beware of possible development of pulmonary hypertension.
- Watch for growth and nutritional issues, especially in patients with esophageal, intestinal involvement, insidious thyroiditis with hypothyroidism, or corticosteroid treatment.
- Comprehensive review of systems and complete physical examination are mandatory and evaluation of systems as previously listed. Referral to rheumatologist is desired to conduct multidisciplinary care and longitudinal follow-up.

REFERRAL

Because MCTD is a complex overlap syndrome, all patients should be evaluated and followed longitudinally by a rheumatologist if possible.

PEARLS & CONSIDERATIONS

COMMENTS

- Anything can happen to these patients—keep your eyes, ears, fingers tuned-in.
- These patients evolve over time, usually into patients with predominantly lupus or scleroderma characteristics.
- Beware of progressive restrictive lung disease and pulmonary hypertension.

PREVENTION

- None is possible to avoid the progression of the signs or symptoms related to the primary disease process.

- No tobacco—it is a vasoconstrictor that aggravates Raynaud's phenomenon.
- Evaluate for antiphospholipid antibodies if contemplating estrogen-containing contraceptives.

PATIENT/FAMILY EDUCATION

- Protect hands (Raynaud's phenomenon)
- Use sun protection (photosensitive rash)
- Use esophageal reflux precautions
- Watch for new symptoms
- Need serial reevaluations by physician
- Maintain all immunizations; except no live virus vaccines if on corticosteroids or other immunosuppressants
- Support groups:
  - Arthritis Foundation. Available online at www.arthritis.org/conditions/DiseaseCenter/ja_other.asp
  - Usually lupus group or possible scleroderma or JRA support group. Available online at www.lupus.org
  - American Juvenile Arthritis Organization. Available online at http://arthritis.about.com/od/mctd/

SUGGESTED READINGS

Michels H: Course of mixed connective tissue disease in children. *Ann Med* 29:359, 1997.

Mier R et al: Long term follow-up of children with mixed connective tissue disease. *Lupus* 5:221, 1996.

Mier R et al: Pediatric-onset mixed connective tissue disease. *Rheum Dis Clin North Am* 31(3):483, 2005.

Singsen BH et al: Mixed connective tissue disease in childhood. A clinical and serologic survey. *J Pediatr* 90:893, 1977.

Tiddens HA et al: Juvenile-onset mixed connective tissue disease: longitudinal follow-up. *J Pediatr* 122:191, 1993.

Yokota S et al: Mixed connective tissue disease in childhood: a nationwide retrospective study in Japan. *Acta Paediatr Japonica* 39:273, 1997.

AUTHOR: **MURRAY H. PASSO, MD**

BASIC INFORMATION

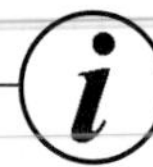

DEFINITION

Molluscum contagiosum is a benign, asymptomatic, self-limited, cutaneous viral infection caused by poxvirus. It affects children, sexually active adults, and immunocompromised individuals.

ICD-9-CM CODE
078.0 Molluscum contagiosum

EPIDEMIOLOGY & DEMOGRAPHICS

- Occurs worldwide
- Spread through direct contact with infected individuals and through autoinoculation
- Also spread through contact with contaminated objects (fomites)
- Most commonly affects preschool and school-aged children
- Higher incidence in warm/tropical countries and more commonly seen with poor hygiene
- Higher association with contact sports, such as wrestling, and use of swimming pools
- Commonly involves the genital area in children and may occasionally be spread by sexual abuse
- Also occurs in young adults in the genital area and thighs as a result of sexual transmission
- Commonly seen in immunosuppressed individuals, occurring in 5% to 18% of patients with human immunodeficiency virus (HIV)
- Incubation period 2 weeks to 6 months
  - Individual lesions last 2 months.
  - Entire episode lasts 9 months to 2 or more years.

CLINICAL PRESENTATION

- Individual lesions are flesh-colored or pearly pink dome-shaped papules.
  - Umbilicated center
  - Sizes ranging from 1 to 5 mm
- May express cheesy, curdlike material from the center
- May occur anywhere on the body
  - Tends to cluster in one or two areas, especially skin folds (axillae, neck, inguinal creases)
- Usually fewer than 20 lesions
  - May see hundreds, especially in immunocompromised individuals
- Usually asymptomatic
  - Pruritus or surrounding dermatitis may develop.
  - Occasionally, lesions become inflamed and bleed.
- May be cosmetically disfiguring, especially in advanced acquired immunodeficiency syndrome (AIDS), when lesions are numerous on the face and scalp
- May develop conjunctivitis if lesions are present around the eyelids

ETIOLOGY

- The molluscum contagiosum virus is a member of the poxvirus (Poxviridae) family and the sole member of the *Molluscipoxvirus* genus.
- The virus is a large, complex, double-stranded DNA virus that replicates in the cytoplasm of cells.
- The virus is especially adapted to the epidermis and infects only human beings.
- Three types of molluscum contagiosum viruses have been identified (i.e., MCV-I, MCV-II, and MCV-III), with no differences with respect to clinical presentation.

DIAGNOSIS (Dx)

DIFFERENTIAL DIAGNOSIS

- Flat warts
- Condyloma acuminata
- Syringoma
- Sebaceous hyperplasia
- Basal and squamous cell carcinoma
- Epidermal inclusion cyst
- Invasive fungal infection (e.g., cryptococcosis) in patients with HIV
- Pyogenic granuloma

WORKUP

- The diagnosis is usually clinically obvious when multiple lesions are present.
- The diagnosis is aided by freezing with liquid nitrogen, which accentuates umbilication.
- Lesions can be removed by curettage or tangential excision.
  - Crushed onto a microscope slide
  - Diagnostic intracytoplasmic inclusion bodies (Henderson-Patterson bodies)

TREATMENT (Rx)

NONPHARMACOLOGIC THERAPY

- Observation—disease is usually self-limited, but may continue to spread.
- Best to avoid overly aggressive or traumatic therapy
- Cryosurgery with liquid nitrogen is effective but limited by pain and blister formation.
- Cryotherapy followed by curettage with a sharp curette is standard and effective treatment.
- Complications of surgical therapy include:
  - Erythema
  - Altered pigment (usually hyperpigmentation)
  - Minor surface depression (usually resolves completely within 3 to 6 months)

ACUTE GENERAL Rx

- Trichloroacetic acid may be caustic to the skin.
- Cantharidin may cause severe blisters.
- Tretinoin may be applied by the patient daily to individual lesions.
- Topical cidofovir causes clearing of molluscum in patients with HIV (reported in several studies).
- Podophyllin is minimally effective.
- Imiquimod 5% cream, applied 5 to 7 days per week, has been shown to be effective in clearing molluscum.
- Treatment with griseofulvin, interferon, and cimetidine have not been shown to be consistently or universally effective.

DISPOSITION

- Patients may be treated every 2 to 4 weeks with topical chemical therapy until resolution.
- Following curettage of all lesions, patients should be observed for local recurrence, which usually occurs within 3 to 4 months; any new lesions can be treated similarly.

REFERRAL

Referral to a dermatologist is appropriate if lesions are numerous, spreading, or cosmetically disfiguring (on face) and if the primary physician is not trained in curettage of molluscum.

PEARLS & CONSIDERATIONS

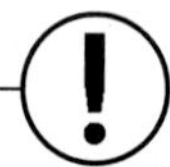

COMMENTS

- It is important to not make the treatment worse than the disease; avoid overly aggressive treatment, especially if painful or traumatic to the patient.
- It can be helpful to pretreat the skin with topical anesthetic (EMLA cream) 1 to 2 hours before curettage or cryotherapy.

PREVENTION

- Avoid known methods of transmission (i.e., contact sports, swimming pools, shared towels).
- Avoid scratching or traumatizing lesions, which can promote spread.

PATIENT/FAMILY EDUCATION

- Patients and parents need to be aware of the infectious nature and avoid methods of transmission: contact sports, swimming pools, shared towels.
- Patients and parents need to be aware of usual spontaneous resolution.
- Patients and parents need to be aware of frequent recurrences, even after successful treatment.

SUGGESTED READINGS

Lewis E et al: An update on molluscum contagiosum. *Cutis* 60:29, 1997.

Ordoukhanian E, Lane A: Warts and molluscum contagiosum. *Postgrad Med* 101:223, 1997.

Severson J, Tyring S: Viral disease update. *Curr Prob Dermatol* 11:37, 1999.

Skinner RB: Treatment of molluscum contagiosum with imiquimod 5% cream. *J Am Acad Dermatol* 47:S221, 2002.

Waugh M: Molluscum contagiosum. *Dermatol Clin* 16:839, 1998.

AUTHOR: **ALLISON L. HOLM, MD**

BASIC INFORMATION

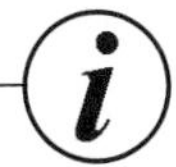

DEFINITION

Motion sickness refers to nausea and malaise resulting from motion, typically while traveling by boat, airplane, train, or automobile.

SYNONYMS

Airsickness
Carsickness
Seasickness

ICD-9-CM CODE
994.6 Motion sickness (also nausea marina)

EPIDEMIOLOGY & DEMOGRAPHICS

- The incidence and severity of symptoms vary with the intensity of the stimulus and the susceptibility of the individual.
- The incidence is as high as 100% in rough seas, 25% during moderate turbulence at sea, but 3% to 4% in the car, less than 1% in airplanes, and less than 0.2% on trains. The incidence of carsickness in children may be higher, but underreported.
- Motion sickness is most common in children 3 to 12 years old.
- More prevalent in females but this has recently been questioned.
- 55% of adults and 50% of children with migraines experience motion sickness.

CLINICAL PRESENTATION

- History reveals characteristic symptoms with motion or perceived motion:
  - Nausea, occasionally with vomiting
  - Malaise
  - Pallor or flushing
  - Sweating
  - Vertigo
  - Younger children may present with ataxia, most commonly gait abnormalities
  - Symptoms resolve when stimulus removed
- Physical exam is generally normal.

ETIOLOGY

- The exact physiologic mechanism is unknown, but it likely involves overload of peripheral receptors (in semicircular canals) as well as vestibular stimulation.
- Neurotransmitter metabolism abnormality.
- Mechanism results in increased gastric and intestinal motility which may produce symptoms of nausea and vomiting.

DIAGNOSIS

Dx

DIFFERENTIAL DIAGNOSIS

- Gastroenteritis
- Vasovagal response
- Presyncope
- Ménière's syndrome, vestibular neuronitis, labyrinthitis
- Benign paroxysmal vertigo
- Hypoglycemia
- Seizure
- Migraine

WORKUP

- History and physical examination should be performed to exclude other diagnoses.
  - Particularly consider migraine.
- Symptoms can be recreated using a stimulus such as a rotating optokinetic drum.
- No laboratory tests or imaging studies are indicated except to exclude other potential causes suggested by history or physical exam.

TREATMENT

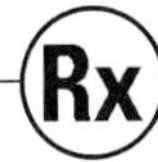

NONPHARMACOLOGIC THERAPY

- Keep children in a central location when traveling on a boat or airplane to reduce head and body movement.
- Focus on a stable horizon or other external object.
- Some studies with adults have suggested that eating less before travel, especially avoiding dairy and foods high in calories, sodium, and protein may reduce the incidence of motion sickness.
- Avoid visual stimuli such as reading, video games, and watching television or videos.

ACUTE GENERAL Rx

- Dimenhydrinate (Dramamine)
  - Sedating and may cause blurred vision, dry mouth, constipation
  - May also cause paradoxic agitation or central nervous system (CNS) stimulation
  - Generally ineffective if administered after the onset of symptoms
  - Dose 1.0 to 1.5 mg/kg/dose every 6 hours.
- Diphenhydramine (Benadryl)
  - Sedating; may cause blurred vision, dry mouth, congestion, constipation, urinary retention, dizziness, confusion
  - May also cause paradoxic agitation or CNS stimulation; rarely seizures
  - Dose 1.25 mg/kg/dose every 6 hours.
- Meclizine (Antivert)
  - Not studied in children under 12 years.
  - Sedating but may cause agitation, blurred vision, dry mouth, constipation, urinary retention, confusion
  - Dose 12.5 to 25.0 mg every 12 hours.
- Promethazine (Phenergan)
  - Sedating and may cause blurred vision, dry mouth, dizziness, confusion
  - May produce extrapyramidal symptoms (dystonic reaction which may generally be relieved with diphenhydramine)
  - Effective even if symptoms have already begun
  - Not approved for children under 2 years.
  - Dose 0.5 mg/kg/dose every 12 hours.
- Scopolamine (Transderm Scop)
  - Not approved for children <12 years.
  - Anticholinergic and side effects may include sedation, blurred vision (pupillary dilation), dry mouth, skin rash, confusion, dizziness, nightmares, hallucinations
  - Dosing is 1.5 mg patch behind ear every 72 hours

COMPLEMENTARY & ALTERNATIVE MEDICINE

- Ginger or ginger root has shown mixed results in motion sickness but does not appear to have any significant adverse effects.
  - Dosing:
    - 3 to 6 years old: 80 mg four times a day
    - 6 to 12 years old: 125 mg four times a day
    - More than 12 years old: 250 mg four times a day
- Acupressure and acupuncture have positive results in adults with postoperative nausea. One study showed benefit for acupressure in seasickness. The few studies in children have mainly been on postoperative nausea and show mixed results.
- One study found biofeedback to be superior to promethazine for motion sickness.
- Green tea is reportedly useful but reliable studies are lacking.

DISPOSITION

- Most patients adapt to continued motion stimulus over a few days.
- Susceptibility generally diminishes with age, but may persist into adulthood.

REFERRAL

As dictated by history and physical exam if symptoms are thought to arise from a cause other than motion sickness.

PEARLS & CONSIDERATIONS

COMMENTS

- Most medications can be sedating and many can cause paradoxic agitation and other significant side effects.
- Advise parents to complete a trial of any planned medications for motion sickness at home prior to travel.
- Consider the possibility of childhood migraine, particularly in patients with severe motion sickness.

PREVENTION

- See "Nonpharmacologic Theraphy."
- Administer medication before beginning travel or exposure to motion.

PATIENT/FAMILY EDUCATION

Numerous patient handouts are available.

SUGGESTED READINGS

Klein JR, Kennedy BC: Children in the wilderness. *In* Auerbach PS (ed): *Wilderness Medicine,* 4th ed. Mosby, 2001, p 1752.
Stauffer WM et al: "Stop the car, Mom I'm going to be sick!" *Contemp Pediatr* 19:43, 2002.
WebMd web site. Available at www.webmd.com/hw/ear_disorders/uF4438.asp

AUTHOR: **MICHAEL K. VISICK, MD**

BASIC INFORMATION

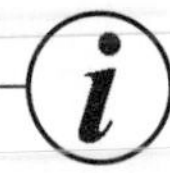

DEFINITION

Mumps is a systemic acute viral illness characterized by swelling of one or both parotid glands.

ICD-9-CM CODES
072.0 Mumps orchitis
072.8 Mumps with complication
072.9 Mumps

EPIDEMIOLOGY & DEMOGRAPHICS

- Humans are the only host.
- The virus is spread by contact with respiratory secretions.
- The disease is generally benign in childhood.
- Severe complications, such as orchitis, may occur in adults.
- The disease should be reported to national regulatory health agencies.
- Death is rare.
- In the prevaccine era, mumps was much more common with winter and spring epidemics every 4 years.
- Little seasonal variation and a 99% decrease in incidence have been noted since the availability of the vaccine.

CLINICAL PRESENTATION

- Incubation period is 14 to 18 days.
- A nonspecific prodrome lasts 1 to 2 days.
- Approximately 20% of patients have subclinical and another 40% to 50% have a mild respiratory illness.
- Parotid swelling bilateral in 70% is the most common clinical manifestation and occurs in 30% to 40% of infections.
- Fever (38.9°C to 39.4°C maximum)
- Anorexia
- Headache
- Vomiting
- Generalized achiness, vague abdominal pain
- Nuchal rigidity (aseptic meningitis)
- Erythema of parotid ducts (Stensen's duct), which open onto the buccal mucosa near the upper second molar, or Wharton's ducts, the ducts of the submaxillary gland, which open at the base of the tongue
- Parotid swelling: swelling over lower jaw and cheek, anterior to auricle, extending behind and under the angle of jaw
- Brawny edema with indiscreet borders
- May be tender to palpation
- Maximum swelling at 3 days
- Resolves slowly after 2 days
- Possible involvement of submaxillary and subungual glands
- May have limited jaw opening

Associated Complications

- Meningoencephalitis
- Epididymitis
- Orchitis (up to 50% of postpubertal males develop this complication). Testicular atrophy and sterility are rare.
- Pancreatitis
- Associated with diabetes mellitus
- Nephritis
- Hearing loss
- Congenital infection
- Increased fetal loss in the first trimester
- No known congenital syndrome

ETIOLOGY

Mumps is an RNA virus of the genus *Paramyxovirus* in the Paramyxovirus family.

DIAGNOSIS

DIFFERENTIAL DIAGNOSIS

- Bacterial parotitis
- Parotid duct stone
- Drug reaction
- Parotid tumor, Sjögren's syndrome
- Other viral causes of parotitis: coxsackie A virus, echovirus, parainfluenza viruses 1, 2, 3, human immunodeficiency virus (HIV).
- Lymphadenopathy (LAN)
  - Anterior cervical and submandibular LAN often confused with parotitis
- Mandibular disease: tumor of jaw (i.e., neuroblastoma), osteomyelitis.
- Consider mumps in the following: meningitis, meningoencephalitis, encephalitis.

LABORATORY TESTS

- Viral isolation from one of the following within first 5 days of illness: saliva, urine, cerebrospinal fluid.
- Serology
  - Positive immunoglobulin M (IgM)
  - Rise in immunoglobulin G (IgG) with paired sera separated by several weeks

TREATMENT

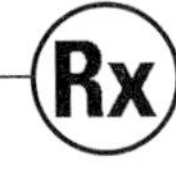

NONPHARMACOLOGIC THERAPY

- Supportive and comfort measures are sufficient in uncomplicated cases of mumps.
- No current antiviral agent is available.
- Postexposure prophylaxis with immunoglobulin is not recommended.

REFERRAL

Consultation with a pediatric infectious disease specialist may be warranted in complicated cases.

PEARLS & CONSIDERATIONS

COMMENTS

- Inapparent infection is more common in adults.
- Classic parotitis is most common in children between the ages of 2 to 9 years.

PREVENTION

- Vaccine—live, attenuated virus.
- Monovalent or in combination (measles-mumps-rubella, preferred)
- The vaccine produces a subclinical, noncommunicable infection
- Antibodies develop in 97% of susceptible children.
- Lifelong immunity
- The first dose should be administered on or after the first birthday.
- A second dose should be given in accordance with vaccine recommendations, preferably between 4 and 6 years of age.
- Vaccinate the adolescent if not previously vaccinated to prevent increased morbidity associated with disease in this group.
- Consider the patient susceptible if born after 1957, without documentation of vaccination, physician-diagnosed illness, or titers confirming infection.
- Adverse events:
  - Most often associated with the measles component of the combination vaccine
  - Fever in 5% to 15%, 7 to 12 days after receiving the vaccine
  - Rashes in 5% of vaccine recipients
  - Transient thrombocytopenia
  - Rare hypersensitivity reactions
  - Aseptic meningitis associated with the Urabe strain but not with the current U.S. strain (Jeryl-Lynn strain)
- Vaccination precautions
  - Minor illnesses with fever are not a contraindication.
  - Egg allergy is not a contraindication to vaccination.
  - History of receiving immunoglobulin (see Measles in Diseases and Disorders [Section]) requires special considerations.
- Immunodeficient host
  - Live virus should not be given to severely immunodeficient children.
  - An interval of at least 3 months should be observed after cessation of any immunosuppressive therapy.
  - High-dose corticosteroids necessitate waiting for an interval of 1 month.
  - HIV infection is not a contraindication unless the child is severely immunocompromised (low CD4 T-lymphocyte counts).
  - Pregnant women should not receive the vaccine.
  - Counsel to avoid conception for 3 months after mumps vaccination.
- Secondary prevention
  - Exclude known infected children from schools and day care.
  - Exclude known susceptible children until vaccination occurs.
  - Exclude unvaccinated children (for religious, medical, or other reasons) at least 26 days from onset of last case.

SUGGESTED READING

Pickering LK: Mumps. *In* Pickering LK (ed) *Red Book: 2003 Report of the Committee on Infectious Diseases*, 26th ed. Elk Grove Village, IL, American Academy of Pediatrics, 2003, pp 439–443.

AUTHOR: **MAUREEN NOVAK, MD**

BASIC INFORMATION

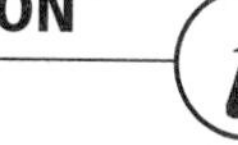

DEFINITION

Munchausen syndrome by proxy (MSBP) is a form of child maltreatment in which caretakers exaggerate, feign, or induce symptoms or illness in children in search of attention and personal gratification for themselves.

SYNONYMS

Factitious disorder by proxy
Meadow's syndrome
Pediatric falsification syndrome
Polle's syndrome

ICD-9-CM CODE
301.51 Munchausen syndrome by proxy (MSBP)

EPIDEMIOLOGY & DEMOGRAPHICS

- Children are affected equally with respect to gender and birth order.
- Perpetrator characteristics are as follows:
  - The patient's mother in 76%
  - Often has training in a medical field
  - May have an affective or personality disorder
  - May have experienced physical or sexual abuse as a child
- Duration from onset of symptoms to diagnosis is months to years.
- Mean age at diagnosis is 20 to 22 months.
- Children 5 years of age with MSBP are likely to have developmental delay.
- 55% of children have other chronic illness.
- One incidence study from Great Britain found the following:
  - 2.8 per 100,000 children younger than 1 year of age
  - 0.5 per 100,000 children younger than 16
- The mortality rate is 6% to 33%.
- 25% of victims' known siblings are dead.

CLINICAL PRESENTATION

- Gathering a meticulous history is crucial; poor history taking has been implicated in contributing to the misdiagnosis of MSBP.
- There is no typical history; the most common presentations include the following:
  - Seizures
  - Bleeding
  - Central nervous system depression
  - Apnea
  - Vomiting or diarrhea
  - Fever
  - Rash
- A few generalizations can be made:
  - The child's medical problems have not responded as expected to therapy.
  - The child's medical course has been unusual in some way.
  - Family history may elicit numerous medical problems that seem implausible.
  - Others have unexplained illness while under the supervision of the caregiver.
- There may be signs of physical abuse, neglect, or failure to thrive.
- Signs and symptoms of child's illness fail to occur in the caregiver's absence.

ETIOLOGY

- Many practitioners believe that MSBP is symptomatic of a psychiatric disturbance in the perpetrator, who acts in a premeditated way, rather than out of acute frustration or rage.
- Some argue that MSBP is a product of many factors:
  - A parent who has the capacity for abuse and the potential to be gratified by the medical system
  - A medical system that is specialized, investigation oriented, fascinated by rare conditions, often ignorant of abusive behaviors, and accepting of reported histories
- Caregivers may do any combination of the following:
  - Give a false story of illness
  - Fabricate a sign of illness
  - Interfere with test results

DIAGNOSIS

Dx

DIFFERENTIAL DIAGNOSIS

- The major obstruction in making the diagnosis is failure to consider MSBP.
- Many medical possibilities may need to be entertained as a cause for the symptoms.

WORKUP

- Hospitalization is required in most cases to protect the child.
- The workup should be individualized, remembering that a thorough history, physical examination, and observation alone may exclude many medical diagnoses.
- Videotaping in the hospital has been helpful; however, legal involvement is suggested if covert taping is planned.
- An empiric trial of foster care may be necessary for diagnosis.

TREATMENT

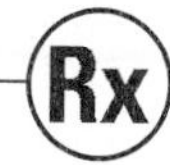

NONPHARMACOLOGIC THERAPY

- Counseling is important for both the patient and the family.
- In most cases of MSBP, removal of the child from the home is recommended.
- Foster care with an unrelated caregiver is preferred to kinship care, where the perpetrator may still have access to the child.

ACUTE GENERAL Rx

Medical therapy is supportive and related to any harm inflicted on the child.

CHRONIC Rx

Long-term counseling may be necessary for both child and perpetrator.

DISPOSITION

- Medical stability and safety of the child must be considered when discussing disposition.
- Mortality and morbidity rates are higher with MSBP than with other forms of child abuse.

REFERRAL

- Consultation with or between specialists is more helpful than referral to specialists.
- Child psychiatry referral may be helpful.
- If MSBP is suspected, a hospital-based child maltreatment team should be involved to ensure the safety of the child and to assist in reporting to state officials.

PEARLS & CONSIDERATIONS

COMMENTS

- MSBP often occurs in isolation, unlike other forms of child maltreatment.
- Anticonvulsants and opiates are the most common nonaccidental poisons used in MSBP.
- 8% of surviving victims of MSBP suffer long-term morbidity as a result of complications of the induced illness or complications from medical procedures.
- Many more develop psychologic difficulties.
- Multidisciplinary team involvement is crucial in MSBP.
  - The team should involve a physician, nurses, and social workers, as well as legal counsel, law enforcement, and a psychologist or psychiatrist.
  - A clinical epidemiologist may be helpful.
  - In the absence of data of commission, relative risk data may be the most compelling evidence available for court proceedings.
- Even with compelling evidence, MSBP is a difficult diagnosis to accept.
- Although diagnosis and intervention is painful for the family, health care providers also find the process extremely stressful and may benefit from counseling.

SUGGESTED READINGS

Child Abuse Evaluation and Treatment for Medical Practitioners. Available at http://www.Child-AbuseMD.com

Child Abuse Prevention Network. Available at http://child.cornell.edu

McClure RJ et al: Epidemiology of Munchausen syndrome by proxy, non-accidental poisoning, and non-accidental suffocation. *Arch Dis Child* 75:57, 1996.

Meadow R: Munchausen syndrome by proxy. *Arch Dis Child* 57:92, 1982.

National Clearinghouse on Child Abuse and Neglect. Available at http://nccanch.acf.hhs.gov

Rosenberg DA: Web of deceit: a literature review of Munchausen syndrome by proxy. *Child Abuse Negl* 11:547, 1987.

Sheridan MS: The deceit continues: an updated literature review of Munchausen syndrome by proxy. *Child Abuse Negl* 27(4):431, 2003.

AUTHOR: **JOELI HETTLER, MD**

BASIC INFORMATION

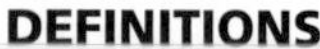

DEFINITIONS

- Muscular dystrophy (MD) is a Degenerative muscle disease causing progressive weakness, loss of ambulation usually by age 12, and death from respiratory and cardiac failure in the second decade of life (Duchenne MD).
- A milder form of the disease is known as Becker muscular dystrophy (BMD) in which the onset of weakness is later, ambulation is still possible beyond age 15, and the progression of weakness is slower.

SYNONYM

Dystrophinopathies

ICD-9-CM CODE

359.1 Muscular dystrophy

EPIDEMIOLOGY & DEMOGRAPHICS

- X-linked recessive inheritance
- Most common muscular dystrophy in children
- Incidence is 1 in 3500 male newborns; about 400 to 600 new cases every year.
- Onset of symptoms: 3 to 5 years (Duchenne); 5 to 15 years or later (Becker)

CLINICAL PRESENTATION

- Early signs include:
  - Delayed walking, toe walking, frequent falls, inability to jump or run, difficulty keeping up with peers
  - Difficulty getting up from a sitting or lying position (Gower's sign)
  - Waddling gait
  - Calf muscle pseudohypertrophy
- Loss of ambulation usually occurs by age 12 in Duchenne MD and after age 15 in BMD.
- Other signs include:
  - Cardiomyopathy
  - Respiratory failure in the late stages
  - Scoliosis
  - Gastric hypomotility
  - Central nervous system manifestations in about one third: delayed speech, decreased verbal ability, impaired intellectual function (nonprogressive)

ETIOLOGY

- Caused by the absence or deficiency of dystrophin, a subsarcolemmal cytoskeletal protein essential for the histologic integrity and membrane function of skeletal muscle
- Mutations in the dystrophin gene (Xp21 band)
- About one third of cases caused by de novo gene mutation while the rest are inherited in an X-linked recessive pattern

DIAGNOSIS

DIFFERENTIAL DIAGNOSIS

- Other muscular dystrophies: limb girdle (LGMD), Emery-Dreifuss, fascio-scapulo-humeral (FSH), myotonic dystrophy I and II
- Congenital myopathies
- Inflammatory myopathy (polymyositis, dermatomyositis)
- Spinal muscular atrophy (SMA)

WORKUP

- Gene test done in peripheral blood sample: dystrophin gene deletion (65%), duplication (5%), or point mutation (30%)
- Muscle biopsy: dystrophic features
- Immunostaining of muscle: decreased or absent dystrophin
- Western blot (on fresh frozen muscle specimen): dystrophin reduced in size or amount (Becker), or absent (Duchenne)
- Electromyocardiogram: myopathic

LABORATORY TEST

- Creatine phosphokinase: markedly elevated (>10 times the upper normal level)

IMAGING STUDIES

- Spine radiographs to monitor scoliosis
- Echocardiogram may show cardiomyopathy

TREATMENT

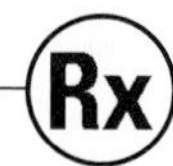

NONPHARMACOLOGIC THERAPY

- Physical therapy, aquatic therapy, occupational therapy: to maintain mobility and independence as long as possible, prevent tendon contractures, provide adaptive equipment at home and school
- Braces: to assist and prolong ambulation
- Psychosocial therapy: to provide support and assistance to patients and families
- Bilevel positive airway pressure supports respiratory function in late stages
- Tracheostomy and ventilatory support in late stages
- Spinal fusion decreases progression of restrictive pulmonary disease and prolong survival. Recommended for curvatures of 35 degrees or more in patients with acceptable pulmonary parameters for surgery.
- Heel cord lengthening improves standing and walking

CHRONIC Rx

- Corticosteroids have been shown to increase strength, improve pulmonary function, and prolong ambulation. Usually start at age 5 years, prednisone 0.75 mg/kg/day
- Angiotensin-converting enzyme inhibitors and β-blockers if needed for cardiomyopathy

DISPOSITION

- Regular visits to neuromuscular center for overall management and corticosteroid treatment
- Also periodic visits to:
  - Cardiologist to monitor for development of cardiomyopathy and therapy
  - Pulmonologist to monitor pulmonary function and initiate ventilatory support
  - Physical therapist: to monitor orthotic device and wheelchair adjustments

REFERRAL

- All patients should be referred to a neuromuscular center with expertise in treating children with muscular dystrophy.
- Muscular Dystrophy Association-(MDA) sponsored clinics are ideal because of a multidisciplinary approach.

PEARLS & CONSIDERATIONS

COMMENTS

- Some general anaesthetics may cause rhabdomyolysis.
- Female carriers can be symptomatic (manifesting carriers).

PREVENTION

- Genetic counseling can be performed for carrier detection and prenatal diagnosis.
- DNA studies on chorionic villus sample done at 6 to 8 weeks postconception.
- DNA, immunoblot, or immunostain tests employed to diagnose affected children can be used for carrier detection.
- Definite carrier: female with more than one son affected or with one son affected and either a brother or maternal uncle affected
- Possible carrier: female with only one affected son or with an affected brother or maternal male relative

PATIENT/FAMILY EDUCATION

- Support groups through the MDA: www.mdausa.org
- Parent Project MD: (1-800-714-kids); www.parentprojectmd.org
- GeneTests. Available at www.geneclinics.org

SUGGESTED READINGS

Brooke MH et al: Duchenne dystrophy: patterns of clinical progression and effects of supportive therapy. *Neurology* 39:475, 1989.

Eagle M et al: Survival in Duchenne dystrophy: improvements in life expectancy since 1967 and the impact of home nocturnal ventilation. *Neuromusc Disord* 12:926, 2002.

Hoffman EP et al: Dystrophinopathies. *In* Karpati G et al (eds): *Disorders of Voluntary Muscle.* Cambridge, Cambridge University Press, 2001, pp 385–432.

Moxley RT et al: Practice parameter: corticosteroid treatment of Duchenne dystrophy: report of the AAN and CNS. *Neurology* 64:13, 2005.

AUTHOR: **EMMA CIAFALONI, MD**

BASIC INFORMATION

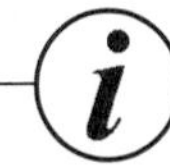

DEFINITION

Myasthenia gravis (MG) is an acquired autoimmune disease in which autoantibodies against the acetylcholine receptor (AChR) at the neuromuscular junction (NMJ) cause impaired neuromuscular transmission, leading to fluctuating weakness of skeletal muscles, causing diplopia, ptosis, dysarthria, dysphagia, and limb weakness. Transient neonatal myasthenia gravis affects 10% to 20% of newborns of myasthenic mothers. Symptoms occur 12 to 48 hours after birth and include generalized muscle weakness and hypotonia, difficulty feeding, feeble cry, ptosis, facial paresis, and respiratory distress. Spontaneous resolution usually occurs within 1 month.

SYNONYMS

Acquired myasthenia
Autoimmune myasthenia
MG
Myasthenia, generalized myasthenia
Ocular myasthenia

ICD-9-CM CODES

358.0 Myasthenia gravis without acute exacerbation; myasthenia gravis not otherwise specified
358.1 Myasthenia gravis with acute exacerbation; myasthenia gravis in crisis

EPIDEMIOLOGY & DEMOGRAPHICS

- MG is the most common disorder of the neuromuscular junction.
- The prevalence is 5 to 14 cases per 100,000 people.
- Onset can occur at any age.
- Girls and young women are more commonly affected than boys and men.
  - The female-to-male ratio is 6:4.
  - The mean age at onset is 28 years among women and 42 years among men.
- Familial acquired MG is rare (1% to 2%).
- Between 10% and 20% of newborns of myasthenic mothers develop transient symptoms.

CLINICAL PRESENTATION

- Muscle weakness and fatigability is improved by rest and exacerbated by sustained exertion, physical and emotional stress, temperature elevation, menses, infections, and certain drugs, such as aminoglycosides, magnesium, β-blockers, and calcium channel blockers (Table 1-16). Spontaneous remission is possible but rare.
- Diplopia and ptosis (i.e., ocular MG) can be the sole symptoms. They are frequently the presenting symptoms and are eventually seen in most patients with generalized MG.
- Different degrees of fluctuating limb weakness (i.e., generalized MG) may be observed.
- The patient may have difficulty with chewing and swallowing.
- The examiner may find slurred speech, flat smile, drooling, jaw weakness, or a droopy face.
- Patients may have shortness of breath, weak cough, or respiratory failure.

ETIOLOGY

- Autoimmune attack on the postsynaptic membrane of the NMJ is mediated by B and T lymphocytes.
- AChR antibody binding to the AChR complex and complement fixation reduce the available binding sites for ACh molecules and damage the postsynaptic membrane.
- Transient neonatal MG is caused by transplacental passive transfer of maternal AChR antibodies.
- MG frequently is associated with thymic hyperplasia, especially in young female patients.
- Thymoma occurs in about 10% of MG cases; it is rare in children.
- Other autoimmune disorders that are frequently associated with MG include pernicious anemia, rheumatoid arthritis, thyroid disease, and systemic lupus erythematosus (SLE).

DIAGNOSIS

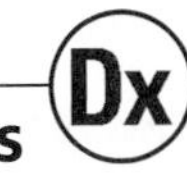

DIFFERENTIAL DIAGNOSIS

- Congenital myasthenic syndromes (caused by genetic abnormalities of the NMJ)
- Infantile botulism
- Mitochondrial diseases (e.g., progressive external ophthalmoplegia [PEO], Kearns-Sayre syndrome)
- Hypothyroidism
- Amyotrophic lateral sclerosis (ALS)
- Guillain-Barré syndrome (GBS)
- Oculopharyngeal muscular dystrophy (a late-onset disease)
- Conversion reaction

WORKUP

- Electrodiagnostic testing includes repetitive nerve stimulation and single-fiber electromyography (SFEMG).
- Tensilon test (i.e., edrophonium chloride) is positive when objective improvement of weakness is observed. Administer 2 mg intravenously and observe for 1 minute; if there is no improvement after 1 minute, an additional 3-mg dose is given. If there is no improvement after 1 minute, the remaining dose of 5 mg is given. Because of potential muscarinic side effects (e.g., bradycardia, bronchospasm), atropine should be readily available.
- The ice test differentiates myasthenic from nonmyasthenic eyelid ptosis. The palpebral fissure increases at least 2 mm immediately after application of ice to the eye and within 2 minutes, ptosis is resolved in 80% of patients with MG.

LABORATORY TESTS

- Serum AChR antibodies (binding, blocking, modulating) are detected in about 80% of generalized and 50% of purely ocular cases.
- Anti-striatal antibody titer is found in late-onset cases or when thymoma is present.
- Anti-MuSK (muscle-specific receptor tyrosine kinase) antibody is present in about 50% to 70% of seronegative MG patients.
- Thyroid function tests are used to evaluate for concomitant thyroid disease (frequently associated with MG).

IMAGING STUDIES

- Chest computed tomography or magnetic resonance imaging is used to rule out thymoma.
- Iodinated contrast agents may exacerbate MG symptoms and should be avoided.

TREATMENT

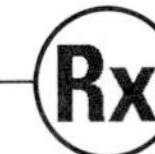

NONPHARMACOLOGIC THERAPY

- Thymectomy is mandatory if thymoma is present. It is recommended for patients 50 years old or younger.
- Plasmapheresis is used for fast improvement, in severe cases, and during myasthenic crises (i.e., respiratory failure).

TABLE 1-16 Drugs to Be Avoided or Used with Caution in Myasthenia Gravis

D-Penicillamine and interferon-α should not be used in myasthenic patients, because they can cause myasthenia gravis (MG).

Botulinum toxin should be avoided.

Increased weakness has occurred in a significant number of MG patients with the following drugs, which should be used only with caution and while monitoring for exacerbation of MG symptoms:

Neuromuscular blocking agents, such as succinylcholine and vecuronium*
Quinine, quinidine, or procainamide
Selected antibiotics, particularly aminoglycosides and ciprofloxacin†
β-Blockers, such as propranolol and timolol maleate eye drops
Calcium channel blockers
Iodinated contrast agents‡
Magnesium salts

*Should be used only by an anesthesiologist familiar with MG.
†Many other antibiotics have been reported to increase MG weakness in some patients.
‡Form of radiographic dye.

ACUTE GENERAL Rx

- Plasmapheresis
- Intravenous immunoglobulin (IVIG)
- Ventilatory support during myasthenic crisis

CHRONIC Rx

- Pyridostigmine (Mestinon)
- Prednisone
- Azathioprine (Imuran)
- Mycophenolate mofetil (CellCept)
- Cyclosporine (Neoral, Sandimmune)

DISPOSITION

- Patients with MG should be regularly followed by a neurologist or neuromuscular specialist.
  - Physicians should monitor patients' muscle strength, respiratory function, bulbar function, response to treatments, and the side effects of long-term immunosuppression.
  - More frequent visits are recommended before operations or periods of stress and intercurrent illnesses, when myasthenic exacerbations may occur.
  - Women of child-bearing age with MG considering pregnancy should seek counseling before pregnancy from their neurologist to maximize clinical improvement, to minimize the use of immunosuppressive drugs, and to be educated about the potential risks to themselves (i.e., MG exacerbation) and the fetus (e.g., transient neonatal MG, arthrogryposis) related to pregnancy, delivery, and the postpartum period.

REFERRAL

- Patients with suspected or definite MG should be referred to a neurologist with experience in the management of this disease or to a neuromuscular specialist.
- Neuromuscular and Muscular Dystrophy Association-sponsored clinics are ideal.

PEARLS & CONSIDERATIONS

COMMENTS

- MG should be strongly considered in a child with new-onset ptosis, diplopia, dysphagia, dysarthria, or muscle weakness that fluctuates from day to day or during the course of the day.
- Check for the potential effect on neuromuscular transmission before prescribing a new drug.

PREVENTION

Avoid exacerbation triggers, such as heat, overexertion, or drugs that impair neuromuscular transmission.

PATIENT/FAMILY EDUCATION

- The Muscular Dystrophy association: www.mdausa.org
- The Myasthenia Gravis Foundation of America has chapters around the country with support group meetings for patients and their families. Their web site (www.mgfa.org) has updated educational material for patients.

SUGGESTED READINGS

Andrews PI et al: Autoimmune myasthenia gravis in childhood. *Semin Neurol* 24:101, 2004.

Ciafaloni E et al: Mycophenolate Mofetil for myasthenia gravis: an open label pilot study. *Neurology* 56:97, 2001.

Ciafaloni E et al: The management of myasthenia gravis in pregnancy. *Semin Neurol* 24:95, 2004.

Ciafaloni E et al: Treatment of myasthenia gravis: current practice and future directions. *Expert Rev Neurother* 2:743, 2002.

Gronseth GS et al: Practice parameter: thymectomy for autoimmune myasthenia gravis (an evidence-based review): report of the quality standards subcommittee of the American Academy of Neurology. *Neurology* 55:7, 2000.

Howard JF et al: Intravenous immunoglobulin for the treatment of acquired myasthenia gravis. *Neurology* 51:30, 1998.

Lindstrom JM et al: Acetylcholine receptors and myasthenia. *Muscle Nerve* 23:453, 2000.

Sanders DB et al: Clinical aspect of MuSK antibody positive seronegative MG. *Neurology* 60:1978, 2003.

AUTHOR: **EMMA CIAFALONI, MD**

BASIC INFORMATION

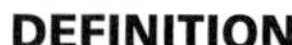
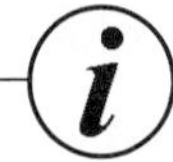

DEFINITION

Mycoplasma pneumoniae is a pleomorphic microorganism with a double-stranded DNA genome and no cell wall that predominantly causes infections in children and adolescents.

SYNONYM

Atypical pneumonia.

ICD-9-CM CODE

483.0 Pneumonia caused by *Mycoplasma pneumoniae*

EPIDEMIOLOGY & DEMOGRAPHICS

- Highest rate of infection is in school-age children with no gender predilection.
- Endemic in large urban areas, especially in temperate climates.
- Can also cause epidemics of infection.
- Transmission is via large droplet, respiratory secretions.
- Spread is slow but occurs during close contact with symptomatic person in acute phase of illness.
- Organisms shed 2 to 8 days before clinical symptoms; present in secretions for more than 4 to 6 weeks
- Incubation: 1 to 4 weeks

CLINICAL PRESENTATION

- Symptoms nonspecific: fever, malaise, headache, cough, upper respiratory tract complaints (pharyngitis, otitis media, myringitis)
- Coryza less common except in young children
- Respiratory disease most common manifestation: atypical and community-acquired pneumonia, bronchitis
  - Cough can persist for more than 4 weeks
  - Can be associated with wheezing especially in those with asthma
  - Pneumonia less common in infants and toddlers (<2 years of age)
  - Rales common on physical exam of children with pneumonia
  - Associated with acute chest syndrome in patients with sickle cell disease
- Systemic manifestations of infection less common but can occur without clinically apparent pulmonary disease: onset 1 day and up to 3 weeks after respiratory symptoms
- Neurologic: encephalitis, meningitis, ataxia, transverse myelitis, polyradiculitis, neuropathy, muscle weakness, Guillain-Barré syndrome, stroke
- Rheumatologic: arthritis, arthralgias
- Hematologic: hemolytic anemia, bone marrow suppression
- Cardiac: myocarditis, pericarditis
- Dermatologic: erythematous maculopapular exanthem, *Erythema multiforme*, Stevens-Johnson
- Gastrointestinal: hepatitis, pancreatitis

ETIOLOGY

- Immunologic response to infection M. pneumoniae includes specific antibody production (immunoglobulin G [IgG], immunoglobulin M [IgM], and immunoglobulin A [IgA]) against organism and specific lymphocyte stimulation in older children.
- Antibody response to diverse antigens
- Etiology of extrapulmonary disease unknown, postulated etiologies include: dissemination/direct invasion; immunologic response to infection; production of neurotoxin (central nervous system disease); vasculopathy/thrombosis

DIAGNOSIS

Dx

DIFFERENTIAL DIAGNOSIS

- Viruses: respiratory syncytial virus, parainfluenza and influenza, adenovirus
- Bacteria: *Streptococcus pneumoniae, Haemophilus influenzae, Bordetella pertussis*
- Others: *Chlamydia psittaci* and *pneumoniae, Coxiella burnetii, Histoplasma capsulatum, Coccidioides immitis, Mycoplasma tuberculosis*
- Of pneumonia: asthma; foreign body aspiration; acute chest syndrome; congestive heart failure/pulmonary edema
- No "gold standard" for diagnosis

LABORATORY TESTS

- Cold agglutinins (IgM autoantibody response to I antigen of red blood cells) correlates with severity of pulmonary disease; however has low specificity
- Specific antibody testing
  - Complement fixation of paired sera to identify fourfold rise in IgG antibody titers.
  - Enzyme-linked immunosorbent assay or immunofluorescence to detect IgM and IgG antibodies, and then rise in titers
- Polymerase chain reaction of nasopharyngeal secretions, blood, cerebrospinal fluid (CSF), urine, tissue
- Culture less useful—organism slow growing
- White blood cell count variable, usually normal
- Erythrocyte sedimentation rate usually elevated
- CSF white blood cell count and protein may be elevated in patients with neurologic disease.
- Increased transaminases in patients with liver involvement; elevated amylase and lipase in patients with pancreatitis
- Positive Coombs test and elevated reticulocyte count in patients with hemolysis, anemia if severe hematologic disease

IMAGING STUDIES

Chest radiograph commonly demonstrates diffuse, bilateral infiltrates. Extent of radiographic findings do not usually correlate with degree of clinical illness.

TREATMENT

Rx

NONPHARMACOLOGIC THERAPY

Supportive care; upper respiratory illness self-limiting

ACUTE GENERAL Rx

- Antibiotics recommended for pneumonia/lower respiratory tract infections caused by *Mycoplasma* although insufficient evidence in literature about efficacy
- Empiric coverage for *Mycoplasma* recommended for children and adolescents with community-acquired pneumonia
- First-line therapy:
  - Macrolides including erythromycin (40 mg/kg/day divided every 6 to 8 hours for 10 days); azithromycin (10 mg/kg/day on day 1, followed by 5 mg/kg/d for 4 days; clarithromycin (15 mg/kg/day divided every 12 hours for 10 days)
  - Tetracycline and doxycycline for children older than 9 years of age
- Second-line therapy: Fluoroquinolones
- Evidence insufficient to support antibiotic therapy for other clinical manifestations
- Consider prophylaxis with macrolide for close household contacts or if at risk for severe disease

DISPOSITION

Home care unless severe disease or severe extrapulmonary manifestations

PEARLS & CONSIDERATIONS

COMMENTS

Most common clinical manifestation of disease involves respiratory tract. Consider *Mycoplasma* in differential of systemic diseases previously delineated.

PREVENTION

Droplet precautions

SUGGESTED READINGS

American Academy of Pediatrics: *Mycoplasma pneumoniae* infections. *In* Pickering LK (ed): *Red Book: 2003 Report of the Committee on Infectious Diseases,* 26th ed. Elk Grove Village, IL, American Academy of Pediatrics, 2003, pp 443–445.

Blasi F: Atypical pathogens and respiratory tract infections. *Eur Respir J* 24:171, 2004.

Broughton RA: Infections due to *Mycoplasma pneumoniae* in childhood. *Pediatr Infect Dis* 5(1):71, 1986.

Cherry JD, Ching N: *Mycoplasma* and *Ureaplasma* infections. *In* Feigin RD, Cherry JD (eds): *Textbook of Pediatric Infectious Diseases,* 5th ed. Philadelphia, Saunders, 2004, pp 2516–2547.

Gavranich JB, Chang AB: Antibiotics for community acquired lower respiratory tract infections (LRTI) secondary to *Mycoplasma pneumoniae* in children. *Cochrane Database Syst Rev* (3):CD004875, DOI:10.1002/14651858.CD004875.pub2, 2005.

Guleria R et al: *Mycoplasma pneumoniae* and central nervous system complications: a review. *J Lab Clin Med* Aug:55, 2005.

Michelow IC et al: Epidemiology and clinical characteristics of community-acquired pneumonia in hospitalized children. *Pediatrics* 113(4):701, 2004.

Neumayr L et al: *Mycoplasma* disease and acute chest syndrome in sickle cell disease. *Pediatrics* 112(1):87, 2003.

Schwartz R, Garty BZ: Variability of arthritis associated with *Mycoplasma pneumonia* infection in children. *Clin Pediatr* 44:633, 2005.

AUTHOR: **MARYELLEN E. GUSIC, MD**

BASIC INFORMATION

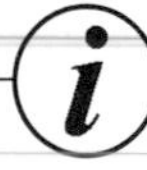

DEFINITIONS

- *Drowning:* death from suffocation in water
- *Near-drowning:* survival, at least temporarily, after suffocation in water
- *Secondary drowning:* death occurring longer than 24 hours after submersion secondary to severe respiratory decompensation (adult respiratory distress syndrome [ARDS], pulmonary edema)
- *Immersion syndrome:* death following submersion in extremely cold water

SYNONYM

Submersion injury: injuries resulting from submersion in water

ICD-9-CM CODES
518.5 Pulmonary insufficiency after trauma and surgery
994.1 Drowning and nonfatal submersion

EPIDEMIOLOGY & DEMOGRAPHICS

- Near-drowning accounts for 8000 deaths per year in the United States.
- It is the second most common cause of accidental death in children.
- Bimodal distribution is noted, most often affecting toddlers and adolescents.
- Toddlers most commonly drown in pools and bathtubs, occasionally in toilets or buckets of water.
- Adolescents most commonly drown in larger bodies of water (e.g., lakes, rivers, oceans).
- Approximately 90% of drownings occur in fresh water.
- About 50% occur in swimming pools.
- Prognosis is poor for patients presenting to the emergency department comatose or with cardiopulmonary resuscitation (CPR) in progress.

CLINICAL PRESENTATION

History

- The following key historical data need to be obtained:
  - Last time seen
  - Estimated length of submersion
  - Any possibility of diving-related injury (e.g., cervical spine injury)
  - Any possibility of other associated trauma
  - Ambient temperatures of water and air
  - Appearance when pulled from water (e.g., limp, blue, apneic, pulseless)
  - Resuscitation efforts at the scene and en route to hospital (e.g., mouth-to-mouth resuscitation, compressions, medications)
  - Estimated length of time until CPR begun, length of CPR
  - Any significant past medical history (e.g., seizures, asthma) or allergies
- Consider abuse or neglect (toddlers)—mechanism proposed in history should match actual physical findings
- Consider associated drug or alcohol intoxication (adolescents)

Physical Examination

- Begin with ABCs (airway, breathing, circulation).
- Careful attention should be given to breath sounds, pulse oximetry, respiratory effort, and mental status.
- Serial examination of respiratory status is most important because patients can rapidly decompensate.

ETIOLOGY

- Approximately 90% involve aspiration of fluid into lungs—usually less than 20 mL/kg.
- About 10% involve "dry drowning"—laryngospasm occurs, preventing aspiration of fluid.
- Fresh water inactivates surfactant, leading to alveolar collapse and pulmonary dysfunction.
- Salt water dilutes surfactant, leading to alveolar collapse and pulmonary dysfunction.
- Both salt and fresh water damage the basement membrane, leading to fluid shifts, ARDS, and pulmonary edema.
- The steps to death progress from aspiration of fluid to pulmonary dysfunction to hypoxemia to anoxic brain injury and cardiac decompensation to death.

DIAGNOSIS

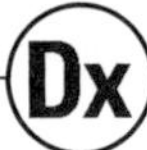

DIFFERENTIAL DIAGNOSIS

- Anoxic encephalopathy
- Cerebral edema
- Spinal cord injury
- Suspected child abuse and neglect
- Alcohol or drug intoxication
- Hypothermia
- Pneumonia, bacterial or viral
- Aspiration pneumonia

LABORATORY TESTS

- Blood should be obtained for a complete blood count, chemistry panel (electrolytes, blood urea nitrogen, creatinine, and glucose), and coagulation studies (prothrombin time, partial thromboplastin time, platelets, fibrinogen, and fibrin split products).
- Urine should be obtained for routine urinalysis and, if indicated, a toxicology screen.
- Monitor continuous pulse oximetry and, if indicated, obtain serial arterial blood gas analysis.

IMAGING STUDIES

- Follow serial chest radiographs.
- If indicated, obtain cervical spine or other skeletal films.
- Computed tomography scan of the brain may be indicated for persistent altered mental status.

TREATMENT

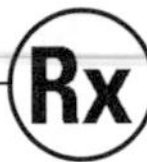

NONPHARMACOLOGIC THERAPY

- Keep the patient warm and dry.
- Intubation and artificial ventilation may be necessary.
- Positive end-expiratory pressure or continuous positive airway pressure is indicated for refractory hypoxemia.
- Extracorporeal membrane oxygenation has occasionally been used as a temporizing measure in extreme cases of refractory hypoxemia.

ACUTE GENERAL Rx

- Give oxygen if warranted.
- Monitor continuous pulse oximetry.
- Nebulized albuterol is indicated for bronchospasm.
- Furosemide (Lasix) may be indicated in the intensive care unit to maintain urine output and decrease fluid overload (cerebral edema).
- Muscle relaxation and sedation may be beneficial during the early phases of artificial ventilation.
- Advance life support drugs as per standard ACLS/PALS/APLS (Advance Cardiac Life Support/Pediatric Advanced Life Support/ Advanced Pediatric Life Support) protocols.
- Steroids (dexamethasone), prophylactic antibiotics, and barbiturates *are no longer routinely recommended.*

DISPOSITION

- Symptomatic patients should be admitted for observation.
- Completely asymptomatic patients may be safely discharged after observation for 4 to 6 hours.
- Patients with altered mental status, unstable vital signs, or significant hypoxemia should be admitted to a pediatric intensive care unit (PICU).

PEARLS & CONSIDERATIONS

COMMENTS

- Asymptomatic patients should be observed for a minimum of 4 to 6 hours.
- Symptomatic patients should be admitted to the hospital.
- Serial examinations are most helpful.
- In toddlers, consider child abuse and neglect.
- In adolescents, consider cervical spine injury and intoxications.
- Deterioration in respiratory function may be sudden and dramatic.

PREVENTION

- *Most drownings are preventable.*
- *Prevention is key!*

- Toddlers should never be left alone near a body of water. This includes not only the swimming pool, but also the bathtub, toilet, or cleaning bucket of water.
- Residential pools should be surrounded on all four sides by a security fence and have an automatic closing security gate with locking latch.
- Parents and families should be taught CPR, particularly if they own a pool.

PATIENT/FAMILY EDUCATION

- Patients and families should be strictly warned against the following activities:
  - Swimming unsupervised
  - Using drugs or alcohol
  - Diving into shallow or unknown waters
- Patients of suitable age should be instructed in swimming and water safety.

SUGGESTED READINGS

Aquatics Safety & Water Rescue. Available at http://www.lifesaving.com

Brain Injury Resource Center. Available at www.headinjury.com/

Byard RW, Donald T: Infant bath seats, drowning and near-drowning. *J Paediatr Child Health* 40:305, 2004.

Department of Boating and Waterways. Available at www.dbw.ca.gov/drown.htm

Drowning Fact Sheet. Available at http://cdc.gov/safeusa/water/water.htm

Drowning Prevention Safety. Available at http://www.preventdrowning.com

Foundation for Aquatic Injury Prevention (FAIP). Available at http://www.aquaticisf.org

Harries M: Near drowning. *BMJ* 327:1336, 2003.

Hwang V et al: Prevalence of traumatic injuries in drowning and near drowning in children and adolescents. *Arch Pediatr Adolesc Med* 157:50, 2003.

Ibsen LM, Koch T: Submersion and asphyxial injury. *Crit Care Med* 30(11 Suppl):S402, 2002.

Immersion Hypothermia & Cold Water Near-drowning. Available at http://scuba-doc.com/hypoth.htm

Peden MM, McGee K: The epidemiology of drowning worldwide. *Inj Control Saf Promot* 10:195, 2003.

Plubrakam R, Tamsamran S: Predicting outcome in pediatric near-drowning. *J Med Assoc Thai* 86(Suppl 3):S501, 2003.

Postgraduate Medicine Symposium on Near-drowning. Available at http://www.postgradmed.com/issues/1998/06_98/thanel.htm

Ross FI et al: Children under 5 years presenting to paediatricians with near-drowning. *J Paediatr Child Health* 39:446, 2003.

Water Safety. Available at http://www.watersafety.org

AUTHOR: **MARK A. HOSTETLER, MD, MPH**

BASIC INFORMATION

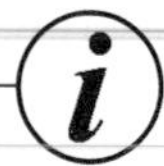

DEFINITION

Neonatal necrotizing enterocolitis (NEC) is an acute coagulation necrosis involving localized and multifocal areas of the small and large bowel mucosa in the newborn, more commonly preterm, infant.

ICD-9-CM CODE

777.5 Necrotizing enterocolitis

EPIDEMIOLOGY & DEMOGRAPHICS

- NEC is primarily a disease of premature infants in modern neonatal intensive care units, but it occurs occasionally in term infants.
- NEC is reported in 6% of infants born at 1500 g or less.
- Age of onset is inversely proportional to gestational age at birth.
- Occurs in first few days in term infants.
- Occurs at several weeks of age in premature infants.
- Peak incidence is at 32 to 33 weeks' gestational age.
- NEC often occurs sporadically in mini-epidemics during times of high nursery census and acuity.
- Additional risk factors include:
  - History of maternal cocaine use
  - Hemodynamically significant patent ductus arteriosus
  - Following double-volume exchange transfusions
  - Perinatal asphyxia

CLINICAL PRESENTATION

History

- Decreased activity, lethargy
- Apnea, bradycardia, tachypnea, temperature instability, hypotension
- Hypoxemia
- Feeding intolerance, residuals, vomiting
- Occult and gross blood in stools
- Increasing abdominal girth

Physical Examination

- Vital sign instability, hypotension
- Decreased activity and tone
- Abdominal wall redness and discoloration
- Abdominal distention, decreased bowel sounds, and tenderness to palpation
- Decreased peripheral perfusion

ETIOLOGY

- Unknown, possibly related to one or more of the following factors:
  - Bacterial invasion or overgrowth
  - Impaired intestinal perfusion
  - Rapid advancement of enteral feedings

DIAGNOSIS

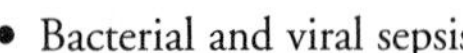

DIFFERENTIAL DIAGNOSIS

- Bacterial and viral sepsis
- Midgut malrotation with volvulus
- Isolated ileal perforation

LABORATORY TESTS

- Complete blood count
  - Low absolute neutrophil count
  - Increased band count
  - Low hematocrit secondary to blood loss
  - Thrombocytopenia
- Metabolic acidosis
- Elevated C-reactive protein
- Blood culture often positive
- May develop disseminated intravascular coagulation with fibrin-split products and abnormally prolonged coagulation (elevated prothrombin time and partial thromboplastin time)

IMAGING STUDIES

- Plain film of abdomen may show:
  - Pneumatosis intestinalis
  - Portal venous gas
  - Intestinal perforation with free air in the peritoneum

TREATMENT

NONPHARMACOLOGIC THERAPY

- Intestinal perforation requires immediate surgical intervention.
- Failure of medical management with persistent metabolic acidosis, hypotension, and thrombocytopenia may require surgical intervention to remove necrotic gut tissue.
- Surgical interventions depend on distribution, extent, and severity of bowel necrosis.
  - Intestinal resection followed by primary intestinal anastomosis or stoma placement.
  - Enterostomy with or without intestinal resection (placement of drains).

ACUTE GENERAL Rx

- Place patient on "nothing-by-mouth" (NPO) orders with low intermittent suction of stomach.
  - Use a double-lumen nasogastric tube (Replogle tube).
  - Maintain NPO orders until at least 7 to 10 days after resumption of normal radiograph.
- Pay careful attention to blood pressure, perfusion, and urine output.
- Administer volume expanders (normal saline, fresh frozen plasma, cryoprecipitate, and blood) to maintain hemodynamic stability and appropriate coagulation profiles.
- Administer packed red cells to maintain hematocrit at 40% to 45%.
- Administer platelet transfusions to maintain platelet count greater than 50,000/mm^3.
- After blood culture is drawn, initiate antibiotic coverage for gram-positive, gram-negative, and anaerobic organisms.
  - Usual choice is a combination of vancomycin, gentamicin, and clindamycin
- Provide parenteral nutrition.

DISPOSITION

- Have the patient complete a 10-day course of antibiotic therapy.
- Maintain NPO status for at least 7 to 10 days after documentation of a normal abdominal radiograph.
- Cholestatic jaundice may result from the prolonged use of total parenteral nutrition.
- Intestinal strictures, usually colonic, may develop.
- Feeding intolerance may develop with reinstitution of feeds.
- Short bowel syndrome may develop after the resection of extensive areas of bowel.

REFERRAL

Infants with NEC should be referred to a regional neonatal center that is staffed with neonatologists, pediatric surgeons, and pediatric radiologists.

PEARLS & CONSIDERATIONS

COMMENTS

"NEC is a riddle wrapped in a mystery inside an enigma."

PREVENTION

Breast milk feedings, when compared with milk formulas, are partially protective for the prevention of NEC.

SUGGESTED READINGS

Henry MC, Moss RL: Current issues in the management of necrotizing enterocolitis. *Semin Perinatol* 28:221, 2004.

Kafetzis DA et al: Neonatal necrotizing enterocolitis: an overview. *Curr Opin Infect Dis* 16:349, 2003.

Pierro A, Hall N: Surgical treatments of infants with necrotizing enterocolitis. *Semin Perinatol* 28:223, 2003.

AUTHOR: **JAMES W. KENDIG, MD**

BASIC INFORMATION

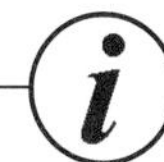

DEFINITION

Nephrotic syndrome (NS) is characterized by proteinuria (>40 mg/m^2/hr), hypoalbuminemia (<2.5 g/dL), edema, and hypercholesterolemia. Primary NS is a disease involving only the kidney, and it is not associated with extrarenal manifestations. Secondary NS occurs as a manifestation of systemic disease that involves the kidney, such as systemic lupus erythematosus (SLE), Henoch-Schönlein purpura (HSP), sickle cell anemia, or uncommonly acute poststreptococcal glomerulonephritis. Primary NS is addressed here.

SYNONYMS

Steroid-resistant nephrotic syndrome
  Diffuse mesangial proliferation
  Focal-segmental glomerulosclerosis (FSGS)
Steroid-sensitive nephrotic syndrome
  Idiopathic nephrotic syndrome
  Lipoid nephrosis
  Minimal change disease
  Nil disease

ICD-9-CM CODES

581.1 Focal segmental glomerulosclerosis (FSGS)
581.1 Membranous glomerulonephritis
581.2 Membranoproliferative glomerulonephritis (MPGN)
581.3 Minimal change nephrotic syndrome (MCNS)
581.9 Nephrotic syndrome, not otherwise specified

EPIDEMIOLOGY & DEMOGRAPHICS

- Age
  - NS affects children of all ages.
  - NS is rare in the first year of life.
  - Congenital NS typically manifests in the first 3 months of life.
- Steroid-sensitive nephrotic syndrome
  - Incidence varies with race, ethnicity, and age.
  - Incidence is estimated at approximately 2 to 2.7 cases per 100,000 children in the United States.
  - Cumulative U.S. prevalence is estimated to be 16 cases per 100,000 children.
- Gender
  - In young children, the male-to-female ratio is 2:1.
  - In adolescents, the male-to-female ratio is 1:1.
- MCNS accounts for 60% to 90% of NS cases among children and most cases among children younger than 7 years.
- In older children, other diagnoses become more prevalent.
- Genetics: increased incidence among family members
- FSGS
  - FSGS accounts for approximately 10% of children with NS.
  - The prevalence of FSGS may be increasing.
  - Approximately 20% of patients are steroid sensitive.

CLINICAL PRESENTATION

History

- Recent history of upper respiratory infection or other viral illness
- History of allergies
- Edema that is dependent
  - Insidious onset; often first noticed in the periorbital region in the morning
  - May be present for weeks
  - Often attributed to allergies
  - Progresses to lower extremities, abdomen, and can become generalized (i.e., anasarca)
- Weight gain
- Changes in urination
  - Decreased urine output
  - Gross hematuria unusual with MCNS
- Respiratory difficulty
  - Suggests pulmonary edema, pleural effusions, or significant abdominal distention
- Anorexia
- Diarrhea resulting from edema of the intestinal wall
- Vomiting
- Abdominal pain
  - May occur with peritonitis and be associated with fever
  - May occur with hypovolemia
  - May occur with rapid development of ascites
  - May occur with thrombosis
- Renal vein thrombosis is associated with gross hematuria and flank pain.
- Headaches
  - May suggest associated hypertension

Physical Examination

- Signs of volume overload
  - Periorbital edema
  - Decreased breath sounds, which suggest pleural effusions
  - Rales
  - Ascites
  - Presacral edema, scrotal or labial edema
  - Peripheral edema
  - Facial edema (difficult to assess when first seeing the child; often helpful to compare the current appearance with a photograph taken before the illness)
- Signs of intravascular volume depletion
  - Tachycardia
  - Hypotension
  - Poor perfusion
  - Dry mucous membranes
  - Orthostatic changes
- Signs of peritonitis
  - Fever
  - Abdominal pain
  - Distention
  - Rebound
  - Guarding
  - Tenderness
  - Absence of bowel sounds
- Signs of skin breakdown
  - Infection can spread quickly in nephrotic children.
- Rash or joint swelling
  - May suggest that the disease is a secondary form of NS

ETIOLOGY

- The cause of primary NS is unknown, but evidence suggests abnormal T-cell function in MCNS.
  - Response to immunomodulatory medications, such as prednisone
  - Relapses often associated with upper respiratory and other minor illness
  - Improves after measles
  - Increased frequency of atopy and allergies in children with MCNS
  - Associated with Hodgkin's lymphoma and non-Hodgkin's lymphoma
- Secondary NS occurs as a complication of other glomerular insults
  - SLE
  - HSP
  - Sickle cell anemia

DIAGNOSIS

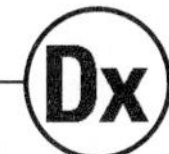

DIFFERENTIAL DIAGNOSIS

- Other renal diseases with edema include acute and chronic renal failure and other nephrotic-nephritic syndromes.
- Other causes of edema include the following:
  - States of protein loss (e.g., protein-losing enteropathy)
  - Decreased protein production (e.g., liver disease, liver failure)
  - Congestive heart failure

LABORATORY TESTS

- Urine studies: evaluation of proteinuria
  - Urinalysis with a 3 to 4+ protein value on the dipstick
  - Spot urine protein-to-creatinine ratio higher than 2.0 considered suspicious in conjunction with hypoalbuminemia
  - Protein excretion on timed urine collection of 40 mg/m^2/hr or more; timed collection not necessarily required for diagnosis
- Hematuria
  - Microscopic hematuria present in about 20% of cases of steroid-responsive NS
  - Gross hematuria unusual
- Microscopic examination of urine sediment may reveal hyaline casts and fat bodies
- Serum studies
  - Low level of total protein
  - Hypoalbuminemia (≤2.5 g/dL)
  - Hyperlipidemia
  - Creatinine
    - Low-normal serum creatinine level suggests hyperfiltration caused by proteinuria.
    - Elevated serum creatinine level may be caused by decreased renal perfusion.

- Hypocalcemia
  - Total calcium level is low because of hypoalbuminemia.
  - Ionized calcium level is typically normal.
- Hemoglobin: may be elevated because of hemoconcentration from intravascular volume depletion.
- Complement
  - The C3 level is normal in idiopathic NS.
  - A low C3 level suggests MPGN.
- Serologies to consider
  - Hepatitis B and C (possibly associated with MPGN and membranous nephropathy)
  - Human immunodeficiency virus (HIV)
  - Antinuclear antibodies (ANAs)

IMAGING STUDIES

- Imaging studies usually are not required.
- Renal ultrasound may show enlarged kidneys caused by interstitial edema.

TREATMENT

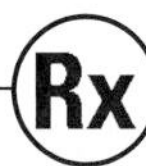

NONPHARMACOLOGIC THERAPY

- Low-salt diet for management of edema
- Recommended daily allowance (RDA) of protein intake for age
- Generally not fluid restricted unless severe hyponatremia
- Low-fat diet

ACUTE GENERAL Rx

- Spontaneous remission may occur within 1 to 2 weeks.
- Screen the patient for infection, including occult infection; place a purified protein derivative (PPD) test, anticipating chronic steroid use.
- Treatment by immunosuppression using corticosteroids
  - Initial episode
    - Prednisone dosage is 2 mg/kg/day or 60 mg/m^2/day (maximum, 80 mg) divided two to three times per day for 4 to 6 weeks.
    - If the patient responds and is in remission, change the regimen to alternate-day steroids (2 mg/kg every other day or 40 mg/m^2 every other day) for an additional 4 to 6 weeks.
    - If the patient continues in remission, steroids are tapered further and discontinued.
    - If the patient is not in remission after 4 to 6 weeks of daily steroids, refer the child to a pediatric nephrologist.
  - Side effects
    - Increased appetite, weight gain, change in appearance, moodiness or behavior changes, hypertension, infection, acne, cataracts, poor growth, osteopenia, peptic ulcers, glucose intolerance, avascular necrosis
    - Rare but serious side effects: pseudotumor cerebri, steroid psychosis, and steroid-related diabetes
- Edema management
  - Judicious use of diuretics (furosemide, 1 to 2 mg/kg) or albumin, or both, may be considered.
  - Monitor electrolytes for hyponatremia and hypokalemia.
  - Risk of severe intravascular volume depletion exists with aggressive diuresis and may be further complicated by development of thromboemboli.
  - Management includes 25% albumin (0.5 to 1 g/kg infused intravenously slowly), and patients should be monitored closely for possible development of congestive heart failure and pulmonary edema.
  - Protocols vary and should be reviewed with a nephrologist.
- Hypertension
  - Management is indicated if blood pressure is persistently greater than 95% for age and height or if the patient is symptomatic.
- Hyperlipidemia
  - Ideal treatment is to induce remission, which leads to resolution of hyperlipidemia.
- Infection prophylaxis
  - Pneumococcal vaccination with Prevnar or Pneumovax, or both, is recommended.
  - For varicella zoster exposure, consider the following:
    - If the antibody status is negative, administer varicella zoster immune globulin (VZIG) or alternative VZIG product, if available, within 96 hours of exposure.
    - Consider adjustment of prednisone dose during the incubation period.
    - If the patient develops chickenpox, begin acyclovir.
    - Varicella zoster vaccine (VZV) should be considered in seronegative children.
    - Some experts recommend immunization after the prednisone dose is less than 2 mg/kg/day or 20 mg/day (if the patient weighs more than 10 kg), whereas others recommend waiting until the patient is off prednisone for 2 weeks, if possible.
    - The Pediatric Nephrology Panel of the National Kidney Foundation Conference on Proteinuria, Albuminuria, Risk, Assessment, Detection, and Elimination (PARADE) has made no recommendations regarding VZV vaccine.
  - Live vaccines should not be given to patients taking high-dose prednisone or other immunosuppressive medications.
- Managing infection
  - Patients are more susceptible to infection because of increased urinary loss of immunoglobulin G (IgG) and complement (factors B and D).
  - In cases of spontaneous bacterial peritonitis, the most common organism is *Streptococcus pneumoniae,* but gram-negative rods such as *Escherichia coli* are also causative.
  - Cellulitis can spread quickly because edema separates fascial planes.
- Thromboembolic management
  - The risk for thrombosis is increased because of urinary loss of antithrombin III, protein C and protein S and because of increased platelet aggregation.
  - Correct the intravascular volume depletion.
  - Mobilization is important.
  - Employ anticoagulation therapy as indicated.
- Consider hospital admission for the following conditions:
  - Hypertension
  - Cardiopulmonary compromise (e.g., congestive heart failure, pleural effusions)
  - Oliguria
  - Severe edema or anasarca
  - Skin breakdown
  - Fever (because of concern for peritonitis, cellulitis, pneumonia, or other generalized infection)
  - Significant intravascular volume depletion
  - Abdominal pain (because of concern for peritonitis, rapid fluid shifts, or renal vein thrombosis)
- A pediatric nephrologist should consider biopsy for the following situations before treatment:
  - Children younger than 1 year or older than 10 years
  - Low level of C3
  - Gross hematuria or significant hypertension
  - Associated renal failure
- A pediatric nephrologist should consider biopsy for the following situations after treatment:
  - Steroid-resistant patient
  - Frequent relapser

CHRONIC Rx

- Relapses are defined as a urine protein excretion level of 2+ or higher on the dipstick for 3 consecutive days.
  - Relapses often occur with illness and may spontaneously remit within a few days.
  - Conservatively manage for a few days with close observation without steroids if the child is otherwise doing well and has no edema.
  - If spontaneous remission does not occur, restart prednisone at 60 mg/m^2/day (maximum, 80 mg), with a divided dose given two to three times per day until urine is protein free for 3

consecutive days. Then change to alternate-day prednisone dosing and begin to taper.
  - Consider alternative immunosuppressive therapies after consultation with or referral to a pediatric nephrologist.
    - If frequent relapser: two or more relapses within 6 months of initial response or four or more relapses in a 12-month period
    - If steroid dependent: two consecutive relapses occurring while on steroids or within 14 days of completion of course
    - If steroid resistant: no response after 8 weeks of prednisone at dose of 60 mg/m^2/day (maximum, 80 mg/day)
  - Alkylating agents (e.g., cyclophosphamide) can be used.
    - The goal is to induce remission and decrease steroid toxicity.
    - They usually are more effective for frequent relapsers compared with steroid-dependent patients.
    - Dosage is 2 mg/kg/day for 8 to 12 weeks.
    - Instruct patients to drink lots of fluid and to void frequently.
    - Monitor the complete blood cell count with a differential count each week.
    - Monitor for hemorrhagic cystitis.
    - Adverse effects include bone marrow suppression, infection, alopecia, infertility (dose related), risk for neoplasm, hemorrhagic cystitis, nausea, and vomiting.
  - Pulse methylprednisolone with or without a cytotoxic agent
  - Cyclosporine
  - Tacrolimus
  - Mycophenolate mofetil
- Hypertension management
  - Angiotensin-converting enzyme (ACE) inhibitors or angiotensin receptor blockers should be considered, because these agents help to decrease proteinuria in addition to controlling blood pressure.
  - Potential adverse effects include increased serum creatinine and potassium levels, angioedema, and fetopathy.
- Hyperlipidemia management
  - Dietary counseling is helpful.
  - Consider the use of a lipid-lowering agent.
- Thromboemboli prophylaxis and management
  - Early treatment of hypovolemia is a preventative measure.
  - Mobilization is useful.
  - Anticoagulation therapy should be started if thrombi occur.
  - The patient may need large doses of heparin because of low levels of antithrombin III caused by urinary loss of the latter.

DISPOSITION

- Nephrotic syndrome can be a chronic illness with remissions and relapses.
  - Thirty percent of patients do not relapse.
  - Between 10% and 20% are infrequent relapsers.
  - Sixty percent are frequent relapsers.
- Long-term prognosis is best predicted by the response to steroids.
  - In MCNS, it may take 1 to 2 weeks to see a response to prednisone therapy.
  - Approximately 90% respond to steroids during the first 4-week course.
  - FSGS is associated with a much higher risk for progression to chronic renal failure.

REFERRAL

All children with NS should be referred to a pediatric nephrologist for consultation and management in conjunction with the primary care physician.

PEARLS & CONSIDERATIONS

COMMENTS

- In patients who have large volumes of dilute urine, a 1+ or 2+ protein level on the dipstick may correspond to the nephrotic range for proteinuria.
- The patient may have total-body fluid overload but have intravascular hypovolemia.

PATIENT/FAMILY EDUCATION

- Monitor urine for remission and relapses.
  - Check urine at home with dipsticks or sulfosalicylic acid (SSA) daily.
  - Remission occurs when the urine test result is negative or indicates only a trace amount of protein for 3 consecutive days.
  - Relapse occurs when urine shows a 2+ or higher protein level by dipstick testing after a period of remission.
- Because relapses tend to occur with illness, check the urine daily during an illness.
  - Daily testing of urine can allow detection of relapse before the patient becomes symptomatic and thereby help decrease morbidity.
- Symptoms and signs requiring medical attention are as follows:
  - Abdominal pain
  - Fever
  - Respiratory distress
  - Decreased urine output
  - Increasing edema
- Review the potential medical complications of NS as outlined previously.
  - Edema is a common problem.
  - Infections include spontaneous bacterial peritonitis (if patients have one episode, the risk of recurrence increases) and cellulitis, which can spread quickly.
  - Thrombosis is a risk when the patient is nephrotic.
  - Intravascular volume depletion should be avoided; acute renal failure can result from severe hypovolemia.
- Review the side effects of medications.
- Discuss chickenpox exposure. Luckily, most children are now immunized at one year and a second varicella vaccination is recommended at school entry.
- Discuss the vaccination schedule.
- Provide low-salt dietary counseling.
- Discuss the natural history and course of disease.
- NS can be a chronic illness with remissions and relapses. The long-term prognosis is best predicted by the response to steroid therapy.

SUGGESTED READINGS

Hogg RJ et al: Evaluation and management of proteinuria and nephrotic syndrome in children: recommendations from a pediatric nephrology panel established at the National Kidney Foundation Conference on Proteinuria, Albuminuria, Risk, Assessment, Detection, and Elimination (PARADE). *Pediatrics* 105:1242, 2000.

Roth KS et al: Nephrotic syndrome: pathogenesis and management. *Pediatr Rev* 23:237, 2002.

AUTHOR: **AYESA N. MIAN, MD**

BASIC INFORMATION

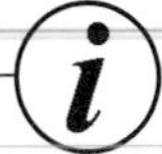

DEFINITION

Neuroblastoma is a highly variable and complex malignancy that arises from primitive neural crest cells populating the adrenal medulla and paravertebral sympathetic ganglion chain. The tumor is highly capricious in its behavior, ranging from spontaneous involution to rapid growth, widespread metastases, and death. Ganglioneuroblastoma and ganglioneuroma are less common, but more benign, differentiated variants of neuroblastoma.

ICD-9-CM CODE(S)
194.0 Neuroblastoma, Unspecified site

EPIDEMIOLOGY & DEMOGRAPHICS

- Neuroblastomas account for approximately 8% to 10% of childhood cancers.
- Incidence is 8 per 1 million per year (500 new cases in the United States annually).
- The median age at diagnosis is 22 months.
  - Younger than 1 year of age: 36%
  - Younger than 4 years of age: 79%
  - Younger than 10 years of age: 97%
- Approximately 65% have a primary tumor in the abdomen or pelvis, 15% in the thorax, and 5% in the neck.
- Approximately 35% of patients have localized disease at presentation; 65% have metastases.

Prognostic Factors

- Predictors of poor outcome: age older than 1 year, stage 4 disease, and a variety of tumor-specific markers (DNA index 1, amplification of *N-MYC* oncogene, poor risk by Shimada pathology classification)
- Predictors of good outcome: age younger than 1 year; stage 1, 2, or 4S disease; tumor-specific markers (DNA index greater than 1, nonamplification of *N-MYC* oncogene)

CLINICAL PRESENTATION

History

- Infants: bluish, bruise-like nodules on the skin, rapid breathing, poor oral intake, distended abdomen
- Older children: abdominal pain and distention but otherwise healthy; cough, shortness of breath with thoracic tumor; leg weakness with paravertebral extension of tumor into spinal canal
- Occasionally, an asymptomatic child is diagnosed by an incidental finding on chest radiograph.
- Metastatic disease: firm, nontender lumps on the neck, bone pain, proptosis, "raccoon eyes," fever, weight loss, malaise
- Paraneoplastic syndromes: jerking of arms and legs (myoclonus), irregular movements of eyes (opsoclonus), diarrhea

Physical Examination

- Infants
  - Respiratory distress
  - Bluish, palpable subcutaneous nodules
  - Massive hepatomegaly
  - Occasionally swollen lower extremities, swollen feet
- Older children
  - Large, firm, nontender or mildly tender abdominal mass
  - Decreased lower extremity strength (with spinal cord compression)
- Metastatic disease
  - Pallor
  - Cachexia
  - Petechiae with bone marrow involvement
  - Horner's syndrome with cervical involvement
  - Firm, nonmobile supraclavicular and cervical adenopathy
  - Proptosis and periorbital ecchymoses with orbital involvement
- Paraneoplastic syndromes
  - Myoclonus
  - Opsoclonus

ETIOLOGY

- Embryonal tumor arising from primitive neural crest cells in the distribution of the adrenal medulla and paravertebral sympathetic chain
- Associated with chromosomal changes, including *N-MYC* oncogene amplification, chromosome 1p deletion, trisomy for 17q
- No known environmental cause
- Familial variants occur but are rare

DIAGNOSIS

DIFFERENTIAL DIAGNOSIS

- Abdominal mass: Wilms' tumor, lymphoma, rhabdomyosarcoma, germ cell tumor
- Lymphadenopathy and bone disease: leukemia, lymphoma, bone metastases
- Diarrhea: infectious causes
- Opsoclonus/myoclonus: primary neurologic disorder

WORKUP

- Bone marrow aspirate/biopsy: may reveal bone marrow disease

Staging

- The most widely used staging system is the International Neuroblastoma Staging System (INSS), based on surgical staging and examination of lymph nodes:
  - Stage 1: completely resected, localized disease
  - Stage 2A: incompletely removed localized tumor
  - Stage 2B: completely or incompletely removed tumor with positive ipsilateral lymph nodes
  - Stage 3: unresectable tumor crossing the midline
  - Stage 4: any primary with distant metastases
  - Stage 4S: localized primary tumor plus metastases to the liver, skin, or bone marrow in a child younger than 1 year of age

LABORATORY TESTS

- Laboratory studies: complete blood count, differential, platelet count, chemistries, lactate dehydrogenase, ferritin
- Urine catecholamine metabolites: urine homovanillic acid and vanillylmandelic acid elevated in 90% to 95% of children with neuroblastoma

IMAGING STUDIES

- Radiograph of the chest and abdomen to assess for calcified mass
- Computed tomography scan of the neck/chest/abdomen/pelvis: calcified mass replacing adrenal gland or along paravertebral sympathetic ganglion chain; extrinsic to kidney; often infiltrative and crossing the midline
- Bone scan/skeletal survey: may reveal lytic lesions caused by bone metastases
- Spine magnetic resonance imaging to assess for spinal cord compression resulting from extension of paravertebral tumor through the neural foramina
- Meta-iodobenzylguanadine (MIBG) scan: nuclear study that detects primary tumor and metastases

TREATMENT

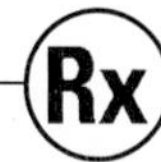

ACUTE GENERAL Rx

- Therapy consists of varying combinations of surgery, radiation, and chemotherapy.
- In addition, newer approaches include high-dose chemotherapy with autologous stem cell rescue, differentiating agents, radiolabeled antitumor monoclonal antibodies, and tumor vaccines.
- Patients are stratified into low-risk, intermediate-risk, and high-risk groups according to age, stage, and *N-MYC* status; treatment is based on the risk group.

Low Risk

- Treatment in this group is generally surgery only.
  - Children of any age with stage 1 disease
  - Children of any age with stage 2 disease (except those more than 1 year old with amplified *N-MYC* and unfavorable histology)
  - Children with 4S disease with nonamplified *N-MYC,* favorable histology, and DNA index greater than 1
- Chemotherapy or radiotherapy in children with stage 4S disease is controversial.

Intermediate Risk

- Treatment is moderately aggressive chemotherapy (cyclophosphamide, doxorubicin, carboplatin [or cisplatin], etoposide).
  - Children younger than 1 year of age with stage 3 or 4 nonamplified *N-MYC*
  - Children younger than 1 year of age with stage 4S nonamplified *N-MYC,*

   - Hospitalization and intravenous antibiotics are reserved for ill-appearing or young children. Consider G-CSF for ill-appearing children (i.e., IVIG and G-CSF are effective for autoimmune neutropenia).
- Congenital neutropenia (e.g., Kostmann's syndrome, cyclic neutropenia, Schwachman-Diamond syndrome)
   - Chronic administration of G-CSF should be given for Kostmann's syndrome and cyclic neutropenia.
   - Antibiotic prophylaxis should be considered for children with an ANC lower than 500/mm^3.
   - Febrile children should be hospitalized and treated with intravenous antibiotics.
   - Use of WBC transfusions is controversial but should be considered for critically ill, febrile children.
- Neonatal neutropenia
   - Treatment to increase the ANC is not necessary in the well infant.
   - Ill infants may benefit from G-CSF administration or WBC transfusion.

DISPOSITION

- Children with acquired neutropenia should have a CBC every few months until the neutropenia resolves, and they should be evaluated for fevers.
- Children with congenital neutropenia should have a CBC every few months, should be evaluated for fevers, and should be monitored for risk of developing leukemia.

REFERRAL

A child with moderate to severe neutropenia should be referred to a pediatric hematologist-oncologist for further evaluation and treatment.

PEARLS & CONSIDERATIONS

COMMENTS

- The classic signs of inflammation (i.e., rubor, calor, dolor, and turgor) may be subtle or absent in neutropenic children.
- A girl with labial cellulitis should have a CBC because this site of infection is unique to neutropenic children.
- Delayed separation of the umbilical cord in a neonate may be associated with neutropenia.

PREVENTION

G-CSF is administered to children with congenital, profound neutropenia.

PATIENT/FAMILY EDUCATION

- Most acquired neutropenias are mild, transient, and not life-threatening.
- Congenital neutropenias are potentially serious, chronic illnesses that require close surveillance to prevent or treat infection, poor dentition, poor growth, and risk of leukemia.

SUGGESTED READINGS

Dinauer MC: The phagocyte system and disorders of granulopoiesis and granulocyte function. *In* Nathan DG, Orkin SH (eds): *Nathan and Oski's Hematology of Infancy and Childhood,* 5th ed. Philadelphia, WB Saunders, 2003.

Korones DN: Neutropenia and lymphopenia. *In* Burg FD et al (eds): *Gellis and Kagan's Current Pediatric Therapy,* 16th ed. Philadelphia, WB Saunders, 1999.

Neutropenia OnLine Forum. Available at www.delphi.com/Neutropenia

The Severe Chronic Neutropenia International Registry. Available at http://depts.washington.edu/registry

AUTHOR: **DAVID N. KORONES, MD**

BASIC INFORMATION

DEFINITION

Obesity is having excess body fat or body weight. There is no one accepted standard definition, and because of the difficulty of measuring body fat and the ranges of heights across age, various criteria have been used. The most common definition uses body mass index (BMI), which is weight in kilograms (kg) divided by height in square meters (m^2). The BMI correlates well with amount of body fat and can be compared with age and gender-matched standards. Obesity or overweight is a BMI greater than the 95th percentile for age and gender; for obese adults, the BMI is greater than 30. At risk for becoming overweight is a BMI between the 85th and 95th percentile for age and gender; for adults, the BMI is between 25 and 30. Using weight-for-height measurements is another way to assess adiposity. Overweight, simple obesity, and morbid obesity are defined as weight-for-height measurements of greater than 110%, 120%, and 140% of expected, respectively. A BMI more than double the 85th percentile is also a definition of morbid obesity.

SYNONYMS

Over fat
Overweight

ICD-9-CM CODES
259.9 Endogenous obesity
278.00 Exogenous obesity
278.01 Morbid obesity

EPIDEMIOLOGY & DEMOGRAPHICS

- Data from sequential cohorts of national datasets have demonstrated that the prevalence and severity of obesity in children and adolescents have increased substantially in the past 3 decades.
- Cycle III of the National Health and Nutrition Examination Survey (NHANES) (1988-1994) found an 11% overall prevalence of overweight (among 6- to 18-year-old subjects) and a 14% prevalence of those who were at risk for overweight.
- Blacks and Mexican Americans have higher rates (range, 14% to 17%) across all age groups and genders compared with whites (range, 10% to 11%), and they have experienced greater increases in prevalence of obesity than whites.
- No consistent associations with socioeconomic status or family education are seen for obesity.
- Trends in obesity demonstrate that the greatest increases have occurred since the mid-1970s.
- Since the 1960s, the prevalence of overweight among children and adolescents has increased twofold to threefold.
- The heaviest cohorts of children have demonstrated the greatest increases in weight recently.
- Obesity is recognized as a serious, chronic medical condition that is associated with a number of conditions causing increased morbidity and mortality.
- Obesity can result in complications in many organ systems, some of which occur during childhood and adolescence, whereas others manifest in adulthood.
- Short-term effects include the following:
    - Orthopedic complications include Blount's disease (i.e., tibia vara), slipped femoral capital epiphyses (30% to 50% of cases are obese), and joint and back pain.
    - Fifty percent of children with benign intracranial hypertension (BIH), previously called pseudotumor cerebri, are obese.
    - Sleep apnea or obesity hypoventilation syndrome occurs (see Obstructive Sleep Apnea & Parasomnias in Diseases and Disorders [Section I]); obstructive and central hypoventilation are seen in morbidly obese patients.
    - Gallbladder disease occurs more commonly in obese patients.
    - Elevated liver enzymes related to nonalcoholic fatty liver disease may progress to steatohepatitis, with late effects of cirrhosis and liver cancer.
    - Obese patients may have endocrine disorders.
        - Polycystic ovary disease (see Polycystic Ovary Syndrome in Diseases and Disorders [Section I])
        - Glucose intolerance and type 2 diabetes mellitus, associated with acanthosis nigricans and hyperinsulinemia (see Diabetes Mellitus Type 2 in Diseases and Disorders [Section I]).
        - Dyslipidemia: higher BMI associated with increased low-density lipoprotein (LDL) cholesterol, plasma triglycerides, and decreased high-density lipoprotein (HDL) cholesterol
    - Obese patients are more likely to have hypertension (see Hypertension in Diseases and Disorders [Section I]).
    - Early adrenarche, pubarche (males and females), and menarche may occur in obese children.
    - Obese children may have accelerated linear growth and bone age, and greater height often leads to unrealistic expectations of maturity by adults and peers.
    - Psychosocial consequences include isolation and stigma, poor self-image and self-esteem, depression, and discrimination based on societal norms for thinness.
    - Binge eating disorder occurs in up to 30% of obese female adolescents.
    - Obesity predisposes to metabolic syndrome (see Metabolic Syndrome in Diseases and Disorders [Section I]).
        - Rates appear to be higher in obese children, particularly those who are moderately or severely obese.
        - Higher levels of C-reactive protein and lower adiponectin levels in these children may represent a heightened risk for cardiovascular disease and diabetes in adulthood.
    - Gastroesophageal reflux disease occurs more often in obese people.
- Long-term effects include the following:
    - Obesity, especially when it occurs or persists until adolescence, tracks into adulthood. Approximately 80% to 85% of obese adolescents become obese adults; persistence is greater for female than for male adolescents.
    - Significant increases in adult morbidity and mortality result from all causes and from specific conditions such as cardiovascular disease (even after controlling for adult weight and smoking history), cancer (i.e., elevated rates of colorectal cancers in men and breast, endometrial, cervical, ovarian, and gallbladder cancers in women), osteoarthritis, osteoporosis, type 2 diabetes, sleep apnea syndrome, and gallbladder and liver disease.

CLINICAL PRESENTATION

History

- Determines potential causes, contributing factors, duration of obesity, and complications
- Abnormal growth or development in early childhood
- Oligomenorrhea or amenorrhea
- Knee pain
- Headaches, blurred vision, and vomiting: suggests BIH
- Daytime somnolence, breathing difficulty or loud snoring during sleep, restless sleep: may all suggest obstructive sleep apnea syndrome
- Abdominal pain
- Abnormal eating patterns, binge eating, and purging: may be signs of eating disorder
- Depressive symptoms (contributing factors to or consequence of obesity); note functioning at school, with family, and with peers to assess degree of social isolation
- History of weight gain from early childhood to present
    - Point when the child began to cross percentiles
    - Early interventions
    - Early events that may have coincided with weight change
    - Any periods of extremely rapid weight gain
    - Crossing more that 1 to 2 BMI units per year: worrisome, as a guideline
- Family history of obesity, diabetes, or cardiovascular disease
- Eating behaviors and diet history
    - Foods eaten daily
    - Patterns of eating
    - Typical meals and snacks

- Weekly consumption of high-caloric, high-fat foods, including take-out or convenience meals, fast foods, and caloric beverages (e.g., juices, regular sodas, sweetened teas)
- Eating when not hungry
- Eating in front of the TV or computer
- Unsupervised eating
- Meal skipping
- How foods are prepared and by whom: can affect risk of obesity
  - Types of snacks available
  - Parental behaviors regarding skipping meals
  - Eating to relieve stress
- Physical activity and exercise habits
  - Organized sports
  - School-based physical education
  - Activities done at home and unorganized outdoor play
- Risk of obesity increased by time spent in sedentary activities, such as watching TV, working or playing on a computer, and playing video games
- Child's behaviors influenced by parental involvement and modeling of active and sedentary patterns
- Ability to overcome obesity influenced by whether the child and parents see obesity as a problem and their readiness to change behaviors

Physical Examination

- Plot height, weight, and calculated BMI percentile according to current BMI graphs for age available from the Centers for Disease Control and Prevention (see BMI Percentile Graphs under Growth in Charts, Formulas, Laboratory Tests and Values [Section IV], also see BMI Nomogram and Calculation Equation in Section IV).
- Triceps skin fold thickness may be helpful if clinician has appropriate way to measure it.
- Body fat distribution should be assessed, concentrating on central versus peripheral adiposity.
  - Central obesity, as one of the criteria of metabolic syndrome (see Metabolic Syndrome in Section I), correlates with higher visceral adiposity, as seen in adults.
  - Central obesity predisposes the individual to a higher risk of cardiovascular disease, particularly if associated with glucose intolerance.
  - Measuring waist circumference and determining whether it is at more than the 90th percentile for age can determine the degree of central adiposity; however, there are no good norms for child and adolescent populations for waist circumference that indicate higher risk, as for adults.
- Ensure that an appropriate-size cuff is used for obtaining blood pressure.
- Dysmorphic features are seen in rare genetic causes, such as Bardet-Biedl syndrome, Cohen syndrome, and Prader-Willi syndrome.
- Acanthosis nigricans (often most apparent at the back of neck, axillae, and intertriginous areas) raises the suspicion of insulin resistance.
- Violaceous striae, truncal obesity (in Cushing's disease), or hirsutism (in hyperandrogenemic anovulatory states) may be seen.
- Blurred optic discs and loss of visual acuity may indicate BIH.
- Abdominal tenderness, especially of the right upper quadrant, suggests liver or gallbladder disease.
- Undescended testicles indicates Prader-Willi syndrome.
- Limited hip range of motion indicates slipped capital femoral epiphysis.
- Lower leg bowing may occur in patients with Blount's disease.
- Sexual maturity rating may be accelerated in obese males and females.

ETIOLOGY

- The cause is multifactorial, representing an interaction between genetic and environmental influences; relative contributions vary among individuals.
- Less than 5% of patients have underlying specific causes, such as an endocrine problem (3%) or a genetic syndrome (2%).
- Familial (genetic) factors have been documented by epidemiologic studies; behavioral and environmental factors are involved. Children and adolescents with one or both obese parents are at significantly higher risk for obesity as adults than those without an obese parent.
- The fat cell theory suggests that fat cells gained early in life, during puberty, or with massive weight gain during adulthood cannot be lost. This supports avoiding overfeeding during infancy, early childhood, and during puberty to prevent obesity.
- Behavioral and lifestyle factors are key contributing factors.
  - Caloric intake is significantly higher in many obese individuals compared with that of nonobese persons.
  - Sedentary lifestyle, physical inactivity, and large amounts of watching TV or playing video or computer games have been implicated.
  - Obese patients often engage in patterns of eating that adversely influence weight, including eating quickly, skipping meals early in the day and eating large quantities late in the day, eating in response to emotional cues rather than when hungry, and eating while watching TV or using the computer.
  - Eating patterns in the United States have shifted dramatically, and many feel that these are in part responsible for obesity prevalence.
  - Thirty percent of food expenditures are for take-out meals, which typically are high in fat and calories.
  - Portion sizes at restaurants and take-out facilities have increased dramatically in recent years.
  - In the past 10 years, soft drink consumption by American children has doubled.
  - The frequency of snacking between meals and children's access to unhealthy fast food and snack items has dramatically increased over the past 2 decades.

DIAGNOSIS Dx

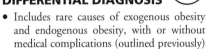

DIFFERENTIAL DIAGNOSIS

- Includes rare causes of exogenous obesity and endogenous obesity, with or without medical complications (outlined previously)
- Exogenous causes
  - Bardet-Biedl and Cohen syndromes
  - Prader-Willi syndrome
  - Hypothyroidism (normal height acceleration precludes this as a diagnosis)
  - Cushing's disease (should see deceleration in linear growth rate)
  - Psychological eating disorder (i.e., bulimia, depression, or binge eating disorder)
- Causes of endogenous obesity
  - Unhealthy eating patterns
  - Low levels of physical activity

WORKUP

- Determine the BMI and percentile.
- Determine whether the patient is overweight (>95th percentile) and in need of a comprehensive medical assessment and intervention.
- If the patient is at risk for overweight (85th to 95th percentile), he or she requires assessment and management if there are signs and symptoms of complications from obesity.
- Detect large recent changes in the BMI.
- Assess concern about weight (see Fig. 1-8).

LABORATORY TESTS

- These tests are of limited value, except for identifying rare children and adolescents with an underlying medical cause and for determining the presence of medical complications of obesity, as outlined previously.
  - Thyroid studies and morning cortisol level, only if clinically indicated
  - Fasting blood glucose and insulin levels
  - Fasting lipid profile: total, LDL, and HDL cholesterol and triglyceride levels
  - Follicle-stimulating hormone (FSH), luteinizing hormone (LH), testosterone (free and total)
  - Liver function studies
  - Chromosome studies

IMAGING STUDIES

- Rarely useful for diagnostic purposes, but helpful when concerned about complications of obesity
  - Ultrasound of gallbladder and liver
  - Electrocardiogram to assess cardiac status
  - Sleep study to rule out sleep apnea syndrome

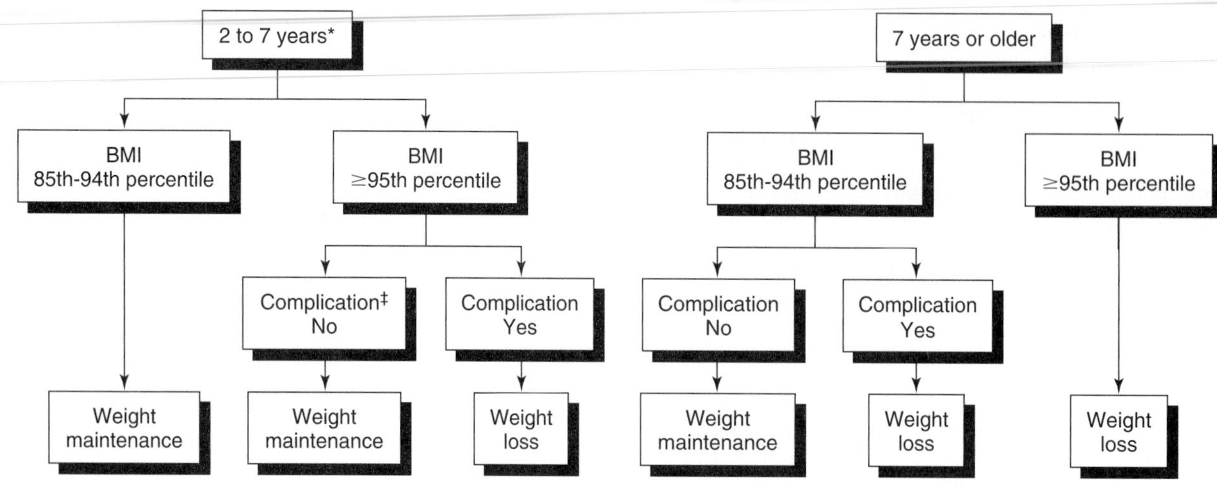

*Indicates that children younger than 2 years should be referred to a pediatric obesity center for the treatment.
‡Indicates complications such as mild hypertension, dyslipidemias, and insulin resistance. Patients with acute complications, such as pseudo-tumor cerebri, sleep apnea, obesity hypoventilation syndrome, or orthopedic problems, should be referred to a pediatric obesity center.

FIGURE 1-7 Recommendations for weight goals. (From Barlow SE, Dietz WH: Obesity evaluation and treatment: expert committee recommendations. *Pediatrics* 102:3, 1998.)

TREATMENT

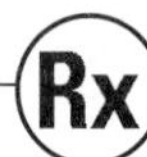

NONPHARMACOLOGIC THERAPY

- The primary goal should be the regulation of body weight and fat through healthy eating and activity levels to provide adequate nutrition for growth and development.
- Weight goal may be maintenance of baseline weight that allows a gradual decline in BMI with linear height growth or weight loss (approximately 1 to 2 pounds per month) (Figure 1-7).
- Secondary goals are to improve any complications and to prevent the development of treatment side effects.
- Principles
  - Numerous studies have documented positive results in treating children and adolescents using individualized programs that integrate several components: dietary modification, exercise, behavior change, and family involvement.
  - Intervention should begin in early childhood, when obesity is identified.
  - Families and children must be ready to make changes; if not, options are to defer treatment or to refer children for counseling for motivational techniques of behavioral change.
  - Education about the short-term and long-term medical consequences of obesity should be included.
  - All family members and caregivers, as well as the child, need to be involved in any treatment program to create new family behaviors that support the child's goals for healthier eating and increased physical activity.
- The need for more independent behaviors among adolescents should be recognized by families.
  - Emphasis is on long-term changes in eating and activity levels rather than a focus on diets or rapid weight loss.
  - Small and gradual changes in behavior are desirable.
  - Use of a team of professionals or referral to a professional, such as a nutritionist, dietician, or counselor, may enhance the success of the treatment.
- Exercise and physical activity
  - Efforts to increase physical activity levels are more successful when families incorporate greater activity into daily routines, such as walking to school or doing active chores, rather than starting formal exercise programs.
  - Making specific efforts to reduce the amount of sedentary activities, such as limiting TV hours, often has the benefit of increasing the child's active time.
- Behavior change methods essential to influencing changes in eating or activity
  - Most methods involve close input by parents in managing the eating behaviors of their children.
  - Behavioral therapy is an essential component.
    - Reduce reinforcements for the child to continue sedentary activities.
    - Provide some choice and control over activities and food choices.
    - Minimize the sense of deprivation.
    - Teach the child how to attend to internal cues of hunger, emotions, and satiety.
  - Additional techniques, such as goal setting and contracting with the child or teen and the parents, self-monitoring of caloric intake and weight, and praise, are all beneficial.
- Family involvement is essential.
  - Includes promoting positive parenting skills
    - Modeling healthy eating behaviors: using praise directed at improved behaviors, not weight loss
    - Being consistent in messages
    - Establishing daily meal times and offering healthy options for snacks and meals
    - Observing the child's behavior
    - Setting limits when necessary
- Dietary modification is needed.
  - Use the U.S. Department of Agriculture's food guidance system (My Pyramid Plan) to adopt a healthy approach to eating. Individualized systems and recommendations are available that depend on the child's age and activity level.
  - Suggest reducing or eliminating high-calorie, calorie-dense foods or substituting with lower-calorie alternatives to reduce caloric intake.
  - The "traffic light diet" approach stresses a balance of high-, medium-, and low-calorie foods, rather than counting calories; this is best for younger children and preadolescents.
- Adjunctive therapies are available.
  - Support groups or group-oriented programs, especially in the context of school programs or health education, may be beneficial for some children and teens and may provide needed peer support.
  - Groups in which parents are also offered separate group meetings are more beneficial than those for children and parents together.

- Commercial programs, such as Jenny Craig and Weight Watchers, are not specifically designed for children and adolescents and have not been evaluated for these ages.
- Bariatric surgery may be an option.
  - Several surgical gastrointestinal procedures are available and are being done more commonly in the pediatric population.
  - The two most common procedures are the Roux-en-Y gastric bypass procedure and the vertical banded gastroplasty.
  - A newer reversible procedure, the Lap-Band, can be done laparoscopically and involves placing a silicone band around the upper segment of the stomach.
  - These procedures are not generally recommended for adolescents and children; they are considered only in cases of extreme obesity, when life-threatening complications are present and when the adolescent has tried and failed to lose weight on standard medical and behavioral programs.
  - A few specialized centers across the country are accruing data on the success and complication rates for surgical treatment of obesity; few long-term outcome data are available.
  - Psychological assessment before surgery is required to ensure that the adolescent will be able to maintain the changes in eating behaviors necessary after surgery (i.e., eating and drinking very small amounts of food more frequently throughout the day) and the postsurgical medication regimens that may be required to avoid complications such as vitamin deficiencies.

ACUTE GENERAL Rx

The therapy for obesity is long-term lifestyle modification.

CHRONIC Rx

- There are no medical therapies that promise long-term significant weight loss reduction in children and adolescents.
  - Because of side effects relative to limited effectiveness and concerns about abuse potential, drugs are not recommended. A variety of anorectic drugs are marketed as weight-loss drugs and are available for adults through prescription, such as methamphetamine HCl (Desoxyn), phendimetrazine tartrate (Bontril, Prelu-2), and phentermine (Fastin and Ionamin).
  - Few studies have been done to assess these anorectic drugs' effectiveness in children and adolescents; relevant studies show few differences between subjects treated with diet control or placebo and medication.
  - Over-the-counter anorectic agents (e.g., Dexatrim) are not effective and are likely to pose risks from side effects and the potential for abuse.
  - Several drugs have been studied in adults and have had limited effectiveness; most are not approved by the U.S. Food and Drug Administration (FDA), nor are they recommended for use in individuals younger than 16 years, although clinical trials are being conducted.
- Sibutramine (Meridia) is a serotonin, norepinephrine, and dopamine reuptake inhibitor, and it has been found to be effective, particularly in individuals on physical activity programs. A serious side effect is hypertension, requiring careful and frequent blood pressure monitoring. Other serotonergic drugs and monoamine oxidase inhibitors should be avoided when using sibutramine.
- Orlistat (Xenical) is a lipase inhibitor that prevents the absorption of dietary fat, and it has been approved as an anti-obesity drug. Side effects include diarrhea, steatorrhea, and malabsorption of fat-soluble vitamins (i.e., A, D, E, and K). Orlistat has been FDA approved for the treatment of obesity; studies of 12- to 18-year-old subjects have documented its effectiveness and safety in this age range, although no studies have tested orlistat in children younger than 12 years.
- Topiramate (Topamax) is an anticonvulsant that has been shown to decrease episodes of binge eating in adolescents with binge-eating disorder or bulimia. The main side effects that can be very problematic include paresthesias, dizziness, somnolence, and slowed thinking.
- Clinical trials evaluating metformin have shown that it may be beneficial in obese adolescents who are at high risk for diabetes, although it does not produce enough weight loss compared with placebo to qualify it as a weight-loss drug.
- Studies have shown fluoxetine, a selective serotonin reuptake inhibitor (SSRI), to be effective in obese individuals meeting the *Diagnostic and Statistical Manual of Mental Disorders* criteria for binge-eating disorder. The SSRIs in general, however, have limited usefulness as long-term anti-obesity drugs unless depression is a comorbid problem.
- Liquid protein-sparing modified fasts (i.e., liquid diets containing 400 to 900 kcal/day) generally provide enough protein and carbohydrates to keep ketosis and protein loss to a minimum.
  - Studies have shown that the 900 kcal/day programs are as effective as the 400 kcal/day fasts and offer better protection from protein loss.
  - These products are prescribed through physician-directed programs that typically combine fasting with nutrition education and behavior modification.
  - Weight loss can be substantial on these programs, but weight regain also is common and substantial.
  - These programs are contraindicated in adolescents who are still actively growing, but they may be recommended in specific cases of extreme obesity and in the presence of secondary complications or comorbid conditions.

COMPLEMENTARY & ALTERNATIVE MEDICINE

- Evidence has demonstrated that several available over-the-counter supplements marketed for weight loss, such as chitosan and guar gum, are not effective.
- Evidence is lacking for the effectiveness of additional supplements such as green tea, chromium, and ginseng.

DISPOSITION

- Obesity should be viewed as a chronic disease that requires ongoing and close follow-up to ensure success in treatment and appropriate management of expected medical consequences.
- Relapse after weight loss is common, and close follow-up can assist patients in managing these relapses.

REFERRAL

- For acute medical complications, refer the patient to a specific subspecialist or pediatric obesity center as needed.
- During the course of treatment, if significant conflict between parents and the child ensues about eating issues or if signs of an eating disorder or depression emerge, referral to a family therapist or individual counselor may be indicated.
- A nutritionist or registered dietician may be best able to assess and make recommendations about caloric intake and requirements, especially in cases in which the provider does not have the time or expertise to do this.

PEARLS & CONSIDERATIONS

COMMENTS

- Because of aromatization of androgens to estrogens that occurs in adipose tissue, obese females have significant amounts of extragonadal estrogen, which may be associated with disruption of normal FSH and LH levels and anovulatory menstrual cycles.
- Because many adolescents may use tobacco as a form of weight control, it is important to ask about this behavior and to counsel the patient regarding adding the risk of tobacco use to the risks associated with obesity.

PREVENTION

- Preventive treatment is ideally provided in the course of routine preventive care when monitoring growth and providing information about the avoidance of excessive intake and the promotion of physical activity.
- For early prevention or intervention, focus on obese parents of infants and young

children, even if the children are currently normal weight.

- For older children and adolescents, focus on those who show early signs of increasing weight.

PATIENT/FAMILY EDUCATION

- The American Dietetic Association's web site (www.eatright.org) provides nutritional information for parents and children.
- The U.S. Department of Agriculture has a web site (www.mypyramid.gov) that provides a wealth of information and interactive programs using the pyramid guidance system. In addition to providing individualized nutrition and physical activity correlated with age, gender, and level of physical activity, it also has an interactive computer game (My Pyramid Blast Off Game) for children between the ages of 6 and 11 years.
- The Weight Control Information Network (www.niddk.nih.gov//nutritiondocs.html) provides general information on weight control, obesity, and nutritional disorders.
- The U.S. Preventive Services Task Force has published recommendations for screening and intervention for overweight in children and adolescents (www.ahrq.gov/clinic/uspstfix.htm).

SUGGESTED READINGS

Barlow SE, Dietz WH: Obesity evaluation and treatment: expert committee recommendations. *Pediatrics* 102:3, 1998.

Department of Health and Human Services: Obesity in childhood and adolescence: assessment, prevention and treatment. *Int J Obesity* 23:2, 1999.

Dietz WH: Health consequences of obesity in youth: childhood predictors of adult disease. *Pediatrics* 101:518, 1998.

Long BJ et al: A multi-site field test of the acceptability of physical activity counseling in primary care: project PACE. *Am J Prev Med* 12:73, 1996.

Ogden OL et al: Prevalence and trends in overweight among US children and adolescents. *JAMA* 288:1728, 2002.

Rollnick S et al: Negotiating behavior change in medical settings: the development of brief motivational interviewing. *J Mental Health* 1:25, 1992.

Weiss R et al: Obesity and the metabolic syndrome in children and adolescents. *N Engl J Med* 350:2362, 2004.

AUTHOR: **SHERYL RYAN, MD**

BASIC INFORMATION

DEFINITION

Obsessive-compulsive disorder (OCD) has recurrent, intrusive, unpleasant thoughts (i.e., obsessions) that do not respond to voluntary suppression, are unrealistic, and not imposed from without. Repetitive behaviors or mental acts (i.e., compulsions) occur in response to these thoughts. For people with OCD, the thoughts or actions can be disabling.

SYNONYM

OCD

ICD-9-CM CODE
300.3 Obsessive-compulsive disorder

EPIDEMIOLOGY & DEMOGRAPHICS

- OCD runs in families and is associated with Tourette's disorder and depression.
- Reported prevalence rates range from 0.2% to 1% in children and up to 3.6% in adolescents.
- Patients tend to conceal symptoms.
- No reliable gender, ethnic, or racial variations have been established; prevalence rates are similar around the world.

CLINICAL PRESENTATION

History

- Developmental rituals are common but usually disappear by 8 to 10 years of age.
- Onset after an untreated streptococcal infection (i.e., pediatric autoimmune neuropsychiatric disorders associated with streptococcal infection [PANDAS]) is reported but controversial.

Physical Examination

- Chapped, red hands from excessive washing
- Patchy hair loss (i.e., trichotillomania)

ETIOLOGY

- There is considerable evidence for a genetic contribution to OCD.
- The possibility of an autoimmune factor is suggested by an apparent but controversial relation to untreated streptococcal infection (PANDAS).

DIAGNOSIS

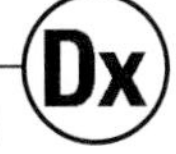

DIFFERENTIAL DIAGNOSIS

- Tourette's movements and tics usually occur without triggering thoughts.
- In pervasive developmental disorder and other developmental disorders, repetitive behaviors are common, but they are unaccompanied by ritualized justification.
- In cases of depression, thoughts may be obsessive and dysphoric, but they do not cause compulsions.
- Obsessions make sense to psychotic patients, but obsessions are understood to be inappropriate by patients with OCD.
- For patients with anorexia and bulimia nervosa, obsessions and compulsions are limited to weight-losing behaviors.

WORKUP

- Patients may acknowledge ritualized behavior only reluctantly.
- Parents may observe washing (85%), repeating (51%), and checking (46%).
- The interviewer-administrated Yale-Brown Obsessive-Compulsive Scale (YBOCS) can be helpful in the evaluation of OCD.
- Self-administered Leyton obsessional inventory (child version) may also be used.

LABORATORY TESTS

Antistreptococcal antibody titers may be elevated.

IMAGING STUDIES

Magnetic resonance imaging (MRI) and positron emission tomography (PET) have revealed intriguing frontal and subcortical abnormalities but are not yet applied clinically.

TREATMENT

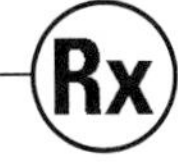

NONPHARMACOLOGIC THERAPY

- Cognitive-behavioral therapy (CBT) works well in older children and adolescents who are willing to undertake it.
- Medication and CBT together are more effective than either alone.

ACUTE GENERAL Rx

- Use of medication without supportive therapy is undesirable.
- Fluoxetine is the selective serotonin reuptake inhibitor (SSRI) of choice for children.
  - Dosages are higher (up to 80 mg daily) than for depression.
  - Begin at 10 mg daily and increase by 10 mg/day every 2 weeks.
  - Improvement is slow but cumulative over several months.
- Clomipramine (up to 3mg/kg) is also effective.
  - Begin at 25 mg daily and increase by 25 mg every 5 to 7 days to a maximum of 100 mg/day.
  - It is less well tolerated because of anticholinergic side effects.
  - Monitor the electrocardiogram for conduction delay.
- Antibiotic treatment of previously untreated streptococcal infection (with elevated antibody titers) may be useful.

CHRONIC Rx

Including cognitive behavioral treatment in the regimen may prevent recurrences.

DISPOSITION

Recurrence is likely if the medication is stopped too soon. It should be continued for at least 1 year and tapered very slowly (i.e., decreased by 25% every 60 days).

REFERRAL

- Refer the patient to a professional who is adept at CBT.
- Refer to a specialist in psychopharmacology because of the probable need for extended treatment.

PEARLS & CONSIDERATIONS

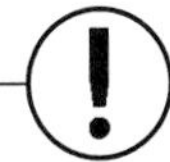

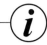

COMMENTS

- OCD treatment (in adults) changes patterns of blood flow in the basal ganglia. This change occurs with CBT, even without medication.
- At least 50% of Tourette's patients develop OCD, and there are overlapping family histories for these disorders.

PREVENTION

There is no reliable information about prevention of OCD.

PATIENT/FAMILY EDUCATION

CBT has a better likelihood than medication alone of preventing recurrence or of forestalling apparent recurrence.

SUGGESTED READINGS

American Academy of Child and Adolescent Psychiatry. Available at www.aacap.org

American Psychiatric Association: *Diagnostic and Statistical Manual of Mental Disorders,* 4th ed. Text Revision.Washington, DC, American Psychiatric Association, 2000, p 943.

Jenike MA: Clinical practice: obsessive-compulsive disorder. *N Engl J Med* 350:259, 2004.

Stein DJ: Obsessive-compulsive disorder [review]. *Lancet* 360:397, 2002.

AUTHOR: **CHRISTOPHER H. HODGMAN, MD**

BASIC INFORMATION

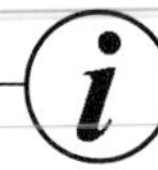

DEFINITION

Obstructive sleep apnea (OSA) is disordered breathing during sleep characterized by periods of partial or complete upper airway obstruction with disruption of normal sleep and ventilatory patterns.

SYNONYM

Upper airway resistance syndrome

ICD-9-CM CODES
780.57 Sleep apnea
780.59 Breathing-related sleep disorder

EPIDEMIOLOGY & DEMOGRAPHICS

- OSA occurs in 1% to 3% of children.
- Of those affected, 75% to 90% are male.
- The incidence has increased over the past 20 years.

CLINICAL PRESENTATION

History

- Snoring (continuous or intermittent, changes with position)
- Mouth breathing, retractions, gasping respirations, pauses in breathing
- Allergic rhinitis
- Behavior disturbances, hyperactivity, declining school performance
- Excessive daytime sleepiness
- Morning headaches
- Enuresis
- Failure to thrive (e.g., poor weight gain)
- Possible history of cor pulmonale or congestive heart failure
  - Shortness of breath
  - Dyspnea
  - Orthopnea
  - Easy fatigue
  - Poor exercise tolerance

Physical Examination

- Tonsillar enlargement
- Boggy nasal turbinates
- Mouth breathing
- Craniofacial anomalies: adenoid facies (i.e., open-mouth posture, flat midface, and dull appearance)
- Body habitus: frequently obese

ETIOLOGY

- The problem may be anatomic, such as a structural blockage of the airway.
- Possible nasal or nasopharyngeal problems include the following:
  - Adenoid hypertrophy
  - Septal hematoma or deviation
  - Choanal atresia or stenosis
  - Nasal polyps or sinonasal tumors
- Oropharyngeal problems include the following:
  - Tonsillar hypertrophy (i.e., pharyngeal or lingual)
  - Macroglossia or glossoptosis
  - Tumors in the floor of the mouth or tongue (especially vascular malformations)
- Laryngeal problems include the following:
  - Laryngomalacia
  - Laryngeal tumors or cysts
  - Laryngeal stenosis (including subglottic stenosis)
- Craniofacial problems (i.e., Down, Crouzon, Apert, and Treacher-Collins syndromes) include the following:
  - Mandibular hypoplasia or retrognathia (e.g., Pierre-Robin sequence)
  - Midface hypoplasia
- Neuromuscular (i.e., poor muscle tone and pharyngeal support) disorders include the following:
  - Cerebral palsy
  - Myotrophic dystrophy
  - Arnold-Chiari malformation
- Miscellaneous problems include the following:
  - Obesity: redundant pharyngeal tissue
  - Mucopolysaccharidoses (Hunter and Hurler's syndrome): nasal congestion, redundant pharyngeal tissue, poor pharyngeal support, fatty soft tissue deposits
  - Achondroplasia: small pharynx, poor muscle tone, relative macroglossia
  - Prader-Willi syndrome: mental retardation, obesity, hypogonadism
  - Gastroesophageal reflux disease: airway irritation and swelling with associated laryngospasm
  - Allergic rhinitis: unresponsive to nasal steroids

DIAGNOSIS

Dx

DIFFERENTIAL DIAGNOSIS

- Primary snoring is caused by increased upper airway resistance with snoring and no discernable symptoms.
- Sleep-disordered breathing is a clinical continuum including upper airway resistance syndrome (UARS), obstructive hypoventilation (OH), and sleep apnea.
- UARS implies increased airway resistance with daytime symptoms.
- OH occurs when upper airway resistance causes elevated $Paco_2$ or decreased Spo_2. No obstructive events are observed.
- Sleep apnea occurs with intermittent but complete upper airway obstruction during sleep.
- Sleep apnea may be obstructive (i.e., blockage of upper airway), central (i.e., decreased respiratory drive from central neurologic origin), or mixed (i.e., central and obstructive apneas).

WORKUP

- The diagnosis is often based on the clinical history and physical examination results.
- Flexible nasopharyngoscopy or laryngoscopy can identify anatomic obstruction.
- Polysomnography monitors oxygen, respirations, air flow, electroencephalogram, sleep stages, and the electrocardiogram.
  - It is done if the diagnosis or severity of the problem is unclear, if no obvious anatomic obstruction is present, or if symptoms are not resolved after initial treatment.
  - Definitions are as follows:
    - Apnea: cessation of airflow for 10 seconds
    - Hypopnea: 50% reduction in air flow with decreased oxygen saturation
    - Respiratory disturbance index: number of apneas (greater than 1 is normal) and hypopneas (apnea-hypopnea index greater than 5 is abnormal) per hour
    - Sleep disturbance index: number of arousals per hour (no normative data; number is nonspecific)
- Home videotapes or cassette recordings may help identify questionable apneic events.
- Overnight home Spo_2 monitor may identify desaturation episodes during sleep.

IMAGING STUDIES

- Cinematic magnetic resonance imaging (MRI) may be performed to identify the obstructive site in complicated cases.
- A lateral airway film can be obtained to identify adenoid hypertrophy.
- A chest radiograph or echocardiogram can identify cor pulmonale and congestive heart failure.

TREATMENT

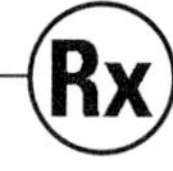

NONPHARMACOLOGIC THERAPY

- Weight loss helps the condition.
- Adenotonsillectomy is often the only intervention necessary.
- Tracheostomy is the gold standard and bypasses the area of obstruction.
- Septoplasty or removal of obstructive nasal tissue can be effective.
- Uvulopalatopharyngoplasty is more commonly used in adults. This process removes excessive uvula and redundant pharyngeal or soft palatal tissue. Tonsillectomy is often performed as well.
- Tongue base reduction, lingual tonsillectomy, and mandibular advancement can be helpful in selected patients.

ACUTE GENERAL Rx

Severe cases may require hospital admission for early intervention.

CHRONIC Rx

- Continuous positive airway pressure (CPAP) is effective but poorly tolerated by some children.
- Treatment of allergy and infection should be considered.

DISPOSITION

- Patients often need to be monitored postoperatively.
- There are risks of respiratory problems and postobstructive pulmonary edema.
- Weight gain, growth hormone normalization, improved behavior, improved quality of life,

and improved school performance have been associated with successful treatment.

REFERRAL

- Otolaryngologists assist in the diagnosis of anatomic obstruction and provide surgical therapy if needed.
- Pulmonologists perform sleep studies, help with the diagnosis of central sleep apnea, and assist in the use of CPAP.

PEARLS & CONSIDERATIONS

COMMENTS

- Not all snoring is OSA. Look for gasping, frequent positional changes, neck extension, or brief awakenings to help differentiate the two.
- Most OSA is caused by adenotonsillar hypertrophy and is easily treated.
- Sleep apnea in children is different from that in adults. Children are less likely to have sustained apneic events but are more susceptible to hypopneas and repeated episodes of desaturation.

PREVENTION

- Avoid obesity.
- Manage allergies if causative.

PATIENT/FAMILY EDUCATION

- Teach parents about pulmonary and cardiac risks if symptoms are severe.
- Provide weight loss education when appropriate.
- Information is available from the American Sleep Apnea Association (www.sleepapnea.org).

SUGGESTED READINGS

Carroll JL: Obstructive sleep-disordered breathing in children: new controversies, new directions. *Clin Chest Med* 24:261, 2003.

Goldstein NA et al: Clinical assessment of pediatric obstructive sleep apnea. *Pediatrics* 114:33, 2004.

Gozal D: Sleep-disordered breathing and school performance in children. *Pediatrics* 102:616, 1998.

O'Brien LA et al: Neurobehavioral implications of habitual snoring in children. *Pediatrics* 114:44, 2004.

AUTHORS: **DAVID R. WHITE, MD** and **CHARLES M. MYER III, MD**

BASIC INFORMATION

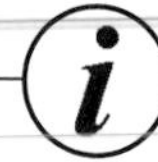

DEFINITION

Occult spinal dysraphism (OSD) is a set of malformations that involve defects of neurulation of the spinal cord or a defect in the skeletal investment of the neural tube, including malformations of all the tissue layers in the midline of the back. OSD involves incomplete vertebral arch formation, usually in the lumbosacral region, with associated neurologic involvement and an unexposed spinal cord (see Meningomyelocele, Syrinx, & Tethered Spinal Cord in Diseases and Disorders [Section I]).

ICD-9-CM CODE
756.17 Occult spinal dysraphism

EPIDEMIOLOGY & DEMOGRAPHICS

- The incidence of OSD in the general U.S. population is unknown.
- The female-to-male predominance is 2:1.

CLINICAL PRESENTATION

History

- Infectious
  - Meningitis caused by multiple organisms or infection that recurs after appropriate treatment may indicate a dermal sinus.
- Urologic or gastroenterologic
  - Enuresis, frequency, urgency
  - Urinary tract infections
  - Bladder or bowel incontinence
  - Constipation
- Orthopedic
  - Abnormal gait
  - Back and leg pain (older children and adolescents)
- Neurologic
  - Lower extremity weakness
  - Decreased spontaneous leg movement (infants)
  - Painless foot burns, ulcers

Physical Examination

- Cutaneous anomalies may occur anywhere along the midline, but they are seen most often in the lumbar region. Combinations of lesions are common.
  - Hair tufts (i.e., hypertrichosis): strong association with diastematomyelia
  - Capillary hemangioma (i.e., pale, flat lesions): often pathologic
  - Lumbosacral dermal sinus: should be distinguished from the common sacrococcygeal pit (see "Pearls & Considerations")
    - A dermal sinus is an opening in the skin that may connect to a subcutaneous tract lined by epithelium, which can be traced to the dura or spinal cord.
    - It is a sign of intradural pathology, and it may become infected and cause meningitis or an intramedullary abscess.
  - Midline or paraspinal masses, such as a lipoma
  - Atretic meningocele or "cigarette burn" sign: thinning of the skin and color changes beneath the skin, resembles a cigarette burn
- OSD may produce orthopedic abnormalities.
  - Foot asymmetry: exaggerated arch, hammer toe
  - Contracted heel cord
  - Leg length discrepancy or asymmetry
  - Progressive scoliosis or kyphosis
- OSD may produce neurologic abnormalities.
  - Absent reflexes (infants), especially the Achilles tendon
  - Decreased rectal sphincter tone
  - Hyperreflexia (older children and adolescents)
  - Asymmetric motor and sensory dysfunction

ETIOLOGY

- Open and closed neural tube defects may be genetically related.
- Some lesions cause caudal traction on the conus medullaris, whereas others cause ventral or dorsal traction. Experimental evidence has shown that traction causes ischemic changes in the spinal cord, which cause neurologic signs and symptoms.

DIAGNOSIS

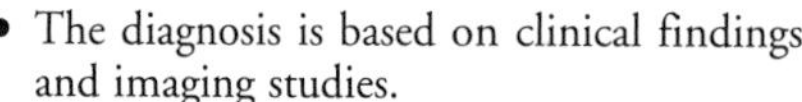

DIFFERENTIAL DIAGNOSIS

- The diagnosis is based on clinical findings and imaging studies.
- Neurologic abnormalities may be in the differential diagnosis for gait disturbances, bowel or bladder dysfunction, and sensory losses or pain.
  - Spinal injury or tumor; spinal cord abscess
  - Diskitis
  - Epidural or subdural spinal bleeding
  - Central nervous system injury (e.g., bleeding, stroke, tumor)
  - Peripheral neuropathies; heavy metal poisoning
- Bone anomalies or injury may be in the differential diagnosis for leg length discrepancy, leg pain, and gait disturbances.

IMAGING STUDIES

- The diagnosis is made with radiographic studies.
- Anteroposterior and lateral plain x-ray films are obtained.
  - Appropriate initial studies
  - Useful for identifying vertebral abnormalities
- Spinal magnetic resonance imaging (MRI) scans
  - Imaging procedure of choice
  - Most likely to detect subtle anatomic abnormalities
- Ultrasound
  - Less sensitive in infants older than 2 months
  - Reader dependent

TREATMENT

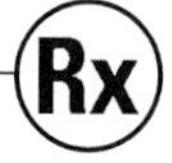

NONPHARMACOLOGIC THERAPY

- Surgery is indicated in symptomatic patients.
- Observation in these cases usually results in neurologic deterioration.

DISPOSITION

- Patients are followed closely for the first 3 to 4 months after surgery and then with annual visits to the pediatric neurosurgeon.
- Repeat MRI scans for asymptomatic patients are of little value.

REFERRAL

Patients should be referred to a pediatric neurosurgeon.

PEARLS & CONSIDERATIONS

COMMENTS

- Coccygeal or sacrococcygeal pits are located in the intergluteal fold over the coccyx; they are of no clinical significance and, if seen in isolation, require no further evaluation.
- Younger children are more likely to present with cutaneous abnormalities, whereas older children are more likely to present with neurologic dysfunction or pain.

PREVENTION

- Women of childbearing age should use periconceptional folate (0.4 mg/day) to help reduce the incidence of neural tube defects.
- If the woman has a previous child or a first-degree relative with any neural tube defects (open or closed), 4 mg of folate daily is suggested.

SUGGESTED READING

Pacheco-Jacome E et al: Occult spinal dysraphism: evidence-based diagnosis and treatment. *Neuroimaging Clin North Am* 13:327, 2003.

AUTHOR: **STEPHANIE SANSONI HSU, MD**

BASIC INFORMATION

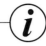

DEFINITION

Osgood-Schlatter disease is a developmental condition of adolescence marked by pain, swelling, and tenderness involving the growing tibial tuberosity. It is more specifically characterized by inflammation of the patellar tendon at its insertion site (apophysitis) on the proximal tibial tuberosity.

SYNONYM

Traction apophysitis of the patellar tendon

ICD-9-CM CODE
732.4 Osgood-Schlatter disease

EPIDEMIOLOGY & DEMOGRAPHICS

- Osgood-Schlatter disease is predominantly a disorder of early adolescent boys (ages 11 to 15 years) and girls (ages 8 to 13 years).
- Prevalence is estimated at 21% of adolescent athletes and 4.5% of nonathletic adolescents.
- The male-to-female ratio is 3:1, but the ratio may be equalizing because of increased participation of girls in sporting activities.
- It is more common among adolescents engaging in athletics requiring repetitive quadriceps contraction.

CLINICAL PRESENTATION

- Anterior knee pain is aggravated by quadriceps stress (e.g., ascending and descending stairs, jumping, running) or by direct pressure on the tibial tuberosity.
- Pain improves with rest.
- Bilateral symptoms are present in 30% of patients.
- There is enlargement of the tibial tuberosity.
- The patellar tendon is thickened.
- There is absence of synovial inflammation or joint effusion.
- Pain increases with quadriceps flexion.
- The quadriceps mechanism and hamstrings are taut.

ETIOLOGY

- Traumatic stress is placed on the proximal tibial tuberosity from repetitive contraction of the patellar tendon by the quadriceps mechanism.
- Repetitive stress causes apophyseal inflammation and heterotopic bone formation at the tibial tuberosity.
- This condition occurs during the developmental period of rapid skeletal growth.

DIAGNOSIS

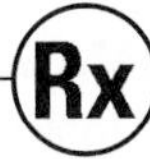

DIFFERENTIAL DIAGNOSIS

- Proximal tibial stress fracture
- Quadriceps tendon avulsion
- Patellofemoral stress syndrome
- Pes anserinus bursitis
- Proximal tibial neoplasm
- Infection (e.g., cellulites, osteomyelitis)
- Patellar tendonitis (Sinding-Larsen-Johansson syndrome)

WORKUP

The diagnosis is typically made on clinical grounds.

IMAGING STUDIES

Anteroposterior and lateral radiographs may be needed to exclude a neoplastic or infectious process.

TREATMENT

Rx

NONPHARMACOLOGIC THERAPY

- Limit activities that stress the patellar tendon.
- Apply ice for short-term relief of pain after activity.
- Practice regular stretching of the quadriceps mechanism and hamstrings.
- Use knee pads to minimize direct trauma.
- Infrapatellar straps or knee braces may partially alleviate symptoms.
- For severe cases not responding to conservative management, more prolonged tendon rest can be achieved with above-the-knee casting for 3 to 6 weeks.
- Surgical excision of the tibial tuberosity or the ossicle in tendon is rarely required.

ACUTE GENERAL Rx

Nonsteroidal anti-inflammatory drugs (NSAIDs) can be prescribed for pain.

CHRONIC Rx

The disorder is typically self-limited.

DISPOSITION

- The disease is generally self-limited, and symptoms may wax and wane.
- Follow-up is dictated by the degree and persistence of symptoms.
- Complications are rare but can include the following:
  - Cosmetic deformity of enlarged tibial tuberosity
  - Patellar tendon avulsion
  - Genu recurvatum resulting from premature fusion of the anterior tibial tubercle and proximal tibia
  - Patellofemoral degenerative arthritis
  - Chondromalacia
  - Uprising of the patella

REFERRAL

- Patients with symptoms not responsive to conservative measures of activity limitation and NSAIDs can be referred to an orthopedic surgeon for bracing or casting.
- Physical therapy may be warranted for some patients.

PEARLS & CONSIDERATIONS

COMMENTS

Corticosteroid injections into the patellar tendon are rarely indicated and may predispose the patient to tendon avulsion.

PATIENT/FAMILY EDUCATION

Normal developmental variation occurs in athletic adolescents.

SUGGESTED READINGS

Bloom OJ, Mackler L: What is the best treatment for Osgood-Schlatter disease? *J Fam Pract* 53:153, 2004.

Dunn J: Osgood-Schlatter disease. *Am Fam Physician* 41:173, 1990.

Kujala U et al: Osgood-Schlatter's disease in adolescent athletes. *Am J Sports Med* 13:236, 1985.

Wall EJ: Osgood-Schlatter disease: Practical treatment for a self-limiting condition. *Physician Sports Med* 26:3, 1998. Available at www.physsportsmed.com

AUTHOR: **JOSEPH A. NICHOLAS, MD**

BASIC INFORMATION

DEFINITION

Osteochondritis dissecans (OCD) is subchondral necrosis of the bone with overlying articular cartilage damage that usually affects the femoral condyles, but it can also involve the patella. Juvenile OCD (JOCD) occurs in skeletally immature persons, and adult OCD occurs after the physis has closed.

ICD-9-CM CODE
732.7 Osteochondritis dissecans

EPIDEMIOLOGY & DEMOGRAPHICS

- The lateral portion of the medial femoral condyle is the classic site (85%) of OCD, although the lateral condyle and patella may be affected.
- OCD is two to four times more common in boys, especially if they are active and athletic (19 of 100,000 girls and 29 of 100,000 boys in one study). The recent increase in the incidence among girls may be associated with increased sports participation by girls.
- OCD most commonly affects 9- to 18-year-old boys and girls.
- It may be an incidental finding on the radiograph.
- There is a better long-term prognosis for JOCD than for adult OCD.

CLINICAL PRESENTATION

- There is a gradual onset (>1 year) of vague, poorly localized knee pain.
- A history of trauma is found in about 50% of cases, but it is unusual to have acute, recent trauma.
- OCD commonly occurs in an athletic child; it is usually activity related but nonspecific.
- Children may experience morning stiffness and stiffness with or after activity.
- A limp may be associated with a "stiff" leg.
- The patient may walk with external rotation of the leg to avoid impingement of the tibial spine on the medial portion of the lateral femoral condyle.
- Grinding, locking, or catching may be caused by a loose or detached lesion; if it occurs, it is generally late in course.
- Rarely is knee swelling reported.
- There are no specific physical findings.
- Tenderness may occur over the involved condyle with the knee flexed. Firm palpation of the femoral condyle, beginning at 90 degrees of flexion and extending the tibia to 30 degrees while holding the limb in internal rotation, may elicit pain (i.e., positive Wilson's sign).
- Pain is relieved when the tibia is externally rotated if OCD occurs in the classic location (i.e., medial portion of lateral femoral condyle).
- These assessments have low sensitivity and specificity.
- Mild effusion is sometimes present.
- The range of motion may be decreased late in the course.

ETIOLOGY

- The cause of OCD is unknown, although many theories exist.
- Trauma or repetitive stress injury in an active, athletic, and growing child or adolescent may cause subchondral bone disturbance or overlying cartilage damage.
- Disruption of a tenuous blood supply with ensuing vascular compromise to the subchondral area is another etiologic theory.
- OCD is more common in growing children.

DIAGNOSIS

DIFFERENTIAL DIAGNOSIS

- Meniscal tear
- Patellofemoral pain syndrome (PFPS)
- Knee joint ligament sprain
- Tumor or bone cyst in the knee area
- Patellar subluxation
- Referred pain from a hip abnormality

IMAGING STUDIES

- Anteroposterior (AP), lateral, and tunnel view radiographs are required for diagnosis.
- The AP view with the knee flexed 20 degrees may be only abnormal radiograph.
  - Notch between distal femoral condyles is visualized.
  - Well-circumscribed subchondral bony separation is a diagnostic finding.
- Irregular or variant ossification or an accessory ossification center is a normal variant sometimes confused with JOCD.
- Magnetic resonance imaging (MRI) is highly sensitive and considered the gold standard. It is used for assessing the size and stage of the lesion.
- Some authorities advocate serial bone scans for diagnosing JOCD.

TREATMENT

NONPHARMACOLOGIC THERAPY

- The goal of treatment is to produce and preserve a stable, normally functioning articular surface.
- For stable (low-stage) lesions, therapy is conservative and nonsurgical.
- Activity modification is warranted if the lesion is not displaced.
- It may be necessary to not bear weight, combined with range-of-motion exercise for 4 to 8 weeks, followed by activity modification for 2 to 6 months.
- If the patient is not healed after 3 to 6 months, surgery may be needed.
  - Commonly done arthroscopically
  - Excision of displaced fragments
  - Internal fixation
  - Bone graft
- For unstable (high-stage) lesions, very large lesions, or in those adolescents approaching skeletal maturity, earlier surgery may be indicated.

ACUTE GENERAL Rx

- Pain medications, such as nonsteroidal anti-inflammatory drugs (NSAIDs), are often warranted.
- There are no specific medications used to resolve fragments.

DISPOSITION

Osteoarthritis is common in patients with JOCD if they are not appropriately treated.

REFERRAL

- Physical therapy or sports medicine consultation may be needed for rehabilitation and physical therapy.
- Refer the patient to an orthopedic surgeon if the diagnosis is unclear, for potential surgical correction, for acute trauma necessitating surgery, and for unresolving pain or dysfunction.

PEARLS & CONSIDERATIONS

COMMENTS

- Infectious, metabolic, and inflammatory diseases of knee, femur, or tibia may manifest with knee pain or effusion.
- All children presenting with knee pain should be evaluated for ipsilateral hip disorders, which can manifest with knee pain.
  - Slipped capital femoral epiphysis
  - Transient (toxic) synovitis of hip
  - Legg-Calvé-Perthes disease

PREVENTION

For asymptomatic OCD, limit the patient's activities until the lesion heals, and treat symptomatic lesions to prevent degenerative arthritis.

PATIENT/FAMILY EDUCATION

The prognosis in JOCD is relatively good.

SUGGESTED READINGS

Cepero S et al: Osteochondritis of the femoral condyles in children and adolescents: Our experience over the last 28 years. *J Pediatr Orthop B* 14:24, 2005.

Hughes JA et al: Juvenile osteochondritis dissecans: A 5 year review of the natural history using clinical and MRI evaluation. *Pediatr Radiol* 33:410, 2003.

Robertson W et al: Osteochondritis dissecans of the knee in children. *Curr Opin Pediatr* 15:38, 2003.

Wall E, Von Stein D: Juvenile osteochondritis dissecans. *Orthop Clin North Am* 34:341, 2003.

AUTHOR: **LYNN C. GARFUNKEL, MD**

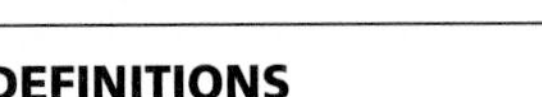

BASIC INFORMATION

DEFINITIONS

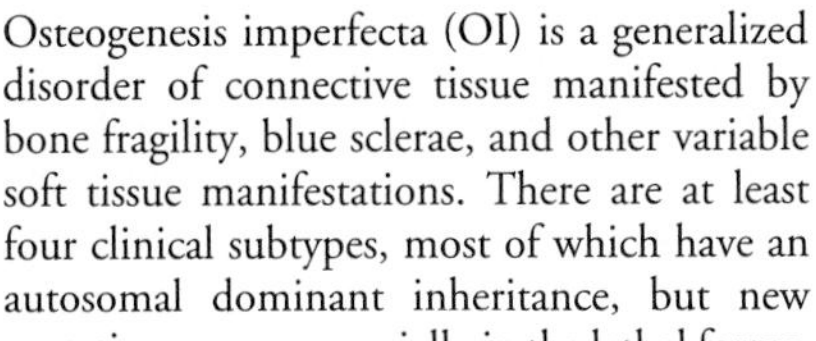

Osteogenesis imperfecta (OI) is a generalized disorder of connective tissue manifested by bone fragility, blue sclerae, and other variable soft tissue manifestations. There are at least four clinical subtypes, most of which have an autosomal dominant inheritance, but new mutations occur, especially in the lethal forms.

- *OI type I*—mildest and most common. Bone fragility, with most fractures caused by mild trauma. Occurs before puberty. The sclerae are blue or have a purple or grayish tint.
- *OI type II*—most severe form and is often lethal in the perinatal period because of respiratory problems. Numerous prenatal fractures result in significant skeletal deformity and contribute to high mortality. Fractures are also sustained during birth. The sclerae are blue or have a purple or grayish tint.
- *OI type III*—bone fragility and severe deformity. Fractures are present at birth. Short limbs and short stature are common. The sclerae are blue in infancy. Respiratory problems caused by rib deformity can be significant. Inheritance appears to be autosomal recessive in most cases.
- *OI type IV*—intermediate between type I and type III in severity. There is bone fragility, mostly before puberty. Short stature can be present, but sclerae are white or near-white. There is mild to moderate bone deformity.
- *Dentinogenesis imperfecta* (brittle teeth) is variable and present in approximately 30% of all types of OI.

ICD-9-CM CODE
756.51 Osteogenesis imperfecta

EPIDEMIOLOGY & DEMOGRAPHICS

- OI type I has an incidence of approximately 4 per 100,000 births.
- OI type II has an incidence of approximately 2.5 per 100,000 births.
- OI type III has an incidence of 1.45 per 100,000 births.

CLINICAL PRESENTATION

History

- Fracture with minimal trauma
- Familial short stature
- Perinatal death (OI type II)
- Presenile hearing loss
- Dentinogenesis imperfecta

Physical Examination

- Blue sclera in types I, II, and III
- Short stature
- Hyperextensible joints
- Hypotonia
- Presenile hearing loss, begins in patients in their 20s and 30s
- Scoliosis
- Deformity
- Brittle teeth
- Barrel chest
- Short limbs

ETIOLOGY

- Reduction or abnormality of procollagen I, resulting in abnormal type I collagen, found in patients with OI type I.
- Mutation in the COL1A1 or the COL1A2 gene loci causes different forms of OI.

DIAGNOSIS Dx

DIFFERENTIAL DIAGNOSIS

- Secondary osteoporosis
- Child abuse
- Hyper-immunoglobulin E (IgE) syndrome

WORKUP

- Skin biopsy
  - Collagen structure is usually normal, but the amount is reduced.
  - Protein and DNA-based studies are done on skin fibroblast culture derived from a skin biopsy sample and can help confirm the diagnosis in most, but not all, cases.
- Prenatal diagnosis
  - High-resolution ultrasound in the second trimester can usually identify fetuses with OI type II and type III. The other forms can sometimes be detected late in the pregnancy.
  - DNA-based prenatal diagnosis using chorionic villus or amniocentesis may be useful in some families.

IMAGING STUDIES

- In types I and IV, radiographs usually show osteoporosis.
- Fractures can be multiple.
- Large calvarium, wormian bones, and hypoplastic dentine are seen.
- Kyphoscoliosis is common.
- In type II, almost no ossification of the skull or wormian bones is found.
- Long bones are short, angulated, and crumpled with thin cortices.
- Ribs show a beaded appearance.
- Multiple fractures are usually seen.
- In type III, severe generalized osteoporosis is seen.
- Wormian bones and severe deossification of membranous skull bones are present.
- Long bones show mild shortening and marked angulation, with metaphyseal and diaphyseal widening.

TREATMENT Rx

NONPHARMACOLOGIC THERAPY

- Fracture prevention (see "Prevention" discussion)
- Dental management in patients with dentinogenesis imperfecta
- Physical therapy and early intervention to maximize mobility in the more severe types of OI
- Management of hearing loss
- Orthopedic care relating to fracture and scoliosis management
- Stapedectomy for hearing loss

CHRONIC Rx

- Growth hormone treatment may be beneficial.
- Bisphosphonates may be beneficial in some situations but they are not yet considered a standard of care.
- Experimental therapy with bone marrow transplantation is being conducted.

DISPOSITION

- Surveillance for hearing impairment and scoliosis

REFERRAL

Referral should be made to the following: genetics, orthopedics, physical therapy, dental (as necessary), and audiology.

PEARLS & CONSIDERATIONS

COMMENTS

- Families with severe postmenopausal osteoporosis should be considered for OI.
- Consider OI in the diagnostic workup of recurrent fractures and suspected child abuse.

PREVENTION

- Avoid high-impact activities to prevent fractures.
- Exercise to promote muscle and bone strength.
- Maintain a healthy diet: appropriate vitamin D, calcium, and phosphate intake.
- Avoid steroid use.

PATIENT/FAMILY EDUCATION

- Types I, II, and IV have an autosomal dominant inheritance. For each pregnancy of affected individuals, there is a 50% chance of having a child with the same condition.
- Affected children from families with no previous history of OI usually have new mutations.
  - Siblings of the affected child would theoretically not be at increased risk.
  - However, gonadal mosaicism in unaffected parents results in an empirical 6% recurrence risk in offspring of such parents.
- OI type III has an autosomal recessive inheritance. Parents of affected children have a 25% recurrence risk for each future pregnancy.

SUGGESTED READINGS

Marini JC et al: Osteogenesis imperfecta. *In* Cassidy SB, Allanson JE (eds): *Management of Genetic Syndromes,* 2nd ed. New York, Wiley-Liss, 2005.

The OI Foundation. Available at www.oif.org

AUTHOR: **CHIN-TO FONG, MD**

BASIC INFORMATION

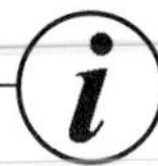

DEFINITION

Osteomyelitis is an infection of bone. It is most commonly caused by pyogenic organisms and rarely by fungi and viruses.

SYNONYM

Bone infection

ICD-9-CM CODES
730.0 Acute osteomyelitis
730.1 Chronic osteomyelitis

EPIDEMIOLOGY & DEMOGRAPHICS

- The incidence is 1 case per 5000 children younger than 13 years. One half of patients are younger than 5 years.
- It is most common in infants and young children. One third of patients are younger than 2 years.
- The male-to-female ratio is 2.5:1.

CLINICAL PRESENTATION

History

- Bone pain (50%) and fever are common.
- In some cases, systemic signs may be minimal, with or without fever.
- Irritability, poor feeding, pseudoparalysis, red or swollen limbs, fever, and malaise may manifest in neonates.

Physical Examination

- Infants and children
  - Limp or refusal to walk
  - Tenderness
  - Limited joint motion
- With extension of infection
  - Local erythema
  - Warmth
  - Swelling more diffuse
- Adolescents
  - Localized point tenderness and limp
  - Decreased use or movement

ETIOLOGY

- Microorganisms are introduced into bone by one of three mechanisms:
  - Hematogenous seeding (most common)
  - Local invasion from contiguous infection
  - Direct inoculation from surgery or trauma
- Bacteria localize to the metaphysis.
- Blood flow may be sluggish in area where nutrient arteries send small terminal branches to terminate in the growth plate. Secondary thrombosis may become a nidus for infection.
- Collection of inflammatory cells and exudate causes the following:
  - Elevation of periosteum and rupture into soft tissue
  - Necrotic bone (i.e., sequestrum)
  - Reparative bone laid down over area (i.e., involucrum)
- Bones with intra-articular metaphysis are predisposed to concomitant septic arthritis when infection ruptures into joint.
  - Hip
  - Shoulder
  - Ankle
  - Elbow
- Common causative bacteria include the following:
  - *Staphylococcus aureus* (70% to 89%), followed by *Streptococcus* (e.g., group A β-hemolytic streptococci, viridans streptococci, *Streptococcus pneumoniae*)
  - Other causes: Enterobacteriaceae, *Salmonella, Kingella kingae*; rarely viruses, fungi, and mycobacteria
  - *Haemophilus influenzae* type b, once common but now greatly decreased in prevalence because of immunization
- Special circumstances are as follows:
  - Sickle cell disease
    - *Salmonella*: 70%
    - *S. aureus*: 10%
    - Gram-negative enterobacteria
  - Neonates
    - *S. aureus*
    - Gram-negative bacteria
    - Group B streptococci
    - Coagulase-negative *S. aureus* (CONS)
    - *Candida albicans*
  - Children younger than 3 years
    - *K. kingae* (32%)
    - *S. pneumoniae* (18%)
    - *S. aureus* (16%)
  - Intravenous drug abusers
    - *Pseudomonas aeruginosa* (especially vertebrae and pelvis)
    - *Serratia marcescens*
  - Facial and cervical osteomyelitis: *Actinomyces* common
  - Superinfection of *S. aureus* osteomyelitis: anaerobes
  - After varicella infection: group A β-hemolytic streptococci
  - Puncture wound of foot (especially through sneaker): *Pseudomonas aeruginosa*
- Femur and tibia are the most commonly affected bones.
  - Predilection for most rapidly growing bones, especially the long bones of lower extremity
  - Occasionally, nontubular bones (e.g., calcaneus) involved

DIAGNOSIS

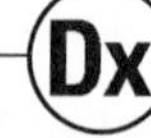

DIFFERENTIAL DIAGNOSIS

- Septic arthritis
- Juvenile arthritis
- Acute rheumatic fever
- Malignancy (e.g., leukemia, Ewing's sarcoma, neuroblastoma)
- Bone infarction (sickle cell)
- Toxic synovitis

WORKUP

- The diagnosis requires two of the following conditions:
  - Purulence of bone
  - Positive blood or bone culture
  - Localized erythema, edema, or both
  - Positive imaging study: radiograph, bone scan, or magnetic resonance imaging (MRI)
    - Cultures of bone (surgically obtained or by needle aspiration) are positive in 80%, and blood cultures are positive in 36% to 67%.

LABORATORY TESTS

- Complete blood cell count (CBC)
  - Leukocytosis with left shift (but may be normal or nearly normal with only a slight left shift)
  - Thrombocytosis (occasionally)
- Erythrocyte sedimentation rate (ESR), a nonspecific sign of inflammation, is usually elevated.
  - Declines 1 to 2 weeks after therapy started
  - Normalizes in 3 to 4 weeks
- C-reactive protein (CRP) level, another marker of inflammation, is usually elevated at presentation and declines within 6 hours of appropriate therapy.

IMAGING STUDIES

- It may take up to 10 to 14 days to see boney change on a radiograph, but it is useful to exclude a fracture or malignancy.
  - Soft tissue swelling (3 days)
  - Obliteration of fat planes (3 to 7 days)
  - Metaphyseal irregularities
  - Periosteal elevation
- Bone scan detects osteomyelitis in the first 24 to 48 hours.
  - Three-phase bone scan with technetium 99m medronate methylene diphosphonate (^{99m}Tc-MDP) may be used.
  - It is useful when the exact site of infection is not certain and when multiple bones may be involved.
  - A *hot spot* is an area of increased uptake in all three phases.
  - A *cold spot* may occur early in course and is an area of decreased uptake caused by bone infarction.
  - Bone scan sensitivity is 90%; specificity is low, 50% sensitivity in neonates.
  - Gallium 67 citrate and indium 111 oxide may be useful if clinical signs are poorly localized.
- White cell scan may be useful.
- Limitations of these studies include time, high radiation dose, and low yield.
- Computed tomography offers excellent bony detail.
  - Reserved for selected cases
  - Helpful in diagnosing spinal and pelvic osteomyelitis
- MRI provides a detailed anatomic picture.

- Prospective sensitivity of 98% and specificity of 75%
- Considered the most sensitive procedure for the diagnosis of osteomyelitis
- Preferred for neonates in whom ^{99m}Tc bone scans may be nondiagnostic
- Useful when the site of bone involvement is apparent clinically
- Delineates subperiosteal or soft tissue collections of exudates that require surgical drainage

TREATMENT

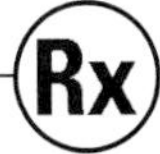

NONPHARMACOLOGIC THERAPY

- Immobilization or splinting of the extremity may help with pain relief and prevention of a pathologic fracture.
- Surgical débridement may be indicated in the following situations:
  - If purulent drainage is found on aspiration of joint or bone
  - If signs or symptoms fail to improve within 48 hours
  - If progressive destruction is visible on the radiograph

ACUTE GENERAL Rx

- Initial management is with parenteral antibiotics after bone aspirate and blood cultures are completed.
- Antimicrobials should cover *S. aureus.*
  - Drugs of choice include β-lactamase–resistant penicillin (e.g., oxacillin, nafcillin), ampicillin-sulbactam, or a first-generation cephalosporin.
  - If methicillin-resistant *S. aureus* (MRSA) is suspected or the patient is penicillin or cephalosporin allergic, use vancomycin.
  - Cefuroxime is empirically used by some with good results.
- *H. influenzae* type b coverage in a very young child includes one of the following:
  - Cefuroxime
  - Ampicillin-sulbactam
  - Third-generation cephalosporin
- Tailor antimicrobials after the organism and sensitivities have been identified.
- The duration of therapy for hematogenous osteomyelitis is controversial.
- Treatment usually lasts for at least 5 to 7 days intravenously. Oral antibiotics are used for 3 to 4 more weeks at two to three times the usual daily recommended dose.
- Consider percutaneously inserted central catheter (PICC) line placement for home intravenous therapy.
- Consider switching to oral antibiotics after the patient is afebrile, local signs and symptoms are reduced, and the patient is maintaining adequate oral intake.
- Check the level of oral antibiotic to ensure absorption and level eightfold to tenfold over the mean inhibitory concentration of organism.

DISPOSITION

- Weekly measurements of CBC, ESR, or CRP should be obtained to follow trends.
- The recommendation to follow peak serial bactericidal titers for a desired titer of 1:8 has been questioned.
- Repeat x-ray films may be indicated in complicated cases or if there is a question about adequate healing.
- Complications include the following:
  - Recurrence
  - Chronic osteomyelitis
  - Leg length discrepancy with lower extremity osteomyelitis
- Risk of complications increases with the following factors:
  - Polymicrobial infection
  - Delay in diagnosis and treatment
  - Short duration of treatment
  - Neonatal age group

REFERRAL

- The patient may be referred to an orthopedic surgeon for management.
  - Bone aspiration
  - Potential need for débridement
- Pediatric infectious diseases specialist for antibiotic management.

PEARLS & CONSIDERATIONS

COMMENTS

- In the neonate, nutrient vessels transverse the growth plate, ending in the epiphysis.
  - These vessels atrophy by 15 to 18 months.
  - More extensive growth plate involvement occurs in neonates.
- Joint aspiration does not significantly alter the bone scan.
- Higher yield is obtained for suspected *K. kingae* when the culture aspirate is deposited directly into a BACTEC bottle.

PATIENT/FAMILY EDUCATION

- Encourage acute and long-term follow-up for monitoring.
- Discuss potential complications.

SUGGESTED READINGS

Floyed RL, Steele RW: Culture-negative osteomyelitis. *Pediatr Infect Dis J* 22:731, 2003.

Karwowska A et al: Epidemiology and outcome of osteomyelitis in the era of sequential intravenous-oral therapy. *Pediatr Infect Dis J* 17:1021, 1998.

Krogstad P: Osteomyelitis and septic arthritis. *In* Feigin R, Cherry J (eds): *Pediatric Infectious Diseases.* Philadelphia, WB Saunders, 2004, pp 713–736.

Moumile K et al: Osteoarticular infections caused by *Kingella kingae* in children: contribution of polymerase chain reaction to the microbiologic diagnosis. *Pediatr Infect Dis J* 22:837, 2003.

Peltola H et al: Simplified treatment of acute staphylococcal osteomyelitis of childhood. *Pediatrics* 99:846, 1997.

Roy DR: Osteomyelitis. *Pediatr Rev* 16:380, 1995.

Sonnen GM, Henry NK: pediatric bone and joint infections: Diagnosis and antimicrobial management. *Pediatr Clin North Am* 43:933, 1996.

AUTHOR: **MEREDITH LANDORF, MD**

BASIC INFORMATION

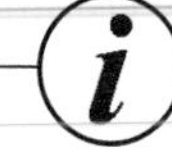

DEFINITION

Osteosarcoma is a neoplasm derived from primitive bone-forming mesenchyme. The pathologic appearance is characterized by the production of osteoid and new bone by spindle-shaped tumor cells. Osteogenic sarcoma is a family of tumors that includes osteosarcoma, chondrosarcoma, and fibrosarcoma.

SYNONYM

Osteogenic sarcoma is a family of tumors to which osteosarcoma belongs.

ICD-9-CM CODE
170.9 Osteosarcoma

EPIDEMIOLOGY & DEMOGRAPHICS

- Osteosarcomas account for 60% of malignant bone tumors.
- The incidence is approximately 5 cases per 1 million children younger than 20 years per year in the United States, with approximately 400 new cases each year.
- The peak incidence is in late adolescence (16 years for females, 18 years for males).
- Males are affected more than females.
- Approximately 90% of osteosarcomas occur in the extremities.
  - The most common site of involvement (approximately 50% of cases) is around the knee, either the distal femur or proximal tibia.
  - Metaphyseal sites of the most rapidly growing bones are more commonly involved.

CLINICAL PRESENTATION

History

- Pain with or without a mass or swelling is reported.
- Systemic symptoms such as fatigue and fever are uncommon.
- Pathologic fractures are rare.

Physical Examination

- Tenderness over the involved bone is elicited.
- A firm mass at the site of involvement is often palpable.

ETIOLOGY

- Most cases are sporadic and have no identified cause.
- The only established environmental cause is ionizing radiation, which is implicated in 3% of cases.
- An association exists with Paget's disease in older patients, with hereditary retinoblastoma, and with Li-Fraumeni syndrome. The *TP53* and retinoblastoma *(RB1)* gene pathways are involved in pathogenesis.
- A relationship exists between rapid growth and the development of osteosarcoma.
- Trauma often brings patients to medical attention, but evidence of a causal relationship is lacking.

DIAGNOSIS

DIFFERENTIAL DIAGNOSIS

- Ewing's sarcoma: second most common tumor occurring in bone
- Other solid malignancies of the extremities: other members of the osteogenic sarcoma family, chondrosarcoma and fibrosarcoma, rhabdomyosarcoma (RMS) or other soft tissue sarcomas, aneurysmal bone cyst, or metastases from RMS or neuroblastoma
- Lymphomas: rarely occur in bone
- Benign bone tumors
- Traumatic lesions
- Infection

WORKUP

- Ideally, biopsy should be done by the orthopedic surgeon who will be performing definitive surgery for local control.
- Approximately 95% of osteosarcomas in children are conventional osteosarcomas of high-grade pathology. They may be osteoblastic, chondroblastic, or fibroblastic based on the predominant type of matrix, although all have osteoid production.
- Other variants, including telangiectatic and small cell osteosarcomas, are also considered high grade.
- Parosteal and periosteal osteosarcomas are rare variants of low-grade and intermediate-grade tumors, respectively, and are rare in children.
- Multiple complex chromosome abnormalities of number or structure have been described.

LABORATORY TESTS

Lactate dehydrogenase and alkaline phosphatase levels are not diagnostic but may indicate tumor burden.

IMAGING STUDIES

- Plain x-ray films of the involved bone (classic "sunburst" pattern is not sensitive or specific)
- Magnetic resonance imaging (MRI) scan of the involved bone
- Bone scan to document the site of disease and assess for bony metastases or synchronous tumors
- Chest radiograph
- Computed tomography (CT) of the chest to evaluate pulmonary metastases

STAGING

- Classification is determined by grade and anatomic extent. Most patients have high-grade tumors with extracompartmental extent, without (stage IIB) or with (stage III) detectable metastases.
- The most common site for metastases is the lungs (85% of patients with metastases).
- Approximately 80% of patients have at least micrometastatic disease.

TREATMENT

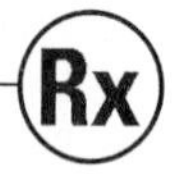

NONPHARMACOLOGIC THERAPY

- Local control requires limb salvage or amputation.
- Radiation therapy is not indicated for first-line therapy of resectable tumors.
  - Potential role in unresectable tumors or for those with tumor at margins of resection
  - Palliative role in cases of progressive disease

ACUTE GENERAL Rx

- Initial chemotherapy usually includes doxorubicin, cisplatin, and methotrexate.
- Ifosfamide and VP-16 are also commonly used active agents.
- Patients are usually treated with neoadjuvant chemotherapy before a definitive surgical procedure is performed.
- Postoperative adjuvant chemotherapy is administered after recovery from surgery.
- Chemotherapy may be adjusted based on the tumor response.
- Targeted therapies, including trastuzumab, targeting epidermal growth factor receptor 2, and imatinib, another tyrosine kinase inhibitor, are being investigated in the treatment of osteosarcoma.

DISPOSITION

- Patients with localized disease have an approximately 70% to 75% 5-year survival rate.
- The overall survival rate for patients with metastatic disease is 20% to 30%.
- Patients with metastatic disease have a better prognosis if metastases can be removed surgically.
- Response to chemotherapy has prognostic significance. Patients with more than 98% tumor necrosis are considered good responders on protocol therapy.
- Plain films and MRI or CT scans of the primary tumor usually are obtained every 3 months for a year, then every 4 to 6 months for 2 years, and then yearly for 10 years. Limb-salvage hardware may cause an artifact on scans.
- Chest radiograph, CT scan of the chest, and bone scan are performed on the same schedule.
- Potential late effects of chemotherapy may include renal glomerular and tubular dysfunction, hearing loss, and cardiomyopathy.
- Patients may experience infectious, traumatic, or other complications of their limb salvage and need long-term follow-up by their orthopedic surgeons.

REFERRAL

Patients should be cared for by pediatric oncologists and by orthopedic surgeons with experience in treating bone tumors.

PEARLS & CONSIDERATIONS

COMMENTS

- Although trauma is not associated with the development of osteosarcoma, patients often present with symptoms after minor injury. Persistent pain should be further evaluated with at least a plain x-ray film.
- Even bone tumors with a benign radiologic appearance should be evaluated by an experienced orthopedic surgeon.
- Patients should be referred to a pediatric oncologist and to an orthopedic surgeon for suspicious lesions.

PREVENTION

No preventive interventions are available.

PATIENT/FAMILY EDUCATION

- Although difficult, the benefits of chemotherapy and aggressive surgical intervention are significant.
- Pediatric oncologists can refer patients and parents to local or national support organizations for children with cancer and their families.
- National organizations include the American Cancer Society and CureSearch, a component of the Children's Oncology Group.
- More information is available at organizational web sites (www.curesearch.org, www.cancer.org).

SUGGESTED READINGS

Halperin EC: Osteosarcoma. *In* Halperin EC et al (eds): *Pediatric Radiation Oncology,* 4th ed. Philadelphia, Lippincott Williams & Wilkins, 2005, pp 291–318.

Link MP et al: Osteosarcoma. *In* Pizzo PA, Poplack DG (eds): *Principles and Practice of Pediatric Oncology,* 4th ed. Philadelphia, Lippincott Williams & Wilkins, 2002, pp 1051–1089.

Marina N et al: Biology and therapeutic advances for pediatric osteosarcoma. *Oncologist* 9:422, 2004.

AUTHOR: **ANDREA S. HINKLE, MD**

BASIC INFORMATION

DEFINITION

Otitis externa is inflammation or infection of the external auditory canal and auricle. Malignant otitis externa refers to temporal bone osteomyelitis.

SYNONYM

Swimmer's ear

ICD-9-CM CODES
380.10 Acute, diffuse, hemorrhagic otitis externa
380.14 Malignant otitis externa
380.15 Mycotic otitis externa
380.23 Chronic otitis externa

EPIDEMIOLOGY & DEMOGRAPHICS

- Uncommon in infants and toddlers
- Accounts for 5% to 20% of pediatric office visits in summer in tropical and subtropical areas

CLINICAL PRESENTATION

- A history of ear pain, fullness, possibly itching, and conductive hearing loss is often associated with recent swimming.
- With malignant otitis externa, the patient often is chronically ill or immunosuppressed.
- Physical examination may reveal erythema and edema of the canal with clear to seropurulent discharge and pain on movement of the tragus of the ear; in severe cases, there can be periauricular swelling.

ETIOLOGY

- Disruption of the normal protective barriers (e.g., hair in the outer part of the canal, cerumen) combined with excessive moisture leads to bacteriologic invasion caused by the following organisms:
  - *Pseudomonas aeruginosa* (most common)
  - *Staphylococcus aureus*
  - Other gram-negative bacteria (e.g., *Proteus, Escherichia coli*)
  - Pathogenic streptococci; rarely, fungi
- Mechanisms that disrupt the barriers include high temperature and humidity, trauma, and alkaline pH.
- Some factors may predispose to these mechanisms.
  - Impacted cerumen
  - Chronic dermatitis (e.g., seborrheic, contact, psoriatic)
  - Perforated otitis media
  - Congenital (e.g., trisomy 21)
  - Acquired narrowing of the canal
  - Immersion baths or swimming
  - Insertion of foreign bodies into the ear canal (e.g., hearing aides, tight fitting ear plugs, cotton swabs or other devices to remove cerumen)

DIAGNOSIS

DIFFERENTIAL DIAGNOSIS

- Furunculosis
- Foreign body
- Serous otitis media
- Acute otitis media
- Bullous myringitis
- Mastoiditis
- Malignancies
- Chronic otorrhea caused by chronic otitis media
- Herpes zoster oticus
- Contact dermatitis

LABORATORY TESTS

- Usually, laboratory tests are not involved in the diagnosis.
- Determination of the erythrocyte sedimentation rate is necessary for excluding malignant otitis externa.

IMAGING STUDIES

Imaging is necessary only for complicated cases in which other diagnoses are being ruled out (e.g., mastoiditis).

TREATMENT

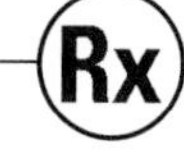

NONPHARMACOLOGIC THERAPY

- Avoid showers, swimming, and excessive exercise until ear edema and pain resolve.
- Lavage and then suction ears with hypertonic saline or 2.5% acetic acid if needed to clear debris, but avoid flushing if the tympanic membrane is perforated.
- Place 2.5% acetic acid solution (i.e., white vinegar, [5% acetic acid] mixed 1:1 with water or rubbing alcohol) in the ear (4 to 6 drops in the ear every 2 hours while awake) during the inflammatory, preinfected stage. Domeboro otic solution (2% acetic acid) can also be used.
- An ear wick can be used to keep the canal patent and to distribute the medicine (needed only in severe cases).
- Surgery is necessary only for severe cases to drain abscesses or for chronic cases that are not responding to medical treatment.

ACUTE GENERAL Rx

- Antibiotic ear drops with or without hydrocortisone may be given.
  - Use 3 or 4 drops of polymyxin or neomycin otic or suspension in the affected ear three to four times per day.
  - Use 3 drops of ciprofloxacin or ofloxacin solution twice daily.
  - Use 1 or 2 drops of an ophthalmic solution such as tobramycin (0.3%) four to six times each day.
- Treat for 5 to 7 days or until 3 days beyond symptom resolution.
- Including hydrocortisone in the drops speeds symptom resolution.
- Analgesics may be given for pain.
- Systemic antibiotics can be used if secondary complications such as cellulitis develop.
  - Cover for staphylococcal organisms with oxacillin or nafcillin.
  - Cover for *P. aeruginosa* if malignant otitis is suspected.

DISPOSITION

Re-examination is needed for severe cases, for lack of resolution, or if the diagnosis is uncertain.

REFERRAL

For treatment failures or severe cases, the patient should be referred to an otolaryngologist.

PEARLS & CONSIDERATIONS

COMMENTS

- Antibiotic ear drops are acceptable even with a perforated eardrum, although there is a small risk of ototoxicity with certain medications (i.e., neomycin). Ofloxacin is the preferred fluoroquinolone ear drop for patients with perforation.
- Neomycin drops may cause severe contact dermatitis, which may confuse the diagnosis.
- Fluoroquinolone drops have the advantage of having better *Pseudomonas* coverage, not causing hypersensitivity, not being ototoxic, and having decreased dosing frequency. Their disadvantages are their cost and the potential risk for causing bacteriologic resistance with repeated use.
- Ophthalmic drops are less acidic than otic drops and may be tolerated better.
- Except for perforated otitis media, treatment is rarely needed for otitis media, even if the tympanic membrane is erythematous.
- In clinical treatment failures, consider Langerhans cell histiocytosis.

PREVENTION

- Silicon earplugs, bathing caps, or oil drops should be used before swimming to keep the ears dry in patients with recurrent otitis externa.
- Dry ears after swimming with a hair dryer (on low setting), and then apply 70% ethyl alcohol drops.
- Use diluted (2% to 2.5%) acetic acid drops in the ear after swimming.
- Avoid manipulation of the ear canal. Do not put anything smaller than an elbow inside the ear.

PATIENT/FAMILY EDUCATION

More information is available on the Internet (www.aafp.org/afp/20010301/927.html).

SUGGESTED READINGS

Beers SL, Abramo TJ: Otitis externa review. *Pediatr Emerg Care* 20:250, 2004.
Guthrie RM: Diagnosis and treatment of acute otitis externa. *Ann Otol Rhinol Laryngol* 108:1, 1999.
Hughes E, Lee J: Otitis externa. *Pediatr Rev* 22:191, 2001.

AUTHOR: **CAROLYN CLEARY, MD**

BASIC INFORMATION

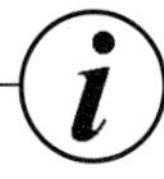

DEFINITION

Otitis media is inflammation of the mucoperiosteal lining of the middle ear cavity. Otitis media may be described as suppurative or serous and as acute or chronic. Complications include extension into the adjacent mastoid air cells, resulting in mastoiditis or perforation of the tympanic membrane with otitis externa. The diagnosis of acute otitis media requires a history of acute onset of symptoms, middle ear effusion, and signs of middle ear inflammation.

SYNONYMS

Acute otitis media
Otitis media with effusion
Serous otitis media
Suppurative otitis media

ICD-9-CM CODES
381.10 Chronic serous otitis media
382.01 Acute otitis media with spontaneous rupture of the tympanic membrane
382.9 Acute otitis media

EPIDEMIOLOGY & DEMOGRAPHICS

- Approximately 90% of children have one episode of acute otitis media by age 2 years.
- Fifty percent of infants in the United States have an episode of acute otitis media by age 6 months.
- About 42% of antibiotics prescribed for children are written to treat otitis media.
- Approximately 2 million surgical procedures are performed each year to place tympanostomy tubes.
- The peak incidence coincides with a peak in the upper respiratory infection rate in the winter months. This pattern may be caused by associated edema and hyperemia of the eustachian tube.
- An increased incidence of the disease is associated with the following factors:
  - Native American or Inuit ethnicity
  - Cleft palate, cleft uvula
  - Craniofacial anomalies
  - Eustachian tube dysfunction
  - Immune deficiencies, such as chronic granulomatous disease, immunoglobulin deficiencies, malignancies, acquired immunodeficiency syndrome, or immune suppression
  - Day-care attendance
  - Down syndrome
  - Connective tissue disorders
  - Passive smoke exposure
- Breastfeeding for at least 6 months is associated with a decreased risk of acute otitis media in the first year of life.

CLINICAL PRESENTATION

History

- Symptoms have an acute onset.
- Fever may be present.
- Otalgia may occur.
- Hearing difficulty may occur.
- In infants and small children, typical symptoms include the following:
  - Irritability
  - Decreased feeding
  - Fever
  - Difficulty sleeping and frequent arousals

Physical Examination

- Immobility of the tympanic membrane
- Bulging tympanic membrane
- Loss of tympanic membrane landmarks
- Hyperemia of the tympanic membrane
- Cloudy or purulent fluid in the middle ear space
- Fever, other signs of systemic illness
- Unsteady gait, suggesting vestibular disturbance
- Hearing loss
- Tympanosclerosis, or scarring of the tympanic membrane, from previous infections

ETIOLOGY

- Poor drainage or obstruction of the eustachian tube leads to accumulation of fluid in the middle ear cavity. This fluid then becomes infected, resulting in otitis media.
- Upper respiratory infections lead to edema and hyperemia of the eustachian tubes, obstructing the drainage of fluid.
- The younger child is anatomically predisposed to ear infections because the eustachian tube is more horizontal than in the adult.
- Causative agents include the following:
  - *Streptococcus pneumoniae*: 25% to 50%
  - *Haemophilus influenzae*: 15% to 30%
  - *Moraxella catarrhalis*: 3% to 20%
  - Viruses, including respiratory syncytial virus (RSV), human rhinovirus, adenovirus, coronavirus, enterovirus, and parainfluenza: 5% to 22%

DIAGNOSIS

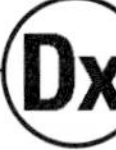

DIFFERENTIAL DIAGNOSIS

- Myringitis
- Otitis externa
- Mastoiditis
- Cholesteatoma
- Otorrhea caused by a foreign body in the canal

WORKUP

- Pneumatic otoscopy
  - An insufflator attached to the otoscope head is used to move the tympanic membrane.
  - Fluid in the middle ear space inhibits this movement.
- Tympanometry
  - Tympanometry incorporates sound energy to determine movement of the tympanic membrane.
  - Abnormal movements indicate abnormal pressures in the middle ear.
  - Tympanometry is used to evaluate and monitor middle ear effusions.
- Spectral gradient acoustic reflectometry
  - Reflected sound waves indicate movement of the tympanic membrane.
  - This method is helpful when a seal of the canal cannot be achieved.
- Tympanocentesis
  - The sample is used for a diagnostic culture.
  - The procedure provides pain relief.
  - It should be considered for the following conditions:
    - In the seriously ill patient with acute otitis media
    - For inadequate response to a second-line antibiotic
    - In the neonate with acute otitis media
    - For immunosuppressed patients
    - For chronic effusion
- For infants younger than 2 months with or without fever, consider further evaluation for extension of the infection and possible sepsis or meningitis.

TREATMENT

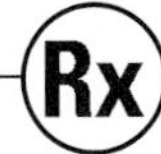

NONPHARMACOLOGIC THERAPY

- Observation without antibiotics may be considered for a previously healthy child 6 months to 2 years old if the illness is not severe and the diagnosis is uncertain. This approach may also be considered for children older than 2 years with a nonsevere illness or an uncertain diagnosis.
- Observation without antibiotics should not be considered for the child who does not have access to a follow-up evaluation in 48 to 72 hours.

ACUTE GENERAL Rx

- Administer amoxicillin (80 to 90 mg/kg/day, divided two times per day) for a 10-day course.
- A 5-day course of antibiotics may be adequate for children older than 2 years.
- Pain relief is achieved with oral analgesics (e.g., acetaminophen, ibuprofen).
- Topical otic analgesics may be used to temporarily ease pain.
- Antihistamines and decongestants have not been useful in the treatment or prevention of otitis media.
- When there may be β-lactamase–positive organisms (e.g., day-care attendance, antibiotics in the previous 30 days) or in cases of severe illness or severe otalgia, a second-line antibiotic may be used. A second-line antibiotic should also be used in children without improvement after 2 to 3 days of the initial therapy.
  - Augmentin: 90 mg/kg of amoxicillin and 6.4 mg/kg of clavulanate, divided two times per day
  - Cefuroxime axetil: 50 to 100 mg/kg/day divided three times per day

- Cefprozil or cefpodoxime
- Azithromycin or clarithromycin
- Ceftriaxone: 50 mg/kg, administered intramuscularly for three daily doses in children unable to tolerate oral medication or in cases of treatment failure with Augmentin
- Clindamycin: 30 mg/kg/day, divided three times daily; may also be used in culture-confirmed pneumococcal disease
- Trimethoprim-sulfamethoxazole
- Fluoroquinolones: oral administration not for routine treatment of otitis media

DISPOSITION

- After the acute infection has been successfully treated, an effusion may persist for 3 months in up to 15% of cases.
- Children should be re-evaluated every 3 months until the effusion resolves. A hearing test is indicated if the effusion persists for 3 months or for any child with language delay, learning problems, or hearing loss.

REFERRAL

- Referral to an otolaryngologist should be considered for any child with four episodes of acute otitis media in a 6- to 12-month period.
- Refer any child with hearing loss to a specialist.
- Bilateral otitis media with effusion persisting for more than 3 months warrants referral.
- Refer a patient with unilateral otitis media with effusion that persists longer than 6 months.

PEARLS & CONSIDERATIONS

COMMENTS

- A red tympanic membrane is not an indication of otitis media without concurrent fluid in the middle ear space. Comparison of ears is useful. The tympanic membrane becomes injected with crying and fever.
- Children have shorter, more horizontal eustachian tubes with less cartilaginous support than adults, and this results in poor ventilatory function. Most children younger than 2 years who spend time in a day-care setting have some middle ear fluid collection with each upper respiratory infection.
- Acute otitis media with purulent conjunctivitis is associated with nontypable *H. influenzae* infection.
- Acute otitis media with hemorrhagic conjunctivitis and pharyngitis may indicate an adenovirus infection.

PREVENTION

The pneumococcal vaccine, a conjugated polysaccharide-protein vaccine, may be a preventive measure.

PATIENT/FAMILY EDUCATION

- Parents should be counseled on the adverse effects of bottle propping, pacifier use after 6 months of age, and passive cigarette smoke exposure in the development of otitis media.
- Breastfeeding for at least 6 months should be recommended to families whose children have recurrent otitis media.
- Day-care attendance is also associated with an increased risk of otitis media.

SUGGESTED READINGS

Subcommittee on Management of Acute Otitis Media, American Academy of Pediatrics and American Academy of Family Physicians: Clinical practice guideline: diagnosis and management of acute otitis media. *Pediatrics* 113:1451, 2004.

Subcommittee on Otitis Media with Effusion, American Academy of Family Physicians, American Academy of Otolaryngology–Head and Neck Surgery, American Academy of Pediatrics: Otitis media with effusion. *Pediatrics* 113:1412, 2004.

AUTHOR: **LORA L. SCHAUER, MD, FAAP**

BASIC INFORMATION

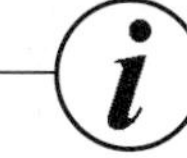

DEFINITION

An ovarian mass is an abnormal growth on one or both ovaries.

SYNONYMS

Adnexal mass
Adnexal tumor
Ovarian cyst
Ovarian tumor

ICD-9-CM CODES
183.0 Ovary, malignant tumor
220 Ovary, benign tumor
620.0 Ovarian cyst (follicular)

EPIDEMIOLOGY & DEMOGRAPHICS

- The incidence of all childhood and adolescent ovarian lesions is 2.6 cases per 100,000 girls per year.
- Sixty-five percent of ovarian masses in this age group are benign.
- In patients younger than 20 years, 58% to 67% of ovarian tumors have germ cell origins.
- Between 20% and 35% of ovarian masses or tumors are epithelial types.
- Approximately 2% to 18% of ovarian masses are sex cord stromal types.
- There does not appear to be a racial or geographic predisposition for ovarian neoplasms.
- Masses can arise at any age, including before birth.

CLINICAL PRESENTATION

History

- The most common presenting symptom is abdominal or pelvic pain; it may be acute or chronic.
- If prepubescent, the pain originates from a mid-abdominal location because the ovaries have not descended deep into the pelvis.
- Increasing abdominal girth and gastrointestinal or urinary symptoms may also occur.
- Ovarian or ovarian mass torsion may be associated with nausea and vomiting.
- Rupture or torsion can mimic an acute abdomen.
- An abdominal mass may be found incidentally.
- Uncommonly, precocious puberty or virilization may be the presenting sign.
- Important information to obtain includes a family or personal history of ovarian masses, pubertal stage, sexual activity, menstrual history (if appropriate), vaginal discharge, fevers, or bowel changes.

Physical Examination

- Vital signs
- Abdominal examination for the following:
  - Palpation of mass
  - Localization of tenderness (if any)
  - Presence or absence of rebound tenderness
  - Referred rebound pain
  - Guarding
  - Rigidity
  - Psoas and obturator signs
  - Bowel sounds
- Pelvic examination for the following:
  - Cultures
  - Size of uterus
  - Location of mass
  - Tenderness
  - Studding or induration of the pouch of Douglas
- Palpation of a mass on rectal examination

ETIOLOGY

- The cause depends on the ultimate tissue diagnosis of the mass.
- Ovarian masses can be cystic or solid, benign or malignant, and they can arise from ovarian tissue or from other tissues that implant on the ovary.
- Those arising from the ovary differentiate from the oocyte, the follicular cells, or the stroma.
- They are classified into functional, epithelial, germ cell, and sex cord stromal types.
- Ovarian cysts are most often caused by normal physiologic processes.

DIAGNOSIS

Dx

DIFFERENTIAL DIAGNOSIS

- Functional benign ovarian cysts are common in infancy and adolescence but less so in prepubertal girls. They are fluid filled on ultrasound and usually resolve with observation.
  - Follicular types result from follicles that did not ovulate but continued to grow.
  - Corpus luteal types result from normal formation of the corpus luteum after ovulation.
  - Theca lutein (rare) types are associated with pregnancy, choriocarcinoma, or molar pregnancy.
- Other tumors are classified by cell derivation; they are solid, any size, and persistent.
- Germ cell tumors are a heterogeneous group derived from primordial germ cell; they often produce tumor markers.
  - Dysgerminoma is the most common malignant germ cell tumor; it is poorly differentiated and rapidly growing. The lactate dehydrogenase (LDH) level is often elevated.
  - Endodermal sinus tumor (yolk sac tumor) is malignant, aggressive, and usually large (>15 cm). It often is associated with an elevated level of alpha-fetoprotein (AFP).
  - Embryonal carcinoma is a highly malignant tumor that may produce β-human chorionic gonadotropin (β-hCG) and AFP. Precocious puberty is sometimes the presenting symptom.
  - Choriocarcinoma is often diagnosed at advanced stage, and it may produce β-hCG.
  - Polyembryoma is rare and very malignant.
  - Teratomas may be mature or immature.
    - Mature cystic teratoma (dermoid cyst) is the most common benign ovarian tumor. It may contain skin, hair, teeth, adipose tissue, brain tissue, or cystic structures.
    - Immature teratoma is a rapidly growing and malignant tumor; 60% have elevated AFP levels.
  - Gonadoblastoma contains germ cell and sex cord stromal elements. These tumors arise in patients with dysgenetic gonads (46,XY).
  - Mixed germ cell tumor is another possible diagnosis.
- Epithelial tumors are rare in children and most common in adults.
  - Serous
  - Mucinous
  - Borderline (low malignant potential)
  - Endometrioma (rare in adolescents with endometriosis)
- Sex cord stromal tumors are made up of granulosa and theca cells and fibroblasts. They frequently produce hormones, and clinical presentation reflects the hormone production.
  - Granulosa cell tumor (juvenile type) occurs in children and produces estrogen. It has a low malignant potential.
  - Thecomas and fibromas are usually benign.
  - Sertoli-Leydig cell tumor (i.e., androblastoma) has a low malignant potential.
- The differential diagnosis includes other causes of abdominal and pelvic masses:
  - Pregnancy
  - Ectopic pregnancy
  - Tubo-ovarian abscess
  - Pelvic kidney
  - Bowel, renal, and adrenal masses

LABORATORY TESTS

- Complete blood cell count
- Urine pregnancy test, if appropriate
- Tumor markers, including the following:
  - β-hCG
  - AFP
  - Carcinoembryonic antigen
  - Cancer antigen 125
  - LDH

IMAGING STUDIES

- The diagnostic test of choice is ultrasound. Abdominal ultrasound is used for younger children and transvaginal ultrasound for adolescents. Ultrasound can determine the following:
  - Location of the mass: ovarian or other sites
  - Size of the mass
  - Consistency of the mass: thin-walled cyst, multiloculated cyst, or solid tumor
- Doppler ultrasound of the ovarian vasculature should be done if torsion is suspected.

- Computed tomography and magnetic resonance imaging rarely add information to the ultrasound results unless a malignancy is strongly suspected.

TREATMENT

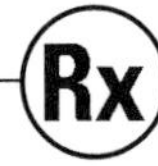

NONPHARMACOLOGIC THERAPY

- The following are treatments for ovarian cysts:
  - In neonates, cysts (even complex cysts) usually are benign and can be followed unless symptomatic.
  - In prepubertal girls, complex cysts should be resected because of the risk of malignancy, and larger simple cysts may require surgery because of the risk of torsion (although this is controversial).
  - In adolescents, cysts are common and often resolve over time.
- If less than 6 cm and simple in appearance, cysts can be observed over a few months for resolution.
- If there is no resolution, the cyst is larger than 6 cm, or it appears to be complex, refer the patient for surgery.
- If simple cysts rupture, transient peritonitis can occur, but it usually resolves within several hours without surgical intervention.
- Corpus luteal cysts are more likely to bleed, rupture, or cause hemoperitoneum, but they may still be managed conservatively if the bleeding stops.
- Mature cystic teratomas usually are treated with surgical resection by laparoscopy or laparotomy.
- Malignant tumors may require combined therapy.
  - Provided the disease is not on the contralateral ovary or uterus, unilateral salpingo-oophorectomy and surgical staging are performed.
  - Every attempt is made to perform conservative surgery.
  - Most patients then receive combination chemotherapy with the BEP (i.e., bleomycin, etoposide, and cisplatin) regimen.
  - Irradiation is sometimes used for persistent disease or recurrence.
- Ovary or ovarian mass torsion is a surgical emergency.

DISPOSITION

- For simple cysts, observation with or without oral contraceptive pills can be done on an outpatient basis for a few months.
- Patients with ruptured simple cysts can be watched in an outpatient (emergency department) setting or in the hospital until symptom resolution while the workup is being completed.
- Hemorrhagic cysts can sometimes be watched in the hospital with serial abdominal examinations.
- Operative management for benign disease is usually done with laparoscopy, but it may require laparotomy.

REFERRAL

Patients with masses that are suspected to be malignant should be referred to a gynecologic oncologist.

PEARLS & CONSIDERATIONS

COMMENTS

- Most ovarian masses in patients younger than 20 years old are benign.
- Ultrasound is the diagnostic test of choice.
- Cysts often can be observed.
- Because functional cysts are unusual in prepubertal girls, the physician must be more aggressive with any ovarian mass identified in this age group.

PATIENT/FAMILY EDUCATION

- Patients with simple cysts who are being observed should understand the following:
  - The benign nature of these cysts
  - The potential for rupture
  - The risk of torsion
  - The likelihood of spontaneous resolution

SUGGESTED READINGS

Brandt ML, Helmrath MA: Ovarian cysts in infants and children. *Semin Pediatr Surg* 14:78, 2005.

Stepanian M, Cohn DE: Gynecologic malignancies in adolescents. *Adolesc Med Clin* 15:549, 2004.

Templemann CL, Fallat ME: Benign ovarian masses. *Semin Pediatr Surg* 14:93, 2005.

von Allmen D: Malignant lesions of the ovary in childhood. *Semin Pediatr Surg* 14:100, 2005.

AUTHOR: **AMY FIX, MD**

BASIC INFORMATION

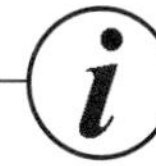

DEFINITION

Pancreatitis is inflammation in the pancreas, which can be acute or chronic. Acute pancreatitis usually resolves without functional sequelae. Chronic pancreatitis involves ongoing structural and functional changes, which may be manifest clinically with chronic, persistent symptoms or recurrent exacerbations. Chronic obstructive pancreatitis can be considered a subset of chronic pancreatitis, and it improves with relief of the obstruction or progresses to chronic pancreatitis if untreated.

ICD-9-CM CODES
577.0 Acute pancreatitis
577.1 Chronic pancreatitis

EPIDEMIOLOGY & DEMOGRAPHICS

- Pancreatitis is not common in children; progression from acute to chronic is rare.
- Risk factors for pancreatitis reflect the causes (see "Etiology"), with the most prevalent being trauma, infection, medications, and genetic or developmental disorders.
- Genetic and developmental disorders involving the pancreas are rare and include hereditary (familial) pancreatitis, cystic fibrosis, and pancreas divisum.
- Hereditary pancreatitis is characterized by recurrent bouts of acute pancreatitis, which can manifest in childhood.
    - Episodes are associated with eventual pancreatic insufficiency and pancreatic cancer later in life.
    - The diagnosis is suggested by a family history and radiographic evidence of pancreatic calcifications.
    - Inheritance pattern is autosomal dominant.
    - Genetic mutations identified in the trypsinogen gene render trypsin resistant to hydrolysis by pancreatic enzymes designed to protect the pancreas from autodigestion initiated by excess trypsin.
    - Screening tests for the mutation are available.
- Cystic fibrosis
    - Chronic pancreatitis has been associated with a specific genotype of cystic fibrosis.
    - Sweat test results are often normal.
    - Diagnosis can be made by identifying specific abnormalities in the genotype and by measuring nasal potential difference (PD), which is abnormally high.
- Pancreas divisum affects pancreatic function.
    - Dorsal and ventral pancreatic ducts do not fuse during development, resulting in drainage of the pancreas through the dorsal duct alone.
    - This is considered a normal variant, but in some individuals, it may cause pancreatitis by obstruction.
    - Management is controversial, can involve surgery or interventional endoscopy.
    - The diagnosis is made by magnetic resonance cholangiopancreatography (MRCP), endoscopic retrograde cholangiopancreatography (ERCP), or endoscopic ultrasound.

CLINICAL PRESENTATION

- Presenting symptoms include the following:
    - Abdominal pain (mild or severe), often worse with meals; vomiting (common); nausea; anorexia
- Predisposing factors may be identified:
    - Drugs or toxins; trauma; infections
- There may be a family history of cystic fibrosis or pancreatitis.
- Physical signs vary with the degree of pancreatic inflammation and systemic involvement.
    - Abdominal tenderness (epigastric); peritoneal signs (rebound, guarding); abdominal distention; decreased or absent bowel sounds; fever (low grade); hypotension, shock; ascites; respiratory distress
- In severe cases, hemorrhagic pancreatitis may occur.
    - Cullen's sign: ecchymoses around the umbilicus; Turner's sign: ecchymoses along the flank

ETIOLOGY

- The exact mechanisms that cause pancreatic inflammation are unclear, but the general process is one of autodigestion resulting from premature activation of proenzymes to active digestive enzymes within the pancreas, beginning with activation of trypsin.
- Etiologies of acute pancreatitis include:
    - The most common cause of acute pancreatitis in adults is cholelithiasis (uncommon in the pediatric population).
    - As many as 50% of pediatric cases of acute pancreatitis are considered idiopathic.
    - Drugs and toxins can cause pancreatitis.
    - Causative infections include viral, bacterial, and parasitic organisms.
    - Mechanical or structural causes include trauma, pancreatic outflow obstruction (e.g., pancreas divisum, strictures, cholelithiasis), bile reflux (e.g., choledochal cyst, strictures, choledocholithiasis), and duodenopancreatic reflux (e.g., duodenal obstruction).
    - Systemic diseases correlating with pancreatitis include vasculitis and inflammatory disorders, autoimmune pancreatitis, sepsis, shock, and Reye's syndrome.
    - Metabolic abnormalities include hypercalcemia, hyperlipidemia, hypothermia, uremia, malnutrition with refeeding, and diabetic ketoacidosis.
    - Genetic disorders include hereditary pancreatitis and cystic fibrosis.
- Etiologies of chronic pancreatitis include:
    - The most common cause of chronic pancreatitis in adults is alcohol.
    - Chronic pancreatitis in children is rare and usually results from hereditary pancreatitis, cystic fibrosis, or a structural abnormality such as pancreas divisum. These conditions cause recurrent bouts of acute pancreatitis that result in chronic inflammation and damage.

DIAGNOSIS

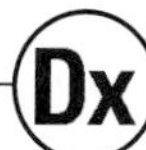

DIFFERENTIAL DIAGNOSIS

- Hepatobiliary disease
    - Hepatitis; hepatic abscess; cholecystitis; cholangitis; biliary colic (choledocholithiasis)
- Peptic acid disease
    - Gastritis; duodenitis; ulcers
- Intestinal disease
    - Appendicitis; perforation or peritonitis; obstruction; acute gastroenteritis
- Renal disease
    - Nephrolithiasis; pyelonephritis

WORKUP

- Step 1: Establish the presence of pancreatitis.
    - Amylase and lipase levels
    - Ultrasound
    - Computed tomography (CT) if ultrasound is not diagnostic
- Step 2: Assess the severity of pancreatic inflammation.
    - Estimates of the severity of pancreatitis have been based on several clinical and laboratory parameters (e.g., Ranson's criteria, APACHE II score), none of which has been validated in children.
    - The following findings are helpful:
        - Clinical signs of hemodynamic compromise and systemic toxicity
        - Laboratory studies, including white blood cell (WBC) count; hemoglobin and hematocrit levels; and concentrations of glucose, electrolytes, blood urea nitrogen (BUN), creatinine, and calcium. Hemoconcentration is a sensitive indicator of severity.
        - CT scan determination of interstitial versus necrotizing pancreatitis (see "Imaging Studies").
- Step 3: Determine the cause of pancreatitis.
    - For the initial episode of acute pancreatitis, if the cause is not apparent by the history and presentation, evaluation should include laboratory tests for metabolic causes (e.g., calcium, triglycerides) and imaging studies (e.g., ultrasound, CT) to rule out obstructive causes.
    - For recurrent pancreatitis, if the cause was not established during the initial episode, the evaluation may include genetic screening for hereditary causes and MRCP or ERCP to further evaluate ductal abnormalities.

LABORATORY TESTS

- The most commonly used tests to establish the diagnosis of pancreatitis are for amylase and lipase levels.
- Amylase levels.
    - The concentration increases within hours of onset of pancreatitis and remains elevated for 4 to 5 days.
    - Other causes of increased amylase include biliary obstruction, intestinal perforation or obstruction, trauma, appendicitis, mesenteric ischemia, parotitis, salivary duct obstruction, and tubo-ovarian disease.

- Lipase levels.
  - Lipase levels are more specific for pancreatitis than amylase levels. The concentration of lipase increases within hours of the onset of pancreatitis and remains elevated for 8 to 14 days.
  - Lipase is better for verifying the presence of pancreatitis later in the course of illness.
  - Nonpancreatic sources of lipase are salivary glands, stomach, and breast milk.
- Diagnosis requires interpretation of results.
  - An increase of at least threefold in both test results is highly suggestive of pancreatitis.
  - The amylase or the lipase level may be falsely normal or falsely elevated in the presence of pancreatitis.
  - Rarely both falsely normal or elevated.
- Other laboratory tests may be useful in assessing severity and determining a cause.
  - Severity: WBC, hemoglobin and hematocrit, glucose, electrolytes, BUN, creatinine
  - Causes: metabolic (e.g., elevated calcium, triglycerides), genetic (e.g., testing for hereditary pancreatitis, cystic fibrosis), autoimmune (e.g., IgG subclasses, such as elevated IgG_4).

IMAGING STUDIES

- Kidney, ureter, and bladder (KUB) examination can suggest the presence of pancreatic inflammation.
  - Nonspecific findings that suggest the presence of pancreatitis include a sentinel loop (i.e., distended loop of small bowel near the pancreas) and the colon cutoff sign (i.e., dilated transverse colon with termination of the gas pattern at the level of the splenic flexure).
- Ultrasound can confirm the presence of pancreatic inflammation and identify potential causes and complications.
  - Usually the initial study performed and can show changes consistent with pancreatitis in 70% to 80% of cases.
  - Identifies potential causes, including stones and biliary tract disease.
  - Identifies complications of pancreatitis, specifically phlegmons and pseudocysts.
- CT is useful if ultrasound is nondiagnostic or does not adequately visualize the pancreas. CT with intravenous contrast is particularly useful for differentiating interstitial from necrotizing (not perfused) pancreatitis.
  - Interstitial pancreatitis is usually milder and sterile.
  - Necrotizing pancreatitis has a higher association with infection and poor outcome.
- ERCP can be used to identify ductal abnormalities and to therapeutically address structural or obstructive causes of pancreatitis such as gallstones. This procedure is not usually performed during the initial episode of pancreatitis unless therapeutic intervention is required.
- Magnetic resonance imaging (MRI) and MRCP are effective tools for assessing pancreatic inflammation and identifying ductal abnormalities.

TREATMENT

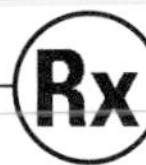

NONPHARMACOLOGIC THERAPY

- Decrease inflammation. Provide supportive care. Assess for and treat complications.

ACUTE GENERAL Rx

- Decrease inflammation. Eliminate any cause or potential contribution to inflammation (e.g., drugs, impacted gallstones).
- Provide supportive care.
  - Close clinical monitoring (in the ICU if pancreatitis is severe) is necessary.
  - Laboratory tests include a complete blood cell count; BUN; liver function tests; and determinations of creatinine, glucose, electrolytes, calcium, and magnesium levels.
  - Eliminate oral intake (i.e., minimize pancreatic exocrine function).
  - Place a nasogastric tube in patients with protracted vomiting or ileus.
  - Provide intravenous fluid hydration and correction of electrolyte imbalances.
  - Administer nutritional support (i.e., parenteral nutrition or nasojejunal feedings) if oral feedings cannot be initiated within a few days.
  - Provide pain management.
- Assess for and treat complications.
  - Metabolic complications include hypocalcemia and hyperglycemia.
  - Infections include phlegmons, fluid collections, and areas of pancreatic necrosis that may become infected, which significantly increases morbidity and mortality.
    - Incidence of infection in necrotizing pancreatitis is 30% to 50%, compared with 1% in interstitial (mild) pancreatitis.
    - In the presence of signs and symptoms of infection, antibiotic therapy with a broad-spectrum antibiotic such as imipenem is recommended.
    - If there is deterioration or no improvement, surgical débridement may be necessary.
  - Pseudocysts are collections of fluid and debris that are encapsulated but that do not contain an epithelial lining.
    - Identified by ultrasound or CT and develop in 10% to 20% of patients with pancreatitis
    - Common in traumatic pancreatitis
    - May require surgical, percutaneous, or endoscopic drainage under certain circumstances

CHRONIC Rx

- Protracted acute, recurrent, or chronic pancreatitis may require ongoing therapy for the following features:
  - Pain; pancreatic endocrine and exocrine insufficiency; nutritional support

DISPOSITION

- When the cause of the pancreatitis is alleviated, most episodes resolve without sequelae.
- Chronic complications may include pseudocysts, chronic pain, and pancreatic insufficiency.
- There is an increased incidence of pancreatic cancer among patients with hereditary pancreatitis.

REFERRAL

- Patients should be referred to a gastroenterologist if they have the following conditions:
  - Mild pancreatitis without a clear cause
  - Obstructive pancreatitis
  - Pancreatitis severe enough to require hospitalization
  - Recurrent or chronic pancreatitis

PEARLS & CONSIDERATIONS

COMMENTS

- Clinical signs and symptoms may be nonspecific, and a high index of suspicion is necessary to make the diagnosis.
- The diagnosis can be established in most cases with amylase and lipase determinations and with ultrasound.
- A family history of recurrent pancreatitis or cystic fibrosis should raise the possibility of pancreatitis in a child with abdominal pain.
- There is no specific treatment for the genetic causes of pancreatitis, and counseling should be provided before moving forward with testing.

PREVENTION

- Avoid medications that have caused pancreatitis.
- Treat underlying metabolic and obstructive causes.

PATIENT/FAMILY EDUCATION

- This condition is not common in children, and specific causes of pancreatic inflammation should be identified and addressed if possible.
- Therapy is supportive and usually includes having no oral intake for a period to rest the pancreas. A nasojejunal tube may also be necessary in the presence of protracted vomiting or an ileus.
- Assessing the severity of the inflammation with clinical observation, laboratory tests, and radiographic study guides subsequent therapy and predictions of outcome.

SUGGESTED READINGS

Etemad B, Whitcomb DC: Chronic pancreatitis: Diagnosis, classification and new genetic developments. *Gastroenterology* 120:682, 2001.

Lowe ME: Pancreatitis in childhood. *Curr Gastroenterol Rep* 6:240, 2004.

National Pancreas Foundation. Available at www.pancreasfoundation.org

North American Society for Pediatric Gastroenterology, Hepatology and Nutrition. Available at www.naspghan.org

Tenner S: Initial management of acute pancreatitis: Critical issues during the first 72 hours. *Am J Gastroenterol* 99:2489, 2004.

AUTHOR: **M. SUSAN MOYER, MD**

BASIC INFORMATION

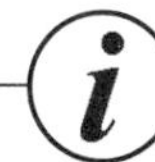

DEFINITION

Parasomnias are undesirable or unpleasant physical phenomena that involve skeletal muscle movement during sleep. Parasomnias are organized into four major categories. Disorders associated with arousal include somnambulism or sleepwalking, somniloquy or sleep talking, and confusional arousals or night terrors. Disorders associated with sleep-wake transition include body rocking; head banging; thumb sucking; and hypnic myoclonia, hypnagogic jerks, or sleep starts. Disorders associated with rapid eye movement (REM) sleep include nightmares, frightening dreams that frequently awaken the child, and REM sleep motor disorder and REM behavior disorders, which are physical dream enactments that occur during sleep. Another parasomnia is sleep bruxism, which is teeth grinding during sleep. (See also Sleep Problems, Nonorganic in this section.)

SYNONYMS

Sleep disorders
Sleep disruption

ICD-9-CM CODES

306.8 Bruxism
307.42 Sleep onset association disorder
307.46 Somnambulism or night terrors
307.47 Nightmare
780.59 Parasomnia

EPIDEMIOLOGY & DEMOGRAPHICS

- Parasomnias occur in most children. Collectively, sleep disturbances are one of the most common complaints of parents to pediatricians.
- For disorders associated with arousal, the exact prevalence of partial arousal disorders is unknown.
  - Symptoms typically begin in early childhood and become progressively less prevalent in adolescents and adults.
  - There is frequently a familial pattern of occurrence.
  - Sleepwalking occurs in 15% to 40% of all children, with onset between 4 and 6 years.
  - Sleep talking usually begins around 3 to 10 years of age and occurs equally in boys and girls.
  - Sleep terrors occur in approximately 3% of all children, with onset between 4 and 12 years, but they affect less than 1% of adults. Sleep terrors occur more commonly in boys than girls.
- For disorders associated with sleep-wake transition, rhythmic movements during sleep occur in approximately two thirds of normal children, with a male predominance.
  - Onset is usually before the first birthday, and complaints typically resolve spontaneously by age 4.
  - Hypnic myoclonia can occur at any age and is considered pathologic only if episodes are excessively frequent or it results in sleep-onset insomnia.
- For disorders associated with REM sleep, the exact lifetime prevalence of nightmares is unknown but likely approaches 100%.
  - Between 20% and 30% of school-age children have at least one nightmare in any 6-month period.
  - Nightmares occur more frequently and have an increased prevalence among children compared with adults.
  - There appears to be no gender predilection or familial predisposition for nightmares.
  - REM sleep motor disorder, or the physical enactment of dreams during sleep, has been described but is rare in children.
- Other parasomnias can affect children.
  - Sleep bruxism can occur at any stage of childhood but usually begins in late childhood or early adolescence and occurs equally in boys and girls.
  - An estimated 50% of children have experienced bruxism, but dental evidence can be identified in only 10% to 20% of the general population.

CLINICAL PRESENTATION

- Most children suffering from parasomnias have no obvious clinical abnormalities during wakefulness. Children are typically medically and developmentally normal but exhibit frightening and disruptive behaviors while sleeping at night.
- Some disorders are associated with arousal.
  - Partial arousal disorders classically arise from slow-wave sleep (SWS) and therefore tend to occur in the first third of the night.
  - The child is apparently awake but does not respond to parental attempts to intervene or console.
  - There is typically amnesia for the events.
  - With somnambulism, the child arises from bed and ambulates. Child may perform complex motor tasks but be unable to negotiate simple obstacles.
  - With somniloquy, the child mumbles or talks in his or her sleep but is usually incomprehensible. The most frequent utterance is "No, no."
  - With confusional arousals, also called nightmares, the child screams inconsolably.
  - Intense sympathetic activity results in mydriasis, diaphoresis, tachycardia, and tachypnea.
- Some disorders are associated with the sleep-wake transition.
  - Rhythmic movement disorders involve stereotypic movements, such as body rocking head banging, and thumb sucking during the transition from wakefulness to sleep.
  - In mild form, these movements may be considered benign developmental events, but they can result in considerable social embarrassment and anxiety, particularly for older and more severely affected children. Bodily injury can occur but is rare.
  - Movements typically occur repetitively at the time of sleep onset and can recur throughout the night during periods of brief awakening and transition back to sleep.
  - Hypnic myoclonia is the occurrence of a single contraction of the postural muscles during the transition from wake to sleep. Parents and children may report body jerks during this time.
  - Hypnic myoclonia is frequently associated with hallucinations that may include the sensation of falling.
- Some disorders are associated with REM sleep.
  - Nightmares classically arise from REM sleep and therefore tend to occur in the latter third of the night.
  - Dreams may be quite complex and frequently involve the perception of credible threat to the child's well-being.
  - There is typically recall of events and circumstances of the dream sequence, although this may be limited by the child's maturational abilities.
  - Body movements during nightmares are rare because of normal REM-associated muscular hypotonia.
  - Nightmares frequently result in emotional upset and anxiety about returning to sleep. However, the intense autonomic activity characteristic of sleep terrors is less prominent.
  - With REM sleep motor disorder, REM sleep motor atonia is impaired, allowing physical enactment of dream sequences, including violent movements, running, or jumping out of bed. Substantial bodily injury may occur during these events.
- Other parasomnias include the following:
  - Bruxism typically presents with morning headache, pain in the jaw area, or tooth hypersensitivity.
  - Forceful tonic or rhythmic jaw clenching results in the irritating sound of tooth grinding.
  - Dental damage; alveolar bone loss; hypertrophy of the masseter, temporalis, and pterygoid muscles; and temporomandibular joint dysfunction can occur.

ETIOLOGY

- Disorders associated with arousal
  - Arousal disorders are caused by partial or incomplete arousal from SWS.
  - Psychopathology is rare in children with arousal disorders.
  - Arousal disorders can be exacerbated by increased sleepiness resulting from irregular sleep schedules, insufficient total sleep quantity, stress, anxiety, environmental factors (e.g., elevated room temperature, noise at night, atypical sleeping

location), fever, pain, bladder distention, and other sleep disorders.
- Disorders associated with sleep-wake transition
  - Sleep-wake transition disorders are typically learned automatisms that function to soothe the child as he or she transitions into sleep. The cause is unknown.
  - Children with autism and pervasive developmental disabilities often exhibit rhythmic movement disorders at sleep onset. Many entirely normal children exhibit these behaviors.
- Disorders associated with REM sleep
  - Occasional nightmares are common during childhood. Frequent or persistent nightmares associated with disturbances in daytime performance warrant investigation into underlying medical or psychological causes.
  - Nightmares are associated with sleep deprivation, irregular sleep schedules, stress, anxiety, environmental factors (e.g., elevated room temperature, noise at night, atypical sleeping location), fever, and pain.
  - Numerous medications trigger nightmares, including catecholamines, β-blockers, antidepressants (particularly bupropion), barbiturates, and alcohol.
  - Nightmares can also occur during withdrawal of antidepressants due to REM rebound.
  - Vivid dreaming occurs during acute alcohol withdrawal as part of the syndrome of delirium tremens (DTs).
  - REM sleep motor disorder is rare in children, and little is known about the etiologic factors in the pediatric population. Most adult cases of REM sleep motor disorder are idiopathic, although neurologic disorders are commonly reported, including narcolepsy, Tourette's syndrome, and various structural, traumatic, and vascular brain injuries.
- Other parasomnias
  - Dental malocclusion may result in bruxism.
  - Bruxism is a characteristic feature of Rett's syndrome.
  - Stress and anxiety are predisposing factors to bruxism.

DIAGNOSIS

DIFFERENTIAL DIAGNOSIS

- Seizures
- Gastroesophageal reflux
- Obstructive sleep apnea syndrome (OSAS)

WORKUP

- A detailed history and physical examination, along with an account of the immediate events, usually lead to a correct diagnosis. Ancillary testing is typically unnecessary. The history should focus on the following information:
  - Typical time of event occurrence
  - Description of behaviors involved
  - Child's responses to parental attempts to intervene
  - Recall of or amnesia for nocturnal events
  - Stereotypic, rhythmic, or repetitive movements during the episodes
  - Symptoms or abnormalities during wakefulness
  - Typical sleep schedule and sleep environment
  - Presence of bedtime rituals
  - Intercurrent illness or medical problems
  - Medication usage or recent discontinuation
  - Psychosocial stressors
- Sleep diaries are useful in determining sleep patterns and current pattern of nocturnal events. Diaries are also useful in following the response to recommended behavioral interventions.
- Attention should focus on habitual snoring because respiratory-induced sleep disruption associated with OSAS may manifest as a parasomnia.

LABORATORY TESTS

- Video nocturnal polysomnography (NPSG) can be useful in demonstrating events.
- Electroencephalography (EEG) can be useful in differentiating parasomnias from nocturnal seizures. The presence of epileptiform activity does not exclude a diagnosis of parasomnia because seizures and parasomnias may coexist.
- PSG can be useful for identification of respiratory events resulting in sleep disruption that may manifest as a parasomnia.
- Characteristic NPSG or EEG findings frequently found in patients with sleep walking and confusional arousals include the following:
  - Sudden or abrupt awakening from SWS
  - Frequent partial arousals during SWS
  - The EEG findings for intrusion of hypersynchronous theta activity into SWS are normal variants and are therefore not diagnostic but can help clarify clinically unclear diagnoses.
  - Somniloquy can occur during any stage of sleep.
  - Typical rhythmic movements occurring during the transition from wakefulness to sleep may be identified in children with rhythmic movement disorders. These movements are notably absent during deeper stages of non-REM and REM sleep.
  - Increased REM density during REM sleep may occur during nightmares followed by abrupt awakening and a prolonged period of wakefulness before return to sleep. Normal muscle atonia is observed during REM sleep.
  - Normal REM sleep associated muscle atonia is absent in patients with REM sleep motor disorder.
  - Rhythmic 1-Hz muscle artifact over the temporalis muscle can be identified in children with bruxism.
- A urine toxicology screen should be obtained if illicit drug use is suspected.

TREATMENT

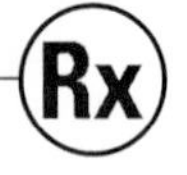

NONPHARMACOLOGIC THERAPY

- Reassurance that the child is normal mentally, neurologically, and developmentally should be provided when appropriate.
- Identify and minimize precipitating causes, including stress and anxiety.
- Effective treatment of OSAS may lead to prompt resolution of symptoms of parasomnias. If symptoms fail to fully resolve, repeat polysomnography is indicated to ensure complete resolution of OSAS.
- Good sleep hygiene remains the cornerstone of therapy.
  - Adequate total amount of sleep for age
  - Consistent bedtime and wake-up time
  - Consistent sleeping location in a quiet, cool, and dark environment
  - Consistent parental response to awakenings
  - Ritualistic and relaxing bedtime routine
- Encourage parents to avoid overinvolvement during events because they may contribute to nocturnal attention-seeking behaviors.
- Limitation of liquid intake and voiding before bedtime may be helpful.
- Scheduled awakenings before the typical time of nocturnal events are controversial but may hasten their resolution.
- Alarms (e.g., bells on a doorknob or gate) to notify a parent that the child has left the bed may be helpful.
- A safe and secure environment is necessary to prevent unintentional injury.
- Use of an occlusive device such as a mouth guard does not prevent bruxism but can protect dentition.

ACUTE GENERAL Rx

- With frequent or injurious nocturnal behaviors, pharmacologic therapy may be indicated, but behavioral measures and effective sleep hygiene should be included.
- Pharmacotherapy should be used for a minimal duration.
  - Be cognizant of daytime hangover effects.
  - Prolonged therapy is associated with tachyphylaxis and dependence.
- Benzodiazepines, including clonazepam, lorazepam, and diazepam, are the most commonly prescribed medications in the treatment of parasomnias.

CHRONIC Rx

- Recommended ritualistic bedtime routines and adherence to strict sleep schedules are frequently in excess of that practiced by the

general population and require substantial effort on the parent's part.
  - Gradual return to a less rigid schedule is allowable and may not result in the recurrence of symptoms, which typically abate with age regardless of therapy.
  - If symptoms recur, nonjudgmental support is necessary.

DISPOSITION

Most parasomnias can be adequately treated with behavioral modifications by the child's general pediatrician in the outpatient setting.

REFERRAL

- OSAS should be accurately diagnosed and treated. (See Obrstructive Sleep Apnea in Diseases and Disorders [Section I].)
  - If symptoms fail to fully resolve, repeat polysomnography is indicated.
  - Noninvasive ventilatory support in the form of continuous positive airway pressure (CPAP) may be necessary to treat residual OSAS.
- If families are unable to accomplish recommended behavioral changes, referral to a behavioral specialist may be necessary.
- Children who fail to respond to behavioral modifications and those with pronounced symptoms (especially those resulting in daytime dysfunction) should be referred to a sleep specialist.
- Children with suspected underlying psychiatric or emotional disturbances should be referred for evaluation and treatment of the emotional disturbance.

PEARLS & CONSIDERATIONS

COMMENTS

- Most parasomnias, although unpleasant and sometimes frightening, are self-limited, benign developmental events and are usually not a sign of more serious pathology.
- OSAS can masquerade as a parasomnia because of the resultant respiratory-induced sleep disruption.
- Behavioral modifications can resolve most sleep disturbances but require significant dedication on the part of parents and their children.
- Short courses of pharmacotherapy in conjunction with behavioral modifications may be necessary.

PREVENTION

- Good sleep hygiene
- Adequate total amount of sleep for age
- Voiding before bedtime

PATIENT/FAMILY EDUCATION

- Reassure parents. Children typically outgrow parasomnias. Most parasomnias are not associated with psychopathology or neurologic abnormalities.
- Educate parents on how to avoid trigger factors.
- Safety measures to limit unintentional injury during nocturnal events include the use of alarm systems, gates, locking exterior doors and windows, and keeping the floor clear of clutter.

SUGGESTED READINGS

Guilleminault C et al: Sleepwalking and sleep terrors in prepubertal children: What triggers them? *Pediatrics* 11:e17, 2003.

Laberge L et al: Development of parasomnias from childhood to early adolescence. *Pediatrics* 106:67, 2000.

MDconsult. Available at http://home.mdconsult.com/das/book/44956218-2/view/1175?sid=342747158

Mindell J, Owens J: *A Clinical Guide to Pediatric Sleep, Diagnosis and Management of Sleep Problems.* Philadelphia, Lippincott Williams & Wilkins, 2003, pp 88–105.

Sheldon SH: Parasomnias in childhood. *Pediatr Clin North Am* 51:69, 2004.

AUTHORS: **HEIDI V. CONNOLLY, MD** and **MARGARET-ANN CARNO, PHD, RN**

BASIC INFORMATION

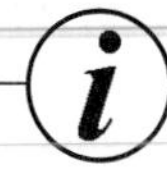

DEFINITION

Patellar subluxation and dislocation (PS/D) occurs almost exclusively laterally from the patella femoral articulation. It is believed by some to be a subset of patellofemoral dysfunction. The patella, a sesamoid bone located within the quadriceps tendon, articulates posteriorly with the femur in the femoral grove and between the femoral condyles.

ICD-9-CM CODE
836.3 Patellar dislocation

EPIDEMIOLOGY & DEMOGRAPHICS

- Essentially all PS/Ds are lateral.
- PS/D occurs in 43 of 100,000 children younger than 16 years old.
- Less than 40% are affiliated with osteochondral fractures.
- Forty-two percent of patella dislocations occur in athletic, active children between 14 and 20 years old. Commonly associated sports include soccer, gymnastics, ice hockey, and dance.
- For 9% to 15% of patients, there is a positive family history (up to 60% in one series).
- No clear gender predilection was found in a large, prospective study, although most reports state that girls are more commonly affected than boys.
- The recurrence rate is 21%, with a threefold increased risk of recurrence for girls compared with boys.
- Associated with joint laxity (hypermobility syndromes)

CLINICAL PRESENTATION

- A dramatic memorable event usually is associated with acute pain at the time of dislocation.
- Most PS/Ds reduce spontaneously.
- Patient may describe "pop" at time of dislocation.
- Acutely swollen knee
  - When medial retinaculum torn during lateral dislocation
  - When associated with osteochondral fracture (up to three fourths of acute dislocations)
- Patients may have tenderness of the medial edge of the patella or the area proximal to the medial femoral epicondyle.
- Positive apprehension may be observed. Passive lateral and medial patellar movements make the patient uncomfortable (see Knee Maneuvers in Charts, Formulas, Laboratory Tests and Values [Section IV]).
- Positive apprehension with stress is pathognomonic for patella instability and tracking malalignment. Pain and contraction of the quadriceps occur when the patella is gently moved laterally while the patient is supine with the leg gently flexed less than 30 degrees.
- If a large effusion occurs after dislocation, hemarthrosis is the most likely cause.
- It is not clear whether an abnormal quadriceps (Q) angle plays any role in the pathology of PS/D.
  - The angle is formed at the center of the patella by the line of pull of the quadriceps tendon and patella tendon.
  - It is measured from the central patella to the anterior superior iliac spine proximally and tibial tuberosity distally.
- A normal Q angle is 15 degrees or less in women and less than 10 degrees in men.
- The Q angle is increased in patients with trisomy 21, patients with other neuromuscular disorders, and those with a high riding or lateral patella.

ETIOLOGY

- The cause is likely multifactorial and associated with bony constraints, ligamentous restraints, and child environmental exposures (see Knee drawing in Charts, Formulas, Laboratory Tests and Values [Section IV]).
- Effects of bony constraints include the following:
  - Trochlear dysplasia: flat intertrochlear groove seen in 30% to 85% of patients with patellar instability
  - Abnormal posterior patella curvature
  - Dysplasia and patellar abnormalities associated with increased femoral anteversion, genu recurvatum, external tibial torsion, foot pronation, and increased patella tilt
  - High patella (patella alta) increases risk
  - Patella entering the femoral groove at a greater degree of flexion, leading to decreased bony constraint of the patella at any degree of flexion
- Lack of bony constraint increases the chance of dislocation.
  - Laxity of medial and lateral patellar ligaments (i.e., vastus mediales obliquus and medial patellofemoral ligament)
  - Tracking abnormality
  - External forces on knee (i.e., internal tibial rotation with valgus stress, planted foot, and quadriceps contraction)

DIAGNOSIS

DIFFERENTIAL DIAGNOSIS

- Acute knee ligament tear, especially the medial cruciate ligament (MCL) or anterior cruciate ligament (ACL), or in combination with an ACL tear
- Meniscal tear
- Osteochondral fractures (i.e., tibial plateau, patella, or femoral condyle)
- Bursitis, synovitis, arthritis
- Patellofemoral pain syndrome (PFPS) possibly confused with subluxation

WORKUP

The workup is based on the history and physical examination findings.

IMAGING STUDIES

- Anteroposterior (AP) and lateral radiographic views
  - AP view is best to evaluate distal femoral physis, proximal tibial physis, and patella.
  - Bipartite patella is an incidental finding; it may become symptomatic after acute trauma.
- Lateral radiograph for patella position and tibial tubercle; measurement of the degree of patella alta
- Sunrise or sulcus view (i.e., merchant, skyline, or axial view)
  - Shows relationship between the patella and distal femur/femoral condyles
  - Tangential radiograph with knee flexed approximately 45 degrees
  - Lack of congruence of the patella femoral joint seen with patella subluxation
- Tunnel or notch view to check for loose bodies
  - AP view with the knee flexed 20 degrees delineates femoral condyles.
  - Femoral condyle lucencies may be seen.
  - Osteochondral fragment may be visualized.

TREATMENT

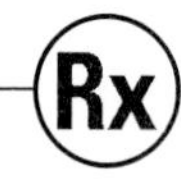

NONPHARMACOLOGIC THERAPY

- Immediate reduction and immobilization with the knee extended for 3 to 6 weeks
- Rest, elevation, ice
- Knee braces for bilateral subluxation possibly helps some
- Knee taping
- Surgical results not uniformly successful, especially for those with an increased Q angle or flat lateral femoral condyle

ACUTE GENERAL Rx

- Nonsteroidal anti-inflammatory drugs for pain
- Manual reduction if not spontaneously reduced or reduced on field
  - Adequate analgesia is imperative; patella dislocation is excruciatingly painful.
  - Flex the hips with the patient in the supine position.
  - Gently extend the knee while pushing the patella medially.

CHRONIC Rx

Long-term therapy consists of quadriceps strengthening and stretching.

DISPOSITION

Most children are able to return to usual activities within 4 to 6 weeks of an acute dislocation.

REFERRAL

- Refer the patient to sports medicine or physical therapy for rehabilitation and exercise training.
- Refer the patient to an orthopedic surgeon for fracture, suspicion of fracture, atypical dislocation (medial) or associated ligamentous injury, or trauma potentially necessitating surgery.
- Consider an orthopedic referral if knee pain does not resolve.

PEARLS & CONSIDERATIONS

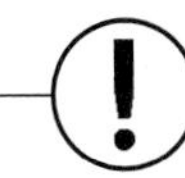

PATIENT/FAMILY EDUCATION

Dislocation recurs in up to 85% of inadequately treated patients.

SUGGESTED READINGS

Beasley LS, Vidal AF: Traumatic patellar dislocation in children and adolescents: treatment update and literature review. *Curr Opin Pediatr* 16:29, 2004.

Fithian DC et al: Epidemiology and natural history of acute patellar dislocation. *Am J Sports Med* 32:1114, 2004.

Geary M, Schepsis A: Management of first-time patellar dislocations. *Sports Med Update* 27:1058, 2004.

Hinton RY, Sharma KM: Acute and recurrent patellar instability in the young athlete. *Orthop Clin North Am* 34:385, 2003.

Moore BR, Bothner J: *Patellar dislocations in children and adolescents.* Up To Date online, 2004.

Roach JW: Knee disorders and injuries in adolescents. *Adolesc Med* 9:589, 1998.

AUTHOR: **LYNN C. GARFUNKEL, MD**

BASIC INFORMATION

DEFINITION

Patellofemoral pain syndrome (PFPS) is one of the anterior knee pain syndromes. It is caused by irritation within the patellofemoral joint. Retropatellar or peripatellar in nature, pain increases after use, on descending or climbing steps, and after prolonged sitting. Patellofemoral dysplasia, patellofemoral dysfunction, patellar tracking abnormalities, runner's knee, and peripatellar pain syndrome are referred to variably and synonymously in orthopedic and sports medicine literature. PFPS must be distinguished from chondromalacia patella (CP), which is disruption and damage of the cartilage of the posterior patella and diagnosed arthroscopically, and CP previously was used synonymously with PFPS.

SYNONYMS

Anterior knee pain (syndrome)
Chondromalacia patella (not synonym but may be found in older literature as synonymous with PFPS)
Patellar tracking abnormality
Patellofemoral dysfunction
Patellofemoral dysplasia
Patellofemoral syndrome
Peripatellar pain (syndrome)
Runner's knee

ICD-9-CM CODES
717.9 Internal derangement of knee
719.46 Patellofemoral syndrome

EPIDEMIOLOGY & DEMOGRAPHICS

- Most common cause of traumatic and nontraumatic knee pain found on presentation to physicians' offices
- Pubertal girls and adults most commonly affected
- Wasting of medial quadriceps common (but also occurs in many chronic knee disorders)

CLINICAL PRESENTATION

- Knee pain may be nonspecific and diffuse; occasionally, pain is medial to or behind the patella.
- Difficulty and pain may occur with descending and climbing stairs and with squatting.
- The theater or movie goers' sign (i.e., inability to sit comfortably with knees flexed for several hours) may be positive.
- Aching may occur after strenuous activity.
- Swelling may occur.
- The patient may have a vague sensation of giving way or sense of locking.
- Focus special attention on the patellofemoral joint for all patients with anterior knee pain syndromes.
- Assess stance and posture, evaluate range of motion, and test ligament stability.
- The patella should face forward while standing upright and while sitting with knees flexed 90 degrees.
- The apprehension test result may be positive.
  - It suggests patellar subluxation or dislocation.
  - Passive lateral and medial patellar movement makes the patient uncomfortable.
  - Pain and contraction of quadriceps occurs when the patella is gently moved laterally while the patient is supine with leg flexed less than 30 degrees.
- A fine grinding or cracking sensation is palpable under patella while the knee is being flexed or extended.
- Mild effusion may be present.
- A large effusion likely indicates hemarthrosis and possibly an osteochondral fracture.
- Quadriceps may be hypotrophied.
- The Q angle may be abnormal. It formerly was thought to play a role, but it may play no role in the symptoms or pathology.
  - The angle is formed at the center of the patella by the line of pull of the quadriceps tendon and patella tendon.
  - It is measured from the central patella to the anterior superior iliac spine proximally and tibial tuberosity distally.
    - Normal: 15 degrees or less in women and less than 10 degrees in men
    - Abnormal: more than 15 degrees, increasing the risk of lateral patellar subluxation
    - Increased in patients with trisomy 21, other neuromuscular disorders

ETIOLOGY

- Multifaceted causes are not completely understood but are believed to involve some or a combination of the following:
  - Overuse or overload (long distance runners)
  - Foot position abnormality
  - Increased Q angle
  - Muscle weakness and inflexibility (i.e., hip muscles, especially quadriceps weakness and hamstring tightness)
  - Tight lateral or weak medial muscles around knee, leading to or exacerbating tracking abnormalities (i.e., abnormality or asymmetry of biomechanical forces)
- Malalignment, with abnormal tracking of patella in the intercondylar groove, may be associated with PFPS.

DIAGNOSIS

Dx

DIFFERENTIAL DIAGNOSIS

- Patellar (jumper's knee) or quadriceps tendonitis
- Sinding-Larsen-Johansson syndrome
- Acute knee injuries (i.e., ligament or meniscal tears)
- Patellar or femoral osteochondritis dissecans
- Patellar, femoral condyle, or tibial plateau fracture
- Chondromalacia patella
- Osgood-Schlatter disease
- Arthritis, prepatellar bursitis
- Tumor or bone cyst in or near knee joint

WORKUP

- Diagnosis is based on clinical features.
- Consider arthroscopy if the presentation is unusual or there is no improvement with appropriate physical therapy; evaluate knee effusions.
- Acute PFPS usually is associated with trauma or bacterial infection.
- Subacute and chronic PFPS usually is associated with neoplastic, rheumatologic, reactive, or metabolic abnormalities.

IMAGING STUDIES

- X-ray examination of the knees usually is normal in PFPS.
- Anteroposterior (AP) and lateral views are used.
  - AP view is best to evaluate distal femoral physis and proximal tibial physis.
  - Bipartite patella is an incidental finding; it may become symptomatic after acute trauma.
- Standing AP view of the entire lower extremity may be used.
  - Assess angular or torsional malalignment.
  - Evaluate femoral anteversion and genu valgum.
- Lateral radiographs are used to assess patella position and tibial tubercle.
- Magnetic resonance imaging may show chondromalacia. However, it is costly and usually not warranted.

TREATMENT

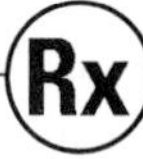

NONPHARMACOLOGIC THERAPY

- The patient should curtail activities that include weight bearing with a flexed knee.
- Muscle-stretching exercises are encouraged for quadriceps, hip adductors, hamstrings, iliotibial band, and calf muscles.
- Promote muscle strengthening, especially for the quadriceps group (including vastus medialis) and hamstrings.
- Patients should modify activity, with gradual resumption when pain free.
- Patients should use ice after activities; it is the safest anti-inflammatory therapy.

ACUTE GENERAL Rx

- Use nonsteroidal anti-inflammatory drugs (NSAIDs) for pain.
- Orthotic support may not be needed.
  - It may provide symptomatic support, although in several well-controlled, studies no improvement was achieved with bracing.
  - There is no evidence that it improves patella tracking.
- Knee taping has been reported (but not studied rigorously) to help some patients with PFPS.

CHRONIC Rx

Ongoing, long-term therapy consists of thigh and leg strengthening and stretching.

DISPOSITION

For many patients with PFPS, a long-term exercise program will be needed.

REFERRAL

- Refer the patient to a sports medicine or physical therapist for rehabilitation or exercise training.
- Refer the patient to an orthopedic surgeon if the diagnosis is unclear, for acute trauma necessitating surgery, and for unresolving pain.

PEARLS & CONSIDERATIONS

COMMENTS

- The most common cause of subacute and chronic knee pain in girls is PFPS.
- Focus special attention on vastus medialis strengthening.
- A neoplasm near the knee may manifest with sports-related trauma.
- Infectious, metabolic, and inflammatory diseases of knee, femur, or tibia may manifest with knee pain or effusion.
- All children presenting with knee pain should also be evaluated for ipsilateral hip disorders, such as slipped capital femoral epiphysis (SCFE), transient (toxic) synovitis of hip, and Legg-Calvé-Perthes disease.

PREVENTION

For many pediatric knee problems, adequate stretch and strengthening with a decrease in repetitive trauma (overuse) can allay problems.

PATIENT/FAMILY EDUCATION

- Most patients with PFPS respond to a nonsurgical approach and benefit from PFPS exercises.
- More information may be obtained from the American Academy of Family Physicians (www.aafp.org/afp/991101ap/99110lb.html).

SUGGESTED READINGS

Davids JR: Pediatric knee: clinical assessment of common disorders. *Pediatr Clin North Am* 43:1067, 1996.

Johnson RP: Anterior knee pain in adolescents and young adults. *Curr Opin Rheumatol* 9:159, 1997.

Juhn MS: Patellofemoral pain syndrome: a review and guidelines for treatment. *Am Fam Physician* 60:2012, 1999.

Lun VMY et al: Effectiveness of patellar bracing for treatment of patellofemoral pain syndrome. *Clin J Sport Med* 15:235, 2005.

Post WR: Patellofemoral pain: results of nonoperative treatment. *Clin Orthop* 436:55, 2005.

Witvrouw E et al: Clinical classification of patellofemoral pain syndrome: guidelines for nonoperative treatment. *Knee Surg Sports Traumatol Arthrosc* 13:122, 2005.

AUTHOR: **LYNN C. GARFUNKEL, MD**

BASIC INFORMATION

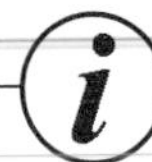

DEFINITION

Patent ductus arteriosus (PDA) is the abnormal persistence of an open lumen in the ductus arteriosus after birth.

SYNONYMS

Patency or persistence of the arterial duct
Persistent ductus arteriosus

ICD-9-CM CODE
747.0 Patent ductus arteriosus

EPIDEMIOLOGY & DEMOGRAPHICS

- Incidence in the preterm infant is strongly influenced by birth weight and gestational age.
- Approximately 45% of infants weighing less than 1700 g and approximately 80% weighing less than 1000 g at birth have clinical signs of PDA.
- Surfactant therapy, resulting in improved lung function and a more rapid decrease in pulmonary vascular resistance, has led to earlier and more frequent clinical emergence of PDA.
- In the term infant, the incidence is approximately 1 case per 2500 live births.
- The female-to-male predominance is approximately 2.5-3:1 for term infants.

CLINICAL PRESENTATION

History

- Preterm: surfactant therapy, labile blood pressure, worsening pulmonary status
- Term infant and older child: highly variable, depending on the size of the shunt
  - Large shunt: failure to thrive, poor feeding associated with tachypnea and diaphoresis
  - Small shunt: asymptomatic

Physical Examination

- Large shunt (term infant and older child)
  - Bounding, poorly sustained pulses, reflecting a wide pulse pressure
  - Hyperdynamic apical impulse with inferolateral displacement
  - Decreased splitting of S_2 (i.e., paradoxical splitting has been documented with a very large shunt)
  - Increased intensity of S_2P_2
  - Harsh, rough, continuous murmur, loudest at left infraclavicular area, with decrescendo during systole
  - May have multiple systolic clicks
- Small shunt (term infant and older child)
  - Normal pulses
  - Normal precordium
  - Normal to slightly decreased splitting of S_2, with normal S_2P_2
  - Grade 2/6 murmur, which is typically still continuous, although the diastolic portion may be difficult to auscultate
- Large shunt (preterm infant)
  - Bounding, poorly sustained pulses (i.e., Ninja pulses) strike fast and fade away.
  - Hyperdynamic apical impulse with an inferior displacement is often visible and palpable in the left paraxiphoid area.
  - A narrowly split S_2 with a prominent S_2P_2 can be identified.
  - The murmur is often nonspecific (or even absent), with the diastolic portion rarely audible.
  - The physical findings are much less reliable in the small (<1200 g) infant, particularly if there is hemodynamic compromise. In this group of patients, the activity and displacement of the left ventricular impulse is the most reliable physical finding in terms of assessing the magnitude of the shunt.

ETIOLOGY

- The exact mechanisms for normal postnatal closure are not fully understood.
- With advancing gestation, the constrictive response to rising Po_2 increases, leading to the high incidence among preterm infants.
- Failure of constriction in the term infant is probably caused by a structural abnormality, with underdevelopment of smooth muscle.
- Increased incidence correlates with maternal rubella infection.
- PDA is more common in individuals born at a high altitude.

DIAGNOSIS

DIFFERENTIAL DIAGNOSIS

- Based on physical findings alone, the differential diagnosis can include the following:
  - Tetralogy of Fallot with pulmonary atresia and large aortic-pulmonary collaterals
  - Coronary cameral fistula
  - Large arteriovenous fistula
- In the older child, the continuous murmur of a venous hum has less variability in intensity during the phases of the cardiac cycle, tends to disappear in the supine position, and can be extinguished by changes in neck position or compression of the jugular vein.

WORKUP

- Electrocardiogram (ECG): depends on the patient's age and the size of the shunt
  - Criteria for left atrial enlargement and left ventricular hypertrophy may be present.
  - In the preterm infant with hemodynamic compromise, repolarization changes consistent with ischemia may be present.

IMAGING STUDIES

- Chest radiograph
  - Cardiomegaly may be identified.
  - Increased pulmonary vascular markings are seen.
  - Signs of pulmonary edema may be present in the preterm infant.
  - Differentiation between worsening lung disease is difficult in the preterm infant.
- Echocardiography: uniformly diagnostic and obviates the need for ECG or a chest radiograph
  - The actual structure can typically be imaged and measured two dimensionally.
  - Color flow mapping demonstrates the direction of shunting, and the width of the jet gives a rough impression of the size of the structure when the acoustic window does not permit optimal imaging.
  - Pulsed or continuous-wave Doppler is helpful in identifying the exact timing of bidirectional shunting.
  - Color flow mapping can detect trivial left-to-right shunts that are not detectable by two-dimensional imaging or by physical examination.

TREATMENT

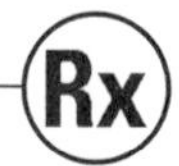

NONPHARMACOLOGIC THERAPY

- Ligation is extremely safe and essentially 100% effective.
- Ligation is the preferred therapy for preterm infants who fail to respond to indomethacin or for whom indomethacin is contraindicated.
- In many institutions, catheter closure with vascular coils is the preferred interventional therapy for infants and children older than 6 months.
  - Proper selection of the patient and the coil is critical because of anatomic variations in the ductus arteriosus.
  - This procedure is less effective for PDAs larger than 3.5 mm in diameter.
  - Newer devices are available for moderate to large PDAs.

ACUTE GENERAL Rx

- Indomethacin has been available since 1976.
- The drug is an effective alternative to surgery and has greatly decreased the need for surgical ligation in preterm infants.
- An initial clinical response may not be permanent, and a second course may be required.
- It is most effective in children younger than 10 days old and in less mature infants.
- Indiscriminate and prophylactic uses are not advisable.
- Early detection and treatment reduce morbidity.
- Renal side effects are usually transient.
- Prolonged treatment, especially in very-low-birth-weight infants, has been associated with an increased risk of necrotizing enterocolitis.

DISPOSITION

- Small PDAs in the preterm infant have a reasonable likelihood of spontaneous closure before the infant is 2 months old.
- Persistence of any hemodynamically important PDA (associated left ventricular enlargement) warrants catheter or surgical intervention.
- Beyond 6 months of age, a PDA large enough to be audible is very unlikely to close and is associated with a sufficient risk of endocarditis to warrant intervention.

REFERRAL

- Most referrals occur in the setting of the neonatal intensive care unit (NICU).
- Outside the NICU, clinical suspicion of even a small PDA (see "Physical Examination") warrants evaluation by a pediatric cardiologist.

PEARLS & CONSIDERATIONS

COMMENTS

- The magnitude of the left-to-right shunt depends on the following:
  - Size of the PDA
  - Relationship of pulmonary and systemic vascular resistance
  - Left ventricular ejection performance
- Each of these factors is highly variable in the extremely preterm infant in the first few days of life.
- After successful treatment with indomethacin, smooth muscle constriction at the origin of the left pulmonary artery may result in a short, high-pitched systolic ejection murmur at the upper left sternal border that radiates to the left axilla.
- The older infant with a hemodynamically important PDA is more predisposed to congestive heart failure than with a comparable shunt at the ventricular level because of the potential for compromise of coronary perfusion due to decreased diastolic aortic perfusion pressure.

SUGGESTED READINGS

Ing R, Sommer R: The snare-assisted technique for transcatheter coil occlusion of moderate to large patent ductus arteriosus: immediate and intermediate results. *J Am Coll Cardiol* 33:6, 1999.

Moss AJ, Adams FH: *Heart Disease in Infants, Children, and Adolescents,* 5th ed. Baltimore, Williams & Wilkins, 1995.

Ramsay JM et al: Response of the patent ductus arteriosus to indomethacin treatment. *Am J Dis Child* 141:294, 1987.

Tammela O et al: Short versus prolonged indomethacin therapy for patent ductus arteriosus in preterm infants. *J Pediatr* 134:552, 1999.

AUTHORS: **R. DENNIS STEED, MD** and **CHARLIE SANG, MD**

BASIC INFORMATION

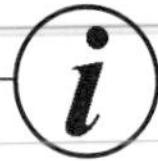

DEFINITION

Pelvic inflammatory disease (PID) encompasses a spectrum of inflammatory conditions of the upper genital tract caused by the spread of microorganisms from the lower genital tract (i.e., vagina and endocervix) to the upper structures of the endometrium, fallopian tubes, or adjacent adnexa. Any combination of endometritis, salpingitis, tubo-ovarian abscess, or pelvic peritonitis is included. Clinical pictures vary from milder forms, such as salpingitis, to more severe presentations, such as tubo-ovarian abscess and pelvic peritonitis.

SYNONYMS

Endometritis
Salpingitis

ICD-9-CM CODES
381.51 Acute salpingitis
614.2 Tubo-ovarian abscess
614.9 Pelvic inflammatory disease
615.9 Endometritis

EPIDEMIOLOGY & DEMOGRAPHICS

- Adolescent age is a strong risk factor for the development of PID; girls between the ages of 15 and 19 years are 10 times more likely to develop PID than those between the ages of 25 and 29 years.
- Increased risk in adolescents is related to numerous factors:
  - Multiple partners
  - Cervical ectopy (presence of columnar epithelium on exocervix), with *Chlamydia trachomatis* and *Neisseria gonorrhoeae* infecting columnar epithelial cells
  - Lower rates of use of barrier contraceptive methods
- PID is a serious consequence of sexually transmitted diseases (STDs) and an important cause of infertility, ectopic pregnancy, and chronic pelvic pain.

CLINICAL PRESENTATION

History

- PID is difficult to diagnose because of the wide variations in clinical signs and symptoms and the lack of precise criteria for diagnosis and treatment.
- Diagnosis is generally made on the basis of clinical findings.
- Specific genitourinary symptoms may include the following:
  - Lower abdominal pain or cramping, with peritoneal signs in severe cases
  - Vaginal discharge
  - Dysuria
  - Any change in previous menses, such as heavier flow, longer duration, or worse menstrual cramping than usual
- Symptoms may be mild or nonspecific (e.g., dyspareunia, abnormal bleeding, vaginal discharge); in these cases, a low threshold for diagnosing PID is important for preventing damage to the reproductive system.
- Although uncommon, systemic signs may be present, such as fever, anorexia, nausea and vomiting, and generalized malaise.
- PID involving gonococcus is more likely to develop within 1 week of menses and to have rapid onset of symptoms.
- Chlamydial or anaerobic PID is more likely to be insidious in onset.
- To generate differential diagnoses, it is essential to confidentially obtain information about sexual activity.

Physical Examination

- Perform a genital examination to look for signs of infection.
- If the following minimum clinical criteria on a genital-pelvic examination are present, the clinician should consider PID:
  - Uterine or adnexal tenderness
  - Cervical motion tenderness
- Additional physical examination findings that can be used to enhance the specificity of these minimum criteria and support the diagnosis of PID include the following:
  - Oral temperature higher than 38.3°C (>101°F)
  - Abnormal cervical or vaginal mucopurulent discharge (see Vaginitis & Cervicitis in Diseases and Disorders [Section I])
- Abdominal examination findings can include the following:
  - Lower abdominal tenderness
  - Peritoneal signs, such as rebound or guarding (in severe cases)
  - Right upper quadrant pain that may be present with associated perihepatitis (i.e., Fitz-Hugh-Curtis syndrome)

ETIOLOGY

- PID is often a polymicrobial infection.
- Sexually transmitted organisms, particularly *C. trachomatis* (25% to 50% of cases) and *N. gonorrhoeae* (33% to 50% of cases) are often implicated.
- Microorganisms that are part of the vaginal flora can also be involved:
  - Facultative anaerobes (i.e., gram-negative rods, *Gardnerella vaginalis, Streptococcus* species including enterococci, and *Haemophilus influenzae*) and anaerobes (i.e., anaerobic streptococci and staphylococci, *Bacteroides* species, and *Actinomyces)* are implicated, especially in cases with tubo-ovarian abscess.
  - Genital mycoplasmas, such as *Ureaplasma urealyticum* and *Mycoplasma hominis,* and cytomegalovirus (CMV) may be implicated as contributing factors in some cases of PID.

DIAGNOSIS

DIFFERENTIAL DIAGNOSIS

- Ectopic pregnancy
- Ovarian cyst (with or without torsion)
- Acute appendicitis
- Endometriosis
- Pyelonephritis
- Septic abortion
- Pelvic thrombophlebitis
- Functional pain

WORKUP

- Obtain a confidential sexual history, including questions about sexual activity, a new sex partner, the number of lifetime sex partners, possible exposure to an STD-infected partner, and presence of STD symptoms. The adolescent must be provided the opportunity to be interviewed confidentially without parent present in the examination room.
- No single history, physical examination, laboratory finding, or other diagnostic procedure is both sensitive and specific for diagnosing acute PID, and combinations of findings generally aid the sensitivity at the expense of specificity, or vice versa.
- The most specific criteria for diagnosing PID may be warranted in certain cases.
  - Endometrial biopsy can provide definitive diagnosis of endometritis.
  - Routine laparoscopy is not recommended, although it provides a definitive diagnosis with findings of hyperemia, edema, or purulent exudate of tubal surfaces.
  - Laparoscopy may be required for the evaluation of treatment failures, to exclude surgical emergencies, or if a tubo-ovarian abscess ruptures or does not respond to medical management within 48 to 72 hours.

LABORATORY TESTS

- Laboratory findings that can be used to support the diagnosis of PID include the following:
  - White blood cells (WBCs) visualized microscopically on smear of vaginal secretions
  - Elevated erythrocyte sedimentation rate (ESR) or C-reactive protein (CRP) concentration
  - Laboratory evidence of *N. gonorrhoeae* or *C. trachomatis* at the cervix (see Cervicitis and *Chlamydia trachomatis* Infections in Diseases and Disorders [Section I])
- Laboratory tests to assist in the diagnoses include the following:
  - Pregnancy test (to exclude ectopic pregnancy)
  - Tests for elevated acute-phase reactants, such as WBC, ESR, or C-reactive protein

IMAGING STUDIES

- Transvaginal ultrasound or magnetic resonance imaging (MRI) techniques may be helpful if the diagnosis is in question, ectopic pregnancy is a strong consideration, or tubo-ovarian abscess is being considered as part of the clinical picture.

- In the presence of PID, ultrasound or MRI may demonstrate increased adnexal volume with thickened, fluid-filled fallopian tubes, free pelvic fluid, or tubo-ovarian complexes.

TREATMENT

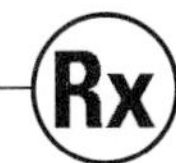

ACUTE GENERAL Rx

- Treatment regimens must provide broad-spectrum coverage of the likely etiologic organisms because PID is often a polymicrobial infection.
- All regimens should be effective against *N. gonorrhoeae* and *C. trachomatis,* even when endocervical tests are negative for these organisms.
- Evidence suggests that providing antibiotic coverage against anaerobes, gram-negative facultative bacteria, and streptococci is essential.
- Treatment should be initiated as soon as the clinical diagnosis is made.
  - Prevention of long-term sequelae correlates with prompt administration of and adherence to appropriate antibiotics.
  - Delays in initiating antibiotic treatment until culture results are available should be avoided.
- Indications for hospitalization are as follows:
  - Consideration for surgical emergency as possible diagnoses
  - Severely ill (e.g., nausea, vomiting, high fever)
  - Pregnancy
  - Tubo-ovarian abscess
  - Failure to tolerate or follow outpatient therapy
  - Failure to respond to outpatient therapy within 48 to 72 hours
- The Centers for Disease Control and Prevention have recommended several regimens.
- Parenteral regimen A
  - Cefotetan (2 g IV every 12 hours) or cefoxitin (2 g IV every 6 hours) plus doxycycline (100 mg IV or PO every 12 hours). (Because intravenous doxycycline is extremely painful, it should be given orally when possible, because oral and intravenous routes provide similar bioavailability.)
  - Parenteral therapy should be continued for 24 hours until clinical improvement is seen, and then oral doxycycline should be continued at 100 mg twice daily to complete 14 days' total therapy.
  - When tubo-ovarian abscess is present, adding clindamycin or metronidazole to the oral doxycycline regimen rather than doxycycline alone for remainder of oral therapy provides more effective anaerobic coverage.
- Parenteral regimen B
  - Clindamycin (900 mg IV every 8 hours) plus gentamicin (IV or IM loading dose of 2 mg/kg body weight), followed by a maintenance dose (1.5 mg/kg) every 8 hours. Single daily dosing of gentamicin may be substituted.
  - Parenteral therapy may be discontinued after 24 hours, if clinical improvement has occurred.
  - After parenteral therapy, doxycycline (100 mg PO twice daily) or clindamycin (450 mg PO four times daily) should be instituted to complete a total of 14 days of therapy.
  - When a tubo-ovarian abscess is present, clindamycin is preferred to doxycycline because of its better anaerobic coverage.
- Alternative parenteral regimens
  - Ofloxacin (400 mg IV every 12 hours) or levofloxacin (500 mg IV once daily) with or without metronidazole (500 mg IV every 8 hours) or ampicillin/sulbactam (3 g IV every 6 hours) plus doxycycline (100 mg IV or PO every 12 hours)
- Oral regimen A (in outpatient settings)
  - Ofloxacin (400 mg PO twice daily for 14 days) or levofloxacin (500 mg PO once daily for 14 days) with or without metronidazole (500 mg PO twice daily for 14 days)
  - Because of the lack of anaerobic coverage with ofloxacin, metronidazole is added to provide coverage.
- Oral regimen B
  - Ceftriaxone (250 mg IM in a single dose) or cefoxitin (2g IM in a single dose) and probenecid (1 g orally in a single dose concurrently) or other parenteral third-generation cephalosporin (i.e., ceftizoxime or cefotaxime) plus doxycycline (100 mg PO twice daily for 14 days) with or without metronidazole (500 mg PO twice daily for 14 days).
- Special considerations
  - Pregnant adolescents with suspected PID should be hospitalized and treated with parenteral antibiotics.
  - It has not been determined whether immunodeficient women infected with human immunodeficiency virus (HIV) require more aggressive therapy than those previously described.

DISPOSITION

- Follow-up
  - Close follow-up of adolescents is essential when they are treated as outpatients.
  - A repeat visit within 48 to 72 hours is necessary; if patients have not demonstrated significant clinical improvement (e.g., defervescence, improvement in clinical symptoms or physical signs), hospitalization, additional diagnostic tests, or surgical intervention may be required.
- Management of sex partners
  - Male sex partners of women with PID should be examined and treated if they have had sexual contact during the 60 days before the onset of the patient's symptoms to reduce the risk of reinfection.
  - Empirical treatment should cover *N. gonorrhoeae* and *C. trachomatis.*

PEARLS & CONSIDERATIONS

COMMENTS

- Most females with PID have mucopurulent cervical discharge or evidence of WBCs on a microscopic evaluation of a saline preparation of vaginal fluid. If the cervical discharge appears normal and no WBCs are found on the wet prep, the diagnosis of PID is unlikely, and alternative causes of pain should be investigated.
- Reported changes in menstrual pattern (e.g., heavier periods, more painful cramps, menses occurring earlier or later than expected) should raise suspicion of early endometrial infection, even in the absence of other symptoms.
- Unilateral adnexal tenderness or swelling suggests tubo-ovarian abscess and other differential diagnoses. Ultrasound can rule out tubo-ovarian abscess.
- The efficacy of the treatment regimens listed have been demonstrated in clinical trials with short-term follow-up; no specific data directly comparing parenteral with oral regimens are available.
- Cervical specimen tests for gonorrhea and chlamydia may be negative because active infection can be restricted to the upper genital tract.
- A positive gonorrheal or chlamydial test result at follow-up more likely indicates reinfection by an untreated sex partner than treatment failure.

PREVENTION

- The most reliable way to avoid STD infection is to abstain from sexual intercourse (i.e., oral, vaginal, or anal sex) or to be in a long-term, mutually monogamous relationship with an uninfected partner.
- When used consistently and correctly, male latex condoms can reduce the risk for STDs.
- Vaginal spermicides containing nonoxynol-9 are not effective in preventing cervical gonorrhea, *Chlamydia*, or HIV infection.
- Contraceptive methods other than male or female condoms do not provide protection against STDs.
- Screening and treating sexually active adolescents for chlamydial infection reduces the incidence of PID (see Cervicitis and *Chlamydia trachomatis* Infections in Diseases and Disorders [Section I]).
- The risks of unprotected sexual intercourse should be explained.
- Infertility rates increase with the number of PID episodes:
  - One episode: 13% to 20%
  - Two episodes: 35%

- Three or more episodes: 55% to 75%
- The risk of ectopic pregnancy is increased 6 to 10 times after one episode of PID.

PATIENT/FAMILY EDUCATION

- Adolescent and parent-appropriate STD information can be found on several web sites (www.iwannaknow.org; www.itsyoursexlife.com; www.kidshealth.org).
- The American Social Health Association (ASHA) offers patient information brochures and online STD information (www.ashastd.org).
- The Centers for Disease Control and Prevention, Division of STD Prevention offers information on its web sites (www.cdc.gov/std/).
  - Disease facts and information: www.cdc.gov/nchstp/dstd/diseaseinfo.htm
  - Personal health questions: www.cdc.gov/nchstp/dstd/personalHealthQuestions.htm
- ETR Associates (pub.etr.org; 831-438-4060) offer patient information brochures.
- Trained health professionals are available at the national STD hotline (800-227-8922) to answer questions and provide referrals 24 hours each day and 7 days per week. All calls are private, personal, and confidential.

SUGGESTED READINGS

Banikarim C et al: Pelvic inflammatory disease in adolescents. *Adolesc Med Clin* 15:273, 2004.

Centers for Disease Control and Prevention: Sexually transmitted disease guidelines, 2002. *MMWR Morb Mortal Wkly Rep* 51(RR-6):42, 2002. Available at www.cdc.gov/STD/treatment/Accessed January 24, 2005.

Ness RB et al: Effectiveness of inpatient and outpatient treatment strategies for women with pelvic inflammatory disease: results from the Pelvic Inflammatory Disease Evaluation and Clinical Health (PEACH) randomized trial. *Am J Obstet Gynecol* 186:929, 2002.

AUTHORS: **SHERYL RYAN, MD, GALE R. BURSTEIN, MD, MPH,** and **KIMBERLY A. WORKOWSKI, MD**

BASIC INFORMATION

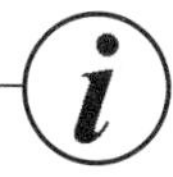

DEFINITION

Pericarditis is a syndrome caused by inflammation (either acute or chronic) of the pericardium, resulting in an increase in the normal volume of fluid surrounding the heart.

SYNONYMS

Pericardial effusion
Postpericardiotomy syndrome

ICD-9-CM CODES
420.90 Acute pericarditis, infective, hemorrhagic (acute nonrheumatic)
420.99 Pericardial effusion, bacteriologic
423.2 Restrictive pericarditis
423.8 Chronic pericarditis
423.9 Cardiac tamponade

EPIDEMIOLOGY & DEMOGRAPHICS

- Primary pericardial disease is uncommon in infants and children.
- The incidence inclusive of all age groups is 3% to 19%.
- Asymptomatic increases in volume of pericardial fluid frequently found when obtaining an echocardiogram for other indications
- The incidence of recurrent pericarditis is 15% to 30%.

CLINICAL PRESENTATION

History
- Acute onset:
  - Sudden onset of malaise, anorexia, dyspnea, orthopnea, chest pain, shoulder pain, abdominal pain
  - Inability to lie supine (pathognomonic of this condition)
- Chronic onset:
  - May be found incidentally.
  - May present as fatigue, general malaise, chest, or abdominal pain.
- There may be a history of recent infectious disease, autoimmune disease, neoplastic disease (or treatment of such), chest trauma/surgery, renal disease, foreign travel, or exposure to incarcerated persons.

Physical Examination
- Ill-appearing or anxious; fever may be present; pallor; dyspnea, tachypnea; refusal to lie supine; tachycardia; decreased blood pressure; pulsus paradoxus (>10 mm inspiratory decline in aortic systolic and pulse pressures) ominous if present; jugular venous distention; pericardial friction rub; distant heart sounds.
- cool or pale extremities
- Hepatomegaly
- In patient with chronic pericardial effusion:
  - There may be no symptoms
  - Incidental chest radiograph finding
  - Rub
  - Distant heart sounds

ETIOLOGY

- Idiopathic (30% in one series)
- Iatrogenic (postpericardiotomy syndrome): surgical procedures such as ASD closure, Fontan procedure, repair of pectus excavatum (23%)
- Trauma (blunt or penetrating chest trauma)
- Neoplastic (33%)
- Connective tissue diseases: arthritis, lupus, inflammatory bowel disease
- Drug-induced: clozapine, herbal remedies (licorice implicated on rare occasions)
- Infectious disease:
  - Bacterial more common in less developed areas (*Meningococcus, Staphylococcus aureus, Streptococcus, Haemophilus influenza*)
  - Viral
  - Tuberculosis
  - Aspergillosis
  - Histoplasmosis
- Chronic recurrent pericarditis more likely with viral and idiopathic causes
- Metabolic or renal disease
- Cardiac transplantation (small donor heart)

DIAGNOSIS

Dx

DIFFERENTIAL DIAGNOSIS

- Myocarditis
- Dilated cardiomyopathy
- Restrictive cardiomyopathy
- Aortic dissection
- Mediastinal mass
- Respiratory illness
- Gastrointestinal illness

WORKUP

Clinical suspicion is paramount.

LABORATORY TESTS

- Complete blood cell count with differential, C-reactive protein, erythrocyte sedimentation rate, antinuclear antibodies, rheumatoid factor, ASO, human immunodeficiency virus
- Bacterial, viral, and mycobacterial fungal cultures (pericardial fluid and blood)
- PPD, thyroid-stimulating hormone (usually hypothyroid)
- Basic metabolic panel, to assess electrolyte status prior to treatment
- 12-lead electrocardiogram for ST segment and voltage changes

IMAGING STUDIES

- Chest radiograph will show cardiomegaly or "water bottle" appearance.
- Use echocardiogram to evaluate pericardial space dimensions, assess right atrial and ventricular collapse, and atrioventricular valve (particularly mitral) inflow signal variability.

TREATMENT

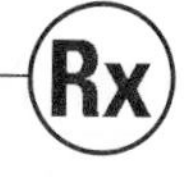

NONPHARMACOLOGIC THERAPY

- The clinical significance of any pericardial effusion depends on hemodynamic compromise and the nature and progression of the underlying disease.
- Surgical intervention is indicated for relief of tamponade or for diagnosis.
  - Pericardiocentesis via needle aspiration or placement of drainage (nephrostomy) tube
  - Surgical pericardial window or "stripping"

ACUTE GENERAL Rx

- It is important to treat the etiology of the pericardial effusion if known.
  - Infection, drug reaction, neoplasm, thyroid disease
- Use symptomatic diuretic therapy judiciously with careful monitoring.
- Anti-inflammatory medications such as high-dose aspirin, ibuprofen, or Naprosyn with appropriate gastrointestinal prophylaxis are often required.
- Corticosteroids are indicated especially if connective tissue disease etiology suspected.
- Colchicine has been used in children with minimal side effects.
- Cyclosporin A has been used, but experience is primarily anecdotal.

CHRONIC Rx

- Treatment of underlying cause imperative.
- Some chronic effusions do not resolve, and need only be followed for evidence of restrictive pericarditis.
- Viral and idiopathic pericarditis may be recurrent and treated at the time of fluid reaccumulation.

DISPOSITION

- Outpatient treatment possible without evidence of hemodynamic compromise.
- Most children, however, are admitted at symptomatic presentation for diagnosis and stabilization.

REFERRAL

- A pediatric cardiologist should always be involved in the care and long-term management of these patients.
- Other subspecialists may be involved based on the primary etiology (rheumatic, infectious, endocrinologic).

PEARLS & CONSIDERATIONS

COMMENTS

- Not all pericardial effusions require intervention—they must be monitored for signs of tamponade.
- Therapy for tamponade is removal of the effusion with simultaneous administration of intravascular fluids.

SUGGESTED READING

Altman CA: Pericarditis. *In* Garson A (ed): *Science and Practice of Pediatric Cardiology.* Baltimore, Williams & Wilkins, 1998, pp 1795–1816.

AUTHOR: **MICHELLE A. GRENIER, MD**

BASIC INFORMATION

DEFINITION

Peritonitis is inflammation of the peritoneal lining of the abdominal cavity.

SYNONYMS

Primary peritonitis
SBP
Spontaneous bacterial peritonitis (SBP)

ICD-9-CM CODES
540.0 With appendicitis
567.2 Bacterial peritonitis, general, generalized acute
567.9 Acute peritonitis

EPIDEMIOLOGY & DEMOGRAPHICS

- Most cases of SBP in children occur in association with nephrotic syndrome or, much less often, cirrhosis.
    - Lower albumin level (<1.5 g/dL) is associated with a higher risk for SBP in children with nephrotic syndrome
- An uncommon cause of acute abdomen, SBP without underlying renal disease, occurs in children younger than 7 years of age.
- A complication of appendicitis is the most common cause of peritonitis in older children.

CLINICAL PRESENTATION

History
- Renal (or liver) disease in most children
- Insidious or rapid onset
- Fever
- Abdominal pain
- Anorexia, vomiting, diarrhea

Physical Examination
- "Toxic" appearance (common)
- Hypotension, tachycardia
- Shallow, rapid respirations
- Absent or decreased bowel sounds
- Rebound tenderness
- Rigid abdomen
- Indwelling catheter

ETIOLOGY

- Primary peritonitis is an infection in the peritoneal cavity without an intra-abdominal source.

The most common organisms include:
- Pneumococci
- Group A streptococci
- Gram-negative enteric organisms
- Staphylococci, coagulase-positive and negative
- Enterococci
- *Candida*
- *Pasteurella multocida*
- *Mycobacteria tuberculosus*

- Secondary bacterial peritonitis is caused by hollow abdominal viscous rupture, mural insufficiency (necrosis), or extension of an intraperitoneal organ infection or abscess.
    - Etiologies include:
        - Ruptured appendix
        - Incarcerated hernia
        - Midgut volvulus
        - Meckel's diverticulum
        - Intussusception
        - Necrotizing enterocolitis
        - Hemolytic uremic syndrome
        - Peptic ulcer disease/ruptured ulcer
        - Traumatic perforation of bowel
        - Other (e.g., meconium in preterm infant)
    - Peritonitis may be seen with genital tract infection from fallopian tube extension of pelvic inflammatory disease (PID).
        - Mixed flora
        - *Neisseria gonococci*
        - Chlamydia
        - Anaerobes
- Foreign bodies (e.g., ventriculoperitoneal shunt, peritoneal dialysis [PD] catheter) are associated with peritonitis.
    - Patients with PD catheters are at risk of gram-positive and gram-negative enteric organism infection.
- Autoimmune or chemical process may lead to noninfectious peritonitis.
    - Systemic lupus erythematosus
    - Mediterranean fever

DIAGNOSIS

DIFFERENTIAL DIAGNOSIS

- Appendicitis with or without perforation, peritonitis, or localized abscess
- PID, Fitz-Hugh-Curtis syndrome (perihepatitis)
- Tubo-ovarian abscess
- Liver, splenic, or renal abscess
- Psoas abscess
- Bowel perforation (traumatic or secondary to necrosis [e.g., necrotizing enterocolitis, strangulated hernias])
- Pneumonia

LABORATORY TESTS

- Complete blood count (CBC) shows increased white blood cell (WBC) count with polymorphonuclear predominance.
- Proteinuria is noted in patients with nephrotic syndrome.
- If known renal or liver disease or ascites, a paracentesis should be done. Findings include:
    - Increased WBC count (>250 cells/mm^3)
    - Increased lactate
    - Decreased pH (<7.35)
    - Positive Gram stain for organisms

IMAGING STUDIES

Upright abdominal film will show free air in patient with ruptured hollow viscus.

TREATMENT

NONPHARMACOLOGIC THERAPY

- Drainage if abscess
- Repair of perforated viscus
- Excision of gangrenous bowel
- Removal of foreign body

ACUTE GENERAL Rx

- Fluid resuscitation should be provided if the patient is unstable.
- Ampicillin or ceftriaxone, and an aminoglycoside should be administered while awaiting definitive culture results and sensitivities.
- Include anaerobic coverage (metronidazole or clindamycin) if secondary peritonitis is suspected (e.g., appendicitis with rupture).
- Antibiotic treatment is generally for 10 to 14 days.

DISPOSITION

- Will depend on primary cause.
- Currently an International Registry has ongoing data collection for analysis of peritonitis in children with PD-related peritonitis to assess the best empiric antibiotic treatment.

REFERRAL

- A nephrologist or gastroenterologist may be involved for underlying disease consultation.
- A pediatric surgeon will be involved for most forms of secondary peritonitis, catheter-related peritonitis, or suspicion of acute abdomen.

PEARLS & CONSIDERATIONS

COMMENTS

- If on underlying renal or liver disease is present, think bowel perforation.
- Treat peritonitis emergently.

PREVENTION

- Assure vaccination (pneumococcal and *Haemophilus influenza*), especially for children with nephrotic syndrome.
- Some evidence exists for using prophylactic antibiotics at time of PD.

SUGGESTED READINGS

Brook I: Microbiology and management of intraabdominal infections in children. *Pediatr Int* 45(2):123, 2003.

Hyans JS: Peritonitis. *In* Behrman RE et al (eds): *Nelson Textbook of Pediatrics.* Philadelphia, WB Saunders, 1998.

Klaus G: Prevention and treatment of peritoneal dialysis-associated peritonitis in pediatric patients. *Periton Dial Int* 25(Suppl 3):S117, 2005.

Shandling B: Peritonitis. *In* Walker WA et al (eds): *Pediatric Gastrointestinal Disease: Pathophysiology, Diagnosis, Management,* 3rd ed. Philadelphia, BC Decker, 2000.

AUTHOR: **LYNN C. GARFUNKEL, MD**

BASIC INFORMATION

DEFINITION

Peritonsillar abscess is a fascial space abscess generally complicating tonsillitis.

SYNONYM

Quinsy

ICD-9-CM CODE
475 Peritonsillar abscess; Peritonsillar cellulitis

EPIDEMIOLOGY & DEMOGRAPHICS

- Peritonsillar abscess is the most common cervical fascial space abscess in pediatric patients.
- The incidence is 30 per 100,000 in the United States among patients 5 to 59 years of age.
- The percentage of patients who are 20 years of age or younger ranges from 33% to 39%.
    - Rare in children younger than age 5 years.

CLINICAL PRESENTATION

History

- From 2 to 4 days of the following:
    - Sore throat
    - Dysphagia
    - Fever
    - Muffled "hot potato" voice

Physical Examination

- Fever, unilateral tonsillar erythema (often without an exudate)
- Bulging of the superior aspect of the tonsil, often with palpable fluctuance
- Uvular deviation
- Trismus
- Fetid breath
- Ipsilateral cervical adenopathy

ETIOLOGY

- A complication of acute tonsillar pharyngeal infection
- Cultures often polymicrobial with aerobes (e.g., *Streptococcus pyogenes,* α-hemolytic streptococci, *Staphylococcus aureus, Haemophilus influenzae*) and anaerobes (e.g., *Bacteroides* species, Fusobacterium, *Prevotella* and *Porphyromonas* species)

DIAGNOSIS

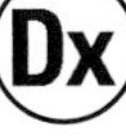

DIFFERENTIAL DIAGNOSIS

- Peritonsillar cellulitis
- Parapharyngeal abscess
- Retropharyngeal abscess
- Tonsillitis

WORKUP

- Clinical differentiation of peritonsillar cellulitis from peritonsillar abscess can be difficult.
- Traditionally, the diagnosis is confirmed by needle aspiration.

LABORATORY TESTS

Culture is not routinely necessary, except for immunocompromised patients, as culture results do not affect management or change the outcome.

IMAGING STUDIES

- Noninvasive imaging techniques of intraoral ultrasound or computed tomography with contrast are reliable in differentiating peritonsillar cellulitis from abscess.
- Intraoral ultrasound is also beneficial for aiding guided-needle aspiration of the abscess.

TREATMENT

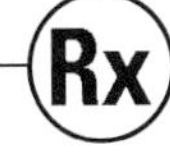

NONPHARMACOLOGIC THERAPY

- Most patients (>80%) can be managed as outpatients.
- Hydration (oral or parenteral) should be maintained.
- Effective drainage of the abscess can be accomplished either by needle aspiration, incision and drainage, or abscess tonsillectomy.
- Studies (see Herzon in "Suggested Readings") suggest that initial surgical management should be needle aspiration because the success rate is 94% and it is believed to be the most cost-effective technique.
- For patients who fail needle aspiration(s), incision and drainage is recommended.
- For the 20% to 30% of children with a history of prior recurrent tonsillitis (two to three episodes of tonsillitis in the past year), the recommended surgical management is either abscess tonsillectomy or needle aspiration, followed by delayed tonsillectomy because these patients seem to be at greater risk for recurrence.

ACUTE GENERAL Rx

- Pain relief
- Antibiotics
    - No clear consensus has been reached regarding penicillin (oral or intravenous) versus broad-spectrum antibiotics, such as clindamycin, penicillin plus metronidazole, or amoxicillin/clavulanate.
- Steroids have not been shown to be beneficial or harmful.

DISPOSITION

- Approximately 4% of patients who are initially managed with needle aspiration require a second aspiration.
- Most recurrences of peritonsillar abscess occur in patients younger than 30 years of age and within 2 months of the initial peritonsillar abscess.

REFERRAL

Refer to otolaryngologist for surgical management.

PEARLS & CONSIDERATIONS

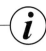

COMMENTS

- Response to parenteral antibiotics in patients who will not tolerate needle aspiration (5% or less) can help differentiate peritonsillar abscess from peritonsillar cellulitis.
    - Patients with cellulitis had improvement of at least one clinical factor (sore throat, fever, trismus, or tonsillar bulge) within 24 to 48 hours of parenteral antibiotics.
    - Children with peritonsillar abscess had no symptomatic change.
- The incidence of abscess within the contralateral tonsil ranges from 2% to 24%.

PREVENTION

Early antimicrobial treatment of streptococcal pharyngitis may decrease the likelihood of developing a peritonsillar abscess.

PATIENT/FAMILY EDUCATION

- Medline Plus Medical Encyclopedia. Available at http://www.nlm.nih.gov/medlineplus/ency/article/000986.htm

SUGGESTED READINGS

Herzon FS: Peritonsillar abscess: incidence, current management practices, and a proposal for treatment guidelines. *Laryngoscope* 105:1, 1995.

Herzon FS, Nicklaus P: Pediatric peritonsillar abscess: management guidelines. *Curr Prob Pediatr* 26:270, 1996.

Johnson RF et al: An evidence-based review of the treatment of peritonsillar abscess. *Otolaryngol Head Neck Surg* 128:332, 2003.

Kieff DA et al: Selection of antibiotics after incision and drainage of peritonsillar abscesses. *Otolaryngol Head Neck Surg* 120:57, 1999.

Scott PM et al: Diagnosis of peritonsillar infections: a prospective study of ultrasound, computed tomography and clinical diagnosis. *J Laryngol Otol* 113:229, 1999.

AUTHOR: **ROBERT R. WITTLER, MD**

BASIC INFORMATION

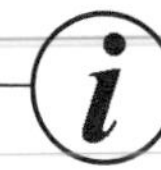

DEFINITION

Pertussis is an acute bacterial respiratory illness usually associated with significant paroxysmal cough, with associated "whoop," caused by *Bordetella pertussis* and less commonly by *Bordetella* parapertussis.

SYNONYM

Whooping cough

ICD-9-CM CODE
033.9 Pertussis

EPIDEMIOLOGY & DEMOGRAPHICS

- Humans are the only known host.
- Transmission is via respiratory secretions.
- Cases are endemic with periodic outbreaks. Epidemics occur in 2- to 5-year intervals, although immunization has controlled disease.
- A 90% transmission rate exists among nonimmune household contacts.
- The highest risk of disease is in young infants and children.
- Pertussis is responsible for 7% of all cough illnesses in adults.
- In the prevaccine era:
  - An attack rate of 157 per 100,000 population existed.
  - Approximately 85% of all cases occurred in children between ages 1 and 9 years, and pertussis was a major cause of mortality in infants.
- In the postvaccine era:
  - Incidence has decreased more than 98%.
  - Epidemic cycles continue in unvaccinated populations, with adolescents and adults remaining a reservoir of infection.
  - Mortality has significantly decreased.
  - Ninety percent of deaths occur in unimmunized infants younger than 6 months old.
  - In the United States approximately 10 deaths per year are caused by pertussis.

CLINICAL PRESENTATION

History

- Incubation is usually 7 to 10 days.
- Catarrhal stage (lasts 1 to 2 weeks)
  - Classically seen in children 1 to 10 years of age
  - Rhinorrhea
  - Lacrimation
  - Mild cough
  - Afebrile
  - Cough severity gradually increases
- Paroxysmal stage (lasts about 4 weeks)
  - Repetitive cough
  - Five to 10 coughs occur per expiration, followed by a large inspiration. Whoop occurs as inhaled air is forced through the narrowed glottis.
  - Paroxysms occur throughout the day and night. Between episodes, patients may appear normal.
- Associated symptoms with cough
  - Cyanosis
  - Eye bulging
  - Tongue protrusion
  - Salivation
  - Lacrimation
  - Posttussive emesis
- Convalescent stage (lasts 1 to 2 weeks)
  - Improvement of coughing spasms
  - Decreased frequency and forcefulness
- Complications
  - Pneumonia
    - Caused by pertussis
    - Secondary bacterial infection
  - Otitis media
  - Apnea
    - Can occur at any time, usually within the paroxysmal phase
  - Seizures
    - Believed to be due to hypoxia
  - Encephalopathy
    - May be caused by *B. pertussis*
    - May be secondary to hypoxia associated with cough
  - Subconjunctival hemorrhage
  - Epistaxis
  - Alveolar hemorrhage or rupture
  - Dehydration
  - Cerebral asphyxia
  - Coma

Physical Examination

- Afebrile
- Observation of classic paroxysms and whoop
- Otherwise usually unremarkable: normal respiratory rate, normal lung examination

ETIOLOGY

B. pertussis is a fastidious, gram-negative, aerobic pleomorphic bacillus.

DIAGNOSIS

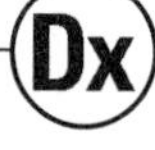

DIFFERENTIAL DIAGNOSIS

- Respiratory syncytial virus bronchiolitis
- Common upper respiratory infection
- Chlamydial pneumonia
- Mycoplasmal pneumonia
- Allergy
- Reactive airway disease
- Apparent life-threatening event (ALTE): an episode that is frightening to the observer and is characterized by some combination of
  - Apnea (central or obstructive)
  - Change in color (pallor, cyanosis, or suffusion)
  - Change in muscle tone (usually diminished)
  - Choking or gagging
  - In some cases, the observer fears that the infant has died.

LABORATORY TESTS

- Leukocytosis with lymphocytosis
  - High white blood cell count (>15,000/mm^3 with 80% lymphocytes)
  - Nonspecific and not sensitive
- Culture
  - Nasopharyngeal mucus from aspiration or on a Dacron swab should be inoculated onto Bordet-Gengou media.
  - Incubation for 10 to 14 days.
  - Recovery is maximal in the early stages of illness, with recovery after the fourth week rare.
  - A positive culture is diagnostic.
  - Negative cultures are common in the following scenarios:
    - In vaccinated patients
    - In patients on antibiotics
    - Late in the illness
- Nonculture methods
  - Direct fluorescent antibody
    - Low sensitivity
    - Variable specificity
    - Culture confirmation
    - Screening purposes only
  - Polymerase chain reaction
    - Rapid
    - Sensitive and specific
  - Serologic methods
    - Heterogeneous antibody response makes use of this test problematic and not diagnostic.

TREATMENT

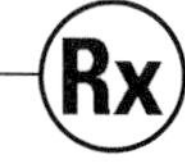

NONPHARMACOLOGIC THERAPY

- Supportive care
- Hydration, oxygenation, nutrition

ACUTE GENERAL Rx

- Antibiotics to decrease further spread
  - Not efficacious in changing course of illness once established
  - Erythromycin (40 to 50 mg/kg/day divided four times a day for 14 days), *or*
  - Azithromycin (10 mg/kg/day the first day and then 5 mg/kg/day days 2 to 5), *or*
  - Clarithromycin (15 mg/kg/day orally in two divided doses for 10 days), *or*
  - Trimethoprim-sulfamethoxazole (10 mg/kg/day of trimethoprim in two divided doses for 14 days); efficacy is unproven
- Insufficient evidence to recommend corticosteroids or β-agonists to decrease coughing
- Treatment of exposed contacts
- Vaccinate contacts younger than 7 years who are unimmunized.
- Chemoprophylaxis should be instituted as follows:
  - Erythromycin for all household contacts regardless of age or immunization status (40 to 50 mg/kg/day divided in four doses; maximum, 2 g/day for 14 days, see alternatives listed previously)

REFERRAL

Pediatric infectious disease consultation may be warranted in complicated cases.

PEARLS & CONSIDERATIONS

COMMENTS

Adolescent vaccination is likely to be recommended soon as a booster dose.

PREVENTION

- Primary prevention
- Whole cell vaccination
  - Suspension of inactivated *B. pertussis* cells with multiple antigens
  - Efficacy: 50% to 90%
  - Immunity persists 3 years and diminishes with time
  - Combined with diphtheria and tetanus toxoids as intramuscular injection
  - Local reactions common
  - Severe systemic reactions: 1 in 1750 doses
    - Convulsions
    - Hypotonic hyporesponsive episodes
    - Acute encephalopathy
- Acellular vaccine
  - Preferred due to decreased vaccine-associated reactions
  - One or more immunogens, but minimal to no endotoxin
  - Combined with diphtheria and tetanus toxoids alone or also with hepatitis B vaccine and inactivated polio virus or with DT and Hib as intramuscular injections
  - Less local and systemic reactions than whole cell vaccine
  - Use same acellular pertussis vaccine product if possible
  - Total of five doses recommended by school entry: first dose at 2 months of age (minimum age is 6 weeks), next two doses at 2-month intervals, fourth dose at 12 to 18 months, and fifth dose at 4 to 6 years of age. (If fourth dose is delayed until after fourth birthday, no fifth dose is necessary. Pertussis immunization is not currently recommended for children older than 7 years of age.)
- Precautions
  - Children who have had well-documented pertussis do not need to continue pertussis immunization schedule.
- In outbreaks, immunization of adult contacts is not yet recommended.
- Adverse immunization reactions:
  - Fever, erythema, induration, and pain at injection site are much less common with acellular pertussis than with the whole cell vaccine.
  - Local reactions are more common after fourth and fifth doses.
- Contraindications to vaccination
  - Anaphylaxis
  - Hypotonic hyporesponsive state within 48 hours
  - Temperature greater than 40.5°C within 48 hours
  - Persistent, inconsolable crying within 48 hours
  - Seizures with or without fever within 3 days
- Deferral of vaccination
  - In children with a progressive neurologic disorder characterized by developmental delay or neurologic findings
  - History of recent seizure until cause is known or seizures are well controlled

PATIENT/FAMILY EDUCATION

- Medline Plus Medical Encyclopedia. Available at http://www.nlm.nih.gov/medlineplus/ency/article/001561.htm
- Vaccine Information for the Public and Health Professionals. Available at http://www.vaccineinformation.org/pertuss/index.asp

SUGGESTED READINGS

Langley JM et al: Azithromycin is as effective as and better tolerated than erythromycin estolate for the treatment of pertussis. *Pediatrics* 114(1):e96, 2004.

Pickering LK: Pertussis. *In* Pickering LK (ed): *Red Book: 2003 Report of the Committee on Infectious Diseases,* 26th ed. Elk Grove Village, IL, American Academy of Pediatrics, 2003, pp 472–486.

Pillay, Swingler G: Symptomatic treatment of the cough in whooping cough. *Cochrane Database Syst Rev* 4:CD003257, 2003.

AUTHOR: **MAUREEN NOVAK, MD**

BASIC INFORMATION

DEFINITIONS

- Streptococcal pharyngitis is the inflammation of the tonsils/pharynx caused by infection with group A streptococcus (GAS).
- Scarlet fever is a systemic illness characterized by a typical "sandpaper" rash that results from erythrogenic toxins produced by GAS.
- Acute rheumatic fever (ARF) is a late, autoimmune complication of GAS infection and is characterized by carditis, arthritis, chorea, erythema marginatum rash, and subcutaneous nodules. (See Rheumatic Fever in Diseases and Disorders [Section I].)
- Acute poststreptococcal glomerulonephritis (APSGN) is an immune complex-mediated complication of GAS infection and is characterized by hematuria, proteinuria, edema, and acute renal failure. (See Glomerulonephritis, Acute in Diseases and Disorders [Section I].)

SYNONYMS

- Scarlet fever
  - Scarlatina (rash)
  - Scarlatiniform eruption
  - Strep rash
  - Streptococcal fever
- Streptococcal pharyngitis
  - Infective sore throat
  - Strep throat

ICD-9-CM CODES

034.0 Streptococcal tonsillitis or pharyngitis
034.1 Scarlet fever
462.9 Pharyngitis
463 Tonsillitis
465.8 Tonsillopharyngitis

EPIDEMIOLOGY & DEMOGRAPHICS

- Acute GAS infection
  - Results from direct contact with respiratory tract secretions from a person infected with GAS.
  - Neither fomites nor household pets are vectors.
  - Epidemic outbreaks occur in crowded conditions.
  - Foodborne outbreaks have also occurred.
  - Incidence is most common among school-age children, but can occur at any age.
  - Occurs more frequently in late autumn, winter, and spring in temperate climates.
  - Communicability is highest during the acute infection, then diminishes over several weeks even without treatment. It abruptly declines within 24 to 48 hours after antibiotic therapy.
  - Asymptomatic prevalence rates of 15% to 50% during outbreaks include both children who are infectious but not ill and those with pharyngeal carriage who are not infectious.
  - Local complications are more likely to occur in untreated patients.
  - Scarlet fever usually occurs with GAS pharyngitis but may be seen with skin infections.
  - Scarlet fever is rare in infancy because of placental transfer of maternal antibody to the toxins and the need for the development of hypersensitivity through prior exposure.
  - Streptococcal toxic shock syndrome, a rare and severe form of scarlet fever with shock and systemic toxicity, has a high mortality rate despite timely and high doses of antibiotics. (See Toxic Shock Syndrome in Diseases and Disorders [Section I].)
  - The incidence of severe, invasive GAS infections (including bacteremia, toxic shock, necrotizing fasciitis, and pneumonia) has increased, although such infections rarely follow GAS pharyngitis.
- Late sequelae of GAS infection: ARF and APSGN
  - The incidence of ARF has declined sharply from 3% in the 1950s to the current attack rate presumed to be as low as 0.3%. Outbreaks of ARF, however, have continued which emphasizes both the importance of accurate diagnosis and of compliance with the recommended duration of therapy.
  - APSGN may follow either GAS throat or skin infection. The latent period for nephritis is longer after skin infection (3 weeks) than after throat infection (10 days).

CLINICAL PRESENTATION

History

- This is a brief, acute illness occurring after a short incubation period (1 to 4 days).
- There is a wide variation in morbidity: subclinical form (30%) to a toxic form (<10%).
- Extreme toxicity is most common in epidemic foodborne outbreaks.
- Acute and sudden onset of fever, sore throat, headache, and abdominal pain that is not associated with diarrhea can occur.
- Absence of other respiratory symptoms (e.g., sneezing, cough, coryza, rhinorrhea, conjunctivitis) is noted in the typical case.
- History of exposure to an infected classmate or other close contact is reported.
- Subsequent symptoms may include halitosis and neck pain and stiffness.
- Clinical manifestations subside in 3 to 5 days unless complications occur.
- Scarlet fever usually presents as a more severe illness with the following symptoms:
  - High fever and mild toxicity
  - Abdominal pain with nausea and vomiting 12 to 24 hours before the onset of rash
  - Appearance of the typical rash on day 2 of the illness
- Young children rarely develop classic acute pharyngitis or scarlet fever.
  - Present with moderate fever and serous, serosanguineous, or mucopurulent rhinitis
  - Illness is more protracted, with persistent low-grade fever, irritability, and anorexia.
  - Referred to as *streptococcal fever* or *streptococcosis*

Physical Examination

- Variable toxicity and fever
- Erythema and inflammation of the posterior pharynx
  - Exudate in 50% to 80% by day 2, whitish to yellowish in color, may be confluent
  - Absence of oral ulcers/vesicles, nasal discharge, conjunctivitis, respiratory signs
- Swollen and tender anterior cervical lymphadenopathy in 30% to 60%
- Palatal petechiae possible
- Pathognomonic rash of scarlet fever
  - Fine, erythematous, confluent punctate rash begins on trunk and spreads peripherally
  - Sandpaper texture, often described as "goose pimples on sunburn"
  - Facial flushing with circumoral pallor
  - Rash fades with pressure
  - Deep red lines, with petechiae in folds of the joints (Pastia lines)
  - Desquamation after 7 to 21 days; commonly on palms and soles but may be diffuse
  - Strawberry tongue (white coated or red in color) with enlarged papillae
- Young children with GAS infection generally have low-grade fever, generalized lymphadenopathy, persistent nasal discharge, and appear ill but not toxic.

ETIOLOGY

- Multiple serotypes of GAS (*Streptococcus pyogenes*) are distinguished by distinctive surface proteins called *M-proteins.*
- GAS associated with tonsillopharyngitis and scarlet fever differs from that causing skin infection.
- Certain serotypes are associated with ARF: The specific rheumatogenic factor has not been identified.
- Other serotypes are associated with APSGN: nephritogenic strains.

DIAGNOSIS

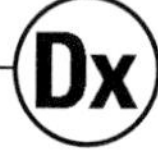

DIFFERENTIAL DIAGNOSIS

- Viral throat infections are more common than GAS and are clinically indistinguishable.
  - Adenovirus
  - Epstein-Barr virus
  - Cytomegalovirus
  - Herpes simplex virus
  - Influenza
  - Parainfluenza

- Coxsackie and possibly other enteroviruses
- Other streptococcal groups (C and G) have been associated with pharyngitis and nephritis but not with ARF.
- Other bacterial infections of the pharynx are uncommon in children, although bacterial cultures can reveal other streptococci (non-β-hemolytic) and *Haemophilus influenzae,* which are generally thought to be normal inhabitants of the upper respiratory tract and need not be treated.

WORKUP

- In the nontoxic child, diagnostic testing should be limited to differentiating GAS infection from viral causes because of the need to treat GAS to prevent complications and sequelae.
- Factors to be considered in the decision to obtain a throat swab for testing in children with pharyngitis are the patient's age, clinical signs and symptoms, the season, and the family and community epidemiology, including contact with a known case or potential exposure to a family member with a history of ARF or APSGN.
- In the rare, toxic child, the extent of the workup depends on the clinical presentation and may include a white cell count and differential, blood and throat cultures, and radiographic studies.
- In a nontoxic child with tonsillitis/pharyngitis and classic scarlet fever, diagnostic evaluation is not thought to be required because the rash is pathognomonic of GAS infection.
- GAS is unlikely in patients younger than 3 years of age and in those with signs of viral infection (e.g., coryza, conjunctivitis, hoarseness, cough, anterior stomatitis, diarrhea, discrete oral ulcers); GAS testing is not recommended in these patients.
- All symptomatic contacts should be tested for GAS, although symptomatic household contacts are often treated presumptively.
- Asymptomatic contacts should be tested only if the contact or a family member of the contact has a history of ARF or APSGN; individuals testing positive under these circumstances should be treated.
- Patients who have repeated episodes of pharyngitis occurring at short intervals and associated with positive cultures or tests for GAS pose a special problem. These individuals are often GAS carriers who are experiencing frequent viral illnesses. Noncompliance or treatment failure should be considered.

LABORATORY TESTS

- Laboratory confirmation of GAS in the form of a throat culture is recommended.
- A specimen should be obtained by vigorous swabbing of the tonsils and posterior pharynx.
- Cultures on sheep blood agar with appropriate use of a bacitracin disk allows a presumptive identification of GAS.
- A false-negative rate of less than 10% is achieved if the swab is obtained and processed properly.
- Several rapid diagnostic tests are available. Most of these tests have high specificity but lower sensitivity.
- A throat culture should be sent in any patient suspected of having GAS who has a negative rapid diagnostic test.

IMAGING STUDIES

- Imaging studies are generally not required for the treatment of GAS infections including those complicated by peritonsillar abscess formation.
- In the rare, toxic child, the extent of the workup depends on the clinical presentation and may include radiographic studies (computed tomography scan of soft tissues of the neck, chest radiographs, and a sinus series).

TREATMENT

Rx

NONPHARMACOLOGIC THERAPY

Medical

- Although GAS infection is a self-limited disease; treatment prevents spread, complications, and latent sequelae and shortens the clinical course.
- A brief delay in initiating antibiotic therapy to process a throat culture does not increase the risk of latent sequelae.
- Infected individuals remain infectious until they have had 24 hours of appropriate therapy; thus they should stay home for that period.

Surgical

- Surgical management in the child with acute GAS tonsillopharyngitis is reserved for the acute complication of associated peritonsillar abscess or deep neck abscess, which may require surgical drainage.
- Tonsillectomy for recurrent GAS infection is not done as commonly as it was in the past.
  - Experts remain conflicted about whether tonsillectomy alters the course of recurrent disease or lessens the possibility of latent sequelae.
  - Only children with more than seven documented episodes of streptococcal tonsillitis in a year or five episodes each in 2 consecutive years should be referred for evaluation for possible tonsillectomy.

ACUTE GENERAL Rx

- Penicillin V is the drug of choice for GAS tonsillopharyngitis and scarlet fever. Amoxicillin is often used instead but offers no microbiologic advantage.
  - The dose is 250 mg (400,000 U) two to three times per day for children and 500 mg two to three times per day for adolescents and adults.
  - Medication should be continued for 10 days to prevent ARF, regardless of the promptness of clinical recovery.
- Intramuscular benzathine penicillin G is also appropriate therapy.
  - It ensures adequate blood concentrations and avoids the problem of compliance, but administration is painful.
  - A single dose of 600,000 U is recommended for children weighing less than 60 pounds and 1.2 million U is recommended for larger children, adolescents, and adults.
  - Mixtures with shorter-acting penicillins (e.g., procaine penicillin) are less painful, as is warming benzathine penicillin G to room temperature before administration.
- Orally administered erythromycin is indicated for patients who are allergic to penicillin.
- Other macrolides (clarithromycin and azithromycin) are also effective.
- Penicillin-allergic individuals can also be treated with a cephalosporin or clindamycin.
- Penicillin- and erythromycin-resistant strains of GAS are uncommon in the United States.
- Tetracycline and sulfonamides should not be used to treat GAS pharyngitis.

CHRONIC Rx

- Generally not applicable as GAS is an acute, self-limited disease.
- GAS carriers are not at risk for latent sequelae and are not infectious, thus they do not require treatment.
- Though some experts recommend oral penicillin prophylaxis during the period of the year of greatest risk for children with recurrent GAS tonsillopharyngitis, this approach should be limited because of concerns about selecting resistant organisms (not GAS).
- Patients with a well-documented history of ARF should be given continuous antibiotic prophylaxis to prevent recurrent attacks.

DISPOSITION

- Most cases of GAS tonsillopharyngitis and scarlet fever can be easily recognized and treated on an outpatient basis by primary care physicians.
- Inpatient treatment may be initially required for toxic-appearing patients suspected of having associated invasive disease.

REFERRAL

- Certain complications (e.g., peritonsillar abscess) may necessitate referral for surgical care.
- Referral of patients for tonsillectomy should be infrequent.
- Patients who develop latent sequelae of GAS infections generally require referral

to a pediatric subspecialist for diagnosis, initial management, and subsequent comanagement.

PEARLS & CONSIDERATIONS

COMMENTS

- Most cases of tonsillopharyngitis in childhood are caused by viruses.
- Clinicians need to detect those cases caused by GAS in order to provide therapy that will lessen both transmission and the possibility of acute and latent complications.
- Diagnostic testing is readily available but should be used with discretion to detect only those patients with disease who need treatment and not those who are carriers.
- Patients with classic scarlet fever can be diagnosed purely on clinical grounds and do not require diagnostic studies.

PREVENTION

- Preventive, prophylactic antibiotics are not indicated for patients at low risk for rheumatic fever.
- Patients with a well-documented history of ARF and those with rheumatic heart disease should be given continuous antibiotic prophylaxis to prevent recurrent attacks.
- Some experts recommend oral penicillin prophylaxis during the period of the year of greatest risk for children with repeated episodes of GAS pharyngitis. The effectiveness of such an approach is unsubstantiated and should be limited because of concerns of antimicrobial resistance.

PATIENT/FAMILY EDUCATION

- Parents should be informed about the following:
  - Natural history, communicability, and usual clinical course of the disease
  - Prompt follow-up if symptoms have not resolved in 3 days
  - The importance of finishing all of the treatment to prevent latent sequelae
  - Recognizing symptoms of the late sequelae of GAS and seeking immediate treatment
- Patients with a history of ARF and their family members must be vigilant and prompt in seeking diagnosis and treatment of possible GAS infection because they are at risk for recurrence.

SUGGESTED READINGS

American Academy of Pediatrics: Group A streptococcal infections. *In* Pickering L (ed): *2003 Red Book: Report on the Committee of Infectious Diseases.* Elk Grove Village, IL, 2003, pp 573–584.

Centers for Disease Control and Prevention. Available at www.cdc.gov/ncidod/dbmc/diseaseinfo/groupastreptococcal_g.http://www.cdc.gov/ncidod/hip/abc/facts39.htm; www.cdc.gov/ncidod/EID/vol2no1/strepyro.htm

Group A streptococcal infections: proceedings of a conference held January 20–22, 1995, in Tampa, Florida. *Pediatrics* 97:S945, 1996.

Kaplan EL: Group A streptococcal infections. *In* Feigin RD, Cherry JD (eds): *Textbook of Pediatric Infectious Diseases.* Philadelphia, WB Saunders, 1992, pp 1296–1305.

Pichichero M: Group A beta-hemolytic streptococcal infections. *Pediatr Rev* 19:291, 1998.

AUTHOR: **LYNN R. CAMPBELL, MD**

BASIC INFORMATION

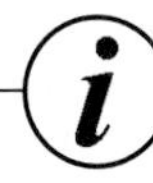

DEFINITION

Pityriasis rosea (PR) is an acute, benign, self-limited skin disorder predominantly affecting adolescents and young adults.

ICD-9-CM CODE
696.3 Pityriasis rosea

EPIDEMIOLOGY & DEMOGRAPHICS

- Slight female predominance, with a female-to-male ratio of 1.2:1
- More common in fall and spring
- Usually occurs in adolescents and young adults (uncommon in children <5 years of age)

CLINICAL PRESENTATION

- There is occasionally a nonspecific prodrome (headache, pharyngitis, lymphadenitis, and malaise).
- Approximately 70% to 80% recall a *herald* patch.
  - Isolated lesion with sharply defined borders. Usually round or oval (2 to 5 cm) with a flat pink or brown center and a red, finely scaled, slightly elevated border.
  - Usually on trunk, upper arms, neck, or thighs, in order of decreasing frequency
- Generalized eruption begins 5 to 10 days after development of the herald patch.
- Spares face (85%), scalp, and distal extremities
- Lesions occur in crops, which may resemble the herald patch but are smaller and more ovoid.
  - These secondary lesions occur on the trunk in a characteristic "Christmas-tree" pattern.
    - The long axis of individual lesions is parallel to the lines of the skin.
    - The trunk of the "tree" is the spine.
  - Secondary lesions have a fine, scaly edge with a tissue-paperlike collarette of scale.
    - Peaks 2 to 7 days after onset of generalized eruption
    - In 25% of cases, lesions are moderately pruritic.
    - Resolution of lesions begins after 2 to 4 weeks.
    - Lesions fade over 4 to 6 weeks.
- Patients may have postinflammatory hypopigmentation or hyperpigmentation (especially in dark-skinned individuals) for weeks to months after healing is complete.
  - Atypical presentation will have an inverse distribution affecting the face, wrists, and extremities but sparing the trunk.
- Young children may have lesions that are papular, vesicular, pustular, urticarial, or purpuric in the early stages.
  - Atypical lesions are more common in very young children, dark-skinned individuals, and pregnant women.
- Children may also have lesions on the face and neck.
  - Uncommonly, the lesions may be found on oral mucosal surfaces.

ETIOLOGY

- The cause is unknown, but a viral etiology is suspected based on the self-limiting course, epidemics with seasonal clustering, and tendency for lifelong immunity.
- Human herpesviruses 6 and 7 (HHV6 and HHV7) and parvovirus B19 are among the specific viruses investigated as causative.

DIAGNOSIS

Dx

DIFFERENTIAL DIAGNOSIS

- The differential diagnosis of the herald patch includes tinea corporis.
- The differential of the secondary eruption includes the following:
  - Drug eruption
  - Seborrheic dermatitis
  - Nummular eczema
  - Guttate psoriasis
  - Secondary syphilis
  - Acute form of pityriasis lichenoides (Mucha-Habermann disease)

WORKUP

- The diagnosis is based on clinical recognition of lesions and distribution pattern.
- The fine, peripheral collarette of scale is characteristic of PR.

TREATMENT

Rx

NONPHARMACOLOGIC THERAPY

- There is no specific therapy for PR. It is a self-limited disease.

ACUTE GENERAL Rx

- Pruritus, if present, may be treated with mild, topical corticosteroids or oral antihistamines.
- Exposure to sunshine or ultraviolet light tends to hasten resolution of lesions but may accentuate postinflammatory hypopigmentation.

DISPOSITION

- The disease is self-limited, including the postinflammatory changes.
- Resolution will not occur for many weeks.
- Patient may need physician note to return to work or school.
- Contagion pattern is not known—there are no recommendations for isolation or exclusion from participation in activities.
- No short- or long-term untoward effect has been identified.

PEARLS & CONSIDERATIONS

COMMENTS

- Similar (and usually smaller) lesions in the typical Christmas-tree distribution follow herald patch.
- Individual lesions have a collarette of fine scale.

SUGGESTED READINGS

Darmstadt GL, Lane A: Diseases of the epidermis. *In* Behrman RE et al (eds): *Nelson Textbook of Pediatrics,* 15th ed. Philadelphia, WB Saunders, 1996.

Drago F et al: Human herpesvirus 7 in patients with pityriasis rosea: electron microscopy investigations and polymerase chain reaction in mononuclear cells, plasma and skin. *Dermatology* 195:374, 1997.

Hurwitz S: *Clinical Pediatric Dermatology,* 2nd ed. Philadelphia, WB Saunders, 1993.

Marcus-Farber BS et al: Serum antibodies to parvovirus B19 in patients with pityriasis rosea. *Dermatology* 194:371, 1997.

Zitelli BJ, Davis HW: *Atlas of Pediatric Physical Diagnosis,* 3rd ed. St. Louis, Mosby, 1997.

AUTHOR: **LISA LOEB COLTON, MD**

BASIC INFORMATION

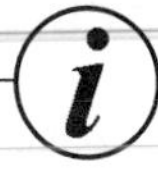

DEFINITION

Pleural effusion is a pathologic collection of fluid between the visceral and parietal pleura in the thoracic cavity.

SYNONYMS

Empyema
Parapneumonic effusion
Sympathetic effusion

ICD-9-CM CODES

012.0 Tuberculous (last digit dependent on laboratory diagnosis) effusion
197.2 Malignant effusion
457.8 Chylothorax
511.1 Bacterial/parapneumonic effusion
511.9 Unspecified effusion
862.29 Traumatic effusion

EPIDEMIOLOGY & DEMOGRAPHICS

- Pleural effusion complicates the cases of at least 2% to 8% of children hospitalized with pneumonia.
- Incidence is declining, presumably due to early recognition and treatment of pneumonia as well as widespread immunization against common organisms *Streptococcus pneumonia* and *Haemophilus influenzae.*

CLINICAL PRESENTATION

- Cough
- Tachypnea
- Fever
- Chest pain
- Respiratory distress
- Fatigue
- Shortness of breath
- Anorexia
- Dullness to chest percussion
- Egophony
- Children with pleural effusion-complicating pneumonia generally fail to clinically improve with initial antibiotic treatment.

ETIOLOGY

The majority of pleural effusions in the pediatric population result from bacterial pneumonia.

- *Streptococcus pneumoniae* represents the most common organism.
- Other infectious etiologies include:
  - *Staphylococcus aureus*
  - *Streptococcus pyogenes*
  - *Enterobacteriaceae*
  - *Anaerobes*
  - *Legionella*
  - *Mycoplasma*
  - *Histoplasma*
  - *Coccidioides*
  - *Aspergillus*
  - *Entamoeba*
  - *Nocardia*
  - *Mycobacterium tuberculosis*
  - *Paragonimus*
- Frequently, the offending pathogen cannot be cultured from the pleural fluid.
- Pleural effusion can also accompany inhaled foreign body and lung abscess.
- Parapneumonic effusion can be divided into three stages:
  - Early/exudative stage or simple parapneumonic effusion with normal fluid pH and glucose.
  - Fibrinopurulent stage in which there is an increase in fibrin and polymorphonuclear cells (PMNs) with a concomitant decrease in glucose and pH and increase in lactate dehydrogenase (LDH).
  - Organizing stage in which fibroblast growth in the parenchymal and visceral pleura results in an inelastic ring or peel. Entrapment of the involved lung develops in this stage.
- Other, noninfectious causes of pleural effusion include:
  - Mediastinal or esophageal disease
  - Neoplasm
  - Tracking of fluid from intra-abdominal sources
    - Pancreatitis
    - Ascites
    - Subphrenic abscess
    - Ventriculoperitoneal shunt
  - Chest trauma
  - Collagen vascular disease
  - Congestive heart failure
  - Septic emboli
- Iatrogenic causes include:
  - Chylothorax—frequently seen as an operative complication of cardiothoracic surgery
  - Malposition or complication of central venous access
  - Ventriculopleural shunt

DIAGNOSIS (Dx)

DIFFERENTIAL DIAGNOSIS

- Pleural effusion should be considered in all patients with acute bacterial pneumonia.
- Parenchymal pulmonary disease
- Thoracic or mediastinal mass
- Careful consideration should be given to underlying diseases (see "Etiology") as a potential cause of pleural effusion and recent invasive procedures that could result in pleural effusion.

LABORATORY TESTS

- Complete blood count
- Blood culture
- Laboratory studies of pleural fluid obligatorily involve thoracentesis with or without additional procedures including thoracostomy tube placement, VATS (video-assisted thoracoscopic surgery), or open thoracotomy. Patients with small, freely flowing effusion may not require thoracentesis. Careful reevaluation, including repeat radiographic studies are obligatory.
- Pleural fluid evaluation in suspected cases of parapneumonic effusion should include:
  - Glucose
  - Protein
  - LDH
  - Culture and gram stain
  - Culture for tuberculosis and acid-fast stain
  - Fungal culture and stain
  - Cell count
  - Cytopathology
- Additional studies of pleural fluid to be considered based on suspected underlying etiology of pleural effusion include:
  - Triglyceride levels
  - Amylase
  - Lipase
  - PPD
- Laboratory studies should include evaluation for underlying collagen, vascular, mediastinal, cardiac, pulmonary, intra-abdominal, or malignant disease depending on clinical suspicion.

IMAGING STUDIES

- Chest radiograph—consider serial radiographs when following small/simple parapneumonic effusions without drainage
- Decubitus chest radiographs
- Thoracic ultrasound—useful to identify loculation, motion, and underlying lung disease
  - May also use as aid for thoracentesis and thoracostomy tube placement
- Computed tomography of the chest—useful to evaluate for pleural thickening, loculations, and to identify underlying pulmonary parenchymal disease

TREATMENT (Rx)

NONPHARMACOLOGIC THERAPY

- Goals of management include selection of appropriate antibiotics, complete pleural drainage, and lung reexpansion.
- Optimal treatment of parapneumonic effusion remains controversial as many children will improve with conservative management alone.
  - VATS and pleural dèbridement are technically easier to perform earlier in the disease process.
  - Failure rates with nonoperative management may be as high as 25%.
  - Duration of illness, length of hospitalization, and cost are lower for children treated with early surgical intervention.
- If nonoperative intervention is selected, frequent clinical and radiographic reevaluation are necessary.
- Failure to improve clinically warrants prompt surgical intervention.

ACUTE GENERAL Rx

- Supplemental oxygen as needed and guided by pulse oximetry
- Ventilatory support for respiratory failure

- For pleural effusion:
  - Antibiotics
  - Thoracentesis
  - Tube thoracostomy with or without fibrinolytic therapy
  - VATS
  - Open decortication
- Treatment of underlying associated conditions often helps to resolve pleural effusion.
- Diet free of long-chain fats can help to resolve chylothorax.

CHRONIC Rx

Follow-up chest radiograph in 3 to 6 months typically shows full resolution of parapneumonic effusion.

DISPOSITION

Children with pleural effusion can be discharged home on oral antibiotics once they have defervesced and are clinically improved.

REFERRAL

Early surgical consultation is recommended.

PEARLS & CONSIDERATIONS

COMMENTS

- Incomplete control of the pleural space is associated with lobular entrapment and reduced long-term pulmonary function.
- Consider fiberoptic bronchoscopy to exclude foreign body as a possibility.

PREVENTION

- Immunization against organisms commonly associated with acute bacterial pneumonia including *S. penumonia* and *H. influenzae.*
- Early recognition of pleural effusion as a common complication of acute bacterial pneumonia can prevent prolonged hospitalization, particularly in the child who fails to respond to antibiotics.

PATIENT/FAMILY EDUCATION

- The vast majority of children who develop a pleural effusion as a complication of community-acquired pneumonia have no underlying immunodeficiency or parenchymal pulmonary disease.
- These children are not at increased risk of complicated pneumonia in the future.
- Lung function, exercise capacity, and chest radiograph return to normal over 3 to 6 months.

SUGGESTED READINGS

Avansino JR et al: Primary operative versus nonoperative therapy for pediatric empyema: a meta-analysis. *Pediatrics* 115(6):1652, 2005.

Campbell JD, Nataro JP: Pleural empyema. *Pediatr Infect Dis J* 18(8):725, 1999.

Colice GL et al: Medical and surgical treatment of parapneumonic effusions. *Chest* 18:1158, 2000.

Thompson AH et al: Randomized trial of intrapleural urokinase in the treatment of childhood empyema. *Thorax* 57:343, 2002.

Weinstein M et al: Effectiveness and safety of tissue plasminogen activator in the management of complicated parapneumonic effusions. *Pediatrics* 113(3):e182, 2004.

Yao CT et al: Treatment of complicated parapneumonic pleural effusion with intrapleural streptokinase in children. *Chest* 125(2):566, 2004.

AUTHOR: **HEIDI V. CONNOLLY, MD**

BASIC INFORMATION

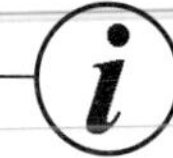

DEFINITION

Pneumonia is an inflammation of the lung caused by a variety of pathogens.

ICD-9-CM CODES
480.9 Pneumonia, viral
481 Pneumococcal pneumonia
482.9 Pneumonia, bacterial, unspecified
483.0 *Mycoplasma pneumonia*
486 Pneumonia, unspecified
487.0 Influenza with pneumonia
507 Pneumonia, aspiration
511.9 Pleural effusion, NOS

EPIDEMIOLOGY & DEMOGRAPHICS

- Pneumonia is more prevalent in the winter months.
- It is more common in younger children.
- Viruses are the most common cause of pneumonia.
- Viral pneumonias are often observed in epidemics.
- Children who are immunocompromised or have underlying lung disease are at greater risk for significant pneumonia.

CLINICAL PRESENTATION

- Pneumonia is often preceded by symptoms of an upper respiratory tract infection.
- Symptoms include fever, malaise, anorexia, and chest pain.
- Cough may be associated with vomiting.
- Some infants may have associated apnea.
- Child may only have nonspecific signs such as fever and general ill appearance.
- Signs suggestive of pneumonia include cyanosis, tachypnea, nasal flaring, retractions, grunting, dullness to percussion of chest, decreased breath sounds, rales, and egophony.

ETIOLOGY

- Determination of the precise cause for pneumonia in children is often difficult.
- More common pathogens include:
  - Virus: respiratory syncytial virus (RSV), parainfluenza, influenza, adenovirus
  - *Mycoplasma pneumoniae*
  - Bacteria: *Streptococcus pneumoniae, Streptococcus pyogenes, Staphylococcus aureus, Streptococcus agalactiae, Haemophilus influenzae* type B
  - *Chlamydia trachomatis, Chlamydia pneumoniae*
  - *Mycobacteria tuberculosis*
- In the immunocompromised patient, also consider organisms such as *Pneumocystis jiroveci, Candida, Aspergillus, Legionella pneumophila,* and cytomegalovirus.
- Other pathogens should be considered if there is history of exposure to certain animals or travel to particular areas.

DIAGNOSIS

DIFFERENTIAL DIAGNOSIS

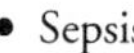

- Sepsis
- Asthma
- Atelectasis
- Bronchiolitis
- Lung sequestration
- Hypersensitivity reaction
- Pulmonary hemorrhage
- Sarcoidosis
- Wegener's granulomatosis
- Foreign body aspiration
- Congestive heart failure
- Malignancy

LABORATORY TESTS

- A complete blood count (CBC) and differential with chest roentgenograph are initial tests.
- Blood cultures are recommended in young, febrile children and children who are seriously ill.
- Sputum for Gram stain and culture in children who can produce an adequate specimen. Most young children, however, cannot provide such a specimen.
- Thoracentesis should be considered if a pleural effusion is present. The specimen is sent for Gram stain and culture, pH, cell count, protein and cytology to differentiate transudate from exudates.
- Bronchoscopy or open lung biopsy (for culture and histology) may be necessary in the evaluation of pneumonia in the seriously ill and immunocompromised patient.

Specific Testing

- Virus:
  - Rapid testing is generally available for RSV and influenza.
  - Shell viral cultures may be read within a few days (used for influenza A and B, RSV, parainfluenza, and adenovirus).
  - Traditional viral cultures are kept longer.
- Bacteria:
  - Gram stain and culture of blood, pleural fluid, and sometimes sputum
  - Antigen testing in urine samples may be helpful for *S. pneumoniae, H. influenzae,* and group B streptococci.
- *M. pneumoniae*:
  - Elevated serum cold agglutinins may be present but test has low specificity.
  - Organism may be cultured in some laboratories.
  - *Mycoplasma*-specific antibody titers may be tested.
- Chlamydia:
  - Organism may be cultured.
  - Antigen testing is available for *C. trachomatis.*
- *M. tuberculosis*:
  - Mantoux skin test (5 TU of PPD) is done for determination of infection.
  - In young children, an early morning gastric aspirate is the preferred specimen for acid-fast stain and culture.
  - Sputum or bronchoscopy specimens may also identify the organism.
- *P. jiroveci*:
  - Sputum samples and specimens obtained by bronchoscopy or lung biopsy are examined for organisms with a silver or fluorescent antibody stain.
- *Candida, Aspergillus*:
  - Organism may be cultured from lung biopsy or observed on histology.
  - Sputum cultures may be difficult to interpret.
- *L. pneumophila*:
  - Organism may be cultured using special media.
  - Urine antigen detection and serology are also available.

IMAGING STUDIES

- Chest radiograph (posterior-anterior and lateral)
- Computed tomography may better delineate chest pathology and may be useful in the severely ill or immunocompromised host.

TREATMENT

ACUTE GENERAL Rx

- Supportive care should be initiated, with maintenance of adequate oxygenation, hydration, nutrition, and fever control.
- Pulse oximetry is helpful to assess level of oxygenation.
- Mechanical ventilation may be necessary in severely ill children.

Antimicrobial Therapy:

Virus: most viral pneumonias are treated symptomatically, but specific antiviral therapy may be beneficial in certain situations.

- RSV: treatment is usually supportive but ribavirin given by aerosol should be considered in some children at high risk for serious RSV disease.
- Influenza: if antiviral drugs are to be used, they should be given within 2 days of onset of illness.
  - Amantadine has activity against influenza A.
  - It is given orally and may have central nervous system side effects.
  - The neuraminidase inhibiters, oseltamivir and zanamivir, may be used for the treatment of influenza A and B.
  - Oseltamivir is given orally to children 1 year of age and older.
  - Zanamivir is given by inhalation to children 7 years of age and older.
  - Cytomegalovirus:
  - Ganciclovir and cytomegalovirus (CMV) intravenous immune globulin (IVIG) have been used in CMV pneumonia in bone marrow transplant patients.
- Bacteria:
  - Numerous antibiotics have activity against the usual bacterial pathogens.
  - Commonly used oral antibiotics include amoxicillin (with or without clavulanate

acid), the second- and third-generation cephalosporins, and the macrolides.
  - Intravenous antibiotics are indicated for children who are seriously ill or vomiting.
  - Treatment for resistant organisms such as methicillin-resistant *S. aureus* (MRSA) should be considered in children with risk factors for such organisms or the critically ill.
  - For the common bacterial pathogens, the duration of antibiotic therapy is usually 10 to 14 days.
  - Longer courses of therapy are often required for children with pneumonia complicated by empyema or abscess, and in the immunocompromised patient.
  - Macrolides and trimethoprim/sulfamethoxazole (TMP/SMX) should not be used for treatment of penicillin-resistant *S. pneumoniae.*
- *M. pneumoniae*:
  - Macrolides (erythromycin, clarithromycin, and azithromycin)
  - Tetracycline may be used in children 8 years and older.
- *C. trachomatis, C. pneumoniae*:
  - Macrolides
  - Tetracycline may be used in children 8 years and older.
- *M. tuberculosis*:
  - Multidrug therapy is given for at least 6 months. Therapy depends on organism sensitivity.
  - Unless drug resistance is suspected, usual therapy consists of isoniazid, rifampin, and pyrazinamide for the first 2 months, followed by isoniazid and rifampin for an additional 4 months.
  - Therapy is extended in children infected with human immunodeficiency virus (HIV).
- *P. jiroveci*:
  - TMP/SMX pentamidine is an alternative drug.
  - The duration of antimicrobial therapy is at least 2 to 3 weeks.
  - Corticosteroids should be considered in children with moderate to severe illness.
- *Candida, Aspergillus*:
  - In children, amphotericin B is typically used for treatment of pneumonia due to *Candida* or *Aspergillus.*
  - Liposomal amphotericin preparations should be considered if there is renal insufficiency, intolerance to amphotericin B, or need for very high dosing.
  - Other drugs that are used to treat *Aspergillus* include voriconazole, itraconazole, and caspofungin acetate.
  - An extended course of therapy is usually required.
- *L. pneumophila*:
  - Azithromycin is the drug of choice.
  - The addition of rifampin is recommended in cases of severe illness, immunocompromised patients, or poor response to macrolide.
  - Doxycycline and TMP/SMX are alternative drugs.

CHRONIC Rx

- Empyemas require drainage.
- Thoracoscopy or thoracotomy with decortication may be necessary.

DISPOSITION

Close follow-up is essential. A repeat chest roentgenograph several weeks after completion of antibiotics helps verify the absence of an underlying abnormality.

REFERRAL

Referral to a pediatric infectious disease or pulmonary specialist is suggested for children with unusual or complicated pneumonias.

PEARLS & CONSIDERATIONS

COMMENTS

- Respiratory viruses are the most common cause of pneumonia.
- The etiologic diagnosis is difficult. Bacterial cultures of upper respiratory tract secretions are usually not helpful. Blood cultures are often not positive.
- Think of pneumonia in febrile children younger than 5 years old with significant leukocytosis (white blood cell count 20,000/mm^3 or higher).

PREVENTION

- Children should receive the usual recommended vaccines unless they have a specific contraindication.
- Other available immunizations for selected high-risk children include vaccines against influenza and meningococcus.
- Penicillin prophylaxis against pneumococcal disease is recommended in many asplenic children.
- Prophylaxis against RSV with palivizumab or RSV-IVIG is recommended for selected young children at risk for severe RSV disease. Refer to current Red Book (see "Suggested Readings") and American Academy of Pediatrics guidelines for specific recommendations.
- Prophylaxis against influenza with antiviral agents may be considered when vaccine is unavailable, contraindicated, or ineffective.
- Children who have infection with *M. tuberculosis*, but without disease, should receive prophylactic isoniazid for 9 months.
- Prophylaxis against *P. jiroveci* with TMP/SMX is indicated in children who are significantly immunocompromised, including some HIV-infected children, some children with primary immunodeficiencies, and some children receiving immunosuppressive therapy.
  - HIV-infected children who have had prior *P. jiroveci* pneumonia usually receive lifelong prophylaxis.
  - Alternative drugs for prophylaxis include pentamidine and dapsone.

PATIENT/FAMILY EDUCATION

- Parents of neonates should be counseled about spread of respiratory viruses and the importance of good hand washing and decreased exposures to ill individuals.
- Children who are immunocompromised or who have certain chronic illnesses should also be appropriately educated about exposures and recommended preventive therapies.

SUGGESTED READINGS

Bachur R et al: Occult pneumonias: empiric chest radiographs in febrile children with leukocytosis. *Ann Emerg Med* 33:166, 1999.

Bradley J: Management of community-acquired pediatric pneumonia in an era of increasing antibiotic resistance and conjugate vaccines. *Pediatr Infect Dis J* 21:592, 2002.

Boyer KM: Nonbacterial pneumonia. *In* Feigin RD et al (eds): *Textbook of Pediatric Infectious Diseases,* 4th ed. Philadelphia, WB Saunders, 2004, pp 286–298.

Klein JO: Bacterial pneumonias. *In* Feigin RD et al (eds): *Textbook of Pediatric Infectious Diseases,* 4th ed. Philadelphia, WB Saunders, 2004, pp 299–310.

Pickering LK (ed): *2003 Red Book: Report of the Committee on Infectious Diseases,* 26th ed. Elk Grove Village, IL, American Academy of Pediatrics, 2003.

AUTHOR: **CAROL A. McCARTHY, MD**

BASIC INFORMATION

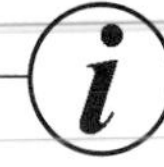

DEFINITION

A spontaneous pneumothorax (PTX) is the abnormal presence of air in the pleural space.

SYNONYM

Collapsed lung

ICD-9-CM CODES
512.0 Tension
512.8 Acute, spontaneous
521.1 Iatrogenic/postoperative/procedural complication
770.2 Newborn
860.0 Traumatic

EPIDEMIOLOGY & DEMOGRAPHICS

- Incidence: 7 to 18 per 100,000 in males; 1 to 6 per 100,000 in females
- Male-to-female ratio of 3:1 to 6:1
- Familial tendency
- Risk factors:
  - Tobacco smoking
  - Tall, thin body habitus
  - Males 10 to 30 years of age
- Recurrence rate:
  - Twenty percent to 30% after first PTX; usually within 2 years and on same side
  - Fifty percent to 60% after the second PTX
  - More than 80% after the third PTX
  - Five percent to 10% risk of contralateral PTX

CLINICAL PRESENTATION

History
- Cardinal manifestation is sudden chest pain; pleuritic, localized pain
- Tachypnea, dyspnea, and tachycardia
- Cough, hemoptysis, and orthopnea less uncommon
- Less than 10% occur during strenuous exercise
- Ipsilateral shoulder pain common

Physical Examination
- Small PTXs (<20%) usually not detectable on physical exam
- Vital signs usually normal except for moderate tachycardia
- Lung examination
  - Hyperresonant to percussion on affected side
  - Decreased or absent breath sounds on affected side
  - Depressed respiratory movement on affected side
- Hypoxemia usually mild when PTX is less than 25%
  - Hypoxemia, when present, caused by shunting
- Hypercapnia rare because underlying lung function is normal

ETIOLOGY

- Primary PTX
  - PTX is most often secondary to rupture of subpleural blebs or bullae on apical portion of upper lobes.
  - Blebs may be secondary to abnormalities of connective tissue, inflammation of bronchioles, or over distention of alveoli.
  - PTX leads to decreased vital capacity and increased alveolar-arterial oxygen gradient and hypoxemia.
- Secondary PTX occurs in patients with preexisting lung disease.
  - Airway disease: asthma, cystic fibrosis, foreign body aspiration
  - Infectious disease: *Pneumocystis carinii* ; anaerobic, gram-negative, or staphylococcal pneumonia; tuberculosis; parasitic
  - Interstitial lung disease
  - Acute lung injury caused by inhaled physical and chemical agents
  - Neoplastic disease
  - Connective tissue disease: Marfan and Ehlers-Danlos syndromes
- Traumatic
  - Complication developing within 24 hours of diagnostic or therapeutic procedures: transbronchial biopsy, central venous line, intubation
  - Mechanical ventilation, barotrauma
  - Penetrating or blunt chest trauma
- Catamenial
  - Recurrent PTX within 48 to 72 hours of menses onset; rare
  - Associated with pelvic endometriosis
- Hamman syndrome
  - During labor and delivery

DIAGNOSIS

DIFFERENTIAL DIAGNOSIS

- Based upon history
  - Pleuritis
  - Asthma
  - Cardiac or psychogenic pain
- Based upon examination
  - Empyema
  - Pleural effusion
  - Bullae or lung cyst
- In neonates
  - Congenital lobar emphysema
  - Congenital adenomatoid malformation
  - Diaphragmatic hernia

IMAGING STUDIES

- Chest radiograph
  - Outer margin of visceral pleura is separated from parietal pleura by lucent gas space devoid of pulmonary vessels or lung markings.
  - In upright position: air collects at the apex
  - Lateral decubitus or expiratory views can detect small air collections.
  - Signs of tension PTX: mediastinal shift, diaphragmatic depression, rib cage expansion
- Chest computed tomography scan
  - Identifies presence of bullae and blebs in patients with recurrent PTX
  - Aids in detecting air collections when radiograph is inconclusive

TREATMENT

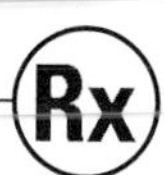

NONPHARMACOLOGIC THERAPY

Observation
- Requires evidence that air leak is sealed
- Generally reserved for asymptomatic patients with less than 20% primary, unilateral PTX
- Serial chest radiographs over 24 hours to ensure no progression
- Gas reabsorbed spontaneously

Surgical
- Thoracentesis or chest tube drainage should be considered for all PTXs 25% or greater, in patients with continued air leak, and in cases of incomplete reexpansion or respiratory distress.
  - Simple aspiration successful in 70% of patients with moderate-sized PTX
  - Needle placed in second anterior intercostal space in midclavicular line
  - Recurrence rate: 25% to 40%
- Chest tube has a success rate of 90% for treatment of first PTX; success rates decrease with recurrences.
  - Insertion is done through the fifth intercostal space in midaxillary line.
  - All secondary PTX should be managed with chest tubes.
  - If duration of PTX is unknown, initial management is through a water seal to minimize risk of reexpansion pulmonary edema; negative pressure is used if lungs fail to reexpand after 12 to 24 hours.
  - Complications include pain, pleural infection, incorrect placement of tube, hemorrhage, and reexpansion pulmonary edema.

ACUTE GENERAL Rx

Medical
- Administration of 100% oxygen
  - Nitrogen is "washed out" of venous blood, increasing the gradient between partial pressure of nitrogen in PTX and venous blood.
  - As nitrogen diffuses out of PTX across this gradient, the total volume of gas in pleural space decreases.
  - Oxygen will accelerate reabsorption by a factor of 4 compared to room air.
  - This procedure is more effective in neonates than in older children.

CHRONIC Rx

Pleurodesis
- Mechanical or chemical pleural abrasion leading to inflammatory response and subsequent adhesion formation
- Goal to achieve adhesion of visceral and parietal pleura in order to obliterate pleural space
- Generally performed after recurrence of PTX, or after first PTX in patients who plan to continue high-risk activities such as flying or diving
- Low success rate in patients with persistent air leak

- Future surgical procedures, such as lung transplantation, may be hampered by this process.
- Most often performed via video-assisted thoracoscopic surgery under general anesthesia; may also be an open procedure
- Recurrence rate: 0.6% to 2.0%

Other Surgical Interventions

- Thoracoscopy indicated for patients who fail noninvasive intervention, have persistent or recurrent PTX, or have risk of significant morbidity should recurrence occur
- Bullectomy: stapling or oversewing of bullae
- Pleurectomy
- Removal of fibrotic "peel"

DISPOSITION

- Those meeting criteria for observation only, may be in hospital or outpatient
  - If outpatient close observation, limited physical activity and ability to obtain emergency services quickly
  - Five percent mortality reported as a result of the development of tension PTX from unrecognized pleural leak
- Those requiring a chest tube: discontinue suction after air leak ceases, continue water seal, remove chest tube if no air leak after 24 hours

REFERRAL

- Pediatric pulmonologist: if PTX is recurrent or to assist with management of primary PTX, or if suspicious of underlying lung disease
- Pediatric surgeon: for all conditions requiring surgical management

PEARLS & CONSIDERATIONS

COMMENTS

- Pleural effusions occur in 20% to 25% of cases.
- In room air, a PTX is absorbed by 1% to 6% per 24 hours.
- PTX is associated with cocaine inhalation and marijuana smoking.
- Tension PTX:
  - Intrapleural pressure greater than atmospheric pressure throughout expiration and often during inspiration
  - More common after traumatic or mechanical ventilation-induced PTX
  - Clinical picture: labored breathing, tachypnea, marked tachycardia, profuse diaphoresis, cyanosis, distended neck veins, tracheal deviation to contralateral side, subcutaneous emphysema, hypotension, displaced point of maximal cardiac impulse
- Bronchopleural fistula:
  - Three percent to 5% of patients with PTX will have persisting air leak.
  - Patients with cystic fibrosis are at increased risk.
  - Surgical intervention is usually required.
- Reexpansion pulmonary edema:
  - Unilateral pulmonary edema following rapid reexpansion of collapsed lung
  - Appears to be caused by increased permeability of pulmonary capillaries damaged by mechanical stress during reexpansion
  - Can occur when PTX is present for more than 3 days and lung is expanded with more than –20 cm water pressure
  - Symptoms usually progress over 24 to 48 hours.

SUGGESTED READINGS

Baumann MH et al: Management of spontaneous pneumothorax: an American College of Chest Physicians Delphi Consensus Statement. *Chest* 119:590–602, 2001.

Panitch H et al: Abnormalities of the pleural space. *In* Taussig L, Landau L (eds): *Pediatric Respiratory Medicine.* New York, Mosby, 1999, pp 1178–1196.

Sahn SA, Heffner JE: Spontaneous pneumothorax. *N Engl J Med* 342:868, 2000.

AUTHOR: **BARBARA A. CHINI, MD**

BASIC INFORMATION

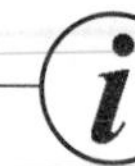

DEFINITION

Polio is an acute viral infection of the brainstem and spinal cord that leads to irreversible motor neuron damage and paralysis. Endemic wild-type viral illness has been eradicated in North America as a result of vaccination.

SYNONYMS

Infantile paralysis
Paralytic polio
Poliomyelitis

ICD-9-CM CODES
045.9 Polio
V04.0 Polio immunization

EPIDEMIOLOGY & DEMOGRAPHICS

- Before widespread immunization, outbreaks of polio occurred in the late summer and fall, with the largest epidemic (more than 57,000 cases) occurring in the United States in 1952.
- 1955: inactivated (Salk) vaccine (IPV) was introduced.
- 1964: trivalent oral (Sabin) vaccine (OPV) was introduced.
- 1978: enhanced-potency inactivated vaccine (E-IPV) was developed.
- 1979: last case of wild-type poliomyelitis was reported in the United States.
- 1999: ACIP voted to change the recommendation for childhood polio vaccination beginning in 2000 to a schedule using only the E-IPV to eliminate the occurrence of vacane associated paralytic poliomyelitis (VAPP). VAPP has been eliminated in the United States as of 2000.
- Outbreaks of polio are still occurring in Nigeria, India, Pakistan, Niger, Afghanistan, and Egypt.

CLINICAL PRESENTATION

History

- VAPP: antecedent administration of OPV from 1 week to 1 month before symptoms; recent administration of DTP (diphtheria, tetanus, pertussis) vaccine may enhance paralysis in active poliovirus infection
- Immunocompromise or exposure to a person recently vaccinated with OPV
- Abortive or aseptic meningitis: nonspecific signs and symptoms of a febrile illness, diarrhea, headache, meningismus, vomiting, and photophobia
- Paralytic poliomyelitis (spinal type): ascending paralysis, may occur without antecedent prodrome, especially in young infants; weakness and paralysis progress through the febrile period of the illness
- Respiratory difficulties occur with paralysis of the intercostal muscles and with bulbar polioencephalitis affecting the brainstem medullary respiratory center.
    - Symptoms include shallow or spasmodic breathing, other cranial nerve involvement, and paralysis of pharyngeal or laryngeal muscles
- Constipation and voiding abnormalities (urinary retention, overflow incontinence)

Physical Examination

- Tremor upon sustained effort may present before weakness.
- Paralysis: muscle tightness and intense muscle pain without true paralysis may be noted early in the presentation.
- Superficial and deep muscle reflexes are absent on the affected side.
- Cranial nerve paralysis presents in the bulbar form.

ETIOLOGY

- Polioviruses are in the group Enterovirus.
- Polio is transmitted by the fecal-oral route.
- Patients are contagious as long as fecal shedding persists, which can be weeks to months.
- Incubation is as follows: 3 to 6 days for mild, nonspecific illness (abortive polio); 7 to 21 days for paralytic polio
- Postpolio syndrome may develop 30 to 40 years after initial childhood infection.

DIAGNOSIS

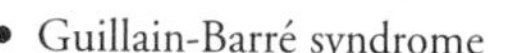

DIFFERENTIAL DIAGNOSIS

- Guillain-Barré syndrome
- Peripheral neuritis (herpes zoster, Bell's palsy, or other etiologies)
- Rabies
- Botulism
- Tetanus
- Transverse myelitis
- Tick paralysis
- Various viral encephalitis/arbovirus infections, including a paralytic form of West Nile virus encephalitis

WORKUP

Nerve conduction studies: asymmetric loss of stretch reflex is the hallmark of poliomyelitis.

LABORATORY TESTS

- Lumbar puncture: cerebrospinal fluid (CSF) may be normal in 10% to 15% of patients, pleocytosis as in viral meningitis
- Viral culture: stool and throat specimens for enterovirus culture, rarely grown from CSF
- Seroconversion by antibody titer to specific serotype

TREATMENT

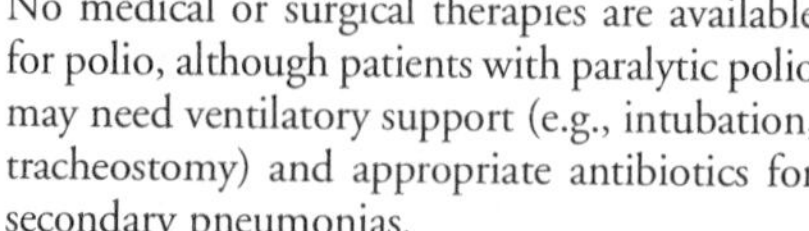

ACUTE GENERAL Rx

No medical or surgical therapies are available for polio, although patients with paralytic polio may need ventilatory support (e.g., intubation, tracheostomy) and appropriate antibiotics for secondary pneumonias.

CHRONIC Rx

- Supportive care for respiratory support, including mechanical ventilation if required
- Nutritional support; physical therapy

PEARLS & CONSIDERATIONS

COMMENTS

- Immunization with IPV has eliminated VAPP in the United States.
- OPV is no longer given in the United States.
- Eradication in other areas of the world of wild-type polio is not complete due to lapses in immunization campaigns.

PREVENTION

- Polio vaccine effectively eradicated wild-type polio in the Western Hemisphere and dramatically reduced circulation in other areas of the world.
- OPV contains live, attenuated poliovirus types 1, 2, and 3 and generates intestinal immunity.
- OPV viruses are excreted in the stool for several weeks after vaccination.
- IPV contains same three virus types which are inactivated with formaldehyde.
- IPV generates high rates of seroconversion but less mucosal immunity than OPV.
- Trace amounts of streptomycin, neomycin, and polymyxin B may be in IPV preparations and may cause rare allergic reactions.
- Both vaccine types are highly immunogenic and effective in preventing polio.
- The only significant adverse reaction to OPV is VAPP, with risk being highest after the first dose (1 case per 760,000 doses) and decreasing with each subsequent dose.
    - For immunocompromised persons, the risk is 3200- to 6800-fold greater.
    - Patients with antibody deficiency syndromes are at highest risk for acquiring VAPP from contact with a vaccinee or from primary vaccination.
- Immunodeficient persons should receive only IPV; household contacts of such persons should also receive only IPV.
- Routinely immunize with IPV at 2, 4, and 6 to 18 months of age, and a booster dose at 4 to 6 years of age.
- OPV would be acceptable in the following circumstances: mass vaccination campaigns to control outbreaks; to eradicate polio in other countries where polio is still endemic
- Any suspected case of poliomyelitis should be reported to state health departments so that investigation can be initiated. If wild-type virus is isolated, OPV may need to be administered in a possible epidemic area. If OPV virus is implicated, no vaccination campaign is necessary because outbreaks with vaccine strains have not been seen.

SUGGESTED READINGS

American Academy of Pediatrics: Poliovirus infections. *In* Pickering LK, Backer CJ, Long SS, McMillan JA (eds): *Red Book 2006 Report of the Committee on Infectious Diseases,* 27th ed. Elk Grove Village, IL, American Academy of Pediatrics, 2006, pp 542–547.

American Academy of Pediatrics, Committee of Infectious Diseases: Poliomyelitis prevention: revised recommendations for use of inactivated and live oral poliovirus vaccines. *Pediatrics* 103:171, 1999.

Centers for Disease Control and Prevention. Available at www.cdc.gov/nip

Recommendations of the Advisory Committee on Immunization Practices: Revised recommendations for routine poliomyelitis vaccination. *MMWR Morb Mortal Wkly Rep* 48:590, 1999.

AUTHOR: **DONNA J. FISHER, MD**

BASIC INFORMATION

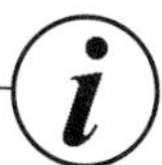

DEFINITION

Polycystic kidney diseases are hereditary disorders involving the development of numerous fluid-filled cysts throughout the cortex and medulla of the kidneys. The following two main types are seen:

- Autosomal dominant polycystic kidney disease (ADPKD)
- Autosomal recessive polycystic kidney disease (ARPKD)

SYNONYMS

Adult polycystic kidney disease (ADPKD)
Infantile polycystic kidney disease (ARPKD)

ICD-9-CM CODES
753.13 ADPKD
753.14 ARPKD

EPIDEMIOLOGY & DEMOGRAPHICS

- ADPKD
  - ADPKD affects approximately 1 in 1000 individuals.
  - Onset usually occurs in adulthood.
  - Fifty percent develop end-stage renal failure by age 60 to 70.
  - All racial groups are affected.
  - Clinical symptoms usually appear in the third to fifth decades of life, although PKD1 may present in childhood. PKD2 tends to have a milder course.
- ARPKD
  - ARPKD affects between 1 in 10,000 and 1 in 55,000 children.
  - Onset usually occurs in infancy and younger childhood.
  - It is invariably associated with congenital hepatic fibrosis.
  - Fifty percent of patients live beyond 10 years of age.

CLINICAL PRESENTATION

History

- ADPKD
  - Positive family history
  - Abdominal and flank pain
  - Gross or microscopic hematuria
  - Urinary tract infections (UTIs)
  - Kidney stones
  - Hypertension
  - Renal cysts may be discovered, even on prenatal ultrasound.
- ARPKD
  - Parents unaffected
  - Respiratory distress
  - Oligohydramnios
  - Spontaneous pneumothoraces
  - Severe hypertension
  - Portal hypertension with age
  - UTIs are common.

Physical Examination

- ADPKD
  - Hypertension
  - Abdominal or flank masses
  - Hepatomegaly (rare)
- ARPKD
  - Flank masses (common)
  - Potter's syndrome (oligohydramnios sequence: flattened nose, micrognathia, low-set ears, pulmonary hypoplasia, limb deformities)
  - Respiratory distress (in the neonatal period)
  - Hypertension (common)
  - Hepatosplenomegaly (usually presents in toddlers to school-age children)
  - Signs of portal hypertension
  - Growth retardation

ETIOLOGY

- Cysts increase in number and size throughout life and compress normal kidney tissue causing inflammation that leads to destruction of renal parenchyma.
- ADPKD: approximately 85% of cases are linked to chromosome 16p and an inherited mutation of one *PKD-1* gene allele.
  - The *PKD-1* gene product, polycystin, is a large membrane-associated protein.
  - A cyst appears to develop from a renal epithelial cell carrying this inherited abnormal *PKD-1* gene when a spontaneous mutation occurs in the other normal, but highly mutagenic, *PKD-1* allele.
  - This leads to two abnormal *PKD-1* genes in the same cell and apparently to cyst formation.
  - Most of the remaining cases are linked to the *PKD-2* gene on chromosome 4q, but a few families appear to have a third form.
- ARPKD: the *PKHD1* gene, encoding the protein fibrocystin (polyductin), is localized on chromosome 6p.
  - Dilated collecting ducts form small fusiform cysts that can enlarge with age.

DIAGNOSIS

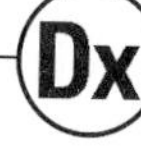

DIFFERENTIAL DIAGNOSIS

- ADPKD
  - Multiple simple renal cysts
  - von Hippel-Lindau disease
  - Tuberous sclerosis
  - Bardet-Biedl syndrome
- ARPKD
  - Bilateral Wilms' tumor
  - Meckel's syndrome
  - Jeune's syndrome
  - Ivemark's syndrome

WORKUP

- ADPKD
  - Diagnosis is made by finding large bilateral renal cysts (may be unilateral early on) in the presence of a family history of ADPKD.
  - In affected families, prenatal and presymptomatic diagnosis can be made by DNA linkage analysis.
  - Documentation of bilateral cysts noted in a parent.
- ARPKD
  - Massively enlarged kidneys are detected at birth or in an older child with congenital hepatic fibrosis.
  - Congenital hepatic fibrosis is invariably found.
  - Renal cysts are absent in parents.
  - DNA mutation analysis available but detects 40% to 80% of individuals with ARPKD.
  - In affected families, prenatal diagnosis can be made by DNA linkage analysis.

LABORATORY TESTS

- ADPKD
  - Urinalysis reveals overt proteinuria in 23% of children. This may portend a worse prognosis.
  - Blood urea nitrogen (BUN), creatinine, electrolytes
  - Urine culture for suspected UTI
  - Consider genetic testing in questionable cases
- ARPKD
  - BUN, creatinine, electrolytes
  - Urine culture for suspected UTI
  - Monitor pulmonary status in newborn period for suspected pulmonary hypoplasia
  - Consider genetic testing

IMAGING STUDIES

- ADPKD
  - Renal ultrasonography detects macroscopic cysts of various sizes.
  - Because the course of ADPKD may be mild and 30% of adults may be unaware that they have the disease, renal ultrasonography should be performed on the parents of a child with bilateral renal cysts and a negative family history of ADPKD.
    - Eighty-three percent of affected individuals will have renal cysts by 30 years of age.
  - Magnetic resonance angiography is used to detect intracerebral aneurysms that may be associated with ADPKD in high-risk older children (those with a family history of ruptured cerebral aneurysm, symptoms suggestive of cerebral aneurysm).
  - Hepatic ultrasound may show hepatic cysts (rare in children, but increase with age).
  - Mitral valve prolapse occurs in 12% of children and may be seen on echocardiogram.
- ARPKD
  - Renal ultrasonography: massive enlargement of the kidneys with loss of corticomedullary differentiation and diffuse markedly increased echogenicity of the renal parenchyma from microcysts; cysts may enlarge as the child grows.
  - Magnetic resonance imaging may have an increasing role in diagnosis.
  - Liver ultrasound may be performed.

TREATMENT

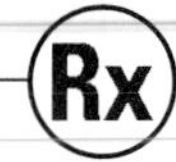

NONPHARMACOLOGIC THERAPY

- No specific treatments are available for either ADPKD or ARPKD.
- Treat symptoms as they arise.
- ADPKD
  - Bed rest, hydration, and analgesics for gross hematuria and cyst hemorrhage
  - Segmental renal arterial embolization for massive bleeding
  - Dialysis for patients reaching end-stage renal failure
- ARPKD
  - Dialysis for patients reaching end-stage renal failure

Surgical

- ADPKD
  - Cyst reduction for chronic pain
  - Cyst drainage for refractory cyst infection
  - Kidney transplantation for patients reaching end-stage renal failure
  - Nephrectomy: may be indicated before transplantation in the face of recurrent UTIs, recurrent severe hematuria, or massively enlarged kidneys interfering with allograft placement
- ARPKD
  - Kidney transplantation for end-stage renal failure
  - Unilateral nephrectomy: suggested for severe respiratory compromise related to compression of the lungs by massively enlarged kidneys

ACUTE GENERAL Rx

- ADPKD
  - Nonsteroidal anti-inflammatory drugs are given for pain control (carefully monitoring renal function).
  - Antibiotics are given for UTIs.
    - Many antibiotics penetrate into cysts poorly, and infections may prove refractory even in the face of sensitive organisms.
    - Trimethoprim/sulfamethoxazole, ciprofloxacin, and tetracyclines tend to gain better entry into cysts than other agents, although the use of the latter agents may be problematic in young children.
    - Prolonged treatment may be required.
- ARPKD
  - Antibiotics are given for UTIs.

CHRONIC Rx

- ADPKD
  - Antihypertensive agents are used for hypertension.
- ARPKD
  - Antihypertensive agents are given for blood pressure control. Several agents may be necessary.

DISPOSITION

- ADPKD
  - Monitor urinalysis and blood pressure closely in at-risk children.
  - A high index of suspicion is required for UTIs and kidney stones.
  - Monitor renal function in patients with known ADPKD.
- ARPKD
  - Monitor renal function.
  - Monitor blood pressure.
  - A high index of suspicion is required for UTIs.
  - Monitor for evidence of hypersplenism (e.g., splenomegaly, anemia, thrombocytopenia) secondary to hepatic disease.

REFERRAL

- Involvement by a pediatric nephrologist should be obtained in the care of children with these disorders.
- Pediatric gastroenterology involvement is needed for children with ARPKD.

PEARLS & CONSIDERATIONS

COMMENTS

- ADPKD
  - Onset of clinical symptoms, extrarenal manifestations, and progression of renal disease can vary significantly, even within families.
- ARPKD
  - Children presenting early tend to have more severe renal involvement and less severe hepatic involvement at presentation than children presenting at an older age.
  - Approximately 30% to 50% die from pulmonary hypoplasia in the newborn period.
  - Twenty-three percent develop bleeding esophageal varices.
  - Approximately 50% of children require antihypertensive treatment by age 5 years.
  - For those surviving the neonatal period, 25% reach end-stage renal failure by age 5 years.

PATIENT/FAMILY EDUCATION

- ADPKD: presymptomatic evaluation and diagnosis may label an at-risk child early on in a disorder that may remain asymptomatic well into adulthood.
- ARPKD: it was initially thought that all patients died in infancy; however, more recent studies have shown that children who survive the neonatal period have a relatively good prognosis (67% are alive without end-stage renal disease at 15 years).
- Support groups:
  - The Polycystic Kidney Research Foundation. Available at www.pkdcure.org
  - The NEPHKIDS web site has information on various kidney diseases with links to an email discussion group for parents of children with kidney disease. Available at http://cnserver0.nkf.med.ualberta.ca/nephkids/
  - Local chapters of the National Kidney Foundation. Available at www.kidney.org

SUGGESTED READINGS

Avni FE et al: Hereditary polycystic kidney diseases in children: changing sonographic patterns through childhood. *Pediatr Radiol* 32:169, 2002.

GeneTests. Available at http://www.genetests.org

Harris PC, Rossetti S: Molecular genetics of autosomal recessive polycystic kidney disease. *Mol Genet Metab* 81:75, 2004.

Kern S et al: Appearance of autosomal recessive polycystic kidney disease in magnetic resonance imaging and RARE-MR-urography. *Pediatr Radiol* 30:156, 2000.

Lee DI et al: Laparoscopic cyst decortication in autosomal dominant polycystic kidney disease: impact on pain, hypertension, and renal function. *J Endourol* 17:345, 2003.

Rossetti S et al: A complete mutation screen of PKHD1 in autosomal-recessive polycystic kidney disease (ARPKD) pedigrees. *Kidney Int* 64:391, 2003.

Tee JB et al: Phenotypic heterogeneity in pediatric autosomal dominant polycystic kidney disease at first presentation: a single-center, 20-year review. *Am J Kidney Dis* 43:296, 2004.

AUTHOR: **WILLIAM S. VARADE, MD**

BASIC INFORMATION

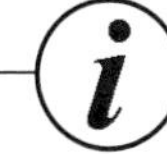

DEFINITION

- Polycystic ovary syndrome (PCOS) describes a broad spectrum of ovarian dysfunction hallmarked by hyperandrogenism and oligomenorrhea. The definition of PCOS is controversial. In 1990, the National Institutes of Health (NIH) defined PCOS as the presence of both:
  - Chronic anovulation *and*
  - Clinical or biochemical evidence of hyperandrogenism, excluding other etiologies.
- The 2003 Rotterdam European Society for Human Reproduction and Embryology and the American Society for Reproductive Medicine (ESHRE/ASRM) broadened the 1990 NIH diagnostic criteria for PCOS. As such, the presence of any two of the three criteria gives the diagnosis of PCOS in women:
  - Polycystic ovaries on ultrasound
  - Oligo-/anovulation
  - Clinical or biochemical evidence of hyperandrogenism, and the exclusion of other etiologies

This diagnosis may be made after the initial 2 to 3 years following menarche because of the common occurrence of anovulatory cycles in pubertal girls. Polycystic ovaries are commonly found in the adolescent female population, and care should be taken in assigning a diagnosis of PCOS in adolescents based upon ultrasound criteria.

SYNONYMS

Functional ovarian hyperandrogenism
Polycystic ovarian disease (PCOD)
Sclerocystic ovarian disease
Stein-Leventhal syndrome
Stein's syndrome

ICD-9-CM CODE
256.4 Polycystic ovary, ovaries

EPIDEMIOLOGY & DEMOGRAPHICS

- PCOS affects 5% to 10% of women of reproductive age.
- Up to 70% of women with PCOS have menstrual cycle abnormalities.
- Up to 70% of women with PCOS are hirsute.
- Approximately 50% of women with PCOS are obese.
- Up to 50% of women with PCOS have insulin resistance.
- Up to 30% of women with PCOS have acne.
- Risk factors include history of premature pubarche, family history of PCOS, Carib-bean-Hispanic ancestry, African American ancestry, and obesity.
- Signs of PCOS begin in adolescence, with a peripubertal onset.
  - Studies suggest that it may be present earlier in life and may have a genetic component.
- PCOS is the most common cause of hyperandrogenism among adolescent girls.

CLINICAL PRESENTATION

History

- Most common presentation: menstrual cycle abnormality, signs and symptoms of hyperandrogenism, and overweightness
- Menstrual history of amenorrhea or oligomenorrhea 2 years or more postmenarche
- History of premature pubarche
- Symptoms of hyperandrogenism (some symptoms are more suggestive of other virilizing disorders)
  - Acne
  - Hirsutism
  - Alopecia
  - Deepening voice
  - Clitoromegaly
  - Increased muscle mass
- Medication and other drug history
- Family history
  - Menstrual abnormalities
  - PCOS
  - Infertility
  - Hirsutism
  - Family ethnicity
  - Diabetes mellitus

Physical Examination

- Should include a search for other causes of hyperandrogenism and menstrual abnormalities such as adrenal disorders, thyroid disorders, prolactinoma, pregnancy, abdominal and pelvic masses, and so forth
  - General appearance: typically overweight, but not always
  - Skin
    - Acne
    - Ferriman-Gallwey Score for Hirsutism (score greater than 6 indicates abnormal hair distribution, score greater than 8 indicates hirsutism) (see Table and Figure)
    - Alopecia
    - Acanthosis nigricans of intertriginous areas such as neck, groin, or axilla
- Pelvic exam (bimanual exam or ultrasound): normal

ETIOLOGY

- The exact cause is unknown.
- Possible mechanisms include:
  - Hyperinsulinism
    - Insulin has a mitogenic effect on ovaries leading to theca cell hyperplasia and subsequent excess androgen production.
    - Insulin inhibits hepatic production of sex hormone binding globulin (SHBG) resulting in higher concentrations of circulating free androgens.
    - Insulin may stimulate adrenal overproduction of androgens.
    - Coincident with the relative insulin resistance during adolescence/puberty
  - Abnormal hypothalamic-pituitary-ovarian function
    - Altered negative feedback regulation of gonadotropin-releasing hormone/luteinizing hormone (GnRH/LH)
    - Increased frequency and amplitude of pulsatile LH secretion
    - Elevated LH levels stimulate ovarian theca cells to secrete excessive amounts of androgen which are converted to estrogens peripherally.
    - Subsequent androgen and estrogen excess
    - Inhibition of follicle-stimulating hormone (FSH) secretion by estrogens
    - Insensitivity of FSH to GnRH stimulation
  - Abnormal ovarian function
    - Arrested follicles produce insufficient FSH resulting in aromatase deficiency and decreased ovarian estrogen production with subsequent androgen excess.
  - Adrenal hyperandrogenism/hyperresponsiveness

DIAGNOSIS

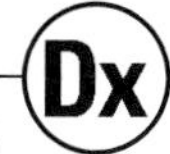

DIFFERENTIAL DIAGNOSIS

- Hyperandrogenism or amenorrhea
- Adrenal tumors
- Chronic illness such as diabetes mellitus
- Congenital adrenal hyperplasia (CAH), nonclassical
- Cushing's syndrome
- Eating disorder
- Exercise-induced amenorrhea
- Hypogonadotropic hypogonadism
- Ovarian tumors
- Pregnancy
- Premature ovarian failure
- Prolactinomas
- Thyroid dysfunction

LABORATORY TESTS

- Fasting lipids–HDL may be low, LDL and Triglycerides may be elevated
- Testosterone may be normal or mild-moderately elevated (current assays for free testosterone are highly variable)
  - Very elevated total testosterone and/or DHEAS: suspect ovarian or adrenal tumor
- Elevated Dihydroepiandrostenedione (DHEAS)
- Normal thyroid-stimulating hormone (TSH) and prolactin
  - Elevated TSH: suspect hypothyroidism
  - Elevated prolactin: suspect prolactinoma
- 17-Hydroxyprogesterone (17-OHP) is less than 200 ng/dl
- Normal fasting gulcose and insulin levels, but may be elevated in concurrent diabetes mellitus (see Diabetes Mellitus, Type II in Diseases and Disorders [Section I])

TABLE 1-17 The Ferriman-Gallwey Hirsute Score for Women

Site	Definition	Grade
Upper lip	A few hairs at the outer margin	1
	A small moustache at outer margin	2
	A moustache extending halfway from outer margin	3
	A moustache extending to the midline	4
Chin	A few scattered hairs	1
	Scattered hairs with small concentrations	2
	Complete cover light	3
	Complete cover heavy	4
Chest	Circumareolar hairs	1
	Circumareolar hairs with mid-line hair	2
	Fusion of circumareolar hairs with mid-line hair giving three-fourths cover	3
	Complete cover	4
Upper back	A few scattered hairs	1
	More than a few scattered hairs but still scattered	2
	Complete cover light	3
	Complete cover heavy	4
Lower back	A sacral tuft of hair	1
	A sacral tuft of hair with some lateral extension	2
	Three-quarter cover	3
	Complete cover	4
Upper abdomen	A few midline hairs	1
	Rather more but still mid-line	2
	Half cover	3
	Complete cover	4
Lower abdomen	A few mid-line hairs	1
	A mid-line streak of hair	2
	A mid-line band of hair	3
	An inverted V-shaped growth	4
Upper arm	Sparse growth affecting not more than a quarter of the limb surface	1
	More than a quarter coverage but still incomplete	2
	Complete cover light	3
	Complete cover heavy	4
Thigh	Sparse growth affecting not more than one fourth of the limb surface	1
	More than one-fourth coverage but still incomplete	2
	Complete cover light	3
	Complete cover heavy	4

- Grade 0 indicates the absence of terminal hair
- Ferriman-Gallwey hormonal hair score = (grade for upper lip) + (grade for chin) + (grade for chest) + (grade for upper back) + (grade for lower back) + (grade for upper abdomen) + (grade for lower abdomen) + (grade for upper arm) + (grade for thigh)
- Interpretation:
  - Minimum hormonal hair score: 0
  - Maximum hormonal hair score: 36
  - The higher the score, the more hirsute the woman.
  - A score more than 6 in a white woman indicates an abnormal hair distribution.
  - Each ethnic group may have a different upper limit of normal.

*Hirsutism in women is measured by the degree of hair growth in nine body regions.
Clinical Dermatology: A Color Guide to Diagnosis and Theraphy by Thomas P. Habif Mosby; 4th ed (October 27, 2003) Chapter 24 Hair Diseases: Table 24-4 The Ferriman-Gallwey Hirsute Score for Women, p 847.

- LH:FSH ratio greater than 2.5-3.0:1
  - LH high (>21 mIU/mL)
  - FSH low to normal
  - Up to 40% of women with PCOS have normal LH/FSH ratio. If suspect premature ovarian failure, FSH would be elevated.
- Other workup for hirsutism may include
  - Fasting cortisol or 24-hour urinary cortisol levels if suspect Cushing's syndrome.
  - Adenocorticotropic (ACTH) hormone stimulation test if 17-OHP is 200 to 1000 ng/dl to rule out late-onset CAH. (see Congenital Adrenal Hyperplasia in Diseases and Disorders [Section I].)

IMAGING STUDIES

- Pelvic or transvaginal ultrasound: classic description of "string of pearls" within the ovary(s) due to the accumulation of small antral follicles with impaired progression to a dominant preovulatory follicle.
- Ultrasound criteria for diagnosis of polycystic ovaries defined as either
  - The presence of 12 or more 2-9 mm diameter follicles in each ovary *or*
  - A single ovarian volume greater than 10 ml.
  - Either criteria must be in the absence of oral contraceptive used and optimally performed between days 3 and 5 of the menstrual cycle.

TREATMENT

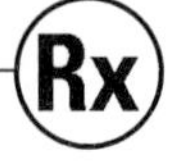

NONPHARMACOLOGIC THERAPY

- Weight loss if overweight or weight management if at risk of overweightness
- Hair removal for existing hair (not as cosmetically effective in the absence of hormonal suppression of regrowth or new hair growth)
  - Laser treatment
  - Electrolysis
  - Depilatories
  - Waxing
  - Bleaching
  - Shaving

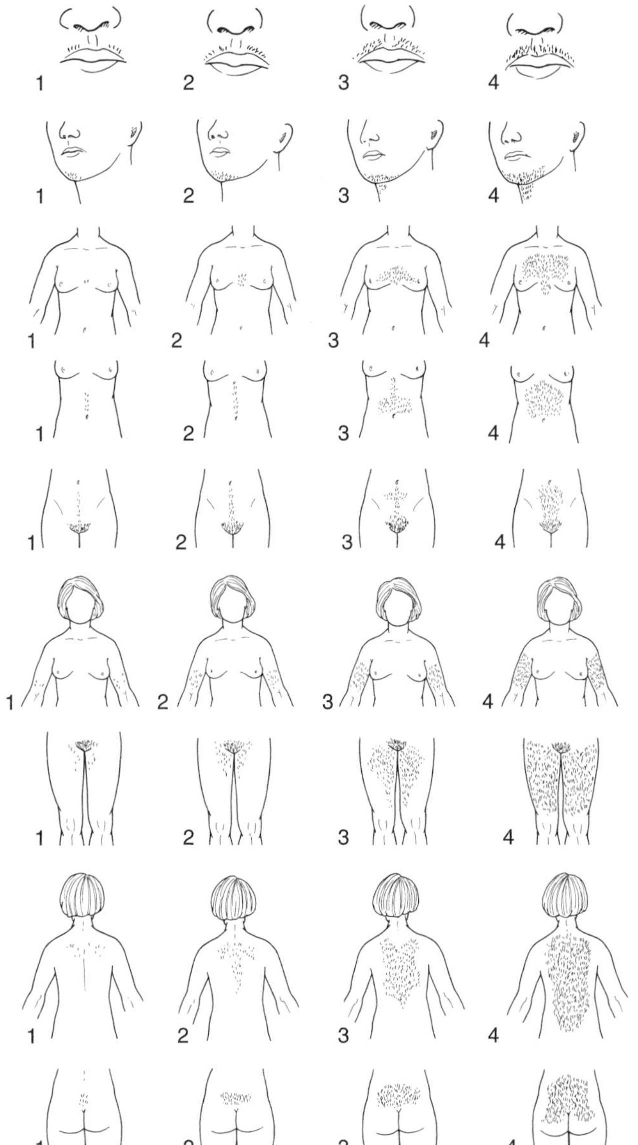

FIGURE 1-8 The Ferriman-Gallwey system for scoring hirsutism. A score of 8 or more indicates hirsutism.

- Smoking cessation
  - Decreases hirsutism secondary to androgens (smoking elevates androstenedione levels)

CHRONIC Rx

- Preferred first-line treatment is combined contraceptive
- Menstrual cycle regulation, androgen reduction, and reduction/prevention of endometrial hyperplasia
  - Combination OCPs, patch, or ring containing 30 to 35 μg ethinyl estradiol and progestins such as norethindrone, norgestimate, desogestrel, or drospirenone (Yasmin)
  - Continuous use of OCP (patch or ring) for 3 to 4 months, followed by 7 days off, may also lessen the increase in LH and testosterone
- Menstrual cycle regulation and reduction/prevention of endometrial hyperplasia
  - Medroxyprogesterone 10 mg daily for 10 to 12 days every 1 to 2 months to promote withdrawal bleeding
  - Depomedroxyprogesterone acetate (Depo-Provera) is not recommended as first-line treatment for menstrual cycle regulation as it can lead to unpredictable cycles and be difficult to manage.
- Androgen reduction (contraception should be used as these are potentially teratogenic)
  - Spironolactone: 100 to 200 mg per day in two divided doses
  - Eflornithine cream (13.9%): apply to affected areas twice daily, at least 8 hours apart
- Acne (see Acne Vulgaris in this section)
  - Benzoyl peroxide (topical gel or cream)
  - Multiple antibiotic regimens (topical or oral)
  - Multiple tretinoin preparations (topical)
  - Accutane
- Other treatment considerations
  - Metformin 500 to 850 mg orally two times per day for hyperinsulinemia, menstrual cycle regulation, increase in sex hormone binding globulin levels, decrease in androgen levels. Its use in adolescents is still being studied.
  - Antihyperlipidemic medication is recommended for adolescents with abnormal lipid profiles.

DISPOSITION

- For adolescents who require OCPs, see the adolescent in 1 month, again at 3 months, and then every 6 months.
- Continue monitoring for cardiovascular risk factors such as glucose intolerance and dyslipidemia.
- Follow-up at appropriate intervals to monitor medication side effects and as needed to support weight loss/weight management efforts and cosmetic effects.

REFERRAL

- Endocrine consultation for associated endocrinopathies
- Dermatology consultation for more severe acne
- Psychological consultation, if indicated
- Reproductive gynecology consultation for infertility issues
- Nutrition/dietician consultation for dietary evaluation and recommendations

PEARLS & CONSIDERATIONS

COMMENTS

- Although ovulatory rate is reduced in PCOS, patients may still become pregnant. Metformin therapy may enhance the ovulatory rate.
- Cyclical progesterone-only therapy may regulate menstrual cycles, but does not address hyperandrogenism.
- Unopposed estrogen in PCOS increases the risk for the following:
  - Endometrial cancer
  - Breast cancer
- In the treatment of hirsutism, noticeable results (decrease in new hair growth) from OCP use may take up to a year and 6 to 9 months with spironolactone.

PREVENTION

- For overweight adolescents, weight management is recommended to ameliorate any associated metabolic abnormalities and to reduce the risk of future comorbidities such as cardiovascular disease.
  - Decreases risk of thromboembolic disease in women who smoke and are taking OCPs

- ○ Decreases risk of cardiovascular disease associated with smoking with caveat that obesity, hyperinsulinism, and hyperandrogenism may independently increase risk of cardiovascular disease

PATIENT/FAMILY EDUCATION

- Explain the diagnosis and cause
- Explain the risk for pregnancy despite chronic oligo-ovulation
- Explain that PCOS is a risk factor for atherosclerosis (dyslipidemia), gestational diabetes mellitus, and diabetes mellitus type 2
- Explain that PCOS is associated with increased rates of subfertility
- Support is available at http://www.pcosupport.org/living/teen/index.php

SUGGESTED READINGS

Driscoll DA: Polycystic ovary syndrome in adolescence. *Ann NY Acad Scie* 997:49, 2003.

Emans SJ: Androgen abnormalities in the adolescent girl. *In* Emans SJ et al (eds): *Pediatric and Adolescent Gynecology,* 5th ed. Philadelphia, Lippincott Williams & Wilkins, 2005, pp 287–333.

Ferriman D, Gallwey JD: Clinical assessment of body hair growth in women. *J Clin Edocrinol* 21:1440, 1961.

Gordon CM et al: *In* Neinstein LS et al (eds): *Adolescent Health Care: A Practical Guide.* Philadlphia, Lippincot Willims & Wikins, 2002, pp 973–993.

Homburg R, Lambalk CB: Polycystic ovary syndrome in adolescence—a therapeutic conundrum. *Hum Reprod* 19(5):1039, 2004.

Legro RS, Azziz R: Androgen excess disorders. *In* Scott JR et al (eds): *Danforths's Obstetrics and Gynecology,* 9th edition. Philadelphia, Lippincott Williams & Wilkins, 2003, pp 663–683.

Rotterdam ESHRE/ASRM-Sponsored PCOS Consensus Workshop Group: Revised 2003 consensus on diagnostic criteria and long-term health risks related to polycystic ovary syndrome. *Fertil Steril* 81(1):19, 2004.

Rotterdam ESHRE/ASRM-Sponsored PCOS Consensus Workshop Group: Revised 2003 consensus on diagnostic criteria and long-term health risks related to polycystic ovary syndrome (PCOS). *Hum Reprod* 19(1):41, 2004.

AUTHOR: **PONRAT PAKPREO, MD**

BASIC INFORMATION

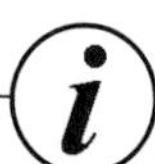

DEFINITION

Posttraumatic stress disorder (PTSD) is a specific psychiatric diagnosis based on abnormal or unusual feelings or behaviors that remain more than 4 weeks after exposure to a traumatic stressor, clustering in three areas that interfere with daily functioning: reexperiencing the trauma, avoiding the stimuli associated with the trauma, and experiencing increased arousal levels.

SYNONYM

PTSD

ICD-9-CM CODE

309.81 Posttraumatic stress disorder

EPIDEMIOLOGY & DEMOGRAPHICS

- In the US, more than 3 million children and adolescents experience some form of trauma annually (e.g., sexual and physical abuse, witnessing violence, natural disasters, house fires, motor vehicle accidents).
- Depending on severity and number of traumatic events, and the level of social/family support, 27% to 100% of children and adolescents develop PTSD with exposure.
- Children exposed to sudden, unexpected, human violence (e.g., domestic violence, homicide, war, terrorism) and those traumatized by a dysfunctional interpersonal relationship (e.g., incest, early neglect) are at greatest risk.
  - As many as 45% to 100% develop PTSD according to some reports.
  - Lifetime prevalence of PTSD higher for children experiencing trauma within the context of an interpersonal relationship (e.g., chronic sexual abuse).
- Exposure to real-life television viewing of traumatic incidents with intense emotion (e.g., Oklahoma City bombings, World Trade Center destruction) can cause PTSD symptoms, especially for populations at higher risk.
- Reportedly, girls are six times more likely to develop PTSD than boys.
- Boys tend to report fewer symptoms than needed to meet criteria for PTSD. However, they exhibit more externalizing behavioral problems subsequent to trauma exposure.
- Younger children who do not have a strong support system or whose life is dramatically changed after a trauma (e.g., house fire necessitating a move, death of a parent) are more susceptible to developing symptoms. They have less control and are more dependent on adults.
- Family history of mental health problems (anxiety disorders, mood disorders, substance abuse, and so forth) and any preexisting mental health diagnoses for the child also place that child at higher risk for developing PTSD.
- Children may have delayed onset of symptoms or change in expression of symptoms as they progress through developmental stages on into adulthood.
- Research is starting to show how early trauma actually alters neurobiologic development.

CLINICAL PRESENTATION

- Infants and toddlers may show the following: attachment problems; sleeping disturbance; separation anxiety; regressive symptoms such as thumb-sucking, loss of newly acquired developmental skills, enuresis; irritability, increased crying, temper tantrums, whining; eating disturbance; generalized anxiety or unrelated fears (e.g., of the dark).
- Preschool and school-age children tend to exhibit:
  - Reenactment of the trauma through play
  - Development of new fears (e.g., fear of the dark, separation anxiety)
  - Nightmares, disrupted sleep
  - Preoccupation with the traumatic event
  - Hyperarousal symptoms (e.g., difficulty concentrating, irritability, angry outbursts)
  - Somatic complaints (e.g., headaches, stomachaches)
  - Restriction in range of expressed emotions (flat affect)
  - Avoidance of situations, places, or people that remind the child of the traumatic event
- Adolescents may experience the aforementioned symptoms in addition to the following:
  - Excessive compliance and withdrawal
  - Increased aggression
  - Seeking premature independence (moving away from home)
  - Sexual acting out behaviors
  - Increased dependence
  - Increased risk for delinquency, substance abuse, and self-endangering reenactment behavior
  - Foreshortened sense of future
- Symptoms that may mask a diagnosis of chronic PTSD include: dissociation, self-injurious behaviors, substance abuse, conduct problems.
- Chronic childhood abuse can disrupt normal biopsychosocial development across many areas such as cognitive skills, regulation of behaviors and emotions, moral development, and interpersonal skills.

ETIOLOGY

- Risk factors for the development of PTSD include:
  - Severity of and length of exposure to the traumatic event(s)
  - Prior history of additional stressors including poor family functioning, poverty, previous exposure to trauma, psychiatric family history, poor physical health
- Typical stressors include the following:
  - Sexual or physical abuse
  - Natural disasters (hurricanes, earthquakes, floods, forest or brush fires)
  - Human-made disasters (plane crashes, bombings, automobile accidents)
  - Violence in school or the community
  - Witnessing domestic violence
- The presence of preexisting psychiatric conditions increases the risk of developing PTSD symptoms.
  - The onset of PTSD often precedes or coincides with development of other psychiatric disorders.
  - According to one study, 80% of adolescents with PTSD meet the criteria for at least one other psychiatric disorder, and 40% had two or more other disorders, especially depression.
- Presentation of symptoms may be triggered by a medical examination (e.g., gynecologic visit for an adolescent who was or is being sexually abused).

DIAGNOSIS

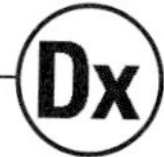

DIFFERENTIAL DIAGNOSIS

- Adjustment disorder: stressor is not extreme in nature.
- Acute stress disorder: posttraumatic symptoms appear and resolve within 4 weeks.
- Simple phobia: avoidance behavior is not limited to trauma-related stimuli.
- Obsessive-compulsive disorder: intrusive thoughts are unrelated to a traumatic event.
- Mood disorder: symptoms present before exposure to the extreme stressor.
- Psychotic disorders: flashbacks associated with PTSD should be distinguished from illusions, hallucinations, and other perceptual disturbances unrelated to the trauma.
- Attention deficit/hyperactivity disorder (AD/HD): hypervigilance, which may appear as distractibility, and hyperarousal present before exposure to trauma.
- Other anxiety disorders: symptoms present before exposure to an extreme stressor.
- Many of these conditions can develop in addition to PTSD, necessitating dual or multiple diagnoses and comprehensive treatment plans.

WORKUP

- At least one of the following reexperiencing symptoms:
  - Recurrent and intrusive distressing memories of the event, including images, thoughts, perceptions, or repetitive play in which traumatic theme(s) occur(s)
  - Recurrent distressing dreams about the trauma or frightening dreams without recognizable content (young children)
  - Acting or feeling as if the trauma were recurring—flashbacks (more common for adolescents), illusions, hallucinations, or trauma-specific reenactment
  - Intense distress at exposure to cues that symbolize or resemble the trauma

- Physiologic reactivity at exposure to internal or external cues that symbolize or resemble the traumatic event
- At least three of the following avoidance/numbing symptoms, which are the most common symptoms for children (not present before the trauma):
  - Efforts to avoid thoughts, feelings, or conversations associated with the trauma
  - Efforts to avoid reminders of the trauma
  - Amnesia for an important aspect of the trauma
  - Diminished interest or participation in normal activities
  - Feelings of detachment or estrangement from others
  - Restricted range of affect (blunted emotions)
  - A foreshortened sense of future (e.g., life will be too short to live to adulthood)
- At least two of the following indications of increased arousal (new since the trauma):
  - Sleep difficulties
  - Irritability or angry outbursts
  - Difficulty concentrating
  - Hypervigilance
  - Exaggerated startle response
- The symptoms from these three categories must be present for at least 1 month and cause clinically significant distress or impairment in functioning.
- Specification of onset and duration of the symptoms of PTSD include the following:
  - Acute: duration of symptoms is less than 3 months
  - Chronic: duration of symptoms is 3 months or longer
  - Delayed onset: at least 6 months have passed between the traumatic event and the onset of symptoms

TREATMENT Rx

NONPHARMACOLOGIC THERAPY

- Outpatient cognitive-behavioral psychotherapy is generally considered the preferred initial treatment, with varying duration depending on the child's and family's needs.
- Essential components to treatment include the following:
  - Psychoeducation for the parents/caretakers and child to help them understand (a) symptoms and course of PTSD, (b) treatment options and how they can help, and (c) realistic goals and expectations for treatment
  - Teaching of specific stress management techniques including deep breathing, thought-stopping, positive self-talk, and positive imagery
  - Direct exploration of the trauma after mastering stress management techniques
  - Identification and correction of inaccurate attributions regarding the trauma (e.g., inappropriate guilt, feeling responsible for the trauma)
  - Inclusion of nonabusing parent(s) or appropriate caretakers in treatment (children often do not share their feelings because it is painful, and they do not want to burden their parents)
  - Addressing grief when loss is experienced

ACUTE GENERAL Rx

- Although there is a need for additional research using controlled medication trials for treatment of children and adolescents with PTSD, pharmacologic intervention should be considered if the child's symptoms are so significant that he or she cannot function.
  - Selective serotonin reuptake inhibitor (SSRI) medications have been shown to help reduce symptoms of anxiety, mood, and reexperiencing symptoms (e.g., flashbacks).
  - Adrenergic agents (e.g., clonidine) target symptoms of hyperarousal and impulsivity. They can be used alone or with an SSRI.
- Established protocols for use of psychoactive medications should be considered as adjunctive treatment for children and adolescents with comorbid psychiatric conditions such as:
  - Mood disorders
  - AD/HD
  - Other anxiety disorders
- Unsuccessful outpatient psychotherapy may also be an indication to consider pharmacologic intervention.
- Referral for psychiatric evaluation is needed for treatment-resistant, complex cases with comorbid conditions.

CHRONIC Rx

Long-term intervention is needed for more persistent, chronic cases of PTSD. The same protocols are used as described with "Acute General Rx."

DISPOSITION

- Close collaboration with mental health professionals and follow-up visits to monitor symptom severity and treatment progress should be maintained.
- Treatment may be more episodic over time, necessitating "booster sessions" of outpatient psychotherapy if symptoms escalate during various developmental stages (e.g., child with sexual abuse history reexperiences symptoms with onset of menses).

REFERRAL

- Referral to a mental health professional is strongly recommended for best treatment.
- Parents may need to seek additional treatment for themselves if they are too traumatized to provide adequate support for their child.

PEARLS & CONSIDERATIONS !

COMMENTS

- The interviewer should follow these guidelines:
  - Be direct while providing a supportive environment.
  - Use developmentally appropriate language with the child.
  - Ask specific questions about symptoms.
- Although some children and adolescents may not meet full criteria for PTSD, cognitive-behavioral therapy should be provided as it may prevent the development of PTSD and lower the risk in adulthood.
- Address the family's need for intervention when indicated.
- Primary care physicians are in a unique position to track PTSD symptoms over time and assess treatment needs as the child develops.

PREVENTION

- Children's Safety Network, National Injury and Violence Prevention Resource Center. Available at www.childrenssafetynetwork.org

PATIENT/FAMILY EDUCATION

- American Academy of Child and Adolescent Psychiatry. Available at www.aacap.org
- Traumatic Incident Reduction. Available at www.healing-arts.org/tir/links.htm#PTSD
- KidsHealth for Parents. Available at www.kidshealth.org/parent/positive/family/ptsd.html
- Focus Adolescent Services. Available at www.focusas.com/PTSD.html

SUGGESTED READINGS

American Psychiatric Association: *Diagnostic and Statistical Manual of Mental Disorders,* 4th ed. Washington DC, American Psychiatric Association, 1994.

Cohen JA: AACAP official action: summary of the practice parameters for the assessment and treatment of children and adolescents with posttraumatic stress disorder. *J Am Acad Child Adolesc Psychiatry* 37:997, 1998.

Cohen JA: Treating acute posttraumatic reactions in children and adolescents. *Biol Psychiatry* 53:827, 2003.

Cooley-Quille MR et al: Emotional impact of children's exposure to community violence: a preliminary study. *J Am Acad Child Adolesc Psychiatry* 34:1362, 1995.

De Bellis MD: Developmental traumatology: the psychobiological development of maltreated children and its implications for research, treatment, and policy. *Dev Psychopathol* 13(3):539, 2001.

Donnelly CL: Pharmacologic treatment approaches for children and adolescents with posttraumatic stress disorder. *Child Adolesc Psychiatric Clin North Am* 12:251, 2003.

Lubit R et al: Impact of trauma on children. *J Psychiatr Pract* 9:128, 2003.

Pfefferbaum B: Posttraumatic stress disorder in children: a review of the past 10 years. *J Am Acad Child Adolesc Psychiatry* 36:1503, 1997.

Pine DS, Cohen JA: Trauma in children and adolescents: risk and treatment of psychiatric sequelae. *Biol Psychiatry* 51:519, 2002.

AUTHOR: **CHRISTINA M. MCCANN, PHD**

BASIC INFORMATION

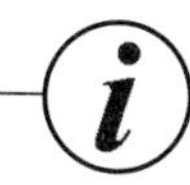

DEFINITION

Posterior urethral valves (PUV) are congenital membranes or tissue folds within the posterior urethra that obstruct urine outflow.

SYNONYM

Congenital obstructing posterior urethral membrane (COPUM)

ICD-9-CM CODE
753.6 Posterior urethral valves

EPIDEMIOLOGY & DEMOGRAPHICS

- Incidence is 1 in 8000 to 1 in 25,000 males.
- Up to one third of children with PUV have renal insufficiency or failure.
  - Present from 11 weeks gestation
  - May present at any age

CLINICAL PRESENTATION

History

- Prenatal
  - Ultrasound showing hydronephrosis
  - Oligohydramnios
  - Ascites (urine)
- Newborn
  - Urine leakage
  - Delayed voiding
- Any age
  - Straining to void
  - Weak or intermittent urinary stream
  - History of urinary tract infections (UTIs)
  - History of gross or microscopic hematuria
- Older child
  - Dysuria
  - Incontinence
  - Enuresis
  - Failure to thrive
- Renal failure

Physical Examination

- Hypertension
- Bladder distention, suprapubic mass
- Leakage of urine with increased abdominal pressure
- Abdominal fluid wave or dullness
- Palpably enlarged kidneys
- Undescended testes
- Patent urachus

ETIOLOGY

- Persistent remnants of the cloacal membrane that normally regresses upon interaction with the mesonephric duct
- The classic description of PUV:
  - Type I, 95%, fibroepithelial leaflets that extend distally from the verumontanum toward the external urinary sphincter
  - Type II, 5%, musculoepithelial folds commonly seen in prune-belly syndrome (PBS)
    - The obstructing nature of this lesion is a point of some controversy.
  - Type III (rare), diaphragm with pinpoint lumen anatomically not in relation to verumontanum
- Current concern about the accuracy of these descriptive categories:
  - A higher incidence of type III valves is noted if endoscopy is performed before catheter passage.
  - There is the implication that type III valves are converted to type I iatrogenically.
    - Catheter passage (likely) causes some alterations in valve appearance.
    - The original description, however, specifies that type III valves lack continuity with the verumontanum.

DIAGNOSIS

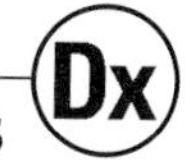

DIFFERENTIAL DIAGNOSIS

- Prenatal
  - PBS
  - Ectopic ureterocele
  - Neurogenic bladder
  - Non-neurogenic neurogenic bladder
  - Megaureter (reflux, obstruction)
- Postnatal based on specific signs or symptoms
  - Dysuria, enuresis, incontinence
    - UTIs
    - Neurogenic bladder
    - Reflex
    - Dysfunctional voiding
    - Constipation
  - Hematuria
    - Glomerular diseases
    - Trauma
    - Cystitis
  - Abdominal mass
    - Wilms' tumor
    - Duplication
    - Hydronephrosis of other causes
    - Lymphoma
    - Neuroblastoma
    - Congenital mesoblastic nephroma

LABORATORY TESTS

- All patients should have serial creatinine measures until consistent value. Levels are obtained every 1 to 3 months.
- Nadir may occur up to 1 year after birth.
- Abnormal values at 1 year are monitored more closely by pediatric nephrology at 6-month intervals through childhood, as the prognosis is more guarded.

IMAGING STUDIES

- Ultrasound of kidneys and bladder
  - Hydronephrosis is often the first sign of abnormality.
    - Seventy percent of infants with PUV have hydronephrosis.
    - Approximately 50% of patients also have other findings, including the following:
      - Megacystis (huge bladder)
      - Oligohydramnios
      - Dilated posterior urethra ("keyhole" sign)
    - Renal dysplasia may be suggested by increased renal parenchymal echogenicity, loss of corticomedullary distinction, and the presence of renal cortical cysts and calcifications.
- Voiding cystourethrogram (VCUG)
  - A fluoroscopic VCUG is done for definitive diagnosis of PUV.
  - In PUV, type I, the posterior urethra is elongated, dilated, and "sausage"-shaped.
  - In contrast, PBS shows a triangular defect.
  - A persistent indentation at the bladder neck (internal sphincter) may be present in either condition.
  - Vesicoureteral reflux occurs in at least 50% of patients.

TREATMENT

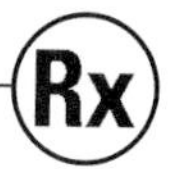

NONPHARMACOLOGIC THERAPY

- Acute management: prenatal
  - In utero treatment of valves with either ablation or vesicoamniotic shunting may be considered in the face of oligohydramnios to aid in pulmonary development.
  - Despite anecdotal successes, universal application of these measures to maximize ultimate renal function awaits a reliable measure of fetal renal potential.
- Acute management: postnatal
  - Many newborns with PUV present with a prenatal diagnosis, pulmonary immaturity, renal insufficiency, or urinary ascites.
  - The initial management depends on bladder drainage via a urethral catheter.
    - Placement in the bladder must be verified.
    - Positioning of the catheter within the urethra, a common occurrence, will not provide adequate decompression of the urinary tract.
      - Creatinine measurement, after the first few days of life, reflects the baby's renal status.
        - A rising value necessitates reassessment of catheter position and degree of hydronephrosis.
        - Surgical drainage may be warranted.
- Valve ablation
  - Once the patient is stable medically, valve ablation (incision, resection, vaporization, disruption) is the primary treatment choice.
  - Endoscopic techniques allow treatment to be performed safely in the 8.0- to 9.5-Fr urethra (approximately 3 mm in diameter).
  - Smaller urethrae can be manipulated with excellent success in trained hands.
- Vesicostomy
  - This procedure is a safe approach to the infant with a small urethra, prior

vesicoamniotic shunt, urinary ascites, or need for other neonatal surgery.
  - Neonates with increasing creatinine levels, progressive hydronephrosis, and poor voiding dynamics, may benefit from vesicostomy even after successful primary valve ablation.
- There is a potential benefit of bladder cycling (i.e., repeated filling and emptying) to maximize bladder function in PUV.
  - These pathophysiologic benefits are still anecdotal.
  - Bladders after vesicostomy still cycle to some degree.

ACUTE GENERAL Rx

- Antibiotics
  - Initially sterile catheters are unlikely to remain sterile after 48 hours.
  - Prophylactic antibiotics (amoxicillin, cephalexin) may not maintain sterility of the urine but may limit colony count and prevent early symptomatic UTI.
  - Periodic instillation of intravesical gentamicin (every other day to achieve minimum inhibitory concentration for *Escherichia coli*) may prevent pyelonephritis when continuous catheterization is prolonged.
  - Antibiotics are not routinely used in children with vesicostomies or in those who are receiving intermittent catheterization.
- Anticholinergics/antimuscarinics
  - Some bladders maintain such high pressures that they adversely affect either renal function or continence.
  - Anticholinergic medications such as oxybutynin, tolterodine, and imipramine may be useful adjuncts in overall care.

DISPOSITION

- Renal function
  - Children with creatinine levels of greater than 1 mg/dL at 12 months of age are likely to develop renal failure.
  - One in ten children demonstrate VURD (valves, unilateral ureteral reflux, renal dysplasia), in which one kidney appears to be sacrificed for the preservation of the contralateral renal unit. The sanctity of the opposite kidney is not absolute.
  - All children require monitoring of their renal status well into adulthood.
- Bladder function
  - Normal bladder function in PUV is rare.
  - Overall, 50% to 80% of boys have their continence delayed significantly.
  - Almost all achieve continence by their teenage years.
  - Detrusor hyperreflexia, poor bladder compliance with small capacity, and myogenic failure all occur with PUV.
    - These conditions may represent sequential stages in the development of bladder dysfunction.
    - Although manageable, bladder dysfunction is a source of considerable long-term disability in PUV.

REFERRAL

The pediatric urologist and nephrologist are critical members of the team in caring for children with PUVs.

PEARLS & CONSIDERATIONS

COMMENTS

- Urinary diversion above the bladder is rarely indicated but may be lifesaving or kidney saving in select cases.
- Transplantation in children with PUV has equal patient and graft survival rates (100% and 81%, respectively) when compared to transplant survival rates for other causes of end-stage renal disease in children.
- Increasing hydronephrosis may be seen despite good surgical results in cases of nephrogenic diabetes insipidus.

PATIENT/FAMILY EDUCATION

- The primary goals are to preserve and maximize renal function.
- PUV is treated with valve ablation, but long-term effects from this congenital lesion, particularly on renal and bladder function, are likely. Follow-up is essential.

SUGGESTED READINGS

Eckoldt F et al: Posterior urethral valves: prenatal diagnostic signs and outcome. *Urol Int* 73(4):296, 2004.

Nguyen HT, Peters CA: The long-term complications of posterior urethral valves. *Br J Urol Int* 83:23, 1999.

Society for Fetal Urology. Available at www.fetalurology.org

Society of Pediatric Urology. Available at www.spu.org

Strand WR: Initial management of complex pediatric disorders: prunebelly syndrome, posterior urethral valves. *Urol Clin North Am* 31(3):399, 2004.

Ylinen E et al: Prognostic factors of posterior urethral valves and the role of antenatal detection. *Pediatr Nephrol* 19(8):874, 2004.

AUTHORS: **ROBERT A. MEVORACH, MD, WILLIAM C. HULBERT, MD,** and **RONALD RABINOWITZ, MD**

BASIC INFORMATION

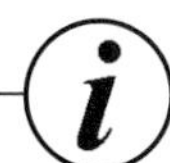

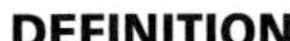

DEFINITION

Puberty is the period during and process by which sexual maturation occurs, leading to reproductive capacity. Gonadarche and adrenarche lead to the acquisition of common secondary sexual characteristics (i.e., thelarche and pubarche). *Thelarche* is the beginning of breast development, which is associated with estrogen effects. *Adrenarche* is the beginning of the maturational increase in adrenal androgen secretion that accompanies and slightly precedes puberty. *Pubarche* is the beginning of pubic hair growth, indicating androgen effects. *Gonadarche* is the beginning of gonadal hormonal activity, which is associated with marked increases in androgens in boys and estrogens in girls. The lower age limits for onset of normal pubertal development, based on small, nonrepresentative samples, have traditionally been defined for girls as 7.5 to 8.5 years old for breast development and 9.5 years for menarche and for boys as 9.0 years old. The age of onset of puberty in girls was reexamined in a large-scale, office-based study (Pediatric Research in the Office Setting [PROS]-American Academy of Pediatrics). Evaluation for precocious puberty (as advised by a statement from Lawson Wilkins Pediatric Endocrine Society) based on the review of the PROS data is now recommended for white girls with breasts or pubic hair before age 7 years, for African American girls with breasts or pubic hair before age 6 years, or for girls with early puberty and rapid pubertal progression (including rapidly advancing bone age), central nervous system (CNS) abnormalities, or behavioral issues associated with the early puberty.

ICD-9-CM CODE

259.1 Precocious sexual development and puberty (includes adrenarche and thelarche)

EPIDEMIOLOGY & DEMOGRAPHICS

- Premature puberty occurs in approximately 4% to 5% of girls using the recommendations from the PROS study.
- Premature pubarche is more common in girls with increased insulin resistance, including those who are obese, have a family history of type II diabetes, and are minorities.
- The rate of premature thelarche is 21 cases per 100,000 patient-years. Sixty percent of cases occur in children between 6 and 18 months old.

CLINICAL PRESENTATION

History

- In cases of true central precocious puberty in girls and boys, the history is compatible with normal, albeit early, puberty.
  - Estrogen effects (girls): unilateral or bilateral breast development, vaginal leukorrhea, growth acceleration, and ultimately menstruation
  - Low-level androgen effects (girls and early puberty in boys): increased body odor, axillary hair, pubic hair, skin oiliness, and mild acne
  - Higher-level androgen effects (boys with middle or late puberty): change in voice, growth acceleration, and facial hair
- Perform a careful review of systems for complaints referable to CNS masses.
- Differentiate premature pubarche or adrenarche from precocious puberty.
  - Increased body odor, pubic hair, and axillary hair in premature pubarche
  - However, no estrogen effects such as breast development, vaginal secretions, or menarche
- Premature thelarche is characterized by the following:
  - Unilateral or bilateral breast development without evidence of other signs of puberty
  - Usually regresses over time
  - Typically occurs in the first 2 years of life

Physical Examination

- True puberty: girls
  - Increased growth velocity occurs early in puberty.
  - Other changes include pubic hair growth, axillary hair, change in color of vaginal mucosa from red to pink, vaginal leukorrhea, and menarche.
  - Café au lait spots are seen in McCune-Albright syndrome (i.e., autonomous ovarian function).
- True puberty: boys
  - Early changes include testicular enlargement (>2.2 cm long), pubic hair, axillary hair, and skin oiliness.
  - Mid-pubertal and later changes include maximum growth acceleration, voice change, penile growth, increase in muscle bulk, and facial hair growth.

ETIOLOGY

- Varies as function of age and gender
- True precocious puberty of central (hypothalamic-pituitary) origin
  - Girls
    - About 95% idiopathic, presumably premature activation of the usual mechanism
    - Other causes: CNS damage from trauma, irradiation, or infection; hypothalamic hamartoma; rarely pineal tumor; hypothalamic mass; optic glioma (often associated with neurofibromatosis type 1 [NF-1])
  - Boys
    - Less likely than girls to be idiopathic
    - Hypothalamic hamartoma most common abnormal finding
    - Other CNS causes: germinomas, astrocytomas, optic nerve gliomas, septo-optic dysplasia, NF-1
- Precocious puberty associated with independent (autonomous) gonadal function
  - Girls
    - Simple ovarian cyst: transient estrogen secretion
    - McCune-Albright syndrome (multiple ovarian cysts) caused by G protein mutation, which results in café au lait spots, polyostotic fibrous dysplasia, and autonomous ovarian estrogen secretion
  - Boys
    - Familial male precocious puberty caused by activating mutation of luteinizing hormone (LH) receptor gene and resulting in increased testosterone levels but only minimal testicular enlargement
- Premature pubarche: androgen effects only (e.g., pubic and axillary hair, adult body odor, acne, skin oiliness) without estrogen effects or other signs of true puberty
  - Girls
    - Premature adrenarche: Mechanism controlling adrenarche is not clear. It is more common in overweight, African American, and Latino girls. Girls who are more severely affected (i.e., have higher androgen levels) often have hyperinsulinism as a result of insulin resistance, which is believed to stimulate adrenal androgen production.
    - Nonclassic congenital adrenal hyperplasia (CAH) is mild enough not to have congenital genital abnormalities.
    - Masculinizing tumors may be the source of hormones.
  - Boys: androgen effects without testicular enlargement (as found in true puberty)
    - CAH results in adrenal production of androgens with subsequent signs of virilization, including growth acceleration, bone age advancement, and pubic hair growth.
- Premature thelarche appears to be caused by subtle overfunctioning of the pituitary-ovarian axis, with mild increases in levels of follicle-stimulating hormone (FSH).

DIAGNOSIS

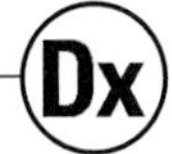

DIFFERENTIAL DIAGNOSIS

It is important to distinguish thelarche, pubarche, autonomous gonadal function, and true (central) puberty because the causes, evaluations, and therapies differ.

LABORATORY TESTS

- Gonadotropins (LH and FSH)
  - Random gonadotropin levels, when measured by standard assays, are often within normal prepubertal range in early puberty.

- Levels of gonadotropins are low in cases of autonomous gonadal function.
- However, random LH levels by ultrasensitive (third-generation) assays above 0.3 IU/L are very highly correlated with active central puberty and with positive gonadotropin-releasing hormone (GnRH) stimulation tests.
- The GnRH stimulation test is helpful in differentiating central precocious puberty from autonomous gonadal function.
  - Rise in LH over FSH after GnRH administration indicates central (hypothalamic-pituitary) activation.
- Estrogen and testosterone
  - These hormone levels are measurably elevated in true puberty.
  - Early-morning levels are typically higher than late-afternoon concentrations and are therefore a more sensitive indicator.
- 17-Hydroxyprogesterone (OHP) and androstenedione levels are often elevated in nonclassic CAH and should be measured in boys with isolated pubarche and in girls and boys with pubarche and advanced bone ages.
- The concentration of dehydroepiandrosterone (DHEA) often is mildly elevated in typical premature pubarche because of premature adrenarche.

IMAGING STUDIES

- It is appropriate to obtain the bone age in all disorders of early puberty and their variations.
  - In true puberty, bone age is advanced significantly beyond chronologic age.
  - In premature adrenarche and premature thelarche, the bone age is not abnormally advanced, although girls with premature adrenarche associated with obesity often have a moderately accelerated bone age.
- Results of magnetic resonance imaging of head with a hypothalamic-pituitary protocol are normal in most pubertal disorders, except those associated with structural abnormalities, such as hamartomas, germinomas, astrocytomas, optic nerve gliomas, or septo-optic dysplasia.
  - This test is not necessary in simple premature adrenarche or in most cases of mildly advanced pubertal development in girls.
- Ultrasound of ovaries and uterus can be helpful in determining whether the pubertal process is active, as indicated by an enlarged uterus and endometrial stripe. It is useful in visualizing solitary ovarian cysts or multiple cysts, as in McCune-Albright syndrome.

TREATMENT

NONPHARMACOLOGIC THERAPY

- Psychologic counseling should be considered for selected children.
- Surgery is useful when a discrete tumor results in precocity, such as a gonadal tumor or some intracranial tumors. Hypothalamic hamartomas usually are not removed.
- Weight control is helpful in overweight children presenting with premature adrenarche.

CHRONIC Rx

- For true central precocious puberty, administration of long-acting GnRH agonists (e.g., long-acting leuprolide acetate [Lupron-Depot]) results in suppression of pituitary gonadotropin secretion.
- For autonomous ovarian function, aromatase inhibitors such as ketoconazole and testolactone have been used, but they are not uniformly or totally effective.
- CAH is treated with hydrocortisone replacement (see Congenital Adrenal Hyperplasia in Diseases and Disorders [Section I]).

DISPOSITION

- The frequency of follow-up depends on the condition and specific circumstances, but in general, careful monitoring of pubertal status every 3 to 6 months is appropriate.
- Re-evaluation of bone age is typically done once yearly unless rapid progression occurs.

REFERRAL

- The decision to consult a pediatric endocrinologist is based on many considerations, including the experience of primary care physician, the age of the child, and the presence of other medical conditions.
- In general, very young children with evidence of true puberty, boys with precocious puberty, children with known or suspected CNS abnormalities, and children with significantly advanced bone ages should be referred.

PEARLS & CONSIDERATIONS

COMMENTS

- A bone age is good to obtain in any situation when there is doubt about whether significant premature development has occurred.
- Obese girls with a small amount of pubic hair, adult body odor, and borderline advanced bone ages rarely have significant, treatable pathology. These girls are often initially thought to have true precocious puberty because, in addition to the aforementioned findings, increased subcutaneous adiposity is often confused with true breast tissue.
- Boys presenting with pubic hair at ages 3 to 8 years may have non–salt-losing CAH and should be evaluated by tests of bone age, serum 17-OHP concentration, and androstenedione level.
- Ages that define precocious puberty are not universally agreed on (Midyett et al, 2003).

PATIENT/FAMILY EDUCATION

- Many cases of premature development wax and wane over time, and the clinical status can unexpectedly change between routine visits.
- Parents should be instructed to notify the physician whenever they notice any significant change in pubertal development in the child who is being monitored.

SUGGESTED READINGS

Herman-Giddens ME et al: Navigating the recent articles on girls' puberty in pediatrics: what do we know and where do we go from here? *Pediatrics* 113:911, 2004.

Kaplowitz P: Clinical characteristics of 104 children referred for evaluation of precocious puberty. *J Clin Endocrinol Metab* 89:3644, 2004.

Kaplowitz P: Precocious puberty: update on secular trends, definitions, diagnosis, and treatment. *Adv Pediatr* 51:37, 2004.

Midyett LK et al: Are pubertal changes in girls before age 8 benign? *Pediatrics* 111:47, 2003.

Root AW: Precocious puberty. *Pediatr Rev* 21:10, 2000.

Wang Y: Is obesity associated with early sexual maturation? A comparison of the association in American boys versus girls. *Pediatrics* 110:903, 2002.

AUTHOR: **CRAIG ORLOWSKI, MD**

BASIC INFORMATION

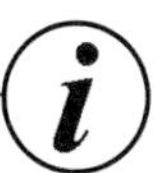

DEFINITION

Premenstrual syndrome (PMS) is a constellation of physical and psychological symptoms that start during the luteal phase of the menstrual cycle or 1 to 2 weeks before the onset of menses. The symptoms usually abate at the onset of menses. Once symptoms of PMS become severe, patients are diagnosed with premenstrual dysphoric disorder (PMDD).

SYNONYMS

PMS
Premenstrual dysphoria
Premenstrual tension

ICD-9-CM CODE

625.4 Premenstrual tension syndromes

EPIDEMIOLOGY & DEMOGRAPHICS

- The prevalence of PMS in adult women ranges from 20% to 40%, with 5% to 10% of women demonstrating severe symptoms.
- The prevalence among adolescents is unknown.

CLINICAL PRESENTATION

History

- Adolescents experience the same symptoms as adult women.
- More than 150 symptoms are described in the literature.
- When obtaining a patient's history, one should include questions about the following physical and psychological symptoms:
  - Physical symptoms
    - Bloating, weight gain
    - Breast soreness
    - Headaches
    - Edema: breasts
    - Abdomen
    - Legs
    - Increased appetite
    - Food cravings
    - Increased acne
    - Constipation
    - Dizziness
    - Fatigue
    - Muscle aches and pain
    - Palpitations
  - Psychological symptoms
    - Irritability
    - Depression
    - Anxiety
    - Mood swings
    - Anger

Physical Examination

- No specific physical findings

ETIOLOGY

- The cause is unknown.
- There are several theories:
  - Change in endocrine homeostasis: progesterone deficiency, hyperprolactinemia, estrogen excess, imbalance of estrogen: progesterone ratio
  - Vitamin B_{12} deficiency
  - Change in glucose metabolism: hypoglycemia
  - Change in neurotransmitters: endorphins, serotonin

DIAGNOSIS

DIFFERENTIAL DIAGNOSIS

- Dysmenorrhea
- Depression and anxiety disorders
- Menstrual-associated migraine
- Cyclic mastalgia

WORKUP

- Diagnosis of exclusion: no other physical or psychological factors are involved.
- This is purely a clinical diagnosis remarkable for history of cyclical onset.
- Symptoms occur over several menstrual cycles.
- Assessment tools include the following:
  - PMS symptom calendar
  - Self-assessment disk
  - Premenstrual Assessment Form (PAF)
  - Prospective Record of the Impact and Severity of Menstrual Symptoms (PRISM)

TREATMENT

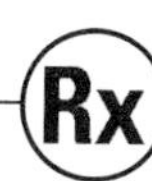

NONPHARMACOLOGIC THERAPY

- Most adolescents do not have symptoms severe enough to warrant medication.
- Dietary changes: avoid salty foods, alcohol, caffeine, chocolate, and concentrated sweets.
  - Increase calcium intake.
- Exercise regularly.
- Maintain a routine sleep schedule.
- Stress management techniques include the following:
  - Biofeedback
  - Self-hypnosis
  - Relaxation

CHRONIC Rx

- Consider the severity of symptoms.
- No consistent benefits with any of the pharmacologic therapies have been proven (only anecdotal).
- Hormonal therapy to inhibit ovulation
  - Combination oral contraceptives
  - Depomedroxyprogesterone acetate (Depo-Provera) 150 mg intramuscularly
- Nonsteroidal anti-inflammatory drugs, especially if the patient also has dysmenorrhea
  - Naproxen 500 mg orally twice per day on days 17 to 28 of menstrual cycle
  - Naproxen sodium 550 mg orally twice per day on days 17 to 28 of menstrual cycle
  - Mefenamic acid 250 mg orally three times per day on days 24 to 28 for bloating, 500 mg orally three times per day on days 19 to 28 for pain
- Vitamin B_6 150 mg orally every day throughout cycle
  - Rare side effect: sensory neuropathy in doses as low as 50 to 200 mg every day over several months
- Consider: benzodiazepine, serotonin reuptake inhibitor, β-blocker, or calcium channel blocker if the adolescent continues with psychological symptoms not relieved by other modalities.
  - Alprazolam 0.25 mg orally two to three times per day for approximately 1 week before menses
  - Prozac 20 to 60 mg orally every day

COMPLEMENTARY & ALTERNATIVE MEDICINE

- Evening primrose oil (γ-linolenic acid) 1.5 g orally two times per day on day 15 to onset of menses
- Chaste berry fruit (Vitex agnus castus) 20 mg daily for mild-to-moderate PMS

DISPOSITION

- No specific follow-up guidelines are available for PMS.
- For adolescents who require oral contraceptives, see the adolescent at 1 month, again at 3 months, and then every 6 months.
- The adolescent should maintain a premenstrual changes calendar.

REFERRAL

Significant mood changes warrant psychological or psychiatric consultation.

PEARLS & CONSIDERATIONS

COMMENTS

- Older adolescents tend to have more intense symptoms than younger adolescents.
- Dysmenorrhea and PMS symptoms are strongly correlated in adolescents.

PATIENT/FAMILY EDUCATION

- Explain the menstrual cycle, possible causes of PMS, and the cyclic nature of PMS.
- Give reassurance.

SUGGESTED READINGS

Braverman PK, Neinstein L: Dysmenorrhea and premenstrual syndrome. *In* Neinstein LS (ed): *Adolescent Health Care: A Practical Guide.* Philadelphia, Williams & Wilkins, 2002, pp 952–965.

Johnson S: Premenstrual syndrome, premenstrual dysphoric disorder, and beyond: a clinical primer for practitioners. *Obstet Gynecol* 104(4):845, 2004.

Kaplan DW, Mammel KA: Adolescence. *In* Hay W et al (eds): *Current Pediatric Diagnosis and Treatment.* New York, Appleton & Lange, 2001.

McEvoy M et al: Common menstrual disorders in adolescence: nursing interventions. *Am J Maternl Child Nurs* 29(1):41, 2004.

AUTHOR: **CAROLYN JACOBS PARKS, MD**

BASIC INFORMATION

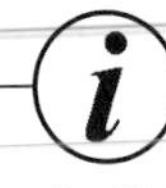

DEFINITION

Prolonged QT syndrome (LQTS) is a familial but clinically and genetically heterogeneous ion channel cardiac disorder leading to syncope, "seizures," and sudden death as a consequence of polymorphic ventricular tachyarrhythmias.

SYNONYMS

Jervell-Lange-Nielsen (J-L-N) syndrome (homozygotic mutations)
Long QT syndrome
Romano-Ward (R-W) syndrome (heterozygotic mutations)

ICD-9-CM CODE
794.31 Abnormal electrocardiogram

EPIDEMIOLOGY & DEMOGRAPHICS

- Incidence is 1 in 10,000 individuals.
- No gender preference exists.
- Inheritance pattern is familial in 80%.
  - Autosomal dominant in R-W syndrome.
  - Autosomal recessive in J-L-N syndrome.
- New mutations occur in 20% of cases.
- Mortality is 5% to 10% per year after onset of symptoms in untreated patients.
- A nearly 10% risk of sudden death as the initial symptom has been reported.

CLINICAL PRESENTATION

History

- Syncope, commonly during physical or emotional stress
- "Seizures" with abrupt onset and paucity of post-event confusion
- Cardiac arrest also related to exercise or emotion
- Sudden death in the same circumstances
- Congenital deafness in most but not all J-L-N patients
- Family history (variable penetrance; QTc may be normal)

Physical Examination

- Often normal
- Bradycardia
- Deafness in J-L-N patients

ETIOLOGY

- LQT_1: gene mutation on chromosome 11 ($KvLQT_1$)
- LQT_2: gene mutation on chromosome 7 (HERG)
  - Gene mutations in LQT_1 and LQT_2 reduce the outward, repolarizing potassium channel function, causing prolongation of the action potential and, consequently, the QT interval.
- LQT_3: gene mutation on chromosome 3 (SCNSA)
  - LQT_3 is caused by persistent or repetitive patency of the inward sodium channel during the plateau phase of the action potential, thereby prolonging the QT interval.
- Newly identified LQT_4, LQT_5, LQT_6, and LQT_7 are caused by potassium channelopathies.

DIAGNOSIS

Dx

DIFFERENTIAL DIAGNOSIS

- Drug-induced QT prolongation (intravenous erythromycin, cisapride, imipramine, pentamidine)
- Mild QTc prolongation related to myocardial ischemia or injury
- Acute central nervous system events
- Cardiomyopathies
- Hypokalemia
- Hypocalcemia
- Hypomagnesemia

LABORATORY TESTS

- QTc: QT corrected for heart rate
  - Bazett's formula:

$$QTc = \frac{QT\ (sec)}{\sqrt{\text{Preceding R–R interval (sec)}}}$$

    - A corrected QT interval more than 460 msec is abnormal.
    - Borderline QTc is 440 to 460 msec.
- Electrocardiogram (ECG) on first-degree relatives; consider other family members as well
- Serum potassium, calcium, magnesium
- Genetic screening for gene mutations (helpful if positive)
- Appearance of T waves may identify type: LQT_1, LQT_2, or LQT_3
- T-wave alternans: appearance of T-wave alternates in a bigeminal pattern
- Polymorphic ventricular tachycardia (PVT): torsades de pointes
- In general, the longer the QTc, the greater the risk of PVT

TREATMENT

Rx

NONPHARMACOLOGIC THERAPY

- Avoidance of competitive sports
- Pacing for native or β-blocker-induced bradycardia
- Left stellate ganglionectomy if medications or pacing insufficient
- Implantable cardioverter-defibrillator if previous therapies insufficient or if syncope or aborted sudden death occurs
- Cardiac transplantation (rarely done)

CHRONIC Rx

- β-blockers (propranolol, nadolol, atenolol)
- Future use of mexiletine for LQT_3
- Avoidance of drugs capable of prolonging the QTc and sympathomimetics
- Avoidance of, and rapid correction of, electrolyte abnormalities

DISPOSITION

All LQTS patients require lifelong cardiac follow-up and therapy.

REFERRAL

All patients with documented or suspected LQTS should be referred to a pediatric cardiologist with expertise in arrhythmias.

PEARLS & CONSIDERATIONS

COMMENTS

- All patients with syncope, atypical "seizures," unexplained life-threatening events, or a family history of premature sudden death should have screening ECGs.
- At present, sufficient evidence to incriminate QTc prolongation as a common etiology of the sudden infant death syndrome (SIDS) is not available, but a few instances of SIDS have been attributed to LQT_2.

PATIENT/FAMILY EDUCATION

- Obtain a list of contraindicated medications from the cardiologist.
- Compliance with therapeutic regimens is essential.
- With appropriate therapy, mortality should be 3% or less per year.
- Future advancements in gene-directed therapy (e.g., potassium channel openers in LQT_1 or LQT_2) should further reduce the risk of symptoms including sudden death.
- Sudden Arrhythmia Death Syndromes Foundation (SADS). Available at www.sads.org

SUGGESTED READINGS

Ackerman MJ: The long QT syndrome. *Pediatr Rev* 79:232, 1998.

Moss AJ et al: ECG T-wave patterns in genetically distinct forms of the hereditary long QT syndrome. *Circulation* 95:2929, 1995.

Schwartz PJ: The long QT syndrome. *In* Camm A (ed): *Clinical Approach to Tachyarrhythmia Series.* Armonk, NY, Futura, 1997.

Zareba W et al: Influence of the genotype on the clinical course of the long-QT syndrome. *N Engl J Med* 339:960, 1998.

AUTHOR: **J. PETER HARRIS, MD**

BASIC INFORMATION

DEFINITION

Pseudotumor cerebri is a diagnosis of exclusion and is defined as headaches with increased intracranial pressure and papilledema in the absence of intracranial mass, hydrocephalus, or abnormal cerebral spinal fluid composition.

SYNONYMS

Benign intracranial hypertension
Idiopathic intracranial hypertension
Meningitis serosa

ICD-9-CM CODE
348.2 Pseudotumor cerebri

EPIDEMIOLOGY & DEMOGRAPHICS

- More prevalent in women with a 2:1 ratio
- General population 1 case per 100,000
- Increased prevalence with obesity to 19.3 cases per 100,000 in women 20 to 44 years of age who are more than 20% above ideal body weight
- Isolated familial cases
- No racial predilection
- Some association with vitamin A overuse and tetracycline use

CLINICAL PRESENTATION

History

- Headaches, either intermittent or permanent. Usually worse in the morning and with recumbent position.
- Unilateral or bilateral blurred vision varying from slight to complete loss of light perception.
- Worse pain with coughing and straining
- Pulsatile tinnitus
- Neck and shoulder pain
- Obesity

Physical Examination

- Papilledema
- Normal neurologic exam
- Visual field defects or decreased visual acuity

ETIOLOGY

Etiology is unknown but possible mechanisms include increased cerebrospinal fluid (CSF) production, decreased CSF absorption, and increased venous sinus pressure.

DIAGNOSIS

DIFFERENTIAL DIAGNOSIS

- Intracranial mass (tumor, bleed)
- Hypothyroidism
- Uremia
- Sleep apnea
- Venous sinus occlusion
- Systemic lupus erythematosus
- Infection
  - Meningitis
  - Encephalitis
- Hydrocephalus

LABORATORY TESTS

- Lumbar puncture
  - Opening pressure greater than 250 mm Hg
  - Normal cytology
  - Slightly reduced protein, otherwise normal chemistries

IMAGING STUDIES

- Computed tomography (CT)
- Magnetic resonance imaging (MRI)
  - Often revealing an empty sella indicating that CSF pressures have been chronically elevated

TREATMENT

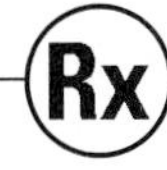

NONPHARMACOLOGIC THERAPY

- Weight loss for obese patients
  - This may include weight reduction surgery for morbidly obese patients. The health benefits from such a drastic measure are far more reaching than just to reduce headaches.

ACUTE GENERAL Rx

- Steroids have been shown to relieve headaches in the short term. Long-term steroids, however, should not be used. Headaches usually resume after steroids are withdrawn.
  - In the case of rapidly progressive visual loss, high-dose intravenous corticosteroids may need to be initiated.
- Nonsteroidal anti-inflammatory drugs (NSAIDs) and other over-the-counter analgesics have not been shown to help.

CHRONIC Rx

Medications

- Carbonic anhydrase inhibitors
  - Acetazolamide—decreases CSF production
  - Taking 500 to 2000 mg/day divided twice daily has been shown to reduce CSF production and exert sufficient decrease in intracranial pressure.
  - Avoid use during pregnancy.
- Diuretics
  - Other classes of diuretic have been tried with varying success.

Lumbar Puncture

- The removal of CSF may relieve headaches for several days to weeks but headaches usually return. Lumbar punctures may need to be repeated but this is usually not a recommended treatment.

Shunt

- Intractable headaches that have not responded to previously mentioned therapies may respond to shunt procedures. These are either ventriculoperitoneal or lumboperitoneal shunts.

Optic Nerve Fenestration

- Creation of a slit in the optic nerve sheath to allow for decompression of this nerve and reversal of papilledema

DISPOSITION

- Often this condition is self-limiting and may spontaneously resolve.
- Fundus photographs may be helpful in follow-up exams.
- Frequent visual acuity testing should be performed.

REFERRAL

Patients should be seen by a neurologist. If possible the neurologist should be one with a special interest in pseudotumor cerebri.

PEARLS & CONSIDERATIONS

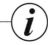

PREVENTION

Weight control may be the only way to attempt to avoid pseudotumor cerebri. Remember there is still an incidence in nonobese patients.

PATIENT/FAMILY EDUCATION

- Intracranial Hypertension Research Foundation, 6517 Buena Vista Drive, Vancouver, WA 98661; email: info@ihrfoundation.org; web site: http://www.IHRFoundation.org; tel: 360-693-4473; fax: 360-694-7062.
- National Organization for Rare Disorders (NORD), P.O. Box 1968 (55 Kenosia Avenue), Danbury, CT 06813-1968; email: orphan@rarediseases.org; web site: http://www.rarediseases.org; tel: 203-744-0100; voice mail 800-999-NORD (6673); fax: 203-798-2291.
- Pseudotumor Cerebri Support Network, 8247 Riverside Drive, Powell, OH 43065; email: ptcduncan@juno.com; web site: http://www.pseudotumorcerebri.com

SUGGESTED READINGS

Binder DK et al: Idiopathic intracranial hypertension. *Neurosurgery* 54:538, 2004.

Idiopathic intracranial hypertension. *In* Goetz: *Textbook of Clinical Neurology,* 2nd ed. New York, Elsevier Publishing, 2003.

Intracranial Hypertension Research Foundation. Available at www.IHRFoundation.org

Mathews MK et al: Pseudotumor cerebri. *Curr Opin Ophthalmol* 14:364, 2003.

AUTHOR: **DAVID CYWINSKI, MD**

BASIC INFORMATION

DEFINITION

Psittacosis is a systemic infection with *Chlamydia* (*Chlamydophila*) *psittaci,* named for psittacine birds. These birds were the organism's earliest identified natural hosts.

SYNONYMS

Bird breeder's disease
Bird fancier's lung
Chlamydiosis
Ornithosis
Parrot fever
Pneumotyphus

ICD-9-CM CODE
073.9 Psittacosis

EPIDEMIOLOGY & DEMOGRAPHICS

- Infection is rare in children.
- Incubation period 5 to 15 days.
- Occurs throughout the world, generally sporadically but outbreaks are seen.
- Transmission occurs from infected birds to humans via the respiratory route by direct contact or inhalation of infectious organisms in aerosolized dust or secretions.
- Birds most commonly infected: parrots, parakeets, finches, turkeys, gulls, pigeons, ducks, and chickens. Most infected birds display minimal symptoms; some may be more severely affected, displaying ruffled feathers, closed eyes, shivering, anorexia, emaciation, dyspnea, serous or mucopurulent ocular or nasal discharge, and diarrhea.
- Infected birds may shed organisms for weeks to months.
- Individuals at greatest risk include pet bird owners, pigeon handlers, pet shop employees, poultry farmers, veterinarians, and poultry abattoir workers.

CLINICAL PRESENTATION

History

- History of bird exposure, which may be brief (up to 25% report no exposure)
- Insidious or abrupt onset of fever, malaise
- Mononucleosis-like syndrome (fever, chills, malaise, pharyngitis, photophobia, myalgia)
- Atypical pneumonia with nonproductive cough, dyspnea, fever, and headache
- Other symptoms may include tinnitus, ataxia, anorexia, nausea, vomiting, abdominal pain, diarrhea, constipation, arthralgias, and rash.

Physical Examination

- Fever, pharyngeal erythema, adenopathy, rales on chest auscultation, and hepatomegaly in more than 50% of patients
- Splenomegaly and bradycardia with typhoidal form
- Less commonly: tachycardia (pericarditis, myocarditis, culture-negative endocarditis) or new murmur; right upper quadrant tenderness and jaundice (hepatitis); cranial nerve palsy, ataxia, neck stiffness (meningitis); diminished/absent reflexes, decreased strength/sensory level (transverse myelitis); joint pain and swelling (reactive arthritis); horder's spots (pink, maculopapular rash resembling rose spots of typhoid fever)

ETIOLOGY

Systemic infection caused by *C. psittaci.*

DIAGNOSIS

DIFFERENTIAL DIAGNOSIS

Viral pneumonia; atypical pneumonia with *Mycoplasma pneumoniae, Chlamydia* (*Chlamydophila*) *pneumoniae,* or *Legionella pneumophila*; infectious mononucleosis; influenza; typhoid fever; Q fever; brucellosis; tularemia; subacute bacterial endocarditis; mycobacterial or fungal pneumonia

LABORATORY TESTS

- Organism may be isolated in cell culture from blood early in infection and from sputum in first 2 weeks of illness. However, isolation is dangerous and thus rarely done.
- Diagnosis is generally confirmed by demonstration of antibodies in patient serum by complement fixation (CF) or by microimmunofluorescence (MIF).
- High CF titers also may result from infection with *C. pneumoniae* and *C. trachomatis;* polymerase chain reaction assay and MIF can distinguish between species.
- Nonspecific laboratory findings include mildly elevated white blood cell count with left shift, eosinophilia, and mildly abnormal transaminases.
- Confirmed case:
  - Clinical illness compatible with psittacosis, ***plus*** Laboratory confirmed by one of the following methods:
  - *C. psittaci* is cultured from respiratory secretions.
  - Antibody against *C. psittaci* is increased fourfold or greater to a reciprocal titer of 32 between paired (i.e., acute- and convalescent-phase) serum samples obtained at least 2 weeks apart, as demonstrated by CF or MIF.
  - Immunoglobulin M antibody against *C. psittaci* is detected by MIF to a reciprocal titer of 16.
- Probable case:
  - Compatible clinical illness, *or*
  - Clinical illness epidemiologically linked to a confirmed case of psittacosis, *or*
  - Single antibody titer of 1:32 (demonstrated by CF or MIF) found in at least one serum sample obtained after onset of symptoms.

IMAGING STUDIES

Chest radiograph (CXR) is abnormal in 75% of patients, with findings striking in comparison to degree of illness; consolidation is seen in single lower lobe in 90% of abnormal CXR. Diffuse miliary or ground-glass appearance and hilar adenopathy are also reported. CXR abnormalities may take weeks to resolve.

TREATMENT

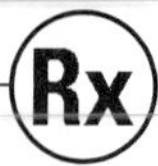

NONPHARMACOLOGIC THERAPY

- Valve replacement for endocarditis

ACUTE GENERAL Rx

- Drug of choice is tetracycline hydrochloride 500 mg orally four times per day or doxycycline 100 mg orally twice a day.
- Alternative therapeutic agents are erythromycin, azithromycin, clarithromycin, and chloramphenicol.
- Due to high probability of relapse after shorter courses of therapy, usual recommended duration is 10 to 21 days, or until patient is afebrile for 10 to 14 days.
- Prolonged antibiotic therapy is indicated for endocarditis.

DISPOSITION

- Symptoms should begin to abate within 24 to 72 hours of initiation of therapy.
- Infection does not confer long-term immunity; reinfection is a possibility.

REFERRAL

- Patients suspected of having psittacosis should be referred to an ID specialist.
- Consultation with veterinarian or state health department may be helpful.
- Contact health department, since psittacosis is a reportable disease in most states.

PEARLS & CONSIDERATIONS

COMMENTS

- Splenomegaly in a patient with acute pneumonitis should raise the diagnostic consideration of psittacosis.
- Person-to-person transmission of psittacosis is uncommon, but can be severe.

PREVENTION

Treat infected birds with tetracycline, chlortetracycline, or doxycycline for ≤45 consecutive days

PATIENT/FAMILY EDUCATION

Pet birds should be purchased from a reputable dealer complying with U.S. Department of Agriculture 30-day quarantine and chlortetracycline treatment regulations.

SUGGESTED READINGS

American Veterinary Medicine Association Compendium of Measures to Control *Chlamydophila psittaci* (formerly *Chlamydia psittaci*) Infection among Humans (Psittacosis) and Pet Birds. Available at www.avma.org/pubhlth/psittacosis.asp

Schlossberg D: *Chlamydophila* (*Chlamydia*) *psittaci* (psittacosis). *In* Mandel GL et al (eds): *Mandell, Douglas, and Bennett's Principles and Practices of Infectious Diseases,* 6th ed. Philadelphia, Elsevier, 2005, pp 2256–2258.

AUTHOR: **LORNA M. SEYBOLT, MD, MPH**

BASIC INFORMATION

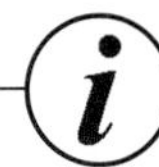

DEFINITION

Psoriasis vulgaris is a chronic skin disorder with a waxing and waning course. Abnormally rapid turnover of the epidermis results in the accumulation of thick scale over sites of frequent trauma and irritation.

Guttate psoriasis is generally subacute inflammation following streptococcal infection.

SYNONYMS

Guttate psoriasis
Psoriasis vulgaris

ICD-9-CM CODE
696.1 Psoriasis vulgaris

EPIDEMIOLOGY & DEMOGRAPHICS

- Approximately 0.5% to 1.5% of the U.S. population is affected.
- The female-to-male ratio in children is 2:1; in adults the ratio is 1:1.
- Psoriasis vulgaris is more common in whites and less common in blacks, Japanese, and North/South American Indians.
- Most cases present during the fall and winter months.

CLINICAL PRESENTATION

- Guttate psoriasis occurs most often in children and young adults.
  - The term is derived from the Latin for *gutta* (a drop), which describes the type of lesions seen.
  - Lesions appear abruptly, often 1 to 2 weeks after a streptococcal infection.
  - Guttate lesions are small (2 to 10 mm), round or oval, erythematous plaques with silvery scale.
  - Guttate lesions are symmetrically distributed over the trunk and proximal extremities.
  - Plaques may be pruritic, painful, or asymptomatic.
  - Streptococcal pharyngitis and streptococcal perianal infections have both been implicated.
  - Guttate psoriasis usually persists for 3 to 4 months and then resolves spontaneously.
- Plaque psoriasis
  - Lesions are sharply demarcated, round, erythematous plaques with silvery scale.
  - Plaque size is highly variable (millimeters to centimeters), but individual lesions are bigger than those seen in guttate psoriasis.
  - Lesions are often symmetrically distributed.
  - Common sites of involvement include the scalp, eyebrows, elbows, knees, umbilicus, genitalia, and gluteal cleft.
  - May be induced in areas of local injury, such as scratches or insect bites (Koebner phenomenon).
  - Nail findings include pitting, oil spots (yellowish brown discolorations), onycholysis (separation of nail plate from nailbed), subungual distal hyperkeratosis (debris), and nail dystrophy (crumbling).

ETIOLOGY

- The exact pathogenesis and relative importance of genetic and environmental factors are still unknown.
- Family studies, epidemiologic studies, and human leukocyte antigen (HLA) studies suggest that psoriasis is genetically determined.
  - The prevalence of psoriasis is higher among first- and second-degree relatives of patients with psoriasis than in the general population.
  - There is an increased frequency of some HLA haplotypes (HLACw6, B13, B17) in patients with psoriasis.
  - Twin studies show higher concordance rates among monozygotic than dizygotic twin pairs.
    - Concordance rates among monozygotic twins are at most 70%, suggesting a role for environmental factors.
- A variety of local and systemic stimuli have been reported to trigger the onset of psoriasis.
  - Medications such as nonsteroidal antiinflammatory drugs, antimalarials, and systemic corticosteroids
  - Pregnancy and use of progesterone-containing oral contraceptive pills
  - Streptococcal infections (especially with guttate psoriasis)

DIAGNOSIS

DIFFERENTIAL DIAGNOSIS

- Plaque psoriasis
  - Seborrheic dermatitis
  - Atopic dermatitis
  - Lichen planus
  - Pityriasis rubra pilaris
- Guttate psoriasis
  - Pityriasis rosea
  - Secondary syphilis

WORKUP

- The diagnosis is usually made on the basis of the characteristic clinical picture.
- Biopsy is rarely needed and should be avoided in children.
- Specific histologic findings can be used if the diagnosis is in question.

TREATMENT

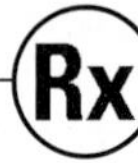

NONPHARMACOLOGIC THERAPY

- Mild soap one to two times per day (e.g., Dove, Purpose, Neutrogena, Basis)
- Thick emollients two to three times per day (e.g., petroleum jelly, Aquaphor ointment, Theraplex emollient, Eucerin cream)

ACUTE GENERAL Rx

- Topical corticosteroids should be applied twice a day to individual plaques for several weeks.
- Oral corticosteroids are contraindicated.
- Patients with severe or extensive disease should be referred to a dermatologist.
- Acute guttate forms, associated with streptococcal infection, should be treated with appropriate antibiotics. The psoriasis sometimes resolves after treatment with antibiotics.

CHRONIC Rx

Usually under care of dermatologist.

DISPOSITION

- Guttate psoriasis is usually limited.
- Psoriasis vulgaris is a lifelong chronic recurring disorder.

PEARLS & CONSIDERATIONS

COMMENTS

- Most patients with guttate psoriasis experience a recurrence of some type of psoriasis within the next 3 to 5 years.
- More than one third of patients with psoriasis experience their first episode by age 20.
- Psoriatic arthritis is rare in children.

PATIENT/FAMILY EDUCATION

See "Pearls & Considerations."

SUGGESTED READINGS

American Academy of Dermatology. Available at www.aad.org

Lewkowicz D, Gottlieb AB: Pediatric psoriasis and psoriatic arthritis. *Dermatol Ther* 17(5):364, 2004.

Marcoux D, Prost Y: Pediatric psoriasis revisited. *J Cutan Med Surg* 6(3):22, 2002.

National Psoriasis Foundation. Available at www.psoriasis.org (patient-oriented).

Sanfilippo AM et al: Common pediatric and adolescent skin conditions. *J Pediatric Adolesc Gynecol* 16(5):269, 2003.

Society for Pediatric Dermatology. Available at www.spdnet.org

AUTHOR: **SUSAN HALLER PSAILA, MD**

BASIC INFORMATION

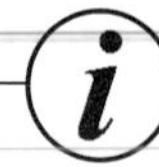

DEFINITION

Pulmonary embolism (PE) is the result of acute blockage of a pulmonary artery by a thrombus formed at another anatomic site, usually a deep vein of the leg.

SYNONYMS

PE
Pulmonary thromboembolism

ICD-9-CM CODE
415.11 Pulmonary embolism

EPIDEMIOLOGY & DEMOGRAPHICS

- The incidence is 1 per 1000 per year, more common in men.
- Risk factors include hypercoagulable state, trauma, immobilization, or intravenous catheter.
- It is rare in children without an intravenous catheter.
- More than 250,000 patients are hospitalized annually in the United States with venous thromboembolism.
- The 3-month mortality rate ranges from 10% to 15%.
- As many as 40% of patients who have deep venous thrombosis (DVT) but no symptoms of PE have small PEs on lung scanning.

CLINICAL PRESENTATION

- Typical symptoms include the *acute* onset of pleuritic chest pain, shortness of breath, cough, and hemoptysis.
- Other symptoms include fever, diaphoresis, wheezing, and syncope.
- Ask about the following risk factors:
  - Surgery within the past 12 weeks
  - Recent immobilization for 3 or more days
  - Previous DVT or PE
  - Fracture and immobilization within the past 12 weeks
  - Strong family history of DVT or PE
  - Cancer, postpartum, and lower extremity paralysis
- Classically tachycardia, tachypnea, and hypoxia
- Other signs may be loud pulmonary component of S_2, murmur of tricuspid insufficiency, right ventricular heave, or evidence of DVT (see Deep Venous Thrombosis in Diseases and Disorders [Section I])

ETIOLOGY

- A thrombus is formed at a distant site (see Deep Venous Thrombosis in Diseases and Disorders [Section I]).
- Pieces of the thrombus detach and travel through the right heart to the pulmonary vasculature.
- The resulting pulmonary arterial obstruction and the release of vasoactive agents by platelets elevate pulmonary vascular resistance.

DIAGNOSIS

DIFFERENTIAL DIAGNOSIS

- Musculoskeletal chest pain (costochondritis)
- Pleurisy
- Cardiac chest pain
- Esophageal spasm
- Pneumothorax

WORKUP

- Available tests include chest computed tomography (CT), ventilation/perfusion lung scanning, Doppler ultrasonography or venography of the legs, and the gold standard of pulmonary angiography.
- Decide whether the patient has a low, moderate, or high pretest probability of PE based on history, physical examination, and results of arterial blood gas (ABG) and electrocardiogram (ECG) as well as more likely alternative diagnoses.
- If the patient has a low pretest probability of PE, a normal chest CT scan or D-dimer blood assay effectively rules out PE.
- If the patient has a high pretest probability of PE, a high-probability lung scan confirms PE.
- If the patient has a moderate pretest probability or the results of the initial test are equivocal or not confirmatory, a series of tests, including compression ultrasonography and venography of the leg, lung scanning, and chest CT, are indicated, reserving invasive pulmonary angiography for the most difficult cases.
- ECG most commonly reveals sinus tachycardia, right ventricular strain, right bundle branch block, or the "$S_I Q_{III} T_{III}$" pattern of large S wave in lead I, and large Q and T waves in lead III.

LABORATORY TEST

ABG reveals respiratory alkalosis with hypoxia.

IMAGING STUDIES

- Chest radiograph is usually normal or shows a small pleural effusion on the affected side. Classically, it has a wedge-shaped infiltrate consistent with pulmonary infarction.
- Echocardiogram will reveal signs of right heart strain or dilation.

TREATMENT

NONPHARMACOLOGIC THERAPY

- Supplemental oxygen and stabilization of vital signs
- Inferior vena caval (Greenfield) filters should be reserved for patients with contraindications to anticoagulation or for patients with recurrent PE on anticoagulation.
  - They do prevent PE in patients with DVT.
  - They carry an increased risk for recurrent DVT after placement.

ACUTE GENERAL Rx

- The mainstay of therapy is anticoagulation with heparin. Low-molecular-weight heparin (LMWH) can be given subcutaneously (1 mg/kg twice a day) and does not need activated partial thromboplastin time monitoring. Outcomes with LMWH are equivalent to those with intravenous unfractionated heparin in PE.
- Oral anticoagulation with warfarin is begun the first day to prevent delays in hospital discharge. A target international normalized ratio (INR) of 2 to 3 is desired.
- Thrombolytic therapy should be reserved for patients with acute, massive PE because bleeding risk is estimated at close to 50%, intracranial hemorrhage is estimated at 1%, and mortality rates are equal to placebo in randomized controlled trials.

CHRONIC Rx

- Oral anticoagulation for at least 1 year is indicated.
- If an underlying irreversible hypercoagulable state is found, lifelong oral anticoagulation is indicated.

DISPOSITION

Hospitalization is indicated until all clinical data are reassuring.

REFERRAL

- If an underlying hypercoagulable state is found, hematology referral is helpful.
- In difficult cases, pulmonary referral is often helpful.

PEARLS & CONSIDERATIONS

COMMENTS

In the presence of a patent foramen ovale or atrial septal defect, paradoxic embolism may occur with signs of systemic arterial embolization, including stroke and threatened limb.

PREVENTION

Early ambulation after surgical procedures, subcutaneous heparin (both LMWH and unfractionated), and pneumatic compression stockings are the mainstays of DVT and PE prophylaxis in high-risk patients.

PATIENT/FAMILY EDUCATION

- Patients should understand that PE is a potentially fatal disease.
- Treatment with anticoagulants reduces the fatality rate to minimal levels.
- Treatment with oral warfarin necessitates intense education about the risks of bleeding (5% per year) and dietary restrictions.

SUGGESTED READING

Wells P et al: Use of a clinical model for safe management of patients with suspected pulmonary embolism. *Ann Intern Med* 129:997, 1998.

AUTHOR: **BRETT ROBBINS, MD**

BASIC INFORMATION

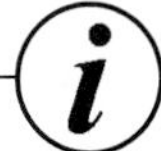

DEFINITION

Pulmonary hypertension is the abnormal elevation of pulmonary arterial pressure or pulmonary vascular resistance. Some authors specify a mean pulmonary arterial pressure greater than 25 mm Hg to define abnormal. Both primary and secondary pulmonary hypertensions occur in children and adolescents. Pulmonary hypertension secondary to longstanding pulmonary over-circulation from congenital heart disease (e.g., unrepaired ventricular septal defect) is called *Eisenmenger syndrome.*

ICD-9-CM CODES
416.0 Primary forms
416.8 Secondary forms

EPIDEMIOLOGY & DEMOGRAPHICS

- Primary (idiopathic) pulmonary hypertension, isolated or familial, is rare in children.
- Incidence in all ages is 2 per 1,000,000 in Western countries.
  - A female preponderance exists.
  - Approximately 5% to 10% of cases are familial with dominant incomplete penetrance pattern.
- One gene for familial primary pulmonary hypertension has been found on chromosome 2q 31–32.
- Mutations in this bone morphogenetic protein receptor type 2 gene (BMPR2) may cause up to 75% of familial forms of primary pulmonary hypertension.
- Reversible pulmonary hypertension secondary to a large left-to-right shunt is not uncommon in patients with congenital heart disease, but Eisenmenger syndrome has become rare since early surgical repair is standard practice.

CLINICAL PRESENTATION

History

- Fatigue and effort intolerance
- Dyspnea and shortness of breath
- Syncope and near sudden death episodes
- Look for family history of the following:
  - Pulmonary hypertension
  - Sickle cell disease
  - Thrombotic disorders

Physical Examination

- Pulmonic component of second heart sound is loud (loud P_2 or loud S_2).
- Cyanosis is usually found only in secondary forms with intracardiac shunting (Eisenmenger syndrome) or severe pulmonary disease (e.g., cystic fibrosis), but oximetry may not be normal in primary forms.
- Lung examination may not necessarily be abnormal in cases of primary pulmonary hypertension.

ETIOLOGY

- Primary forms include the following:
  - Primary or idiopathic pulmonary hypertension
  - Familial pulmonary hypertension
- Secondary forms include the following:
  - Increased pulmonary blood flow from congenital heart lesions
    - Ventricular septal defect
    - Atrioventricular septal defect
    - Patent ductus arteriosus
    - Isolated atrial septal defect can result in pulmonary hypertension, but usually only after many decades.
  - Irreversible pulmonary hypertension (with cyanosis); occurs after years of increased pulmonary blood flow; also referred to as Eisenmenger syndrome
  - Pulmonary venous obstruction
    - Obstructed anomalous pulmonary venous return
    - Pulmonary veno-occlusive disease
    - Cor triatriatum (obstructive left atrial membrane)
  - Left-sided heart failure
    - Dilated cardiomyopathy
    - Mitral valve stenosis or severe incompetence
  - Chronic pulmonary emboli or infarction
    - Collagen vascular diseases, including scleroderma, systemic lupus erythematosus, and systemic juvenile rheumatoid arthritis
    - Protein S deficiency and other thrombophilias
    - Ventriculoatrial shunts for hydrocephalus
    - Sickle cell anemia
  - Other conditions
    - Human immunodeficiency virus infection
    - Anorexic drug use
    - Cocaine abuse
    - High-altitude exposure
  - Chronic parenchymal lung disease
  - Chronic airway obstruction
  - Musculoskeletal disorders with hypoventilation
  - Pulmonary hypertension resulting from lung disease, airway obstruction, or hypoventilation often termed *cor pulmonale*
    - This indicates right ventricular hypertrophy or signs of right-sided heart failure secondary to lung or airway disease.
    - Etiologies of cor pulmonale are discussed in Cor Pulmonale in Diseases and Disorders (Section I).

DIAGNOSIS

Dx

DIFFERENTIAL DIAGNOSIS

See "Etiology."

WORKUP

- Right ventricular hypertrophy on electrocardiogram may suggest pulmonary hypertension.
- Echocardiography may be diagnostic if significant pulmonary hypertension can be demonstrated and cardiac causes of pulmonary hypertension (e.g., left-to-right shunts, pulmonary venous obstruction, left ventricular failure) are ruled out. Diagnosis is usually first established by echocardiography.
- Cardiac catheterization documents elevated pulmonary arterial pressure and excludes the secondary causes noted previously.

LABORATORY TESTS

- If family history suggests inherited disorders causing pulmonary emboli, pulmonary infarction, or venous thromboses the following test should be considered:
  - Hemoglobin electrophoresis is done to look for sickle cell disease (SS).
- Obtain protein S, protein C, and antithrombin levels. The role of other thrombophilic disorders may be considered, including abnormal factor V (factor V Leiden or factor V Arg 506→Gln mutation) and the G20210A mutation in the prothrombin gene.

IMAGING STUDIES

- Chest radiography and pulmonary function testing may exclude serious lung disease causing secondary pulmonary hypertension.
- In some cases, radionuclide perfusion studies may be needed to diagnose or exclude multiple pulmonary emboli.

TREATMENT

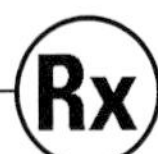

NONPHARMACOLOGIC THERAPY

- Lung transplantation is an option but has significant short- and long-term risks.
- Palliative atrial septostomy may alleviate symptoms of syncope or resuscitated sudden death and serve as a bridge to transplantation.
- Secondary forms of pulmonary hypertension may respond well to therapeutic interventions (e.g., surgical closure of cardiac shunts) before irreversible vascular changes occur.

CHRONIC Rx

- Pulmonary vasodilator therapy
  - Home oxygen treatment
  - Oral calcium channel blocker treatment (e.g., nifedipine) probably useful only if acute response to vasodilators during catheterization is present (a minority of patients)
  - Oral endothelin receptor blockers (e.g., bosentan)
  - Oral phosphodiesterase type 5 inhibitors to increase intravascular nitric oxide (e.g., sildenafil)
  - Continuous intravenous or subcutaneous prostacyclin analogue infusions (e.g., epoprostenol, treprostinil)

  - Inhaled prostacyclin analogues (e.g., iloprost)
- Anticoagulation/chronic warfarin treatment if possible thrombotic or embolic component

DISPOSITION

- Use of the World Health Organization (WHO) classification system of functional impairment may be useful to follow course and treatment response.
  - Class I: no limitation of physical activity
  - Class II: slight limitation of activity with normal exertion
  - Class III: marked limitation with less than normal exertion
  - Class IV: symptoms with any physical activity or at rest
- The distance walked during 6 minutes has become a standard measuring tool for symptom quantification in pulmonary hypertension.
  - The patient is allowed to walk at any pace and rest as needed.
  - Patient is encouraged to walk as far as possible along a measured hallway for 6 minutes.
  - Distance walked has been correlated with severity of disease, prognosis, and with drug efficacy.

REFERRAL

- Specialized, usually intensive, follow-up of children with severe pulmonary hypertension is indicated, especially those with primary pulmonary hypertension.
- Referral to a lung transplantation center may be warranted.

PEARLS & CONSIDERATIONS

COMMENTS

- For primary pulmonary hypertension, the prognosis is much worse than for secondary forms; 2- to 3-year survival with current treatment is approximately 50%.
- For some secondary forms, the prognosis may be as poor as with primary pulmonary hypertension (e.g., progressive pulmonary vein stenosis not amenable to surgical repair). Other secondary forms may have significantly better long-term prognosis (e.g., Eisenmenger syndrome in which survival into the fourth and fifth decades is possible).
- Patients with Eisenmenger physiology and unrepaired congenital heart disease have a longer survival than those with no heart disease and severe primary pulmonary hypertension.
- Right-to-left shunting across intracardiac defects causes cyanosis but may prevent or delay sudden death caused by a sudden lack of systemic cardiac output during periods of increased pulmonary hypertension.
- Syncope is an ominous sign and may predict sudden death.
- Ten percent to 30% of young adults with sickle cell anemia may have pulmonary hypertension.

PREVENTION

Detection of congenital heart disease has prevented most cases of Eisenmenger syndrome but pulmonary hypertension in older adults from undetected atrial septal defect may continue to be a problem.

PATIENT/FAMILY EDUCATION

- Pulmonary Hypertension Association. Available at www.phassociation.org

SUGGESTED READINGS

American College of Chest Physicians. Available at www.chestjournal.org/content/vol126/1_suppl/

Executive summary from the World Symposium on Primary Pulmonary Hypertension 1998. Available at www.who.int/ncd/cvd/pph.html

Haworth SG: Primary pulmonary hypertension in childhood. *Arch Dis Child* 79:452, 1998.

PHCentral. Available at www.phcentral.org/med/links.html

Pulmonary Hypertension Association. Available at www.phassociation.org

Rosenzweig E, Barst R: Idiopathic pulmonary arterial hypertension in children. *Curr Opin Pediatr* 17(3):372, 2005.

Rosenzweig EB et al: Effects of long-term bosentan in children with pulmonary arterial hypertension. *J Am Coll Cardiol* 46(4):69, 2005.

AUTHOR: **DAVID W. HANNON, MD**

BASIC INFORMATION

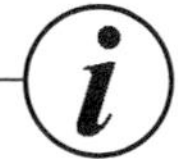

DEFINITION

Pulmonary stenosis, or more generally, right ventricular outflow track (RVOT) obstruction, is an anatomic blockage to right ventricular output. Obstruction can occur at multiple levels, including subvalvar (infundibular), valvar, or supravalvar stenosis of the main pulmonary artery or branch pulmonary arteries. These lesions can occur in isolation or in combination. The most severe form is pulmonary atresia.

SYNONYMS

Double-chambered right ventricle
Infundibular pulmonary stenosis
Peripheral pulmonary stenosis (PPS)
Right ventricular outflow track

ICD-9-CM CODES
746.0 Pulmonary valve anomaly, unspecified
746.01 Congenital pulmonary atresia
746.02 Congenital stenosis of the pulmonary valve
746.83 Infundibular (subvalvar) pulmonic stenosis
747.3 Anomalies of pulmonary artery (e.g., supravalvar pulmonary stenosis or atresia, peripheral pulmonic stenosis)

EPIDEMIOLOGY & DEMOGRAPHICS

- RVOT obstruction occurs in 25% to 30% of all congenital heart disease.
- RVOT obstruction is rarely familial.
- RVOT obstruction is associated with some genetic syndromes.
  - Supravalvar pulmonary stenosis (pulmonary artery stenosis): Williams syndrome (i.e., infantile hypercalcemia syndrome), Alagille syndrome, and congenital rubella syndrome
  - Valvar pulmonary stenosis: Noonan's syndrome
- Infundibular pulmonary stenosis is rarely an isolated anomaly; it usually is associated with tetralogy of Fallot.

CLINICAL PRESENTATION

History

- Neonatal critical or severe pulmonary valve stenosis or atresia
  - Manifests shortly after birth with cyanosis caused by right-to-left atrial level shunting
  - Right-sided congestive heart failure
- Noncritical pulmonary valve stenosis
  - Murmur usually heard at birth or shortly thereafter
  - Rarely symptomatic
- Subvalvar (infundibular) obstruction: rarely an isolated anomaly
- Supravalvar pulmonary stenosis (pulmonary artery stenosis): usually seen with recognizable syndromes such as Williams syndrome or congenital rubella syndrome
- Peripheral pulmonary artery stenosis: nonpathologic murmur heard in newborns through approximately 8 months old

Physical Examination

- Neonatal critical or severe pulmonary valve stenosis or atresia
  - Generalized cyanosis
  - Tachypnea without distress
  - Marked hepatomegaly
  - Peripheral edema: usually seen in periorbital area in infants
  - Peripheral pulses—normal unless cardiac output severely diminished.
- Cardiac examination of a critical infant
  - May have ejection murmur in the pulmonic area
  - May have murmur of tricuspid valve regurgitation
  - May have continuous murmur of patent ductus arteriosus
  - Ejection click uncommon in neonates
  - Pulmonic component of second sound at base usually absent
- Examination of a patient with noncritical pulmonary valve stenosis
  - Well-developed, well-nourished child
  - Normal pulses and perfusion
- Cardiac examination of a patient with noncritical pulmonary valve stenosis
  - Ejection (crescendo-decrescendo) murmur heard at the upper left sternal border
  - Murmur increases in intensity and peaks later in systole as the severity of the obstruction progresses
  - Prominent ejection click heard unless the valve is significantly dysplastic
  - Pulmonic component of second heart sound at the base delayed and diminished, may be absent
- Subvalvar (infundibular) obstruction
  - Systolic ejection murmur heard at the middle to upper left sternal border that peaks in midsystole
  - No ejection click
  - Pulmonic component of second heart sound usually normal
- Supravalvar pulmonary stenosis (i.e., pulmonary artery stenosis)
  - Systolic ejection murmur heard high along the left sternal border typically transmitted into the lung fields
  - No ejection click
  - Pulmonic component of second heart sound at base may be accentuated
  - Assess for syndromes (e.g., Williams syndrome, congenital rubella)
- Peripheral pulmonary artery stenosis (i.e., branch pulmonary artery stenosis)
  - Physiologic murmur often heard in infants
  - Soft ejection murmur, more prominent over lung fields with radiation into the axilla and back
  - No ejection click
  - Murmur typically gone by 8 months to 1 year of age

ETIOLOGY

- RVOT obstruction may develop in utero from altered patterns of fetal blood flow.
- Subvalvar obstruction represents hypertrophied infundibular muscle or isolated intraventricular muscle bands.
- Pulmonary valve stenosis may have a normal annulus diameter, but commissural fusion of the leaflets creates a narrowed orifice.
- In severe or critical neonatal pulmonic valve stenosis, the valve annulus may be hypoplastic and the valve leaflets thickened, dysplastic, and immobile, or the valve may be atretic with no opening.
- Supravalvar pulmonary stenosis may be a localized narrowing of the artery or arteries or may be generalized hypoplasia of the distal pulmonary arterial tree.

DIAGNOSIS

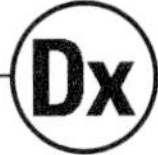

DIFFERENTIAL DIAGNOSIS

- Careful attention to location and characteristics helps differentiate pulmonary stenosis from other systolic murmurs.
  - Aortic stenosis murmur is heard at the middle left sternal border and aortic region.
  - Ventricular septal defect murmur is heard at the lower left sternal border and is harsh and holosystolic.
  - Shunting defects (e.g., atrial septal defect) have a soft flow murmur rather than true ejection.

WORKUP

- Neonatal critical or severe pulmonary valve stenosis or atresia
  - Electrocardiogram: variable findings
    - Right ventricular hypertrophy or left ventricular hypertrophy (if hypoplastic right ventricle)
    - Right atrial enlargement
  - Chest radiograph
    - Marked cardiomegaly
    - Prominent right atrium
    - Diminished pulmonary blood flow
  - Echocardiogram
    - Identifies site of obstruction
    - Measure pulmonary annulus
    - Estimate gradient across the valve
    - Assess ventricular size and function
    - Identifies atrial level shunting (e.g., foramen ovale, atrial septal defect) and direction of flow
    - Identifies abnormal coronary artery communications with the right ventricle
  - Cardiac catheterization and angiocardiography
    - Delayed until response to prostaglandin infusion
    - Typically performed only if intervention indicated (e.g., balloon valvuloplasty)

- Provides additional specific anatomic details (i.e., coronary anatomy)
- Noncritical pulmonary valve stenosis
  - Electrocardiogram: right ventricular hypertrophy that increases with increasing right ventricular hypertension, increasing degree of obstruction
  - Chest radiograph
    - Normal heart size
    - Prominent pulmonary artery segment reflecting post-stenotic dilation
    - Normal pulmonary blood flow
    - Apex possibly rounded and uptilted off the diaphragm
  - Echocardiogram
    - Localizes obstruction
    - Estimation of gradient
    - Anatomy of valve leaflets (e.g., thin, mobile, doming)
    - Size and function of right ventricle
  - Cardiac catheterization and angiocardiography: performed only if intervention indicated (i.e., balloon valvuloplasty)
- Subvalvar (infundibular) obstruction
  - Electrocardiogram, chest radiograph, echocardiogram, catheterization, and angiography per primary diagnosis (e.g., tetralogy of Fallot)
- Supravalvar pulmonary stenosis
  - Chest radiograph: similar to noncritical pulmonary valve stenosis but without prominent pulmonary artery segment
  - Electrocardiogram and echocardiogram: similar to noncritical pulmonary valve stenosis
  - Cardiac catheterization and angiography
    - Indicated to delineate anatomy of obstruction
    - May be performed in conjunction with balloon angioplasty or stent implantation

TREATMENT

NONPHARMACOLOGIC THERAPY

- Noncritical pulmonary stenosis
  - Routine follow-up with mild degrees of obstruction
  - No activity restriction needed
  - Subacute bacterial endocarditis prophylaxis not required

ACUTE GENERAL Rx

- For neonatal critical or severe pulmonary valve stenosis or atresia, use immediate prostaglandin infusion to reopen the ductus arteriosus and increase pulmonary blood flow.
- For subvalvar and supravalvar pulmonary stenosis, treatment is based on the primary diagnosis.

CHRONIC Rx

- Neonatal critical or severe pulmonary valve stenosis or atresia
  - Balloon valvuloplasty is used for some infants; therapy is individualized.
  - Balloon valvuloplasty may not be performed in the following conditions.
    - Tricuspid annulus is too small.
    - Pulmonic annulus is too small.
    - Right ventricle is too small for adequate function.
  - Surgical pulmonary valvotomy or valvectomy and RVOT reconstruction with placement of systemic-to-pulmonary shunt may be indicated in patients with hypoplastic right-sided structures.
- Noncritical pulmonary valve stenosis: severe obstruction
  - Definitive therapy with balloon valvuloplasty.
  - Surgical valvotomy is indicated when valvuloplasty unsuccessful (i.e., dysplastic valves).
- Supravalvar pulmonary stenosis (i.e., main pulmonary artery stenosis)
  - Stenosis may be amenable to balloon dilation or primary stenting.
  - Surgery is delayed until the obstruction becomes severe.
- Anatomic peripheral pulmonary artery stenosis (i.e., branch pulmonary artery stenosis)
  - It is a difficult condition to treat.
  - It may be amenable to balloon dilation or primary stenting, or both.
  - Surgical repair is difficult.

DISPOSITION

- Neonatal critical or severe pulmonary valve stenosis or atresia
  - Long-term follow-up is required.
  - Repeat intervention depends on the initial catheter or surgical intervention and the size of right-sided structures.
  - Pulmonary valve replacement may be required.
- Noncritical pulmonary valve stenosis
  - Follow-up is needed for possible restenosis, although it rarely occurs.
  - Subacute bacterial endocarditis (SBE) prophylaxis is indicted in selected cases.

REFERRAL

All patients with suspected RVOT obstruction should be referred to a cardiologist for diagnosis and management.

PEARLS & CONSIDERATIONS

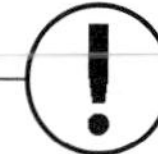

COMMENTS

- Presence of a systolic ejection murmur at birth may signify a ventricular outflow tract obstruction.
- A long and late-peaking systolic ejection murmur suggests severe obstruction.
- An ejection click signifies a thin, mobile valve and signifies valvar stenosis.
- Physical growth is excellent with pulmonic stenosis.
- Ejection murmurs have a crescendo-decrescendo pattern.
- Location of the murmur is critical for differentiating the cause.
  - Pulmonary valve stenosis murmur is heard at the upper left sternal border.
  - Infundibular pulmonary stenosis murmur is heard at the middle upper left sternal border.
  - Supravalvar pulmonary stenosis murmur is heard at the high left sternal border, with radiation into the lung fields.

PATIENT/FAMILY EDUCATION

- The prognosis for pulmonary valve stenosis after balloon valvuloplasty or surgery is excellent.
- The need for repeat intervention is uncommon if the initial intervention was performed after early infancy.
- The prognosis is less favorable for nonvalvular obstruction.
  - It depends on associated defects and anatomy.
  - Subacute bacterial endocarditis (SBE) prophylaxis is required for complex cases.
- Activity restriction depends on residual RVOT obstruction.

SUGGESTED READINGS

American Heart Association. Available at www.americanheart.org

Congenital Heart Information Network. Available at www.tchin.org/pdheart.htm

Emedicine. Available at www.emedicine.com

Heart Center Online. Available at www.heartcenteronline.com

Moss, Adams: *Heart Disease in Infants, Children and Adolescents including the Fetus and Young Adult,* 6th ed. Baltimore, MD, Williams & Wilkins, 2001, pp 820–863.

Park MK: *Pediatric Cardiology for Practitioners,* 4th ed. Mosby, St. Louis, 2002, pp 155–158.

Pediheart. Available at www.pediheart.org

AUTHOR: **DANIEL E. MIGA, MD**

BASIC INFORMATION

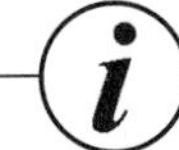

DEFINITION

Hypertrophic pyloric stenosis (HPS) is an acquired condition in which the circumferential muscle of the pyloric sphincter becomes thickened, resulting in elongation and obliteration of the pyloric channel.

SYNONYMS

Congenital hypertrophic pyloric stenosis
HPS
Pyloric stenosis (PS)

ICD-9-CM CODE

750.5 Congenital hypertrophic pyloric stenosis; pyloric stenosis; hypertrophic, infantile pyloric stenosis

EPIDEMIOLOGY & DEMOGRAPHICS

- Incidence 2 to 4 cases per 1000 live births.
- 4:1 male-to-female predominance.
- More than 90% of cases are sporadic.
- Between 7% and 10% of cases are familial.
  - A mother who had HPS as an infant transmits the risk of developing HPS to her offspring (19% for boys and 7% for girls).
  - A father who had HPS as an infant transmits a lower risk of developing HPS to his offspring (5% for boys and 2.5% for girls).
  - Siblings of patients with HPS are 15 times more likely to have HPS than children without any affected siblings. First-born males are not necessarily more frequently afflicted than other siblings.
- Associated anomalies are rare.

CLINICAL PRESENTATION

- 2 week and 2 month old infant.
- Several days to weeks of projectile, nonbilious emesis is reported.
- Emesis can have a coffee grounds appearance or be blood streaked as a result of gastritis or esophagitis.
- History of formula changes.
- Parents report infant hunger.
- Weight loss or no weight gain may be seen.
- Signs/symptoms of dehydration.
- A palpable "olive" is felt just under the epigastrium.
  - If palpated, there is no need for further diagnostic tests.
  - Palpation of this pyloric mass is extremely difficult in an agitated, crying infant with a full stomach.
- Diagnostic aids to physical examination:
  - Pass a nasogastric tube to empty stomach.
  - Quiet the child by allowing him or her to suck on a "sweet" pacifier.
  - Apply firm, gentle, steady pressure with flat part of first three or four digits.
  - Hold the infant's legs gently flexed at the knees and hips.
  - For right-handed examiners, the legs are held up at the ankles with left hand. Right hand is placed between the legs with the fingertips in the epigastrium.
  - Apply pressure posteriorly toward the vertebral bodies until the child strains and flexes the abdominal muscles. Pressure should be kept steady until the child relaxes. The common mistake is to relax pressure when the child strains.
  - Gentle palpation under the epigastrium reveals an acorn-like mass that rolls under the fingers with respirations and palpation.
  - Do not mistake the edge of the liver or the rectus muscle for the olive.
- Examination may take 15 to 30 minutes; be patient.

ETIOLOGY

- No direct cause has been confirmed.

DIAGNOSIS

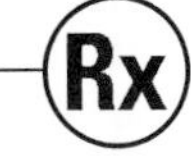

DIFFERENTIAL DIAGNOSIS

- The differential diagnosis of nonbilious emesis in nonfebrile infants includes the following: pylorospasm; feeding or milk intolerance; gastroesophageal reflux disease; salt-wasting adrenogenital syndrome; central nervous system conditions resulting in elevated cerebrospinal fluid pressures (hydrocephalus, subdural hemorrhage).
- Less common diagnoses include duodenal or antral webs and gastric tumors.

LABORATORY TESTS

- Hypochloremic, hypokalemic, metabolic alkalosis
- Acidosis with significant dehydration
- Unconjugated hyperbilirubinemia: common, probably resulting from decreased hepatic glucuronosyltransferase activity

IMAGING STUDIES

- Historically, the diagnostic test of choice was an upper gastrointestinal series.
  - HPS is confirmed by finding a narrowed pyloric channel, known as the *string* sign.
  - Shouldering of the pyloric muscle with bulging into the proximal duodenum is also common.
- The gold standard for now is an ultrasound.
  - Pyloric muscular wall thicker than 3 to 4 mm.
  - Channel longer than 14 to 17 mm.
  - Together, these measurements have a >90% positive predictive value.

TREATMENT

NONPHARMACOLOGIC THERAPY

- Surgical pyloromyotomy.
- Surgery may be performed through several types of incisions, including umbilical, right upper quadrant, and supraumbilical.
- Laparoscopic pyloromyotomy is performed in many institutions.
- Laparoscopic and umbilical approaches may offer a cosmetic advantage, and the laparoscopic procedure may decrease time to feeding tolerance.
- Regardless of the operative approach chosen, successful treatment of HPS ensures that the hypertrophied muscle is split the entire length of the pylorus.
- Incomplete myotomy can result in failure to relieve symptoms and may require reoperation.

ACUTE GENERAL Rx

- The first step in treatment should be rehydration and correction of abnormal electrolytes.
- Most surgeons and anesthesiologists would agree to proceed with an operation when the HCO_3 level is less than 30 mEq/L and the chloride level is more than 100 mEq/L.

DISPOSITION

- Postoperatively, patients are not fed for 2 hours.
- They begin on small volumes of formula or breast milk.
- Volume is increased over 12 to 16 hours, until baby is taking maintenance feeds.
- Children may vomit once or twice postoperatively. Emesis is often projectile.
- Parents are encouraged to continue with the feeding regimen.

REFERRAL

Babies suspected of having HPS should be referred to a pediatric surgeon for evaluation.

PEARLS & CONSIDERATIONS

COMMENTS

- HPS should be considered in infants treated for formula intolerance who fail to improve.
- Infants with persistent nonbilious emesis should be evaluated by a pediatric surgeon or have an abdominal ultrasound.

SUGGESTED READINGS

Murphy SG: Hypertrophic pyloric stenosis. *In* Mattei P (ed): *Surgical Directives: Pediatric Surgery.* Philadelphia, Lippincott Williams & Wilkins, 2003, pp 269–272.

Puri P, Lakshmanadass G: Hypertrophic pyloric stenosis. *In* Puri P (ed): *Newborn Surgery.* New York, Arnold, 2003, pp 389–398.

AUTHOR: **RICHARD A. FALCONE, JR., MD**

BASIC INFORMATION

DEFINITION

Rabies is a viral infection of the central and peripheral nervous systems, causing encephalitis with or without paralysis that is uniformly fatal.

SYNONYMS

Hydrophobia
Mad dog disease

ICD-9-CM CODES
071 Rabies
V01.5 Rabies exposure
V04.5 Rabies immune globulin
V04.5 Rabies vaccinations

EPIDEMIOLOGY & DEMOGRAPHICS

- In the United States, terrestrial rabies is most common in raccoons on the eastern coast and in skunks, foxes, coyotes, and dogs on the Texas-Mexican border.
- Bat (avian) rabies is widespread in the 49 continental states but does not occur in Hawaii.
- Five antigenic variants of rabies strains exist in the United States.
  - The single raccoon strain is predominant.
  - One case of human rabies has resulted from the raccoon rabies strain in the United States.
- Domestic animals usually succumb to the strain predominant in their geographic region.
- The only rodent in the United States that can carry rabies long enough to transmit it to humans is the groundhog.
- Other small rodents and lagomorphs (e.g., rabbits, hares) usually die before transmitting the virus to humans.
- Cats are the most common domestic animals reported by health departments as being rabid. There are a high number of unvaccinated strays, with possible contacts to bats and other mammals.
- Since 1980, most endemic rabies cases in humans have been associated with bats.
  - From 1990 to 2002, bat strains of rabies virus were associated with 27 of 36 cases of human rabies in the United States.
  - Other cases have been associated with dog or animal bites in travelers returning from abroad, especially in countries where wild canine rabies is endemic.

CLINICAL PRESENTATION

History

- Determine the nature of the interaction with the animal. Was the attack provoked or unexpected? Was there any strange animal behavior? Was the animal typically nocturnal but out during the daytime?
- Determine vaccination status of animal.
- Document the nature of the presentation of illness in the animal and possible human case.
- The most common type in humans is the *furious form.* Classic symptoms include paresthesias at the site of the bite, hypersalivation, hydrophobia, and spasms and contractions of the neck muscles. This form is also common in cats.
  - Many animals, including bats, exhibit "dumb" rabies (i.e., paralytic form).
  - Both forms progress to paralysis of pharyngeal and respiratory muscles, seizures, and coma, with death occurring in 1 to 3 weeks.
  - Rabies postexposure prophylaxis should be given in a true exposure instance no matter how old the injury.

Physical Examination

- Examination of a patient who has been bitten by an animal should include:
  - Localization and documentation of the extent of the wound
  - Neurologic examination looking for signs of altered mental status, anxiety, hyperactivity, or bizarre behaviors with interspersed calm periods
  - Autonomic instability: hypertension, hypersalivation, hyperthermia, and hyperventilation
  - Muscle fasciculations, priapism, and focal or generalized convulsions
- Paralysis may be present only in the bitten limb at first, but it usually becomes diffuse and may ascend (similar to Guillain-Barré syndrome).

ETIOLOGY

- Rabies is caused by the rabies virus: genus *Lyssavirus,* family Rhabdoviridae.
- It is a bullet-shaped RNA virus with three major components:
  - Surface glycoprotein (G protein)
  - Outer envelope protein (M or matrix protein)
  - Nucleocapsid
- Transmitted by bite or saliva of an infected mammal or by contamination of mucosa or skin lesions by infectious material.
- Any mammal can carry and potentially transmit rabies, but it is usually transmitted by carnivorous species and bats.
- Transmission of the virus in saliva through mucous membranes, open wounds, or scratches is possible but rarely documented.
- Human-to-human transmission has occurred with corneal transplants and solid organ transplants.
- Cases have been reported in humans exposed to aerosols of bat guano in caves or aerosolized laboratory strain virus.
- When the rabies virus enters muscles, it replicates locally; then it is transported through peripheral sensory nerves to the spinal ganglia, where it replicates and travels up the spinal cord to the brain. The virus migrates to the gray matter of the brain, predominantly in the neurons of the limbic system, midbrain, and hypothalamus. Efferent nerves transport the virus to the acinar glands of the submaxillary salivary glands, where it achieves high concentrations.
- This transit time is presumably shorter if the initial wound is severe with a high load of virus and is close to the head.
- The incubation period in human beings is from 5 days to many years; the average is 1 to 3 months before the onset of symptoms.

DIAGNOSIS

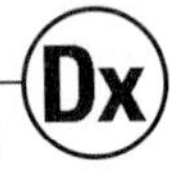

DIFFERENTIAL DIAGNOSIS

- Other encephalitides should be ruled out, especially herpes simplex encephalitis, because it is treatable.
- Guillain-Barré syndrome, transverse myelitis, and poliomyelitis may manifest with similar paralytic features.
- Rigidity of tetanus contractions are more prolonged; mental status is usually normal.
- Rule out other forms of epilepsy and poisoning with atropine-like compounds.

LABORATORY TESTS

- Brain biopsy with immunohistochemical or fluorescent antibody staining is definitive. Wild animals that have been captured after biting should be euthanized and have testing of the unfixed brain tissue done by state health departments.
- Skin or corneal biopsy for similar specific stains.
- A rise in specific neutralizing antibodies by rapid fluorescent focus inhibition test (RFFIT) is often not documented in true rabies cases because the victims succumb before mounting a response. This test is more useful to ascertain serostatus in immunized animals and humans.
- Viral culture of saliva, cerebrospinal fluid, and brain can be done in specialized laboratories.

TREATMENT

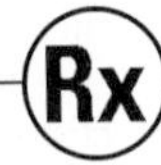

ACUTE GENERAL Rx

- Secondary complications, such as bacterial superinfection and tissue destruction, may occur.
- Coma may last for hours to months with active intensive care support.
- Cardiac arrhythmias, myocarditis, and further autonomic dysfunction lead to cardiopulmonary arrest.

DISPOSITION

Rabies is almost always fatal. A few cases of survival have been reported with late administration of vaccine or in combination with experimental therapies such as ribavirin and interferon.

REFERRAL

Questions about who needs prophylaxis may be directed to public health officials and infectious disease consultants.

BASIC INFORMATION

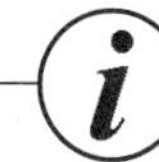

DEFINITION

Renal tubular acidosis (RTA) is a disorder in which a defect in secretion of protons by the proximal and/or distal nephron of the kidney results in bicarbonate wasting (proximal) or reduced acid secretion (distal). As a consequence, a persistent non-anion gap (hyperchloremic) metabolic acidosis develops. The serum anion gap, [Na] − ([Cl] + [HCO_3]), is normally 8 to 12 mEq/L in adults and 20% to 30% higher in infants.

SYNONYMS

Type 1 or classic RTA (i.e., distal renal tubular acidosis [DRTA])
Type 2 RTA (i.e., proximal renal tubular acidosis [PRTA])
Type 3 RTA (i.e., no longer considered a distinct entity)
Type 4 RTA (i.e., hyperkalemic distal renal tubular acidosis)

ICD-9-CM CODES
276.2 Acidosis
588.89 Acidosis, renal, tubular (distal or proximal) (Other specified disorders resulting from impaired renal function)

EPIDEMIOLOGY & DEMOGRAPHICS

- Incidence of DRTA is 1 in 10,000 people; PRTA is less common.
  - Although primary RTA is recognized to be a rare disease, referrals to exclude RTA are much more common than the incidence of the disease.
  - As a referring diagnosis, primary RTA accounted for 6% of renal consultations in children of Venezuela.
- Most cases present in infancy.
- There is no sex predominance in DRTA or in Type 4 RTA.
- DRTA may be inherited as an autosomal dominant or recessive trait.
  - Autosomal recessive DRTA often presents in infancy, whereas autosomal dominant DRTA may not present until adolescence or young adulthood.
  - Mutations in the genes encoding carbonic anhydrase II, kidney anion exchanger 1 (kAE1), and subunits of the renal proton pump (H^+-ATPase) have been identified in patients with DRTA.
- DRTA is almost always permanent.
- Isolated PRTA is more common in males.
- Isolated PRTA may be transient.
- Genetically transmitted PRTAs include autosomal dominant and recessive forms.
- PRTA (with ocular abnormalities) may be caused by inactivating mutations in the Na/HCO_3 cotransporter gene (SLC4A4).
- PRTA may also be associated with other genetically transmitted disorders, such as osteopetrosis with carbonic anhydrase II deficiency.
- Inherited defects leading to Type 4 RTA are due to aldosterone deficiency or resistance.
  - Congenital adrenal hyperplasia with salt wasting
  - Isolated hypoaldosteronism
  - Pseudohypoaldosteronism (defect at the aldosterone receptor level)

CLINICAL PRESENTATION

- DRTA presentation often includes recurrent vomiting and dehydration, poor feeding, constipation, failure to thrive, and metabolic acidosis.
  - There is usually growth retardation.
  - There may be associated nephrocalcinosis, renal stones, rickets, or osteomalacia.
  - Hypokalemia is frequent, and when severe can lead to severe muscle weakness.
  - Kussmaul respiration due to acidosis-induced stimulation of respiration can be seen.
  - Sensorineural deafness is often found with genetic forms of DRTA in which the vacuolar proton pump is mutated.
  - Secondary causes include autoimmune and tubulointerstitial diseases, chronic rejection of renal transplantation, associated genetic diseases (including Type 1 glycogen storage disease, Ehlers-Danlos syndrome, hereditary elliptocytosis, sickle cell anemia, medullary cystic disease, and obstructive uropathy), and certain drugs including amphotericin B, lithium, vanadate, and analgesics.
- PRTA presentation includes growth retardation, recurrent vomiting, failure to thrive, but rarely problems with stones or nephrocalcinosis; bone disease does not occur unless there is phosphate wasting.
  - PRTA may be an isolated defect.
  - It is often associated with multiple tubular dysfunction (e.g., Fanconi syndrome, renal glucosuria, phosphate or amino acid wasting, hypouricemia) or
  - As part of such diseases as cystinosis, Wilson's disease, tyrosinemia, hereditary fructose intolerance, Lowe syndrome, galactosemia, glycogen storage disease, metachromatic leukodystrophy, galactosemia, toxins/drugs (including ifosfamide, gentamicin, cadmium, and lead), and mitochondrial myopathies.
- Rickets may be seen with DRTA and with phosphate-wasting forms of PRTA.
- Hypokalemia is usually seen with PRTA and DRTA.
- Type 4 RTA is either isolated or appears in patients with renal parenchymal disease.
  - Manifestations of acidosis (as noted above), hyperkalemia, and renal salt wasting may be prominent.
  - Type 4 RTA may be transient in infancy and early childhood.
  - Type 4 RTA may also result from tubular damage resulting from obstructive nephropathy, tubulointerstitial nephritis (methicillin nephrotoxicity), sickle cell disease, kidney transplant rejection, and lupus nephritis.
  - Type 4 RTA also results from drugs that interfere with sodium channel function (amiloride, trimethoprim), aldosterone (spironolactone), and sodium pump activity (cyclosporine).
- Impaired growth is usually manifested by a decrease in body length below the 5th percentile; this may be followed by a fall in weight below the 5th percentile.
- Signs of volume depletion (dehydration) are often seen with DRTA and in some forms of salt-wasting Type 4 RTA.
- Muscle wasting because of increased muscle breakdown and a tendency to hypoalbuminemia can be seen.
- Central nervous system and cardiac depression may result from very severe acidosis.

ETIOLOGY

- PRTA is caused by an impaired capacity of the proximal tubule to reabsorb bicarbonate (via a reduced rate of sodium-dependent proton secretion or sodium-bicarbonate exit across the basolateral membrane or by decreased cytosolic carbonic anhydrase [CA] II activity).
- DRTA is caused by impaired distal proton secretion and failure to acidify the urine (via a disorder of the renal proton pump).
- Hyperkalemic DRTA (Type 4) is usually caused by an insufficiency of aldosterone synthesis or resistance to aldosterone effect because of a defect in the receptor, or tubular damage. Hyperkalemia is often out of proportion to the degree of renal impairment.

DIAGNOSIS

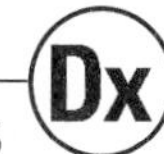

DIFFERENTIAL DIAGNOSIS

- Normal anion gap metabolic acidosis with hypokalemia
  - Gastrointestinal loss of bicarbonate (diarrhea, fistula, ureteroenterostomy, ureterosigmoidostomy).
  - Renal loss of bicarbonate (acetazolamide, hyperparathyroidism).
  - Classic proximal and distal RTA.
  - Post correction of chronic hypocapnia.
  - Rapid intravenous hydration with 0.9% (normal) saline.
- Normal anion gap metabolic acidosis with normo- or hyperkalemia
  - Drugs (acidifying agents, such as NH_4Cl, arginine chloride, $CaCl_2$, $MgSO_4$, cholestyramine resin, $MgCl_2$, Sulfamylon)
  - Hyperalimentation (excessive cationic amino acids)
  - Hypoaldosteronism
  - Tubular resistance to aldosterone
- Elevated anion gap metabolic acidosis
  - Uremic acidosis
  - Ketoacidosis (starvation or fasting, diabetic ketoacidosis, ethanol intoxication)
  - Lactic acidosis (tissue hypoxia, muscular exercise, ethanol ingestion, systemic causes, inborn errors of metabolism)

- Toxins (methanol, ethylene glycol, salicylates, paraldehyde)

LABORATORY TESTS

- Obtain measurements of serum Na, K, Cl, HCO_3, BUN, creatinine, blood pH, and $PaCO_2$.
- Estimate GFR from Schwartz formula (GFR [ml/min/1.73 m^2] = 0.55 × height [cm]/ serum creatinine [mg/dl]).
- Calculate serum anion gap = [Na] − ([Cl] + [HCO_3]).
- Obtain fresh spot urine or urine under oil for measurement of pH: normally less than 5.5 when serum bicarbonate is reduced.
  - With classic hypokalemic DRTA urine pH is greater than 5.5; with proximal RTA urine pH is less than 5.5 when serum HCO_3 is below threshold and greater than 5.5 when above bicarbonate threshold.
  - With Type 4 (hyporeninemic hypoaldosteronism) urine pH is less than 5.5 and with tubular resistance urine pH is greater than 5.5.
- Obtain measurements of urine electrolytes (in mEq/L) for calculation of urine net charge (formerly urine anion gap, which gives an estimate of urinary ammonia excretion) = urine Na + urine K − urine Cl, with normal value near zero mEq/L (urine pH should be <7.0)
  - Urine net charge of −30 to 0 (implies high urinary ammonia): indicates sufficient renal ammonium excretion during acidosis, and so consider causes such as GI bicarbonate loss, PRTA, acetazolamide.
  - Urine net charge greater than 0 (implies low urinary ammonia): indicates renal cause such as DRTA and Type 4 RTA.
  - Urine osmolal gap is helpful in infants, when the urine net charge is positive, or if it is unclear whether increased excretion of unmeasured anions is responsible: measured urine osmolality (mosmol/kg) − calculated urine osmolality (in mosmol/kg) from 2 × {[Na (mEq/L) + K (mEq/L)] + urea (mg/dl)/2.8 + glucose (mg/dl)/18}/2 = twice the urine ammonium excretion (in mosmol/kg). An osmolal gap value of 30 to 50 mosmol/kg represents an ammonium excretion that would be appropriate for metabolic acidosis.
- Bicarbonate titration: slowly raise serum bicarbonate concentration by infusing 0.5 to 1 mEq/kg/h.
  - Calculate fractional excretion of bicarbonate (FE HCO_3 = urine HCO_3/ serum HCO_3 × serum creatinine/urine creatinine × 100) at different serum bicarbonate levels; normally FE HCO_3 is less than 1%.
  - Urine pH and fractional excretion of bicarbonate are relatively constant in DRTA.
  - Urine pH and fractional excretion of bicarbonate rise at subnormal serum bicarbonate levels in PRTA.
  - If there is bicarbonate wasting at subnormal levels of serum bicarbonate (FE HCO_3 >5%), check for urinary phosphate wasting (FE PO_4 >20%).
  - Urine pCO_2 as indicator of distal acidification: under conditions of bicarbonate titration, measure urine and blood pCO_2: normal U-B pCO_2 greater than 20 mm Hg, and U-B less than 20 indicates reduced rate of distal acid excretion.
- A 24-hour urine test for calcium, creatinine, citrate, potassium, and sodium: hypercalciuria, hypocitraturia, and potassium wasting are associated with DRTA; sodium wasting may be seen with aldosterone-dependent (Type 4) RTA.
- Summary of tests:
  - PRTA, below HCO_3 threshold: urine pH less than 5.5, urine net charge negative, U-B pCO_2 greater than 20 mm, normal urine calcium and citrate excretion, normal or low serum potassium; FE HCO_3 greater than 15% at normal serum HCO_3 levels.
  - DRTA: urine pH greater than 5.5, urine net charge positive, FE HCO_3 less than 5%, U-B pCO_2 less than 20 mm, high urine calcium and low urine citrate excretions, normal or low serum potassium.
  - Type 4 RTA
    - Hypoaldosteronism: urine pH less than 5.5, urine net charge positive, FE HCO_3 less than 15%, UB pCO_2 less than 20 mm, normal urine calcium and citrate excretions, hyperkalemia, probable abnormalities in plasma renin and/or aldosterone concentrations.
    - Tubular resistance: urine pH greater than 5.5 and normal renin and aldosterone values.

IMAGING STUDIES

Ultrasonography of the kidney may show nephrocalcinosis or renal calculi in undiagnosed or untreated DRTA.

TREATMENT

ACUTE GENERAL Rx

- Correct blood pH to 7.2 or serum bicarbonate to 10 mEq/L using intravenous sodium bicarbonate over several minutes to a few hours. Calculate dose assuming a bicarbonate space of 0.5 L/kg. The dose is 0.5 × weight in kg × (10 − actual serum bicarbonate in mEq/L).
- Hypokalemia and hypocalcemia should be corrected before correcting the acidosis to prevent severe muscle weakness, respiratory muscle paralysis, arrhythmias, or painful tetany during bicarbonate infusion.

CHRONIC Rx

- Sodium bicarbonate is effective therapy and corrects acidosis caused by any form of RTA.
- A preferred alternative is citrate of sodium or potassium, which is converted by the liver to bicarbonate.
  - Citrate is more palatable than bicarbonate and not associated with side effects related to excessive gastrointestinal gas.
  - Potassium citrate does not result in the volume expansion caused by sodium salts, which becomes very important in the treatment of PRTA.
  - Citrate can be given as a liquid (e.g., Bicitra, Polycitra, or Polycitra-K, Alza Pharmaceuticals) or as an extended-release tablet (10 mEq, Urocit-K, Mission Pharmacal).
    - Bicitra provides 1 mEq/ml of sodium and potential alkali.
    - Polycitra provides 2 mEq/ml of potential alkali, half as sodium and half as potassium.
    - Polycitra-K provides 2 mEq/ml of potential alkali, 2 mEq/ml as potassium.
- Initial alkali therapy for RTA
  - DRTA: 2 to 4 mEq/kg/day, but may have to increase dose to accommodate the acidosis generated from "catch-up" growth.
  - PRTA: 5 to 20 mEq/kg/day, but may need to combine with low salt diet if large doses of sodium bicarbonate are utilized.
  - Type 4 RTA: 1 to 4 mEq/kg/day
- Additional treatment for Type 4 RTA
  - Hyperkalemia: restrict potassium intake, furosemide 1 to 2 mg/kg/day and/or chlorothiazide 10 to 20 mg/kg/day; may also be necessary to use cation-exchange resin (sodium polystyrene sulfonate, Kayexalate) at 0.5 to 1 gm/kg once or twice daily.
  - Mineralocorticoid therapy for aldosterone deficiency: fludrocortisone 0.05 to 0.15 mg/m^2/day.

COMPLEMENTARY & ALTERNATIVE MEDICINE

- Mineral waters containing oil of peppermint, carbonate of soda, and citric acid
- Aqua soda containing sodium bicarbonate and sodium citrate

DISPOSITION

- Some cases of infantile PRTA and Type 4 RTA may remit spontaneously.
- Alkali treatment may be required for life; failure to continue treatment of DRTA is likely to result in renal damage because of nephrolithiasis.
- Alkali therapy should maintain serum bicarbonate at greater than 22 mEq/L
  - Treatment with sodium salts alone will cause hypokalemia.
  - DRTA with hypokalemia responds well to potassium citrate.
  - PRTA responds well to a mixture of sodium and potassium citrate.
  - PRTA may require concomitant thiazide diuretic treatment to reduce volume expansion caused by sodium citrate.

- In PRTA with Fanconi syndrome, additional management of phosphate, sugar, and amino acid wasting may be required.
- The effects of therapy should be monitored monthly for the first 6 months.
  - Monitor closely serum bicarbonate, urinary calcium/creatinine ratio (in DRTA), and linear growth.
  - Catch-up growth and growth spurts will require increased dosage.
  - Giving a larger dose of alkali at bedtime is based on the rationale that growth hormone secretion is maximal during sleep and that the optimal correction of metabolic acidosis during this period will have a significant beneficial effect.
- In DRTA obtain annual ultrasonographic imaging of the kidneys to monitor nephrocalcinosis.

REFERRAL

- A formal diagnosis of any form of RTA should be referred to a pediatric nephrologist.
- Subsequent management of alkali therapy can be shared with the pediatric nephrologist, provided that growth is maintained and there is no risk of nephrolithiasis/ nephrocalcinosis.

PEARLS & CONSIDERATIONS

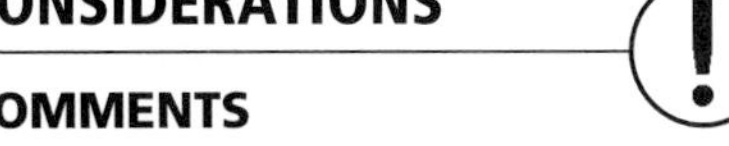

COMMENTS

- The astute clinician will take advantage of spontaneous acidosis to examine renal acidification (urine pH, net charge, etc.).
- It is important for volume contraction and electrolyte disorders to be corrected before formal testing of renal acid and bicarbonate handling.
- Low serum bicarbonate can be a laboratory artifact when a small amount of blood (1 ml) is obtained with difficulty and stored in a large-capacity tube (10 ml) before measurement. Serum bicarbonate should agree to within 10% of the bicarbonate concentration calculated from simultaneous venous or arterial blood gas.
- Urine pH measurement is not useful in the absence of a near-simultaneously obtained serum bicarbonate or blood pH.
- DRTA, as well as an inborn error of metabolism, should be considered when a patient presents with hyperammonemia and severe acidosis (acidosis leads to increased ammonia synthesis, but there is inadequate renal excretion with the high urine pH of DRTA).
- Gastroesophageal reflux has been observed with severe DRTA; electrolytes should be checked when such reflux is refractory to therapy.
- Urine net charge is inaccurate when there is a large concentration of non-chloride anions (e.g., ketoacids, penicillin, salicylate).
- Urine citrate excretion is decreased in DRTA (leading to kidney stone formation and nephrocalcinosis), and successful treatment of DRTA increases urinary citrate excretion.

SUGGESTED READINGS

Carlisle EJF et al: Renal tubular acidosis (RTA): recognize the ammonium defect and pHorget the urine pH. *Pediatr Nephrol* 5:242, 1991.

DuBose TD Jr, McDonald GA: Renal tubular acidosis. *In* DuBose TD Jr, Hamm LL (eds): *Acid-Base and Electrolyte Disorders: A Companion to Brenner & Rector's The Kidney.* Philadelphia, Elsevier Science, 2002, pp 189–206.

Gregory MJ, Schwartz GJ: Diagnosis and treatment of renal tubular disorders. *Semin Nephrol* 18:317, 1998.

Igarashi T et al: Molecular basis of proximal renal tubular acidosis. *J Nephrol* 15:S135, 2002.

Karet FE: Inherited distal renal tubular acidosis. *J Am Soc Nephrol* 13:2178, 2002.

McSherry E et al: Renal tubular acidosis in infants: the several kinds, including bicarbonate-wasting, classic renal tubular acidosis. *J Clin Invest* 51:499, 1972.

Nash MA et al: Renal tubular acidosis in infants and children. *J Pediatr* 80:738, 1972.

National Kidney Foundation web site. Available at www.Kidney.org

National Kidney and Urologic Diseases Information Clearinghouse web site. Available at www.Kidney.NIDDK.NIH.gov

Nicoletta JA, Schwartz GJ: Distal renal tubular acidosis. *Curr Opin Pediatr* 16:194, 2004.

AUTHOR: **GEORGE J. SCHWARTZ, MD**

BASIC INFORMATION

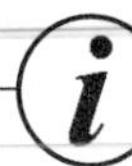

DEFINITION

Respiratory syncytial virus (RSV) infection or bronchiolitis is an acute, wheezing-associated illness in early life preceded by an upper respiratory infection, resulting in obstruction of small airways.

SYNONYM

RSV bronchiolitis

ICD-9-CM CODE

466.1 Acute bronchiolitis

EPIDEMIOLOGY & DEMOGRAPHICS

- Humans are the only source of infection.
- Incidence in the United States is 11.4 cases per 100 children in the first year of life.
- More than 50% of all infants will be infected with RSV by the end of the first year of life, and in day-care settings, almost 100% of infants are infected with RSV by the end of the first year of life. Most infants are infected by the end of the second year of life.
- RSV occurs in yearly epidemics occurring in winter and early spring.
- The male-to-female ratio is 1.5:1 for hospitalized patients. The infection rate is similar for males and females.
- Transmission occurs predominantly from direct contact and large-particle aerosols rather than small-particle aerosols.
- Viral shedding occurs 1 to 2 days before symptoms and continues for 1 to 2 weeks after symptoms abate.

CLINICAL PRESENTATION

History

- Upper respiratory infection with rhinorrhea and cough may occur for several days and be associated with a low-grade fever.
- Cough may become increasingly productive, with increasing respiratory distress.
- Decreased feeding may be reported.
- Hypoxemia occurs in severe cases, although cyanosis usually is not evident.
- Apnea may occur in former premature infants and infants younger than 4 months.
- Associated otitis media caused by RSV or bacteria can occur.

Physical Examination

- Tachypnea and tachycardia may be found.
- A hyperinflated chest may be associated with increased anteroposterior diameter, hyperresonance on percussion, or intercostal retractions.
- Wheezing is often detectable without a stethoscope.
- Wheezing, inspiratory and expiratory crackles, and prolonged expiration are found on auscultation.
- The liver and spleen may be palpable because of a hyperinflated chest.

ETIOLOGY

- RSV is an enveloped RNA paramyxovirus.
- Group A and B organisms often circulate concurrently. The clinical and epidemiologic differences between the two groups and their importance are not clear.

DIAGNOSIS

DIFFERENTIAL DIAGNOSIS

- Broadly, all causes of wheezing must be considered. RSV infection often is difficult to differentiate from asthma, especially if it is the first episode of wheezing.
  - Gastroesophageal reflux with aspiration
  - Foreign body aspiration
  - Vascular rings
  - Congestive heart failure
  - Cystic fibrosis
  - Pertussis or pertussis syndromes
- Bronchiolitis may also be caused by influenza, parainfluenza, adenovirus, and rhinovirus. *Chlamydia* pneumonia can manifest with cough and wheezing with rales.

WORKUP

- Diagnosis is based on a combination of clinical and epidemiologic findings.
- Chest radiographs may not be helpful in distinguishing RSV from other respiratory viral infections or even bacterial causes.

LABORATORY TESTS

- Nasopharyngeal washings or a nasal plus a pharyngeal swab combined in one transport media vial is the most effective means of collecting a sample.
- Viral isolation by culture is the standard, but technical difficulties, cost, and increased time to detection are disadvantages compared with more rapid tests. Sensitivity of viral culture isolation ranges from 60% to 97%, depending on laboratory experience; specificity is almost 100%.
- Direct fluorescent antibody testing of nasal or nasopharyngeal washes or aspirates is the most sensitive rapid method of detecting RSV, but sensitivity depends on laboratory experience.
- Less technical kit immunoassays for rapid diagnosis are available and are commonly used in laboratories. Most assays demonstrate sensitivity between 80% and 90% compared with culture.
- Reverse-transcriptase polymerase chain reaction (RT-PCR) assays have been developed to detect RSV, which in research laboratories appear to be the most sensitive method for detection of RSV in respiratory secretions, but these assays are not widely available for clinical use.

IMAGING STUDIES

Chest radiographs typically show hyperinflation with flattened diaphragms and hyperlucency of the parenchyma, prominent bronchovascular markings, and multiple areas of atelectasis (most commonly in the right upper and middle lobes), which are difficult to differentiate from infiltrates.

TREATMENT

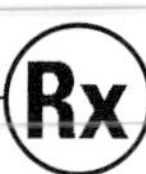

NONPHARMACOLOGIC THERAPY

Oxygen and supportive care with fluid replacement are the mainstays of treatment.

ACUTE GENERAL Rx

- Although used often, bronchodilators, including nebulized epinephrine and β_2-agonists, have not demonstrated consistent effectiveness in many studies.
- Many studies have not demonstrated benefit from oral, inhaled, or parenteral corticosteroids for first-time wheezers.
- Ribavirin is the only specific treatment approved for use in children hospitalized with RSV infection. Use of ribavirin is controversial because of its high cost in association with conflicting effectiveness in some outcome measures, such as length of hospitalization.

DISPOSITION

- Mortality rates for hospitalized patients range from 1% to 3%, although the rate increases for patients who have underlying cardiac, pulmonary, or immunodeficient conditions.
- RSV infection, especially in infants who are hospitalized with lower respiratory tract disease, is associated with subsequent recurrent wheezing or other respiratory problems; it is not necessarily causal.
- Reasons for this association are not clear but likely multifactorial, including atopic predisposition, genetic susceptibility to airway responsiveness, and perhaps concomitant viral infections or environmental pollutants.

REFERRAL

Severe cases may necessitate referral to a pediatric pulmonologist.

PEARLS & CONSIDERATIONS

COMMENTS

- Auscultatory examination findings change throughout the episode.
- Apnea occurs early or at onset of the disease process.
- Secondary bacterial infections rarely occur (1.2%).
- Reinfection can occur within the same season.

PREVENTION

- Eliminate exposure to cigarette smoke.
- Decrease exposure to settings where RSV or other respiratory viruses may be transmitted (e.g., child care centers, large crowds).
- Emphasize hand hygiene, especially in a household with older siblings.
- Immunize infants at 6 months for influenza.
- For certain high-risk patients, two immunoprophylaxis options are available that decrease hospitalization rates but do not

significantly decrease mortality rates. (Refer to the suggested reading of American Academy of Pediatrics policy statement for details on indications of immunoprophylaxis use.)

- RSV immune globulin intravenous (IGIV, RespiGam) is a polyclonal hyperimmune globulin from donors with high serum titers of RSV-neutralizing antibody.
- Palivizumab (Synagis) is a humanized murine monoclonal antibody with neutralizing and fusion inhibitory activity against RSV. Palivizumab is preferred over RSV IGIV because of easier administration, safety, and effectiveness.
- Immunoprophylaxis should be considered for children at least 2 years old who have chronic lung disease needing medical therapy.
- Immunoprophylaxis may benefit infants of 32 weeks' gestation who do not have chronic lung disease and infants of 32 to 35 weeks' gestation who have multiple risk factors for exposure or acquisition of RSV.
- Palivizumab should be considered in 2-year-old infants and children who have hemodynamically significant cyanotic and acyanotic congenital heart disease, depending on the degree of physiologic cardiovascular compromise. Recipients of palivizumab had a 45% decrease in rate of RSV-related hospitalization compared with the placebo group.
- Immunoprophylaxis should be started at the start of RSV season, which is usually the beginning of November in the Northern Hemisphere. The last dose should be given in March, which will provide protection until April. No more than five doses should be given during the entire RSV season.
- Neither RSV IGIV nor palivizumab are effective for treatment of RSV disease.

SUGGESTED READINGS

American Academy of Pediatrics Committee on Infectious Diseases and Committee on Fetus and Newborn Policy Statement: Revised indications for the use of palivizumab and respiratory syncytial virus immune globulin intravenous for the prevention of respiratory syncytial virus infections. *Pediatrics* 112:1442, 2003.

Feltes TM et al: Palivizumab prophylaxis reduces hospitalization due to respiratory syncytial virus in young children with hemodynamically significant congenital heart disease. *J Pediatr* 143:532, 2003.

Hall CB: Respiratory syncytial virus. *In* Feigin RD, Cherry JD (eds): *Textbook of Pediatric Infectious Diseases.* Philadelphia, WB Saunders, 2004, pp 2315–2341.

Hall CB, McCarthy CA: Respiratory syncytial virus. *In* Mandell GL et al (eds): *Principles and Practice of Infectious Diseases.* New York, Churchill Livingstone, 2004, p 155.

Henderson FW et al: Respiratory-syncytial-virus infections, reinfections and immunity. *N Engl J Med* 300:530, 1979.

The Impact-RSV study group: Palivizumab, a humanized respiratory syncytial virus monoclonal antibody, reduces hospitalization from respiratory syncytial virus infection in high-risk infants. *Pediatrics* 102:531, 1998.

Meissner HC et al: Revised indications for the use of palivizumab and respiratory syncytial virus immune globulin intravenous for the prevention of respiratory syncytial virus infections. American Academy of Pediatrics Technical Report. *Pediatrics* 112:1447, 2003.

UpToDate Online. Available at www.utdol.com

AUTHORS: **SHARON F. CHEN, MD** and **CAROLINE B. HALL, MD**

BASIC INFORMATION

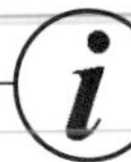

DEFINITION

Retinoblastoma is a malignant tumor of neuroepithelial origin that arises from the embryonic neural retina. It is the most common ocular tumor of childhood.

ICD-9-CM CODE
190.5 Retinoblastoma

EPIDEMIOLOGY & DEMOGRAPHICS

- Retinoblastoma occurs in 1 per 14,000 to 34,000 live births (i.e., 200 to 350 cases per year in the United States).
- Approximately 65% to 80% of cases are unilateral; 20% to 35% are bilateral.
- The median age of detection for bilateral disease is 4.5 months; for unilateral disease, the median age is 22 months.
- Most cases are detected by age 3 years.
- Although only 10% of patients have a family history, 25% to 40% of cases are familial (inherited). There are three possibilities:
  - Parent has retinoblastoma.
  - Parent has the retinoblastoma gene *(RB1)* but is asymptomatic.
  - Parent has new germline mutation of the *RB1* gene.
- The 5-year overall survival rate is approximately 90%, higher for children with local disease and much lower for children with advanced local disease or metastatic disease.

CLINICAL PRESENTATION

History

- Most commonly, parents notice something in the eye (i.e., leukocoria) or notice a "white reflex" in a flash picture.
- Less commonly, the parents describe a "lazy eye" (i.e., esotropia or exotropia).
- Approximately 10% of patients have a family history of retinoblastoma.

Physical Examination

- Leukocoria
- Less often esotropia, orbital inflammation, hyphema, fixed pupil, or heterochromia iridis
- Ophthalmologic examination
  - White-yellow-pink mass with associated tortuous vessels
  - Retinal detachment or vitreous hemorrhage
  - Vitreous seeding of tumor
  - Multifocal, bilateral masses

ETIOLOGY

- All tumors are associated with a mutation in the *RB1* gene, located on chromosome 13q14. The *RB1* gene is a tumor suppressor gene, a gene whose function is to stop cell division.
- Patients with familial retinoblastoma have an inherited mutation in one *RB1* gene and develop retinoblastoma when there is a spontaneous mutation in the second gene of the pair.
- Patients with nonfamilial retinoblastoma develop spontaneous mutations in both *RB1* genes.

DIAGNOSIS

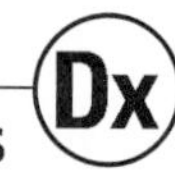

DIFFERENTIAL DIAGNOSIS

- The diagnosis is usually straightforward and can be made based on the ophthalmologic examination findings without a biopsy.
- For a mass, the differential diagnosis includes the following:
  - Hamartoma
  - Granuloma
  - Uveitis
  - Emboli caused by subacute bacterial endocarditis
- For retinal detachment, the differential diagnosis includes the following:
  - Coats' disease
  - Retinopathy of prematurity
  - Persistent hyperplastic vitreous

WORKUP

- Ophthalmologic examination is performed with the patient under anesthesia to assess for vitreous seeding, multifocal disease, bilateral disease.
- Because retinoblastoma is usually confined to the orbits and is essentially a curable disease, the most commonly used staging system is based on the likelihood of saving vision in the affected eye or eyes.
  - Group I (very favorable): single or multiple tumors less than 4 disc diameters (1 disc diameter = 1.5 mm)
  - Group II (favorable): single or multiple tumors 4 to 10 disc diameters
  - Group III (doubtful): any tumor anterior to the equator or single lesion more than 10 disc diameters
  - Group IV (unfavorable): multiple tumors, some more than 10 disc diameters; any tumor extending anterior to the ora serrata
  - Group V (very unfavorable): large tumors involving more than one half of the retina; vitreous seeds
- There is no universal agreement on a system for staging disease beyond orbit. One proposed system is the St. Jude Children's Research Hospital staging system:
  Stage 1: tumor confined to the retina
  Stage 2: tumor confined to globe, involving up to or beyond cut end of optic nerve
  Stage 3: extraocular extension into the central nervous system, including tumor cells in cerebrospinal fluid
  Stage 4: distant metastases
- Adverse prognostic factors include the following:
  - Tumor involvement in optic nerve beyond lamina cribrosa or beyond cut end of optic nerve
  - Tumor involvement in scleral emissaria veins and episcleral tissues
  - Trilateral retinoblastoma (i.e., retinoblastoma plus ectopic retinoblastoma in the pineal region)
  - Distant metastases

LABORATORY TESTS

- Complete blood cell count, differential cell count, platelet count, blood chemistries
- Lumbar puncture (indicated for patients with locally advanced or metastatic disease)
- Bone marrow aspirate and biopsy (indicated for patients with locally advanced or metastatic disease)

IMAGING STUDIES

Head computed tomography or magnetic resonance imaging is used to assess extension of disease through the optic nerve and the presence of a pineal region tumor (i.e., trilateral retinoblastoma).

TREATMENT

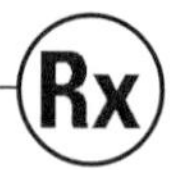

NONPHARMACOLOGIC THERAPY

- The goal of therapy is cure.
- Because the disease is so often localized and curable, a second goal is preservation of vision.
- Enucleation is reserved for the following cases:
  - Unilateral retinoblastoma when the eye is blind
  - Bilateral retinoblastoma when one eye is blind
  - Glaucoma with visual loss
  - Local recurrence uncontrolled by less aggressive measures
- Photocoagulation "burns" vessels around small tumors.
  - This is effective for tumors less than 4.5 mm in diameter.
  - It is not effective when the tumor is near the optic disc, near the macula, or in the vitreous because of the risk of vision loss.
- Cryotherapy is indicated for small tumors anterior to the equator or for recurrences after radiotherapy. It is sometimes given with chemotherapy.
- Radioactive plaque application (i.e., radiation implant) is done for tumors 2 to 16 mm in diameter.
- External beam radiation is indicated for multifocal tumors, tumors too close to the optic nerve or macula, larger tumors, and vitreous seeding. Efforts are being made to avoid or delay radiotherapy (particularly in patients with familial retinoblastoma) because of the risk of a second malignancy.

ACUTE GENERAL Rx

- Chemotherapy is increasingly recognized as an effective adjunct to other approaches. Chemotherapy alone seldom cures this disease.
- Chemotherapy may be an effective adjunct in infants with multifocal disease. It allows for reduction of the tumor size with subsequent use of local therapies and avoidance or delay in external beam radiotherapy.

- Chemotherapy is indicated for children with large tumors in whom there is some hope of preserving vision and for children with metastatic disease.
- Effective agents include carboplatin, VP-16, cyclophosphamide, and vincristine.

DISPOSITION

- Recommended follow-up includes examination under anesthesia periodically over the first 5 years, with decreasing frequency over time.
- Late effects include second malignancies and ocular complications.
- The risk of a second malignancy in children with retinoblastoma is high.
    - Risk is greatest for children with familial retinoblastoma who received external beam radiotherapy.
    - Risk increases with increasing dose of radiation, with younger age at irradiation, and with treatment with cyclophosphamide.
    - Most second malignancies are in the radiation field and include osteosarcoma, fibrosarcoma, and other spindle cell neoplasms.
        - Overall risk of second malignancy with 50 years' follow-up is as high as 50% in cases of familial retinoblastoma; it is only 5% for children with sporadic retinoblastoma.
        - With 40 years' follow-up, there is a 30% mortality rate from second malignancy for patients with familial retinoblastoma who received irradiation (versus 6% for those who did not receive irradiation).
- Ocular complications include increased risk of cataracts, decreased tearing, and orbital bone hypoplasia with external beam irradiation.

REFERRAL

Children with retinoblastoma should be evaluated and treated by an ophthalmologist with experience in treating this disease, and treatment should be done in conjunction with a pediatric oncologist and pediatric radiation oncologist.

PEARLS & CONSIDERATIONS

COMMENTS

- Familial retinoblastoma usually occurs in infants and is usually multifocal and bilateral.
- Although only 10% of children with retinoblastoma have a family history of the disease, another 15% to 30% have inherited disease.
- Children with familial retinoblastoma have an increased risk of ectopic pineal region retinoblastoma (i.e., trilateral retinoblastoma).

PREVENTION

- An infant with a family history of retinoblastoma should undergo periodic screening ophthalmologic examinations under anesthesia to look for retinoblastoma.
- Infants and children with retinoblastoma should continue to undergo screening examinations under anesthesia to look for recurrent or new lesions.
- Genetic counseling should be a part of the evaluation of the families of children with retinoblastoma, and siblings should be examined for the disease.

PATIENT/FAMILY EDUCATION

- Retinoblastoma is a very curable disease, and treatment goals are aimed at preservation of vision as well as cure.
- A child can have familial retinoblastoma even without a family history of the disease.
- Children with familial retinoblastoma are at increased risk for second malignancies.
- Parent's Guide to Understanding Retinoblastoma: www.retinoblastoma.com/guide.htm

SUGGESTED READINGS

CancerNet: Retinoblastoma (PDQ) Treatment–Health Professionals. Available at www.cancernet.nci.nih.gov

Halperin EC et al: Retinoblastoma. *In* Halperin EC et al (eds): *Pediatric Radiation Oncology,* 4th ed. Philadelphia, Lippincott Williams & Wilkins, 2004.

Hurwritz RL et al: Retinoblastoma. *In* Pizzo PA (ed): *Principles and Practice of Pediatric Oncology,* 4th ed. Philadelphia, Lippincott Williams & Wilkins, 2002.

AUTHOR: **DAVID N. KORONES, MD**

BASIC INFORMATION

DEFINITION

Retropharyngeal abscesses are deep neck infections involving the retropharyngeal space or the parapharyngeal (lateral pharyngeal) space.

SYNONYMS

Deep neck infections
Parapharyngeal abscesses
  Lateral pharyngeal abscess
  Pharyngomaxillary abscess
  Pterygomaxillary abscess
Pharyngeal space abscess
Retropharyngeal abscesses
  Posterior visceral space abscess
  Retroesophageal space abscess
  Retrovisceral space abscess

ICD-9-CM CODES
478.24 Abscess, lateral pharyngeal
478.25 Abscess, retropharyngeal

EPIDEMIOLOGY & DEMOGRAPHICS

- Retropharyngeal infections are at least 10-fold more common in children than parapharyngeal (lateral pharyngeal) infections.
- Limited data suggest that the frequency of retropharyngeal space infections may be increasing.
- Because the retropharyngeal nodes tend to atrophy with age, retropharyngeal abscesses primarily occur in young children.
  - In one review, 75% of the patients were younger than 5 years, and the median age was 36 months.
  - Other studies indicate that approximately 55% of infections occur in children younger than age 2 years, with 35% occurring in those younger than age 1 year.
  - These infections may occur in older children and adults.
- Parapharyngeal (lateral pharyngeal) infections are most likely to occur in older children, adolescents, and adults.

CLINICAL PRESENTATION

History

- With both retropharyngeal and parapharyngeal space infections, there is often a history of a preceding upper respiratory tract infection.
- Children with infection in the retropharyngeal space may present with:
  - Fever
  - Restlessness
  - Limited motion of the neck
  - Neck posturing or stiffness
  - Sore throat
  - Poor oral intake
  - Dysphagia or pain on swallowing
  - Drooling
  - Dyspnea
  - Muffled speech and cry
  - Stridor (relatively uncommon)
- Children with parapharyngeal space infections often have many of the same symptoms as those with retropharyngeal space infections.

Physical Examination

- Children with a retropharyngeal space infection may demonstrate these findings:
  - Fever
  - Pain or stiffness with active or passive movement of the neck
  - Torticollis
  - Midline or unilateral swelling of the posterior pharynx
  - Evidence of pharyngitis
  - Ipsilateral, mildly tender cervical adenopathy
  - Evidence of respiratory distress, including tachypnea and stridor
  - Variably toxic appearance
  - Trismus is uncommon, unlike the child with a peritonsillar abscess or cellulitis
- Children with a parapharyngeal infection may have the following:
  - Fever
  - Tender, high cervical mass
  - Perimandibular induration and erythema
  - Medial displacement of the lateral pharyngeal wall and inferior tonsillar pole
  - Drooling
  - Evidence of respiratory distress, including tachypnea and stridor
  - Variable degree of toxicity
- When there is involvement of the anterior (muscular) compartment, there may be trismus from irritation of the internal pterygoid muscle.
- When there is involvement of the posterior compartment, there may be evidence of involvement of some cranial nerves (IX through XII) or the cervical sympathetic chain.
- Evidence of Horner's syndrome (e.g., meiosis, ptosis, ipsilateral anhidrosis of the face, enophthalmos)
- Decreased gag reflex and dysphagia
- Ipsilateral vocal cord paralysis and lingual deviation

ETIOLOGY

- Retropharyngeal space infections in children usually result from suppurative adenitis of lymph nodes in this location.
  - Most patients have had a recent episode of nasopharyngitis, adenoiditis, or otitis media.
  - Other possible sources of infection include traumatic perforation from a foreign body, endotracheal intubation, or endoscopy; dental abscess; petrositis; dental procedures; peritonsillar abscess; vertebral body osteomyelitis; and extension of infection from the parapharyngeal (lateral pharyngeal) space.
- Infections of the parapharyngeal (lateral pharyngeal) space may arise from several sources, including the following:
  - Bacterial pharyngitis
  - Mastoiditis
  - Otitis media
  - Peritonsillar abscess
  - Petrositis
  - Cervical adenitis
  - Infection in the submandibular or parotid salivary glands
  - Infection in the tongue
  - Penetrating trauma
  - Foreign bodies
  - Extension from a retropharyngeal abscess
- Retropharyngeal and parapharyngeal space infections often involve mixed flora with a combination of aerobic and anaerobic bacteria.
- The most common aerobic isolates include α- and γ-hemolytic streptococci, group A β-hemolytic streptococci, and *Staphylococcus aureus.*
- Less common aerobic bacteria isolated include *Haemophilus* species, *Moraxella catarrhalis, Streptococcus pneumoniae, Bartonella henselae,* and members of the Enterobacteriaceae family.
- Prominent anaerobic bacteria isolated include *Bacteroides* species, *Peptostreptococcus* species, and *Fusobacterium* species.
- Rarely, *Mycobacterium tuberculosis,* the atypical mycobacteria, or fungi have been linked to these infections.

DIAGNOSIS

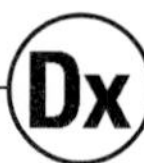

DIFFERENTIAL DIAGNOSIS

- Retropharyngeal space and parapharyngeal space infections must be distinguished from the following:
  - Cervical lymphadenitis
  - Peritonsillar abscess
  - Viral laryngotracheobronchitis (i.e., croup)
  - Bacterial tracheitis
  - Epiglottitis
  - Prevertebral abscess
  - Each other

LABORATORY TESTS

- The white blood cell count is usually elevated, with a predominance of polymorphonuclear leukocytes.
- Blood cultures are rarely positive.
- Gram stain and aerobic and anaerobic cultures should be done on any material obtained at the time of needle aspiration or incision and drainage.

IMAGING STUDIES

- Computed tomography (CT) of the neck, with or without administration of a contrast agent, has become the imaging study of choice for patients suspected of having a deep neck infection. Its advantages over conventional radiography include the following:

- Ease of interpretation in the presence of normal variation in the appearance of the soft tissues of the neck with neck position and phases of respiration
- Accurate determination of the extent of the infection, including involvement of adjacent spaces
- Visualization of vascular structures to detect potential complications (e.g., venous thrombosis)
- Potential differentiation of cellulitis from abscess
  - Abscess formation is suggested by the presence of a low-attenuation homogeneous area surrounded by ring enhancement with contrast agent.
  - The ability of CT to predict the presence of pus at surgery or aspiration has a false-negative rate of 13% and false-positive rate of 10%.

- Conventional anteroposterior (AP) and lateral radiographs of the neck, if done, should be taken in true lateral position for the lateral film, with the neck in extension and during full inspiration.
  - In retropharyngeal space infections, the lateral neck radiograph may demonstrate the following:
    - Increased thickness of the prevertebral soft tissues exceeding the AP diameter of the contiguous vertebral bodies or thickening of the retropharyngeal space (at C2) of more than 7 mm or the retrotracheal space (at C6) of more than 14 mm
    - Presence of air or an air-fluid level in the soft tissues
    - Loss or reversal of the normal cervical lordotic curvature
    - Presence of a foreign body
  - In parapharyngeal space infections, the AP and lateral neck radiographs may also reveal ipsilateral pharyngeal fullness and obliteration of the pyriform sinus.

TREATMENT

Rx

NONPHARMACOLOGIC THERAPY

- Patients with deep neck infections must be monitored carefully for the development of respiratory distress from upper airway obstruction.
- If significant respiratory distress develops, the patient should be transferred to a pediatric intensive care unit, and an otolaryngologist experienced in the management of these infections should be consulted if consultation was not obtained earlier.
- Endotracheal intubation to secure the airway may occasionally be necessary pending incision and drainage of an abscess in the operating room.
- Previously, 10% to 25% of patients with retropharyngeal and parapharyngeal infections were thought to be cured with medical (antibiotic) therapy alone, but it is now recognized that many (most in some studies) with these infections, including those who have abscesses identified by CT scan, will respond to antibiotic therapy alone.
- Patients who have CT scan findings consistent with cellulitis, without abscess formation, almost always respond to empirical antibiotic therapy directed against the usual pathogens. Needle aspiration can be performed in an effort to recover the etiologic agent, but it is not essential and usually not done.
- Patients who appear to have an abscess by CT scan and who have significant respiratory compromise, hemorrhage, subcutaneous emphysema, or cranial nerve involvement should be taken to the operating room to secure the airway, if not done earlier, and undergo incision and drainage of the abscess.
- Patients who appear to have an abscess by CT scan but do not have significant respiratory compromise, hemorrhage, subcutaneous emphysema, or cranial involvement can be managed in two ways:
  - Needle aspiration is safer in a patient with a parapharyngeal (lateral pharyngeal) abscess than in one with an abscess in the retropharyngeal location.
    - Parenteral antibiotic therapy is administered, and the patient's response to therapy can be assessed clinically, with or without follow-up CT scans.
    - If an unsatisfactory response occurs, repeat needle aspiration or, more commonly, incision and drainage can be performed.
  - Empirical antibiotic therapy is directed against the most likely pathogens, and the patient is monitored with or without a follow-up CT scan.
    - Obtaining a follow-up CT scan is not essential if the patient is improving clinically.
    - If no improvement occurs in 48 hours or if there is progression of infection, a drainage procedure is mandatory.
    - The second approach is favored by most with experience in managing these infections.
- Patients with retropharyngeal abscesses who require surgical drainage can usually have the procedure done with a transoral approach.
  - Some patients may need drainage by an external approach if there is extension laterally toward the great vessels or if insufficient improvement occurs after an initial transoral approach.
  - Patients with lateral pharyngeal abscesses who require surgical drainage usually have the procedure done with an external approach.

ACUTE GENERAL Rx

- Empirical antibiotic therapy of deep neck infections is directed at the usual offending pathogens.
- If aspiration or incision and drainage become necessary, antimicrobial therapy can be altered on the basis of results of the Gram stain, as well as aerobic and anaerobic bacterial cultures of abscess contents.
- Combination of ampicillin and the β-lactamase inhibitor sulbactam (Unasyn) is considered the regimen of choice.
- Clindamycin is an acceptable alternative in penicillin-allergic patients.
  - *Staphylococcus aureus* may demonstrate inducible resistance to clindamycin.
  - Clindamycin is not active against gram-negative aerobic bacteria, which are occasionally isolated.
- An alternative antibiotic regimen includes an expanded-spectrum cephalosporin combined with an agent effective against anaerobes, such as clindamycin or metronidazole.
- Antimicrobial therapy is given intravenously.
  - After sufficient improvement, a change to a suitable oral agent is reasonable.
  - For patients who have been treated with ampicillin-sulbactam (Unasyn), amoxicillin-clavulanate (Augmentin) is usually used.
- Therapy is usually continued for 10 to 14 days, with hospitalization recommended until the patient's condition has improved sufficiently that oral antibiotic therapy can be initiated.

DISPOSITION

- Patients require close follow-up after therapy is instituted to assess whether they are responding adequately. This is particularly true for patients who are initially managed medically, without surgical intervention. If improvement is not seen within 48 hours or if infection progresses, a drainage procedure is indicated.
- Patients should be monitored closely for the development of one or more of the potentially serious complications of deep neck infections, including the following:
  - Severe upper airway obstruction resulting in significant respiratory distress
  - Rupture of the abscess into the pharynx or trachea, resulting in asphyxiation, empyema, or lung abscess
  - Suppurative descending mediastinitis
  - Thrombophlebitis with thrombosis of the internal jugular vein
  - Erosion of the carotid or vertebral arteries, resulting in hemorrhage
  - Palsies of cranial nerves VI, IX, X, XI, or XII
  - Horner's syndrome
  - Septic pulmonary emboli

REFERRAL

- In view of the potential for airway compromise and other serious complications of deep neck infections, patients with these infections should be hospitalized at facilities where they can be monitored closely and complications are appropriately handled.

- Patients require ready access to a pediatric intensive care unit and to an infectious disease specialist and an otolaryngologist experienced in the medical and surgical management of these infections.

PEARLS & CONSIDERATIONS

COMMENTS

- A deep neck infection should be considered in a child with a preceding upper respiratory infection or oral or neck trauma who develops fever, irritability, limited motion of the neck, torticollis, dysphagia, drooling, dyspnea, muffled speech or cry, stridor, neck swelling, or displacement of the posterior or lateral pharyngeal wall.
- CT of the neck has evolved as the imaging modality of choice in assessing these infections.
- Patients should be hospitalized and receive parenteral antibiotic therapy initially; some patients require surgical drainage, but most respond to antibiotic therapy alone.

PATIENT/FAMILY EDUCATION

Patients and their families should be informed about the seriousness of these infections, the need for close monitoring after antibiotic therapy is initiated, and the potential need for surgical drainage.

SUGGESTED READINGS

Broughton RA: Nonsurgical management of deep neck infections in children. *Pediatr Infect Dis J* 11:14, 1992.

Craig FW, Schunk JE: Retropharyngeal abscess in children: clinical presentation, utility of imaging, and current management. *Pediatrics* 111:1394, 2003.

Goldstein NA, Hammerschlag MR: Peritonsillar, retropharyngeal, and parapharyngeal abscesses. *In* Feigin RD et al (eds): *Textbook of Pediatric Infectious Diseases,* 5th ed. New York, WB Saunders, 2004, pp 178–185.

Lalakea M, Messner AH: Retropharyngeal abscess management in children: current practices. *Otolaryngol Head Neck Surg* 121:398, 1999.

Lee SS et al: Retropharyngeal abscess: epiglottitis of the new millennium. *J Pediatr* 138:435, 2001.

McClay JE et al: Intravenous antibiotic therapy for deep neck abscesses defined by computed tomography. *Arch Otolaryngol Head Neck Surg* 129:1207, 2003.

Sichel JY et al: Nonsurgical management of parapharyngeal space infections: a prospective study. *Laryngoscope* 112:906, 2002.

AUTHOR: **ROBERT A. BROUGHTON, MD**

BASIC INFORMATION

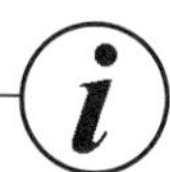

DEFINITION

Rhabdomyolysis results from skeletal muscle cell injury or cell death with release of the intracellular contents into the circulation. Rhabdomyolysis is caused by a variety of factors, and severity ranges from asymptomatic elevations of muscle enzymes to life-threatening cases involving extreme enzyme elevation, electrolyte abnormalities and acute renal failure. Increased serum intracellular contents such as myoglobin, creatinine kinase (CK), potassium, phosphorus, aspartate transaminase, uric acid, and lactate dehydrogenase (LDH) serve as clinical markers for the syndrome. The classic triad of muscle weakness, myalgias, and darkened urine may be present in severe cases.

SYNONYMS

Meyer-Betz disease

Myoglobinuria (much less descriptive for the clinical syndrome)

ICD-9-CM CODE

728.88 Rhabdomyolysis

EPIDEMIOLOGY & DEMOGRAPHICS

- Incidence in childhood is unknown.
- Rhabdomyolysis affects about 1 in 10,000 people in the United States, with a slightly greater incidence among men.
- Among adults presenting with acute renal failure, 8% to 15% of cases were attributed to rhabdomyolysis.

CLINICAL PRESENTATION

- Localized or diffuse myalgias (in 50%)
- Focal muscle weakness (with severe muscle damage)
- Red- or tea-colored urine
  - It may be caused by myoglobinuria.
  - It is an inconsistent finding because it may resolve by the time of presentation, even with persistent CK elevation.
- Renal failure causes; volume depletion; renal ischemia; tubular obstruction (i.e., pigment casts); tubular injury (i.e., toxicity of the breakdown product of myoglobin, ferriheme, which is accentuated by acidic urine)

ETIOLOGY

- Damage to muscle cell and membrane results in liberation of intracellular contents.
- Many causes exist, including the following:
  - Trauma: blunt trauma, electrical injury, burns, prolonged immobilization
  - Exercise: induction of the syndrome by strenuous exercise
  - Toxins (46% to 80% of cases): alcohol, drugs of abuse, medications (e.g., statins), envenomation
  - Metabolic causes: inborn disorders affecting carbohydrate or lipid metabolism, thyroid dysfunction, diabetic ketoacidosis, electrolyte abnormalities
  - Infections: influenza, human immunodeficiency virus (HIV), herpes simplex virus (HSV), many other viruses and bacterial infections
  - Environmental causes: hyperthermia, hypothermia
  - Muscle abnormalities: myopathies, polymyositis, dermatomyositis

DIAGNOSIS

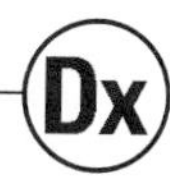

DIFFERENTIAL DIAGNOSIS

- A significant overlap exists between the cause and the differential diagnosis.
  - Autoimmunity: polymyositis, dermatomyositis
  - Genetic disorders: muscular dystrophies, abnormal carbohydrate or lipid metabolism
  - Infection: pyomyositis, abscess

LABORATORY TESTS

- An abnormal serum CK level is considered the gold standard for diagnosis.
  - This test is the most sensitive marker of myocyte injury.
  - CK-MM fraction accounts for at least 95% of elevated CK levels; CK-MB fraction accounts for the remainder.
  - Some sources suggest that five times the normal level of CK is required for diagnosis.
  - Conflicting data exist about whether CK levels correlate with disease severity.
- Urinalysis with microscopy reveals tea-colored urine.
  - Dipstick is positive for blood.
  - No (or few) red blood cells (RBCs) are seen on microscopic evaluation.
  - Muddy casts are also seen.
- Serum electrolytes may reveal an anion-gap metabolic acidosis, hyperkalemia, hypocalcemia, hyperphosphatemia, and elevated blood urea nitrogen (BUN) and creatinine levels.
- Serum and urine myoglobin levels are not reliable markers for diagnosis because of rapid clearance of myoglobin from plasma and poor correlation of myoglobinuria with myoglobinemia. Fifty percent of patients with rhabdomyolysis have myoglobinuria.
- Further studies are guided by the workup for the specific cause.

IMAGING STUDIES

Magnetic resonance imaging may be useful for the diagnosis; it has 90% to 95% sensitivity.

TREATMENT

ACUTE GENERAL Rx

- Treat the underlying disease.
- Treat electrolyte abnormalities.
- Prevent or manage acute renal failure.
  - Early aggressive therapy appears to lower the risk of complications.
  - Administer intravenous fluids (e.g., saline) at a rate to maintain high urine output to ensure sufficient flow to the kidneys.
- The suggested intravenous rates are 100 to 300 mL/hr in adults (i.e., one to two times maintenance).
  - Some suggest administration of sodium bicarbonate to maintain a urine pH higher than 6.5.
  - Consider dialysis for patients who do not respond to fluid therapy and for those in renal failure.
- Damaged muscles are at risk for capillary leak with secondary third-spacing and potential compartment syndrome.

DISPOSITION

- After renal function has normalized and the underlying cause has been addressed, the patient can be discharged.
- Patients with exercise-induced rhabdomyolysis should be counseled against vigorous exercise.
- Patients with alcohol or drug-induced rhabdomyolysis should be counseled against the use of alcohol or drugs; etiologic medications should be discontinued.

REFERRAL

Referral to a nephrologist is indicated for any evidence of renal failure.

PEARLS & CONSIDERATIONS

COMMENTS

- The classic triad of muscle weakness, myalgias, and darkened urine is *not* present in most patients, especially early in the disease.
- CK is present in the serum immediately after muscle injury and peaks within 36 to 48 hours.
- Myoglobinuria occurs only in the presence of rhabdomyolysis, but rhabdomyolysis may occur without detectable myoglobin in the urine.
- The urine may be tea-colored, with a dipstick positive for blood but few RBCs.
- Acute renal failure is the primary determinant of morbidity and mortality.
- The serum creatinine level is elevated to a greater extent than BUN because of creatinine release from injured muscle.
- Levels of CK, phosphate, albumin, and potassium or the presence of sepsis or hypotension may have some value as a predictive tool for renal failure.
- Suspect rhabdomyolysis in any patient with a history of prolonged immobilization or unconsciousness.

PREVENTION

For those with underlying known predisposition, avoid precipitants.

SUGGESTED READINGS

Coco TJ, Klasner AE: Drug-induced rhabdomyolysis. *Curr Opin Pediatr* 16:206, 2004.

Melli G et al: Rhabdomyolysis: an evaluation of 475 hospitalized patients. *Medicine (Baltimore)* 84:377, 2005.

Miller ML: Rhabdomyolysis. *In* Rose BD (ed): *UpToDate.* Waltham, MA, 13.3, 2006.

Russell TA: Acute renal failure related to rhabdomyolysis: pathophysiology, diagnosis and collaborative management. *Nephrol Nurs J* 32:409, 2005.

AUTHOR: **SUSANNE E. TANSKI, MD**

BASIC INFORMATION

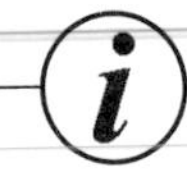

DEFINITION

Rhabdomyosarcoma is a neoplasm derived from primitive mesenchymal cells of striated muscle lineage. It may occur anywhere in the body, including sites that do not normally contain striated muscle.

SYNONYMS

RMS
Soft tissue sarcomas

ICD-9-CM CODE

171.9 Rhabdomyosarcoma

EPIDEMIOLOGY & DEMOGRAPHICS

- Rhabdomyosarcoma is the most common soft tissue sarcoma.
- It accounts for 3.5% of malignancies in children younger than 15 years and 2% of cancers in adolescents 15 to 19 years old.
- The incidence is approximately 4 or 5 cases per year per 1 million children younger than 20 years.
- Approximately 350 new cases are diagnosed each year in the United States.
- Incidence among males is greater than that among females.
- Incidence among blacks and Asians is less than among whites.
- Approximately 60% to 70% of patients are younger than 10 years; a second smaller incidence peak occurs in early to middle adolescence.

CLINICAL PRESENTATION

History

- Approximately 35% of rhabdomyosarcomas arise in the head and neck region, 24% in the genitourinary tract, 19% in extremities, and the remainder in truncal and other sites.
- A mass or swelling develops, with or without pain, or a disturbance of normal body function occurs because of the presence of a mass (e.g., bowel or bladder dysfunction).
- Orbital masses usually manifest with proptosis, limited eye movement, or diplopia.
- Nasopharyngeal tumors often manifest with nasal discharge, which may be bloody.
- Bladder tumors may manifest with hematuria or difficulty voiding.
- Tumors of the female genital tract may manifest with vaginal discharge or extrusion of tumor.
- Tumors in parameningeal sites with central nervous system extension may manifest with cranial nerve palsies or with headache and vomiting.
- Systemic complaints such as fatigue or weight loss may occur.

Physical Examination

- A mass may be palpable; it is usually firm with indistinct margins.
- The mass may be tender or nontender.
- No mass may be apparent on examination.
- Examination may reveal only signs as described in the history (e.g., proptosis, limited extraocular movements, cranial nerve palsies).
- Lymphadenopathy may be palpable if rhabdomyosarcoma has metastasized to lymph nodes.
- Tenderness may be elicited in sites of bony metastases.

ETIOLOGY

- Most cases of rhabdomyosarcoma are sporadic.
- No environmental risk factors have been identified.
- Rhabdomyosarcoma is associated with neurofibromatosis, Beckwith-Wiedemann syndrome, and Li-Fraumeni syndrome.
- Insulin-like growth factor II may play a role in pathogenesis.
- Molecular lesion may involve lack of activity of MyoD family of proteins, which function to commit mesenchymal cells to a skeletal muscle lineage.

DIAGNOSIS

Dx

DIFFERENTIAL DIAGNOSIS

- Other malignancies
  - Other soft tissue sarcomas
  - Other round blue cell tumors, which include neuroblastoma, lymphoma, and Ewing's sarcoma family of tumors
  - Wilms' tumor
  - Germ cell tumors
- Trauma
- Benign tumors
- Infection manifesting with signs, symptoms, or mass lesions similar to rhabdomyosarcoma

WORKUP

- Biopsy of a mass is done after appropriate radiologic evaluation.
- Sampling of regional lymph nodes is required for paratesticular and extremity lesions and may be indicated for other locations.
- Pathologic examination includes the following:
  - Embryonal type: more than 50% of cases, more likely in genitourinary sites and orbital sites, more common in younger children. Botryoid tumors are polypoid variants. A characteristic loss of heterozygosity is seen at 11p15.
  - Alveolar type: 25% of cases; more often in extremity and trunk primaries, and more common in adolescent patients. Characteristic chromosomal translocations include t(2;13) and t(1;13).
  - Undifferentiated sarcomas express no lineage markers and are traditionally treated with rhabdomyosarcoma regimens.
- Staging includes the following guidelines:
  - Stage 1 to 4 is determined by clinical and radiologic evaluation, based on location with favorable and unfavorable sites, size of primary greater or less than 5 cm, evidence of lymph node involvement, and presence or absence of metastases.
  - Orbital, head and neck except parameningeal, and nonbladder, nonprostate genitourinary sites are favorable sites.
- Grouping is done for surgical assignment and based on extent of resection.
  - Group I: completely resected tumor
  - Group II: microscopic residual disease at the margins of the tumor or in regional lymph nodes
  - Group III: unresectable or incompletely resected tumor with gross residual disease
  - Group IV: metastatic disease

LABORATORY TESTS

- No diagnostic laboratory test is available.
- Baseline complete blood cell count and chemistries, including renal and liver function tests, should be obtained.

IMAGING STUDIES

- Computed tomography (CT) or magnetic resonance imaging (MRI) for the primary tumor
- Metastatic evaluation
  - Chest CT
  - Skeletal survey
  - Bone scan
  - Bilateral bone marrow aspirates and biopsies
  - Cerebrospinal fluid cytology for parameningeal tumors
  - Regional lymph node imaging for paratesticular and extremity tumors

TREATMENT

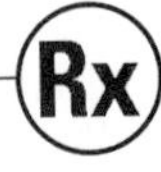

NONPHARMACOLOGIC THERAPY

- Radiation therapy is indicated for patients with group II to IV tumors with embryonal histology and group I to IV tumors with alveolar histology. New methods of radiation therapy may be indicated to minimize late effects on surrounding normal tissue.
- Surgical resection should be performed if possible, but the cosmetic result and function need to be considered in assessing resectability. Fewer than 20% of patients have tumors that can be completely excised with disease-negative margins.

ACUTE GENERAL Rx

- Chemotherapy includes the following:
  - Vincristine and actinomycin D for lower-risk disease, with cyclophosphamide added for higher-risk disease.
  - Other active agents include ifosfamide, VP-16, doxorubicin, topotecan, and irinotecan. Studies are focusing on the benefit of topotecan and irinotecan added to front-line therapy.

- Targeted therapies and other new agents are being investigated for high-risk and relapsed disease.
- A role for high-dose therapy with autologous peripheral blood stem cell rescue in metastatic or recurrent disease has not been defined but continues to be studied.

DISPOSITION

- Prognostic factors include age, stage, group, and histology.
- Patients with low-risk disease, including group I or II and group III, stage 1 embryonal histology have the best outcome, with an 88% survival rate at 3 years.
- Patients with intermediate-risk disease, including group I to III alveolar histology; group III, stage 2 or 3; or group IV and age younger than 10 years, have a 55% to 76% survival rate at 3 years.
- Other patients with group IV metastatic disease continue to fare poorly, with a 20% rate of 3-year survival.
- More than 80% of patients who relapse have a poor prognosis. Patients with initial stage 1 and group I tumors with embryonal histology and local relapse have the best potential for cure. Relapses after 5 years are rare.
- CT or MRI of the primary tumor site is generally performed every 3 months during the first year off therapy and then repeated at increasing intervals. Surveillance chest CT and bone scans are performed on the same schedule.
- Late effects of irradiation depend on the radiation field and surgical intervention, but they may include the following:
  - Hypoplasia of the radiated bone or soft tissue
  - Linear growth impairment
  - Growth hormone deficiency
  - Bowel or bladder dysfunction
  - Infertility; sexual and reproductive dysfunction
  - Second malignancies, including skin, thyroid, brain, bone, and breast tumors
- Late effects of chemotherapy usually result from cyclophosphamide and may include the following:
  - Infertility
  - Renal tubular dysfunction
  - Secondary malignancies, including leukemia and bladder cancer

REFERRAL

- Patients should be referred to pediatric specialists, including pediatric surgeons, pediatric oncologists, and pediatric radiation therapists.
- Patients should ideally be cared for at institutions that enroll patients in cooperative group protocols.

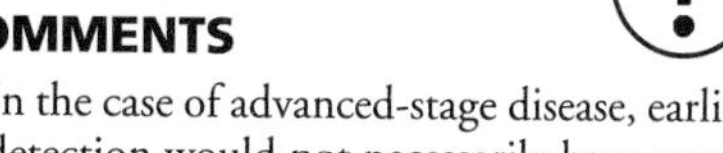

PEARLS & CONSIDERATIONS

COMMENTS

- In the case of advanced-stage disease, earlier detection would not necessarily have correlated with lower-stage disease.
- Malignancy should be considered in the differential diagnosis of usually benign conditions such as epistaxis, chronic sinusitis or otitis, and persistent pain.
- Boys should be encouraged from an early age to report any change in testes.
- Patients at the highest risk for developing secondary malignancies are those with neurofibromatosis or a family history of cancer.

PATIENT/FAMILY EDUCATION

- Although difficult, the benefits of chemotherapy, radiation therapy, and surgery are significant.
- Pediatric oncologists can refer patients and parents to local or national support organizations for children with cancer and their families. National organizations include the American Cancer Society and CureSearch, a component of the Children's Oncology Group.
- More information is available on the Internet (www.curesearch.org; www.cancer.org).

SUGGESTED READINGS

Friedmann AM et al: Rhabdomyosarcoma. *In* Halperin EC et al (eds): *Pediatric Radiation Oncology,* 4th ed. Philadelphia, Lippincott Williams & Wilkins, 2004, pp 319–346.

Meyer WH, Spunt SL: Soft tissue sarcomas of childhood. *Cancer Treat Rev* 30:269, 2004.

Wexler LH et al: Rhabdomyosarcoma and the undifferentiated sarcomas. *In* Pizzo PA, Poplack DG (eds): *Principles and Practice of Pediatric Oncology.* Philadelphia, Lippincott Williams & Wilkins, 2002, pp 939–971.

AUTHOR: **ANDREA S. HINKLE, MD**

BASIC INFORMATION

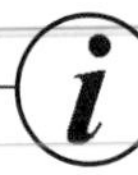

DEFINITION

Rheumatic fever is an acute, noninfectious, inflammatory sequela to a virulent group A β-hemolytic streptococcal pharyngitis, with joint, skin, subcutaneous, and cardiac symptoms appearing 2 to 3 weeks after infection. Neurologic symptoms of choreoathetosis are generally delayed by weeks to months.

ICD-9-CM CODES
390 Acute rheumatic fever (ARF)
391 Acute rheumatic fever with carditis
392 Rheumatic (Sydenham's) chorea

EPIDEMIOLOGY & DEMOGRAPHICS

- Rheumatic fever was formerly epidemic in inner-city, crowded, lower-class neighborhoods. Now it is sporadic, clinically milder, and more common in middle class, suburban, and rural areas. The reasons for the change are not known.
- Rheumatic fever was formerly more severe. It now occurs with fewer joints involved, less severe carditis clinically, but more valve involvement as determined by echocardiography. It is difficult to interpret these finding in view of the introduction of the echocardiogram.
- Five percent of children with ARF are younger than 5 years.

CLINICAL PRESENTATION

- Modified Jones criteria are used for the diagnosis. The clinical diagnosis of ARF requires two major criteria or one major criteria plus two minor criteria as well as evidence of a recent streptococcal infection.
- Major criteria
  - Arthritis
    - Abrupt onset of hot, red, swollen, very tender middle-sized joints
    - Involvement of elbows, wrists, knees, and ankles
    - Less common involvement of other joints
    - Arthritis typically multiple and migratory individual joints resolve without residual in 24 hours as other joints are affected
    - More common in young children
  - Carditis
    - Mitral valve involvement is most common.
      - Acute annular valvulitis with dilation leading to mitral insufficiency or regurgitation
      - Pansystolic, pure-toned, high-pitched murmur at the apex
      - Accentuated by maneuvers that increase systemic vascular resistance, such as hand grip or squat
      - Important not to confuse with normal vibratory (Still's) murmur (i.e., early and midsystolic; musical and low-pitched with multiple overtones; heard at the lower left sternal border)
    - Aortic insufficiency is the second most common cardiac abnormality.
      - Early diastolic, high-pitched murmur with a metallic echoing quality over the middle sternum to the middle to lower left sternal border
      - Important not to confuse with the diastolic component of a venous hum (i.e., more hollow; heard below the right clavicle; completely eradicated by maneuvers that affect venous inflow, such as change in head position, lying supine, jugular vein distention)
    - Severe degrees of mitral or aortic regurgitation may lead to left-sided congestive heart failure.
    - Tricuspid or pulmonic valve involvement is rare.
    - Pericarditis is not encountered in the absence of valvular dysfunction.
  - Chorea
    - A progressive increase in uncontrolled and uncontrollable writhing and choreiform movements (i.e., St. Vitus dance)
      - Particularly involves the extremities
      - Facial grimacing or truncal choreiform movements also seen
      - Progressive clumsiness
    - Irritability and mood swings
    - Prolonged course of weeks to months
    - Eventual resolution without neurologic residual effects
  - Erythema marginatum
    - Evanescent, migratory, reasonably symmetric, smoothly irregular rash
    - Primarily over the trunk and proximal extremities
    - Pale pink borders and clear centers
    - More commonly observed in young children but almost never occurs without carditis or arthritis
    - Considered diagnostic for acute rheumatic fever
  - Subcutaneous nodules
    - Small, lentil-sized, nontender nodules beneath the skin
    - Found on extensor surfaces of joints and occiput
    - Almost never occurs in the absence of carditis
    - Alone, do not establish the diagnosis of rheumatic fever
- Minor criteria
  - Arthralgia: similar to arthritis except without objective findings of inflammation
  - Fever: moderate
  - Family history: usually positive for another family member with acute rheumatic fever

ETIOLOGY

- Follows group A β-hemolytic streptococcal pharyngitis
- Genetic component present
- Specific pathologic pathway unknown

DIAGNOSIS

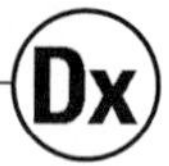

DIFFERENTIAL DIAGNOSIS

- Rash
  - Urticaria
  - Viral exanthems
  - Serum sickness
  - Acute streptococcal infection
  - Staphylococcal scalded skin syndrome
  - Toxic shock syndrome
- Arthritis and arthralgias
  - Septic joint
  - Juvenile rheumatoid arthritis
  - Serum sickness
  - Any collagen vascular disease
  - Postviral arthritis
- Cardiac findings
  - Cardiomyopathy
  - Myocarditis, endocarditis
  - Congenital valve abnormalities
  - Systemic lupus erythematosus

LABORATORY TESTS

- Laboratory data
  - White blood cell (WBC) count: moderate elevation to 12,000 to 18,000 cells/mm^3, with little if any left shift
  - Erythrocyte sedimentation rate (Westergren method): elevated
    - Without carditis, 60 to 80 mm/hr
    - With carditis, more than 100 mm/hr
  - Evidence of a preceding virulent streptococcal pharyngitis required for diagnosis
    - Elevated antistreptolysin O (ASO) titer or elevated streptozyme level
    - Positive throat culture
    - Positive culture in a sibling helpful
- Electrocardiogram
  - Tachycardia
  - Loss of sinus arrhythmia with carditis
  - Prolonged PR interval: indicative of vagus nerve involvement, not carditis
  - Left atrial or left ventricular enlargement

IMAGING STUDIES

- Chest radiograph
  - Usually normal
  - If significant carditis, evidence of left atrial and left ventricular dilation
  - May show pulmonary venous congestion
- Echocardiography
  - Useful for confirming valve leak and assessing significance
    - Holosystolic for mitral regurgitation
    - Holodiastolic for aortic regurgitation if used to establish the diagnosis
    - Mild echocardiographic valvular insufficiency: may be normal
  - Left ventricular size
  - Myocardial function

- Difficult to assess minimal degrees of valve dysfunction

TREATMENT

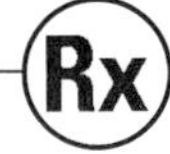

NONPHARMACOLOGIC THERAPY

- Bed rest, formerly considered essential, should probably be continued during the period of acute inflammation.
  - Improves comfort of patients with arthritis
  - Decreases cardiac demands in patients with carditis

ACUTE GENERAL Rx

- A full therapeutic course of an antistreptococcal antibiotic should be administered to eradicate any remaining streptococci.
  - Oral penicillin V
    - Children: 250 mg two to three times daily for 10 days
    - Adolescents and adults: 500 mg two to three times daily for 10 days
  - Benzathine penicillin (one dose intramuscularly)
    - The dose is 600,000 units for children who weigh less than 60 pounds
    - The dose is 1.2 million units for children who weigh more than 60 pounds
- Anti-inflammatory therapy with aspirin (100 mg/kg/day), divided in four doses, may be given.
  - This is adequate therapy for all except patients with severe carditis.
  - Therapy is continued until signs of active inflammation have disappeared.
  - Decrease dosage if needed to avoid symptoms of abdominal pain or tinnitus.
- Patients with severe or life-threatening carditis and congestive heart failure should be treated with prednisone (2 mg/kg/day, divided in four doses) and conventional treatment for heart failure (see Congestive Heart Failure in Diseases and Disorders [Section I]).

CHRONIC Rx

- All patients who have had acute rheumatic fever should receive antistreptococcal prophylaxis.
  - No carditis with initial episode: prophylaxis for 5 years or until age 21 years
  - Carditis with no residual heart disease: prophylaxis into adulthood or at least 10 years
  - Both groups need careful throat culturing and treatment for any sore throat and fever.
  - Carditis with residual heart disease: prophylaxis at least until age 40, possibly lifelong
- Consider the choice of antistreptococcal prophylactic regimens:
  - Intramuscular benzathine penicillin: 1.2 million units monthly
    - Excellent antistreptococcal protection
    - Therapeutic for acquired infection
    - Painful
  - Oral penicillin V: 250 mg twice daily
    - Requires patient cooperation, difficult to enforce
    - Well tolerated
  - For penicillin-sensitive patients, sulfadiazine or sulfisoxazole daily
    - Children who weigh less than 60 pounds: 0.5 g
    - Children who weigh more than 60 pounds: 1.0 g
  - Penicillin- and sulfa-sensitive patients: 250 mg of erythromycin twice daily
- Antibacterial prophylaxis at times of possible bacteremia is needed in the presence of rheumatic heart disease. The drug chosen should be different from the prophylactic antistreptococcal agent.
- Careful attention to protection against infective endocarditis is needed for patients with residual rheumatic heart disease, particularly for those who have required artificial valve implantation. Choose an antibiotic in conformity with the American Heart Association recommendations (see Endocarditis Prophylaxis in Prevention [Section V]).

REFERRAL

Acute and long-term follow-up by a cardiologist is appropriate.

PEARLS & CONSIDERATIONS

COMMENTS

- Normal sinus arrhythmia is lost during acute rheumatic carditis.
- Mitral regurgitation murmurs increase in intensity with isometric contraction, such as a hand grip or squat.
- Aortic valve regurgitation is best heard over the sternum and the left ventricular cavity. It is accentuated by leaning forward, by holding the breath in deep expiration, and by crouching on hands and knees (the same is true for rheumatic pericarditis).
- A patient with rheumatic chorea has the following conditions:
  - When told to raise the hands over the head, the patient has the palms facing out, which is not seen normally.
  - The patient demonstrates milkmaid's grip, a rhythmic squeezing of the fingers when grasping an object.
  - Rheumatic chorea may be one sided, a condition called hemichorea.
  - Handwriting may deteriorate severely in patients with rheumatic chorea.
  - Choreiform movements may be brought out or intensified by intention, holding the hands with fingers spread and counting backward from 10 to 1.
  - Chorea rarely occurs with the other manifestations of acute rheumatic fever.
- Acute rheumatic arthritis is extremely painful.
- Recurrent episodes of rheumatic fever are usually similar to the first (i.e., if there is carditis during the first episode, subsequent episodes are likely to have carditis).
- Modern rheumatic fever is significantly different, with less severe arthritis, fewer joints involved, and more identification of carditis if echocardiography findings are used as diagnostic. However, mitral or aortic regurgitation should be more than the clinically insignificant, mild valve insufficiency commonly seen in modern echocardiographic studies.

PATIENT/FAMILY EDUCATION

- Patients with rheumatic arthritis and rheumatic chorea recover without residual effects.
  - Patients remain susceptible to recurrences, particularly in first 3 years after the initial episode.
  - Patients should receive antistreptococcal prophylaxis during that time.
  - Emphasize appropriate throat culturing and lifelong therapy for illnesses with fever and sore throat.
- Patients with rheumatic carditis may recover or have significant cardiac damage.
  - Mitral valve regurgitation may progress to mitral valve stenosis.
  - Aortic valve regurgitation may progress and is uncommonly accompanied by aortic stenosis.
  - Surgical repair or valve replacement may be needed.
  - Cardiac damage is more severe with each recurrent episode.

SUGGESTED READINGS

Dajani AS et al: Prevention of rheumatic fever. *Circulation* 78:1082, 1998.

Narula J et al: Diagnosis of acute rheumatic carditis. *Circulation* 100:1576, 1999.

Tani LY et al: Rheumatic fever in children younger than 5 years: is the presentation different? *Pediatrics* 112:1065, 2003.

Veasy LG: Rheumatic fever—T. Duckett Jones and the rest of the story. *Cardiol Young* 5:293, 1995.

AUTHORS: **CHLOE ALEXSON, MD** and **J. PETER HARRIS, MD**

BASIC INFORMATION

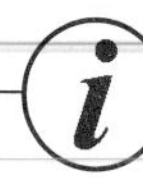

DEFINITION

Rickets is a failure in mineralization of growing bone or osteoid tissue, with characteristic changes of the growth plate cartilage in children before closure of the growth plate.

ICD-9-CM CODE
268.0 Rickets

EPIDEMIOLOGY & DEMOGRAPHICS

- Fortification of infant formulas and routine supplementation of infants with vitamin D have significantly decreased the incidence of rickets during the first 2 to 4 years of life.
- Data on the prevalence of rickets among children are not available; however, between 1986 and 2003, of the 166 cases of nutritional rickets in 22 published studies reported in U.S. children between the ages of 4 and 54 months, 83% were black, 96% were breastfed, and only 5% had vitamin D supplementation during breastfeeding.
- At-risk populations include the following:
  - Unsupplemented, exclusively breastfed infants for extensive periods
  - Formula-fed infants in countries where infants' milk is not supplemented with vitamin D
  - Infants fed macrobiotic or strictly vegetarian diets
  - Children who have restricted outdoor activities or clothing that precludes sun exposure
  - Poorly fed infants and children
  - Children who escape regular medical surveys
  - Children born to vitamin D-deficient mothers

CLINICAL PRESENTATION

- Skeletal changes, muscular hypotonia, and bone pain are the main features of vitamin D deficiency during infancy.
- Osseous changes of rickets can be recognized only after several months of vitamin D deficiency. Florid rickets can appear toward the end of the first and during the second year of life.
- Early skeletal signs of rickets include the following:
  - Wrist and costochondral enlargement (rachitic rosary) are the most reliable signs of rickets.
    - High sensitivity, 72% and 76%, respectively
    - Specificity, 81% and 64%, respectively for active rickets
  - Craniotabes (i.e., thinning of the outer table of the skull)
  - Large anterior fontanelle with delayed closure (not specific)
- Signs of advanced rickets include the following:
  - Deformities of the head with frontal bossing and parietal or occipital flattening
  - Deformities of the chest: pigeon chest, Harrison's groove
  - Deformities of the spinal column and pelvis: scoliosis, kyphosis, lordosis, coxa vara
  - Bowlegs or knock-knees and overextension of the knee joints (caused by relaxation of ligaments)
- Other clinical signs include failure to thrive, delayed tooth eruption, and delay in standing or walking.

ETIOLOGY

- Abnormalities of vitamin D
  - Nutritional deprivation
    - Low-birth-weight infants
    - Intestinal malabsorption
    - Anticonvulsant drugs (e.g., phenytoin)
    - Chronic renal disease
  - Metabolic defects
    - Absence of renal 25-hydroxyvitamin D1α−hydroxylase
    - Abnormal 1,25 $(OH)_2D$ receptor
- Calcium deficiency
  - Nutritional deprivation
    - Preterm infants
    - Low dietary calcium intake after weaning (i.e., weaning diet with minimal dairy content)
  - Malabsorption
  - Excessive loss: hypercalciuria
- Phosphorus deficiency
  - Nutritional deprivation
  - Hyperphosphaturia: familial hypophosphatemia
- Hypophosphatasia
  - Perinatal, infantile, childhood, adult forms
  - Pseudo-hypophosphatasia

DIAGNOSIS

DIFFERENTIAL DIAGNOSIS

- Nonrachitic craniotabes: physiologic, hydrocephalus, osteogenesis imperfecta
- Enlargement of costochondral junction
  - Scurvy
  - Chondrodystrophy
- Epiphyseal lesions
  - Congenital epiphyseal dysplasia
  - Cytomegalic inclusion disease
  - Syphilis
  - Rubella
  - Copper deficiency
- Other metabolic disturbances with osseous lesions resembling rickets
  - Hereditary or acquired hyperphosphaturia
  - Hypophosphatasia
  - Gastrointestinal malabsorption
  - Renal diseases (e.g., primary renal tubular acidosis, type II proximal)

WORKUP

- Diagnosis is based on a history of inadequate sunshine exposure and intake of vitamin D.
  - Often observed in blacks or immigrant populations who are breastfeeding for prolonged periods
  - Seen in cultures in which extensive clothing cover precludes sun exposure
- Clinical findings are listed in the previous sections.
- The diagnosis is confirmed chemically and by radiographic examination.
- Screening high-risk infants for subclinical rickets (no clinical evidence for rickets) by using wrist films paired with 25-hydroxyvitamin D levels (deficiency <12 ng/mL) can be a secondary prevention method of vitamin D-deficiency rickets.

LABORATORY TESTS

- Serum minerals
  - Normal or low serum calcium
  - Low serum phosphorus (<4 mg/dL)
- Elevated serum alkaline phosphatase level
- Serum 25-hydroxyvitamin D: low in vitamin D deficiency but normal in metabolic disturbances of vitamin D metabolism

IMAGING STUDIES

- Wrist radiograph of the distal ends of the long bones
  - Widened, cupped, and frayed
  - Decreased shaft density
  - Increased distance of distal ends to the metacarpal bones

TREATMENT

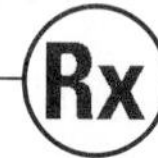

ACUTE GENERAL Rx

- In countries where follow-up care is difficult, a traditional dose of 5 mg (200,000 IU) of vitamin D (i.e., single-day, large-dose therapy) is repeated in 3 months.
  - Care should be taken to observe for hypercalcemia if there is concomitant high calcium intake.
  - Hypocalcemia and hypophosphatemia may occur if there is insufficient mineral intake with high-dose vitamin D therapy.
  - A lower dose of vitamin D is preferable because of possible side effects.
- Sufficient calcium is needed for correction of the demineralization defect and to avoid the complication of hypocalcemia.
  - Children should have daily intakes of calcium of at least 1 g per day during the first months of treatment by dietary intake or oral calcium supplements.
  - In children with very low serum calcium levels (<7.0 mg/dL), if large doses of vitamin D are given, calcium infusion may be needed from a few hours before the first administration of vitamin D,

not to exceed daily total doses of 50 mg/kg/day, up to normalization of serum calcium to avoid the occurrence of clinical signs of hypocalcemia.

CHRONIC Rx

- Cure of simple rickets is achieved with doses of 400 to 800 IU/day (10 to 20 µg/day) of vitamin D for 3 to 6 months, resulting in the following:
  - An increase of serum 25$(OH)_2$D and correction of calcium and phosphorus within 6 to 10 days
  - Normalization of parathyroid hormone levels within 1 to 2 months
  - Normalization of alkaline phosphatase activity
  - Healing of radiologic signs of rickets within 3 to 6 months, depending on the severity of the deficiency

DISPOSITION

- If therapy is appropriate, healing begins within a few days and progresses slowly until normal bone structure is restored.
- Enlargement of the epiphyses of the long bones disappears only after months or years of treatment.
- Severe bowing of the legs may disappear within several years without osteotomies.
- In developing countries, intercurrent infections (i.e., pneumonia, tuberculosis, and enteritis) may cause the death of rachitic children.

PEARLS & CONSIDERATIONS

COMMENTS

- Rickets and osteopenia in preterm infants are usually unrelated to vitamin D deficiency.
  - These conditions are related to calcium and phosphate deficiency.
  - Phosphate deficiency is of particular concern in preterm infants who are fed human milk.

PREVENTION

- New vitamin D intake guidelines for healthy infants and children were issued by the American Academy of Pediatrics in 2003. All infants, including those who are exclusively breastfed, should have a minimum intake of 200 IU of vitamin D per day beginning during the first 2 months of life, and it should be continued throughout childhood and adolescence because adequate sunlight exposure is difficult to determine for a given individual.
- To prevent rickets and vitamin D deficiency, an intake of 200 IU per day of vitamin D is recommended for the following:
  - All breastfed infants unless they are weaned to at least 500 mL per day of vitamin D-fortified formula or milk
  - All nonbreastfed infants who are ingesting less than 500 mL per day of vitamin D-fortified formula or milk
  - Children and adolescents who do not get regular sunlight exposure, do not ingest at least 500 mL per day of vitamin D-fortified milk, or do not take a daily multivitamin supplement containing at least 200 IU of vitamin D
- Prevention in preterm infants requires fortification of formula or human milk with calcium and phosphate. Commercial mineral-fortified formulas or milk fortifiers are available.
- Although regular sun exposure is the physiologic way to prevent vitamin D deficiency, there is new awareness of the hazards of ultraviolet-B light exposure in childhood (age when direct sunlight exposure initiated) and subsequent development of skin cancer in adulthood.
- Because of growing concerns about sunlight and skin cancer, limited exposure to ultraviolet light is recommended by the American Academy of Pediatrics (2003):
  - Infants younger that 6 months should be kept out of direct sunlight.
  - Minimize sunlight exposure for children's activities by using protective clothing and sunscreens.

PATIENT/FAMILY EDUCATION

- The new American Academy of Pediatrics guidelines to provide a minimal intake of 200 IU of vitamin D per day for all infants, beginning in the first 2 months of life, should be emphasized in the education of all families, particularly the families of children at greatest risk of vitamin D deficiency (i.e., exclusively breastfed or dark-skinned infants).
- Children should be weaned to a diet adequate in vitamin D and calcium.
- The higher risk of rickets among young, breastfed, black children should be emphasized.

SUGGESTED READINGS

Garabedian M, Ben-Mekhbi H: Rickets and vitamin D deficiency. *In* Holick MF (ed): *Vitamin D: Physiology, Molecular Biology, and Clinical Applications.* Totowa, NJ, Humana Press, 1999, pp 273–286.

Gartner LM et al: Prevention of rickets and vitamin D deficiency: new guidelines for vitamin D. *Pediatrics* 111:908, 2003.

Koo WWK, Tsang RC: Building better bones: calcium, magnesium, phosphorus, and vitamin D. *In* Tsang RC (ed): *Nutrition during Infancy: Principles and Practice,* 2nd ed. Cincinnati, OH, Digital Educational Publishing, 1997, pp 175–207.

Wharton B, Bishop N: Rickets. *Lancet* 362:1389, 2003.

AUTHORS: **RAN NAMGUNG, MD, PHD** and **REGINALD TSANG, MD, MBBS**

BASIC INFORMATION

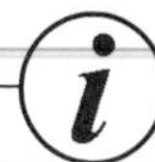

DEFINITION

Rocky Mountain spotted fever (RMSF) is an infection caused by *Rickettsia rickettsii.* RMSF is the most common rickettsial illness in the United States. It is a multisystem disease with significant mortality if untreated.

SYNONYM

RMSF

ICD-9-CM CODE

082.0 Rocky Mountain spotted fever

EPIDEMIOLOGY & DEMOGRAPHICS

- Ticks are the vector and the reservoir of *R. rickettsii* in nature (i.e., the dog tick, *Dermacentor variabilis,* in the eastern two thirds and western coast of the United States; the wood tick, *Dermacentor andersoni,* in the Rocky Mountain states; and other ticks in Mexico, Central America, and South America).
- Modes of transmission include the following:
  - Tick bites, with transmission from the tick's salivary glands after at least 6 to 10 hours of attachment
  - Rarely, by direct contact with tick fluid during removal of an attached tick
- Incidence and prevalence:
  - RMSF is strongly seasonal. Approximately 90% of all cases occur between April and September; 43% are in May and June. However, 10% of cases are sporadic, and they have been described in every month, although winter cases are more likely in the southern United States.
  - About 500 to 1000 cases per year are reported in the United States; 15 to 20 fatalities are reported per year, but the true incidence is thought to be twofold to threefold higher.
  - The overall annual incidence rate in the United States is 0.22 cases per 100,000 people. About two thirds of the U.S. total caseload are children younger than 15 years; the peak incidence is in children 5 to 9 years old (0.37 cases per 100,000 children).
  - RMSF is strongly geographic. Although first described in Rocky Mountain states, most U.S. cases occur in the Southeast (especially North and South Carolina, Georgia, Virginia, and Maryland) and the lower Midwest (Oklahoma, Missouri, Arkansas, and Tennessee).
  - Case distribution with focal restriction to small islands or hot spots in individual rural counties or even urban neighborhoods is well documented.
  - Risk factors and affected groups are as follows:
    - Age 5 to 9 years
    - Exposure to wooded areas with high grass
    - Exposure to dogs with ticks
    - Residence in or travel to known endemic areas during April to September
  - Risk factors for fatal outcome include the following:
    - Failure to receive tetracycline or doxycycline for therapy
    - Delay in treatment beyond fifth day of illness
    - Age older than 40 to 60 years
    - Atypical symptoms (e.g., lack of visible rash, lack of tick bite history; in some studies, black patients have higher risk of fatal illness, which may be due to the difficulty in visualizing their rash)

CLINICAL PRESENTATION

- History and physical examination findings
  - Residence in or travel to an endemic area, with dog exposure or tick bite (50% to 60%)
  - Fever (80% to 90%): commonly higher than 38.9°C; almost uniformly present after the third day
  - Severe headache (80% to 90%): may be difficult to assess in young children
  - Myalgia (80%)
  - Nausea and vomiting (50% to 60%)
  - Rash
    - Appears after 2 to 3 days; on day 1, 14% of patients; by day 3, 42% of patients; by day 6, 80% to 95% of patients
    - Begins as blanching, erythematous, 1- to 4-mm macules on ankles and wrists, moving inward (centripetally) to trunk; palms, and soles, which are involved in 50% to 80%; within a few days, macules progress to maculopapules and then nonblanching petechiae
    - Rash less likely to be recognized in blacks and, in some reports, older men
- Classic triad of fever, rash, and history of tick bite eventually evident in 60% to 90% of cases, but only in 3% to 18% of cases at the initial physician visit (i.e., the history and physical examination must be repeated serially if RMSF is suspected)
- Incubation period: mean of 7 days after tick bite (range, 2 to 14 days)
- Complications as disease progresses:
  - Widespread vasculitis, edema; may progress to skin necrosis
  - Encephalitis: confusion, lethargy or stupor, delirium, coma, cerebrospinal fluid lymphocytic pleocytosis (25% to 30%)
  - Noncardiogenic pulmonary edema, adult respiratory distress syndrome (10% to 20%)
  - Cardiac arrhythmia
  - Coagulopathy, gastrointestinal hemorrhage
  - Anemia (especially severe in patients with glucose-6-phosphate dehydrogenase deficiency)
  - Death: usually occurs at 8 to 15 days after onset if no treatment is given or if treatment is begun too late
  - Possible long-term complications in survivors: gangrene and loss of limbs; impaired hearing, motor, and intellectual function; and incontinence

ETIOLOGY

R. rickettsii: a small, gram-negative, obligately intracellular bacterium, which infects endothelial cells lining small vessels in all major tissues and organs.

DIAGNOSIS

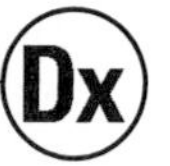

DIFFERENTIAL DIAGNOSIS

- Early RMSF
  - Enteroviral infection
  - Ehrlichiosis
  - Infectious mononucleosis
  - Scarlet fever
  - Gastroenteritis
  - Acute abdomen
  - Leptospirosis
  - If late in the year, influenza
- Later RMSF (after 3 to 5 days)
  - Meningococcemia
  - Ehrlichiosis
  - Other rickettsial illnesses (e.g., murine typhus)
  - Measles
  - Immune complex vasculitis
  - Thrombotic thrombocytopenic purpura

WORKUP

- Diagnosis is based on the history and physical examination findings. Culture is not routinely available.
- Common nonspecific laboratory abnormalities include the following:
  - Thrombocytopenia (<150,000/µL in 67% of cases)
  - Normal white blood cell count with left shift
  - Hyponatremia (<134 mEq/L in 50% to 80%)
  - Elevated levels of transaminases

LABORATORY TESTS

- Serologic tests become positive only after 7 to 10 days or more of illness, long after the time at which treatment should be begun.
  - The standard assay is indirect immunofluorescent antibody titer (IFA) in serum.
    - Sensitivity is 94% to 100%, and specificity is almost 100%.
    - Titers of more than 1:64 are usually detectable after 7 to 10 days of illness.
    - A fourfold rise in IFA antibody titer in paired acute and convalescent samples or a single titer of more than 1:64 in

the presence of a compatible illness is considered diagnostic for RMSF.
  - Other antibody tests (e.g., latex agglutination, enzyme immunoassay, polymerase chain reaction assay) are available, but they are less standardized or perform less well. None reveals antibodies earlier than the IFA test.
  - The classic Weil-Felix agglutination titers have poor sensitivity and specificity (<70% to 80%) and are no longer suggested for use.
- Direct immunofluorescence staining of vascular endothelium in skin-punch biopsies is used for detection of *R. rickettsii.*
  - Sensitivity of 70% to 90%; highly specific
  - Useful only in patients with rash
  - Very few reliable laboratories capable of correctly performing this assay
  - Theoretical advantage of rapid diagnosis precluded by the time spent obtaining and shipping a proper specimen to a reliable laboratory

TREATMENT

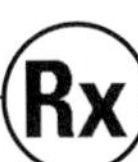

NONPHARMACOLOGIC THERAPY

Intensive care support may be required.

ACUTE GENERAL Rx

- Empirical antimicrobial therapy for RMSF is necessary because delaying treatment until confirmation of the diagnosis can lead to death. The only drugs proved to be effective in the treatment of RMSF are tetracyclines, including doxycycline, and to a lesser extent, chloramphenicol.
- Doxycycline is now considered the drug of choice for RMSF, even in children younger than 8 years old.
  - Practitioners and parents *should not* be unduly concerned with the small, theoretical risk of tooth staining by doxycycline therapy of young children. Doxycycline appears to bind teeth less than tetracycline, especially when used in the comparatively brief regimens suggested for RMSF.
  - In contrast, practitioners and parents *should* be concerned with the greater risk of fatal RMSF if doxycycline therapy is not provided. Doxycycline is also the drug of choice for ehrlichiosis, which may be a diagnostic consideration in patients thought to have RMSF—another reason for choosing doxycycline.
  - Chloramphenicol (familiar to older practitioners as the past drug of choice) is no longer recommended for therapy of RMSF. Its toxicities are multiple (e.g., dose-related bone marrow suppression, idiosyncratic aplastic anemia, gray-baby syndrome in ill children who may have decreased hepatic function), and the oral formulation is no longer available in the United States.
- Doxycycline dosage is 4 mg/kg/day in two divided doses, up to a maximum of 100 mg two times per day (may be administered orally or, if seriously ill, intravenously).
- Therapy is recommended for 7 days or until the patient is afebrile for more than 2 days (whichever is longer); some practitioners treat as long as 14 days.

PEARLS & CONSIDERATIONS

COMMENTS

- Pitfalls in the diagnosis of RMSF include the following:
  - Waiting too long to see if a petechial rash develops before diagnosis
  - Not eliciting a history of travel or exposure to ticks (or even pet dogs with ticks), although absence of tick exposure or a bite does not exclude RMSF (only 60% sensitive)
  - Mistaking early gastrointestinal symptoms of RMSF for gastroenteritis
  - Not using doxycycline to treat RMSF because of inappropriate concerns about cosmetically perceptible teeth staining
- Children in the southeastern or south-central United States with an RMSF-like illness characterized by few or no macular lesions, rare to absent petechiae, and relatively more prominent leukopenia, may have ehrlichiosis.
  - *Ehrlichia* are rickettsia-like bacteria that are transmitted by the bite of the Lone Star tick, *Amblyomma americanum,* or the deer tick, *Ixodes scapularis* (i.e., the Lyme disease tick), depending on the *Ehrlichia* species and region of the country.
  - Doxycycline treats RMSF and ehrlichiosis.
- Lyme disease is not transmitted by ticks that carry *R. rickettsi,* although a related borrelial infection, Southern tick-associated rash illness, may be.

PREVENTION

- Careful checking for ticks and removal of entire tick without crushing may prevent RMSF transmission.
- Wearing long clothing, applying insect repellent when outdoors, and spraying tick repellent on pet dogs are also appropriate preventive measures.
- Even in endemic areas, most ticks are not infected with rickettsia; prophylactic antibiotics are not indicated for asymptomatic individuals after a bite.
- No vaccine is available.

PATIENT/FAMILY EDUCATION

- Centers for Disease Control and Prevention (disease information topic "A to Z" list): www.cdc.gov/az.do

SUGGESTED READINGS

American Academy of Pediatrics: Rocky Mountain spotted fever. *In* Pickering LK (ed): *2003 Red Book: Report of the Committee on Infectious Diseases,* 26th ed. Elk Grove Village, IL, American Academy of Pediatrics, 2003.

Edwards MS, Feigin R: Rickettsial diseases. *In* Feigin RD et al (eds): *Textbook of Pediatric Infectious Diseases,* 5th ed. Philadelphia, WB Saunders, 2004.

Masters EJ et al: Rocky Mountain spotted fever: a clinician's dilemma. *Arch Intern Med* 163:769, 2003.

Thorner AR et al: Rocky Mountain spotted fever. *Clin Infect Dis* 27:1353, 1998.

Walker DH, Raoult D: *Rickettsia rickettsi* and other spotted fever group rickettsiae (Rocky Mountain spotted fever and other spotted fevers). *In* Mandell GL et al (eds): *Mandell, Douglas, and Bennett's Principles and Practice of Infectious Diseases,* 6th ed. Philadelphia, Elsevier, 2005.

AUTHOR: **GEOFFREY A. WEINBERG, MD**

BASIC INFORMATION

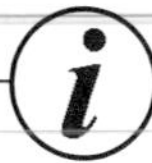

DEFINITION

Rotator cuff syndrome (RCS) is defined as an obstruction of the subacromial or supraspinatus outlet space, anatomically defined by the acromion, coracoacromial arch, and acromioclavicular joint above and the humeral head and glenoid below. Obstruction of the subacromial or supraspinatus outlet space most commonly results in supraspinatus tendon pathology. RCS is classified as primary, secondary, or internal.

SYNONYMS

Rotator cuff injury
Shoulder impingement syndrome (SIS)

ICD-9-CM CODE
726.1 Rotator cuff syndrome

EPIDEMIOLOGY & DEMOGRAPHICS

- In the pediatric population, RCS is seen most often in athletes whose sport involves repetitive overhead motions (e.g., baseball pitch, tennis serve, volleyball serve or hit, swimming strokes).
- Most of these young athletes present with underlying glenohumeral instability, which leads to secondary RCS. Primary RCS is seen more often in adults older than 35 years.
- Anatomic variation of the acromion can contribute to RCS: hooked (type III) more so than curved (type II) more so than flat (type I).

CLINICAL PRESENTATION

History

- Gradual increase in shoulder pain with overhead activities suggests RCS.
- Pain may be difficult for the patient to localize. Many patients point to a diffuse area around the deltoid muscle.
- Pain with the humerus in forward flexion and internal rotation suggests impingement.
- Pain with the humerus in abduction and external rotation suggests anterior glenohumeral instability and laxity.

Physical Examination

- Inspect the entire shoulder girdle and scapula for a muscle mass or bony asymmetry. Palpate the acromioclavicular joint for separation and the clavicle for fractures. Palpate the biceps, supraspinatus, and subscapularis tendons for tenderness.
- Test the strength of the rotator cuff muscles: supraspinatus, infraspinatus, teres minor, and subscapularis.
- Test active and passive ranges of motion, including forward flexion, abduction, external and internal rotation, adduction, and extension. A painful arc between 70 and 120 degrees of abduction suggests impingement.
- Provocative testing for impingement signs includes the following:
    - Neer test: Standing behind or beside the patient, passively elevate (forward flexion) the arm while stabilizing the scapula with downward digital pressure on the coracoacromial arch. A positive test result demonstrates pain with increasing arm elevation.
    - Hawkins-Kennedy test: Passively elevate (forward flex) the arm to 90 degrees in adduction and then forcibly internally rotate the humerus. A positive test result elicits pain.
- Tests for instability signs include the following:
    - Sulcus sign: Grasp the patient's elbow and apply inferior traction. Dimpling of the skin subjacent to the acromion suggests glenohumeral instability.
    - Apprehension sign: With the patient supine to stabilize the scapula, slowly move the patient's arm into an abducted and externally rotated position. Apprehension and guarding with continued abduction and external rotation is a positive test result. Easing of the patient's apprehension by direct posterior pressure on the anterior proximal humerus (i.e., simulating relocation of the glenohumeral joint that presumably partially dislocated with the previous abduction and external rotation) is a positive relocation test result that suggests glenohumeral instability.
- Refer to the web site references (see "Suggested Readings") for illustrations to assist in the physical examination.

ETIOLOGY

- Primary RCS is indicated by hooked (type III) acromion anatomy, acromioclavicular inferior osteophytes, coracoacromial ligament hypertrophy, subacromial bursal thickening and fibrosis, and repetitive overhead activity.
- Secondary RCS seems to result from underlying subtle glenohumeral joint instability. The process starts as repetitive stresses on the dynamic glenohumeral stabilizers, which leads to fatigue of the rotator cuff muscles, which then leads to anterior superior movement of the humeral head. The abnormally located humeral head obstructs the supraspinatus outlet space leading to supraspinatus tendinopathy.
- Internal impingement syndrome is caused by partial undersurface (i.e., posterior aspect) tears of the supraspinatus tendon, usually seen in athletes with repetitive throwing motions.

DIAGNOSIS

Dx

DIFFERENTIAL DIAGNOSIS

- Anterior subluxation of the shoulder
- Suprascapular nerve injury
- Acromioclavicular joint separation
- Cervical spine pathology

WORKUP

A thorough history and physical examination can indicate rotator cuff pathology associated with RCS. Studies such as plain radiographs and magnetic resonance imaging (MRI) can rule out other shoulder pathology or may help confirm the diagnosis of RCS.

IMAGING STUDIES

- Plain radiographs include an anteroposterior view of the glenohumeral joint, internal rotation view of the humerus with a 20-degree upward angulation to show the acromioclavicular joint, an axillary view to rule out subtle signs of instability, and a supraspinatus outlet view (if <7 mm, higher risk for impingement).
- MRI can detect tendon degeneration, partial rotator cuff tears (especially with contrast agent), inflammation, edema, hemorrhage, and scarring.

TREATMENT

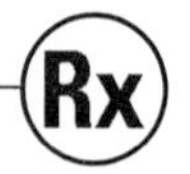

NONPHARMACOLOGIC THERAPY

- Acute-phase rehabilitation
    - Goals are to relieve pain and inflammation, prevent muscle atrophy, and reestablish nonpainful range of motion.
    - Eliminate activities that cause pain.
    - Start active rest: "Rest" from the inciting activity or sport, but to prevent muscle atrophy, begin range of motion (i.e., strengthening activities), including range-of-motion exercises performed below shoulder level and isometric strengthening exercises (see references in "Suggested Readings").
- Recovery-phase rehabilitation
    - Goals are to normalize range of motion, perform symptom-free activities of daily living, and improve neuromuscular control and muscle strength.
    - This phase should be done under the supervision of a physical therapist, especially for the young athlete, who will need to start a sport-specific interval program to gradually transition to full participation.
- Maintenance phase
    - Goals are to maintain proper warm-up, stretching, and strengthening techniques to prevent a repeat injury.
    - This phase should be started under the supervision of a physical therapist and continued by the patient with a consistent home exercise program.
- Surgery indications
    - In general, surgical intervention is not considered until a supervised rehabilitation program has been attempted for at least 3 to 6 months and the patient continues to be disabled.

ACUTE GENERAL Rx

Nonsteroidal anti-inflammatory medications can be used to help alleviate the initial pain and inflammation.

DISPOSITION

- Conservative therapy with a supervised rehabilitation program is successful for 60% to 90% of patients.
- If there is no improvement after 3 months of rehabilitation, re-evaluate the situation.

REFERRAL

- Refer to a physical therapist for supervised rehabilitation program.
- Refer to a sports medicine specialist for recurrent problems in the young athlete.
- Refer to an orthopedic surgeon for surgical indications.

PEARLS & CONSIDERATIONS

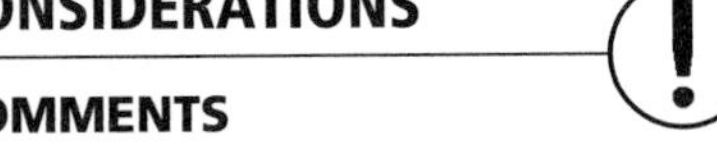

COMMENTS

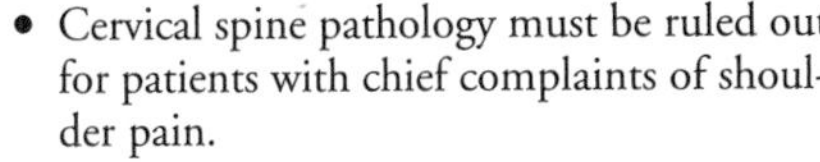

- Cervical spine pathology must be ruled out for patients with chief complaints of shoulder pain.
- RCS and rotator cuff disease affect athletes at a younger age compared with the general population.

PREVENTION

- Continuing a home exercise program, started under the supervision of a physical therapist, is critical to prevent repeat injury.
- In a supervised program, young athletes should transition to full participation with gradual increases of intensity and frequency of activity to prevent repeat injury.

PATIENT/FAMILY EDUCATION

Young athletes whose sport involves repetitive overhead motions should be educated on the proper techniques for warm-up, stretching, and strength maintenance of rotator cuff muscles and parascapular muscles.

SUGGESTED READINGS

Almekinders LC: Overuse injuries in the upper extremity: impingement syndrome. *Clin Sports Med* 20:491, 2001.

American Academy of Family Physicians (AAFP): http://familydoctor.org/268.xml (exercises for acute rehabilitation, with illustrations).

American Academy of Family Physicians (AAFP): http://familydoctor.org/265.xml (rotator cuff exercises for strengthening, with illustrations).

American Academy of Family Physicians (AAFP): www.aafp.org/afp/980215ap/fongemie.html (online version of Fongemie AE et al: Management of shoulder impingement syndrome and rotator cuff tears. *Am Fam Physician* 57:667, 1998, physical examination, with illustrations).

Bielak KM, Henderson JM: Shoulder injuries. *In* Birrer RB (ed): *Sports Medicine for the Primary Care Physician.* Boca Raton, FL, CRC Press, 2004, p 411.

Chang WK: Shoulder impingement syndrome. *Phys Med Rehabil Clin North Am* 15:493, 2004.

UpToDate Online: www.utdol.com (search "shoulder impingement syndrome," includes illustrations of the physical examination).

AUTHOR: **SHARON F. CHEN, MD**

BASIC INFORMATION

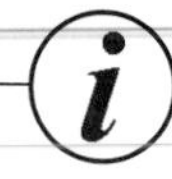

DEFINITION

Rubella is a mild viral disease characterized by a rash, generalized lymphadenopathy, and fever. Congenital rubella syndrome consists of anomalies of the ophthalmologic, cardiac, auditory, and neurologic systems.

SYNONYMS

German measles
Three-day measles

ICD-9-CM CODES
056.9 Rubella without mention of complication
771.0 Congenital rubella

EPIDEMIOLOGY & DEMOGRAPHICS

- In the era before a vaccine, rubella circulated in an epidemic pattern of 6- to 9-year cycles.
- The last pandemic period in the United States was in 1964.
- The virus is transmitted by droplet secretions or direct contact with infected human or contaminated fomites.
- The peak incidence is in late winter and early spring.
- Approximately 25% to 50% of infections are asymptomatic.
- Maximum infectivity occurs from 5 days before and continues for 5 to 6 days after the rash starts.
- The incidence has decreased by 99% from the prevaccine era. Vaccination started in 1966 to 1968.
- The incubation period for postnatal rubella is 14 to 21 days (usually 16 to 18 days).
- The attack rate was highest in 5- to 9-year-old children.
- The incidence is high among preschool children.

CLINICAL PRESENTATION

History

The patient's immunization status should be determined.

Physical Examination

- Postnatal illness
  - Prodromal complaints include malaise, fevers (rarely beyond first day of rash), and anorexia for a few days.
  - Rash is erythematous and maculopapular; it starts on the face, with centrifugal spread toward the hands and feet. It involves the entire body during first day, begins to fade the next day, and lasts 3 to 5 days.
  - Lymphadenopathy (suboccipital, postauricular, and cervical) precedes the exanthem and may last several weeks.
  - Complications may include arthritis, arthralgia, encephalitis, thrombocytopenia, and rarely, myocarditis and pericarditis.
- Congenital rubella has the following features:
  - The disease occurs as a result of in utero infection during the first trimester of pregnancy.
  - Fetal infection may be subacute or chronic, and it may result in abortion, stillbirth, or malformations.
  - Congenital anomalies include the following:
    - Auditory: sensorineural deafness
    - Cardiac: patent ductus arteriosus, peripheral pulmonary artery stenosis
    - Neurologic: behavioral problems, meningoencephalitis, mental retardation
    - Ophthalmologic: cataracts, retinopathy, congenital glaucoma

ETIOLOGY

Rubella is an RNA virus classified as a *Rubivirus* of the Togaviridae family.

DIAGNOSIS

DIFFERENTIAL DIAGNOSIS

- Febrile illness with rash
  - Measles
  - Toxoplasmosis
  - Scarlet fever
  - Roseola
  - Parvovirus B19 (i.e., fifth disease)
  - Adenoviruses
  - Enteroviruses
  - Other common respiratory viruses

LABORATORY TESTS

- The virus can be isolated from the throat, blood, urine, or cerebrospinal fluid. Laboratory technicians need to know to look for rubella virus in a cell culture (no longer done routinely).
- Acute and convalescent serology is determined by enzyme immunoassay and latex agglutination assays for group A rubella virus antigen detection. A fourfold or greater rise in titer or seroconversion is diagnostic.
- Rubella-specific immunoglobulin M (IgM) antibody testing is available.
  - Useful in babies with intrauterine growth retardation and nonimmune mothers
  - Mothers with suspected rubella during pregnancy

TREATMENT

ACUTE GENERAL Rx

- No specific therapy is available.
- Symptomatic therapy is indicated.

REFERRAL

Refer the patient with congenital rubella to a cardiologist, otolaryngologist, ophthalmologist, or neurologist as needed.

PEARLS & CONSIDERATIONS

COMMENTS

- Rubella is now rare in immunized children.
- Consider the diagnosis in underimmunized and older populations.
- Rubella is the third childhood febrile exanthem. Measles and scarlet fever are first and second, respectively.

PREVENTION

- Live-virus rubella immunization (RA 27/3 strain) is usually combined with measles and mumps vaccines (MMR).
- Serum rubella antibody develops in 95% of vaccine recipients after a first dose at 12 months of age or older.
- Two doses of measles vaccine are recommended. The second dose should be given at 4 to 6 years and no later than 11 to 12 years of age.

PATIENT/FAMILY EDUCATION

- Immune status should be assessed in early pregnancy.
- Seronegative pregnant women should be immunized in the postpartum period.

SUGGESTED READINGS

American Academy of Pediatrics. Rubella. *In* Pickering LK, Baker CJ, Long SS, McMillan JA (eds): *Red Book: 2006 Report of the Committee on Infectious Diseases,* 27th ed. Elk Grove Village, IL, American Academy of Pediatrics, 2006, pp 574–579.

Centers for Disease Control and Prevention (CDC): Control and prevention of rubella: evaluation and management of suspected outbreaks, rubella in pregnant women, and surveillance for congenital rubella syndrome. *MMWR Morb Mortal Wkly Rep* 50:1, 2001.

Centers for Disease Control and Prevention. Available at www.cdc.gov

Cherry JD: Rubella virus. *In* Feigin RD, Cherry JD (eds): *Textbook of Pediatric Infectious Diseases,* 5th ed. Philadelphia, WB Saunders, 2004, pp 2134–2154.

AUTHOR: **CYNTHIA CHRISTY, MD**

BASIC INFORMATION

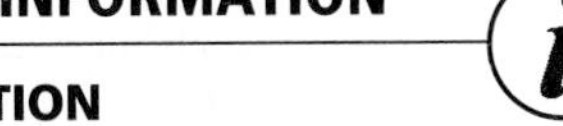

DEFINITION

Nontyphoidal *Salmonella* can cause gastroenteritis and invasive infections (e.g., osteomyelitis, sepsis, bacteremia). Typhoid fever is a bacteremic, febrile illness that results in variable clinical manifestations, including chronic carriage, moderate self-limited illness, shock, or death.

SYNONYMS

Enteric fever
Salmonella sepsis

ICD-9-CM CODES
002.0 Typhoid
003.9 *Salmonella*

EPIDEMIOLOGY & DEMOGRAPHICS

- Approximately 50,000 cases of nontyphoidal *Salmonella* occur each year in the United States.
- More than 500 cases of typhoid fever occur per year in the United States. They are usually returning foreign travelers.
- The peak incidence is in infants, children younger than 5 years, and adults older than 70 years.
- The incidence is higher in the warmer months.
- Bacteria are excreted in the stool for a mean of 5 weeks (longer in children younger than 5 years), but they can be present for up to a year.
- Chronic carriers (i.e., excretion for more than 1 year) often have gallbladder disease.
- The incubation period for gastroenteritis is 6 to 72 hours (mean, 24 hours).
- The incubation period for typhoid fever is 3 to 60 days (usually 7 to 14 days).
- There are several risk factors for acquiring *Salmonella* infections.
    - Decreased gastric acid production may predispose to gastroenteritis.
    - Impaired cellular immunity may be a result of chronic granulomatous disease, cancer, immunosuppressive therapy, or human immunodeficiency virus (HIV) infection.
    - Patients with sickle cell disease have an increased risk for *Salmonella* osteomyelitis.
    - Age younger than 12 months is a risk factor.
    - Concurrent infections include malaria, schistosomiasis, and bartonellosis.

CLINICAL PRESENTATION

History

- Gastroenteritis
    - Abrupt onset of nausea, vomiting, and crampy abdominal pain, followed by watery diarrhea that may contain blood or mucus.
    - Fever occurs in fewer than 70% of patients.
    - Symptoms typically persist for 7 days in healthy children but longer in infants and immunocompromised children.
- Nontyphoidal bacteremia
    - Fever, chills
    - More common in infants and immunocompromised children
- Typhoid fever bacteremia
    - Stepwise, insidious development of fever over approximately 1 week
    - May occur with constipation or diarrhea
    - Headache, lethargy, malaise, myalgia, abdominal pain
    - Mental status changes; intestinal hemorrhage and possible perforation
- Extra-intestinal focal infections
    - Often occur at anatomic abnormalities or areas of previous trauma
    - Osteomyelitis, suppurative arthritis, meningitis, brain abscess, others

Physical Examination

- Gastroenteritis
    - Abdominal pain in periumbilical or right lower quadrant
    - Reactive arthritis after gastroenteritis
- Nontyphoidal bacteremia
    - Toxic appearance, signs of shock (e.g., tachycardia, pallor, poor perfusion, hypotension)
    - High incidence of jaundice, likely due to hemolysis
- Extra-intestinal focal infections: per individual infections
- Typhoid fever bacteremia
    - Children may have a toxic appearance, fever, and signs of shock.
    - Infants and young children may have less impressive examination findings, similar to a "viral illness."
    - Hepatosplenomegaly and rose spots occur in the second week of illness. Rose spots, seen in 5% to 20% of patients, are 2- to 4-mm erythematous macules on the trunk and abdomen that may occur in crops. They may also occur with nontyphoidal *Salmonella*.

ETIOLOGY

- Salmonellae are non–spore-forming, motile, usually non–lactose-fermenting, gram-negative rods.
    - A single species, *Salmonella enterica*, is represented.
    - However, serotypes are often referred to as species (i.e., *S. enterica* ser. Typhi is often written *S. typhi*)
- Transmission is through ingestion of the organism.
    - Bacteria invade the intestinal wall and may enter the bloodstream.
    - Gastrointestinal inflammation results in fecal leukocytes.
- Bacteremia can lead to sepsis, typhoid fever, or focal invasive infections.
- Nontyphoidal *Salmonella* is associated with animal reservoirs, including reptiles, chickens, turkeys, pigs, and cattle.
- *S. enterica* ser. Typhi has no animal reservoir; infection is caused by contact with food or water contaminated with human feces.

DIAGNOSIS

DIFFERENTIAL DIAGNOSIS

- Viral gastroenteritis: rotavirus, astrovirus, adenovirus, caliciviruses (Norwalk agent), hepatitis A
- Bacterial gastroenterocolitis: *Campylobacter, Shigella, Escherichia coli,* staphylococcal food poisoning, *Vibrio* species, *Yersinia*
- Parasitic infections: *Giardia, Cryptosporidium, Entamoeba histolytica,* others
- Other causes: antibiotic-associated colitis, chemical colitis, appendicitis, inflammatory bowel disease

LABORATORY TESTS

- Culture of *Salmonella* from stool, blood, urine, or foci of infection is diagnostic.
- Blood culture should be obtained for all febrile or toxic-appearing patients.
- Serologic tests are not recommended (i.e., high false-positive and false-negative rates).
- Fecal leukocytes are usually present (often mononuclear cells with *S. enterica* ser. Typhi).
- Serotyping is important only in an outbreak evaluation. *S. enterica* ser. Typhi is group D.

IMAGING STUDIES

- Abdominal imaging if intra-abdominal complications are suspected.
- Musculoskeletal imaging if osteomyelitis is suspected.

TREATMENT

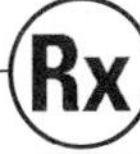

NONPHARMACOLOGIC THERAPY

- Rehydration and electrolyte management are the mainstays of therapy.
- Hospitalize patients who are toxic, severely dehydrated, or immunocompromised.

ACUTE GENERAL Rx

- Gastroenteritis
    - Antibiotics are *not recommended* for noninvasive gastroenteritis in low-risk patients because they may prolong the carrier state and do not speed the resolution of symptoms.
    - Antibiotics may be warranted for patients at highest risk of bacteremia or complications: infants younger than 3 months, immunocompromised patients, patients with chronic gastrointestinal disease, and patients with hemoglobinopathy.

- Antimotility agents are *not recommended* because they may worsen disease.
- Treatment of invasive disease
  - Bacteremia: 10 to 14 days of therapy; provide parenteral therapy for severely ill patients.
  - Bacteremia in patients with HIV: 4 to 6 weeks of therapy may help prevent relapse.
  - Osteomyelitis: Treat for 4 to 6 weeks; use surgical intervention as indicated.
  - Meningitis: Treat for at least 4 weeks with a third-generation cephalosporin.
  - Typhoid fever: Treat for 2 to 3 weeks; many patients can be managed as outpatients. Fever can persist for 5 to 7 days after the bacteremia has cleared. Give corticosteroids for typhoid fever with severe mental status changes. Antibiotic choice is based on the travel history.
    - Strains in Latin America and sub-Saharan Africa are usually sensitive to amoxicillin (100 mg/kg/day in four divided doses) or trimethoprim-sulfamethoxazole (TMP-SMX) (8 mg/kg of TMP, 40 mg/kg of SMX per day in two divided doses).
    - Strains in Asia and northeast Africa are commonly resistant and require a third-generation cephalosporin.
    - Fluoroquinolones are more effective than cephalosporins. There is extensive worldwide pediatric experience using quinolones for this life-threatening infection, although they are not approved for use in children.
  - Relapse is common, even with appropriate antibiotic therapy.

CHRONIC Rx

Chronic (≥1 year) *S. enterica* ser. Typhi carriage may be eradicated by high-dose amoxicillin and probenecid or fluoroquinolones.

DISPOSITION

- Follow-up cultures are indicated only for infection control.
- Patients with *S. enterica* ser. Typhi should be excluded from child care until cultures are negative.
- Contacts of patients with symptomatic *S. enterica* ser. Typhi should be screened, and infected individuals should be excluded from child care.
- Contacts of patients with nontyphoidal *Salmonella* do not need to be screened.
- Children recovering from nontyphoidal *Salmonella* do not need follow-up stool cultures; they can return to child care when asymptomatic.

REFERRAL

- All documented cases of *Salmonella* should be reported to the local health department.
- Refer complicated or severely ill patients to pediatric infectious disease or pediatric gastroenterology specialists.

PEARLS & CONSIDERATIONS

COMMENTS

The inoculum size determines the incubation period, symptoms, and severity.

PREVENTION

- Isolation and contact precautions should be instituted for diapered and incontinent children.
- Infected individuals should be excluded from food handling.
- No vaccine is available for nontyphoidal *Salmonella.*
- Consider vaccinating household contacts of chronic carriers and children traveling in endemic areas with prolonged exposure.
  - Ty21a live-attenuated vaccine (oral) is approved for children older than 6 years.
    - Do not administer while patients are taking antibiotics or are immunocompromised.
    - The capsule form is taken every other day for four doses; a booster is required every 5 years.
  - Vi capsular polysaccharide vaccine (intramuscular) is for children older than 2 years.
    - Single intramuscular dose
    - Booster required every 2 years

PATIENT/FAMILY EDUCATION

- Use proper hand washing and food preparation techniques, and sanitize water supplies.
- Discourage keeping reptiles as pets.

SUGGESTED READINGS

American Academy of Pediatrics. *Salmonella* infections. *In* Pickering LK, Baker CJ, Long SS, McMillan JA (eds): *Red Book: 2006 Report of the Committee on Infectious Diseases,* 27th ed. Elk Grove Village, IL, American Academy of Pediatrics, 2006, pp 579–584.

Centers for Disease Control (CDC). Available at http://www.cdc.gov/ncidod/diseases/submenus/subsalmonella.htm; http://www.cdc.gov/ncidod/diseases/submenus/subtyphoid.htm

Cleary TG: *Salmonella* species. *In* Long SS et al (eds): *Principles and Practice of Pediatric Infectious Disease.* New York, Churchill Livingstone, 2003, pp 830–835.

AUTHOR: **MELANIE WELLINGTON, MD**

BASIC INFORMATION

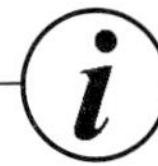

DEFINITION

Scabies is a skin infestation by small parasites called itch mites *(Sarcoptes scabiei).* The term is derived from the Latin word *scabere,* meaning "to scratch."

ICD-9-CM CODE
133.0 Scabies

EPIDEMIOLOGY & DEMOGRAPHICS

- Humans are the main infection source through close human physical contact.
- Transmission from dogs and other animals is rare.
- Infants and young children have a more varied presentation.
- Approximately 50% to 66% of family members will become clinically infected.
- Scabies affects all socioeconomic levels, ages, genders, and races.
- Delayed type IV hypersensitivity reaction occurs 10 to 30 days after exposure. If sensitized from a previous infection, symptoms may begin within 1 to 4 days after reinfection, but the reaction usually is not as severe.

CLINICAL PRESENTATION

- Intensely pruritic rash appears worse at night.
- Household members often report similar symptoms.
- Severity varies within a household.
- The classic lesion is a slightly raised and fairly linear burrow ranging from a few millimeters to a centimeter. A black dot (i.e., mite) is seen at the leading edge.
- It is typically located in the webs of fingers and toes and on the sides of hands and feet.
- Children younger than 5 years are often infected from head to toe, including palms and soles, with eczematous lesions.
- Older children and adults have lesions in the webs of fingers, axillas, flexor surfaces of arms, belt line, nipples, buttocks, and genitals. Facial involvement is rare.
- Secondary lesions commonly are the result of scratching and possibly of secondary infection.
  - Crusted papules
  - Vesicles
  - Pustules
  - Excoriations
  - Eczematous areas

ETIOLOGY

- The female mite burrows into stratum corneum, sucking tissue for nutrition.
- She lays 40 to 50 eggs over 4 to 6 weeks.
- Immune-mediated sensitivity to mites, their feces, and eggs causes the intense pruritic reaction.

DIAGNOSIS

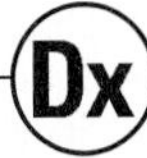

DIFFERENTIAL DIAGNOSIS

- Atopic dermatitis (common misdiagnoses, especially in infancy)
- Papular urticaria
- Acropustulosis of infancy
- Dyshidrotic eczema on hands
- Impetigo (although may have impetiginized scabies)

WORKUP

- Usually based on clinical examination findings
- Scabies scraping
  - Locate a burrow.
  - Put a drop of mineral oil on the lesion.
  - Scrape with a No. 15 blade to produce a speck of blood.
  - Scrape several lesions and place them on a slide, place a cover slip on top, and examine under low power for presence of mites, eggs, or scybala.

TREATMENT

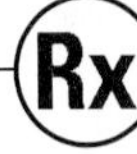

NONPHARMACOLOGIC THERAPY

- Prior use of topical steroids may produce some improvement and mask clinical findings.
- When it is difficult to identify a burrow for scraping, apply a washable marker over the web spaces and rinse with water. Retained ink after rinsing may identify a burrow.
- Norwegian scabies (i.e., keratotic scabies) is an intense infestation with widespread crusted hyperkeratotic lesions. It is uncommon and generally occurs in disabled or immunocompromised patients.
- Resolution of all lesions should be seen within 4 weeks after treatment.

ACUTE GENERAL Rx

- Permethrin (5%) can be used.
  - Apply from head (including scalp) to toe, leave on for 8 to 14 hours, and then rinse.
  - This product may be used in children older than 2 months of age.
- A 1% gamma benzene hexachloride lotion (Lindane or Kwell) can be used.
  - Apply for 8 to 12 hours and then rinse.
  - This lotion is less preferable because of central nervous system toxicity with prolonged skin contact.
  - Use is contraindicated in persons with a seizure disorder, infants (<2 years old), and pregnant women.
- For infants younger than 2 months and for pregnant women, use 5% and 10% precipitate sulfur in petrolatum applied for 3 consecutive nights and rinsed 24 hours later.
- Ivermectin is an oral agent that has been used to treat severe cases but does not have U.S. Food and Drug Administration (FDA) approval for the treatment of scabies.
- Treat all household contacts.
- It may be necessary to cover infants' and toddlers' hands and body with clothing to prevent licking of the scabicide.
- Oral antihistamines can be used in children older than 1 year for their antipruritic effect; it is worth trying to decrease itching and scratching.
- Topical corticosteroids are worth trying to relieve pruritus, but use only after the scabicide treatment is complete.

DISPOSITION

A follow-up visit in 2 weeks may be warranted to assess the success of therapy.

REFERRAL

Refer to a dermatologist for severe cases or cases refractory to treatment.

PEARLS & CONSIDERATIONS

PATIENT/FAMILY EDUCATION

- Instructions on the use of scabicides should be clear.
- Emphasize the need to treat all close household contacts.
- Persistence of itching 1 to 2 weeks after successful treatment is normal because of the sensitivity to degenerating mites.
- Vacuum furniture and mattresses.
- Wash in hot water the bed linens, towels, and clothing worn next to the skin in the past 4 days, including jackets, sweaters, and hats. Isolate nonwashable items for 3 to 4 days; mites will die after 3 days without human contact.
- Children may return to day care or school 24 hours after treatment.

SUGGESTED READINGS

American Academy of Pediatrics. Scabies. *In* Pickering LK, Baker CJ, Long SS, McMillan JA (eds): *Red Book: 2006 Report of the Committee on Infectious Diseases,* 27th ed. Elk Grove Village, IL, American Academy of Pediatrics, 2006, pp 584–587.

Huynh TH, Norman RA: Scabies and Pediculosis. *Dermatol Clin* 22:7, 2004.

Pomeranz AJ, Fairley JA: The systematic evaluation of the skin in children. *Pediatr Clin North Am* 45:61, 1998.

AUTHOR: **KRISTEN SMITH DANIELSON, MD**

BASIC INFORMATION

DEFINITION

Idiopathic scoliosis (IS) is a three-dimensional abnormality of the spine that includes abnormal lateral curvature, angulation, and rotational deformities with no clear underlying cause. Scoliosis is defined radiographically by a lateral spine curvature of more than 10 degrees Cobb angle. Scoliosis is a common complication of some neuromuscular and vertebral abnormalities. Other forms of spinal deformity include kyphosis and Scheuermann's kyphosis.

SYNONYMS

Crooked back
Spinal deformity

ICD-9-CM CODE

737.30 Scoliosis

EPIDEMIOLOGY & DEMOGRAPHICS

Infantile (Birth to 3 Years), Rare

- Most likely to resolve spontaneously (75%)
- Accounts for less than 1% of cases
- More common in boys
- Associated with plagiocephaly, bat-ear deformity, congenital muscular torticollis, developmental dysplasia of the hip, and mental retardation
- Inguinal hernia in 7.5%
- Congenital heart disease in 2.5%
- Curve to left most common in infantile scoliosis

Juvenile (3 to 10 Years)

- Mimics adolescent scoliosis with right curve predominance, increased incidence in girls
- Accounts for 10% to 20% of cases
- Course may be severe, but not uniformly

Adolescent (Older than 10 Years)

- Also called idiopathic scoliosis (IS) and accounts for up to 90% of all scoliosis
- Two percent to 3% prevalence of curves greater than 10 degrees in 16-year-olds
- Up to 2% prevalence of curves greater than 20 degrees
- Approximately 0.2% prevalence of curves greater than 30 degrees and 0.1% prevalence of curves greater than 40 degrees.
- Female-to-male ratio of 5:1 to 10:1 for significant curves
- Right thoracic most common (right scapula protrudes medially, right shoulder rotated forward)
- No increased risk of early mortality in mild to moderate adolescent IS
- Dominant or multiple gene inheritance pattern likely
- Increased risk in offspring of parent with IS
- High concordance rates in monozygotic twins

CLINICAL PRESENTATION

History

- Age at onset is typically during puberty in IS.
- Onset can be gradual or sudden.
- Sudden onset is atypical for IS.
- Sudden onset may indicate trauma, infection, or tumor of the spine.
- Age to menarche and Tanner staging helps to predict progression (the earlier the onset of scoliosis, the higher the chance of progression).
- Back pain suggests another diagnosis.
- Other congenital anomalies suggest diagnosis is not IS.
  - Scoliosis common with neuromuscular disorders (myopathic or neuromuscular scoliosis)
  - Increased association of spine deformities seen with congenital cardiac and urologic abnormalities
  - Spinal defects may follow radiation to chest or abdomen
- Family history
  - Genetic associations
  - Marfan's syndrome
  - Osteogenesis imperfecta
  - Neurofibromatosis
  - IS in relatives increases risk

Physical Examination

- Rib protuberance found on one side.
- Less than 10-degree curvature is normal.
- Flexibility of spine measured with twisting and rotation: stiffness indicates irritating lesions (e.g., spondylolysis, spinal cord tumor).
- Posture: shoulder and pelvic symmetry should be noted. Characteristic findings include:
  - One shoulder higher than other
  - Shoulder blade prominence on one side
  - Uneven waist
  - Hip higher on one side
  - Leg length inequality may lead to secondary scoliosis that corrects with shoe lifts.
  - Plumbline, dropped from T1 spinal process, should be 2.7 cm or less from gluteal cleft.
- Angle of trunk rotation is measured with a scoliometer (an inclinometer).
  - Adam's forward-bend test: patient bends forward with knees extended, arms extended and palms touching until the spine is parallel to the floor. (See Scoliosis in Charts, Formulas, Laboratory Tests and Values [Section IV].)
    - Observe patient from back and side, looking for rib hump.
    - Scoliometer measurement (at apex of curve) of more than 7 degrees is abnormal.
- Skin pigmentation, spinal skin dimpling, or nevi over spine may indicate underlying abnormality.
  - Neurofibromatosis
  - Spinal dysraphism
- Gait should be assessed and is generally normal with IS.
- Neurologic examination important and generally normal with IS.
- Ankle clonus, Babinski, or abnormal abdominal reflexes indicate spinal abnormality.
- Asymmetry may indicate an intraspinal process.
  - Intraspinal tumor
  - Lipoma
  - Syringomyelia, hydromyelia
  - Tethered cord
  - Neurofibromatosis
  - Muscle weakness
  - Cavus foot indicates neurologic process.
- Longitudinal height measurements seated and standing
  - Upper:lower body segment length and arm span (increased arm span in Marfan's syndrome)

ETIOLOGY

- The cause is unknown and, hence, the term *idiopathic.* Unsubstantiated hypotheses include:
  - Differential growth rate as a result of growth hormone secretion abnormalities
  - Central nervous system (CNS) abnormalities of proprioception and vibratory sensation
  - Insufficiency of costovertebral ligaments and biomechanical abnormalities
  - Asymmetric weakness of spinal support muscles, possibly caused by calcium transport defect resulting from abnormal calmodulin
  - Collagen abnormality
- Forms related to underlying neuromuscular abnormalities caused by the inability to maintain posture because of muscle weakness or laxity
  - Osteogenesis imperfecta (OI)
  - Muscular dystrophy
  - Cerebral palsy
- Bony anomalies rarely responsible for scoliosis
  - Vertebral collapse (e.g., resulting from leukemia)
  - Injury of vertebrae
- Progression of IS depends on the amount of linear growth left after diagnosis. The younger the age at diagnosis and the higher the degree of angular deformity, the more likely it is that the curve will progress. Progression more likely with the following:
  - Young age at diagnosis
  - Lower Risser sign (rating of skeletal maturity) at diagnosis
    - Risser 0–1 with spinal curve less than 20 degrees: 22% progressed
    - Risser 4–5 and same curve abnormalities: less than 2% progressed
    - Risser 0–1 with curve 20 to 30 degrees: 68% progressed
    - Risser 4–5 with this larger curve: 23% progressed
  - Longer time to onset of menarche from diagnosis
  - Female gender
- Large curves, greater than 50 degrees, often progress, even in skeletally mature.

DIAGNOSIS

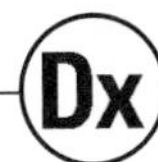

DIFFERENTIAL DIAGNOSIS

- Tethered cord
- Neuromuscular diseases
  - Muscular dystrophy
  - Spinal muscular atrophy
  - Cerebral palsy
  - Familial dysautonomia
- Neurofibromatosis
- Spinal tumors, lipoma
- Vertebral body bony anomalies or fractures
- Connective tissue disorders
- Marfan's syndrome
- Ehlers-Danlos syndrome
- Homocystinuria
- Syringomyelia, hydromyelia
- Leg length discrepancy
- Osteogenesis imperfecta
- Klippel-Feil syndrome

IMAGING STUDIES

- Standing anteroposterior and lateral radiograph of entire spine—occiput to sacrum (See Scoliosis in Charts, Formulas, Laboratory Tests and Values [Section IV].)
- Pelvic radiograph to determine Risser stage (used as an assessment of skeletal maturity) and chance of progression.
- Risser grades signify degree of ossification of iliac apophysis which is predictable from anterolateral to posterior medial.
  - 0: no ossification
  - 1: up to 25% ossification
  - 2: 26% to 50% ossification
  - 3: 51% to 75% ossification
  - 4: 76% to 100% ossification
  - 5: complete bony fusion
- Seated radiograph if patient is not ambulatory.
- If leg length discrepancy, blocks should be used under feet to assess true spinal curvature.
- Special views may be warranted as directed by orthopedic surgeon or neurosurgeon.
- Computed tomography, magnetic resonance imaging, or computed tomographic myelography:
  - Performed in infantile scoliosis because of the significant association with CNS abnormalities.
  - Can be used to visualize for spinal dysraphism.
  - New or progressive neurologic abnormalities require investigation.
- Congenital deformity
  - Approximately 25% associated with genitourinary (GU) anomalies, so consider GU visualization
  - Associated with cardiac disease 10% to 15% of the time
- Bone scan
  - May be used in patients with pain if source of symptoms is not obvious.

TREATMENT

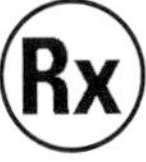

NONPHARMACOLOGIC THERAPY

- Follow-up every 4 to 6 months if greater than 10-degree curve in skeletally immature child or adolescent.
- No specific exercises are beneficial.
- For kyphosis, reassurance and observation or exercise are generally indicated.
- If greater than 40-degree curvature, surgical correction is recommended.
- If greater than 50-degree curvature, even if skeletally mature, surgery is also recommended, since even after maturity large angle curves progress.
- Anterior fusion, posterior fusion, or both, may be done depending on degree of curvature and skeletal maturity.
- Instrumentation without spinal fusion with progressive rod lengthening may be appropriate for infantile scoliosis.

ACUTE GENERAL Rx

- If 20- to 30-degree curvature or greater and more than 5 degrees of progression, bracing is indicated.
- If initial curve is greater than 25 degrees, even without evidence of progression, some would brace, especially in the skeletally immature patient.
- Bracing does not change torsional deformities such as rib prominence.
  - Bracing is 40% effective in adolescents with thoracic curves.
  - Under-arm brace is worn 23 hours per day.
  - Girls are weaned from brace gradually when skeletal maturity is reached (Risser score of 4 or higher) and 2 years past menarche.
  - Boys are treated until achieving a Risser score of 5 as progression may continue for longer.
- If scoliosis is associated with other processes, other specific treatments may be needed.

DISPOSITION

- The patient must be followed by orthopedic surgeon and pediatrician until progression is no longer occurring.
- Social isolation, lower marriage rate, and limited job opportunities noted in up to 19% of women with curves greater than 40%.
- No increased prevalence of back pain is noted compared with that of the general population.
  - Back pain, however, is common after fusion.
- Secondary rib and sternum rotational displacement persists.
- Restrictive lung disease has been observed, but only with marked scoliosis of more than 100 degrees in the absence of kyphosis.
- Cardiac restriction (very rare except in infantile scoliosis).
- Degenerative joint disease is increased only in those whose vertebrae shift translaterally in thoracolumbar and lumbar curves.
- Neurologic function interference is extremely rare.

REFERRAL

- Orthopedic surgeon for large, progressive, or atypical courses
- Orthopedic referral for any cases of preadolescent scoliosis

PEARLS & CONSIDERATIONS

COMMENTS

- Rapid onset or progression of scoliosis indicates a neurologic or vertebral process.
- Idiopathic adolescent scoliosis should be neither painful nor activity limiting.

PREVENTION

Bracing may halt progression, but it does not improve curvature.

PATIENT/FAMILY EDUCATION

- This is a common abnormality.
- IS is not generally associated with pain or neurologic abnormalities.
- Activity restriction is not indicated for most patients with idiopathic adolescent scoliosis.
- National Scoliosis Foundation, 5 Cabot Place, Stoughton, MA 02072; 800-NSF-myback; 718-341-6333; email: scoliosis@aol.com

SUGGESTED READINGS

KidsHealth. Available at www.Kidshealth.org/teen/health_problems/diseases/scoliosis.html

Lonstein JE: Scoliosis, surgical versus nonsurgical treatment. *Clin Orthop Rel Res* 443:248, 2006.

Reamy BV, Slakey JB: Adolescent idiopathic scoliosis: review and current concepts. *Am Fam Physician* 64:111, 2001.

AUTHOR: **LYNN C. GARFUNKEL, MD**

BASIC INFORMATION

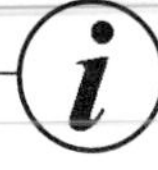

DEFINITION

Scorpions are arachnids that sting with the *telson,* the tip of their flexible tail.

ICD-9-CM CODE
989.5 Toxic effect of venom

EPIDEMIOLOGY & DEMOGRAPHICS

- There were approximately 14,400 scorpion stings reported in the desert areas of the southwestern United States in 2003. These states are Arizona, New Mexico, Texas, and Nevada.
- Ten stings were associated with major sequelae.
- The last verified death from a scorpion sting in the United States was that of a 5-month-old child in 1968.
- Children under 16 years of age are most commonly affected.
- Scorpions are endemic in the southwestern United States, and most live above ground in wood piles and in crevices.
- Scorpions have a negative response to high-intensity light, they also hide in shoes, blankets, or clothing left on the floor during daylight hours, as well as under tents.
- **The *Centruroides exilicauda,* the only potentially lethal scorpion in the United States, is fluorescent under ultraviolet light and can be located with a Wood's lamp.**

CLINICAL PRESENTATION

- Immediate and severe local pain and paresthesias
- No erythema, swelling, or blistering
- Pain and paresthesias may progress to remote sites
- Cranial nerve dysfunction demonstrated as blurred vision, disconjugate gaze, nystagmus, slurred speech, and hypersalivation
- Skeletal neuromuscular dysfunction characterized by restlessness, fasciculations, opisthotonos, and jerking movements often mistaken for seizures
- Tachycardia and hypertension
- Respiratory distress from respiratory muscle incoordination and failure
- Nausea, vomiting, rhabdomyolysis, and metabolic acidosis are possible

ETIOLOGY

- *C. exilicauda* is the potentially lethal scorpion found in the United States.
- Other U.S. species cause only minor local reactions.
- Venom contains neurotoxins that produce systemic effects of hypertension, cranial nerve, and skeletal motor dysfunction as well as paresthesias and pain.

DIAGNOSIS

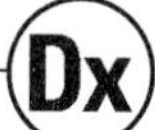

DIFFERENTIAL DIAGNOSIS

- Insect sting or bite
- Spider bite
- Animal bite

WORKUP

- History of residing in or travel to the southwestern United States
- Characteristic immediate severe pain without surrounding erythema or swelling
- Exaggerated pain with tapping over the envenomated area (tap test)

LABORATORY TESTS

- Complete blood cell count to examine for evidence of hemolysis
- Coagulation studies looking for venom-induced coagulopathy and hypofibrinemia
- Creatine kinase and a urinalysis to assess for rhabdomyolysis
- Spirometry should be followed to assess diaphragmatic function
- An electrocardiogram may be abnormal in more than half of envenomated children. Typically, sinus tachycardia is noted, but QTc prolongation and T-wave abnormalities are also seen.

IMAGING STUDIES

- Chest radiograph to evaluate for unilateral pulmonary edema

TREATMENT

Rx

NONPHARMACOLOGIC THERAPY

- Ice pack applied for 30 minutes each hour
- Elevation
- Tourniquets are controversial

ACUTE GENERAL Rx

- Airway management is most important particularly in young children, whose smaller diameter airways lead to an increased chance of respiratory difficulty.
- In small children, the risks of antivenin administration are overshadowed by the risks of an untreated *C. exilicauda* sting. Prompt antivenin administration may prevent endotracheal intubation.
- In adults, most symptoms are minor and short-lived (12 to 48 hours). The risks of antivenin administration may outweigh the risks of envenomation.
- Antivenin reverses cranial nerve and somatoskeletal symptoms, but not pain and paresthesias.
- Risk of anaphylaxis with antivenin administration requires intensive observation and readiness with epinephrine, intravenous fluids, and antihistamines.
- Avoid narcotics, barbiturates, benzodiazepines, or other potent analgesics. These medications are generally ineffective in these cases and can lead to apnea and loss of protective airway reflexes.
- Topical anesthetics tend to be more helpful than narcotic analgesics.

DISPOSITION

Patients are closely monitored until a patent airway is ensured and neurologic symptoms are stable.

REFERRAL

Referral to a pediatric tertiary care center may be necessary in severe cases for administration of antivenin and intensive care monitoring.

PEARLS & CONSIDERATIONS

!

COMMENTS

- Airway compromise is of greatest concern in children under 1 year of age.
- Airway management is the first step in the care of scorpion stings.
- Lack of swelling and erythema at the sting site as well as exaggerated pain to a firm finger tap indicates a sting by *C. exilicauda,* the only native scorpion associated with systemic sequelae.

PREVENTION

- Prevention is of extreme importance in reducing morbidity and mortality from scorpion envenomation.
- Remove dead wood, firewood, and leaves.
- Clothing, shoes, and camping gear left outside should be shaken before being used.
- Footwear is recommended in scorpion-prone areas.
- *C. exilicauda* is fluorescent under ultraviolet light and can be easily located in the dark using a Wood's lamp.

PATIENT/FAMILY EDUCATION

- Advise patients regarding the risk and signs of scorpion stings as well as reasonable preventive measures.
- Additional information regarding treatment and prevention of scorpion stings is available at www.desertusa.com/oct96/du_scorpion.html

SUGGESTED READINGS

Bond GR: Snake, spider, and scorpion envenomation in North America. *Pediatr Rev* 20:147, 1999.

Connor A, Seldon B: Scorpion Envenomation. *In* Auerbach PS (ed): *Wilderness Medicine: Management of Wilderness and Environmental Emergencies.* St. Louis, Mosby, 1995, pp 831–841.

Desert USA. Available at www.desertusa.com

Holve S: Treatment of snake, insect, scorpion, and spider bites in the pediatric emergency department. *Curr Opin Pediatr* 8(3):256, 1996.

Litovitz TL et al: 2003 Annual Report of the American Association of Poison Control Centers Toxic Exposure Surveillance System. *Am J Emerg Med* 22(5):378, 2004.

Lovecchio F, McBride C: Scorpion envenomations in young children in central Arizona. *J Toxicol Clin Toxicol* 41(7):937, 2003.

Schexnayder SM, Schexnayder RE: Bites, stings, and other painful things. *Pediatr Ann* 29(6):354, 2000.

AUTHORS: **MARK RODDY, MD** and **ROBERT J. FREISHTAT, MD, MPH**

BASIC INFORMATION

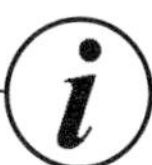

DEFINITION

Seborrheic dermatitis is a subacute or chronic inflammatory disorder confined to the sebaceous gland–rich skin of the head, the trunk, and occasionally, the intertriginous areas.

SYNONYMS

Cradle cap
Dandruff
Seborrhea

ICD-9-CM CODE
690.10 Seborrheic dermatitis

EPIDEMIOLOGY & DEMOGRAPHICS

- Seborrheic dermatitis is a common disorder with a bimodal age distribution (early infancy and adulthood).
  - It may be two separate entities.
  - Adult disease may begin in puberty.
  - Equal frequency in seen in both sexes in infancy.
  - There is no racial predilection.

CLINICAL PRESENTATION

- Pruritus is not a major feature.
- Skin exposed to saliva (i.e., perioral and anterior neck crease) is often affected.
- The scalp, flexural creases, and diaper area are typically involved in infants.
- Erythematous plaques may have sharply defined borders.
- Small, erythematous papules with fine scale may be scattered around larger plaques.
- Scalp lesions are thick, yellowish plaques with white scales.

ETIOLOGY

- The cause remains unknown.
- Seborrheic dermatitis coincides with periods of sebaceous gland activity, implicating sebum in the pathogenesis.

DIAGNOSIS

DIFFERENTIAL DIAGNOSIS

- Atopic dermatitis
- Psoriasis
- Langerhans cell histiocytosis (Letterer-Siwe disease)
- *Candida albicans* diaper dermatitis
- Irritant diaper dermatitis
- Acrodermatitis enteropathica

WORKUP

The diagnosis is usually made on the basis of the characteristic clinical picture.

TREATMENT

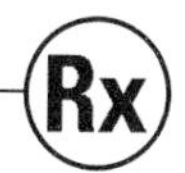

NONPHARMACOLOGIC THERAPY

- Daily shampooing of the scalp and face with mild shampoo is recommended.
- Keratolytic shampoos (containing sulfur or salicylic acid) may be used for thick scales on the scalp.

ACUTE GENERAL Rx

Mild topical corticosteroids may be given in short courses when the dermatitis is unresponsive to shampooing.

REFERRAL

Refer the patient to a dermatologist when the condition does not respond to the use of shampoo and a mild topical corticosteroid.

PEARLS & CONSIDERATIONS

COMMENTS

- Severe seborrheic syndrome with generalized exfoliative erythroderma may be seen in a variety of congenital immunodeficiency syndromes.
- Patients with human immunodeficiency virus (HIV) infection or acquired immunodeficiency syndrome (AIDS) may have more severe disease, which can be refractory to therapy.

SUGGESTED READINGS

American Academy of Dermatology. Available at www.aad.org
Elewski BE: Clinical diagnosis of common scalp disorders. *J Investig Dermatol Symp Proc* 10:190, 2005.
Gee BC: Seborrheic dermatitis. *Clin Evidence* 12:2344, 2004.
Society for Pediatric Dermatology. Available at www.spdnet.org

AUTHOR: **SUSAN HALLER PSAILA, MD**

BASIC INFORMATION

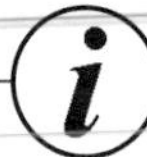

DEFINITIONS

- An epileptic seizure is defined as manifestation(s) of epileptic (excessive or hypersynchronous), usually self-limited activity of neurons in the brain.
- Epileptic disorder is a chronic neurologic condition characterized by recurrent epileptic seizures.
- A focal (partial) seizure is one whose initial semiology indicates, or is consistent with, initial activation of only part of one cerebral hemisphere.
- A generalized (bilateral) seizure is a seizure whose initial semiology indicates, or is consistent with, more than minimal involvement of both cerebral hemispheres.
- Unprovoked seizures are afebrile and without any clear precipitating cause (e.g., head injury, infection, hypoglycemia, etc.).

SYNONYMS

Generalized tonic-clonic seizure
Grand mal
Petit mal

ICD-9-CM CODES

345.90 Epilepsy, unspecified
780.3 Convulsive seizure

EPIDEMIOLOGY & DEMOGRAPHICS

- Five percent of population has at least one unprovoked seizure.
- The incidence of epilepsy is 40 to 70 per 100,000 with a peak incidence in the first 10 years of life and a second peak in late adulthood.
- Fifty percent of epilepsy develops before age 15 years.
- Prevalence is 4 to 6 cases per 1000 children.

CLINICAL PRESENTATION

Clinical Presentation Depends on Type of Seizures

- Partial seizures
  - Simple partial seizure
    - Consciousness is not impaired.
    - Usually very brief with motor, somatosensory, psychic, or autonomic features
    - There may be transient motor weakness following the seizure.
  - Complex partial seizures
    - Most common seizure type in children and adults
    - "Complex" refers to impairment in consciousness
    - May start as simple partial seizure and progress or may begin as complex seizure
    - May last 30 to 60 seconds
    - Frequently include automatisms, such as finger movements or lip smacking
    - May evolve into secondary generalized seizures
- Generalized seizures
  - Abrupt onset
  - Alteration of consciousness
  - Bilateral
  - Absence seizures
    - Brief (<10 seconds)
    - Most untreated children have more than 10 seizures a day, some may have hundreds
    - Typically consist of staring and impaired consciousness
    - May include tonic, atonic, and clonic components
  - Myoclonic, clonic, tonic, or atonic ("drop" attacks)
  - Tonic-clonic seizures
    - Most generalized tonic-clonic seizures in children are secondarily generalized partial seizures.
    - Presence of aura or initial behavioral arrest or change suggests focal onset.

Relevant Medical History (Following a Seizure)

- When possible, obtain history from someone who witnessed the event. Obtain details from start to end of event (ictus) with attention to:
  - Duration
  - Focality at onset and presence of lateralizing findings during seizure
  - Facial features, including appearance of eyes (open, rolled back, deviated), facial twitching, drooling
  - Position and behavior of extremities
    - Rhythmic jerking or sustained postures more typical of seizures
    - Flailing and thrashing movements are unusual
  - What occurred during the "postictal" (after seizure) period.
    - Sleepy, normal, any transient focal weakness (Todd's paralysis)
  - Determine patients' recollection of event.
  - Patient's recent health
    - Acute illness, toxin exposure, triggers for hypoglycemia or other metabolic derangements, trauma
- If this is the first seizure or the seizure history is unknown, promptly assess.

Physical Examination

- If the patient is having a seizure with motor manifestations (convulsions), assess airway, and other vital signs.
- Make sure the patient is lying either on back or side with head cushioned.
- Most seizures resolve on their own within 5 minutes and at that time normal breathing should resume.
- Once the patient is stable and seizure has stopped:
  - Look for conditions needing emergency management—head injury, obtundation, infection, acute ingestion.
  - Other findings that suggest specific etiologies:
    - Dysmorphic features
    - Large or small head circumference, bulging fontanelle
    - Skin findings may suggest neurocutaneous syndromes
      - Tuberous sclerosis—hypopigmented macules, adenoma sebaceum, subungual fibromas
      - Neurofibromatosis—café au lait spots, neurofibromas
      - Sturge-Weber syndrome—facial port-wine stain, glaucoma

ETIOLOGY

- Epileptic seizures are caused by hypersynchronous neuronal discharges from many different conditions, including:
  - Central nervous system malformation
  - Genetic and hereditary factors (e.g., benign rolandic epilepsy, idiopathic generalized tonic-clonic seizures, benign familial neonatal convulsions, juvenile myoclonic epilepsy)
  - Head trauma
  - Neoplasm or space-occupying lesion
  - Cerebrovascular disease
  - Metabolic disease (such as urea cycle defects, disorders of amino acid and organic acid metabolism, B_6 dependency, mitochondrial diseases)
  - Infections (meningitis, encephalitis, brain abscess)
  - Toxins

DIAGNOSIS

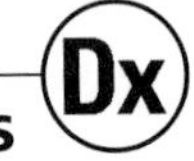

DIFFERENTIAL DIAGNOSIS

- Any condition associated with recurrent abnormal movements, transient altered awareness, or episodic symptoms can be confused with seizures.
- Paroxysmal movements
  - Tics, benign sleep myoclonus, paroxysmal choreoathetosis, self-stimulation/masturbation
- Loss of tone or consciousness or transient altered awareness
  - Syncope, narcolepsy, daydreaming, attention deficit/hyperactivity disorder, migraine
- Behavior disorders
  - Head banging, rage attacks, breath-holding spells
- Sleep disorders
  - Night terrors, sleep walking, nightmares
- Psychiatric disorders
  - Hallucinations, fugue, panic attack
- Specific disorders with episodic events
  - Hypoglycemia, hypocalcemia, periodic paralysis, cardiac arrhythmias, gastroesophageal reflux, tetralogy spells, intoxication, vertigo

WORKUP

- An electroencephalogram (EEG) should be done after the first unprovoked seizure.
  - It should include awake and asleep tracings, if possible.
  - Depending on the age of the patient, hyperventilation and photic stimulation should be performed.
- Interictal EEGs show abnormalities in only 60% of patients with epilepsy.
- Epileptiform discharges are those EEG waves with abnormal morphology that are seen in patients with epilepsy.
  - They include sharp waves, spikes, and spike-wave complexes.

- In general, localization (focal or generalized) is more important than appearance.
- Slowing of EEG wave frequency is a nonspecific finding that may indicate an underlying encephalopathy.
- Unless a seizure occurs during an EEG, the presence of epileptiform discharges does not provide a diagnosis of seizures or epilepsy. The information from the EEG must be combined with the details of the seizure presentation, medical history, and exam. The EEG is helpful in determining:
  - Seizure type
  - Need for further imaging
  - Epilepsy syndrome
  - Risk for recurrence

LABORATORY TESTS

- Based on clinical history, consider glucose, calcium, and phosphorus.
- In infants with seizures or in older children with suggestive clinical history, assess for a metabolic disturbance.
  - Serum amino acids, urine organic acids, biotinidase, ammonia, lactate and pyruvate, other genetic studies are based on the clinical diagnosis.

IMAGING STUDIES

- Magnetic resonance imaging (MRI) is the preferred study for evaluating focal seizures, recurrent seizures, and focal EEGs.
  - May not be indicated with a single seizure, primary generalized epilepsy, or typical presentations of "benign" epilepsies such as benign rolandic epilepsy with centrotemporal spikes.
- In emergent situations, computed tomography (CT) may be more readily available and is useful for diagnosing acute intracranial injury.
  - Emergent neuroimaging should be done for:
    - Any child with postictal focal deficit or altered sensorium that does not resolve within several hours of seizure
    - High suspicion of central nervous system trauma
    - Increased intracranial pressure
  - CT in nonemergent situations may be helpful if MRI is unavailable.

TREATMENT

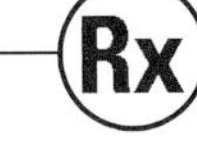

NONPHARMACOLOGIC THERAPY

- Avoid specific triggers such as sleep deprivation and fever.
  - Some seizures may be triggered by light, reading, or minor trauma.
- Ketogenic diet is a restrictive high-fat diet that may be recommended in those children who have refractory seizures or intolerable side effects to medication.
  - Initiation of this diet requires strict adherence by patient and family as well as close monitoring by dieticians and neurologists experienced in this treatment.

Epilepsy Surgery

- Reserved for children with focal seizures unresponsive to anticonvulsant therapy
- Assessment and treatment in tertiary centers where detailed studies aid in localization
- Types of surgery (depending on indication and seizure type): lobectomy, hemispherectomy, corpus callosotomy, multiple subpial transections
- Vagal nerve stimulation
  - Indicated as adjunct therapy to reduce frequency of seizures in individuals older than 12 years of age with partial-onset seizures that are refractory to antiepileptic medications
  - Works by intermittent stimulation of vagal nerve via surgically implanted battery and electrodes

ACUTE GENERAL Rx

- Generally consists of supportive care.
- In the case of prolonged seizures (status epilepticus) emergency management is required and intravenous anticonvulsants are used to stop seizures.

CHRONIC Rx

- In general, no treatment after the first single unprovoked seizure.
  - If the EEG and history suggest a potentially catastrophic epilepsy syndrome, such as infantile spasms, treatment is initiated promptly.
- Medication choice depends on seizure type, epileptic syndrome, and age of patient.
  - Partial epilepsy syndromes (e.g., complex partial epilepsy) are treated with agents such as carbamazepine, oxcarbazepine, and phenytoin.
  - Primary generalized epilepsy syndromes (e.g., childhood absence epilepsy, juvenile myoclonic epilepsy) are treated with "broader spectrum" anticonvulsants such as divalproex sodium, lamotrigine, or ethosuximide, which can also be used to treat refractory partial epilepsy syndromes.

Examples:

- Partial epilepsy: a 10-year-old girl has a history of two partial seizures consisting of arrest in activity without loss of muscle tone and unilateral motor symptoms lasting for 20 seconds. An EEG shows occasional focal left temporal spikes; the MRI is normal. A reasonable medication to use to prevent recurrent seizures might be carbamazepine or oxcarbazepine.
- Generalized epilepsy: a teenage boy has frequent episodes of brief staring during the day which last only a few seconds. He also has had one generalized tonic-clonic seizure lasting 10 seconds. His EEG shows multifocal spike-wave discharges and his EEG is normal. A reasonable medication to initiate would be divalproex sodium or lamotrigine.

DISPOSITION

- Goal of anticonvulsant therapy is to stop recurrent seizures.
- Follow-up is frequent by phone or in clinic until the medical treatment proves effective.
- If seizure free for 2 years, consider weaning from anti-epileptic drugs.
- Careful monitoring of psychosocial adjustment of family and patient is advised.

REFERRAL

Patients with recurrent afebrile seizures can be referred to a pediatric neurologist.

PEARLS & CONSIDERATIONS

COMMENTS

- Seizures often occur with eyes open, though the eyes may be described as rolled back or deviated.
  - Events that occur with eyes closed may be sleep behaviors and not seizures.
- The use of video-EEG monitoring of seizures is helpful in evaluating frequent seizure-like behaviors.

PREVENTION

- Factors that may exacerbate seizures include fever, undue stress, or lack of sleep.
- Careful consideration of other medications that may potentially lower the seizure threshold (e.g., bupropion) is warranted.

PATIENT/FAMILY EDUCATION

- Educate parents and child about causes and treatment for epilepsy.
- Careful education is needed concerning medication side effects, interactions, and necessity for compliance.
- Review first aid for seizures: loosen clothing around neck, remove harmful objects from environment, maintain airway.
- Patient is cautioned to refrain from swimming and bathing alone.
- Patient may participate in all sports, including contact sports, using appropriate protective equipment.
- Check state laws concerning driving and epilepsy.
- Alert teachers and school officials, review first aid, monitor for learning disorders.

SUGGESTED READINGS

The Epilepsy Foundation (also known as the Epilepsy Foundation of America). Available at www.epilepsyfoundation.org

Hirtz D et al: Practice parameter: evaluating a first non-febrile seizure in children: report of the quality standards subcommittee of the American Academy of Neurology, the Child Neurology Society, and the American Epilepsy Society. *Neurology* 55:616, 2000.

Hirtz D et al: Practice parameter: treatment of the child with a first unprovoked seizure: report of the quality standards subcommittee of the American Academy of Neurology and the Practice Committee of the Child Neurology Society. *Neurology* 60:166, 2003.

AUTHOR: **JENNIFER M. KWON, MD**

BASIC INFORMATION

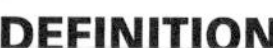
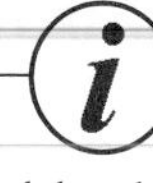

DEFINITION

Serotonin syndrome is characterized by the triad of altered mental status, autonomic dysfunction, and neuromuscular abnormalities. It is a predictable consequence of excess serotonergic agonism of the central nervous system (CNS) receptors and peripheral serotonergic receptors that produce this spectrum of clinical findings from barely perceptible to lethal.

SYNONYM

Serotonergic syndrome

ICD-9-CM CODE

333.99 Serotonin syndrome

EPIDEMIOLOGY & DEMOGRAPHICS

- First described in 1955; increase in use of serotonergic agonists likely the cause of recent increase in reported cases.
- Sixty percent of patients present within 6 hours after initial dose, an overdose, or a change in dose of prescription serotonergic drug.
- Serotonin syndrome is estimated to occur in 14% to 16% of patients who overdose on selective serotonin reuptake inhibitors (SSRIs).
    - Also noted after starting a serotonergic agent and within 5 to 6 weeks after discontinuing fluoxetine, sertraline, paroxetine, or monoamine oxidase inhibitors (MAOIs)
- 2002 Toxic Exposure Surveillance System:
    - 99,860 incidences of exposures to antidepressant
    - 46,244 incidences of exposures to SSRIs
        - 7349 (16%) with moderate to major toxic effects
        - 93 (0.2%) deaths
    - Serotonin syndrome not explicitly listed as an outcome
    - Described in all ages (newborns to elderly)
        - Majority (75.6%) between ages of 22 and 50 years
        - 14.6% in patients 0 to 21 years
        - Male to female ratio of 1:1.7
        - Has been described after a single 60 mg dose of fluoxetine (Prozac) in a child
- Risk factors
    - Taking two or more medications that increase CNS serotonin levels
    - Addition of another medication metabolized by the cytochrome P450 isoenzymes
    - Recent changes in dosage(s) of serotonergic drugs
- Slow metabolizer of SSRIs (~7% of population)

CLINICAL PRESENTATION

History

- Prescription serotonergic agents available to patient or in household
- Antidepressants: SSRIs, MAOIs, tricyclic antidepressants (TCAs)
- Other drugs associated with serotonin syndrome:
    - Analgesics
    - Antiemetics
    - Migraine medications
    - Anticonvulsants
    - Antibiotics
- Overdose or missing pills
- Recent additions or changes in dosages
- Over-the-counter (OTC) medication history
    - Cold medications: dextromethorphan
    - Dietary aides: L-tryptophan
    - Herbal remedies: St. John's wort, ginseng
- Illicit drug use
- Suicidal tendencies or depression
- Family history of intolerance of serotonergic medications

Physical Examination

- Mental status
    - Agitation
    - Delirium
- Autonomic hyperactivity
    - Hypertension
    - Tachycardia
    - Mydriasis
    - Diaphoresis
    - Active bowel sounds
    - Diarrhea
    - Hyperthermia, minimum temperature greater than 38°C
- Neuromuscular dysfunction
    - Hyperreflexia
    - Inducible clonus
    - Myoclonus
    - Ocular clonus
    - Spontaneous clonus
    - Peripheral hypertonicity
    - Shivering
    - Seizure
    - Akathisia
    - Ataxia
    - Nystagmus
- Tremor, restlessness, and rigidity are prominent symptoms in newborns.
- Hypertonicity, rigidity, and high-grade fever (>38.5°C) are prominent features in life-threatening cases of serotonin syndrome.

ETIOLOGY

- Serotonin neurons in the CNS are found primarily in the midline raphe nuclei in the brainstem from the midbrain to the medulla.
    - Rostral end regulates wakefulness, affective behavior, food intake, thermoregulation, migraine, emesis, and sexual behavior.
    - Lower pons and medulla regulate nociception and motor tone.
    - In periphery, serotonin regulates vascular tone and gastrointestinal motility.
- Serotonin syndrome probably results from excessive stimulation of 5-HT_{1A} and 5-HT_2 serotonin receptors.
- It is usually a result of administration of a serotonin agonist to a patient who is already taking a medication capable of increasing the effects of the serotonin pathway.
- Possible serotonin potentiating interactions include:
    - Increase serotonin synthesis
        - L-tryptophan
    - Decrease serotonin metabolism
        - Isocarboxazid
        - Phenelzine
        - Selegiline
        - Tranylcypromine
    - Increase serotonin release
        - Amphetamines
        - Cocaine
        - Reserpine
        - Methylenedioxymethamphetamine (MDMA or ecstasy)
    - Increase serotonin uptake
        - Tricyclics
        - SSRIs
        - Doxepin
        - Nefazodone
        - Trazodone
        - Amphetamines
        - Cocaine
        - Dextromethorphan
        - Meperidine
        - Venlafaxine
    - Direct serotonin receptor agonists
        - Buspirone
        - Lysergic acid
        - Diethylamide (LSD)
        - Sumatriptan
    - Nonspecific increase in serotonin activity
        - Lithium
        - Dopamine agonists
        - Amantadine
        - Bromocriptine
        - Bupropion
        - Levodopa

DIAGNOSIS

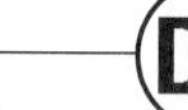

- Multiple diagnostic criteria
- Hunter Serotonin Toxicology Criteria algorithm—84% sensitive, 97% specific
    - Step 1: serotonergic agent administered in the past 5 weeks?
    - If yes, Step 2: any of the following symptoms?
        - Tremor and hyperreflexia
        - Spontaneous clonus
        - Hypertonia, temperature greater than 38°C, and either ocular clonus or inducible clonus
        - Ocular clonus and either agitation or diaphoresis
        - Inducible clonus and either agitation or diaphoresis
    - If yes to Step 1 and any of the symptoms listed in Step 2 = serotonin syndrome

- If no to Steps 1 or 2 = *not* serotonin syndrome
- Clonus is the most important sign in this algorithm.
- Rule out other possible causes, especially neuroleptic malignant syndrome (NMS)
- If neuroleptic agent started or dosage changed prior to the onset of symptoms consider NMS rather than serotonin syndrome

DIFFERENTIAL DIAGNOSIS

- Neuroleptic malignant syndrome
- Malignant hyperthermia
- Catatonia
- Infection
  - Meningitis, tetanus, septicemia
- Encephalitis
  - Infectious or metabolic
- Dystonic reaction
- Hyperthyroidism
- Stiff-man syndrome
- Poisonings/overdoses
  - Anticholinergics, LSD, MDMA or ecstasy, amphetamines, cocaine, lithium, MAOIs, phencyclidine (PCP), salicylates, water hemlock, strychnine, 2,4-dichlorophenoxyacetic acid, dinitrophenol, pentachlorophenol

WORKUP

- No specific laboratory or imaging studies

TREATMENT

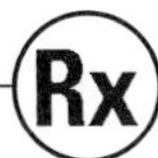

NONPHARMACOLOGIC THERAPY

Discontinue offending medications.

ACUTE GENERAL Rx

- Discontinue offending medications.
- Supportive—intravenous fluids as needed
- Neuromuscular abnormalities
  - Hyperreflexia and tremor without hyperpyrexia—consider benzodiazepine
  - For hyperthermic patients with a temperature greater than 41.1°C consider immediate sedation, neuromuscular paralysis, and orotracheal intubation
- Agitation
  - Consider benzodiazepine (i.e., diazepam).
  - Avoid physical restraints which may contribute to mortality by increasing muscle activity and thereby lactic acidosis and hyperthermia.
- Autonomic instability
  - Hypotension
  - Low dose of sympathomimetic amine (i.e., norepinephrine)
    - May get a dramatic response if MAOIs have been ingested since monoamine oxidase limits intracellular concentration of epinephrine and norepinephrine
  - Hypertension
    - Consider short-acting agents such as nitroprusside or esmolol.
    - Avoid long-acting β_2 agents such as propanolol.
      - May worsen hypotension of autonomic instability by preventing tachycardia
      - Masks tachycardia which can be used to determine the persistence of symptoms
- Hyperthermia
  - Immediate paralysis with nondepolarizing agent (i.e., vecuronium)
  - Avoid succinylcholine—arrhythmia risk associated with hyperkalemia, a consequence of rhabdomyolysis.
  - Antipyretics ineffective
  - Serotonin antagonists may be considered in severe cases.
    - More studies are needed to determine safety and efficacy.
    - Cyproheptadine—via nasogastric tube
    - Atypical antipsychotics—sublingual olanzapine or intramuscular chlorpromazine
  - Avoid bromocriptine and dantrolene.
    - Used to treat NMS
    - May exacerbate serotonin syndrome and may lead to death

DISPOSITION

- Mild to moderate cases often resolve within 24 to 72 hours.
- Some patients require mechanical ventilation.
- Mortality rate approximately 12%

PEARLS & CONSIDERATIONS

COMMENTS

- A high degree of suspicion is needed to make the diagnosis.
- Rapid progression to death occurs unless offending agents are stopped and supportive care is initiated.
- It is important to distinguish from NMS since the therapies used to treat one can lead to death in the other.
- Hyperthermia is secondary to muscular contractions, therefore serotonin syndrome is best treated with paralysis when temperature exceeds 41°C; not responsive to antipyretics.
- Use chemical sedation and avoid physical restraints for agitation.

PREVENTION

- Reconsider the use of two or more serotonergic medications.
- Consider using less serotonergic alternatives.

PATIENT/FAMILY EDUCATION

- Patient/parent education on symptoms of serotonin syndrome
- Educate about OTC medication interactions.

SUGGESTED READINGS

Boyer EW, Shannon M: Current concepts in the serotonin syndrome. *N Engl J Med* 352:1112, 2005.

Dunkley AH, Whyte IM: The Hunter Serotonin Toxicity Criteria: simple and accurate diagnostic decision rules for serotonin toxicity. *QJM* 96:635, 2003.

Gillman PK: The serotonin syndrome and its treatment. *J Psychopharmacol* 13:100, 1999.

Hemeryck A, Belpaire F: Selective serotonin reuptake inhibitors and cytochrome p-450 mediated drug-drug interactions: an update. *Curr Drug Metabolism* 3:13, 2002.

Sternbach H: The serotonin syndrome. *Am J Psychiatry* 148:705, 1991.

AUTHOR: **S. NICHOLE FEENEY, MD**

BASIC INFORMATION

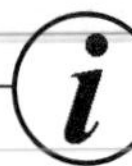

DEFINITION

Serum sickness is a systemic vasculitis induced by a type III hypersensitivity reaction to a foreign antigen.

ICD-9-CM CODE
999.5 Serum sickness

EPIDEMIOLOGY & DEMOGRAPHICS

- Incidence varies depending on the specific antigen; for each antigen the quoted rates vary greatly.
- Currently, antibiotics are the leading cause of serum sickness; among antibiotics, cefaclor and penicillin are associated with the highest incidence.
- Incidence and severity increase with age and higher doses of medication.
- Horse serum is associated with a high incidence of severe serum sickness.

CLINICAL PRESENTATION

- Symptoms begin 4 to 21 days after administration of the antigen.
    - If previously sensitized to the antigen, symptoms may begin within 1 to 2 days.
- Following injections, the first symptom is erythema and pain at the injection site.
- Rash is typically the first systemic sign.
    - Begins as an erythematous rash with serpiginous border, often along the junction of the palmar and dorsal surfaces of the hands and feet.
    - The rash may progress into generalized urticaria or morbilliform-like lesions.
- Common complaints include low-grade fever, malaise, myalgia, arthralgia, arthritis of multiple joints (typically involving the hands and feet), generalized pruritus, edema of hands and feet, and gastrointestinal symptoms.
- Lymphadenopathy near the injection site is common.
- Retinal and palpebral hemorrhages may occur.

ETIOLOGY

- Serum sickness is a type III hypersensitivity reaction in which immune complexes are deposited on endothelial tissue and initiate an inflammatory process.
- Known antigens include but are not limited to equine sera (including Centruroides antivenom, which is produced in horses), drugs, human gamma globulin, Hymenoptera stings, and hepatitis viruses.

DIAGNOSIS

DIFFERENTIAL DIAGNOSIS

- Lupus erythematous or other systemic vasculitis
- Erythema multiforme
- Urticaria

LABORATORY TESTS

- Commonly noted laboratory data include the following:
    - Hematology: thrombocytopenia, initial leukocytosis followed by leukopenia, eosinophilia (typically late in course)
    - Nephrology: proteinuria, hemoglobinuria, microscopic hematuria
    - Immunology: elevated erythrocyte sedimentation rate, decreased C3 and C4 levels
- Skin biopsy of lesions: immune deposits of immunoglobulin M, immunoglobulin G, immunoglobulin E, and C3; perivascular infiltration of lymphocytes, histiocytes and rarely neutrophils

TREATMENT

ACUTE GENERAL Rx

- Discontinue suspect medications.
- Typically serum sickness has a 7- to 10-day self-limited course that requires only symptomatic treatment with antihistamines and nonsteroidal anti-inflammatory drugs.
- Severe cases respond well to prednisone 1 to 2 mg/kg/day for 7 to 14 days.

DISPOSITION

- For typical self-limited cases, no follow-up is necessary once symptoms resolve.
- Rare complications include Guillain-Barré syndrome, permanent neuritis (most commonly involving the brachial plexus), myocarditis, arteritis of coronary arteries, laryngeal edema, and pleuritis.

REFERRAL

The majority of cases can be managed by a primary care physician with appropriate referrals for complications.

PEARLS & CONSIDERATIONS

COMMENTS

- Horse serum is associated with the highest incidence and most severe symptoms.
- Currently most reactions are secondary to drugs and are relatively benign.
- There is currently no means of predicting which patients will develop serum sickness.
- Some experts believe that administering prophylactic antihistamines may reduce the rate of serum sickness.

PATIENT/FAMILY EDUCATION

Exposure to the same antigen may trigger another episode of serum sickness.

SUGGESTED READINGS

Calabrese LH, Duna GF: Drug-induced vasculitis. *Curr Opin Rheum* 8:34, 1996.

Erffmeyer JE: Serum sickness. *Ann Allergy* 56:105, 1986.

Naguwa SM, Nelson BL: Human serum sickness. *Clin Rev Allergy* 3:117, 1985.

AUTHOR: **CHRISTOPHER COPENHAVEN, MD**

BASIC INFORMATION

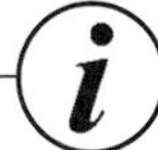

DEFINITION

Sexual abuse occurs when a child is exposed to or engaged in sexual activities in which the child cannot give consent, or are coercive in nature, or violate the law, or when there is a developmental asymmetry among the participants. The perpetrator is generally an older or more mature person. The sexual activities may include any of the following: fondling of genitalia or breasts, oral-genital contact, vaginal or anal penetration, exploitation in pornography or prostitution, exhibitionism, or voyeurism.

SYNONYMS

Molestation
Rape
Sexual assault

ICD-9-CM CODES
995.53 Sexual abuse
V71.5 Alleged sexual abuse

EPIDEMIOLOGY & DEMOGRAPHICS

- Sexual abuse accounts for approximately 10% of all abuse cases.
- In the mid-1990s there were approximately 200,000 cases of child sexual abuse per year. This number has fallen to just under 100,000 cases in 2003.
- Approximately one in three reports of child abuse are substantiated.
- Estimated incidence of sexual abuse occurring in childhood: women: 12% to 25%, men: 8% to 10%.
- Perpetrators:
  - Ninety percent are males (at least 20% are adolescents).
  - Up to 90% are known to the victims (approximately one third are relatives).
- Age of onset: most common in school-age children but occurs at all ages.
  - Occurs in all socioeconomic groups.

CLINICAL PRESENTATION

History

- Sexual abuse classically develops along the following pattern:
  - The victim is engaged in a relationship with the perpetrator.
  - Sexual interaction is gradually established.
  - Secrecy is established through threats or rewards.
  - Disclosure may occur depending on the receptiveness of the caretakers.
  - Suppression may occur if abuse is not disclosed or when there is inadequate therapy.
- Focus on the genitourinary system (rectal or genital bleeding or other complaints) as well as behavioral issues (phobias, sleep disorders, etc.).
- Use a non-leading interview style with attention to the child's spontaneous utterances.
- Anatomically correct dolls or line drawings may be helpful to the experienced interviewer.

Physical Examination

- If the physical examination is done within 72 hours of the sexual assault:
  - A rape protocol should be performed which includes the collection of forensic material.
  - Physical exam findings (e.g., tears of the hymen or abrasions) are more likely to be discovered (though not common) at this time than if the exam is done after 72 hours.
- If more than 72 hours from the abusive episode, the exam should include:
  - A thorough pediatric examination, noting signs of trauma (digital or speculum exams are unnecessary in the prepubertal child)
  - Genital examination using the supine and often also the knee-chest positions in females
  - Anal evaluation should be performed, though signs of trauma uncommon
  - Visualizing the hymen: with the child supine, gentle traction on the lower portion of the labia majora with moderate separation in an outward, slightly downward motion
    - Hymenal appearance: annular, crescentic, redundant, septate, and imperforate
    - Transverse diameter of the opening varies with position; its measurement should not be used for diagnostic purposes
  - Foley catheter technique may be helpful to visualize the hymen in adolescents.
    - A Foley catheter with a 10 mL balloon is inserted into the vagina. The balloon is then inflated and retracted slowly until the edges of the hymen are contacted and thereby better visualized. The balloon is then deflated and the catheter removed.
  - Colposcopy is helpful.
    - Tears, abrasion, or other trauma are present in only a small percentage of cases.
- Signs of trauma should be documented, preferably by photographs or by detailed illustrations.
- Most children proven to be sexually abused have normal examinations or nonspecific findings.
- Minor variations of the hymen or anus are often seen in nonabused children.
- A normal exam should not deter a physician from reporting a suspicion of sexual abuse.

ETIOLOGY

- Why children are sexually abused is unclear.
- There is no classic profile for a sexually abused child.
  - Factors that place a child at greater risk include: substance abuse (in the victim's immediate environment, especially by a potential perpetrator), home violence, mental or physical disability in the child, female gender, age (preadolescence and early school-age), and a parenting situation where one or both parents do not live with the child.
- Whether the abuse is within the family or occurs outside the family structure, there are moral and social mores that must be overcome by the perpetrator in a setting where the child is not adequately protected or supervised.

DIAGNOSIS

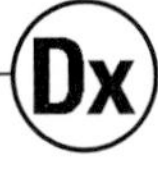

DIFFERENTIAL DIAGNOSIS

- Based largely on the history which may or may not be supported by physical findings
- Genital findings may be caused by the following:
  - Lichen sclerosis
  - Prolapsed urethra
  - Streptococcal cellulitis (perianal or perineal)
  - Hemangiomas
  - Straddle injuries
  - Molluscum contagiosum
- Anal findings including fissures or dilation; they may be caused by the following:
  - Postmortem dilatation
  - Crohn's disease
  - Constipation
  - Neurogenic problems

WORKUP

- Screening for sexually transmitted diseases (STDs) should be considered in following situations:
  - Historical factors: perpetrator with STD, patient with STD or genital discharge, sibling with STD, or other high-risk situations such as prostitution or multiple perpetrators
- Examination factors: vaginal discharge, genital or anal injuries, adolescent age group
  - The most common STDs are gonorrhea, *Chlamydia*, genital warts.
- Interpretation of positive tests for STDs and their relationship to sexual abuse, excluding congenital infections are as follows (*note:* confirmatory testing is generally required):
  - Gonorrhea, syphilis, human immunodeficiency virus (HIV), *Chlamydia*: diagnostic of abuse (if not acquired from birth; rare cases of nonsexual transmission excluded)
  - *Trichomonas*: highly suspicious for abuse
  - Genital warts, genital herpes: suspicious for abuse
  - Bacterial vaginosis: inconclusive for abuse

- Material collected for forensic analysis includes:
  - Swabs of mouth, rectum, vagina, and any suspicious staining on skin (identified by an ultraviolet light source)
  - Swabs of mouth, rectum, and vagina should also be performed to evaluate for STDs
  - Swabs of all bite marks
  - Saliva or blood specimen of victim for a DNA standard
  - Collection of underwear and any clothing and linens with suspicious staining
  - Collection of combed pubic hair (before the genital examination is performed) as well as plucked (preferred by most crime labs) or cut pubic hair for hair standards
- Expected results: forensic evidence is most likely to be recovered when collected close to the time of assault, ideally within 12 to 24 hours. It is not useful to attempt collection of forensic evidence after 72 hours.
- Interpretation of abnormal results:
  - Definitive evidence of sexual contact: sperm, seminal fluid, or pregnancy
  - Highly suspect for sexual contact: acute injuries of the genitalia or an STD

LABORATORY TESTS

- Laboratory evaluation is centered on STDs.
- See previous "Workup" section.
- Prevalence of STDs: 2% to 7%

TREATMENT

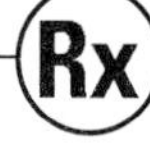

NONPHARMACOLOGIC THERAPY

- Mental health assessment and therapy
- Surgical intervention when significant vaginal or rectal injuries require repair

ACUTE GENERAL Rx

- STDs should be treated with appropriate agents when identified.
- STD prophylaxis is acceptable in sexually active adolescents.
- Postexposure prophylaxis (PEP) with antiretroviral therapy should be considered for the victim of sexual abuse with high-risk exposures including:
  - Perpetrator known to be HIV-positive
  - High-risk contact (highest with receptive anal or vaginal intercourse)
  - Repeated sexual encounters with a high-risk perpetrator
- Other considerations for PEP should include:
  - Consultation with local infectious disease expert
  - Length of time since exposure (must be started within 72 hours)
  - Effectiveness of PEP and its toxicity
- PEP may be started while waiting for HIV test results and expert consultation.
- Emergency contraception should be discussed with adolescent if less than 72 to 120 hours since assault (approved by U.S. Food & Drug Administration for use within 72 hours but potentially effective up to 120 hours after coitus).
  - Testing for pregnancy prior to emergency contraception and prophylactic antibiotics is prudent.

CHRONIC Rx

- Ongoing mental health support as necessary

DISPOSITION

- Positive tests require follow-up for test of cure.
- Repeat testing for HIV and syphilis may be necessary.
  - Syphilis: retest at 1 month and at 3 months
  - HIV: retest at 4 to 6 weeks, 12 weeks, and 6 months
- Patients with acute injuries may benefit from a repeat examination to demonstrate healing.

REFERRAL

- Acute rape cases should be seen immediately.
- Less acute cases of abuse should be evaluated in a judicious manner and are likely better evaluated at a child abuse center than an emergency department.
  - Medical personnel are mandated reporters by law in suspected or known cases of sexual abuse in all states.
  - Be familiar with your jurisdiction's reporting agencies and state child abuse reporting statutes.
  - Detailed and legible medical records, drawings, or photographs should be recorded.

PEARLS & CONSIDERATIONS

COMMENTS

- It is normal for there to be no abnormal findings on the physical exam after sexual abuse.
- The Health Insurance Portability and Accountability Act (HIPAA) does not preempt child abuse reporting laws.

PATIENT/FAMILY EDUCATION

- Caretakers should understand that protecting the child from further abuse is paramount.
- Mental health therapy is critical for the patient and often for the family as well.
- The child should be informed of his or her normal exam or the likelihood that his or her body will heal to a normal state if injuries are present.

SUGGESTED READINGS

American Academy of Pediatrics (Policy Statement) Committee on Adolescence: Emergency contraception. *Pediatrics* 116(4):1026, 2005.

American Professional Society on the Abuse of Children (APSAC). Available at http://www.apsac.org/

Atabaki, Paradise: The medical evaluation of the sexually abused child: lessons from a decade of research. *Pediatrics* 104:178, 1999.

Center for Disease Control and Prevention. Available at http://www.cdc.gov

Havens PL, Committee on Pediatric AIDS: Postexposure prophylaxis in children and adolescents for nonoccupational exposure to human immunodeficiency virus. *Pediatrics* 111(6):1475, 2003.

Kellogg N, Committee on Child Abuse and Neglect: The evaluation of sexual abuse in children. *Pediatrics* 116(2):506, 2005.

Reece RM: *Child Abuse: Medical Diagnosis and Management.* Philadelphia, Lippincott Williams & Wilkins, 2001.

Tennyson Center for Children at Colorado Christian Home. Available at www.childabuse.org

AUTHORS: **CHARLES SCHUBERT, MD** and **KATHI MAKOROFF, MD**

BASIC INFORMATION

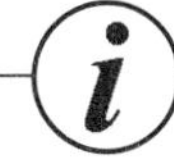

DEFINITION

Shigellosis is a gram-negative bacillary dysentery caused by members of the genus *Shigella* (family Enterobacteriaceae).

SYNONYM

Bacillary dysentery

ICD-9-CM CODE

004 Shigellosis

EPIDEMIOLOGY & DEMOGRAPHICS

- Approximately 25,000 cases are reported annually in the United States.
- Shigellosis is spread from human feces by the fecal-oral route. No natural animal reservoirs are known.
- Most commonly a pediatric disease infecting children 6 months to 5 years of age.
  - Crowded areas with poor hygiene and sanitation are predisposing factors.
- It is most commonly transmitted from person to person.
  - Ingestion of contaminated food and water and contact with a contaminated object can transmit *Shigella.* Transmission also can occur with anal intercourse.
  - Houseflies are considered vectors, transporting infected feces.
- Foodborne transmission represents 20% of *Shigella* transmission in the United States.
  - Shigellosis accounts for 2% of foodborne illness-related hospitalizations and 0.8% of total foodborne illness deaths.
- **Transmission in feces ceases when the organism is no longer present in stool, which usually occurs within 4 weeks of illness. *Shigella* carriers are rare, but they can have intermittent bouts of the disease and can harbor the organism for more than 1 year.**

CLINICAL PRESENTATION

- Incubation period is usually 2 to 4 days.
- Shigellosis classically presents with crampy abdominal pain; rectal burning; and multiple small, bloody, mucoid bowel movements. Severity can vary greatly and may or may not include constitutional symptoms.
- Fever presents in 40% of cases. The classic presentation of blood and mucus in the stool is seen in only 33% of cases.
- Children usually have mild infections lasting 1 to 3 days (7 days in adults).
- It is often biphasic:
  - Phase one is secondary to enterotoxin.
    - Symptoms include fever, watery diarrhea, and abdominal pain.
  - Phase two is secondary to invasion of colonic epithelium, leading to tenesmus and small-volume bloody stools.
- A variety of extraintestinal manifestations may be seen: bacteremia; colonic perforation; neurologic (not related to direct central nervous system infection) manifestations are particularly common in children and include seizures and meningismus.
- Fulminant toxic encephalopathy (ekiri) is rare.
  - Hemolytic uremic syndrome (usually from *Shigella dysenteriae* type 1)
  - Reiter's syndrome or asymmetric large joint arthritis: may develop 2 to 3 weeks after onset (*Shigella flexneri*)

ETIOLOGY

- Shigellosis is caused by nonmotile, gram-negative, nonencapsulated rods, usually non–lactose-fermenting and non–gas-producing.
- *Shigella* are serologically grouped (A to D) on the basis of the carbohydrate antigen of their lipopolysaccharide.
  - Group A: *S. dysenteriae*—10 serotypes (widespread in rural Africa and the Indian subcontinent)
  - Group B: *S. flexneri*—14 serotypes (most common in tropical countries, second most common in the US)
  - Group C: *Shigella boydii*—18 serotypes (uncommon in the US)
  - Group D: *Shigella sonnei*—1 serotype (causes most shigellosis in the US; mildest disease)

DIAGNOSIS

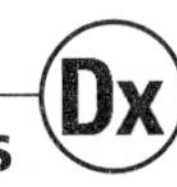

DIFFERENTIAL DIAGNOSIS

- Invasive (bacterial) diarrheal illnesses include the following:
  - *Salmonella, Campylobacter,* and *Yersinia*
  - Invasive amoebic illness (*Entamoeba histolytica*)
  - Colonic mucosal-damaging organisms, including *Escherichia coli* O157:H7
- Subacute illness can be confused with ulcerative colitis.

LABORATORY TESTS

- Methylene blue wet mount of stool can help identify erythrocytes and sheets of polymorphonuclear cells, but it is not specific for *Shigella.*
- Rectal swabs or fecal specimens can be sent for culture. This organism is fastidious, and samples should be placed in fecal transport medium or cultured directly within 2 to 4 hours.
- Blood cultures are rarely helpful because bacteremia is uncommon in immunocompetent hosts.

TREATMENT

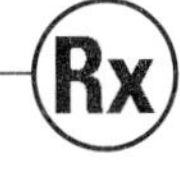

NONPHARMACOLOGIC THERAPY

- Rehydration and electrolyte management

ACUTE GENERAL Rx

- Medical management is indicated in most cases. With dysentery, antibiotics shorten the duration of diarrhea and eliminate organisms from stool. In mild illness, antibiotics can help limit spread.
- For shigellosis of unknown susceptibility or ampicillin-resistant strains, trimethoprim-sulfamethoxazole (TMP-SMX) is the drug of choice. Azithromycin, ceftriaxone, and fluoroquinolones (especially ciprofloxacin) are good alternatives.
- *Shigella* acquired from developing countries is more likely to have multiple resistances (often plasmid-acquired) and may be resistant to TMP-SMX, ampicillin, and increasing the fluoroquinolones.
- A 5-day course of antibiotics is usually considered adequate therapy. Longer therapy may be necessitated in immunocompromised children (7 to 10 days).

DISPOSITION

The disease is usually self-limited. Hydration/electrolyte disturbances may require close monitoring.

PEARLS & CONSIDERATIONS

COMMENTS

- Narcotic-related antimotility agents may prolong excretion and course of symptoms.
- Symptoms of mild diarrhea and cramps may persist after adequate treatment secondary to mucosal injury.

PREVENTION

- Infected individuals should not return to food preparation occupations or child care until treatment has been provided and diarrhea has ceased.
- Symptomatic contacts of infected individuals (whether child care providers or household contacts) should be cultured.
- Multiple vaccines are in advanced clinical phases:
  - A conjugate *S. sonnei* vaccine developed by the National Institutes of Health (NIH) has been in phase III trials.
  - Live-attenuated *S. flexneri* 2a strains are being tested by Walter Reed Army Institute of Research, Pasteur Institute of Paris, and the Center for Vaccine Development, University of Maryland.

PATIENT/FAMILY EDUCATION

Handwashing, as well as control measures for sanitary water and food handling, should be emphasized.

SUGGESTED READINGS

Basualdo W: Randomized comparison of azithromycin versus cefixime for treatment of shigellosis in children. *Pediatr Infect Dis J* 22(4):374, 2003.

Centers for Disease Control and Prevention. Available at www.cdc.gov/ncidod

Green S, Tillotson G: Use of ciprofloxacin in developing countries. *Pediatr Infect Dis J* 16:150, 1997.

United Nations Initiative for Vaccine Research. Available at www.who.int/vaccine_research/

AUTHOR: **GUS GIBBONS EMMICK, MD**

BASIC INFORMATION

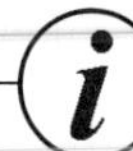

DEFINITION

Short bowel syndrome refers to a foreshortened bowel with subsequent nutrient malabsorption. Neither the absolute length nor the percent of resection or reduction in surface area is part of the definition.

SYNONYM

Short gut (syndrome)

ICD-9-CM CODES
579.2 Blind loop syndrome
579.3 Short bowel syndrome

EPIDEMIOLOGY & DEMOGRAPHICS

- No known ethnic distribution
- Prematurity (necrotizing enterocolitis)
- True incidence unknown

CLINICAL PRESENTATION

History
- Previous bowel resection
- Poor weight gain
- Diarrhea
- Multiple nutrient deficiency states

Physical Examination
- Muscle wasting
- Abdominal distention
- Succession splash
- Scars from previous surgery

ETIOLOGY

Any disease or abnormality that decreases the absorptive area of the intestines can lead to short bowel syndrome.
- Inflammatory diseases
  - Crohn's disease
  - Necrotizing enterocolitis
  - Radiation enteritis
- Anatomic disorders
  - Bowel atresia
  - Volvulus
  - Gastroschisis
  - Omphalocele
  - Hirschsprung's disease
  - Congenital short bowel
- Vascular insufficiency
  - Thrombosis
  - Volvulus
  - Vascular disease

DIAGNOSIS

Dx

DIFFERENTIAL DIAGNOSIS

- Steatorrhea: fecal fat coefficient of absorption less than 90%
  - Liver disease
  - Pancreatic insufficiency (cystic fibrosis)
- Impaired xylose absorption
- Malabsorption from disaccharidase deficiency
  - Low-pH stools with positive reducing substances
- Chronic infections: can present with short gutlike syndrome
  - Acquired immunodeficiency syndrome (AIDS)
  - Parasites
- Celiac disease
- Milk-protein intolerance

IMAGING STUDIES

Radiographic demonstration of shortened gut must be abnormal, but extent of resection varies.

TREATMENT

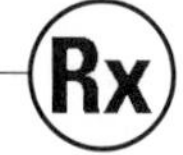

NONPHARMACOLOGIC THERAPY

- Consider tapering enteroplasty or intestinal lengthening procedure (Bianchi procedure) in the case of dilated bowel with bacterial overgrowth when otherwise unable to advance feedings or manage condition medically.
- Do not attempt artificial valves, reverse segments, or other means designed to reduce intestinal transit in children because these procedures often induce bacterial overgrowth.
- Consider intestinal transplantation only in the presence of irreversible liver disease or life-threatening recurrent sepsis or loss of central venous access.

ACUTE GENERAL Rx

- Parenteral nutrition
  - Use exclusively only for 1 to 2 weeks.
  - Institute enteral feedings as early as possible.
  - Monitor volume and electrolyte losses in diarrheal stool.
    - Replace milliliter per milliliter with solution containing electrolyte concentrations equal to losses.
- Enteral nutrition
  - Begin early.
  - Begin slowly.
  - Use continuous infusions, not bolus feedings.
  - Use amino acid or protein hydrolysate formula, preferably with a high percentage of long-chain fat content to stimulate gut adaptation and reduce osmotic fluid losses.
  - Advance enteral and decrease parenteral nutrition in an isocaloric fashion on a daily basis.
    - Base transition on tolerance, with periodic adjustments for growth and metabolic needs.
    - Use weight gain as the primary end point, not calculations of needed caloric intake.
- Monitoring
  - Stool output is primary end point for advancing or reducing enteral feedings.
  - Do not monitor stool fat content.
  - Do not monitor for occult blood, but observe for gross blood.
  - Advance enteral feedings as long as stool or ostomy output is reasonable (<20 to 40 mL/kg/day).
  - Monitor electrolytes, minerals, trace minerals, vitamins, and liver enzymes based on institutional total parenteral nutrition (TPN) guidelines.
  - Monitoring for nutritional deficiencies becomes more crucial once TPN is discontinued.
- Dietary therapy
  - Use amino acid or hydrolysate formula during the first year to reduce the risk of allergic inflammation in the gut.
  - Start infant on solids at a normal developmental age, but begin feedings with meat because high fat content will reduce osmotic stool losses and increase the stimulus for adaptation of the bowel.
  - Avoid hypertonic liquids (e.g., Kool-Aid, juices, soda).
  - Introduce oral feedings of liquids and solids early (i.e., during the first 2 to 3 weeks) in small quantities to stimulate sucking and swallowing reflexes.
- Once TPN has been weaned:
  - Monitor carefully for deficiencies of minerals and fat-soluble vitamins.
  - Use continuous enteral infusion during the nighttime and bolus or oral feeding during the daytime as a transition to oral feeding.
  - Avoid hypertonic beverages and high-carbohydrate diets.
  - Avoid high oxylate-containing foods, such as chocolate.
  - Caloric needs may rise during puberty, necessitating transient return to parenteral nutrition.

CHRONIC Rx

Complications
- TPN liver disease
  - Prevent with aggressive use of enteral feedings, avoidance of septic episodes, and treatment of small bowel bacterial overgrowth.
  - Ursodeoxycholic acid has been used but has not been definitively shown to be helpful.
- Nutritional deficiency states
  - Fat-soluble vitamins (A, D, E, K) and minerals, such as calcium, magnesium, and zinc, are the most common deficiencies.
  - Usually deficiencies develop after patient has been weaned from parenteral nutrition.
  - B_{12} deficiency is common with extensive ileal resection and requires parenteral or nasal therapy.
- Biliary tract disease
  - Gallstones
  - More common in TPN-dependent patients who are intolerant of enteral feedings
  - Often requires cholecystectomy if present

- Small bowel bacterial overgrowth
  - This is common if motility is slow or the bowel is dilated.
  - Diagnosis is based on increased urine indicans, elevated breath hydrogen after glucose administration, increased serum d-lactate level.
  - Bacterial overgrowth is common but usually only a problem when inflammation exists; therefore, culture demonstration of increased bacterial organisms is not generally helpful.
  - Demonstration of inflammation in the distal small bowel endoscopically is often suggestive of pathologic bacterial overgrowth and may respond to anti-inflammatory therapy (i.e., aspirin, glucocorticosteroids).
- Anastomotic ulcerations
  - May result in severe blood loss and anemia
  - Require endoscopic diagnosis
  - Medical therapy usually not helpful; often requires resection

DISPOSITION

- Patients with less than 40 cm of small bowel at the time of neonatal resection and those who lack an ileocecal valve may have a poor prognosis for becoming independent of parenteral nutrition.
- Patients with less extensive resection may eventually, over a period of years, no longer need parenteral nutrition.
  - If patients are not independent of parenteral nutrition by age 5 years, they will likely need lifelong parenteral nutrition.
- Intestinal transplantation has been advocated for children with irreversible TPN liver disease, loss of central venous access, or severe recurrent sepsis.
  - The prognosis for long-term survival off TPN is little better than 50% with transplantation.
  - Long-term parenteral nutrition in the stable patient probably carries a better ultimate prognosis.

REFERRAL

Web Sites

- Healthtouch Online. Available at www.healthtouch.com
- MCW HealthLink. Available at www.Healthlink.mcw.edu
- National Institute of Diabetes & Digestive & Kidney Diseases. Available at www.niddk.nih.gov/health/digest/summary/shortbo/shortbo.htm

PEARLS & CONSIDERATIONS

COMMENTS

- If a patient is previously doing well and then starts doing poorly with no changes, look for bacterial overgrowth or nutritional deficiency states.
- Avoid antidiarrheal agents such as loperamide in children with stasis and bacterial overgrowth.
- Encourage use of diets high in fat and low in simple carbohydrates.

SUGGESTED READINGS

Buchman AL et al: AGA technical review on short bowel syndrome and intestinal transplantation. *Gastroenterology* 124(4):1111, 2003.

Dabney A et al: Short bowel syndrome after trauma. *Am J Surg* 188(6):792, 2004.

DiBaise JK et al: Intestinal rehabilitation and the short bowel syndrome: part 1. *Am J Gastroenterol* 99(7):1386, 2004.

DiBaise JK et al: Intestinal rehabilitation and the short bowel syndrome: part 2. *Am J Gastroenterol* 99(9):1823, 2004.

Matarese L et al: Intestinal Failure and Rehabilitation: A Clinical Guide. *In* Vanderhoof JA, Young RJ (eds): *Antimicrobials and probiotics.* New York, CRC Press, 2005, pp 177–186.

Thompson JS et al: Short bowel syndrome and Crohn's disease. *J Gastrointest Surg* 7(8):1069, 2003.

Vanderhoof JA et al: New and emerging therapies for short bowel syndrome in children. *Paediatr Drugs* 5(8):525, 2003.

Vanderhoof JA, Young RJ: Enteral nutrition in short bowel syndrome. *Semin Pediatr Surg* 10(2):65, 2001.

AUTHORS: **JON A. VANDERHOOF, MD** and **ROSEMARY J. YOUNG, RN, MS**

BASIC INFORMATION

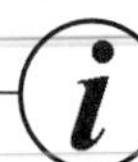

DEFINITION

Short stature is defined as height below the third percentile or greater than two standard deviations (SD) below the mean height for chronologic age.

SYNONYM

Dwarfism—severe form of short stature with height less than three standard deviations below the mean.

ICD-9-CM CODE
783.4 Short stature

CLINICAL PRESENTATION

History

- Prenatal history—maternal infection, consumption of alcohol, drugs
- Pattern of growth (height and weight) including birth weight and length in relation to gestational age
- Family history—parental heights, onset of puberty of parents and immediate relatives
- Profile of patient's pubertal development including onset of breast development, menarche, onset of testicular and penile enlargement and pubic hair
- Nutrition
- Evidence of systemic disease—gastrointestinal, cardiac, pulmonary, renal
- Drug administration—steroids, methylphenidate
- Neurologic symptoms especially headache, visual disturbance, recent history of enuresis
- Psychosocial milieu

Physical Examination

Full physical examination with special emphasis on the following:

- Accurate measurements of height, weight, head circumference, arm span, upper and lower body segments
- Assess nutritional state, fat distribution
- Abnormal pigmentation of the skin
- Dysmorphic features
- Pubertal stage
- Complete neurologic exam including funduscopy and visual fields
- Examination of the thyroid gland

ETIOLOGY

Normal Variant

- Familial or genetic short stature
  - Normal or relatively small weight and length at birth
  - Onset and progression of puberty is normal
  - Final adult height, short, but appropriate for parental heights
  - Bone age consistent with chronologic age
- Constitutional delay of growth and adolescence
  - Growth velocity may be decreased in the first 2 to 3 years of life ("catch down") but normal thereafter
  - Delayed skeletal growth and maturation and delayed onset of puberty
  - Final adult height and progression of sexual development are normal
  - Often with family history of delayed growth and onset of sexual development

Pathologic Causes of Short Stature

- Proportionate—normal upper/lower body segment ratio for age
  - Endocrinopathies—usually associated with increased weight-to-height ratio
- Growth hormone (GH) deficiency/insensitivity
- Hypothyroidism
- Cushing's syndrome
  - Malnutrition
  - Gastrointestinal pathology—malabsorption, inflammatory bowel disease, celiac disease
  - Renal disease—renal tubular acidosis, chronic renal failure, nephrogenic diabetes insipidus
  - Other chronic diseases—cardiac, pulmonary, liver, chronic infection
  - Intrauterine growth retardation
- Infants with birth weight ≤2 SD from the mean for gestational age, sex, and race
- Causes include placental insufficiency, fetal infections, teratogens, and chromosomal abnormalities
- Disproportionate—abnormal upper/lower body segment ratio for age
  - Skeletal dysplasia—achondroplasia, hypochondroplasia
  - Metabolic bone disease—rickets
  - Abnormalities of vertebral bodies
- Associated with dysmorphic features
  - Trisomy 21 (Down syndrome)
  - Prader-Willi syndrome
  - Turner syndrome
    - Short stature is the most consistent and sometimes the only clinical sign
  - Russell-Silver syndrome

Idiopathic Short Stature

- By definition, "short stature" whose cause is not defined after appropriate workup. Some cases of familial/genetic short stature and even constitutional delay of growth and development may masquerade as idiopathic short stature.
- Most recent Food and Drug Administration (FDA)-approved indication for treatment with recombinant human growth hormone (rhGH) when basic criteria are met:
  - Height ≤2.25 SD from mean for age and sex
  - Still unfused growth plates
  - No other cause for short stature

DIAGNOSIS

Dx

DIFFERENTIAL DIAGNOSIS

Diagnostic Approach

- Growth curve analysis
  - Reliability of measurements
  - Inaccurate plotting of measurements on the growth chart and measurement error are common reasons for misdiagnosis of growth disorders and inappropriate referral.
  - Height velocity (see Figure 1-9)
    - This is the most important aspect of growth evaluation.
    - Accurate determination requires a minimum of 6 months of observation.
    - Normal height velocity for chronologic age at any absolute height is unlikely to be associated with pathologic causes.
    - Normal average yearly growth rates: 8 cm at 2 years, 7 cm at 3 years, 5 to 6 cm from 4 to 9 years
  - Absolute height
    - Bears some relationship to the likelihood of pathologic condition.
    - Absolute height of 3 SDs below the mean is more likely to be pathologic than height of 1 SD below the mean.
  - Weight-to-height ratio
    - Endocrine disorders are usually associated with relatively preserved weight gain or frank obesity in a short child.
    - Systemic disorders (gastrointestinal, renal, pulmonary, cardiac, and so forth) are associated with greater impairment of weight gain than linear growth.
- Other helpful parameters:
  - Target height (mean parental height):
    - Males = (father height (cm) + mother height (cm) + 13) ÷ 2
    - Females = (father height (cm) + mother height (cm) −13) ÷ by 2
    - Child's height is appropriate for the family if the projected adult height is within 8 cm of the target height.
  - Upper to lower segment body ratio:
    - Lower segment is measured from symphysis pubis to the floor
    - Upper segment = height − lower segment
    - Useful to assess whether the short stature is proportionate or disproportionate
    - Mean U/L ratio: 1.7 (birth), 1.3 (3 years), 1.0 (after 7 years), 0.9 (adult)

LABORATORY TESTS

- Well-nourished or obese child with deceleration in linear growth
  - Thyroid-stimulating hormone (TSH) and free T_4—elevated TSH and low free T_4 indicate primary hypothyroidism.
  - Insulin-like growth factor-I (IGF-I, somatomedin-C) and insulin-like growth factor binding protein-III (IGF-BP)—low levels are suggestive of GH deficiency.
  - Provocative GH stimulation test (arginine-insulin tolerance test) is the accepted "gold standard" method for confirming the diagnosis of GH deficiency.
  - Urinary free cortisol level—if suspecting Cushing's syndrome
- Thin child with deceleration of linear growth
  - Complete blood cell count and sedimentation rate—helpful to identify patients

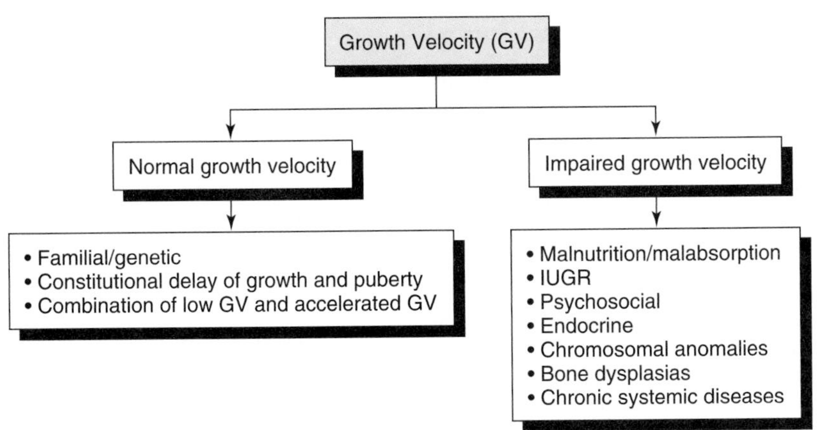

FIGURE 1-9 Growth velocity.

with inflammatory bowel disease or chronic inflammatory process
  - Urinalysis, serum creatinine, and electrolytes—to exclude renal disorder
  - Sweat chloride test—indicated if suspecting cystic fibrosis
  - Serum calcium, phosphorus, alkaline phosphatase—to exclude subtle forms of rickets or other disorders of mineral metabolism
- Short child with dysmorphic features or disproportionate short stature:
  - Karyotype: should be obtained if features suggest chromosomal abnormalities or a syndrome. Also indicated in most female children with short stature to exclude Turner syndrome even in the absence of classical physical stigmata.
  - Skeletal dysplasia radiologic survey—especially in disproportionate short stature

IMAGING STUDIES

Bone age—skeletal maturity assessment done by comparing the appearance of epiphyseal centers on radiography with age-appropriate published standards. Has both diagnostic and prognostic implications.

Diagnostic Implications
- Delayed bone age
  - Normal variant: constitutional delay of growth and development
  - Pathologic variants:
    - Endocrine disorders: GH deficiency, hypothyroidism, Cushing's syndrome
    - Malnutrition
    - Chronic diseases: renal, cardiac, pulmonary, gastrointestinal
- Bone age consistent with chronologic age
  - Normal variant: familial/genetic short stature
  - Pathologic variants:
    - Dysgenetic/syndromic short stature
    - Bone dysplasia

Prognostic Implications
- Used to predict final adult height. Normal or advanced bone age in a child with short stature is of greater concern than delayed bone age. Linear growth will continue until epiphyseal fusion is complete.

TREATMENT

Rx

CHRONIC Rx
- If specific cause is identified, treat the underlying disease
- Specific hormone replacement for hypothyroidism and GH deficiency
- Turner syndrome—consider GH treatment
- Constitutional delay of growth and adolescence
  - Reevaluate every 6 to 12 months
    - Treatment with short course of testosterone is an option in some patients.
- Approved indications for GH treatment in short stature (date of FDA approval in parentheses)
  - Growth hormone deficiency (1985)
  - Chronic renal insufficiency (1993)
  - Turner syndrome (1996)
  - Prader-Willi syndrome (2000)
  - Small for gestational age without catch-up (2001)
  - Idiopathic short stature (non-GH deficient short stature) (2003)

PEARLS & CONSIDERATIONS

COMMENTS
- Deceleration of height velocity after 2 to 3 years of life indicates pathology unless proven otherwise.
- Systemic disorders are usually associated with greater impairment of weight gain than linear growth.
- For a short child with preserved weight gain, think of endocrine disorders.
- Longitudinal determination of height velocity is the most important factor in evaluation of short stature.

PATIENT/FAMILY EDUCATION
- Little People of America, National Headquarters, Box 745, Lubbock, TX 79408; (888) 572-2001; www.lpaonline.org
- Human Growth Foundation, Inc., 997 Glen Cove Avenue, Glen Head, NY 11545; (800) 451-6434; www.hgfound.org
- Turner Syndrome Society of the United States, 1313 Southeast 5th Street, Suite 327, Minneapolis, MN 55414; (800) 365-9944; www.turner-syndrome-us.org

SUGGESTED READINGS

Lifshitz F, Botero D: Worrisome growth. *In* Lifshitz F (ed): *Pediatric Endocrinology,* 4th ed. Philadelphia, Saunders, 2003, pp 1–35.

Rosenfeld RG, Cohen P: Disorders of growth hormone and insulin-like growth factor secretion and action. *In* Sperling MA (ed): *Pediatric Endocrinology,* 2nd ed. Philadelphia, Saunders, 2002, pp 211–288.

AUTHORS: **RAM K. MENON, MD** and **OSCAR ESCOBAR, MD**

Section I DISEASES AND DISORDERS

BASIC INFORMATION

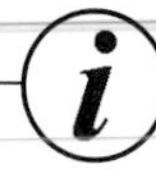

DEFINITION

The term *sickle cell disease* describes hemoglobin SS (Hb SS), hemoglobins resulting from the production of Hb S in concert with another abnormal hemoglobin (e.g., Hb SC, SD, SO), and the sickle β-thalassemia syndromes in which Hb S is accompanied by either reduced (β^+) or absent (β^0) production of normal adult hemoglobin (Hb Sβ thalassemia). Vaso-occlusion and chronic hemolytic anemia characterize the disease.

SYNONYM

Sickle cell anemia applies to Hb SS

ICD-9-CM CODE
282.60 Sickle cell anemia

EPIDEMIOLOGY & DEMOGRAPHICS

- Annual incidence of sickle cell anemia in the United States: 1 per 500 African American births; 1 per 1000 to 1400 Hispanic American births. Incidence rate in the United States is approximately 1 in 500, or 0.20%.
- Prevalence of sickle cell anemia in the United States: 72,000 people with sickle cell anemia. There are 2 million carriers; 1 in 12 African Americans is a carrier. Prevalence rate for sickle cell anemia is approximately 1 in 3777, or 0.03%.
- Sickle cell disease has a recessive inheritance pattern. For example, if the sickle mutation (S trait) is carried by both parents, there is a 25% chance of an offspring having Hb SS, a 50% chance of the essentially benign condition S trait, and a 25% chance of having normal hemoglobin (Hb AA).
- Many states provide universal hemoglobinopathy screening shortly after birth.
- The disease severity is quite variable.

CLINICAL PRESENTATION

- Anemia (and reticulocytosis) generally presents in Hb SS by 4 months of age and is not detected in the newborn.
  - Baseline anemia intensified with aplastic crises or splenic sequestration, two potentially life-threatening events
- Pain crises
  - These are experienced as deep, throbbing pains, usually without physical findings.
  - Children younger than 5 years may experience pain in the form of the "hand-foot syndrome," with swelling and tenderness of hands or feet.
- Increased susceptibility to infection with encapsulated organisms
- Acute chest syndrome with pulmonary infiltrate; restrictive lung disease
- Symptoms of stroke; cognitive abnormalities
- Short stature prior to puberty, evidence of delayed sexual maturation
- Scleral icterus, cholelithiasis, acute pancreatitis
- Hyposthenuria (usually seen by age 3) with urinary frequency and enuresis; papillary necrosis, nephrotic syndrome, priapism
- Cortical thinning, aseptic necrosis of femoral/humoral heads with pain on weight bearing or with rotation of hip or arm, bony distortion secondary to bone marrow expansion, osteomyelitis
- Skin ulcers
- Nonproliferative retinopathy with adjacent hemorrhage, proliferative retinopathy stages 1 to 5. Retinal neovascularization may result in blindness, vitreous hemorrhage, retinal detachment; hyphema.
- Systolic flow murmur, pulmonary hypertension
- Splenomegaly in infants and children; also seen in adolescents with Hb SC or $S\beta^+$
- Neurologic deficits secondary to overt stroke
- Cognitive deficits secondary to overt or silent stroke

ETIOLOGY

- A single nucleotide change (A to T) in the β-globin gene results in substitution of valine for glutamic acid in the sixth position of the β-globin chain of hemoglobin; this change leads to the synthesis of Hb S.
- When exposed to low oxygen tension, Hb S tends to polymerize within the red cell, resulting in alterations of membrane shape and function, increased cell density, and reduced deformability.
- Distorted "sickled" cells obstruct blood flow in small vessels, leading to tissue ischemia (vaso-occlusion).
- Red cell alterations lead to reduced cell life span (hemolytic anemia).
- Young reticulocytes express receptors that make them more adherent to endothelial cells lining blood vessels; increases in cytokines enhance these interactions.
- Abnormalities of clotting are noted and may contribute to stroke, chest crises, and the like.

DIAGNOSIS

DIFFERENTIAL DIAGNOSIS

- Other causes of anemia, primarily hemolytic

LABORATORY TESTS

- Preferably on child and his or her parents; interpret with aid of a hematologist, if possible (following ranges apply to children older than 5 years):
  - Complete blood count (CBC): Hb (g/L) = 6 to 11 (SS), 6 to 10 ($S\beta^0$ thalassemia), 9 to 12 ($S\beta^+$ thalassemia), 10 to 15 (SC)
  - Indices: mean corpuscular volume (fL) = more than 80 (SS), less than 80 ($S\beta^0$ thalassemia), less than 75 ($S\beta^+$ thalassemia), 75 to 95 (SC)
  - Reticulocyte count (%) = 5 to 20 (SS, $S\beta^0$ thalassemia), 5 to 10
  - Blood film: sickle cells, targets, Howell-Jolly bodies, nucleated red cells, polychromasia
  - Solubility test (e.g., the Sickledex): positive in sickle cell trait, disease; negative in Hb C, D, O, and so forth, β-thalassemia trait
  - Hemoglobin electrophoresis, quantitative measurements of Hb A_2 and F

IMAGING STUDIES

- Regular (at least yearly, after age 2) transcranial Doppler ultrasound screening to assess stroke risk
- Magnetic resonance imaging (MRI) or computed tomography (CT) if stroke suspected
- Other studies relevant to symptoms (i.e., chest radiograph, so forth)

TREATMENT

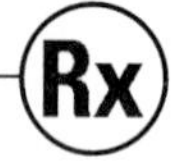

ACUTE GENERAL Rx

Anemia

- Red cell transfusion may be needed when anemia is exacerbated by aplastic crises or splenic sequestration. Consult a hematologist to avoid hyperviscosity or volume overload. For repeated splenic sequestration crises, chronic transfusion or splenectomy may be indicated.
- Patient should be transfused preoperatively (consult a hematologist for guidelines) if general anesthesia is to be used.

Infection

- Examine the child and obtain cultures and appropriate laboratory studies.
- Emergently treat any febrile or ill-appearing child with antibiotics effective against *Streptococcus pneumoniae* and *Haemophilus influenzae.*
  - Use additional antibiotic in areas where resistant organisms are identified.
  - National Institutes of Health (NIH) guidelines for admission are as follows:
    - Temperature higher than 40°C
    - Seriously ill appearance
    - Hypotension
    - Poor perfusion and dehydration
    - Pulmonary infiltrate
    - Corrected white blood cell count of more than 30,000/mm^3 or less than 5000/mm^3
    - Platelet count less than 100,000/mm^3
    - Hemoglobin less than 5 g/dL
    - History of *S. pneumoniae* sepsis
    - Admit all children whose follow-up cannot be guaranteed.
- If treated as an outpatient:
  - Examine the child and obtain cultures and appropriate laboratory studies.
  - Give ceftriaxone intravenously or intramuscularly.
  - Have patient return within 24 hours; have the child return sooner if ill appearing.

- Administer a second dose of ceftriaxone to all patients at 24 hours.
- If blood cultures are negative at 48 hours, may discontinue antibiotics or treat identifiable source orally.

Pain

- Home therapy: provide hydration, nonsteroidal anti-inflammatory drugs, and if needed, oral pain medications such as codeine or morphine.
- Emergency room: if unable to control pain at home, administer intravenous hydration and morphine.
- Inpatient setting: continued therapy as an inpatient may be required.
  - Anticipate pain with regular, not as-needed, dosing.
  - Patient-controlled analgesia pump to administer morphine may be useful.
  - Carefully monitor oxygen saturation and provide a bedside spirometer, as patient may develop acute chest syndrome.
  - Behavioral modification techniques and hypnosis may be helpful.

Acute Chest Syndrome: Admit to Hospital

- Treat with ceftriaxone and azithromycin.
- Carefully monitor oxygen saturation, may need oxygen supplementation.
- May require transfusion
- Bedside spirometer helpful
- May benefit from bronchodilators

Stroke: Immediate Intervention in an Intensive Care Unit

- Administer an exchange transfusion under the supervision of a hematologist.
- The goal is to reduce the Hb S level to less than 20%.
- Subsequent chronic transfusion therapy will be needed.

CHRONIC Rx

Regular visits to a comprehensive sickle cell disease center and primary physician are needed.

- Immunizations
  - Standard series, including hepatitis B and Prevnar series
  - Pneumovax vaccine (age 2 years and again at age 4 to 6 years)
  - Meningococcal vaccine (age 2)
  - Annual influenza vaccine
- Penicillin prophylaxis: 125 mg orally two times per day until age 3 years, then 250 mg orally two times per day
- Folic acid:
  - Age 2 to 6 months: 0.1 mg
  - Age 6 to 12 months: 0.25 mg
  - Age 1 to 5 years: 0.5 mg
  - Age 5 years or older: 1 mg orally per day
- Regular laboratory studies, including a full CBC, reticulocyte count, platelet count, urinalysis, tests of liver and kidney function, hepatitis/human immunodeficiency virus antibodies if transfused, and tests to assess pulmonary status
- Regular (at least yearly) transcranial Doppler (TCD) ultrasound screening to assess stroke risk
- For patients with frequent debilitating pain or repeated chest crises, consider hydroxyurea therapy (under the guidance of a hematologist).
- For children who have experienced an overt ischemic stroke, chronic transfusion therapy to maintain the hemoglobin S level below 30%
- Children with TCD velocities above 200 cm/second should be offered chronic transfusion therapy.
- Consider bone marrow transplantation in young children with matched sibling donor.

REFERRAL

Regular visits to dentist and ophthalmologist are needed. Patient may require referral to a pediatric nephrologist, cardiologist, pulmonologist, orthopedist, urologist, neurologist, gastroenterologist, or surgeon for evaluation and treatment of various complications.

PEARLS & CONSIDERATIONS

COMMENTS

The documented decrease in the mortality rate for children with sickle cell disease is likely related to preventive strategies, including early diagnosis, penicillin prophylaxis, comprehensive care, and the recognition and treatment of life-threatening events.

PREVENTION

- As described previously under "Chronic Rx"

PATIENT/FAMILY EDUCATION

- Anticipatory guidance should be age- and syndrome-appropriate.
  - Topics for discussion and reinforcement include:
    - Need to seek medical attention for fever or ill appearance
    - Regular penicillin administration
    - Appropriate hydration
    - Thermometer use
    - Spleen palpation
    - Recognition of signs of sequestration, aplastic crises, stroke, priapism, aseptic necrosis, and chest crises
- Genetic counseling and diagnostic testing should be made available to all families of children with sickle cell disease.
- Emphasis should be on preventing complications.
- Support groups: Sickle Cell Disease Association of America, Inc.; local chapters in many cities

SUGGESTED READINGS

Adams RJ et al: Prevention of first stroke by transfusions in children with sickle cell anemia and abnormal transcranial Doppler ultrasonography. *N Engl J Med* 339:5, 1998.

Miller ST et al: Prediction of adverse outcomes in children with sickle cell disease. *N Engl J Med* 342:83, 2000.

National Institutes of Health, National Heart, Lung, and Blood Institute, Division of Blood Diseases and Resources: *The Management of Sickle Cell Disease,* 4th ed. (NIH Publication No. 02-2117). Bethesda, MD, National Institutes of Health, 2002.

Stewart MJ, Nagel RL: Sickle cell disease. *Lancet* 364:1287, 2004.

Zimmerman SA et al: Sustained long-term hematologic efficacy of hydroxyurea at maximum tolerated dose in children with sickle cell disease. *Blood* 103:2039, 2004.

AUTHOR: **NORMA B. LERNER, MD**

BASIC INFORMATION

DEFINITIONS

- *Acute bacterial sinusitis:* bacterial infection of the paranasal sinuses lasting less than 30 days in which symptoms resolve completely.
- *Subacute bacterial sinusitis:* bacterial infection of the paranasal sinuses lasting between 30 and 90 days in which symptoms resolve completely.
- *Recurrent acute bacterial sinusitis:* episodes of bacterial infection of the paranasal sinuses, each lasting less than 30 days and separated by intervals of at least 10 days during which the patient is asymptomatic.
- *Chronic sinusitis:* episodes of inflammation of the paranasal sinuses lasting more than 90 days. Patients have persistent residual respiratory symptoms such as cough, rhinorrhea, or nasal obstruction.
- *Acute bacterial sinusitis superimposed on chronic sinusitis:* patients with residual respiratory symptoms develop new respiratory symptoms. When treated with antimicrobials, these new symptoms resolve, but the underlying residual symptoms do not.

SYNONYMS

Acute rhinosinusitis
Acute sinusitis
Infectious sinusitis
Rhinosinusitis

ICD-9-CM CODES
461.0 Acute maxillary sinusitis
461.1 Acute frontal sinusitis
461.2 Acute ethmoidal sinusitis
461.3 Acute sphenoidal sinusitis
461.8 Other acute sinusitis
461.9 Acute sinusitis, unspecified

EPIDEMIOLOGY & DEMOGRAPHICS

- Upper respiratory infections (URIs) are the most common clinical problems for primary practitioners who care for children.
- Approximately 5% to 10% of URIs in early childhood are complicated by acute sinusitis.

CLINICAL PRESENTATION

History

- Bacterial sinusitis causes a spectrum of nonspecific symptoms and is likely under diagnosed.
- Classic symptoms reported in adults include nasal congestion, purulent rhinorrhea, postnasal drainage, facial or dental pain, headache, hyposmia, and cough.
- Unlike adults, children do not usually report sinus congestion, pain, or headache.
- Some children may not even appear to be ill, and if fever is present, it is low grade.
- Some children may have a cold that seems more severe than usual, with high fever, purulent and copious nasal discharge, periorbital swelling, and facial pain.
- Important symptoms in a child could include daytime and nighttime cough (particularly when first lying down) and nasal discharge. A persistent daytime cough is often the symptom that brings a child to medical attention.

Physical Examination

- In general, for children younger than 10 years of age, the physical examination is of little value in making a specific diagnosis of acute sinusitis.
- *Visualization*—nasal mucosa: characterize nasal secretions, polyps, and the structure of the nasal septum; inspect tympanic membranes because concomitant otitis media is common.
- *Palpation*—check tenderness over maxillary and frontal sinuses; tap maxillary teeth with tongue blade.
- *Transillumination* is best when determined to be either normal or absent; difficult in children younger than 10 years of age.
- When present, periorbital swelling, facial tenderness, and malodorous breath (in the absence of dental disease and nasal foreign body) are probably the most specific findings in acute sinusitis.

ETIOLOGY

- Infants have patent maxillary and ethmoid sinuses, which continue to grow until late adolescence. Sphenoid sinuses begin development at 2 years of age. Frontal sinuses begin to form by 6 years of age and complete development by 12 years.
- During an acute viral respiratory tract infection the epithelium of the sinus ostia and ostiomeatal complex undergo inflammatory response:
    - Altered ciliary function
    - Increased secretory activity
- Obstruction of an ostium during an acute viral process creates the conditions for a secondary bacterial infectious sinusitis.
- Sinusitis occurring in the first week of a respiratory infection is usually viral in origin.
- In patients with acute sinusitis, about 75% of maxillary sinus aspirates contain bacteria, usually *Streptococcus pneumoniae,* nontypeable *Haemophilus influenzae,* or *Moraxella catarrhalis.* Group A streptococcus or *Staphylococcus aureus* may also be present.
- These organisms are also common in patients with chronic sinusitis, although *S. aureus,* coagulase-negative staphylococci, α-hemolytic streptococci, and enteric bacilli are more common in this condition.
- Fungal infections may rarely be observed as a nonfulminant, chronic sinusitis in older children and adolescents.
- Conditions that predispose children to chronic sinusitis include the following:
    - Allergic and nonallergic rhinitis
    - Anatomic abnormality of the ostiomeatal complex
    - Nasal anatomic variations (septal deviation, concha bullosa)
    - Cystic fibrosis
    - Common variable immunoglobulin deficiency
    - Immunoglobulin A (IgA) deficiency
    - Ciliary dyskinesia, Kartagener syndrome, Young syndrome
    - Aspirin sensitivity
    - Acquired immunodeficiency syndrome (AIDS)
    - Bronchiectasis
    - Cocaine abuse
    - Wegener's granulomatosis
    - Rhinitis medicamentosa

DIAGNOSIS

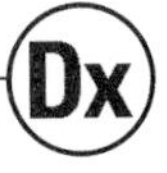

DIFFERENTIAL DIAGNOSIS

- Infectious: acute viral infection, acute or chronic bacterial sinusitis
- Allergic: seasonal allergic rhinitis perennial allergic rhinitis
- Vasomotor: idiopathic (vasomotor rhinitis), abuse of nose drops (rhinitis medicamentosa), drugs (reserpine, guanethidine, prazosin, cocaine)
- Mechanical: foreign body, polyps, tumor, deviated septum, central nervous system leak, enlarged tonsils and adenoids
- Hormonal: pregnancy, hypothyroidism, hyperthyroidism

WORKUP

- The diagnosis of acute bacterial sinusitis is based on clinical criteria in children who present with upper respiratory symptoms that are either persistent or severe.
    - Persistent symptoms are those that last longer than 10 to 14 days.
    - Severe symptoms include temperature ≥ 102°F and purulent nasal discharge present concurrently for at least 3 to 4 days in a child who seems ill.
    - The child who seems toxic should be hospitalized.
- Current indications for maxillary sinus aspiration include the following (typically with subspecialty referral):
    - Failure to respond to multiple courses of antibiotics
    - Severe facial pain
    - Orbital or intracranial complications
    - Evaluation of an immunocompromised host

IMAGING STUDIES

- Imaging studies are not necessary to confirm a diagnosis of clinical sinusitis in children ≤ 6 years of age.
- The need for radiographs as a confirmatory test in acute sinusitis in children older than 6 years with persistent symptoms and for all children with severe symptoms is controversial. A normal radiograph can be powerful evidence in ruling out acute bacterial sinusitis. However, given the difficulties in performing these studies, the American College of Radiology has suggested that

the diagnosis of acute uncomplicated sinusitis should be made on clinical grounds alone.

- Computed tomography (CT) scans of the paranasal sinuses should be reserved for patients in whom surgery is being considered as a management strategy.

TREATMENT

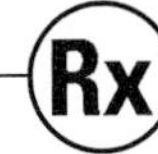

ACUTE GENERAL Rx

- Antibiotics are recommended for the management of acute bacterial sinusitis to achieve a more rapid clinical cure.
- Clinicians should consider use of the most narrow-spectrum agent that is active against the most likely pathogens. Risk factors to consider for penicillin-resistant *Streptococcus pneumoniae* (PRSP) include:
  - Day care attendance
  - Recent receipt of antimicrobial therapy (<30 days)
  - Age less than 2 years
  - Exposure to environmental tobacco smoke
- One approach recommended by Cincinnati Children's Hospital Medical Center:
  - In the child with no risk factors for PRSP standard dose amoxicillin (45 mg/kg/day in 2 divided doses) or Augmentin (with standard dose amoxicillin component) may be considered as initial therapy.
  - In children with risk factors for PRSP, high-dose amoxicillin (80 to 90 mg/kg/day in 2 divided doses) or Augmentin (with high-dose amoxicillin component) should be used as first-line therapy.
  - Augmentin with high-dose amoxicillin (if not used as initial therapy), cefuroxime, cefpodoxime, cefprozil, and cefdinir are reasonable considerations as second-line agents.
  - Once therapeutic response has been demonstrated, the selected therapeutic agent should be continued for a minimum of 10 to 14 days.
  - If no improvement occurs or if there is worsening of symptoms after 72 hours with a first- or second-line agent, a second- or third-line agent should be considered. Third-line agents include clindamycin and cefixime.
  - In the penicillin-allergic patient, second- or third-line agents, in addition to the macrolides, and new anilides or trimethoprim-sulfamethoxazole (TMP-SMX) may be considered.
  - Toxic-appearing children who demonstrate poor tolerance of oral intake may require initial parenteral therapy either as an outpatient or during a short inpatient stay. Reassessment of such patients after initial stabilization may avoid unnecessary imaging and referral early in the course of therapy.
- Adjuvant therapies (saline irrigation, antihistamines, decongestants, mucolytic agents, and topical corticosteroids) are not recommended as part of standard care because of controversial and limited efficacy data.

REFERRAL

The complications of acute bacterial sinusitis usually involve either the orbit:

- Periorbital cellulitis
- Orbital cellulitis
- Subperiosteal orbital abscess

Or the central nervous system:

- Frontal lobe abscess
- Potts puffy tumor (osteomyelitis of frontal bone)
- Venous sinus thrombosis
- Meningitis
- Epidural empyema
- Subdural empyema
- Intracerebral abscess

Children with complications or suspected complications of acute bacterial sinusitis should be treated promptly and aggressively. This should include referral to an otolaryngologist possibly with the consultation of an infectious disease specialist and neurosurgeon.

PEARLS & CONSIDERATIONS

COMMENTS

- Sinusitis is insidious in children, and concurrent otitis media is common.
- Quantitative sweat chloride tests for diagnosis of cystic fibrosis should be considered in children with nasal polyps or colonization of the nose and sinuses with *Pseudomonas* species.

PATIENT/FAMILY EDUCATION

- Medline Plus: Sinusitis. Available at http://www.nlm.nih.gov/medlineplus/sinusitis.html

SUGGESTED READINGS

American Academy of Pediatrics Subcommittee on Management of Sinusitis and Committee on Quality Improvement: Clinical practice guideline: management of sinusitis. *Pediatrics* 108(3):798, 2001.

Cincinnati Children's Hospital Medical Center: *Evidence-based clinical practice guideline for children with acute bacterial sinusitis in children 1 to 18 years of age.* Cincinnati Children's Hospital Medical Center, April 27, 2001.

Lau J et al: *Diagnosis and treatment of uncomplicated acute sinusitis in children: Evidence Report/Technology Assessment No. 9(Suppl).* (AHRQ Publication No. 01-E005.) Rockville, MD, Agency for Healthcare Research and Quality, 2000.

Oxford LE, McClay J: Complications of acute sinusitis in children. *Otolaryngol Head Neck Surg* 133:32, 2005.

AUTHOR: **MARC A. RASLICH, MD**

BASIC INFORMATION

DEFINITION

Sleep problems include difficulty initiating sleep, difficulty sleeping through the night, disturbance in the amount or timing of sleep (including refusal and night wakings), and abnormal behaviors. Night terrors are a partially awake, partially asleep state that usually include fearful talking or thrashing and are not usually remembered in the morning. Nightmares are fearful dreams that usually result in awakening and a memory of the dream. Sleep talking and sleepwalking are also considered nonorganic sleep problems. (See Obstructive Sleep Apnea & Sleep-Disordered Breathing and Parasomnias in Diseases and Disorders [Section I]).

SYNONYMS

Sleep disorders
Sleep disruption

ICD-9-CM CODES

307.40 Nonorganic sleep disorder, unspecified
307.41 Transient disorder of initiating or maintaining sleep
307.42 Persistent disorder of initiating or maintaining sleep
307.43 Transient disorder of initiating or maintaining wakefulness
307.44 Persistent disorder of initiating or maintaining wakefulness
307.45 Phase-shift disruption of 24-hour sleep-wake cycle
307.46 Somnambulism or night terrors
307.47 Other dysfunction of sleep stages or arousal from sleep
307.48 Repetitive intrusions of sleep
307.49 Other sleep disorder

EPIDEMIOLOGY & DEMOGRAPHICS

- Sleep disorders are some of the most common complaints of parents to pediatricians.
- Frequent night waking occurs in 25% of 6- to 12-month-olds and 20% of 1- to 2-year-olds.
- Difficulty settling occurs in 50% of 4-year-olds.
- Nightmares occur in 5% of 1-year-olds and up to 39% of 4-year-olds (generally, estimates range from 25% to 50% of children).
- Night terrors or sleep terrors occur in 1% to 6% of children (usually at 18 months to 6 years of age).
- Sleep talking occurs in about 8% of 4- and 5-year-olds.
- Estimates of sleepwalking range from 1% to 15% (persistent sleepwalking may occur in as many as 2.5% of children).

CLINICAL PRESENTATION

History

- Familial causes of nonorganic sleep problems are uncommon.
- Questions to ask include:
  - Are there evening activities and a bedtime ritual?
  - How are difficulties at bedtime handled?
  - What are the time and length of waking?
  - What are the time, ease, and spontaneity of morning waking?
  - What is the daytime schedule for weekdays and weekends?
  - What are the timing and length of daytime sleeping?
  - How do the parents view the problem?
- History of snoring may be suggestive of obstructive sleep apnea.
- Determine whether the child experiences sleep terrors.
- Determine whether the child experiences sleepwalking.
- Obtain a description of the sleep environment: noise (TV), lighting, with other people (parents, siblings), pets.
- Ask about medications and other medical conditions.
- Ask about recent illnesses.
- Determine whether there is a history of seizures.

Physical Examination

- No abnormalities are expected in physical exam of nonorganic sleep problems.
  - Nasal air flow
  - Tonsil size
  - Neurologic examination

ETIOLOGY

- Physical factors such as upper respiratory infections or injuries may lead to a temporary sleep problem.
- Developmental factors such as separation anxiety may also be a cause.
- Behavioral factors include overly dependent children and overly involved parents.
  - Other possible behavioral etiologies include anxiety, depression, and posttraumatic stress.
- Environmental and interactional factors include:
  - Bedtime and nighttime feedings
  - Use of objects that are associated with falling asleep, such as pacifiers, and presence of parents at bedside when falling asleep
  - Parents who have difficulty setting limits
  - Family stresses

DIAGNOSIS

DIFFERENTIAL DIAGNOSIS

- Diagnosis is based on the history, with physical examination used to rule out other abnormalities.
- Obstructive sleep apnea is often caused by enlarged tonsils and adenoids in children.
- Seizure disorder, anxiety, or depression may be present.

WORKUP

- Have parents keep a sleep log (diary) for at least 1 week to obtain the current pattern of difficulties. Parents should report:
  - Time child falls asleep
  - Time of awakenings
  - Time of return to sleep
  - Time of final awakening in the morning
  - Naps during the day
- A polysomnogram and the multiple sleep latency test may be useful if no other explanation is obtained for a child with a significantly shorter nighttime sleep pattern (< 5 hours) and no additional daytime sleep.
  - These devices are not typically needed for general nonorganic sleep difficulties.

TREATMENT

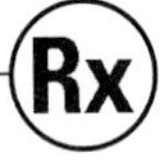

NONPHARMACOLOGIC THERAPY

- Difficulty initiating sleep
  - Set limits.
    - This is done by a gradual ignoring procedure.
    - Increase length of time before each return to child's room.
    - Spend a brief time in room to reassure the child.
- Difficulty with nighttime waking
  - Review sleep associations.
  - Assist the child in self-soothing behaviors.
  - Good sleep hygiene is essential.
  - Consistent schedule
  - Consistent pattern
  - Wait for progressively longer periods before checking on, or briefly visiting with, the child.
- Night terrors
  - Explain that they are not harmful. Night terror is most scary to those who are awake.
  - Night terrors occur in a sleep state that is not a dream state (non-rapid eye movement [REM]).
  - Child usually has no memory of the event.
  - Night terrors last minutes to half an hour.
  - Parents should provide protection if the child is thrashing wildly.
  - Usually terrors resolve in days to months.
  - If left alone and simply watched, child will normally return to normal sleep and calm after a few minutes.
- Nightmares
  - These are managed by comforting the child.
  - Any additional discussion about the nightmare should occur during the day.
  - Nightmares can be caused by watching scary TV shows or movies or by family stress.
  - Eliminate or manage stress to help prevent future nightmares.

- Sleep phase-shift
  - These are managed by an incremental shift back to the normal night shift, then rigidly adhering to the schedule.
- Transient sleep problems
  - Generally no need for specific treatment.

ACUTE GENERAL Rx

- Benadryl use for sleep initiation has been recommended and may result in brief, limited improvement.
- Melatonin has also been used for temporary assistance in sleep initiation.
- For serious sleep terrors (high frequency or extreme disruption to family), benzodiazepines or tricyclic antidepressants may be (cautiously and temporarily) considered.

REFERRAL

- Most sleep problems are well managed behaviorally.
  - If difficulty persists, a behavioral specialist can be consulted.
  - Organic sleep problems should be treated and referred as medically indicated.
- Concerns of serious emotional disturbance related to sleep problems should be referred for evaluation of the emotional disturbance.

PEARLS & CONSIDERATIONS

COMMENTS

- Behavioral solutions of sleep problems can lead to other successful behavioral changes.
- Common nonorganic sleep problems can often be relieved through behavioral interventions in 2 weeks or less.
- Sleep initiation and nighttime waking solutions using a progressive ignoring procedure allow parents to gain control. However, if success is not attained within a few days, referral to a behavioral specialist may be necessary.
- Solving basic sleep problems should be presented to parents as a way of providing the child with appropriate developmental guidance.

PREVENTION

Anticipatory guidance about normal sleep patterns, positive sleep associations, good sleep hygiene or habits, and good behavioral limit-setting can significantly reduce or prevent sleep problems.

PATIENT/FAMILY EDUCATION

- Focus on understanding of the following:
  - Normal patterns and length of sleep based on age (well described in detail by Ferber, 1985)
    - Length of sleep ranges from about 15 hours of total sleep time for a 3-month-old (10 hours at night and five 1-hour naps), to 13 hours for a 2-year-old (1 or more hour during naps), to 11 hours for a 5-year-old, and 8 to 9 hours for a teenager.
    - Normal sleep patterns are cyclic, moving between awake or partially awake, light non-REM, deep non-Rem, and REM sleep.
    - More deep sleep occurs early in the night and near morning, while more light sleep and dreaming occur in the middle of the night.
  - The stages of sleep:
    - Deep non-REM. This is the deepest sleep.
    - Light non-REM. A lighter version of the deepest sleep.
    - REM sleep. This is where dreaming occurs.
  - The normal occurrence of nightly partial awakenings:
    - Partial awakenings: Child may get up if this is after light sleep or dreaming; if after deep non-REM the child may sleepwalk, sleep talk, or have night terrors.
  - Sleep associations and how to establish bedtime rituals with positive sleep associations
  - Use of "transitional object" (e.g., a special toy or favorite blanket) to assist a child in falling asleep
- Typically, nighttime feedings are not needed after 3 months of age.
- By 6 months of age, most children are capable of sleeping through the night.

SUGGESTED READINGS

American Academy of Sleep Medicine. Available at www.asda.org

Blum NJ, Carey WB: Sleep problems among infants and young children. *Pediatr Rev* 17:87, 1996.

Ferber RA: *Solve Your Child's Sleep Problems.* New York, Simon & Schuster, 1985.

Ferber RA, Kryger MH (eds): *Principles and Practice of Sleep Medicine in the Child.* Philadelphia, WB Saunders, 1995.

National Sleep Foundation. Available at www.sleepfoundation.org

Pantley E: *The No-Cry Sleep Solution.* New York, McGraw-Hill, 2002.

Weissbluth M: *Healthy Sleep Habits, Happy Child.* New York, Ballantine Books, 2005.

AUTHOR: **ROGER A. YEAGER, PHD**

BASIC INFORMATION

DEFINITION

Slipped capital femoral epiphysis (SCFE) is the most common adolescent orthopedic hip disorder. It is characterized by the displacement of the capital femoral epiphysis from the femoral neck through the physeal plate (growth plate).

SYNONYMS

Physiolysis of the hip
SCFE
Slipped upper femoral epiphysis

ICD-9-CM CODES

732.2 Slipped upper femoral epiphysitis
732.9 Epiphysitis

EPIDEMIOLOGY & DEMOGRAPHICS

- Prevalence ranges from 0.2 per 100,000 in eastern Japan to 10.08 per 100,000 in the northeastern United States.
- Male-to-female ratio is 1.5:1.0.
- Relative racial frequency is 1.0 for whites, 4.5 for Pacific Islanders, 2.2 for blacks, 1.05 for Amerindians, 0.5 for Indonesian-Malay peoples, and 0.1 for Indo-Mediterranean peoples. Differences are theoretically based on mean body weight for each racial group or variability in acetabular depth in each racial group.
- Mean age of presentation is 12 years in girls (usually prior to menarche) and 13.5 years in boys (usually prior to Tanner stage IV).
- Main risk factor is obesity (= 90% weight for age and gender).
- Other risk factors include endocrine abnormalities, especially hypothyroidism and growth hormone deficiency; genetic disorders, such as Down syndrome and Rubinstein-Taybi syndrome; and renal failure.

CLINICAL PRESENTATION

History

- Usual presentation is nonradiating pain and altered gait.
  - Pain is increased with physical activity.
  - Pain may be chronic or intermittent.
- Fifteen percent of children and adolescents initially present with thigh or knee pain.
- The *chronic* pattern of presentation is the most common, defined by intermittent symptoms for longer than 3 weeks. Other pattern presentations include *preslip*, defined by pain but no displacement of the epiphysis, *acute*, and *acute-on-chronic*.
- Presentation with bilateral disease occurs in 20% of cases.
- In unilateral disease, the contralateral hip may be affected in 30% to 60% of cases.

Physical Examination

- Affected leg is usually held in an externally rotated position.
- *Stable* SCFE (slip) is defined by the patient walking or weight bearing; *unstable* SCFE is defined by inability to bear weight even with crutches.
- Gait is usually antalgic in unilateral SCFE. Gait is waddling in bilateral SCFE.
- With moderate to severe SCFE (displacement greater than one third of the diameter of the femoral neck), atrophy of the upper thigh and gluteal muscles may be present, sometimes associated with a Trendelenburg gait.
- Anterior hip may be tender to palpation.
- Abduction and external rotation of the affected leg when the hip is passively flexed from an extended position is highly suggestive of SCFE.

ETIOLOGY

- The proximal femur distal to the physis (growth plate) is displaced anterolaterally and superiorly in relation to the femoral head.
- It is unclear what factors weaken the physeal plate, but factors may include: normal periosteal thinning and widening of the physis (especially in periods of rapid growth), obesity (which increases mechanical strain on physis), genetic predisposition, endocrine and metabolic disorders that cause abnormal growth and mineralization of cartilage, trauma, inflammatory changes

DIAGNOSIS

Dx

DIFFERENTIAL DIAGNOSIS

- Legg-Calvé-Perthes disease
- Avascular necrosis of femoral head
- Juvenile rheumatoid arthritis
- Septic joint
- Bone tumors

LABORATORY TESTS

Pursue appropriate testing for endocrine disorders, especially hypothyroidism, or renal failure if clinically indicated.

IMAGING STUDIES

- Plain radiographs usually diagnose SCFE.
  - Anterior-posterior (AP) and lateral views of both hips should be obtained.
  - Lateral views can be frog-leg or cross-table lateral.
  - The latter view may be better for acute unstable presentations as further manipulation may worsen the slip.
- Positive findings on plain radiographs show posterior displacement of the femoral epiphysis: ice cream slipping off cone. Early findings include widening and irregularity of the physis with thinning of the proximal epiphysis.
- Magnetic resonance imaging (MRI) may be useful for early symptomatic preslips that demonstrate normal plain radiographs. The MRI may demonstrate widening of the physis with surrounding edema.

TREATMENT

Rx

NONPHARMACOLOGIC THERAPY

- All patients should be promptly referred to a pediatric orthopedic surgeon and should avoid bearing weight until evaluation.
- All patients with unstable SCFE and most patients with bilateral SCFE should be admitted to the hospital for bed rest and complete avoidance of weight bearing to avoid further slippage.
- Treatment of SCFE is a surgical procedure, usually with screw fixation: stabilization of the physis with a single cannulated screw placed in the center of the epiphysis.
- Prophylactic pinning of the contralateral hip in unilateral SCFE presentations is controversial.

DISPOSITION

- Crutches are usually needed for 6 to 8 weeks postsurgery.
- Thirty percent to 60% of patients with unilateral SCFE will have a contralateral slip. The majority of patients will present within 18 months from diagnosis of the first slip. Many of the contralateral slips are asymptomatic, so close follow-up with the orthopedic surgeon is important.
- Complications of SCFE include osteonecrosis of the femoral head and chondrolysis (narrowing of the joint space and loss of articular cartilage). Both complications increase the risk of developing osteoarthritis.
- Prognosis is related to severity of the slip. Increasing severity of the slip increases risk of complications.

REFERRAL

All patients with SCFE should be immediately referred to an orthopedic surgeon pediatric hip experience.

PEARLS & CONSIDERATIONS

!

COMMENTS

- In children with unilateral SCFE and underlying endocrine disorders, the contralateral hip will be affected in up to 100% of cases.
- Initial presentations of SCFE may only be symptoms of isolated thigh or knee pain. The physician must remember to also evaluate the hip, as a delay in diagnosis of SCFE can worsen the prognosis.
- Consider underlying endocrine, renal, or genetic disorders in children with SCFE who are younger than 10 years old, older than 16 years old, or are less than 50th percentile for weight.

SUGGESTED READINGS

Hubbard AM: Imaging of pediatric hip disorders. *Radiol Clin North Am* 39:721, 2001.

Kehl DH: Slipped capital femoral epiphysis. *In* Morrissey RT, Weinstien SL (eds): *Pediatric Orthopedics.* Philadelphia, Lippincott Williams & Wilkins, 2001, pp 999–1033.

Loder RT: The demographics of slipped capital femoral epiphysis: an international multicenter study. *Clin Orthop* 322:28, 1996.

Reynolds RA: Diagnosis and treatment of slipped capital femoral epiphysis. *Curr Opin Pediatr* 11:80, 1999.

Wells D et al: Review of slipped capital femoral epiphysis associated with endocrine disease. *J Pediatr Orthop* 13:610, 1993.

AUTHOR: **SHARON F. CHEN, MD**

BASIC INFORMATION

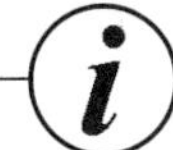

DEFINITION

Snake bites are particularly important in children. The clinical course of a child after a snake bite tends to be more severe than that of an adult, because children receive a larger per kilogram dose of venom.

SYNONYM

Snake bite

ICD-9-CM CODE
989.5 Toxic effect of venom

EPIDEMIOLOGY & DEMOGRAPHICS

- In the United States in 2003, 3000 poisonous and 3800 nonpoisonous or assumed nonpoisonous snake bites were reported.
- In children, 702 poisonous and 771 nonpoisonous bites were reported.
  - Bites associated with major sequelae were 153, including 2 resulting in death.
- Male adolescents and adults are most commonly bitten.
- While most bites occur in desert areas of the southwestern United States and Mexico, snake bites occur throughout North America as poisonous snakes are either indigenous or kept as exotic pets.
- More than 95% of poisonous snake bites are caused by rattlesnakes, copperheads, and cottonmouths, known as pit vipers or *Crotalidae.*

CLINICAL PRESENTATION

Local Symptoms

- Usually significant pain from the moment of envenomation
- Variable local edema
- Fang marks may be visible
- Ecchymosis at site
- Bullae (fluid-filled or hemorrhagic)
- Necrosis develops
- Possible compartment syndrome

Systemic Symptoms

- Tender regional lymphadenitis
- Nausea
- Metallic taste in mouth
- Muscle fasciculations
- Generalized bleeding (from intravenous sites and wound)
- Hypovolemic shock

***Elapidae* Envenomations: Coral Snakes and Cobras**

- Neurotoxic effects of numbness, tremors, salivation, ptosis, dysarthria
- Delayed dyspnea and respiratory paralysis

ETIOLOGY

- *Crotalidae* venom causes increased permeability of capillary membranes, leading to extravasation of electrolytes, albumin, and red cells into the envenomated site. Hemolysis and edema occur, followed by hypotension.
- *Elapidae* envenomations (coral snakes) cause neurotoxic effects.

DIAGNOSIS

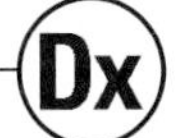

DIFFERENTIAL DIAGNOSIS

- Snake bite
- Spider bite
- Anaphylaxis
- Sepsis

WORKUP

- History of witnessed bite
- Localized pain and inflammation
- Nausea
- Metallic taste or fasciculations
- Numbness or other neurologic manifestations

LABORATORY TESTS

- Check for electrolyte abnormalities: metabolic panel
- Look for coagulopathy: complete blood cell count with platelet count, prothrombin time, fibrinogen

TREATMENT

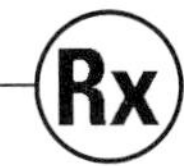

NONPHARMACOLOGIC THERAPY

- Minimize movement (may splint bitten extremity).
- Remove restrictive clothing and jewelry.
- Apply a circumferential rubber band (not a tourniquet) to occlude venous and lymphatic drainage of venom.
- Do not put ice on wound or attempt to suck out venom orally.
- Assess severity and rapidity of progression of local edema by performing serial extremity circumference measurements every 20 to 30 minutes.
- Edema increasing at a rate greater than 0.5 cm/hour is rapid enough to cause concern for inadequate distal perfusion.
- Surgical consultation is mandatory for any concern for adequacy of distal perfusion or development of compartment syndrome.

ACUTE GENERAL Rx

Therapy is aimed at managing local tissue damage, capillary leak syndrome, and possible coagulopathic and neurotoxic venom effects.

- Provide intravenous fluid resuscitation.
- Administer narcotic analgesia.
- Tetanus booster if more than 5 years since last tetanus immunization or patient is not fully immunized.
- Rapid proximal progression of swelling or the presence of coagulopathy or other systemic findings indicates the need for antivenin administration.
- Call 1-800-222-1222 to consult the regional poison center for instructions regarding administration of antivenin.
- Anaphylaxis can occur with antivenin administration.
- Delayed serum sickness reactions almost universal after antivenin administration.

CHRONIC Rx

- Serum sickness, manifested by urticaria, pruritus, arthralgias, and swollen joints, may be treated with corticosteroids until all symptoms have subsided for 24 hours.
- Physical therapy is indicated during the recovery phase.

DISPOSITION

When pain is managed with oral narcotics and edema and systemic symptoms have ceased the patient may be discharged.

REFERRAL

Referral to a tertiary care center is necessary in severe cases for administration of antivenin and intensive care monitoring.

PEARLS & CONSIDERATIONS

COMMENTS

- Maintain vital signs and close monitoring.
- Ensure distal extremity perfusion.
- Consult the regional poison center for indications and instructions regarding antivenin administration.

PREVENTION

- Do not handle snakes unless familiar with their identification and management.
- Avoid the known habitats of snakes, including areas that snakes seek for protection (rocks, caves, fallen trees, rocky ledges).
- Wear adequate protective clothing.
- Avoid walking at night in snake-infested areas. Most venomous snakes avoid sunlight.
- Additional information regarding treatment and prevention of snake bites is available at http://www.fda.gov/fdac/features/995_snakes.html

SUGGESTED READINGS

Bond GR: Snake, spider, and scorpion envenomation in North America. *Pediatr Rev* 20:147, 1999.

Hodde D, Tecklenburg FW: Bites and stings. *In* Fleisher GR, Ludwig S (eds): *Textbook of Pediatric Emergency Medicine,* 4th ed. Philadelphia, Lippincott Williams & Wilkins, 2000, pp 979–998.

Litovitz TL et al: 2003 Annual Report of the American Association of Poison Control Centers Toxic Exposure Surveillance System. *Am J Emerg Med* 22(5):378, 2004.

McKinney PE: Out-of-hospital and interhospital management of crotaline snakebite. *Ann Emerg Med* 37(2):168, 2001.

Sullivan JB et al: North American venomous reptile bites. *In* Auerbach PS (ed): *Wilderness Medicine: Management of Wilderness and Environmental Emergencies.* St. Louis, Mosby, 1995, pp 680–707.

AUTHORS: **MARK RODDY, MD** and **ROBERT J. FREISHTAT, MD, MPH**

BASIC INFORMATION

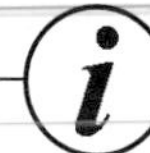

DEFINITION

Hereditary spherocytosis is the most common inherited abnormality of the red cell membrane that can cause hemolytic anemia.

SYNONYM

Hereditary spherocytosis

ICD-9-CM CODE
282.0 Hereditary spherocytosis

EPIDEMIOLOGY & DEMOGRAPHICS

- Hereditary spherocytosis affects approximately 1 in 5000 individuals.
- It is most common in people of Northern European ancestry.

CLINICAL PRESENTATION

History

- Affected individuals may have minimal hemolysis and therefore are not diagnosed as children, or they may have a severe hemolytic anemia presenting with pallor, jaundice, fatigue, and exercise intolerance.
  - Newborn patients can present with anemia and hyperbilirubinemia.
    - Hemolysis may be more prominent in the newborn because hemoglobin F binds 2,3-diphosphoglycerate (DPG) poorly.
    - This increase in free 2,3-DPG destabilizes spectrin-actin-protein 4.1 interactions in the red blood cell (RBC) membrane which in turn leads to more rapid RBC breakdown.
  - Because of the shortened red cell life span, patients are susceptible to aplastic crises associated with parvovirus and other infections.
  - Pigmentary (bilirubin) gallstones may form as early as age 4 to 5 years.
    - At least 50% of unsplenectomized patients ultimately form gallstones.
- Positive family history of jaundice, anemia, or gallbladder stones may be reported.

Physical Examination

- Pallor; tachycardia; icterus; after infancy, the spleen is usually enlarged; right upper quadrant tenderness (bilirubin cholelithiasis)

ETIOLOGY

- Hereditary spherocytosis is transmitted as an autosomal dominant and, much less often, as an autosomal recessive disorder.
- As many as 25% of patients have no previous family history.
- Spheroid red cells most commonly result from abnormalities of spectrin or ankyrin, structural proteins of the red cell membrane.
  - Gene defects corresponding to these protein abnormalities have been described.
- The protein abnormalities cause a loss of membrane surface area without a proportional loss of cell volume.
  - These spherocytic red cells have decreased deformability, and are destroyed prematurely in the spleen.

DIAGNOSIS

DIFFERENTIAL DIAGNOSIS

- Other inherited disorders of the red cell membrane include hereditary elliptocytosis, hereditary stomatocytosis, and hereditary pyropoikilocytosis.
  - Distinguished from each other by evaluating the blood film for distinctive morphology
- Immune hemolysis also may cause a large number of spherocytes on the blood film.
  - Distinguished from hereditary spherocytosis by a positive direct Coombs (antiglobulin) test indicating immunoglobulin on the red cell surface
- Rare causes of spherocytosis include thermal injury, clostridial septicemia with exotoxemia, and Wilson disease, each of which may present as a hemolytic anemia.

WORKUP

The diagnosis of hereditary spherocytosis is suggested by the presence of a positive family history, splenomegaly, reticulocytosis, and spherocytosis of red cells.

LABORATORY TESTS

- The hemoglobin level is usually 6 to 10 g/dL, depending on individual severity, but can be in the normal range.
- The mean corpuscular volume (MCV) is normal and the mean corpuscular hemoglobin concentration (MCHC) is often increased.
- The reticulocyte percentage is increased to 6% to 20%.
- Spherocytes are found on the blood film, usually accounting for 15% to 20% of cells.
- The presence of spherocytes in the blood can be confirmed by an osmotic fragility test (however the osmotic fragility test is not specific for hereditary spherocytosis and may be abnormal in immune and other hemolytic anemias).
- A Coombs test should be performed to ensure that the clinical findings are not secondary to immune hemolytic anemia.
- Other evidence of hemolysis may include elevated indirect bilirubin and decreased haptoglobin.
- As a research tool, the specific protein abnormality can be established in 80% of patients by RBC membrane protein analysis using gel electrophoresis.

IMAGING STUDIES

Gallstones may be seen on abdominal ultrasonography.

TREATMENT

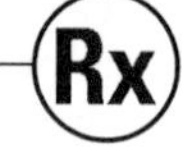

NONPHARMACOLOGIC THERAPY

Hematocrit and reticulocyte percentage should be obtained early during febrile illnesses to detect aplastic crises. It is important to know the patient's baseline values.

ACUTE GENERAL Rx

Transfusion may be needed for aplastic crises.

CHRONIC Rx

- Patients with hereditary spherocytosis who maintain a hemoglobin greater than 10 g/dL and a reticulocyte percentage less than 10 should be treated expectantly with folic acid 1 mg daily.
- In infants with severe anemia (hemoglobin <10g/L), chronic transfusion therapy may be necessary to delay splenectomy until at least 2 years of age in order to reduce the high risk of postsplenectomy sepsis.
- Splenectomy eliminates hemolysis in hereditary spherocytosis but should be delayed if possible until after 6 years of age to minimize risk of postsplenectomy sepsis.
- Splenectomy should be reserved for:
  - Patients who cannot sustain hemoglobin of 10 g/L or who have poor growth or cardiomegaly.
  - Those who have experienced repeated aplastic crises.
  - Those with markedly enlarged spleens who may be at risk for splenic rupture or who have abdominal discomfort or early satiety.
- Vaccines for encapsulated organisms such as *Pneumococcus, Meningococcus,* and *Haemophilus influenzae* type b should be administered before splenectomy and prophylactic oral penicillin V administered thereafter.

DISPOSITION

- Hematocrit and reticulocyte percentages should be monitored every 6 to 12 months.
- Immunizations for encapsulated bacteria before splenectomy and penicillin prophylaxis after splenectomy are recommended.

REFERRAL

- Pediatric hematology

PEARLS & CONSIDERATIONS

COMMENTS

- These patients are at risk for aplastic crisis.
- They may also develop early cholelithiasis.

PATIENT/FAMILY EDUCATION

Because of the susceptibility to aplastic crises associated with parvovirus and other infections, families should contact a health care provider when the child experiences febrile illnesses.

SUGGESTED READINGS

Bolton-Maggs PBH et al: Guidelines for the diagnosis and management of hereditary spherocytosis. *Br J Haematol* 126:455, 2004.

Hassoun H, Palek J: Hereditary spherocytosis: a review of the clinical and molecular aspects of the disease. *Blood Rev* 10:129, 1996.

Nathan DG, Orkin SH (eds): *Nathan and Oski's Hematology of Infancy and Childhood,* 6th ed. Philadelphia, WB Saunders, 2003.

AUTHORS: **JILL S. HALTERMAN, MD, MPH** and **GEORGE B. SEGEL, MD**

BASIC INFORMATION

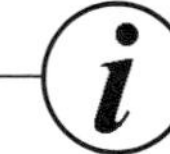

DEFINITION

Spiders belong to the class Arachnida, which includes animals with four pairs of legs and no wings or antennae.

SYNONYM

Spider envenomation

ICD-9-CM CODE

989.5 Toxic effect of venom

EPIDEMIOLOGY & DEMOGRAPHICS

- Overall, death and long-term morbidity resulting from spider bites are very rare.
- Most spider bites cause no more than a local reaction, although the bites of two species of spiders in the United States can sometimes cause severe symptoms.
  - Brown recluse (*Loxosceles reclusa)* spider
  - Black widow (*Latrodectus mactans* and *Latrodectus hesperus*) spider
- **Brown recluse** is brown with a yellow, violin-shaped marking on the dorsal cephalothorax.
  - Located mostly in southern and midwestern states
  - Infest dark, quiet areas (i.e., woodpiles, storage sheds, attics, and closets)
  - Do not bite humans unless provoked, such as when they are trapped between one's skin and clothing or a bed sheet
- **Black widow** has a red or yellow hourglass-shaped marking on its abdomen.
  - Only the female black widow can envenomate humans
  - Located throughout the entire United States except Alaska
  - Prefer to live and build their webs in warm, dry, dark areas
  - ***Latrodectus mactans* is found in the eastern United States and *Latrodectus hesperus* in the western United States**

CLINICAL PRESENTATION

- **Brown recluse**
  - Bite is usually painless initially or causes only mild stinging.
  - After an hour, the site develops an erythematous, urticarial rash (pruritic and edematous). Edema of facial bites can be extensive.
  - The center of the bite, which begins as a pale-blue macule with an inflammatory halo, becomes purpuric and then vesicular.
  - It may progress to necrosis, a process called *necrotic arachnidism*. It should be noted that necrotic skin lesions not due to brown recluse spider bites are frequently misdiagnosed as *necrotic arachnidism.*
  - Induration at the site and regional lymphadenopathy may be present.
  - Young children are at the greatest risk for systemic symptoms which may include nausea, vomiting, arthralgias, muscle aches or spasms, hemolysis, thrombocytopenia, hemoglobinuria, renal failure, shock, and altered mental status.
  - Resolution of the skin lesion may take months.
- **Black widow**
  - Bite begins with a pinprick sensation at the site.
  - The bite develops into a wheal with a pale center although the local reaction is usually not very pronounced. Skin necrosis does not occur.
  - Within an hour, muscle cramping spreads throughout the body.
  - Abdominal pain can be severe and may be confused with an acute abdomen.
  - Systemic symptoms peak at 3 hours and are mild in the majority of patients. The most common symptoms are abdominal pain, hypertension, myalgias or muscle spasms, anxiety, and agitation. Signs of autonomic instability (i.e., tachycardia, fever, salivation, diaphoresis, vomiting, bronchorrhea, ptosis, and priapism) may also occur.
  - Symptoms resolve slowly without antivenom and may take 2 days.
  - Headaches and other vague symptoms may persist for weeks without antivenom.
  - Long-term outcomes are very favorable.

ETIOLOGY

- Spider venom has many different components and, depending on the species, may contain enzymatic proteins, which cause local tissue destruction, or neurotoxins which can cause the systemic manifestations such as diffuse pain, muscular contractions, and autonomic instability.
- In addition, venom components can have hemolytic effects, inhibit coagulation, or stimulate platelet aggregation leading to thrombosis.

DIAGNOSIS

DIFFERENTIAL DIAGNOSIS

- Witnessing the spider bite and a description of the spider's appearance are keys to making a definitive diagnosis.
- Knowing the region of the United States where the bite occurred may also help exclude specific species.
- Location of the bite often occurs at the entry points of clothing such as shirt cuffs and collars or the groin region in patients wearing shorts. Multiple lesions suggest a parasitic insect bite rather than a spider bite.
- The change in a bite lesion over time or the presence of associated systemic symptoms or signs may also help determine the involved species.
- Other conditions to consider:
  - Infections (i.e., fungal, bacterial, or viral infection, especially herpes simplex and zoster)
  - Snake bites or other insect bites and stings
  - Foreign body reactions
  - Burns
  - Systemic conditions that predispose to focal skin lesions (e.g., diabetes mellitus, leukemia, lupus erythematous)

LABORATORY TESTS

- Laboratory tests may be useful for identifying complications in patients exhibiting systemic signs or symptoms of spider envenomation.
- Complete blood cell count may show anemia or signs of hemolysis in brown recluse bites.
  - This hemolytic anemia is associated with a negative Coombs test.
- Prothrombin time and partial thromboplastin time may identify a coagulopathy.
- Urinalysis and serum creatinine may be obtained to look for hemoglobinuria and renal failure which are sometimes associated with hemolytic anemia.

TREATMENT

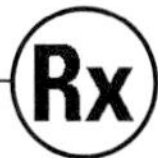

NONPHARMACOLOGIC THERAPY

- Basic treatment for all spider bites should include wound care and symptom control.
- Wound care includes: cleaning, application of ice, elevation of wound site.
- Tetanus immunization status should be updated in all patients with a spider bite.
- **Brown recluse bites**
  - Early wound excision is controversial and has not been shown to improve outcomes.
  - Cosmetic issues predominate after the initial period.
  - Skin grafting is common later.

ACUTE GENERAL Rx

- Emphasis should be on symptom control: analgesics for pain and antipruritics for itching.
- Almost all cases will have good outcomes without any additional medical treatment.
- Antibiotic therapy is not indicated unless a secondary cellulitis is suspected.
- **Brown recluse bites**
  - No specific medical treatments have been proven to change the clinical course.
  - Oral dapsone may inhibit skin necrosis but prospective human trials demonstrating its efficacy are lacking.
  - Corticosteroids are controversial. Their benefit has not been proven and they are generally not recommended.
  - Role of anti-venom is unclear.

TABLE 1-18 **Signs and Symptoms of Spider Bites**

Etiology	Demographics	History	Physical Examination
Brown recluse Disease: loxoscelism Toxin: phopholipase D Size: ~25 mm	Midwest through Texas, southern U.S.	Painless bite, rarely catch spider; thin spider body with "violin" shape on its back	Two fang marks; initial purpuric urticarial macule becomes vesicular; central necrosis late
Black widow Disease: latrodectism Toxin: neurotoxin	Most common in southern U.S., occasionally in northern climates	Pinprick bite sensation; red hourglass on its back; usually bite after web is disturbed	Two fang marks; target lesion early; sore lymph nodes and severe muscle and abdominal pain
Tarantula Size: 10-50 mm	Southwest U.S.	Large and hairy; bite after provoked; hairs can cause hives themselves	Two fang marks; wheal and flare; local pain; usually short-lived symptoms
Running spider Yellow sac spiders Toxin: necrotic Size: 5-12 mm	Indoors throughout the U.S., especially in northeast U.S.	Yellow sack on back; localized irritation	Two fang marks; wheal and flare; necrotic crust; nausea
Hobo spider Toxin: necrotic Size: ~10-18 mm	Pacific northwest	Found in sheet webs in the home; headaches and nausea	Warm swelling at site turns to blistering and necrosis
Wolf spider Nonvenomous Size: 14-15 mm	Very common in North America; many are nocturnal	Dark in color	Two fang marks; wheal and flare
Black jumping spider Nonvenomous Size: 5-15 mm	Common in North America; diurnal	Bright colors	Two fang marks; wheal and flare; local urticaria

- **Black widow bites**
  - Anti-venom causes a rapid resolution of symptoms but its use is limited because of the possibility of severe anaphylactic reactions and serum sickness.
  - Anti-venom is indicated only for extreme hypertension or uncontrollable pain. Skin testing should be performed prior to use because of the high occurrence of anaphylactic reactions.
  - Narcotic pain management with morphine should be initiated.
  - Intravenous calcium is falling out of favor because of its transient effect.
  - Benzodiazepines or muscle relaxants are useful adjuncts to analgesia for muscle spasms.
  - Nitroprusside or anti-venom can be provided for persistent hypertension after adequate pain relief.

DISPOSITION

- All patients should be monitored initially for signs of anaphylaxis.
- Patients with systemic signs, symptoms, or complications should be admitted to the hospital.
- Follow-up for wound reevaluation may be necessary to monitor for signs of infection.

REFERRAL

Referral of a brown recluse spider bite to a plastic surgeon is prudent.

PEARLS & CONSIDERATIONS

COMMENTS

- Anaphylaxis, although rare, is a possibility as with any bite or sting.
- Death or long-term morbidity from spider bites is extremely rare.
- Proper identification of the spider is helpful in predicting systemic symptoms.
- Wound care and pain relief are the foundations of therapy.

SUGGESTED READINGS

Boyer LV et al: Spider bites. *In* Auerbach (ed): *Wilderness Medicine,* 4th ed. St. Louis, Mosby, 2001, pp 807–838.

Diekema DS, Reuter DG: Arthropod bites and stings. *Clin Pediatr Emerg Med* 2:3, 2001.

Isbister GK: Necrotic arachnidism: the mythology of a modern plague. *Lancet* 364:549, 2004.

Sams HH: Necrotic arachnidism. *J Am Acad Dermatol* 44:4, 2001.

Saucier JR: Arachnid envenomation. *Emerg Med Clin North Am* 22:2, 2004.

AUTHORS: **JEFFREY BLAKE, MD** and **ROBERT J. FREISHTAT, MD, MPH**

BASIC INFORMATION

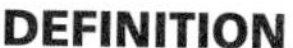
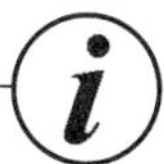

DEFINITION

Spinal muscular atrophy (SMA) is an inherited neuromuscular disorder resulting in anterior horn cell degeneration with resultant disuse and atrophy of voluntary muscles.

- The classic infantile disease (type I) presents before age 5 months and is generally severe, leading to death before 2 years of age.
- A milder form (type III) may present after age 3 years and progress slowly, with survival into adulthood.
- An intermediate form is also relatively common (type II), typically presents between 3 and 24 months of age, and is associated with a variable prognosis.
- An adult-onset form (type IV) typically presents after age 35 and progresses more slowly, usually sparing bulbar and respiratory function.

SYNONYMS

SMA type I—Werdnig-Hoffman disease, acute SMA
SMA type II—subacute, proximal SMA
SMA type III—Kugelberg-Welander disease, Wohlfart-Kugelberg-Welander disease, chronic SMA
SMA type IV—adult-onset SMA

ICD-9-CM CODES

335.0 Werdnig-Hoffman disease
335.1 Spinal muscular atrophy (SMA), nonspecified
335.11 Kugelberg-Welander disease
335.19 Other—adult spinal muscular atrophy

EPIDEMIOLOGY & DEMOGRAPHICS

- Frequency is approximately 1 in 10,000.
- Carrier frequency is 1 in 50.
- SMA is the most common genetic cause of death in infancy.

CLINICAL PRESENTATION

History

- Progressive weakness: generalized, including bulbar muscles, in the acute forms; more proximal muscle weakness in the chronic forms.
- Delayed or absent motor milestones or loss of motor milestones/skills

Physical Examination

Weakness, hypotonia, respiratory and bulbar weakness, hyporeflexia, fasciculations, especially tongue and fingers, occasional skeletal deformities, scoliosis

ETIOLOGY

- Homozygous mutations occur in the telomeric survival motor neuron (SMN1) gene on chromosome 5q13.
- The most common mutation (90% to 95%) is a homozygous deletion of exon 7.
  - The abnormal gene product fails to self-oligomerize into nuclear bodies called *gems*.
  - These gems appear to be important in mRNA processing.
- Genotype-phenotype correlations are under study. The phenotype is usually consistent within a given family (i.e., when one child is affected with the type I form, subsequent affected siblings are highly likely to also present with the type I form).
- A centromeric survival motor neuron (SMN2) pseudogene nearby on the same chromosome complicates genetic analysis, especially heterozygote prediction.
  - The product of the SMN2 pseudogene typically skips exon 7. However, it now appears that the pseudogene can make a small amount of normal SMN protein.
  - There is some evidence that the amount of normal SMN protein made by the SMN2 gene can modify the severity of SMA, with those who make more normal protein having a milder course.
- Another nearby gene locus, the neuronal apoptosis inhibitory protein (NAIP), appears deleted in half of severe SMA type I cases, and NAIP locus may also be involved in modification of SMA phenotype.

DIAGNOSIS

DIFFERENTIAL DIAGNOSIS

- Congenital myotonic dystrophy
- Maternal myasthenia gravis
- Acquired anterior horn cell disease (e.g., poliomyelitis, which is usually asymmetric)
- Kennedy spinal-bulbar neuronopathy
- Amyotrophic lateral sclerosis
- Muscular dystrophies

LABORATORY TESTS

- Muscle biopsy is usually definitive and shows large, round atrophic fibers and clumps of hypertrophic type Ia fibers.
- Genetic testing (white blood cell DNA) is now available for diagnosis but not for carrier testing. This test has a sensitivity of approximately 95%.
- Creatine kinase normal to slightly elevated.
- Nerve conduction velocity and cerebrospinal fluid protein are normal.
- Sensory nerves are normal.

TREATMENT

NONPHARMACOLOGIC THERAPY

Careful attention should be paid to pulmonary toilet and nutritional needs.

CHRONIC Rx

- Clinical trials of drugs such as indoprofen, valproic acid, and phenylbutyrate are in variable stages of planning or execution. These show promise in some individuals to increase the amount of SMN protein made by the SMN2 gene. Information on clinical trials can be found on the Muscular Dystrophy Association and Families of Spinal Muscular Atrophy SMA web sites listed under "Patient/Family Education".
- Treatment with antibiotics for respiratory illnesses should be initiated.
- Influenza immunization should be provided yearly beginning at 6 months of age (or first fall-winter period after patient is 6 months).
- Some families have elected intubation and long-term ventilation for children with type I disease, a controversial choice.

DISPOSITION

- Follow-up depends on the age, rate of progression, and severity of symptoms.
- Disease is usually rapidly fatal in infants.
- Older patients with milder disease may have slow progression with variable, occasionally even relatively normal, survival.

REFERRAL

- Neurologist will most likely make diagnosis.
- Diagnosis and management may require the assistance of a geneticist, nutritionist, gastroenterologist, pulmonologist, respiratory therapist, and nursing care specialist.
- The local muscular dystrophy association clinic may be of assistance.

PEARLS & CONSIDERATIONS

COMMENTS

- Weakness and areflexia or hyporeflexia should prompt serious concern for SMA.
- Fasciculations, especially tongue fasciculations, are highly suggestive of SMA.
- The understanding of the molecular genetic pathophysiology of SMA is evolving at a rapid rate. The reader is referred to the genetic literature or Online Mendelian Inheritance in Man for periodic updates.

PATIENT/FAMILY EDUCATION

- Genetic counseling is important for affected individuals and family members. Inheritance is autosomal recessive in most cases. As noted, heterozygote detection may be difficult. Prenatal diagnosis, including preimplantation diagnosis, has been accomplished in a few cases.
- Phenotype (severity of disease) appears to cluster in families.
- Nutritional, pulmonary, and habilitative issues should be addressed early.
- Course and progress can be anticipated and reviewed, and planning for long-term care should begin at diagnosis.
- Support groups include:
  - Families of Spinal Muscular Atrophy, 800-886-1762; www.fsma.org
  - Muscular Dystrophy Association, 800-572-1717; www.mdausa.org

SUGGESTED READINGS

Brahe C et al: Phenylbutyrate increase SMN gene expression in spinal muscular atrophy patients. *Eur J Hum Genet* 13:256, 2005.

Dreesen JC et al: Preimplantation genetic diagnosis of spinal muscular atrophy. *Mol Hum Reprod* 4:881, 1998.

Families of Spinal Muscular Atrophy. Available at www.fsma.org

Gubitz AK et al: The SMN complex. *Exp Cell Res* 296:51, 2004.

Muscular Dystrophy Association. Available at http://www.mdausa.org

Prior T et al: Homozygous SMN1 deletions in unaffected family members and modification of the phenotype by SMN2. *Am J Med Genet* 130A:307, 2004.

Sumner C et al: Valproic acid increases SMN levels in spinal muscular atrophy patient cells. *Ann Neurol* 54:647, 2003.

AUTHOR: **GEORGIANNE ARNOLD, MD**

BASIC INFORMATION

DEFINITION

Staphylococcal scalded skin syndrome (SSSS) is a blistering skin disease caused by exfoliative (epidermolytic) toxins of some strains of *Staphylococcus aureus.*

SYNONYMS

Pemphigus neonatorum
Ritter disease (first described by Gottfried Ritter von Rittersheim in the 19th century as *dermatitis exfoliativa infantum*)
Scalded skin syndrome
SSSS
Staphylococcal epidermal necrolysis

ICD-9-CM CODES
695.1 Scalded skin syndrome
695.81 Ritter disease

EPIDEMIOLOGY & DEMOGRAPHICS

- SSSS usually occurs in neonates, infants, and young children.
  - Perianal, perineal, and periumbilical lesions are common in neonates.
  - Children usually have extremity lesions.
  - Very ill infants and children have diffuse skin involvement.
- Fewer than 50 cases reported in adults.
- May occur in outbreaks (in nurseries) or as isolated disease.
- Immature renal function with reduced ability to clear bacterial exotoxin may be the reason why neonates are susceptible.
- Renal or immunologic dysfunction may lead to disease in adults.
- White children are more susceptible than black children.
- Most (62%) cases in children are in those <2 years old, 98% are <6 years.
- Mortality rate is <4% in pediatric cases but >50% in the adult population.
- *Ritter disease* is the term used to describe generalized SSSS in neonates.
- Pemphigus neonatorum is a milder, self-limited disease of infants causing few blisters.

CLINICAL PRESENTATION

History

- Neonatal presentation: febrile illness presents at 3 to 16 days of life.
  - Rapid skin changes with redness, blistering, and peeling are noted.
  - Skin changes: diffuse or focal with periumbilical or perianal distribution.
- Older children may have local or diffuse disease. Early febrile stage followed by generalized erythema
  - Rapid onset of flaccid blister formation
  - Peeling of large sheets of skin

Physical Examination

- Children can look well or toxic with diffuse erythema.
- Fever
- Generalized erythema for <10 to 18 hours
- Skin diffusely tender
- Rapid development of flaccid bullae and vesicles that rupture, leaving painful, denuded red base
  - Positive Nikolsky sign: gentle pressure or force on intact skin leads to blister formation at plane of cleavage within upper epidermis.
  - Develops over large areas.
  - Common in flexural creases of hands, buttocks, and feet.
- Perioral erythema, cracking, crusting, and peeling is common with sparing of the mucous membranes.
- Conjunctival erythema is common.
- In neonates with mild or limited disease the bullae may be periumbilical or perineal.

ETIOLOGY

- Responsible *S. aureus* usually belong to phage group II. Approximately 5% of *S. aureus* isolates produce exfoliative toxins. About 32% of patients with exfoliative toxin-producing strains develop SSSS.
- The exfoliative toxin reaches skin via circulation after initial localized infection (nose, throat, umbilicus, and so forth).
- There are three serologic forms of staphylococcal epidermolytic toxins but only two linked to SSSS: ET-A and ET-B.
  - Both bullous impetigo and SSSS are associated with ET-A and ET-B.
  - SSSS is more associated with ET-B and bullous impetigo is more commonly associated with ET-A.
  - There are less neutralizing antibodies to ET-B in general population.
- Toxins cause intraepidermal lysis at the granular layer of the epidermis.
- No or few inflammatory cells are involved.

DIAGNOSIS

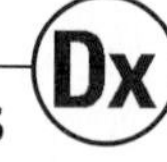

DIFFERENTIAL DIAGNOSIS

- Bullous impetigo (may be a limited form of SSSS)
- Toxic epidermal necrolysis (TEN), also known as *Lyell disease:* usually drug-induced (cleavage is deeper, below epidermis)
- Stevens-Johnson syndrome, also known as *erythema multiforme major*
- Epidermolysis bullosa (congenital bullous disorder)
- Burn (sunburn, chemical burn, other thermal cause)
- Listeriosis
- Staphylococcal or streptococcal scarlet fever
- Cellulitis
- Atopic dermatitis
- Staphylococcal toxic shock syndrome
- Kawasaki disease

WORKUP

- Clinical recognition of blistering exanthem, with sparing of the mucous membranes, and prominent perioral pattern of crusting

LABORATORY TESTS

- Blisters themselves usually culture negative.
- Other areas may be culture positive: umbilicus, conjunctivae, breast, nasopharynx, blood (rare)

TREATMENT

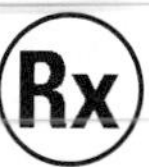

NONPHARMACOLOGIC THERAPY

- Keep exposed denuded skin covered and clean.
- Isolation is recommended, especially in nursery settings.

ACUTE GENERAL Rx

- Antistaphylococcal antibiotics
  - β-Lactamase-resistant penicillins, *or*
  - First-generation cephalosporins (not in jaundiced newborn, however)
  - Recent increase in methicillin (nafcillin)-resistant *S. aureus* (MRSA, NRSA) may lead to changes in recommendations for initial antibiotic treatment.
- Fever control
- Fluid support if necessary

DISPOSITION

- Fluid losses through skin can be significant.
- Recovery is generally rapid in the absence of secondary infection.

REFERRAL

- Rarely indicated
- Dermatology consultation if diagnosis is questionable
- Intensive care or burn unit for infants and children with large denuded areas

PEARLS & CONSIDERATIONS

COMMENTS

- Differentiating from TEN is critical because SSSS requires antibiotic therapy.
- Classic purulent nasal discharge with distinctive perioral cracking.
- No mucous membrane involvement in SSSS.

PREVENTION

- Surveillance of potential carriers especially in nurseries: good handwashing, meticulous umbilical cord care

PATIENT/FAMILY EDUCATION

Full re-epithelialization without scarring usually takes 1 to 2 weeks.

SUGGESTED READINGS

Farrell AM: Staphylococcal scalded-skin syndrome. *Lancet* 354:880, 1999.
King RW, deSant VP: SSSS. eMedicine. Available at www.emedicine.com/EMERG/topic782.htm
Ladhani S, Evans RW: Staphylococcal scalded skin syndrome. *Arch Dis Child* 78:85, 1998.
Ladhani S, Joannou C: Difficulties in diagnosis and management of the staphylococcal scalded skin syndrome. *Pediatr ID J* 19:819, 2000.
Patel GK, Finley AY: Staphylococcal scalded skin syndrome: diagnosis and management. *Am J Clin Derm* 4(3):165, 2003.
Pollack S: Staphylococcal scalded skin syndrome. *Pediatr Rev* 17:18, 1996.
Yamasaki O et al: Clinical manifestations of staphylococcal scalded skin syndrome depend on serotypes of exfoliative toxins. *J Clin Microbiol* 43(4):1890, 2005.

AUTHOR: **LYNN C. GARFUNKEL, MD**

BASIC INFORMATION

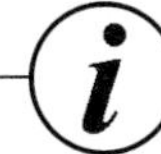

DEFINITION

Stevens-Johnson syndrome (SJS) is an exfoliative dermatitis with severe erosions of at least two mucosal surfaces, including extensive necrosis of oral and nasal mucosa and purulent conjunctivitis but less commonly involving vaginal, urethral, gastrointestinal, or respiratory mucous membranes.

SYNONYM

Erythema multiforme major

ICD-9-CM CODES
695.1 Erythema multiforme major, Stevens-Johnson syndrome

EPIDEMIOLOGY & DEMOGRAPHICS

- The exact incidence is unknown.
- Peak incidence is in the second decade of life.
- SJS is more common in the spring and summer.

CLINICAL PRESENTATION

- Between 1 and 14 days after a prodrome of malaise with fever or other flulike symptoms, there is an abrupt onset of symmetric, red macules that progress to central blistering and potentially extensive epidermal necrosis.
- The extent of skin involvement varies.
- Lips develop hemorrhagic crusts, with loss of the mucosa and severe stomatitis.
- Purulent conjunctivitis with photophobia and pseudomembrane formation may develop.
- Anogenital mucosa also may be involved.
- Esophageal, respiratory, and nasal mucosa are occasionally involved.
- Generalized lymphadenopathy and hepatosplenomegaly are usually present.
- Signs of dehydration (e.g., tachycardia, hypotension) may be observed.
- Signs of electrolyte abnormalities (e.g., edema, arrhythmias) may be seen.

ETIOLOGY

- Drugs are a major precipitating factor, although many other factors have been implicated.
- Nonsteroidal anti-inflammatory drugs (e.g., ibuprofen, naproxen) are the most common offenders, followed by sulfonamides, anticonvulsants (i.e., hydantoins and barbiturates), penicillins, tetracycline, and doxycycline.
- It has been postulated that in children with drug-induced SJS, genetic differences in detoxification of drugs may be responsible.

DIAGNOSIS

DIFFERENTIAL DIAGNOSIS

- Kawasaki disease
- Acute graft-versus-host disease
- Staphylococcal scalded-skin syndrome
- Paraneoplastic pemphigus

WORKUP

- The diagnosis is usually made on the basis of the characteristic prodrome followed by the abrupt onset of extensive areas of mucocutaneous necrosis, with at least two mucosal sites involved.
- Children develop fluid and electrolyte imbalances.

LABORATORY TESTS

- A complete blood cell count can demonstrate leukocytosis (65% of patients), eosinophilia (20%), and anemia (15%).
- All children with SJS have an increased erythrocyte sedimentation rate.

TREATMENT

NONPHARMACOLOGIC THERAPY

- Prolonged hospitalization in a burn or intensive care unit is usually necessary.
- All possible offending agents should be stopped.
- Protection from secondary infection includes wound dressing and burn care.
- Ophthalmologic care is closely monitored by an ophthalmologist.
- Pulmonary toilet must be monitored.

ACUTE GENERAL Rx

- Provide fluid and electrolyte management. This involves intravenous volume and electrolyte repletion, maintenance, and ongoing loss replacement.
- Nutritional supplementation is critical.
- Pain management should be provided.
- Use of systemic steroids is controversial and contraindicated in some cases.

CHRONIC Rx

- Possible early skin grafting or use of biologic dressings
- Physical therapy to prevent contractures

PEARLS & CONSIDERATIONS

COMMENTS

SJS is often complicated by dehydration, electrolyte imbalance, and secondary bacterial infection of skin, mucosa, or lungs, as well as cutaneous scarring and dyspigmentation.

SUGGESTED READINGS

American Academy of Dermatology. Available at www.aad.org

Carder KR: Hypersensitivity reactions in neonates and infants. *Dermatol Ther* 18:160, 2005.

Prendiville J: Stevens-Johnson syndrome and toxic epidermal necrolysis. *Adv Dermatol* 18:151, 2002.

Shin HT, Channg MW: Drug eruptions in children. *Curr Probl Pediatr* 31:207, 2001.

Society for Pediatric Dermatology. Available at www.spdnet.org

AUTHOR: **SUSAN HALLER PSAILA, MD**

BASIC INFORMATION

DEFINITION

Strabismus is misalignment or deviation of the eyes and does not refer to visual acuity.

SYNONYMS

Convergent/divergent strabismus
Esotropia
Exotropia
Lazy or wandering eye
Squint
"Wall-eyed", "cross-eyed"

ICD-9-CM CODES
378.0 Esotropia
378.1 Exotropia
378.5 Paralytic strabismus
378.7 Other specified strabismus
378.9 Unspecified disorder of eye movements (strabismus NOS)

EPIDEMIOLOGY & DEMOGRAPHICS

- Strabismus affects 3% to 5% of children in North America.
  - Esotropia (eyes deviate inward—nasally) found in 72%
  - Exotropia (eyes deviate outward—temporally) in 23%
  - Vertical strabismus in 5%
- Strabismus has no gender predilection.
- Risk factors for strabismus include:
  - Prematurity
  - Family history in a first- or second-degree relative
  - Cerebral palsy
  - Chromosomal disorders
  - Prenatal drug exposure
  - Major head trauma
  - Structural eye defects
- Congenital cases are diagnosed from birth to 6 months of age.
- Acquired cases generally occur before 6 years of life.
- The earlier the diagnosis after onset, the better the prognosis.

CLINICAL PRESENTATION

- All children should be screened for strabismus at routine well-child visits.
- Historical elements include: the age of onset, history of progression, constancy versus intermittency, history of other associated neurologic symptoms, and whether the eye misalignment is the same in all gaze positions (comitant) or differs by gaze position (noncomitant).
- Nonparalytic (most common type)—includes esotropia and exotropia. In this type there is an absence of identifiable neurologic/mechanical deficit in the ocular muscle.
  - Infantile (congenital) esotropia—onset by 6 months of age
  - Accommodative esotropia—onset usually 18 months to 4 years
  - Infantile exotropia—onset by 6 months (rare)
  - Acquired—presents with squinting, diplopia, and eyestrain
- Paralytic—cranial nerves III, IV, or VI may be affected by congenital, traumatic, infectious, ischemic, or compressive processes leading to a paretic or palsied eye muscle.
- Syndromic strabismus—caused by anomalies of extraocular muscles or adjacent tissues (e.g., Duane's, Möbius, or Brown syndrome).
- Physical examination should focus on the following:
  - Visual acuity of each eye or fixation preference (up to 50% of patients with strabismus have reduced vision)
  - Ocular motility (oblique muscle overreaction which may lead to A or V pattern increasing exotropia on upward gaze strabismus, nystagmus)
  - Corneal light reflex test (Hirschberg test):
    - If reflex is centered on both pupils, eyes are aligned.
    - If reflex is displaced temporally, the eye is esotropic.
    - If reflex is displaced nasally, the eye is exotropic.
  - Cover/uncover test—examiner covers one eye to evaluate the uncovered eye. Test is used to diagnose a manifest strabismus (tropia).
    - If no movement, eyes are aligned.
    - If the uncovered eye moves out to take up fixation, the eye is esotropic.
    - If the uncovered eye moves in to take up fixation, the eye is exotropic.
  - Alternate cover test—examiner rapidly covers and uncovers each eye. This test may detect phorias (latent deviations) as well as tropias. Phoric deviations are diagnosed when the cover is removed and movement is seen in that eye. Small phoric deviations diagnosed with this test may not be of clinical significance.

ETIOLOGY

- The etiology of strabismus depends on the type.
- The cause of nonparalytic strabismus (most common type) is unknown, but may be due to either anomalies of motor innervation to the extraocular muscles, or anomalies of binocular vision and fusion.

DIAGNOSIS

DIFFERENTIAL DIAGNOSIS

- Pseudostrabismus
  - Wide nasal bridge gives esotropic appearance (pinch skin over bridge and note symmetric light reflexes and ocular alignment).
  - Hypertelorism gives exotropic appearance (note symmetric light reflexes and ocular alignment).

IMAGING STUDIES

- No imaging studies are generally needed for nonparalytic strabismus.
- Neuroimaging may be required for atypical or acquired cases to rule out pathology.

TREATMENT

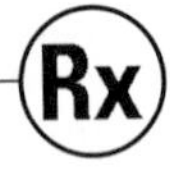

NONPHARMACOLOGIC THERAPY

- Potential therapies depend on the type of strabismus and include glasses, miotic eyedrops, prisms, eye exercises, and surgery.
  - Congenital esotropia usually requires surgery (usually after age 6 months).
  - Accommodative esotropia usually requires glasses and less often surgery.
  - Infantile exotropia requires surgery.
  - Acquired exotropia may require surgery, depending on severity.
  - Amblyopia (visual loss) is common with strabismus and requires treatment (see Amblyopia in Disease and Disorders [Section I]).

DISPOSITION

Follow-up is determined by the eye specialist and depends on the type of strabismus, presence of amblyopia, and method of treatment.

REFERRAL

All patients with eye deviation that has not resolved by 3 months of age require referral to an eye care provider.

PEARLS & CONSIDERATIONS

COMMENTS

- Children do not outgrow strabismus.
- Children usually do not complain of diplopia.
- Early detection and treatment yield the best outcome.

PREVENTION

- Strabismus usually cannot be prevented.
- Complications, however, can be avoided with prompt diagnosis and referral.

SUGGESTED READINGS

American Academy of Pediatrics—Policy Statement, Committee on Practice and Ambulatory Medicine and Section of Ophthalmology: Eye examination in infants, children, and young adults by pediatricians. *Pediatrics* 111:902, 2003.
Hertle R: *Pediatric Eye Disease Color Atlas and Synopsis.* New York, McGraw-Hill, 2002.
Ticho B: Strabismus. *Pediatr Clin North Am* 50:173, 2003.

AUTHOR: **DANIEL YAWMAN, MD**

BASIC INFORMATION

DEFINITION

- "Disorders in the rhythm of speech, in which the individual knows precisely what he or she wishes to say, but at the same time is unable to say it because of an involuntary, repetitive prolongation or cessation of sound." (*International Classification of Diseases,* The World Health Organization, 1977, p. 202).
- Developmental stuttering is brief periods of stuttering that cease by the time a child enters school. In general, these are repetitions of whole words and phrases; they may include simple comments and changes to previously spoken thoughts. Part-word repetitions and sound prolongations occur much less commonly.

SYNONYMS

Acquired stuttering
Developmental stuttering
Dysfluency
Idiopathic or pathologic stuttering
Stammering

ICD-9-CM CODE
307.0 Stammering and stuttering

EPIDEMIOLOGY & DEMOGRAPHICS

- Stuttering onset is between toddlerhood and puberty.
  - Peak onset is between 2 to 5 years of age.
  - Mean age of onset is 5 years, with a median age of 4 years.
- There is a genetic role in stuttering. The specific mode or modes of transmission, however, are unknown.
- A higher concordance for stuttering is observed in monozygotic twins (77%) than in dizygotic same-sex twins (32%) or same-sexed siblings (18%).
- First-degree relatives of people who stutter have more than a threefold higher risk of developing stuttering than the general population.
- Male relatives of female stutterers are at the highest risk of stuttering, with a greater than fourfold risk observed.
- The severity of stuttering is not related to the extent of the family history of stuttering.
- For men who ever stuttered, 9% of their daughters and 22% of their sons will stutter.
- For women who ever stuttered, 17% of their daughters and 36% of their sons will be affected.
- The prevalence of stuttering in prepubertal schoolchildren is 1% but generally drops in postpubertal schoolchildren.
  - The prevalence seems to remain constant from school entry to age 12 and declines slowly thereafter.
  - The prevalence after puberty is 0.8%.
- The prevalence in children is elevated because of the high incidence of developmental dysfluency.
- The male-to-female ratio is approximately 3:1 overall but increases with age.
- Stuttering is present in all cultures, races, languages, and historical periods.
- The incidence varies among cultures and socioeconomic groups, being more common in the upper socioeconomic classes (this may be a function of increased surveillance of this group).
- Famous people who stuttered include Moses, Aristotle, Sir Isaac Newton, Winston Churchill, John Updike, King George VI, James Earl Jones, Marilyn Monroe, and Jimmy Stewart.
- Almost 80% of school-age children who stutter recover fluency spontaneously or with minimal speech therapy by the age of 16 years.
  - Even with more severe stuttering, the prognosis is favorable if treatment starts early.
  - The outcome is less favorable for those who continue to stutter into adulthood.
  - Left handedness may predict chronic stuttering.

CLINICAL PRESENTATION

History

- Obtain past medical history of perinatal asphyxia or trauma, associated seizure disorder, cerebral palsy, head trauma, or cerebral vascular injury.
- Establish:
  - Age of onset of stuttering
  - Whether onset of stuttering developed gradually or abruptly
  - History of articulation or phonologic disorder diagnosed in patient's speech
  - History of learning disability, reading disorder, or attention deficit disorder
  - History of anxiety disorder
  - Patient's awareness of dysfluencies
- Family history of stuttering in a twin or first-degree relative increases the risk.
- If stuttering is present when singing, whispering, speaking together in a group, or when the patient cannot hear his or her own voice, this usually results in fluent speech.

Physical Examination

- Assess the type and degree of word dysfluencies.
  - More than 90% of stuttering occurs on the initial syllable of the utterance.
  - The incidence is greater on words starting with consonants, words located early in a sentence, and longer words.
- In general, there is concern if the child has five or more "breaks" per 100 words spoken.
- "Breaks" may include any of the following:
  - Whole word, phrase, or syllable repetitions and sound prolongations
  - Presence of silent pauses before, after, or within a word
  - Inappropriate articulating postures
- Also make note of the following:
  - Normal or excessive speaking rate
  - Tendency toward more dysfluencies in response to stress
- Assess the stutterer's and parents' attitude toward the problem.
- A certified speech and language pathologist with an expertise in fluency disorders should perform the formal evaluation.
- A thorough evaluation of oral motor skills, auditory acuity, and language level is indicated, in addition to the child's speech performance.

ETIOLOGY

- The cause remains unknown, or at least controversial.
- Subtle neurophysical dysfunctions are believed to disrupt the precise timing required to produce speech.
  - Studies suggest an association with oversecretion of dopamine.
- Stutterers have difficulty coordinating air flow, articulation, and resonance. Small asynchronies are even found in stutterers' fluent speech.
- Perinatal brain damage is the only environmental factor known to be associated with some cases of idiopathic stuttering.
  - Perinatal brain damage is also associated with epilepsy, cerebral palsy, and other neurologic syndromes.
  - All are associated with stuttering at a higher-than-expected prevalence rate.
- Deafness is the only "factor" resulting in a reduced prevalence of stuttering.
- Acquired stuttering may develop in a previously fluent speaker after brain injury (trauma or cerebrovascular accident). The symptoms are clinically identical to idiopathic stuttering.

DIAGNOSIS

DIFFERENTIAL DIAGNOSIS

- Developmental stuttering
- Idiopathic stuttering
- Acquired stuttering

WORKUP

- A certified speech and language pathologist should perform a formal evaluation after the appropriate referral.
- The presence of repetitions, together with prolongations, is necessary and sufficient for the disorder to be diagnosed.
- Referral to a speech-language pathologist is indicated if a child meets the following criteria:
  - Has consistent stuttering behaviors
  - Has been stuttering at least 3 months
  - Demonstrates tension or struggle behavior when stuttering
  - Is aware that his or her speech pattern is abnormal—this may be noted as early as 3 years of age but full awareness is not usually reached until 5 years.
- Referral is also necessary if the child's parents show great concern about the problem, regardless of the child's awareness or secondary behaviors.

- Speech and language development is delayed in stutterers by about 6 months.
- Articulation errors are three times more common in children who stutter.
  - Errors are noted before the child's stuttering behaviors.
  - Errors are independent of the age of onset of the stuttering.
- Intelligence tests have revealed a significantly lower score for stutterers compared with nonstutterers (half a standard deviation). Both verbal and nonverbal tests of intelligence have demonstrated the same difference.
- Stutterers have been described as having "difficulty with social adjustment," but this condition is probably a consequence rather than a cause of stuttering.

TREATMENT

Rx

NONPHARMACOLOGIC THERAPY

- The only true cure for stuttering appears to be one's childhood spontaneous remission (80%).
- Mild stuttering can be self-limited, but behaviorally oriented therapy is effective in young children.
- Delaying direct stuttering therapy for the "mild" stutterer may actually interfere with their ability to establish fluency.
- Many practitioners believe that speech therapy for stuttering should begin with the onset of stuttering to maximize the efficiency and cost-effectiveness of therapy.
- The Lidcombe Program of Early Stuttering Intervention, developed at the University of Sydney, Australia, is one formal program that has provided positive outcomes for preschoolers who stutter.
- More severe stuttering requires speech therapy directed at the behavioral, cognitive, and affective aspects of speech, as well as counseling.
- There are seven speech environments in which stuttering frequency can be immediately reduced or eliminated: (1) choral speech, (2) lipped speech, (3) prolonged speech and delayed auditory feedback provided by an ear-level prosthetic device, (4) rhythmic speech, (5) shadowing, (6) singing, and (7) slowed speech.
- Several treatment methods increase the fluency of stutterers' speech: (1) prolonged speech, (2) precision fluency-shaping, (3) rhythmic speech, (4) airflow therapy, (5) electromyogram (EMG) biofeedback of the speech musculature, and (6) attitude change. Of these methods, only prolonged speech, precision fluency-shaping strategies, and EMG biofeedback have been shown critically to provide long-lasting fluency.

ACUTE GENERAL Rx

- Haloperidol (Haldol) and risperidone (Risperdal), both dopamine antagonists, have demonstrated consistent improvement in stuttering in double-blind studies.
  - Haldol, however, cannot be used long term, because of its unacceptable side effects.
- Recently, olanzapine (Zyprexa), also a dopamine antagonist, has been shown to reduce the symptoms of stuttering, but further research is needed.

DISPOSITION

- In general, the goal of speech therapy is to establish and maintain the feeling of fluency control, rather than to attain an arbitrarily determined level of fluency.
- "Self-acceptance" is the treatment of choice of the National Stuttering Project rather than working to directly change the stutterers' speech behaviors.

REFERRAL

- Speech and language specialist for diagnosis and therapy in prolonged cases
- Developmental behavior specialist, especially if there are associated developmental or behavioral difficulties

PEARLS & CONSIDERATIONS

COMMENTS

How to Talk to People Who Stutter

- Try not to finish sentences for people who stutter. This can make them feel more frustrated, and you might not say the same words they were thinking.
- Avoid saying things such as "relax" and "slow down." It doesn't help.
- Be extra patient, especially on the telephone, which can be the hardest place to talk smoothly.
- If you didn't understand what was said, say, "I'm sorry, I didn't get that." This is always better than just pretending to understand or making a wild guess.
- Use a relaxed tone of voice yourself, and don't talk extra slowly or loudly. There is nothing wrong with the hearing of people who stutter!
- Keep eye contact with stutterers; don't drop your eyes in discomfort or embarrassment, because this will only make them feel worse.
- Show in every way that you are listening to what the stutterer is saying, not how he or she is saying it.

PREVENTION

- When dysfluencies are first detected in children parents are commonly advised to speak more slowly to children and avoid interrupting them, in an effort to decrease the number of dysfluent events. These strategies however have not been proven to help.
- Stuttering Prevention Programs: 519-675-0449 or 905-682-6388; email: twray@prevent-stuttering.com

PATIENT/FAMILY EDUCATION

- Stuttering Foundation of America, P.O. Box 11749, 3100 Walnut Grove Road, Suite 603, Memphis, TN 38111; 800-992-9392; www.stutteringhelp.org
- National Stuttering Project, 5100 E. La Palma Avenue, #208, Anaheim Hills, CA 92807; 800-364-1677.
- The National Center for Stuttering, The National Stutterer's Hotline: 800-221-2483; email: executivedirector@stuttering.com; web site: www.stuttering.com

SUGGESTED READINGS

American Speech-Language-Hearing Association. Available at www.asha.org

Guitar B, Conture EG: *The Child Who Stutters: To the Pediatrician,* 3rd ed. (Publication No. 0023). Memphis, TN, Stuttering Foundation of America, 2004, pp 1–16.

National Center for Stuttering. Available at www.stuttering.com

Nippold MA, Rudzinski M: Parents' speech and children's stuttering: a critique of the literature. *J Speech Lang Hear Res* 38:978, 1995.

Onslow M et al: An operant intervention for early stuttering. The development of the Lidcombe program. *Behav Modif* 25(1):116, 2001.

Starkweather CW, Givens-Ackerman J: *Stuttering.* Austin, TX, Pro-ed Inc, 1997.

Stuttering Foundation of America. Available at www.stutteringhelp.org

Weir E, Bianchet S: Developmental dysfluency: early intervention is key. *CMAJ* 170(12):1790, 2004.

AUTHOR: **DOROTHY M. DELISLE, MD**

BASIC INFORMATION

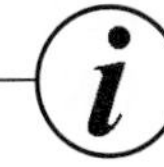

DEFINITION

Tetralogy of Fallot (TOF) is a form of congenital heart disease characterized by a ventricular septal defect (VSD), an "overriding" aorta, right ventricular outflow tract obstruction (RVOTO), and right ventricular hypertrophy.

SYNONYMS

Fallot's
Fallot's tetralogy
Tet
TOF

ICD-9-CM CODE
745.2 Tetralogy of Fallot

EPIDEMIOLOGY & DEMOGRAPHICS

- TOF is the most common of the cyanotic congenital heart diseases.
- TOF affects 10% of children with congenital heart disease.
- The prevalence is 3.53 cases per 10,000 live births.
- There is a slight predominance of TOF in boys.

CLINICAL PRESENTATION

- Presentation depends on the severity of the RVOTO and the amount of pulmonary blood flow.
- Loud murmurs of pulmonic stenosis at the upper left sternal border associated with a single second heart sound are common.
- If the pulmonary blood flow is significantly limited, the patient will be cyanotic.
- Soft, continuous murmurs from aorta-pulmonary collateral arteries are common in patients with TOF and pulmonary atresia.

ETIOLOGY

- The cause of congenital heart disease is presumably heterogeneous and may depend on the interaction between genetic predisposition and environmental factors.
- Microdeletions of chromosome region 22q11 are frequently found in patients with TOF who have certain craniofacial anomalies.
  - Velocardiofacial syndrome
  - Sometimes found in patients with TOF not suspected to have a chromosome abnormality

DIAGNOSIS

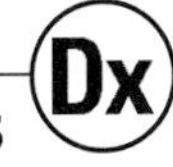

DIFFERENTIAL DIAGNOSIS

Any cyanotic heart disease with obstruction between the ventricle and the pulmonary artery can cause cyanosis and a murmur at the upper left sternal border.

WORKUP

- Chest radiography may show a small main pulmonary artery segment, decreased pulmonary vascular markings, and an upturned cardiac apex. These abnormalities give the appearance of a boot-shaped heart.
- In some patients, cardiac catheterization is necessary to make an accurate preoperative diagnosis, but most centers operate without catheterization.

IMAGING STUDIES

- The diagnosis is made by echocardiography.
- Chest radiography is useful, as previously described.

TREATMENT

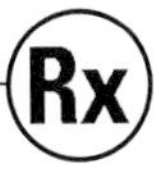

NONPHARMACOLOGIC THERAPY

- The therapy for TOF is surgical correction.
- Surgical repair involves closure of the ventricular septal defect and opening the right ventricular outflow tract.
- Timing of surgery depends on the severity of the RVOTO and on the protocols of the operating center.
- Operative mortality should be significantly less than 5%.
- In some patients with very small pulmonary arteries, palliation with an aorta-pulmonary shunt may be necessary to improve pulmonary blood flow and to increase pulmonary artery size.
- Balloon dilatation of the pulmonary valve has also been used to increase pulmonary blood flow and encourage pulmonary artery growth.

ACUTE GENERAL Rx

During a hypercyanotic tetralogy spell, pushing the knees to the chest can increase systemic vascular resistance, which then increases pulmonary blood flow.

CHRONIC Rx

Rarely, patients who are inoperable because of size or other concerns may benefit transiently from β-blockers.

DISPOSITION

- General pediatric care should occur.
- The patients should receive antibiotics at times of endocarditis risk.
- Cardiology follow-up of patients after repair of TOF continues for life.
- Pediatric cardiologists and eventually physicians expert in the management of adults with congenital heart disease should follow these patients carefully for development of arrhythmias, right ventricular dysfunction, and the need for additional surgical intervention, such as replacement of the pulmonary valve.

REFERRAL

Referral to a pediatric cardiologist is indicated for diagnosis and appropriate timing of a surgical referral.

PEARLS & CONSIDERATIONS

COMMENTS

- Patients with TOF and good pulmonary arteries should do very well, and the operative mortality should be low.
- If the pulmonary arteries are small, the outlook is not as optimistic.
- Consider whether the child may have endocarditis before antibiotic administration. If endocarditis is a possibility, obtain a blood culture before starting antibiotics.

PREVENTION

Intrauterine diagnosis is possible, but there is no known prevention.

PATIENT/FAMILY EDUCATION

More information about congenital defects can be found on the Internet (http://www.tmc.edu/thi/congenit.html#Congenital defects main page).

SUGGESTED READINGS

EMedicine. http://www.emedicine.com/radio/topic685.htm

Kirklin JW et al: Morphologic and surgical determinants of outcome events after repair of tetralogy of Fallot and pulmonary stenosis. *J Thorac Cardiovasc Surg* 103:706, 1992.

Momma K et al: Tetralogy of Fallot associated with chromosome 22q11 deletion. *Am J Cardiol* 76:618, 1995.

Shinebourne EA, Anderson RH: Fallot's tetralogy. *In* Anderson RH et al (eds): *Paediatric Cardiology.* London, Churchill Livingstone, 2002, pp 1213–1250.

AUTHOR: **MICHAEL E. MCCONNELL, MD**

BASIC INFORMATION

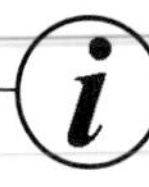

DEFINITION

Thalassemia is a heterogeneous group of autosomal recessive genetic disorders characterized by decreased or absent synthesis of globin chains, leading to anemia and microcytosis. Clinically, there are two major forms: α-thalassemia and β-thalassemia.

SYNONYMS

α-Thalassemias
- αα/αα (i.e., normal)
- αα/α– (i.e., silent α-thalassemia)
- αα/–– or α–/α– (i.e., α-thalassemia trait)
- α–/–– (i.e., hemoglobin [Hb] H disease)
- ––/–– (i.e., hydrops fetalis, incompatible with extrauterine life)

β-Thalassemias
- β/β (i.e., normal)
- β/– (i.e., β-thalassemia trait or β-thalassemia minor)
- –/– (i.e., β-thalassemia major, Cooley's anemia, or Mediterranean anemia)

ICD-9-CM CODE
282.4 Thalassemia

EPIDEMIOLOGY & DEMOGRAPHICS

- Thalassemias are found in regions of the world previously endemic for malaria.
- β-Thalassemia has the highest incidence in the Mediterranean basin.
- α-Thalassemia has the highest incidence in Southeast Asia, particularly Laos and Thailand.
- Between 2% and 3% of blacks have α-thalassemia trait.

CLINICAL PRESENTATION

- Ethnicity (see "Epidemiology & Demographics"), family history of anemias, and transfusion dependence may be reported.
- Children with hydrops fetalis die in utero by 30 weeks' gestation.
- Children with β-thalassemia major present with severe anemia at 1 to 2 years old.
- Children with severe thalassemia syndromes (i.e., β-thalassemia major or Hb H disease) have pallor and hepatosplenomegaly.

ETIOLOGY

Several hundred different genetic defects have been described that affect the structure of the α and the β globin genes or the regulation of their expression.

DIAGNOSIS

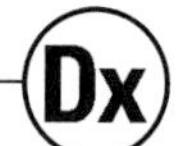

DIFFERENTIAL DIAGNOSIS

Consider diseases that cause microcytic anemia, including iron deficiency, lead poisoning, sideroblastic anemia, and Hb E disease.

LABORATORY TESTS

- Includes complete blood cell count (CBC), smear, and Hb electrophoresis
- CBC results
  - Anemia (e.g., Hb of 10 to 11 g/dL in β-thalassemia trait)
  - Microcytosis (e.g., mean corpuscular volume [MCV] in high 60s in β-thalassemia trait)
  - Mentzer index (MCV/red blood cell [RBC]) can be less than 11.5 in β-thalassemia trait and greater than 13.5 in iron deficiency)
  - Red cell distribution width (RDW) elevated in iron deficiency and Hb H disease, but not in β-thalassemia trait
- Peripheral blood smear reveals microcytosis and hypochromia.
- Hemoglobin electrophoresis
  - β-Thalassemia trait: elevated HbA_2 (>3.5%)
  - α-Thalassemia: Hb Barts (i.e., excess γ-globin chains) at birth and Hb H (i.e., excess β-globin chains) in older children

TREATMENT

NONPHARMACOLOGIC THERAPY

- For mild anemia, no therapy is warranted.
- Splenectomy for hypersplenism causes an increased requirement for RBC transfusions in patients with β-thalassemia major.

CHRONIC Rx

- Children with β-thalassemia major require regular RBC transfusions.
- Iron chelation with subcutaneous Desferal (deferoxamine, 5 to 7 days/wk) is needed to prevent increasing iron overload from chronic transfusions.
- Oral chelators are under clinical investigation.
- Bone marrow transplantation can be curative.

COMPLEMENTARY & ALTERNATIVE MEDICINE

Ingestion of tea with meals decreases the absorption of dietary iron.

REFERRAL

The diagnosis and care of children with severe thalassemia syndromes is best performed by pediatric hematologists.

PEARLS & CONSIDERATIONS

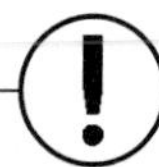

COMMENTS

- Hb Barts and Hb H indicate α-thalassemia and are both "fast-moving" hemoglobins.
- Clinical severity of thalassemia syndromes can be affected by the inheritance of glucose-6-phosphate dehydrogenase (G6PD) deficiency or abnormal hemoglobins (e.g., Hb E, Hb S).
  - G6PD deficiency can make the hemolysis worse.
  - Sickle/β-thalassemia is clinically quite similar to homozygous hemoglobin SS (sickle cell) disease and hemoglobin SC (sickle C) disease.
- The lack of the αα/–– genotype makes the prevalence of Hb H disease and hydrops fetalis rare in Mediterranean and black American populations.

PREVENTION

- Screen family members of affected individuals.
- Provide patient education.
- Prenatal diagnosis of thalassemia syndromes is available in the United States and in countries where thalassemia is prevalent.

PATIENT/FAMILY EDUCATION

- Genetic counseling is important. The risk of having affected fetuses when both parents have β-thalassemia trait is 1 in 4 (i.e., autosomal recessive inheritance).
- Chronic transfusion therapy leads to iron overload and eventual death from heart failure or cirrhosis unless compliance with chelation is maintained.
- The Thalassemia Action Group (129-09 26th Avenue, Flushing, NY 11354; 718-321-2873) is a support group for patients with thalassemia syndromes.
- The Ahepa Cooley's Anemia Foundation (1909 Q Street N. West, Washington, DC 20009; 202-232-6300) can provide information.
- Cooley's Anemia Foundation (129-09 26th Ave., Flushing, NY 11354; 800-522-7222; www.cooleysanemia.org) is a national nonprofit organization dedicated to serving patients with all forms of thalassemia.

SUGGESTED READINGS

Olivieri NF: The β-thalassemias. *N Engl J Med* 341:99, 1999.

Orkin SH, Nathan DG: The thalassemias. *In* Nathan DG et al (eds): *Nathan and Oski's Hematology of Infancy and Childhood,* 6th ed. Philadelphia, WB Saunders, 2003.

AUTHOR: **JAMES PALIS, MD**

BASIC INFORMATION

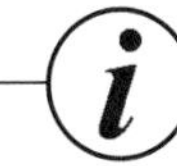

DEFINITION

Superficial thrombophlebitis is a thrombosis of a superficial vein with accompanying inflammatory reaction.

SYNONYM

Phlebitis

ICD-9-CM CODE
451.89 Thrombophlebitis

EPIDEMIOLOGY & DEMOGRAPHICS

This is almost entirely a disorder of adults with lower extremity venous incompetence.

CLINICAL PRESENTATION

- Pain, erythema, and swelling in a distinct vein
- Commonly occurs in veins after phlebotomy or venous access

ETIOLOGY

- Contributing factors are the three elements of Virchow's triad: intimal damage, stasis, and hypercoagulability.
- Thrombophlebitis usually occurs in varicose veins of the leg as a result of stasis of blood.
- Occasionally, local trauma (e.g., intravenous catheters) may play a role, especially if the affected vein is normal.

DIAGNOSIS

Dx

DIFFERENTIAL DIAGNOSIS

- Concomitant deep venous thrombosis occurs in approximately 5% of patients, so it is important to evaluate the patient for this disorder (see Deep Venous Thrombosis in Diseases and Disorders [Section I]).
- Cellulitis, calciphylaxis, and lymphangitis can mimic this disorder.

WORKUP

Search for underlying predisposing factors such as trauma and hypercoagulable states, particularly if the vein is otherwise normal.

LABORATORY TESTS

- If no predisposing conditions are present, investigating for hypercoagulable states is important.
- Consider the prothrombin time (PT), partial thromboplastin time (PTT), protein C, protein S, antithrombin III, lupus anticoagulant, activated protein C resistance, and prothrombin gene mutation.

IMAGING STUDIES

Ultrasound of the affected limb is important to rule out concomitant deep venous thrombosis.

TREATMENT

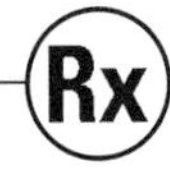

NONPHARMACOLOGIC THERAPY

Apply warm compresses and elevate the affected limb.

ACUTE GENERAL Rx

- Use nonsteroidal anti-inflammatory drugs (NSAIDs).
- Antibiotics have no role.

CHRONIC Rx

- If recurrent, treat venous stasis with compression stockings.
- If an underlying hypercoagulable state is found, long-term anticoagulation is indicated.

DISPOSITION

- Resolution usually occurs within 1 to 2 weeks from institution of the conservative measures outlined.
- The patient should be monitored for the development of deep venous thrombosis.

REFERRAL

- This disorder can easily be diagnosed and treated by a primary care physician.
- If a hypercoagulable state is found, referral to a hematologist is helpful.
- If chronic venous stasis is problematic, referral to a vascular surgeon is helpful.

PEARLS & CONSIDERATIONS

COMMENTS

- Medications most commonly associated with chemical phlebitis are nafcillin, diazepam, pentobarbital, and contrast media.
- Superficial thrombophlebitis that occurs in several distinct areas over a short period is called *migratory superficial phlebitis.* It may signal an underlying malignancy, especially pancreatic or gastric cancer.

PREVENTION

Elevation of the legs and simple compression stockings to decrease dependent edema and varicose veins of the legs can be helpful.

PATIENT/FAMILY EDUCATION

Elevation of the affected limb and mobilization are important to prevent the development of deep venous thrombosis.

SUGGESTED READING

Bounameaux H, Reber-Wasem M-A: Superficial thrombophlebitis and deep vein thrombosis. *Arch Intern Med* 157:1822, 1997.

AUTHOR: **BRETT ROBBINS, MD**

BASIC INFORMATION

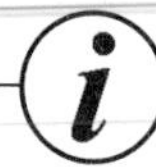

DEFINITION

Tinea capitis is a fungal infection of the scalp, hair shaft, and pilosebaceous apparatus.

SYNONYM

Ringworm of the scalp

ICD-9-CM CODE
110.0 Tinea capitis

EPIDEMIOLOGY & DEMOGRAPHICS

- Tinea capitis is the most common dermatophytosis of childhood.
- It generally is a disease of prepubertal children between 2 and 10 years old.
  - Rarely affects infants
  - Rarely occurs in postpubertal individuals
- Spread of infection has been demonstrated in households.
- Outbreaks have been reported in schools and child-care centers.
- The incidence in the United States is increasing.
- This condition is much more common in blacks.
- Asymptomatic carriage may be an important reservoir for infection.

CLINICAL PRESENTATION

History

- Usually, a caretaker notices hair or scalp changes such as patchy hair loss, scaly scalp, or pustular lesions.
- The child or parents may first notice enlarged occipital lymph nodes.

Physical Examination

- Scalp scaling is present.
- Infected areas are round or oval and sometimes irregular.
  - Individual patches are 1 to 6 cm in diameter.
  - Multiple patches are common.
- Lesions may coalescence, with formation of gyrate patterns.
- Broken-off hairs, 1 to 3 mm above the scalp, may be seen.
- Partial alopecia may occur.
- This condition may cause associated pustulation, suppuration, or kerion formation.
- Lymphadenopathy, usually occipital and posterior cervical, may be very prominent, even with mild scalp disease.
- "Black dot" ringworm is a form characterized by multiple, small, circular patches of alopecia. The hairs are broken off at the surface of the scalp, resulting in a dot appearance; darker hairs are seen on lighter skin surfaces.
- A kerion is a sharply demarcated, inflammatory, indurated, boggy, granulomatous tumefaction.
  - It is a form of immune response to the fungus, but secondary staphylococcal infection may also complicate the picture.
  - It is usually not painful.
  - The onset of kerion is acute, and it can become large; however, usually only one area is involved.

ETIOLOGY

- *Trichophyton tonsurans* causes 95% of cases in North and South America.
- The second most common cause in the United States is *Microsporum canis,* which is zoophilic and can be acquired by contact with infected animals such as pet cats and dogs.
  - In some areas of the United States, specifically Arizona, *M. canis* is the most common cause.
  - *M. canis* is also the most common cause worldwide.
- Other dermatophytes such as *Microsporum audouinii, Microsporum gypseum, Microsporum ferrugineum, Trichophyton mentagrophytes, Trichophyton violaceum, Trichophyton schoenleinii, Trichophyton verrucosum, Trichophyton soudanense,* and *Trichophyton rubrum* also cause tinea capitis.

DIAGNOSIS

DIFFERENTIAL DIAGNOSIS

- Seborrheic dermatitis
- Atopic dermatitis
- Psoriasis
- Alopecia areata
- Traumatic alopecia: trichotillomania, traction alopecia
- Pseudopelade
- Folliculitis decalvans
- Impetigo
- Lesions of systemic lupus erythematosus (i.e., discoid lupus)
- Syphilis
- Histiocytosis
- Scleroderma

WORKUP

- The clinical presentation is fairly distinctive, but other diagnoses can mimic tinea capitis, and confirmation of the diagnosis is generally advised.
- Wood's lamp examination is generally not helpful because *T. tonsurans* and *T. violaceum* do not fluoresce.
  - Hairs infected by *M. audouinii* and *M. canis* produce a brilliant green fluorescence.
  - Those infected by *T. schoenleinii* produce a pale green fluorescence.

LABORATORY TESTS

- Potassium hydroxide (KOH) preparations can be useful for immediate confirmation of infection, but the sensitivity and specificity depend on the experience of the individual performing the test and the morphology of the lesion scraped.
  - False-negative and false-positive results occur.
  - Culture is recommended.
- To obtain a fungal culture, rub several areas of the scalp with a clean, disposable toothbrush or sterile cotton swab, and inoculate onto an antibiotic-enriched mycologic media.

TREATMENT

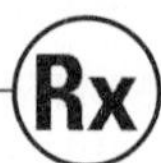

ACUTE GENERAL Rx

- Unlike tinea corporis, cruris, and pedes, systemic antifungal therapy is *always* required for tinea capitis because topical therapies do not penetrate deeply enough into the hair follicle to adequately eradicate infection.
- Griseofulvin has been the standard therapy since 1958.
  - The starting dose of the standard micronized griseofulvin is 20 to 25 mg/kg/day, given once daily for 8 weeks (some patients require a longer treatment course).
  - This dosage is higher than that recommended in several standard references.
  - It is absorbed more rapidly when ingested along with fatty foods.
  - An ultra-micronized griseofulvin dispersed in polyethylene glycol has twice the bioavailability, allowing the dosage to be one half of the micronized form.
- When griseofulvin is not tolerated or is ineffective, there are some alternatives, but these agents cannot be recommended as first-line therapy until further comparison studies are done and more is known about their safety in children.
  - Itraconazole: 5 mg/kg/day given once daily with food for 4 weeks
  - Fluconazole: 6 mg/kg/day for 3 to 4 weeks
  - Terbinafine: effective and safe in studies at a dosage of 4.5 to 6 mg/kg/day (up to 250 mg/day) for 4 to 6 weeks; available only in a pill form and not as efficacious for *M. canis* infection
- Use of adjunctive sporicidal topical agents, such as 1% or 2.5% selenium sulfide or 2% ketoconazole shampoo, twice weekly can limit the spread of infectious spores and may improve appearance.
- Simultaneous use of antifungal shampoo (containing selenium sulfide or ketoconazole) by family members of infected children is advisable as preventive therapy and to eliminate the carrier state. Apply for 5 to 10 minutes three times each week.
- Appropriate therapy of kerion is controversial:
  - Despite the puslike appearance, antibiotics are not usually necessary. Use of oral antistaphylococcal medications can be considered if severe with tenderness, multiple pustules, or abscesses or if other areas of scalp show clear evidence of impetigo or pyoderma.
  - Oral prednisone, 1 mg/kg/day for 10 days or longer, may be helpful in patients with

severe kerion (controversial); it increases patient comfort and may prevent scarring alopecia.
  - Incision and drainage are not indicated because loculations are small and the septa thick.

DISPOSITION

- Check the patient taking griseofulvin after 6 weeks of therapy to determine effectiveness and to decide length of therapy.
- If there are no signs of disease (i.e., scalp is totally normal), The Committee on Infectious Diseases of the American Academy of Pediatrics recommends continuing therapy for 2 weeks after resolution of symptoms, so in this case, for a total of 8 weeks.

REFERRAL

Consider a dermatologic referral for diagnostic questions or treatment failure.

PEARLS & CONSIDERATIONS

COMMENTS

- Tinea capitis may resemble seborrheic or atopic dermatitis and be misdiagnosed for months. In this situation, diffuse or patchy dandruff-like scaling is present, but alopecia or inflammation is minimal or absent.
- Widespread tinea corporis, particularly when it is on the face, neck, or upper chest, can be a sign of occult scalp tinea infection or asymptomatic carriage.
- Although kerions often heal with treatment of the underlying fungus, scarring alopecia is a possible complication if the inflammation is severe and diagnosis is delayed.
- Although oral ketoconazole is used occasionally in pediatrics, it is not recommended for treatment of tinea capitis. Because of the risk of hepatotoxicity, the expense of the drug, the lack of superiority to griseofulvin in controlled studies, and the emergence of other more promising antifungal agents, oral ketoconazole is not the preferred treatment choice.
- When using selenium sulfide shampoo as adjunctive treatment of tinea capitis, there is no difference between the 2.5% and 1% preparations in time required to produce a negative surface culture. The 1% solution is less expensive.

PREVENTION

Avoid sharing combs, pillows, and head gear because the organism has been cultured from fomites and is likely responsible for spread.

PATIENT/FAMILY EDUCATION

- Stress the need for prolonged (usually 8 weeks) course of therapy.
- Advise that griseofulvin be taken with fatty foods (e.g., milk, ice cream).
- It is not necessary to shave the scalp.

SUGGESTED READINGS

Blumer JL: Pharmacologic basis for the treatment of tinea capitis. *Pediatr Infect Dis J* 18:191, 1999.

Feigin RD, Cherry JD (eds): *Textbook of Pediatric Infectious Diseases*, 5th ed. Philadelphia, WB Saunders, 2004.

Howard RM, Friedin IJ: Dermatophyte infections in children. *In* Aronoff SC (ed): *Advances in Pediatric Infectious Diseases*, vol 14. St Louis, Mosby, 1999.

Hurwitz S: *Clinical Pediatric Dermatology*, 2nd ed. Philadelphia, WB Saunders, 1993.

Lobato MN, Vugia DJ: Tinea capitis in California: a population-based study of a growing epidemic. *Pediatrics* 99:551, 1997.

Roberts BJ, Friedlander SF: Tinea capitis: a treatment update. *Pediatr Ann* 34:3, 2005.

Weston WL et al: *Color Textbook of Pediatric Dermatology*, 2nd ed. St Louis, Mosby, 1996.

AUTHOR: **LARRY DENK, MD**

BASIC INFORMATION

DEFINITION

Tinea corporis is a superficial dermatophyte fungal infection of the glabrous skin. Several areas of the body are excluded in the definition and have other names, such as the scalp (i.e., tinea capitis), bearded areas (i.e., tinea barbae), the groin (i.e., tinea cruris), hands (i.e., tinea manuum), feet (i.e., tinea pedis), and nails (i.e., onychomycosis).

SYNONYMS

Body ringworm
Ringworm

ICD-9-CM CODE

110.5 Tinea corporis

EPIDEMIOLOGY & DEMOGRAPHICS

- Tinea corporis is often acquired by close person-to-person contact, as occurs in a household, day care, or school.
- The index case may have tinea corporis, capitis, or pedis.
- Contact with domestic animals, particularly young kittens and puppies, is a common cause.
- There have been several reports of epidemics among high school wrestlers (i.e., tinea gladiatorum).
- Individuals with certain immunologic abnormalities, such as atopic dermatitis, presumably caused by a decreased cell-mediated delayed sensitivity and an increased humoral (IgE) response, are particularly prone to chronic and recurrent dermatophyte infections.

CLINICAL PRESENTATION

History

- A round lesion that may be expanding is discovered by a caretaker or the patient.
- The area may be mildly pruritic.
- There are no associated systemic symptoms.

Physical Examination

- The classic lesion is annular, oval, or circinate. It is minimally inflamed, with a sharply defined papulovesicular border and often with some central clearing.
- The lesions typically begin as red papules or pustules that rupture and evolve to form papulosquamous lesions.
- These lesions then spread out from the periphery as new vesicles form and begin to clear centrally.
- Over a period of weeks, the patches may expand up to 5 cm in diameter.
- The pattern can vary and may mimic many conditions. Lesions may be eczematous, vesicular, pustular, and less often, granulomatous.
- Sites of predilection include the nonhairy areas of the face, trunk, and limbs.
- Lesions are usually solitary but can be multiple.
- Inappropriate treatment with topical steroids decreases the inflammation and alters the clinical appearance while the infection persists, a condition referred to as *tinea incognito*.
- An uncommon but distinctive variant of tinea is a deeper granulomatous folliculitis and perifolliculitis disorder (i.e., Majocchi's granuloma).
  - Usually occurs on one lower leg or dorsum of a foot
  - Nodular lesions: sometimes several in one area
  - Often occurs on the legs of girls who shave their legs closely and get an infected ingrown hair
  - Caused by *Trichophyton rubrum* or *Trichophyton mentagrophytes*
  - Primary focus: diffuse *T. rubrum* infection of the foot

ETIOLOGY

- The species of dermatophyte causing tinea corporis depends on the source of the infection.
- *T. rubrum* is the most common cause worldwide, probably because it spreads from the feet of those with tinea pedis.
- In areas where tinea capitis is endemic, tinea corporis is more commonly caused by *Trichophyton tonsurans,* the most common cause of tinea capitis.
- *Microsporum canis* is the usual cause if the spread is from a pet.
- Other causative dermatophytes include *Microsporum audouinii, T. mentagrophytes, Trichophyton verrucosum,* and *Epidermophyton floccosum.*

DIAGNOSIS (Dx)

DIFFERENTIAL DIAGNOSIS

- Candidiasis
- Contact dermatitis
- Early cellulitis
- Erythema annulare centrifugum
- Erythema chronicum migrans
- Erythema multiforme
- Erythrasma
- Fixed drug eruptions
- Granuloma annulare
- Nummular eczema
- Psoriasis
- Sarcoidosis
- Seborrheic dermatitis
- Syphilis
- Systemic lupus erythematosus
- Herald patch of pityriasis rosea
- Tinea versicolor
- Vitiligo

WORKUP

- Diagnosis is usually made on clinical grounds.
- Wood's light examination is not helpful in the diagnosis of suspected lesions on glabrous skin unless the lanugo hairs are infected.

LABORATORY TESTS

- Confirm by potassium hydroxide (KOH) microscopic wet-mount examination.
  - Obtain a large amount of fine scale by gentle scraping of the edge of a lesion with the belly of a No. 15-blade scalpel or the edge of a glass slide.
  - Mount onto the center of the slide, add 1 or 2 drops of 20% KOH, apply a coverslip (gently press down with the eraser end of a pencil to crush the scales), and examine under low power.
  - True hyphae are seen as long, branching, often septate rods of uniform width that cross the borders of epidermal cells.
  - Cotton fibers, cell borders, or other artifacts may be misinterpreted as positive findings.
- Obtain a fungal culture of skin lesions if the result of direct microscopy is negative and clinical suspicion is high.

TREATMENT

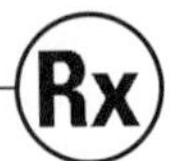

ACUTE GENERAL Rx

- Topical therapy is adequate for most cases of tinea corporis.
  - Apply to lesions twice daily for at least 4 weeks.
  - An imidazole cream such as miconazole (Micatin, Monistat-Derm) or clotrimazole (Lotrimin, Mycelex) is usually recommended because both are inexpensive, available over the counter, and relatively free of side effects.
  - Other available imidazole creams include ketoconazole (Nizoral), econazole (Spectazole), sulconazole (Exelderm), and oxiconazole (Oxistat).
- Although clearing and relief from any associated pruritus is often seen within the first 7 to 10 days after initiation of therapy, topical treatment with the imidazoles should continue for a minimum of 2 to 3 weeks after the affected area is clinically clear.
- If therapy with any of the aforementioned agents fails, clinicians should prescribe 1% terbinafine cream (Lamisil), a fungicidal allylamine derivative.
  - Terbinafine is also given twice daily but for a shorter time, only until clinical signs and symptoms are significantly improved (usually 1 to 2 weeks).
  - Terbinafine does not cover *M. canis.*
- Topical corticosteroids are generally unnecessary. However, a *mild* steroid cream may be used twice daily for a few days for relief in those with pruritus or severe inflammation.
  - Combination antifungal and steroid creams are *not* indicated.
  - The duration of steroid application should be brief.
  - Antifungal application is prolonged.
- Some cases of tinea corporis require systemic therapy: patients with widespread or deep-seated follicular lesions (i.e., Majocchi's

granuloma), those with associated tinea capitis, and immunocompromised hosts.
- Griseofulvin (20 mg/kg/day) given once daily with fatty foods for 3 weeks is usually adequate. If there is associated tinea capitis, continue the same dose for 6 to 8 weeks (see Tinea Capitis in Diseases and Disorders [Section I]).
- Itraconazole is also very effective for systemic treatment of tinea corporis and cruris.

DISPOSITION

- Recheck in 2 weeks to ensure that the area is improving.
- If no response has occurred, the diagnosis is incorrect, or a resistant dermatophyte has been encountered.

REFERRAL

A dermatology referral should be considered for resistant cases or when the diagnosis is unclear.

PEARLS & CONSIDERATIONS

COMMENTS

- The term *fungus infection* incorporates disorders caused by tinea (i.e., dermatophyte) and yeasts (e.g., *Candida*). They are not synonymous and have different responses to fungal agents.
  - Topical nystatin is effective against candidal infection but ineffective in the treatment of a tinea (dermatophyte) infection.
  - Tolnaftate (Tinactin) and undecylenic acid (Gordochom) are beneficial in the management of dermatophytoses such as tinea pedis, tinea cruris, and tinea corporis, but they are ineffective against disorders resulting from candidal infection.
  - Many agents treat both types of infection. These include ciclopirox (Loprox), clotrimazole (Lotrimin), econazole (Spectazole), ketoconazole (Nizoral), miconazole (Micatin, Monistat-Derm), oxiconazole (Oxistat), and sulconazole (Exelderm).

PREVENTION

- Minimize spread to close contacts by frequent hand washing, adequate treatment of the index case, and avoidance of clothes sharing.
- Keep the lesion covered between medication applications until it shows signs of improvement.
- Have any family pet with tinea treated.

PATIENT/FAMILY EDUCATION

- Emphasize the generally benign and common nature of the infection, but also explain the need for prolonged therapy to cure the infection.
- It is mildly contagious.
- Instruct the patient or caregiver to apply topical agent to the entire lesion plus about a 1 cm border beyond it.

SUGGESTED READINGS

Berg D, Erickson P: Fungal skin infections in children. New developments and treatments. *Postgrad Med* 110:83, 2001.

Feigin RD, Cherry JD (eds): *Textbook of Pediatric Infectious Diseases,* 5th ed. Philadelphia, WB Saunders, 2004.

Howard RM, Frieden IJ: Dermatophyte infections in children. *In* Aronoff SC (ed): *Advances in Pediatric Infectious Diseases,* vol 14. St Louis, Mosby, 1999.

Hurwitz S: *Clinical Pediatric Dermatology,* 2nd ed. Philadelphia, WB Saunders, 1993.

Weston WL et al: *Color Textbook of Pediatric Dermatology,* 2nd ed. St Louis, Mosby, 1996.

AUTHOR: **LARRY DENK, MD**

BASIC INFORMATION

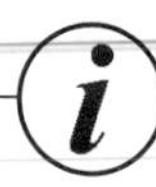

DEFINITION

Tinea cruris is an extremely common superficial dermatophyte fungal infection of the groin and upper thighs.

SYNONYMS

Jock itch
Ringworm of groin

ICD-9-CM CODE
110.3 Tinea cruris

EPIDEMIOLOGY & DEMOGRAPHICS

- Occurs primarily in adolescent and adult males
- More common and more symptomatic in hot, humid weather
- More common in obese individuals
- More common in athletes because of sweating and chafing in the region
- Commonly associated with tinea pedis

CLINICAL PRESENTATION

History

- Eruption noted by the individual or an intimate partner.
- Itching or burning sensation may be severe.
- Vigorous physical activity, chafing, and wearing of tight-fitting clothing such as athletic supporters, jockey shorts, wet bathing suits, panty hose, or slacks may contribute to the development of tinea cruris.

Physical Examination

- Erythematous, scaly, sharply demarcated rash in the groin, possibly with central clearing.
- The eruption is usually bilaterally symmetric on the upper inner thighs and intertriginous folds of the groin area in a half-moon shape. Occasionally, it extends to the perianal region, buttocks, and abdomen.
- A vesiculopustular border may be present.
- The scrotum, penis, or labia are usually spared or more mildly involved. By comparison, *Candida* will usually involve scrotum, penis, or labia.
- Excoriation may occur as a consequence of the patient's scratching.

ETIOLOGY

The groin is infected by one of several fungi: *Trichophyton rubrum, Trichophyton mentagrophytes,* or *Epidermophyton floccosum.*

DIAGNOSIS

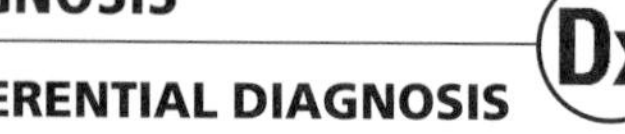

DIFFERENTIAL DIAGNOSIS

- *Candida albicans* infection
- Intertrigo
- Seborrheic dermatitis
- Psoriasis
- Primary irritant or allergic contact dermatitis
  - Diaper dermatitis in infants
  - Medication application
- Erythrasma
- Tinea versicolor
- Erysipelas or perianal strep infection

WORKUP

- Diagnosis is based on clinical presentation.
- Wood's light examination is negative. This differentiates tinea from erythrasma, which has a coral-red fluorescence.

LABORATORY TESTS

- Can confirm diagnosis by KOH microscopic examination of scrapings.
- Fungal culture generally is not necessary.

TREATMENT

NONPHARMACOLOGIC THERAPY

- Reduce chafing and irritation is by wearing loose-fitting cotton underclothing.
- The obese patient should lose weight.
- Bland absorbent powder such as ZeaSorb AF medicated powder can reduce perspiration and friction.

ACUTE GENERAL Rx

- Topical therapy is usually adequate.
- Apply to lesions twice daily for at least 4 weeks. There are many choices.
  - An imidazole cream such as miconazole (Micatin, Monistat-Derm) or clotrimazole (Lotrimin, Mycelex) is usually recommended because both are inexpensive, available over the counter, and relatively free of side effects.
  - Other available imidazole creams include ketoconazole (Nizoral), econazole (Spectazole), sulconazole (Exelderm), and oxiconazole (Oxistat).
- Although clearing and relief from any associated pruritus is often seen within the first 7 to 10 days after initiation of therapy, topical treatment with the imidazoles should continue for a minimum of 2 to 3 weeks after the affected area is clinically clear.
- If therapy with any of these agents fails, clinicians should prescribe 1% terbinafine cream (Lamisil), a fungicidal allylamine derivative.
- Terbinafine is also given twice daily but for a shorter time, only until clinical signs and symptoms are significantly improved (usually 1 to 2 weeks).
- Topical corticosteroids are generally unnecessary. However, a *mild* steroid cream may be used twice daily for a few days for relief in those with pruritus or severe inflammation.
  - Combination antifungal and steroid creams are *not* indicated.
  - The duration of steroid application should be brief.
  - Antifungal application is prolonged.
- Failure to treat concomitant tinea pedis usually results in prompt recurrence.
- Oral therapy may be indicated for lesions that are resistant or recur frequently and can be treated with either oral griseofulvin or itraconazole, as described in Tinea Corporis in Diseases and Disorders (Section I).

DISPOSITION

Recheck the patient in 2 weeks.

REFERRAL

Consider a dermatology referral for resistant cases or diagnostic questions.

PEARLS & CONSIDERATIONS

COMMENTS

- The term *fungus infection* incorporates disorders caused by tinea (i.e., dermatophyte) and yeasts (e.g., *Candida*). These conditions are not synonymous and have different responses to therapy.
- Topical nystatin (Mycostatin) is effective against candidal infection but ineffective in the treatment of a dermatophyte infection.
- Tolnaftate (Tinactin) and undecylenic acid (Gordochom) are beneficial in the management of dermatophytoses (i.e., tinea pedis, tinea cruris, and tinea corporis) but are ineffective against candidal infection.
- Many agents treat both types of infection. These include ciclopirox (Loprox), clotrimazole (Lotrimin), econazole (Spectazole), ketoconazole (Nizoral), miconazole (Micatin, Monistat-Derm), oxiconazole (Oxistat), and sulconazole (Exelderm).
- Erythrasma is a fairly common chronic superficial dermatosis of the crural area caused by *Corynebacterium minutissimum.*
  - The treatment can be topical erythromycin, clindamycin, miconazole, or Whitfield ointment or a 10- to 14-day course of oral erythromycin.
  - Erythrasma can coexist with a dermatophyte infection.

PREVENTION

- Bathe or shower then thoroughly dry the groin area after athletic activity (including swimming) or any activity that causes sweating.
- Avoid prolonged exposure of the groin to tight-fitting, wet, or sweaty clothes.

PATIENT/FAMILY EDUCATION

- Offer reassurance regarding the generally benign and common nature of the disorder.
- Advise that recurrences are common.

SUGGESTED READINGS

Feigin RD, Cherry JD: *Textbook of Pediatric Infectious Diseases,* 5th ed. Philadelphia, WB Saunders, 2004.

Howard RM, Frieden IJ: Dermatophyte infections in children. *In* Aronoff SC (ed): *Advances in Pediatric Infectious Diseases,* vol 14. St Louis, Mosby, 1999.

AUTHOR: **LARRY DENK, MD**

BASIC INFORMATION

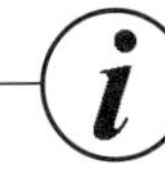

DEFINITION

Tinea versicolor is a superficial fungal infection of the skin caused by the yeast *Malassezia furfur.*

SYNONYM

Pityriasis versicolor

ICD-9-CM CODE

111.0 Tinea versicolor

EPIDEMIOLOGY & DEMOGRAPHICS

- Worldwide distribution; more common in humid and tropical climates
- Increased incidence in adolescence and young adulthood
- More commonly recognized in the summer, because hypopigmented lesions become more evident when the normal skin is darkened by sun and the lesions fail to tan
- Factors that seem to favor the overgrowth of *Malassezia:* pregnancy, excessive sweating, occlusion, malnutrition, immunosuppression, high plasma cortisol levels, oral contraceptives, and excess heat and humidity

CLINICAL PRESENTATION

- Hypopigmented lesions can be red or hyperpigmented and usually occur on the chest and trunk, neck, and upper arms.
- Onset is insidious.
- Patients generally are asymptomatic, but some complain of mild pruritus.

Physical Examination

- Multiple oval, macular, and patchy lesions with fine scales are seen.
- Lesions may be hypopigmented or hyperpigmented (i.e., fawn-colored or brown), depending on the patient's complexion and exposure to sunlight.
- Occasionally, lesions are salmon-pink or reddish.
- The lesions are usually distributed over the upper portions of the trunk (most common), neck, proximal arms, and occasionally, the face or other areas.
- Facial lesions are more common in children; the forehead is the most common facial site.
- Lesions may coalesce to involve a large contiguous area.
- Lesions can become lighter than the surrounding skin in summer and relatively darker during winter.
- Infections caused by *M. furfur* may manifest with follicular papules or pustules involving the same areas.

ETIOLOGY

- The infection is caused by proliferation of *M. furfur,* a lipophilic yeast that is a normal inhabitant of the skin flora.
- Under certain predisposing conditions, the yeast form undergoes a dynamic change to a pathogenic mycelial form associated with clinical disease.
- Nomenclature of these yeasts is confusing.
  - *Pityrosporum ovale* and *Pityrosporum orbiculare* were previously used to distinguish *M. furfur* with an oval or round shape, respectively.
  - Occasionally, the term *Pityrosporum* is used instead of *Malassezia.*

DIAGNOSIS

DIFFERENTIAL DIAGNOSIS

- Dermatophyte infections (tinea corporis); eczema; melasma (formerly referred to as *chloasma*); pityriasis alba; pityriasis rosea; postinflammatory hypopigmentation; seborrheic dermatitis; secondary syphilis; vitiligo

WORKUP

- The eruption is usually distinctive, and the diagnosis can often be made on clinical grounds.
- Tinea versicolor demonstrates a green-yellow, copper-orange, bronze, or blue-white fluorescence under Wood's light.
- The diagnosis can be confirmed by potassium hydroxide wet mounts of cutaneous scrapings. Hyphae and thick-walled budding spores in grapelike clusters are seen under the microscope (i.e., spaghetti and meatballs pattern).
- Fungal cultures are unsatisfactory because the organism is difficult to grow on culture media.

TREATMENT

ACUTE GENERAL Rx

- Tinea versicolor generally responds to a variety of topical preparations.
- Selenium sulfide (2.5%) shampoo (Selsun, Exsel) is a convenient, inexpensive, rapid, and highly effective mode of therapy.
  - Apply a thin layer to the entire affected area overnight once each week for 4 weeks, followed by once each month for 3 months to help prevent recurrences.
  - The preparation is washed off in the morning by bath or shower, at which time all night clothes, bedding, and undergarments should be changed.
  - For the unusual patient who experiences irritation from the overnight application, an alternative is to apply the same 2.5% selenium sulfide solution for only 10 to 30 minutes nightly for 2 weeks.
- Ketoconazole (2%) shampoo applied to affected areas for 10 minutes for 3 consecutive days is an alternative.
- Topical antifungal medications (e.g., miconazole, oxiconazole, ciclopirox, terbinafine, clotrimazole) can be applied twice daily for 2 to 4 weeks. They are effective but more expensive because of the large surface area to be covered.
- Oral treatment is reserved for individuals with resistant or recurrent infection. Effective agents include the following:
  - Ketoconazole: 200 mg/day for 5 days
  - Fluconazole: 400 mg as a single dose 1 day and repeated in 1 week
  - Itraconazole: 200 mg/day for 5 to 7 days

CHRONIC Rx

For some individuals, monthly application of selenium sulfide topically may keep fungal growth in check.

DISPOSITION

- The prognosis is good, with death of the fungus usually occurring within 3 to 4 weeks of treatment.
- Recurrences are common, especially during the hot and humid months.

REFERRAL

Consider referral to a dermatologist for resistant cases or if the diagnosis is uncertain.

PEARLS & CONSIDERATIONS

COMMENTS

- *Malassezia (Pityrosporum)* species have also been associated with seborrheic dermatitis, folliculitis, and steroid acne.
- Patients with tinea versicolor occasionally have concomitant folliculitis, seborrheic dermatitis, and acne vulgaris.
- Some systemic antifungals (e.g., ketoconazole, fluconazole) work by being secreted in the sweat. If prescribing these systemic antifungals, advise exercise about 1 hour after taking the medicine so that the patient will sweat and leave the sweat in contact with the skin for 8 to 12 hours.
- Itraconazole is secreted in sebum and does not require sweating for effectiveness.
- Systemic terbinafine is not effective against *Malassezia.*

PREVENTION

- Tinea versicolor is mildly contagious, and measures should be taken to prevent spread to family members and close contacts.
- Some experts advise monthly application of the 2.5% selenium sulfide shampoo to prevent recurrence.

PATIENT/FAMILY EDUCATION

- Patients should be informed that the hypopigmented areas will not disappear immediately after therapy. It may take several months to return to normal pigmentation, even after eradication of the fungus.
- Recurrences are common.

SUGGESTED READINGS

Assaf RR, Weil ML: The superficial mycoses. *Dermatol Clin* 14:57, 1996.

Feigin RD, Cherry JD: *Textbook of Pediatric Infectious Diseases,* 5th ed. Philadelphia, WB Saunders, 2004.

Hurwitz S: *Clinical Pediatric Dermatology,* 2nd ed. Philadelphia, WB Saunders, 1993.

Ljubojevic S et al: The role of *Malassezia furfur* in dermatology. *Clin Dermatol* 20:179, 2002.

Weston WL et al: *Color Textbook of Pediatric Dermatology,* 2nd ed. St. Louis, Mosby, 1996.

AUTHOR: **LARRY DENK, MD**

BASIC INFORMATION

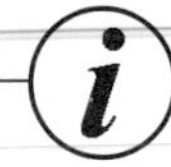

DEFINITION

Torticollis is unilateral contraction of the lateral cervical [sternocleidomastoid (SCM)] muscles resulting in rotation of the head and neck with associated head tilt. Torticollis may be congenital or acquired.

SYNONYMS

Stiff neck
Wry neck

ICD-9-CM CODES
723.5 Intermittent or spastic/torticollis NOS
754.1 Congenital
767.8 Due to birth injury

EPIDEMIOLOGY & DEMOGRAPHICS

- Congenital torticollis occurs in 0.4% of live births.
- Males more frequently affected than females

CLINICAL PRESENTATION

Clinical Torticollis
History

- Infant prefers to keep head turned to one side.
- May not be noticed at birth, but usually detected within the first month of life.
- Infant may have a birth history remarkable for breech presentation or forceps delivery.
- Other orthopedic disorders—metatarsus adductus, congenital hip dysplasia, talipes equinovarus—occur in up to 20% of cases.

Physical Examination

- Tight SCM muscle, often with palpable, hard, olive-like mass in the midsection of the cervical muscle
  - Palpable between ages 4 and 6 weeks
  - Typically regresses by 4 to 6 months, leaving only contracture and fibrotic thickening of the involved muscle
- Head tilt in the direction of the muscle involved with chin turned away from the contracted side
- Later findings include facial asymmetry and plagiocephaly (flattening on affected side)
- Assess for other orthopedic abnormalities that may be associated with torticollis (e.g., congenital hip dysplasia)
- Assess for associated ophthalmologic and neurologic abnormalities

Acquired Torticollis
History

- Assess for history of trauma, recent or concurrent illness, drug exposure.
- Associated neurologic symptoms such as dizziness, unsteadiness, or abnormal eye movements seen with paroxysmal torticollis of infancy, idiosyncratic responses to some medications, as well as central nervous system (CNS) tumor, destructive process, or structural lesion

Physical Examination

- Tight SCM muscle with head tilt in the direction of the muscle involved and chin turned away from the contracted side
- Lymphadenopathy (cervical adenitis, tonsillitis, retropharyngeal infection)
- In the absence of obvious infection, careful neurologic and ophthalmologic examinations are essential.

ETIOLOGY

Congenital Torticollis

- May be secondary to mechanical constraint in utero or, less often, birth trauma
- Related most commonly to neuromuscular abnormality with fibrotic shortening of the SCM
- Less commonly related to underlying bony anomalies (of the atlas, odontoid, or atlantoaxial articulation), skin web (pterygium colli), central nervous system disorder (e.g., involving cranial nerve XI at origin in cervical spinal cord or exit from base of skull)

Acquired Torticollis

- Secondary to an acute process resulting in spasm of the SCM muscle
  - Most cases are related to ligamentous or muscular injuries, sudden onset follows minor injury, strenuous activity, or sudden position change.
  - Inflammatory or infectious causes include tonsillitis, cervical adenitis, or retropharyngeal abscess causing cervical node enlargement and irritation of surrounding muscles.
  - Atlantoaxial rotational subluxation can occur secondary to trauma or in children with underlying conditions that predispose to atlantoaxial instability (trisomy 21, bone dysplasia, Morquio syndrome).
- Reversible torticollis (apparent torticollis without SCM muscle shortening)
  - Idiosyncratic response to phenothiazines, metoclopramide, or haloperidol (dystonic reaction)
  - Paroxysmal torticollis of infancy
    - Rare
    - Associated with vestibular dysfunction
    - Presents at age 2 to 8 months with associated distress, pallor, possible eye rolling/deviation, and ataxia
  - Sandifer syndrome with arching and posturing secondary to gastroesophageal reflux
- Pseudotorticollis
  - Secondary to abducens or other oculomotor palsies, spasmus nutans, or congenital nystagmus—head tilt is a mechanical compensation that allows for one visual image (prevents diplopia).
- Progressive torticollis
  - Infratentorial tumor
  - Structural lesions: colloid cyst of the third ventricle, syringomyelia
  - Sarcoma with invasion and entrapment of cranial nerves
  - Basal ganglia dysfunction or destruction (e.g., Wilson disease with destruction secondary to copper deposition)
  - Myositis of the SCM

DIAGNOSIS

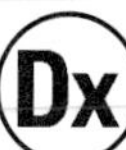

DIFFERENTIAL DIAGNOSIS

Congenital Torticollis

- Other causes of neck masses in region of the SCM muscle
  - Cystic hygroma
  - Branchial cleft cyst
  - Underlying vertebral or neurologic abnormalities
  - Vertebral dislocation
  - Klippel-Feil syndrome with failure of normal vertebral segmentation of the cervical spine
  - Sprengel's deformity with congenital elevation of the scapula

Acquired Torticollis

See preceding "Etiology."

WORKUP

Congenital Torticollis

- Most patients require only a careful physical examination.
- When a cervical muscle mass is not palpable or torticollis is not responding to therapy, plain films of the neck should be obtained to look for cervical bony abnormalities (e.g., hemivertebrae). Magnetic resonance imaging (MRI) should be done for patients with complicated cervical anomalies.
- In cases of plagiocephaly without obvious torticollis, consider evaluation for craniosynostosis.

Acquired Torticollis

- A careful physical examination and history will dictate further workup for acute torticollis.
  - Cervical spine films or imaging studies may be required in cases of trauma.
  - Barium swallow or pH probe may be useful in cases of suspected gastroesophageal reflux (Sandifer syndrome).
  - Computed tomography (CT) of the neck may be useful if a retropharyngeal abscess is suspected.
- Progressive torticollis
  - MRI and radiographic imaging of the head and neck
  - Slit-lamp examination for Kayser-Fleischer corneal ring; serum tests to assess for Wilson disease
  - Creatinine phosphokinase to rule out myopathy

TREATMENT

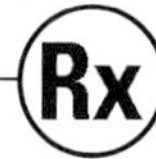

NONPHARMACOLOGIC THERAPY

Congenital Torticollis

- Passive stretching involves lateral flexion of the head to the side opposite the torticollis and rotation of the chin to the affected side; supervision by a physical therapist is helpful.
- The infant should be placed in relation to objects of interest so that active head turning to the unaffected side is encouraged.

- In certain cases with significant secondary plagiocephaly, treatment with a fitted plastic helmet may remedy the plagiocephaly.
- Most cases resolve by 1 year of age.
- Surgical referral is indicated if not resolved by 1 year of age for potential lengthening of the SCM muscle.

Acquired Torticollis

- When torticollis is secondary to muscle spasm, strain, or intervertebral disk calcification, local heat may be helpful.
- Patients with atlantoaxial subluxation require referral to an orthopedic or neurologic surgeon.

ACUTE GENERAL Rx

- Analgesics and muscle relaxants can be given in cases due to muscle spasm or strain.
- Appropriately treat the underlying cause (e.g., systemic antibiotics for infection).

REFERRAL

Congenital Torticollis

- Refer patients with any of the following:
  - Failure to improve after 2 to 3 months of conservative treatment
  - Presence of anomalies of the skull or cervical spine
  - Abnormal neurologic or ophthalmologic examinations
    - Failure to resolve by 1 year of age

Acquired Torticollis

- Refer patients with any of the following:
  - Presence of anomalies of the skull or cervical spine
  - Progressive torticollis or failure to respond to conventional therapy
  - Abnormal neurologic or ophthalmologic examinations

PEARLS & CONSIDERATIONS

COMMENTS

- Head tilt toward the muscle involved with the chin turned to the opposite side.
- In congenital torticollis, early detection and treatment with stretching exercises can promote resolution of craniofacial abnormalities.
- A careful history and clinical examination focusing on the neck with neurologic, and ophthalmologic examinations will differentiate causes and allow appropriate diagnosis and management.

PATIENT/FAMILY EDUCATION

Congenital Torticollis

- See "Nonpharmacologic Therapy" for stretching exercises and infant positioning.
- Resolution of torticollis before 1 year of age can lead to a resolution of facial asymmetry.

SUGGESTED READINGS

Braun MA: Torticollis. *In* Dershewitz RA (ed): *Ambulatory Pediatric Care,* 3rd ed. Philadelphia, Lippincott Williams & Wilkins, 1999.

Griffin LY (ed): *Essentials of Musculoskeletal Care,* 3rd ed. Rosemont, IL, American Academy of Orthopedic Surgeons and the American Academy of Pediatrics, 2005.

Rosenstein BJ: Torticollis. *In* Hoekelman RA (ed): *Primary Pediatric Care,* 4th ed. St. Louis, Mosby, 2001.

AUTHOR: **LAURA JEAN SHIPLEY, MD**

BASIC INFORMATION

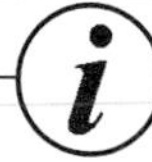

DEFINITION

Tourette syndrome (TS) is a chronic neuropsychiatric condition with onset in childhood characterized by the presence of motor and vocal tics that have been present for more than 1 year and that have changed in type, anatomic location, and severity over time. Affected individuals often have behavioral characteristics that include features of obsessive-compulsive disorder (OCD) or attention deficit/hyperactivity disorder (AD/HD), or both.

SYNONYMS

Gilles de la Tourette syndrome
Tourette disorder

ICD-9-CM CODE
307.23 Tourette syndrome

EPIDEMIOLOGY & DEMOGRAPHICS

- Up to 25% of children have tics at some time during childhood.
- Up to 3% of children have motor tics lasting more than 1 year.
- Between 0.1% and 1% of children have TS.
- Onset is before 18 years of age.
- Peak age of onset is between 5 and 7 years.
- TS is more common in boys than girls by 4:1 to 8:1.
- An autosomal dominant pattern of inheritance is observed in many families, but the genetics are complex.

CLINICAL PRESENTATION

History

- Tics are stereotyped, repetitive, involuntary movements that most commonly involve the face, head, neck, upper extremities, or a combination of these areas.
- Tics typically begin at about the time a child is entering school, but they may start in the toddler years.
- Tics may be simple movements or noises, or they may be more complex ensembles of movements or words.
  - Simple motor tics: sudden, brief, meaningless movements such as eye blinking, eye movements, grimacing, head jerks, arm jerks, tooth clicking, finger movements, kicks
  - Complex motor tics: slower, longer, more purposeful movements such as sustained looks, facial gestures, biting, touching objects or self, gestures with hands, gyrating and bending, copropraxia (obscene gestures)
  - Simple vocal tics: sudden, meaningless sounds or noises such as throat clearing, barking, coughing, spitting, clacking, hissing, many other sounds
  - Complex vocal tics: sudden, more meaningful utterances such as syllables, words, phrases, or statements; may also have echolalia and coprolalia
- The most common tics are eye blinking, face wrinkling, and sniffing.
- Coprolalia is uncommon, occurring in less than 10% of cases.
- If tics persist more than 1 year, they may increase in severity over a few years and then decrease.
- Tics typically change over time, with cessation of some tics and appearance of new tics. They also change severity over time, usually increasing in association with stress or excitement.
- Peak severity occurs between 9 and 11 years of age.
- Up to 50% of patients have resolution of tics in adulthood.
- When present, AD/HD symptoms typically precede the onset of tics.
- When present, obsessive-compulsive features may precede or follow the onset of tics.
- In many cases, AD/HD or obsessive-compulsive symptoms are more bothersome than are tics.
- A family history of tics and obsessive-compulsive features are common.
- A rare association with preceding streptococcal infection has been hypothesized but not proved.

Physical Examination

- Results of the general physical examination are normal.
- The neurologic examination findings are normal, except for the presence of tics. Tics may not be seen in the office.
- When in doubt, viewing a home video can help confirm the diagnosis.

ETIOLOGY

- Tics are familial in most cases, but a specific cause is unknown.
- Tics may accompany other neurologic disorders, but this is uncommon, and other neurologic signs or symptoms would usually be present.

DIAGNOSIS

Dx

DIFFERENTIAL DIAGNOSIS

- Transient tic disorder (tics present <1 year)
- Chronic motor tics disorder (motor tics present >1 year without vocal tics)
- Other movement disorders: chorea, myoclonus, dystonia
- Seizures
- Stereotypies (i.e., repetitive, patterned, rhythmic involuntary movements that do not change in type over time)

WORKUP

- Careful history, including psychiatric history for comorbid AD/HD, OCD symptoms, and anxiety
- Detailed family history
- Neurologic examination
- Diagnosis based entirely on the history and examination

TREATMENT

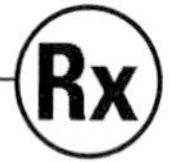

NONPHARMACOLOGIC THERAPY

- Education of patient, family, and school personnel about TS and its manifestations
- Specific educational modifications, especially during times of increased tic severity
- Educational modifications for comorbid AD/HD if present
- Cognitive-behavioral therapy may be helpful for OCD symptoms if present.
- Supportive psychotherapy as indicated

ACUTE GENERAL Rx

- Symptoms should be treated if they are causing distress to the child.
- It is important to identify what symptoms are causing impairment (e.g., tics, AD/HD, OCD).
- Treatment is indicated only if symptoms are significantly interfering with the patient's functioning.
- All available pharmacologic treatments are for symptomatic therapy only.
- Some medications have proven efficacy for tics.
  - α-Adrenergic receptor agonists (e.g., clonidine, guanfacine)
  - Typical neuroleptics (e.g., haloperidol, pimozide)
  - Atypical neuroleptics (e.g., risperidone)
  - Benzodiazepines (e.g., clonazepam)

CHRONIC Rx

- Treatment duration should be reassessed periodically to determine if the target symptoms have improved enough to consider withdrawing the medication.
- Chronic treatment is determined by the persistence and severity of the symptoms.
- Caution should be exercised with long-term use of neuroleptics because of the risk of tardive dyskinesia.

DISPOSITION

- For many children, education and reassurance is sufficient.
- For children with functional or psychosocial impairment, a multidisciplinary team, including the pediatrician; child neurologist, developmental pediatrician, or psychiatrist; psychologist; and educational specialist, is most effective at case management.
- When comorbid features (e.g., AD/HD, OCD, anxiety) are present, referral to a child neurologist, developmental pediatrician, or child psychiatrist with expertise in TS is recommended.
- Collaboration between provider, school, and family is essential.
- Recognize the waxing and waning course of tics to avoid unnecessary frequent medication changes.

- Watch for signs of increasing depression or anxiety.

REFERRAL

When comorbid features (e.g., AD/HD, OCD, anxiety) are present, referral to a child neurologist, developmental pediatrician, or child psychiatrist with expertise in TS is recommended.

PEARLS & CONSIDERATIONS

COMMENTS

- Tics are very common during childhood. In most cases, they are transient and do not cause difficulty. Even when chronic, many children do not require medical treatment.
- It is important that the child meet the full diagnostic criteria before making the diagnosis of TS.
- After the diagnosis of TS is made, the first course of treatment is education.
- It can be difficult to distinguish between complex tics and compulsions. When in doubt, a child with complex tics versus compulsions should be referred to a TS expert.
- Tics are involuntary. They are sometimes misinterpreted as intentional oppositional behavior, and it is important to help school personnel understand the nature of the tics.

PATIENT/FAMILY EDUCATION

- Most patients do not progress to severe forms depicted by media.
- Waxing and waning severity of symptoms is to be expected.
- The child may need specific educational accommodations.
- Parents serve a very important advocacy role.
- Learning disabilities may be associated with TS.
- Local support groups are extremely helpful for family and patients.
- The Tourette Syndrome Association (www.tsa-usa.org) has local chapters in many areas.

SUGGESTED READINGS

Kurlan R (ed): *Handbook of Tourette's Syndrome and Related Tic and Behavioral Disorders.* New York, Dekker, 2005.

Kurlan R et al: Prevalence of tics in schoolchildren and association with placement in special education. *Neurology* 57:1383, 2001.

Kurlan R, Kaplan EL: The pediatric autoimmune neuropsychiatric disorders associated with streptococcal infection (PANDAS) etiology for tics and obsessive-compulsive symptoms: hypothesis or entity? Practical considerations for the clinician. *Pediatrics* 113:883, 2004.

Leckman JF: Tourette's syndrome. *Lancet* 360:1577, 2001.

Robertson M: Tourette syndrome, associated conditions and the complexities of treatment. *Brain* 123:425, 2000.

AUTHOR: **JONATHAN W. MINK, MD, PHD**

BASIC INFORMATION

DEFINITION

Toxic shock syndrome (TSS) is an uncommon but life-threatening bacterial infection often characterized by sudden onset of high fever, diarrhea, vomiting, headache, muscle aches, local pain, and multiorgan dysfunction. The staphylococcal and streptococcal types of TSS are caused by release into the bloodstream of bacterial toxins that trigger a rapid immune reaction, producing the symptoms of toxic shock.

ICD-9-CM CODES
040.89 Toxic shock
041.00 *Streptococcus*
041.11 *Staphylococcus aureus*
041.19 *Staphylococcus*, other

EPIDEMIOLOGY & DEMOGRAPHICS

- Description of both syndromes occurred in the 1980s.
- Streptococcal TSS has a moderately high incidence at 0 to 4 years, with increased risk with advancing age beyond young adult. Males may be predominately affected. Blacks may be more susceptible to invasive group A streptococcal disease. Patients with chronic diseases (e.g., human immunodeficiency virus [HIV] infection, cancer, diabetes) are at increased risk, as are those with certain acute illness (particularly pediatric patients with varicella), although most patients previously were healthy.
- Staphylococcal TSS has no age or sex predominance. Nonmenstrual cases have no clear sex predominance. The incidence may be increasing slowly. Healthy individuals with normal immune systems are usually affected.
- Patients probably lack immunity to virulence factors and have predisposing conditions.
- Secondary cases are rare.

CLINICAL PRESENTATION

- Streptococcal TSS often begins with severe, localized pain at the infection site, but it may begin with influenza-like symptoms (20%).
  - Mental status is altered in 55% of patients.
  - Invasive infection is almost invariably present, although symptoms of pneumonia, sinus infections, or pharyngitis may be observed.
- Staphylococcal TSS begins with nonspecific constitutional symptoms for 2 to 3 days; fever follows, and diarrhea and orthostasis may develop early.
  - Menstrual staphylococcal TSS now represents a minority of TSS cases, almost exclusively occurring with tampon use but rarely with intrauterine device use.
  - Nonmenstrual TSS can occur in association with the following:
    - Burns
    - Empyema
    - Focal tissue infections (e.g., impetigo, abscess, varicella lesions)
    - Nasal packing
    - Osteomyelitis
    - Pneumonia
    - Postoperative settings, including in relation to surgical implants
    - Postpartum (i.e., endometriosis or mastitis)
    - Septic arthritis
    - Sinusitis

Physical Examination

- TSS generally manifests with fever, tachycardia, tachypnea, and hypotension.
- Streptococcal TSS usually occurs in association with invasive infection, complicating 8% to 14% of invasive streptococcal infections, especially necrotizing fasciitis (up to 70% of cases). Local findings are generally present and progress rapidly.
  - Staphylococcal TSS infection site findings are generally unimpressive but may include tissue infections, pneumonia, sinus tenderness, joint or bony findings, or incisional infection.
  - Less common sources include peritonitis, otitis, epiglottis, meningitis, cellulitis (especially with varicella), pelvic infections, endocarditis, osteomyelitis, and pharyngitis (rare).
  - Generalized erythema (less commonly patchy) is common with the staphylococcal form; it is less common with the streptococcal form. Palms and soles are usually involved, and the rash may have flexor accentuation.
  - Mucosal hyperemia, conjunctival hemorrhages, "strawberry tongue," and aphthous ulcers are more common in staphylococcal TSS.
  - Bullae are more common with streptococcal TSS.
  - Later evidence of anasarca from interstitial fluid losses is possible with both syndromes.

ETIOLOGY

- TSS is a systemic inflammatory response syndrome resulting from toxin-mediated effects on the immune system. It requires a conducive environment for toxin production, a susceptible host, and specific toxin-producing strains of certain microbes.
- Staphylococcal toxins TSST-1, enterotoxins B and C, or streptococcal pyrogenic exotoxins A and B probably act as superantigens to suppress certain protective cellular immune responses and to enhance production of cytokines and tumor necrosis factor (TNF). This inflammatory cascade bypasses conventional immune activation sequences.

DIAGNOSIS

Dx

- Streptococcal TSS case definition
  - Isolation of group A streptococci (groups B, C, F, and G also reported) from sterile site (if from nonsterile site, it is a probable case)
  - Hypotension: systolic blood pressure 90 mm Hg or lower in adults, less than the 5th percentile for age in children
  - Organ system involvement, including at least *two* of the following:
    - Renal system: creatinine level elevated twice the upper limit of normal for age (twice the baseline if preexisting elevation), or 2 mg/dL or more
    - Hematologic system: platelets 100,000/mm^3 or less or disseminated intravascular coagulation
    - Hepatic system: transaminase or bilirubin levels twice the upper limits of normal or twice the baseline if underlying liver disease
    - Respiratory system: acute respiratory distress syndrome (ARDS), acute pulmonary edema, or pleural effusion with hypoalbuminemia
    - Skin: generalized erythematous macular rash; may desquamate, tissue necrosis, including necrotizing fasciitis, myositis, or gangrene
- Staphylococcal TSS case definition
  - Temperature 38.9°C (102.0°F) or higher
  - Diffuse erythroderma or polymorphic maculopapular rash
  - Desquamation of the palms and soles 1 to 2 weeks after syndrome onset
  - Hypotension: systolic blood pressure less than 90 mm Hg or less than the 5th percentile in children *or* a drop in systolic blood pressure 10 mm Hg or more from lying to sitting position *or* orthostatic syncope
  - Involvement of three or more of the following organ systems:
    - Gastrointestinal system: vomiting or diarrhea at onset
    - Musculoskeletal system: myalgias or creatinine phosphokinase (CPK) greater than twice the upper limits of normal or higher
    - Mucous membrane hyperemia: conjunctival, oropharyngeal, or vaginal
    - Renal system: blood urea nitrogen (BUN) or creatinine level greater than twice the upper limit of normal *or* pyuria of 5 or more white blood cells per high-power field without evidence of a urinary tract infection
    - Hepatic system: transaminase or bilirubin levels twice the upper limits of normal
    - Hematologic system: platelet count of 100,000/mm^3 or less
    - Central nervous system: disorientation or altered consciousness without focal signs (in the absence of fever or hypotension)
    - Cardiopulmonary system: ARDS, pulmonary edema, new-onset second- or third-degree atrioventricular block, evidence of myocarditis
    - Negative culture results (e.g., throat, cerebrospinal fluid [CSF], urine), except positive blood culture for *S. aureus*

- Negative serology results for Rocky Mountain spotted fever, leptospirosis, and rubeola

DIFFERENTIAL DIAGNOSIS

- Acute rheumatic fever
- Disseminated Epstein-Barr virus or fungal infection
- Gram-negative sepsis
- Heat stroke
- Kawasaki disease
- Legionnaire's disease
- Leptospirosis
- Lyme disease
- Meningococcemia
- Recalcitrant erythematous desquamating disorder (associated with acquired immunodeficiency syndrome)
- Rocky Mountain spotted fever
- Scarlet fever and other exanthems
- Staphylococcal scalded skin syndrome
- Stevens-Johnson syndrome
- Systemic juvenile rheumatoid arthritis
- Systemic lupus erythematosus
- Toxoplasmosis
- Typhus

LABORATORY TESTS

- Electrolytes, calcium, creatinine, and BUN
- Complete blood cell count and coagulation studies
- Blood and urine cultures; consider CSF studies
- CPK
- Urinalysis
- Liver function tests, pancreatic function tests
- Oxygen saturation; consider arterial blood gases
- Electrocardiogram
  - Troponin testing
  - Echo for hemodynamically unstable patient
- Frequent metabolic acidosis secondary to poor perfusion
- Leukocytosis with prominent left shift is expected and anemia are often seen
- Abnormal coagulation study results for 40% of patients
- Hypokalemia and hypocalcemia are common; hyponatremia is less common.
- Hypoalbuminemia is common.
- Bacteremia in most streptococcal cases but rare in staphylococcal TSS (69% to 97%)

IMAGING STUDIES

Obtain a chest radiograph.

TREATMENT

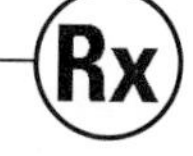

NONPHARMACOLOGIC THERAPY

- Provide supplemental oxygen at high concentrations; consider intubation based on clinical condition.
- Provide aggressive fluid resuscitation with normal saline (may consider colloid preparations in the later stages).
- Consider central access and hemodynamic monitoring to guide further resuscitation.
- The patient may require correction of coagulopathy with fresh frozen plasma, platelets, or cryoprecipitate, or some combination.
- Anemia may require transfusion of packed red blood cells.
- Correct electrolyte abnormalities as needed.

ACUTE GENERAL Rx

- For streptococcal cases
  - Clindamycin with high-dose penicillin G is administered intravenously.
  - Intravenous immune gamma globulin (IVIG) may result in dramatic improvement (1 to 2 g/kg initial dose, then 0.5 g/kg/day up to 5 days).
  - Consider dexamethasone for refractory shock.
  - Seventy percent of patients require surgical débridement, fasciotomy, laparotomy, hysterectomy, or amputation, depending on site of origin and degree of necrosis.
- For staphylococcal cases
  - Clindamycin is given intravenously; add vancomycin, a first-generation cephalosporin, or antistaphylococcal penicillin (e.g., nafcillin); antistaphylococcal β-lactam antibiotics *may* enhance toxin production.
  - IVIG (0.5 g/kg) may be given.
  - Steroids have been recommended for refractory cases, but evidence to support their use is lacking.
- Consider vasopressors for shock refractory to fluid resuscitation. Dopamine may be supplemented with norepinephrine if needed.
- Ceftriaxone may need to be added to cover meningitis (until a definite diagnosis is made) or doxycycline for Rocky Mountain spotted fever and leptospirosis.
- Consider sodium bicarbonate if the patient is severely acidotic (pH less than 7.1) and has a worsening acid-base status despite appropriate fluid resuscitation and ventilatory correction.
- Consider acetaminophen for antipyresis.
- Consider anti-TNF antibody.

DISPOSITION

All patients with suspected TSS should be admitted to an intensive care unit.

REFERRAL

Early consultation with a pediatric intensivist is recommended. Surgical consultation may be necessary for streptococcal infections.

PEARLS & CONSIDERATIONS

COMMENTS

- Few signs of infection are present at the originating site of staphylococcal TSS. Significant findings are usually present at the infected site of streptococcal TSS.
- Streptococcal TSS may manifest with early-onset shock and organ failure without the typical rash.
- Mortality is much higher for streptococcal (30% to 70%) than staphylococcal (<3% in menstrual, 6% to 9% in nonmenstrual) TSS.
- Renal dysfunction precedes shock in TSS (unlike shock from sepsis).
- Most patients improve significantly within 48 to 72 hours with treatment.
- Evidence of ARDS or refractory hypotension is a poor prognostic indicator.

PREVENTION

- Few preventive measures are available.
  - Avoidance of tampon use
  - Reducing duration of nasal packing to a few days (possibly with use of antibiotic prophylaxis)
  - Appropriate treatment of wounds and burns

PATIENT/FAMILY EDUCATION

- Completion of a full 10-day course of antibiotics helps reduce the rate of relapse; 30% to 40% of inadequately treated staphylococcal TSS cases relapse.
- Controversy exists about whether household contacts of streptococcal TSS cases should receive prophylaxis.

SUGGESTED READINGS

Darenberg J et al: Intravenous immunoglobulin G therapy in streptococcal toxic shock syndrome: a European randomized, double-blind, placebo-controlled trial. *Clin Infect Dis* 37:333, 2003.

Baxter F et al: Severe group A streptococcal infection and streptococcal toxic shock syndrome. *Can J Anesth* 47:1129, 2000.

Stevens DL: The toxic shock syndromes. *Infect Dis Clin North Am* 10:727, 1996.

McCormick JK et al: Toxic shock syndrome and bacterial superantigens: an update. *Ann Rev Microbiol* 55:77, 2001.

Working Group on Severe Streptococcal Infections: Defining the group A streptococcal toxic shock syndrome: rationale and consensus definition. *JAMA* 269:390, 1993.

AUTHORS: **JOHN L. HICK, MD** and **KAREN L. RESCH, MD**

BASIC INFORMATION

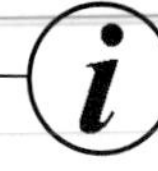

DEFINITION

Toxoplasmosis is a parasitic infection caused by the single-celled organism *Toxoplasma gondii.* Normally asymptomatic, it may produce severe ocular and central nervous system sequelae in immunocompromised hosts (e.g., patients with human immunodeficiency virus [HIV], transplant and chemotherapy recipients) and transplacentally infected infants.

SYNONYMS

Toxo
Toxoplasma

ICD-9-CM CODES
130.0-130.9 Toxoplasmosis
760.2 Maternal toxoplasmosis, affecting fetus or newborn
771.2 Other congenital infections

EPIDEMIOLOGY & DEMOGRAPHICS

- Toxoplasmosis is ubiquitous, occurring worldwide. More than 60 million people in the United States are infected.
- The incidence of congenital infection is estimated as 1 case per 1000 to 10,000 live births.
- The risk of transplacental transmission is highest in third trimester; the risk of severe sequelae is highest if infection occurs in the first trimester.
- Reactivation of latent infection may occur in immunocompromised hosts.

CLINICAL PRESENTATION

- The incubation period is 4 to 21 days (average, 7 days).
- Infection acquired after birth is usually asymptomatic but may cause generalized, self-limited flulike symptoms (e.g., malaise, muscle aches, lymphadenopathy).
- Congenital infection is asymptomatic at birth in 70% to 90% of cases.
- There is often a maternal history of cat exposure (e.g., cat litter box, gardening) or eating undercooked meat.
- Symptoms at birth may include maculopapular rash, microcephaly, intrauterine growth retardation, jaundice, seizures
- Late manifestations of congenital infection include visual impairment (common), developmental delay, spasticity, hydrocephalus, seizures, learning disabilities
- Rare manifestations include pneumonitis, myocarditis, pericarditis

ETIOLOGY

- *T. gondii* is a protozoan parasite. Although cat species are the definitive host, it may encyst in the tissue of virtually all mammals.
- Infection is generally by oral or parenteral routes, specifically from the following:
  - Oocysts in cat feces contaminating a litter box or garden soil
  - Eating or improperly handling raw meat, especially lamb, pork, or venison
  - Maternal-fetal transmission from a recently infected (or immunocompromised) mother
  - Rarely, from donated blood or organs

DIAGNOSIS

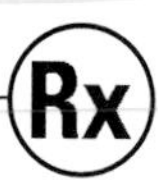

DIFFERENTIAL DIAGNOSIS

- Other STORCH (i.e., **s**yphilis, **t**oxoplasmosis, **o**ther, **r**ubella, **c**ytomegalovirus, **h**erpes simplex virus) infections, especially syphilis and cytomegalovirus
- Neonatal sepsis or aseptic meningitis
- Other lymphadenopathic disease (e.g., lymphoma, infectious mononucleosis)
- Other hemolytic disease (e.g., erythroblastosis fetalis)
- Other ocular disease (e.g., idiopathic chorioretinitis, colobomatous defect, intraocular hemorrhage, retinoblastoma, glioma)

WORKUP

- Signs and symptoms of infection can be protean and nonspecific.
- Workup includes serology, imaging studies, and ophthalmologic examination.
- Neonatal evaluation includes funduscopic examination for necrotizing retinitis (i.e., cotton-wool patches or punched-out pigmented lesions) and assessment of HIV-positive patient

LABORATORY TESTS

- Maternal infection. Serology: simultaneously assay immunoglobulin G (IgG) plus immunoglobulin M (IgM) or immunoglobulin A (IgA)
- Fetal infection
  - Polymerase chain reaction (PCR) or antigen detection on amniotic fluid (very sensitive at 18 weeks' gestation)
  - Parasite isolation from amniotic fluid or blood cells (i.e., mouse inoculation)
  - Serology: enzyme immunoassay for IgM or IgA
- Neonatal infection
  - Serology: sequential IgG, double-sandwich IgM or IgA
  - Parasite isolation from cord, placenta, or peripheral blood (i.e., mouse inoculation)
  - PCR on buffy coat or CSF pellet
- HIV-positive patients
  - Serology: IgG
  - PCR or antigen detection from blood (buffy coat), biopsy tissue, or CSF pellet

IMAGING STUDIES

- Fetal infection: serial cranial ultrasound for dilated lateral ventricles
- Neonatal: computed tomography of the head for intracranial calcifications or hydrocephalus

TREATMENT

NONPHARMACOLOGIC THERAPY

If chorioretinitis does not respond to systemic antimicrobials (with or without steroids), photocoagulation may be indicated and, rarely, vitrectomy or lens removal.

ACUTE GENERAL Rx

- Asymptomatic, immunocompetent adults and children 5 years old or older do not require treatment.
- Women infected with *T. gondii* $\leq$ 6 months before pregnancy do not require treatment.
- Pregnant women require treatment if they have recently become infected with *T. gondii* or are immunocompromised (i.e., HIV positive) and infected with *T. gondii*
- All infections in neonates and immunocompromised individuals should be treated.
- Treatment during pregnancy includes:
  - First trimester: spiramycin (available only from the U.S. FDA)
  - After 17 weeks: pyrimethamine-sulfadiazine and calcium leucovorin
- Neonatal and congenital infections are treated with pyrimethamine-sulfadiazine plus calcium leucovorin for at least 1 year.
- HIV-positive and immunosuppressed patients are treated as follows:
  - Pyrimethamine-sulfadiazine plus calcium leucovorin for active infection.
  - Trimethoprim-sulfamethoxazole is used for prophylaxis of inactive infections.
  - Clindamycin or atovaquone plus pyrimethamine may be substituted for sulfadiazine in sulfa-sensitive individuals.
  - Zidovudine (AZT, Retrovir) may compromise the efficacy of pyrimethamine-sulfadiazine treatment.
- Isolated chorioretinitis is treated as follows:
  - Pyrimethamine-sulfadiazine plus calcium leucovorin is given for 1 month.
  - If infection involves the macula or optic nerve head, steroids may be added.

DISPOSITION

- Patients taking pyrimethamine require complete blood cell count with platelets biweekly for signs of marrow suppression.
- Congenital infections require close ophthalmologic, audiologic, and neurologic follow-up, as well as serial brain imaging for signs of obstructing hydrocephalus.
- These children often need special services for developmental delays.

REFERRAL

Infectious disease specialist.

PEARLS & CONSIDERATIONS

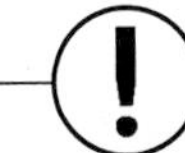

PREVENTION

- Patient education.
- Pregnant, prepregnant, and immunocompromised individuals should avoid handling cat litter boxes, sand, or garden soil and avoid handling or eating raw and undercooked meat. If performing these high-risk activities, always wear gloves and wash hands thoroughly with soap and water afterward. Keep cats indoors, and feed them only dry or canned prepared foods

SUGGESTED READINGS

Abramowicz M et al (eds): *Drugs for parasitic infections, In The Medical Letter On Drugs and Therapeutics.* New Rochelle, NY, The Medical Letter, August 2004, pp 1–12. Available at: http://www.medletter.com/freedocs/parasitic.pdf

Centers for Disease Control and Prevention (CDC). Available at www.cdc.gov (keyword search: toxoplasmosis).

AUTHOR: **D. STEVEN FOX, MD, MSc**

BASIC INFORMATION

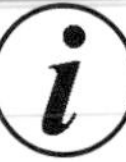

DEFINITIONS

Tracheomalacia and laryngomalacia are disorders of the trachea and larynx that cause them to be abnormally collapsible as a result of the loss of structural integrity or low muscle tone. In tracheomalacia, softening of the tracheal rings makes them unable to maintain airway patency, particularly during expiration. Tracheomalacia may also occur from bulging of the muscular posterior wall of the trachea anteriorly into the airway lumen. More commonly encountered, laryngomalacia is caused by the softness of laryngeal structures and is more likely to cause inspiratory symptoms. These conditions are closely related to the less commonly encountered tracheobronchomalacia and bronchomalacia.

ICD-9-CM CODES

519.1 Tracheomalacia, unspecified
748.3 Laryngomalacia or tracheomalacia, congenital

EPIDEMIOLOGY & DEMOGRAPHICS

- The two most common causes of stridor in infants
- Difficult to assess incidence because of the spectrum of disease
- Twice as common in males
- Presentation usually between birth and 2 months

CLINICAL PRESENTATION

- Usually begins within the first few days of life, rarely as late as 3 months
- Symptoms worst with upper respiratory infections, exertion, supine position, or feeding
- Often positional; prone position often associated with improved breathing abilities
- Often associated with wheezing, dyspnea, hoarseness, aphonia, or chronic cough
- In severe cases, possible poor weight gain and cyanotic episodes
- Coarse wheezing worse on expiration in tracheomalacia, worse on inspiration in laryngomalacia
- Stridor with laryngomalacia
- Prolonged expiratory phase with tracheomalacia
- Croupy cough with tracheomalacia
- In severe cases, chest retractions (possibly causing chest wall deformity)
- Apnea, bradycardia, cyanosis ("dying spell") with feeding seen (also seen in patients with esophageal anomaly repairs who have persistent tracheomalacia)

ETIOLOGY

- Several causes are possible.
    - A congenital process of uncertain origin that results in diffuse softness of the upper airway system
    - A congenital process of uncertain origin that results in a loss of the normal tone that resists collapse of structures into the airway
    - A congenital process brought about by abnormal development of the embryonic foregut and vasculature, which results in localized weakening of the tracheal rings
    - A weakness brought about by an impinging structure such as a vascular ring, tracheoesophageal fistula, atretic esophagus, or tracheostomy tube

DIAGNOSIS

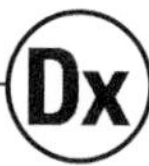

DIFFERENTIAL DIAGNOSIS

- Airway tumor
- Bifid epiglottis
- Brachial cleft cyst, thyroglossal duct remnant, mucous retention cyst
- Congenital goiter
- Dysfunctional suck or swallow
- Epiglottic or laryngeal atresia
- Esophageal atresia
- Gastroesophageal-induced edema of the larynx
- Intraluminal or laryngeal webs
- Laryngeal cartilaginous or vocal cord anomalies
- Laryngeal cysts
- Laryngeal edema from trauma or aspiration
- Laryngocele
- Laryngotracheoesophageal cleft
- Lymphoma
- Macroglossia
- Mandibular hypoplasia syndromes (e.g., Pierre-Robin syndrome)
- Neonatal tetany
- Paradoxical vocal cord motion
- Severe generalized laryngeal or tracheal chondromalacia (e.g., Ehlers-Danlos syndrome)
- Tracheobronchomalacia, bronchomalacia
- Tracheoesophageal fistula
- Vascular ring

WORKUP

- The diagnosis may be made presumptively by the history and physical examination results.
- Direct laryngoscopy may reveal laryngomalacia.
- Bronchoscopy may reveal the severity and extent of weakness in tracheomalacia.

IMAGING STUDIES

- Chest radiograph to exclude some vascular anomalies
- Echocardiography or computed tomography (CT) for severe cases
- Rarely, angiography, fluoroscopy, or cone CT to elucidate certain vascular or dynamic abnormalities

TREATMENT

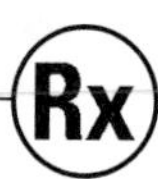

NONPHARMACOLOGIC THERAPY

Positioning may help breathing.

CHRONIC Rx

Antireflux treatment to minimize edema of the laryngeal structures if clinical signs of gastroesophageal reflux.

DISPOSITION

Verification of resolution is made by clinical examination.

REFERRAL

Depending on the cause, involvement of a radiologist, otolaryngologist, or cardiothoracic surgeon may be warranted.

PEARLS & CONSIDERATIONS

COMMENTS

- Most patients have a congenital form, which usually resolves by 18 months, although some predisposition to airway illnesses (e.g., croup) may persist for years.
- Presence of expiratory symptoms helps to differentiate tracheomalacia from laryngomalacia, which is usually inspiratory.

PATIENT/FAMILY EDUCATION

- Most cases spontaneously resolve.
- Most important parameters to monitor are respiratory status, feeding, and growth.

SUGGESTED READINGS

Altman KW et al: Congenital airway anomalies in patients requiring hospitalization. *Arch Otolaryngol Head Neck Surg* 125:525, 1999.

Altman KW et al: Congenital airway anomalies requiring tracheotomy: a profile of 56 patients and their diagnoses over a 9 year period. *J Pediatr Otorhinolaryngol* 41:199, 1997.

Bibi H et al: The prevalence of gastroesophageal reflux in children with tracheomalacia and laryngomalacia. *Chest* 119:409, 2001.

Downing GJ, Kilbride HW: Evaluation of airway complications in high risk preterm infants: application of flexible fiberoptic airway endoscopy. *Pediatrics* 95:567, 1995.

Geggel RL: Conditions leading to pediatric cardiology consultation in a tertiary academic hospital. *Pediatrics* 114:e409–e417, 2004.

Myer CM, Cotton RT: Airway obstruction. *In A Practical Approach to Pediatric Otolaryngology.* Chicago, Year Book Medical Publishers, 1988, pp 169–205.

Virtual Children's Hospital Electric Airway. Available at www.vh.org/pediatric/provider/pediatrics/ElectricAirway/Text/TracheoLaryngo.html

AUTHOR: **CHRISTOPHER F. BOLLING, MD**

BASIC INFORMATION

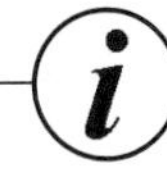

DEFINITION

Transfusion reactions include urticaria, fevers, and hemolysis caused by antibodies in the recipient directed against components of the transfused product, including antigens on the red blood cells (RBCs) themselves, plasma proteins, or antigens on contaminating white blood cells or platelets.

SYNONYMS

Acute hemolytic reactions
Delayed hemolytic reactions
Febrile nonhemolytic reactions
Transfusion-related acute lung injury
Urticarial reactions

ICD-9-CM CODE
999.8 Transfusion reaction

EPIDEMIOLOGY & DEMOGRAPHICS

- Febrile nonhemolytic reactions occur as often as 1 in 100 units of RBCs transfused.
- Urticarial reactions occur as often as 1 in 1000 units of RBCs transfused.
- Delayed hemolytic reactions occur as often as 1 in 1000 units of RBCs transfused.
- Transfusion-related acute lung injury has an estimated frequency of 1 in 10,000 units of RBCs transfused, and it is more likely to occur in the setting of sepsis.
- Acute hemolytic reactions occur 1 in 250,000 to 1 in 1,000,000 units of RBCs transfused and are usually caused by administrative or clerical errors (i.e., misidentification of the blood sample tested or misidentification of the recipient receiving the transfusion).

CLINICAL PRESENTATION

- Febrile nonhemolytic reactions can be associated with shortness of breath, pain in the chest, back or neck pain, fevers, tachypnea, and hypertension.
- Urticarial reactions can occur on a first transfusion and cause pruritus and hives.
- Delayed hemolytic transfusion reactions occur 3 to 14 days after a transfusion and are characterized by fever, jaundice, and hemoglobinuria.
- Transfusion-related acute lung injury causes dyspnea within 4 hours of a transfusion and is characterized by hypoxia and respiratory distress.
- Acute hemolytic reactions occur early in the course of the transfusion, with chills, chest and flank pain, nausea, dyspnea, tachycardia, hematuria, and hypotension, potentially leading to shock and death.

ETIOLOGY

- Febrile nonhemolytic reactions are caused by antibodies in the recipient directed against donor plasma proteins or antigens on contaminating white blood cells or platelets.
- Urticarial reactions are thought to be caused by recipient allergies to donor plasma proteins.

DIAGNOSIS

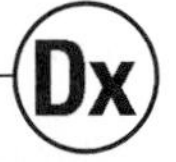

DIFFERENTIAL DIAGNOSIS

- The onset of fever in the setting of an RBC transfusion may be caused by the following:
  - Acute nonhemolytic reactions (clinically benign)
  - Acute hemolytic reactions (potentially life-threatening)
  - A coincidental febrile illness
  - Bacterial contamination of the transfused product

LABORATORY TESTS

- With the guidance of the blood bank, the workup should include the following:
  - A Coombs test is used to look for RBC antibodies.
  - Measure hemoglobin on pretransfusion and post-transfusion blood samples to look for evidence of ongoing hemolysis.
- Measure hemoglobinuria on a urine sample as evidence of acute hemolysis; a negative result rules out an acute hemolytic transfusion reaction.
- Delayed hemolytic transfusion reactions cause anemia (complete blood cell count) and an increase in indirect bilirubin but no hemoglobinemia.

TREATMENT

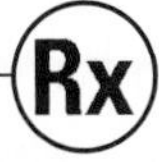

ACUTE GENERAL Rx

- Febrile nonhemolytic reactions: Stop the transfusion and assess for evidence of hemolysis. It is usually possible to complete the transfusion.
- Urticarial reactions: Stop the transfusion temporarily. If the urticaria improves within 30 minutes, resume the transfusion.
- Delayed hemolytic reactions: Treat the anemia with transfusion therapy.
- Transfusion-related acute lung injury: Provide supportive care, including ventilatory support as needed.

DISPOSITION

- Urticarial reactions: Monitor carefully for evidence of anaphylaxis, including laryngeal edema, bronchospasm, or vascular collapse.
- Delayed hemolytic reactions: Treat the anemia that develops.
- Transfusion-related acute lung injury: Admit to the hospital for supportive care.
- Acute hemolytic reactions: Admit to the hospital to monitor intake and output and renal function.

REFERRAL

- The blood bank should be notified immediately of any transfusion reactions.
- Chronic transfusion therapy of patients with thalassemia major or sickle cell disease should be managed by pediatric hematologists.

PEARLS & CONSIDERATIONS

COMMENTS

Patients with sickle cell disease who are on chronic transfusion programs are at increased risk for developing antibodies to minor group antigens that can cause delayed hemolytic transfusion reactions.

PREVENTION

Microaggregate filters can decrease the risk of nonhemolytic transfusion reactions by removing white blood cells.

PATIENT/FAMILY EDUCATION

- Obtain informed consent before transfusion therapy is initiated.
- Make the patient aware of the potential for a delayed transfusion reaction, which can cause anemia and jaundice.

SUGGESTED READINGS

Goodnough LT et al: Transfusion medicine. *N Engl J Med* 340:438, 1999.

Sloop GD, Friedberg RC: Complications of blood transfusion: how to recognize and respond to noninfectious reactions. *Postgrad Med* 98:159, 1995.

AUTHOR: **JAMES PALIS, MD**

BASIC INFORMATION

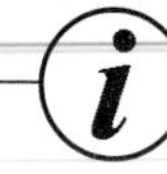

DEFINITION

Transient synovitis of the hip is an acute, nonspecific, self-limited inflammation of the synovial membrane of the hip joint.

SYNONYMS

Acute transient epiphysitis
Coxitis fugax
Coxitis serosa seu simplex
Intermittent hydrarthrosis
Irritable hip
Observation hip
Phantom hip
Reactive synovitis
Toxic synovitis
Transitory coxitis
Transitory synovitis

ICD-9-CM CODE
727.0 Transient synovitis of the hip

EPIDEMIOLOGY & DEMOGRAPHICS

- Transient synovitis is the most common cause of hip pain in children 3 to 8 years old.
- Average age of onset is 6 years, but it can occur in infancy through adolescence.
- A child has a 3% risk for developing transient synovitis at some point.
- There is no seasonal preference.
- Right and left hip involvement occurs equally.
- It is usually unilateral (<5% of cases are bilateral).
- The male-to-female ratio is 2:1.
- The incidence among blacks is much lower than in other groups.

CLINICAL PRESENTATION

History

- The presenting complaint is acute onset of unilateral hip pain in an otherwise healthy child.
- Pain typically occurs in the ipsilateral groin or hip area or is referred to the anterior thigh or knee.
- Associated limp, antalgic gait, or refusal to bear weight may be seen.
- Approximately 50% of patients present after 1 to 3 days of symptoms.

Physical Examination

- The affected extremity is held in a flexed and externally rotated position.
- There is restricted range of motion at the hip, especially with abduction and internal rotation.
- The child's temperature rarely exceeds 38°C (100.4°F).

ETIOLOGY

- No definitive cause is known for transient synovitis.
- Hypotheses include association with the following:
    - Active or recent infection
    - Allergic hypersensitivity
    - Preceding trauma

DIAGNOSIS

DIFFERENTIAL DIAGNOSIS

- Acute rheumatic fever
- Diskitis
- Juvenile rheumatoid arthritis
- Legg-Calvé-Perthes (LCP) disease
- Osteomyelitis of pelvis or femur
- Psoas abscess
- Septic arthritis
- Slipped capital femoral epiphysis (SCFE)
- Trauma
- Tuberculous arthritis
- Tumor

WORKUP

Transient synovitis is a diagnosis of exclusion.

LABORATORY TESTS

- Complete blood cell count with a differential cell count (usually less than 11,000/mm^3 and may be elevated in septic arthritis)
- Erythrocyte sedimentation rate (ESR) (usually less than 20 mm/hr)
- Blood culture if septic arthritis or osteomyelitis is suspected
- Joint aspiration if septic arthritis is suspected (>90% polymorphonuclear leukocytes in septic arthritis)
- Purified protein derivative if tuberculous arthritis is suspected

IMAGING STUDIES

- Anteroposterior and frog-leg view radiographs of the pelvis (usually normal; rule out LCP disease and SCFE)
- Ultrasound of the hip joint
    - Not routinely required
    - May be used to monitor resolution of effusion or in conjunction with needle aspiration of the joint

TREATMENT

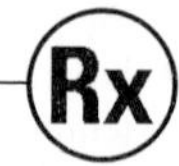

NONPHARMACOLOGIC THERAPY

- Bed rest and no weight bearing are recommended until the pain resolves and full joint motion returns, usually in 3 to 10 days.
- Rest is followed by period of abstinence from strenuous activities involving the hip.
- Routine joint aspiration is not recommended.
- Joint aspiration is done to rule out other causes of hip pain in questionable cases.

ACUTE GENERAL Rx

- Oral nonsteroidal anti-inflammatory agents may be given for pain relief.
- Avoid use of aspirin because of the association with Reye's syndrome.
- Antibiotics and steroids are not routinely recommended.

DISPOSITION

- If pain or a limp persists for more than 10 days, reevaluate.
- Check the child's temperature regularly to monitor for fever.
- Some authorities recommend repeat radiographs at 6 months to detect LCP disease.

PEARLS & CONSIDERATIONS

COMMENTS

- Suspect septic arthritis if the child has severe pain or spasm with movement of the hip, tenderness on palpation, temperature higher than 38°C (100.4°F), or ESR greater than 20 mm/hr. Presence of any two of these criteria is 95% sensitive and 91% specific for septic arthritis.
- Use the clinical prediction rule to differentiate between septic arthritis and transient synovitis. With a history of fever (>38.5°C), no weight-bearing, ESR greater than 40 mm/hr, and serum white blood cell count of more than 12,000 cells/mm^3, the predicted probability of septic arthritis is 93% to 99%.
- An association between the development of LCP disease and transient synovitis has been reported (range, 0% to 17%; average 1.5%).

PATIENT/FAMILY EDUCATION

- Noncompliance with the treatment regimen is associated with a longer duration of symptoms and increased risk for recurrence.
- Twenty-one-year follow-up in some studies has shown that the radiologic changes are not associated with functional limitations.

SUGGESTED READINGS

Kocher MS et al: Validation of a clinical prediction rule for the differentiation between septic arthritis and transient synovitis of the hip in children. *J Bone Joint Surg Am* 86:1629, 2004.

Twee TD: Transient synovitis as a cause of painful limps in children. *Curr Opin Pediatr* 12:48, 2000.

AUTHOR: **INDRA KANCITIS, MD**

BASIC INFORMATION

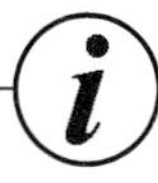

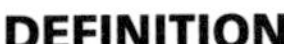

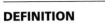

DEFINITION

Transposition of the great arteries (TGA) is defined by a discordant ventriculoarterial connection in which the aorta originates from the right ventricle and the pulmonary artery arises from the left ventricle, resulting in systemic and pulmonary circulations in parallel rather than in series.

SYNONYMS

Complete transposition
D-transposition
Transposition of the great vessels (TGV)

ICD-9-CM CODE
745.1 Transposition of the great arteries

EPIDEMIOLOGY & DEMOGRAPHICS

- The incidence is 3 cases per 10,000 live births. TGA occurs in 2.5% to 5.0% of infants born with congenital heart disease.
- TGA usually is sporadic and nonfamilial. It has a male-to-female ratio of 2:1.
- This is the most common type of cyanotic cardiac malformation in the first month of life.
- Some form of communication between the systemic and pulmonary circulations (e.g., patent foramen ovale, fossa ovalis atrial defect, ventricular defect, patent ductus arteriosus [PDA]) is essential for early survival.
- The mortality rate is greater than 90% by 1 year in untreated patients.
- In simple transposition, there is a patent foramen ovale and a PDA, which subsequently close.
- Associated defects include the following:
  - Ventricular septal defect (VSD): 20%
  - Large atrial septal defect: 10%
  - VSD and pulmonary stenosis: 5%
- Extracardiac malformations are uncommon and usually minor.

CLINICAL PRESENTATION

History
- Generally no interference with fetal well-being
- Cyanosis: may be mild initially but rapidly progresses
- Tachypnea and exertional dyspnea

Physical Examination
- Cyanosis
- Tachypnea usually without but occasionally with dyspnea
- Single or narrowly split, accentuated second heart sound
- Usually no murmur unless pulmonary stenosis is present
- Otherwise normal, but with a large VSD as a complicating lesion, mild cyanosis with congestive heart failure developing at 2 to 6 weeks dominates the clinical picture

ETIOLOGY

An abnormality of conotruncal development is related to differential conal absorption and abnormal aortopulmonary septation.

DIAGNOSIS

DIFFERENTIAL DIAGNOSIS

- Cyanotic malformations (i.e., right-to-left shunting) of the heart with increased pulmonary blood flow
- Pulmonary hypertension of the newborn

LABORATORY TESTS

- Blood gas determinations reveal hypoxemia and a low-normal carbon dioxide tension (e.g., 32 to 35 mm Hg).
- Electrocardiogram reveals normal right ventricular dominance in neonates.

IMAGING STUDIES

- Chest radiograph reveals an abnormal silhouette.
  - Egg-on-side pattern
  - Narrow pedicle
  - No visible conus
  - Increased pulmonary blood flow
  - Mild cardiomegaly
  - Lung hyperinflation
- Echocardiography reveals the following:
  - Side-by-side great vessels
  - Anterior aorta arising from the right ventricle
  - Posterior pulmonary artery from the left ventricle
  - Size, patency of fossa ovalis, ductus
  - Associated lesions: VSD, pulmonary valve stenosis
  - Distribution of coronary arteries
- Catheterization or angiography is done if questions persist about the coronary artery distribution or pattern or associated anomalies.

TREATMENT

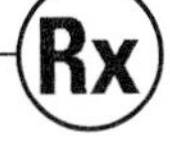

ACUTE GENERAL Rx

- Prostaglandin E_1 infusion to maintain ductal patency
- Balloon atrial septostomy if a restrictive atrial communication is present
- Early arterial switch procedure (i.e., great arteries and coronary arteries) within the first 2 weeks of life
- Rarely, an atrial switch procedure (Mustard or Senning operation) because of a coronary artery pattern precluding coronary transfer

DISPOSITION

- Lifelong follow-up by a cardiologist is necessary.
- Lifelong infective endocarditis prophylaxis is needed.
- Short- and long-term survival after an arterial switch procedure is 95% or more.
- Postarterial switch problems are unusual, but late aortic insufficiency may occur.
- If an atrial switch procedure has been performed, there is a substantial risk for atypical atrial flutter and other atrial arrhythmias, sudden death, and right or systemic ventricular failure, with a cumulative survival rate of 80% at 20 years of follow-up.

REFERRAL

All patients with suspected TGA should be referred immediately to a pediatric cardiologist.

PEARLS & CONSIDERATIONS

COMMENTS

- Suspect TGA in an infant with deep cyanosis, increased pulmonary blood flow, and an unusual cardiac silhouette.
- Arterial saturation is related to the size of the atrial communication and the amount of pulmonary blood flow.

PATIENT/FAMILY EDUCATION

- The risk of recurrence is very low.
- Intelligence after an early arterial switch should be in the normal range.
- This malformation may preclude some competitive sports as the child grows.
- Local chapters of Helping Hearts or related parental organizations provide support and information.

SUGGESTED READINGS

Helbing WA et al: Long-term results of atrial correction for transposition of the great arteries. *J Thorac Cardiovasc Surg* 108:363, 1994.
Karl TR et al: Arterial switch operation. *Tex Heart Inst J* 24:322, 1997.
Kirklin JW et al: Clinical outcomes after the arterial switch operation for transposition. *Circulation* 86:1501, 1992.
Rigby ML, Chan K-Y: The diagnostic evaluation of patient with complete transposition. *Cardiol Young* 1:26, 1991.

AUTHOR: **J. PETER HARRIS, MD**

BASIC INFORMATION

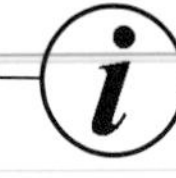

DEFINITION

Trichomoniasis is an infection of the genitourinary system (i.e., vagina, urethra, and periurethral glands) with the flagellated protozoa *Trichomonas vaginalis.*

SYNONYM

Trich
Trich vaginitis (TV)

ICD-9-CM CODES
131.0 Urogenital trichomoniasis
131.01 Trichomonal vulvovaginitis
131.02 Trichomonal urethritis

EPIDEMIOLOGY & DEMOGRAPHICS

- Prevalence among teenagers varies from 8% to 34%.
- Peak prevalence occurs between 16 and 35 years of age.
- Onset of symptoms varies from several days to weeks.
- An estimated 7.4 million new cases occur each year in men and women in the United States.

CLINICAL PRESENTATION

History

- Perineal pruritus (60% to 75%)
- Bothersome and irritating vaginal discharge (50%)
- Dysuria (20%)
- Dyspareunia
- Asymptomatic (up to 25% of females and 90% of males)

Physical Examination

- Frothy gray, green, or yellow vaginal discharge of various consistencies (pH >4.5)
- Diffuse vulvitis
- Colpitis macularis or "strawberry spots"—(i.e., petechiae on the cervix) not always present

ETIOLOGY

- Sexually transmitted infection by the protozoan *T. vaginalis*
- Evidence showing nonsexually transmitted infections can occur with trichomonads surviving in wet sponges or towels for up to 1.5 hours

DIAGNOSIS

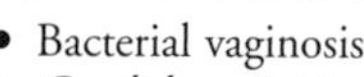

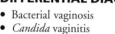

DIFFERENTIAL DIAGNOSIS

- Bacterial vaginosis
- *Candida* vaginitis
- *Chlamydia* cervicitis
- Gonococcal cervicitis
- Nongonococcal urethritis
- Nonspecific vaginitis

LABORATORY TESTS

- Wet-mount microscopy has a sensitivity of approximately 60% to 70%. This is the most practical means for rapid diagnosis.
- Culture methods (gold standard) have a sensitivity of 95%, and results are available in 3 to 7 days.
- In-pouch TV culture system has a sensitivity of 85.7%; it is easier and faster than the ordinary culture method.
- Pap smear has a sensitivity of 33% to 79%; it is unreliable because of the high false-positive rate.
- Immunofluorescence methods have a sensitivity of 85% and specificity of 99%. Enzyme immunoassay has a sensitivity of 82% and specificity of 73%.

TREATMENT

ACUTE GENERAL Rx

- First-line treatment with metronidazole (2 g taken orally one time) has an approximate 90% cure rate.
- Alternative therapy consists of metronidazole (500 mg taken orally twice daily for 7 days) which has an approximate 90% cure rate.
- Another alternative therapy is metronidazole vaginal gel (one applicator used intravaginally twice daily for 5 days) which has an approximate 50% cure rate.

CHRONIC Rx

- If infection continues, repeat treatment with a 7-day course of metronidazole and perform culture for sensitivities.
- For treatment failure, use metronidazole (2 g taken orally once daily for 5 days).

DISPOSITION

A follow-up visit is necessary if patients remain or become symptomatic.

REFERRAL

For persistent infection, consider referral to a specialist.

PEARLS & CONSIDERATIONS

COMMENTS

- If untreated in pregnancy, ongoing infection is associated with premature rupture of the membranes, postpartum endometritis, prematurity, and low birth weight.
- There is no evidence of teratogenesis or mutagenesis associated with metromidazole use during pregnancy.
- Single-dose therapy is associated with more side effects than longer treatment regimens.

PREVENTION

Safe sex practices include abstinence from sex and condom use with sexual contact to prevent contracting sexually transmitted diseases.

PATIENT/FAMILY EDUCATION

- Trichomoniasis increases the risk of human immunodeficiency virus (HIV) transmission.
- Patients who are infected with HIV should receive the same treatment as uninfected patients.
- Sexual contacts must be treated (2 g of metronidazole taken orally in a single dose).
- While taking metronidazole, patients must not drink alcohol, which can cause a disulfiram-like reaction (e.g., abdominal cramping, nausea, vomiting).

SUGGESTED READINGS

Centers for Disease Control and Prevention (CDC): Sexually transmitted diseases treatment guidelines 2002. *MMWR Morb Mortal Wkly Rep* 51(RR-6):6, 2002.

Centers for Disease Control and Prevention (CDC). Available at www.dpd.cdc.gov/dpdx/HTML/Trichomoniasis.htm

Emans SJ: Vulvovaginal complaints in the adolescent. *In* Emans SJ et al (eds): *Pediatric and Adolescent Gynecology,* 4th ed. Philadelphia, Lippincott, 1998, 423–456.

Forna F, Gulmezoglu AM: Interventions for treating trichomoniasis in women [review]. *Cochrane Database Syst Rev* (4):CD000218, 2004.

Patel SR et al: Systematic review of diagnostic tests for vaginal trichomoniasis. *Infect Dis Obstet Gynecol* 8:248, 2000.

AUTHOR: **NICOLE L. MIHALOPOULOS, MD, MPH**

BASIC INFORMATION

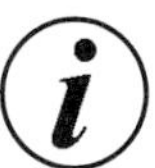

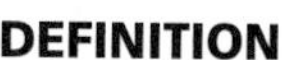

DEFINITION

Tuberculosis (TB) is a disease characterized by active replication of *Mycobacterium tuberculosis* complex. Children with pulmonary TB have chest radiographic changes and may or may not have clinical symptoms or physical examination abnormalities. Latent TB infection (LTBI) is an infection with *M. tuberculosis*, but the organism is in a latent or dormant state. The patient has a skin test result that is positive for TB but a normal chest radiograph and no signs or symptoms of tuberculosis.

SYNONYMS

Consumption
LTBI
Scrofula (i.e., mycobacterial disease in a peripheral lymph node)
TB

ICD-9-CM CODES

010.01 Primary tuberculosis (often used to code for LTBI)
011.6 Tuberculosis pneumonia (any form)
012.1 Tuberculosis of intrathoracic lymph nodes
017.2 Peripheral scrofula
795.5 Positive tuberculosis TB skin test (TST) without active tuberculosis (nonspecific)
V01.1 Exposure to active tuberculosis

EPIDEMIOLOGY & DEMOGRAPHICS

- One third of the world's population is infected with *M. tuberculosis.*
  - Incidence is highest in Asia, Africa, Eastern Europe, and Latin America.
  - Prevalence of infection increases incrementally with age (i.e., with accumulated risk of exposure).
- Active tuberculosis after infection is highest in the first year of life.
  - Children younger than 1 year old have a 40% risk of developing active disease if infected.
  - This is in contrast to the population as a whole, who have only a 10% lifetime risk of reactivation to active disease.
- Other populations at increased risk of activation after infection:
  - Adolescents (especially girls)
  - Recently exposed or infected individuals (50% of the risk of activation is in the first 2 years of infection)
  - Recent immigrants (<5 years in the United States)
  - Those with various immunocompromising medical conditions (e.g., human immunodeficiency virus [HIV] infection, cancer, chronic immunosuppressive therapy, diabetes mellitus, renal failure)
- In the United States, most children with TB are foreign born, children of immigrant families, and other minorities.
- Of 922 U.S. children younger than 15 years and diagnosed with TB in 2003, 432 (47%) were Hispanic, 118 (13%) were Asian, and 261 (28%) were black.

CLINICAL PRESENTATION

- More than 50% of U.S. children diagnosed with active TB are asymptomatic. Most are identified because they were evaluated after known exposure to a contagious adolescent or adult with active pulmonary or laryngeal TB.
- Symptomatic children may have sluggish weight gain or weight loss, cough, fever, malaise, bone or joint pain, or symptoms of meningitis.
- Physical examination abnormalities are scant in children with pulmonary TB. Even children with impressive radiographic changes may have only modest lung findings on examination.
  - Infants are more likely to have fever, rales, and increased work of breathing.
  - Adolescents have disease more typical of an adult presentation, with fever, cough, weight loss, night sweats, and rales with decreased breath sounds, dullness to percussion, or egophony.
- Lymphadenopathy is the most common extrapulmonary finding.
  - Intrathoracic lymphadenopathy is common and is symptomatic only if there is significant compression on a bronchus or erosion through the bronchial wall (i.e., endobronchial TB).
  - Scrofula (i.e., peripheral mycobacterial lymphadenopathy) caused by TB is more often found in older children. It most typically occurs in the cervical node chains and is characterized by gradual lymph node enlargement, skin discoloration, skin thinning, and eventual skin breakdown.
- Meningitis and military TB are the next most common sites of extrapulmonary TB and are more often associated with fever and systemic symptoms. Meningitis caused by TB is more indolent than that caused by other bacteria and viruses.
- TB can occur in other body parts, including bone, joints, skin, and kidneys.

ETIOLOGY

- Inhalation of *M. tuberculosis* causes most TB cases.
- Much less commonly, ingestion of unpasteurized milk products containing *M. bovis* causes TB (with a propensity to cause lymphatic disease).
- Rarely, newborns may be infected congenitally or during the birth process.

DIAGNOSIS

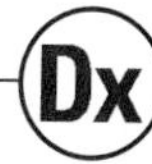

DIFFERENTIAL DIAGNOSIS

- Community acquired pneumonia
  - Bacterial pneumonia, including lung abscess and necrotizing pneumonia
  - Viral pneumonia
- Intrathoracic lymphadenopathy
  - Coccidiomycosis
  - Other fungal infections
  - Viral infections
  - Nontuberculous mycobacterial infections
  - Malignancies
- Subacute peripheral adenopathy
  - Scrofula caused by nontuberculous mycobacteria
  - Cat-scratch disease
- Meningitis
  - Bacterial
  - Viral
  - Fungal

WORKUP

- Tuberculin skin test (TST) performed by the Mantoux method and read by an experienced clinician 48 to 72 hours later for induration.
- Interpretation should be based on risks of exposure or risks for active disease.
- The TST is considered positive at an induration greater than 5 mm for the following groups:
  - Children or adolescents in close contact with a known or suspected infectious case of TB
  - Children or adolescents with suspected TB disease (i.e., finding on the chest radiograph consistent with active or previously active TB; clinical evidence of TB disease)
  - Children or adolescents who are immunosuppressed (e.g., receiving immunosuppressive therapy, with immunosuppressive conditions such as HIV infection)
- The TST is considered positive at an induration of more than 10 mm for children or adolescents at increased risk of disseminated disease:
  - Those younger than 4 years
  - Those with concomitant medical conditions (e.g., Hodgkin's disease, lymphoma, diabetes mellitus, chronic renal failure, malnutrition)
  - Children or adolescents at increased risk for exposure to cases of TB disease
  - Those born in a country with a high prevalence of TB
  - Those who travel to a country with a high prevalence of TB
  - Those with parents born in a country with a high prevalence of TB

- Those frequently exposed to adults with risk factors for TB disease (e.g., adults who are HIV infected or homeless, users of illicit drugs, those who are incarcerated, migrant farm workers)
- The TST is considered positive at an induration of more than 15 mm for children older than 4 years with no risk factors.
- Children with no risk factors for TB and without clinical concern for TB should not be skin tested.
- Twenty percent of children with active TB have negative TB skin test results at the time of presentation. Infants and children with disseminated disease are more likely to have a false-negative TST result.

LABORATORY TESTS

- HIV serology should be performed for any individual diagnosed with active TB.
- For children too young to submit spontaneous or induced sputum for AFB smear and culture, first morning gastric aspirates provide the highest yield (but still less than 50% for three sequential specimens).
  - The first specimen collected has the very highest yield and should be undertaken very carefully.
  - See www.nationaltbcenter.edu for detailed instructions.
- Cerebrospinal fluid (CSF) should be collected for children suspected of having TB meningitis and is usually collected for children with miliary and congenital TB. CSF should be submitted for routine studies, as well as a generous volume for AFB smear, culture, and polymerase chain reaction.
- Cultures of other appropriate specimens (e.g., blood, urine, biopsy of lymph nodes, bone) should be collected in the event of extrapulmonary TB.
- Bronchoalveolar lavage (BAL) is reserved for patients for whom the diagnosis is not established and other diagnoses are entertained.

IMAGING STUDIES

- Frontal and lateral chest radiographs with best possible technique and expert interpretation are required for all cases of positive TST and suspected TB. Radiographic abnormalities include the following:
  - Infiltrate in any lobe
  - Enlarged lymph nodes (hilar, mediastinal, paratracheal are most common)
  - Atelectasis, particularly associated with an obstructive lymph node
  - Cavities, most commonly in adolescents
  - Pleural effusion, more common in adolescents
  - Isolated calcified granulomata: *not* findings of active TB; frequently seen in LTBI
- Computed tomography is most appropriate for extrapulmonary TB and cases of pulmonary disease for which the diagnosis of TB is uncertain.

TREATMENT

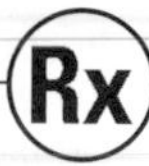

NONPHARMACOLOGIC THERAPY

- Treatment of active tuberculosis should be undertaken by or in close consultation with a pediatric TB expert.
- Patients thought to have active TB should be reported to the local health jurisdiction within 1 working day.
- Every effort should be made to identify the source case and to collect cultures to ascertain susceptibility results and to guide therapy.

ACUTE GENERAL Rx

- Treatment of LTBI is indicated for all children and adolescents.
- First-line treatment is 9 months of daily isoniazid (INH): 270 doses within a 12 month period.
- Rifampin (RIF) is given daily for 6 months in the event of known INH-resistant, RIF-susceptible disease or in the event of severe INH intolerance.
- Most children tolerate INH very well and overcome mild side effects.
  - Use tablets (crushed or fragmented into vehicle if needed) rather than the liquid.
  - Dose at bedtime.
  - Anticipate an early period of mild gastrointestinal upset.
- Children should be monitored monthly for compliance, signs and symptoms of active TB, and evidence of toxicity.
  - Hepatotoxicity is rare in children, and routine liver function testing is not indicated.
  - Families should look for early symptoms of hepatotoxicity (i.e., anorexia, malaise, and abdominal pain).
  - Patients should stop INH and report for evaluation if symptoms of hepatotoxicity develop.
- Vitamin B_6 supplementation is required only for exclusively breastfed infants, children who are malnourished or take a milk- and meat-deficient diet, or those with symptoms of peripheral neuropathy.
- Concurrent use of some antiepileptic drugs may affect drug levels and the risk for toxicity.
- For treating active TB in most parts of the United States, rates of INH resistance exceeds 4%.
  - Empirical therapy with four TB drugs is indicated after culture collection.
  - INH, RIF, pyrazinamide, and ethambutol are usually given daily for 2 months by directly observed therapy (DOT).
  - Patients are monitored for treatment adherence, toxicity, and complications.
  - If the patient is doing well clinically, a chest radiograph should be repeated at 2 months.
- If the radiograph is improved (or not worse), adherence is good, and the isolate is pan-susceptible, the patient should complete 6 months of therapy with INH and RIF twice weekly by DOT.
- If the radiographic picture has worsened, the following possibilities should be considered in consultation with an expert in pediatric TB:
  - Poor adherence
  - Drug-resistant TB
  - Malabsorption
  - Mechanical obstruction by a lymph node leading to collapse or postobstructive pneumonia
  - Incorrect diagnosis of TB
  - Intercurrent disease with community-acquired pneumonia or reactive airways disease
- Extrapulmonary TB sometimes requires longer therapy, as does drug-resistant TB, and expert consultation is all the more important.

DISPOSITION

- Serial monitoring includes the following:
  - Obtain a repeat chest radiograph at 2 months into treatment.
  - Oversee the continuation phase to finish 6 months of therapy (usually with INH and RIF twice weekly by DOT).
  - Obtain another chest radiograph at the completion of therapy (COT).
  - If the COT radiograph is normal, the patient can be followed serially by the primary caregiver for signs and symptoms of TB.
  - If the COT radiograph is significantly better but not normal (more than one half of pediatric TB radiographs are not normal at the end of successful therapy), repeat the radiograph at 4 months and 1 year after therapy is completed. If the radiograph continues to improve, the patient can be followed symptomatically during well-child care. If the chest radiograph worsens, consult a pediatric TB expert.

REFERRAL

Children with active TB should be managed by the most expert physician or clinic available.

PEARLS & CONSIDERATIONS

COMMENTS

- TB skin tests should be used to screen only children at high risk for infection or disease.
- All children diagnosed with LTBI deserve treatment.
- A negative skin test result does not rule out active TB disease.
- The diagnosis of active TB is based on clinical, radiographic, and demographic information. A positive TB culture from sputum or gastric aspirate definitively diagnoses

active TB, but a negative culture *never* rules out active TB.

PREVENTION

- Two strategies are used to prevent TB in children.
  - Routine risk factor screening is done by pediatric providers at each well-child visit; TB skin testing is done only for at risk children and as part of complete evaluation and treatment of infected children.
  - The most productive and effective prevention of TB in children is prompt diagnosis and treatment of adults with active TB.
    - Assessment of young children exposed to individuals with active TB includes TB skin testing, focused history, physical examination, and chest radiography.
    - Children identified during this process with active TB are treated promptly with multidrug therapy.
    - Children with LTBI are treated with INH to prevent development of active TB.
- Young children exposed to a contagious case of TB without active TB and with a negative skin test result frequently deserve prophylactic therapy to treat early LTBI and prevent rapid advancement to active TB.
  - These children should undergo repeat TST 3 months after the source case is not contagious or contact is broken.
  - If the skin test result is still negative, the INH therapy can be stopped.
  - If the skin test result has converted to positive, 9 months of INH treatment for LTBI should be completed.

PATIENT/FAMILY EDUCATION

Because of fears and misconceptions, families of children with active TB require extensive education and counseling.

SUGGESTED READINGS

Francis J: Curry National Tuberculosis Center. Available at www.nationaltbcenter.edu

Loeffler AM: Pediatric tuberculosis. *Semin Respir Infect* 18:272, 2003.

Pediatric Tuberculosis Collaborative Group: Targeted tuberculin skin testing and treatment of latent tuberculosis infection in children and adolescents. *Pediatrics* 114:1175, 2004.

AUTHOR: **ANN M. LOEFFLER, MD**

BASIC INFORMATION

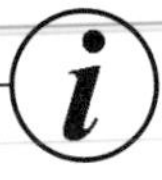

DEFINITION

Tuberous sclerosis (TS) is a neurocutaneous syndrome inherited in an autosomal dominant fashion. It is characterized by skin lesions (angiofibromas, hypopigmented macules), tumors (hamartomas) of the nervous system (cortical tubers, subependymal nodules, giant cell astrocytomas), and seizures. Kidney cysts and tumors (angiomyolipomas), cardiac tumors (rhabdomyomas), pulmonary cystic and fibrotic disease, and rectal polyps may also be seen.

SYNONYMS

Bourneville's disease
Epiloia

ICD-9-CM CODE
759.5 Tuberous sclerosis

EPIDEMIOLOGY & DEMOGRAPHICS

- Estimated prevalence of 1 in 6000 newborns
- Occurs in all races and ethnic groups, and in both genders
- The second most common neurocutaneous syndrome seen in children (after neurofibromatosis)
- Autosomal dominant inheritance but two thirds of cases are sporadic and represent new mutations

CLINICAL PRESENTATION

- Seizures, especially infantile spasms
- Developmental delay/mental retardation
- Unusual skin lesions
  - Ash leaf spots: hypopigmented macules, often elliptical in shape
  - Multiple café au lait spots in many patients as well
  - Adenoma sebaceum: facial angiofibromas less than 0.5 cm in diameter, pink to red in color, seen in bilaterally symmetric distribution on the face around the nose and cheeks
  - Shagreen patch: large patch of fused fibromas on the trunk in approximately 25% of patients with TS
  - Ungual fibromas: fleshy growths along the nailbed
  - Polygonal hypopigmented macules ("thumbprints"): most common but least specific skin lesions
  - Confetti-type hypopigmented macules pathognomonic for TS
    - *Note:* Visualization of all hypopigmented skin lesions is enhanced by ultraviolet/Wood's lamp illumination
- Teeth: characteristic diffuse small pits in the enamel
- Eye
  - Hypopigmented areas in the iris occasionally seen
  - Whitish yellow choroidal hamartomas around the optic nerve head on funduscopic examination
- Heart: symptoms of congestive heart failure possible (rare)
- Kidney: hypertension or hematuria (rare)
- Lungs: difficulty breathing, rales (rare)

ETIOLOGY

- Caused by mutations in one of two genes: TSC1 and TSC2.
- Only one of the genes needs to be affected for TS to be present.
- The TSC1 gene, discovered in 1997, is on chromosome 9 and produces a protein called *hamartin.*
- The TSC2 gene, discovered in 1993, is on chromosome 16 and produces the protein *tuberin.*
- Scientists believe these proteins act as tumor growth suppressors, agents that regulate cell proliferation and differentiation.

DIAGNOSIS

DIFFERENTIAL DIAGNOSIS

- Neurofibromatosis
- Incontinentia pigmenti
- Linear sebaceous nevus syndrome
- Neurocutaneous melanosis

WORKUP

- In most cases the first clue to recognizing TS is the presence of seizures or delayed development.
- In other cases, the first sign may be the characteristic skin lesions.
- Diagnosis of the disorder is based on a careful clinical examination in combination with imaging studies. Doctors should carefully examine the skin for the wide variety of skin features, the fingernails and toenails for ungual fibromas, the teeth and gums for dental pits or gum fibromas, and the eyes for hypopigmented areas or retinal hamartomas. A Wood's lamp or ultraviolet light may be used to locate the hypomelanotic macules which are sometimes hard to see on infants and individuals with pale or fair skin.
- In infants TS may be suspected if the child has cardiac rhabdomyomas or seizures (infantile spasms) at birth.
- Diagnostic criteria for TS according to a 1998 consensus panel convened by the National Institutes of Health and Tuberous Sclerosis Alliance are listed in Table 1-19.

LABORATORY TEST

No current genetic testing is widely available.

IMAGING STUDIES

- Computed tomography (CT) or magnetic resonance imaging (MRI) of the brain
- Ultrasound of the heart, liver, and kidneys, which may show tumors in those organs

TREATMENT

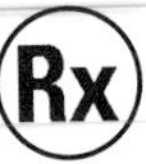

NONPHARMACOLOGIC THERAPY

- Educational and behavioral therapies are important in the management of developmental delays and mental retardation.
- Surgery, including dermabrasion and laser treatment, may be useful for treatment of skin lesions.
- Surgical treatment for nervous system or other tumors is usually not undertaken until symptoms from a growing tumor appear.

ACUTE GENERAL Rx

No specific or curative treatment for TS is available.

CHRONIC Rx

Medical treatment of seizures and other complications is the same as if TS were not present.

DISPOSITION

- The prognosis for individuals with TS depends on the severity of symptoms. Those individuals with mild symptoms generally do well and live long productive lives, while individuals with the more severe form may have serious disabilities or complications, even death.
- With appropriate medical care, most individuals with the disorder can look forward to normal life expectancy.
- Because TS is a lifelong condition, individuals need to be regularly monitored by a doctor to make sure they are receiving the best possible treatments.
- Developmental status and school performance should be followed closely. Neurodevelopmental testing should be considered at school entry for children who have not yet been tested.
- In persons with a diagnosis of TS, brain MRI is generally recommended every 1 to 3 years.
- Renal imaging is also recommended periodically.

REFERRAL

- Due to the many varied symptoms of TS, care by a clinician experienced with the disorder is recommended.
- Most children with TS are referred to a neurologist. Other subspecialty referrals, including cardiology, nephrology, dermatology, and neurosurgery, may be warranted.

PEARLS & CONSIDERATIONS

COMMENTS

- About 25% of children with infantile spasms have TS.

TABLE 1-19 **Revised Diagnostic Criteria for Tuberous Sclerosis Complex**

Major Features	Minor Features
• Facial angiofibromas or forehead plaque	• Multiple randomly distributed pits in dental enamel
• Non-traumatic ungual or periungual fibroma	• Hamartomatous rectal polyps
• Hypomelanotic macules (more than three)	• Bone cysts
• Shagreen patch (connective tissue nevus)	• Cerebral white matter migration lines
• Multiple retinal nodular hamartomas	• Gingival fibromas
• Cortical tuber	• Non-renal hamartoma
• Subependymal nodule	• Retinal achromic patch
• Subependymal giant cell astrocytoma	• "Confetti" skin lesions
• Cardiac rhabdomyoma, single or multiple	• Multiple renal cysts
• Lymphangiomyomatosis	
• Renal angiomyolipoma	

Definite TS: Either 2 major features or 1 major feature with 2 minor features
Probable TS: One major feature and one minor feature
Possible TS: Either 1 major feature or 2 or more minor features

- Seizures occur in about 70% of people with TS.
- The eye findings, although helpful diagnostically, are not symptomatic.
- Dental pitting is seen in virtually all patients by the time they reach adulthood.
- Fifty percent to 60% of people with TS have learning and developmental problems ranging from mild areas of difficulty to severe disabilities (25%).
- Some children with TS, usually those who have a mental disability, are also diagnosed with autism. There appears to be a connection between TS and autism that is not understood. Current research is exploring this link.

PATIENT/FAMILY EDUCATION

- The risk of a child having TS if one parent is affected is 50%.
- Generally, the severity of various symptoms changes little over the years. If a child is mildly affected, the child is likely to remain mildly affected as he or she matures.
- Parents should be educated regarding the common manifestations of TS and the necessity for periodic screening.
- The Tuberous Sclerosis Alliance has resources and information for patients and families, including family support, financial planning, and self-advocacy. Web site: www.tsalliance.org
- Many cities and states have their own TS support groups. Neurologists often are aware of the support groups in the local area.

SUGGESTED READINGS

National Institute of Neurological Disorders and Stroke Tuberous Sclerosis Fact Sheet. Available at www.ninds.nih.gov/disorders/tuberous_sclerosis/detail_tuberous_sclerosis.htm

Tuberous Sclerosis Alliance. Available at www.tsalliance.org

AUTHOR: **JEFFREY M. KACZOROWSKI, MD**

BASIC INFORMATION

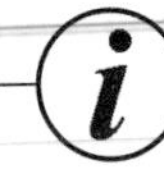

DEFINITION

Turner syndrome is a chromosomal condition in females in which the complete or partial absence of a second normal X chromosome results in short stature and ovarian failure.

SYNONYMS

Ulrich-Turner syndrome
XO genotype

ICD-9-CM CODE
758.6 Turner syndrome

EPIDEMIOLOGY & DEMOGRAPHICS

- The incidence is 1 in 1500 to 1 in 2500 liveborn females among all racial groups.
- It affects approximately 3% of all females conceived, with only about 1% of these conceptions surviving to term.

CLINICAL PRESENTATION

History

- Mild intrauterine growth retardation is followed by normal height increase from birth until approximately 3 years.
  - After age 3, there is a progressive decrease in growth velocity until 14 years of age.
  - Adolescent growth is prolonged because of delayed epiphyseal fusion. The final expected height typically falls between 142.0 and 146.8 cm (46 to 48 inches).
- Primary amenorrhea and infertility may occur.
- Prenatal diagnosis of Turner syndrome is becoming more common with increasing prenatal testing in advanced maternal age.
  - Turner syndrome is not associated with advanced maternal age per se.

Physical Examination

- All ages
  - Triangular faces
  - Ptosis, strabismus
  - Posteriorly rotated ears
  - Short stature
  - Shield chest, increased inter nipple distance
  - Short fourth metacarpal
  - Madelung deformity of the radius: cubitus valgus (increased carrying angle at the elbows)
  - Nail dysplasia
- Newborn period
  - Congenital lymphedema: puffy hands and feet, webbed neck
  - Low posterior hairline
- Infancy
  - Heart murmur
  - Decreased peripheral pulses and capillary refill
- Childhood
  - Short stature
  - Hypertension
- Adolescence
  - Delayed or absence of puberty
  - Pigmented nevi

ETIOLOGY

- With conventional chromosomal studies, about 50% of Turner syndrome patients show a 45,X pattern.
- Mosaicism of 45,X with other cell lines such as 46,XX, 46,XY, or 47,XXX are common.
- Structural abnormalities of an X chromosome (deletions, rings, or translocations), either isolated or mosaic with a 45,X or 46,XX cell line, are also seen.
- With modern cytogenetic techniques, mosaicism is increasingly being detected.
- The short stature in Turner syndrome appears to be caused by the absence of one copy of the SHOX gene, which is located on the short arm of the X chromosome.

DIAGNOSIS

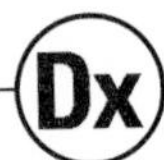

DIFFERENTIAL DIAGNOSIS

- Noonan syndrome affects both males and females and consists of Turner-like physical features, predominantly right-sided cardiac defects (e.g., pulmonic stenosis, asymmetric hypertrophy of the septum), and generally more significant developmental disabilities.
- Pure gonadal dysgenesis consists of a group of Mendelian disorders in which affected individuals are phenotypically female but may have 46,XX or 46,XY chromosomal pattern.
- Mixed gonadal dysgenesis is associated with the presence of a testis on one side and a streak gonad on the contralateral side. Most patients with this disorder have a 45,X/46,XY chromosomal pattern.
- An isolated SHOX gene defect results in short stature and the skeletal manifestation of Turner syndrome, but it is not associated with primary amenorrhea or lymphedema.

WORKUP

- Routine chromosome study
- Fluorescence in situ hybridization (FISH) or other DNA-based methods may be used to define more complex alterations.
- Cardiac evaluation including echocardiography
  - Aortic coarctation: approximately 20%
  - Bicuspid aortic valve: approximately 50%
- Endocrine evaluation
  - Primary hypothyroidism (10% to 30%), thyroiditis
  - Glucose intolerance
  - Delayed puberty and primary amenorrhea
- Renal ultrasound for anomalies
  - Horseshoe kidney
  - Ectopic kidneys
  - Double collecting system
- Prenatal diagnosis
  - Aided by ultrasound
    - Thickened nuchal folds
    - Cystic hygroma
    - Renal anomalies
    - Cardiac anomalies
    - Definitive diagnosis done by chromosomal analysis on chorionic villus or amniocytes

TREATMENT

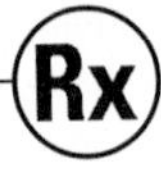

NONPHARMACOLOGIC THERAPY

- Support stocking for lymphedema
- Maintain physical activity to avoid obesity
- Education intervention as needed
- Repair of aortic coarctation if needed
- Ophthalmologic intervention for ptosis and strabismus if needed
- Plastic surgery
- Some families elect to have plastic surgery to correct dysmorphic features
- Myringotomy tube placement if needed
- Prophylactic gonadectomy for all women with Turner syndrome with a Y chromosome

ACUTE GENERAL Rx

- Growth hormone replacement therapy (usually with a weak anabolic agent such as oxandrolone) beginning between 2 to 5 years of age, until bone age exceeds 15 years
- Estrogen replacement beginning in adolescent years to promote the development of secondary sexual characteristics
- Thyroid replacement as needed
- Medication for attention deficit and hyperactivity may be needed

DISPOSITION

- Blood pressure monitoring
- Annual monitoring of thyroid function and glucose tolerance
- Monitoring of luteinizing hormone and follicle-stimulating hormone during adolescent years
- Annual check for scoliosis
- Hearing evaluation
- Monitoring for lymphedema, which may persist for months and even recur
- Monitoring for gastrointestinal bleeding resulting from mesenteric vascular abnormalities or inflammatory bowel disease
- Dietary management, exercise, and weight control
- Screen for learning disability, especially for deficits in attention, mathematical and visuospatial organization skills
- Psychological support for patient and family as needed
- Cardiac, otolaryngologic, ophthalmologic follow-up as needed

REFERRAL

- Cardiology
- Endocrine
- Genetics
- Developmental intervention as needed

- Nephrology, otolaryngology, ophthalmology, dermatology, plastic surgery as needed

PEARLS & CONSIDERATIONS

COMMENTS

- Because of the consistent presence of short stature and the variability of the other findings, which often manifest only during certain age windows, any girl with unexplained short stature should be evaluated for Turner syndrome by chromosome analysis.
- Approximately 10% of patients with Turner syndrome go through puberty spontaneously. The presence of pubic and axillary hair does not rule out primary ovarian failure.
- In prepubertal girls, the position of nipples lateral to the midclavicular line usually indicates increased inter-nipple distance.
- When Turner syndrome is diagnosed, cytogenetic results should be evaluated carefully for the presence of a covert Y chromosome.
    - DNA-based studies may be needed for this purpose.
    - The presence of a Y chromosome increases the risk for gonadoblastoma and dysgerminoma to 15% to 25%, necessitating prophylactic gonadectomy.
- Cheek-swab and Barr-body analysis are not acceptable for the diagnosis of Turner syndrome.
- There is a tendency for keloid formation in patients with Turner syndrome, which should be taken into account when plastic surgery or removal of pigmented nevi is considered.

PREVENTION

- Prophylactic antibiotics before dental procedure for patients with cardiac anomalies
- Aggressive treatment of middle ear disease to prevent conductive hearing loss

PATIENT/FAMILY EDUCATION

- For teenagers, sex education counseling should be done to emphasize that primary amenorrhea is not enough reason not to practice "safe sex."
- For late teens and young adults, counseling about modern reproductive technologies such as egg donation program should be done.
- Intelligence is usually normal except in patients with unusual chromosomal variants, such as a ring X chromosome.

SUGGESTED READINGS

American Academy of Pediatrics Committee on Genetics: Health supervision for children with Turner syndrome. *Pediatrics* 111:692, 2003.

Rosenfeld RG: *Turner Syndrome: A Guide for Physicians.* The Turner Syndrome Society, Genetic Mason Medical Communications, Inc., 1992.

Saenger P: Turner's syndrome. *N Engl J Med* 335:1649, 1996.

Turner Syndrome Society of Canada. Available at www.TurnerSyndrome.ca/

Turner Syndrome Society of the United States. Available at www.turner-syndrome-us.org/

AUTHOR: **CHIN-TO FONG, MD**

BASIC INFORMATION

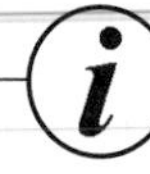

DEFINITION

Ureteropelvic junction obstruction (UPJO) is a congenital resistance to the transport of urine from the renal pelvis into the proximal ureter.

SYNONYM

Ureteral valves—upper

ICD-9-CM CODE
753.21 Congenital obstruction of ureteropelvic junction

EPIDEMIOLOGY & DEMOGRAPHICS

- Prenatal ultrasound diagnosis of hydronephrosis occurs in 1% of all births.
  - Approximately 50% of these patients have hydronephrosis at their postnatal examination.
- UPJO
  - Incidence is 1 per 20,000: sporadic, but familial tendency.
  - Male-to-female ratio is 2:1 to 4:1.
  - There is a 15% to 40% incidence with horseshoe ectopic kidney.
  - One third of patients with UPJO have the abnormality bilaterally.
    - Degree of obstruction varies between kidneys
  - Approximately 10% are associated with vesicoureteral reflux.

CLINICAL PRESENTATION

History
- Prenatal hydronephrosis
- Younger than 18 months old
  - Visible abdominal mass
  - Failure to thrive
  - Fever
  - Emesis
  - History of urinary tract infection
  - History of renal calculi
  - Hematuria
- Abdominal pain

Physical Examination
- Palpable abdominal mass (may transilluminate)
- Hypertension uncommon (0.1%)

ETIOLOGY

- The ureteropelvic junction (UPJ) is a normal site of relative narrowing of the urinary collecting system.
  - UPJOs are partial blockages that commonly result in some degree of hydronephrosis.
  - This hydronephrosis, in turn, may pose a risk to ultimate renal function.
  - Obstructions are dynamic and may regress, progress, or remain unchanged over time.
  - UPJOs may lie on a pathophysiologic continuum from the functionally irrelevant extrarenal pelvis, to the uniformly nonfunctioning multicystic dysplastic kidney (MCDK).
- Specific causes include:
  - Intrinsic narrowing: 75%
    - Aperistalsis
    - Smooth muscle deficiency
  - Ureterovascular tangles: 15%
  - High, abnormal ureteral insertion: 7%
  - Periureteral fibrosis: 3%
  - Ureteral valve: rare
  - Accessory renal artery may be coincident, but is not a sufficient causative agent.

DIAGNOSIS

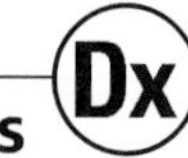

DIFFERENTIAL DIAGNOSIS

- Prenatal hydronephrosis
  - MCDK
  - Vesicoureteral reflux
  - Ureterovesical junction obstruction
  - Megacalycosis
  - Multiple renal cysts
- Abdominal mass
  - MCDK
  - Congenital mesoblastic nephroma
  - Wilms' tumor
  - Neuroblastoma

WORKUP

- Prenatally detected
  - Serum creatinine after 5 days of life to reflect baby's renal status

IMAGING STUDIES

- Ultrasound: renal and bladder
  - Hydronephrosis without ureterectasis should be present.
  - Assess for duplication anomaly (lower-pole UPJO is more common), parenchymal thickness, and presence of corticomedullary differentiation.
  - Hydronephrosis is graded from 0 to 4 using the Society for Fetal Urology (SFU) scale (see "Suggested Readings").
  - Early ultrasound, within first few days of life, may underestimate grading because of the relative decrease in urine output in the newborn.
  - Solid masses should be defined by this study.
- Nuclear medicine scanning
  - Radionuclide scans are used to assess relative function and drainage of the kidneys.
  - Technetium 99m-diethylenetriamine-pentaacetate (^{99m}Tc-DTPA) is filtered and therefore is used to calculate the glomerular filtration rate (relative function is calculated from this data).
  - "Well-tempered renogram" has been advocated by the SFU to provide some standardization and thus the ability to compare outcomes for advocated treatments (see link to SFU in "Suggested Readings" for reference and protocol).
  - MAG-3 is cleared primarily by tubular secretion, with a small component filtered.
    - This can be used to estimate renal plasma flow (relative function is calculated).
    - Furosemide administration is used to assess poor drainage.
    - Defines areas of parenchymal loss.
  - Technetium 99m-dimercaptosuccinic acid (^{99m}Tc-DMSA) and glucoheptonate bind to proximal tubular cells.
    - Assess relative functional parenchyma.
    - Furosemide administration is used to assess drainage.
    - Defines areas of parenchymal loss.
- Voiding cystourethrogram
  - 10% incidence of vesicoureteral reflux in UPJO series.

TREATMENT

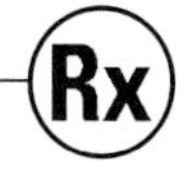

NONPHARMACOLOGIC THERAPY

- Observe the patient.
- Most cases of hydronephrosis, from prenatally detected UPJO, resolve upon continued follow-up postnatally.
- Some authors have advocated "aggressive observation" of all UPJOs.
  - Only one in four cases require surgery; requisite events include:
    - Symptoms
    - Gross loss of function
    - Urinary tract infections
  - Optimal observation should not allow a 10% rate of renal injury to be incurred.
  - Application of this approach should be with care, in the well-counseled family.

Surgical
- Pyeloplasty
  - The surgical principle is removal or bypass of the site of blockage.
  - Drains, splints, nephorostomy rubes (direct catheter drainage of the affected renal pelvis), and timing of repair are a matter of surgeon prefference.
  - This procedure is successful in more than 90% of patients treated.
  - Laparoscopic and robotic surgery are currently replicating "open-surgical" techniques effectively.
- Endopyelotomy
  - An incision is made at the site of blockage as visually defined through an endoscope or under fluoroscopy.
  - The instrument for incision may be inserted retrograde via the urethra/bladder/ureter or via a direct puncture into the renal pelvis through the kidney.
  - This procedure is successful in less than 80% of patients treated.
  - In cases of failed initial pyeloplasty, endopyelotomy is the procedure of choice and carries a success rate of up to 91%.

ACUTE GENERAL Rx

- Antibiotics
  - One in three children with UPJO will have an associated urinary tract infection at some point.

- Because the adverse effect of low-dose antibiotic prophylaxis is minimal, routine use of amoxicillin in neonates and nitrofurantoin or trimethoprim-sulfamethoxazole in infants is reasonable.
- Use of antibiotics in older children is best guided by cultures and manner of presentation.

DISPOSITION

- Follow-up is dictated by therapy.
- One of three functionally unobstructed kidneys will show persistent hydronephrosis.
- Long-term follow-up is mandatory in all children with UPJO, regardless of grade, to ensure renal preservation and no increase in obstruction.

REFERRAL

- Prenatal consultation with the pediatric urologist is highly encouraged.
- All patients with prenatal hydronephrosis should be evaluated by a pediatric urologist and those with bilateral findings (or UPJO in solitary kidneys) should be seen within 48 hours of birth.

PEARLS & CONSIDERATIONS

COMMENTS

- Approximately 33% of patients with kidneys with more than 12 mm of maximal renal pelvis diameter after 24 weeks of gestation require eventual pyeloplasty.
- Hematuria following minor trauma should bring UPJO into the differential.
- Abdominal pain with UPJO is localized to the kidney whether in an orthotopic or ectopic location.
- Renal dysplasia may be noted on ultrasound as small cysts or echogenic foci within the parenchyma. This may influence therapeutic decisions.

PATIENT/FAMILY EDUCATION

- The goal of therapy is to ensure optimal function of the involved kidney.
- The grade of hydronephrosis does not correlate with degree of obstruction.
- Laparoscopy and robotic surgery are becoming options for surgical repair under certain conditions.

SUGGESTED READINGS

Kim DS et al: Elastin content of the renal pelvis and ureter determines post-pyeloplasty recovery. *J Urol* 173(3):962, 2005.

Munver R et al: Laparoscopic pyeloplasty: history, evolution and future. *J Endourol* 18(8):748, 2004.

Nelson CP et al: Contemporary trends in surgical correction of pediatric ureteropelvic junction obstruction: data from the nationwide inpatient sample. *J Urol* 173(1):232, 2005.

Society for Fetal Urology (SFU). Available at www.fetalurology.org

Society of Pediatric Urology. Available at www.spu.org

AUTHORS: **ROBERT A. MEVORACH, MD, WILLIAM C. HULBERT, MD,** and **RONALD RABINOWITZ, MD**

BASIC INFORMATION

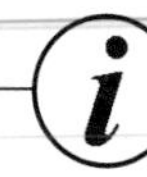

DEFINITION

Urethritis is inflammation of the urethra as a result of a variety of infectious and noninfectious causes.

SYNONYMS

Urethral inflammation
Urethral irritation

ICD-9-CM CODES
098.0 Gonococcal infection, acute, of lower genitourinary tract
098.2 Gonococcal infection, chronic, of lower genitourinary tract
099.3 Reiter's disease
099.40 Nonspecific urethritis
099.41 *Chlamydia trachomatis*

EPIDEMIOLOGY & DEMOGRAPHICS

- Urethritis is most common in the sexually active male; it is only occasionally seen in the prepubertal child.
- Gonococcal urethritis is the most commonly reported sexually transmitted disease in the United States, accounting for 35% of adolescent males and men evaluated for urethritis.
- The incidence of gonococcal urethritis is decreasing, but the incidence of nongonococcal urethritis (NGU) is increasing.

CLINICAL PRESENTATION

History
- Adolescents and older children: dysuria, itching, and discharge
- Sexual activity
- Young children and infants: crying concomitant with voiding, urinary retention
- Use of bubble bath, irritating soaps or lotions, non-cotton underwear, sexual abuse, poor hygiene in younger child

Physical Examination
- It is often difficult to differentiate gonococcal from nongonococcal urethritis based on symptoms and signs alone.
- Penile/urethral discharge, which is often purulent, mucoid, and yellow-green, is easily expressed; discharge may also be scant and clear.
- Erythematous, edematous urethral and periurethral tissues may be noted.

ETIOLOGY

- Infectious: local invasion of infectious (gonococcal or nongonococcal) organisms into urethral lining cells with subsequent host inflammatory response
  - Gonococcal urethritis is caused by *Neisseria gonorrhoeae.*
  - NGU is most commonly caused by *Chlamydia trachomatis;* less commonly it is caused by *Ureaplasma urealyticum* and *Mycoplasma genitalium.*
  - Approximately 20% to 30% of NGU cases are caused by organisms such as *Haemophilus* species, *Bacteroides* or other anaerobes, genital mycoplasmas, *Candida albicans, Trichomonas vaginalis,* herpes simplex virus, human papillomavirus, or pinworm infestation.
    - Genital infection with these organisms most commonly presents as urethritis in males and cervicitis in females.
- Noninfectious: physical (e.g., non-cotton underwear in young girls, sexual abuse) or chemical (e.g., bubble bath, soaps, lotions, powders) irritation

DIAGNOSIS

DIFFERENTIAL DIAGNOSIS

- Meatitis
- Balanitis
- Vaginitis
- Cervicitis

LABORATORY TESTS

- Document the presence of urethritis with any of the following:
  - Mucopurulent or purulent discharge in males
  - Gram stain of urethral discharge showing more than 5 white blood cells (WBCs) (preferred method of diagnosis) per oil immersion field on a gram-stained smear of urethral secretions
  - Positive leukocyte esterase test on first-void urine or microscopic exam of first-void urine with more than 10 WBCs per high-power field
  - Intracellular (within polymorphonuclear leukocytes) gram-negative diplococci in a gram-stained urethral discharge specimen for gonorrhea
    - Newer DNA amplification assays (polymerase chain reaction [PCR] and ligase chain reaction) for *N. gonorrhoeae* and *C. trachomatis* are largely replacing traditional cultures because of their greater sensitivity and ease and convenience of patient sample collection.
- For males with urethritis who have a purulent discharge:
  - Perform Gram stain on urethral discharge.
  - Send swab of discharge for PCR test for *N. gonorrhoeae* and *C. trachomatis.*
  - With both *N. gonorrhoeae* and *C. trachomatis,* treat for infection.
- For males with urethritis but no discharge:
  - Send first 15 mL of a first-voided urine for PCR test for *N. gonorrhoeae* and *C. trachomatis.*
  - Send urine for urinalysis and urine culture.
  - Defer therapy until test results for *N. gonorrhoeae* and *C. trachomatis* are available, except in patients unlikely to return for follow-up evaluation, in which case treatment should be given for both gonorrheal and chlamydial infection.
- If opted for, culture *N. gonorrhoeae* on Thayer-Martin medium/chocolate agar:
  - Males: proper culture is obtained by inserting a small, non-cotton swab 2 to 3 cm into the urethra and plating the specimen immediately onto appropriate culture media.
  - Females: proper culture is obtained by first wiping the exocervix and then placing a non-cotton swab into the cervical os and rotating the swab several times; the specimen is then immediately plated onto appropriate culture media.
- *C. trachomatis* culture: the swab is placed into *Chlamydia* transport media.
- Viral culture should be done for herpes simplex when suspected.

TREATMENT

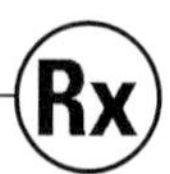

ACUTE GENERAL Rx

- Patients infected with *N. gonorrhoeae* are often coinfected with *C. trachomatis* and are most often treated for both organisms presumptively, especially when follow-up cannot be ensured.
- In populations in which coinfection rates are low, patients may be treated for gonorrhea and tested for *Chlamydia* if follow-up is ensured.
- Recommended regimens for the treatment of gonococcal urethritis are as follows:
  - Cefixime 400 mg orally in a single dose, *or*
  - Ceftriaxone 125 mg intramuscularly in a single dose, *or*
  - Ciprofloxacin 500 mg orally in a single dose, *or*
  - Ofloxacin 400 mg orally in a single dose, *or*
  - Levofloxacin 250 mg in a single dose
- Plus, if chlamydial infection is not ruled out:
  - Azithromycin 1 g orally in a single dose, *or*
  - Doxycycline 100 mg orally twice a day for 7 days
- Recommended regimens for the treatment of NGU are as follows:
  - Azithromycin 1 g orally in a single dose, *or*
  - Doxycycline 100 mg orally twice a day for 7 days
    - Alternative regimens include the following:
      - Erythromycin base 500 mg orally four times a day for 7 days, *or*
      - Erythromycin ethylsuccinate 800 mg orally four times a day for 7 days, *or*
      - Ofloxacin 300 mg orally twice a day for 7 days, *or*
      - Levofloxacin 500 mg once a day for 7 days

- Recommended regimens for the treatment of recurrent or persistent urethritis are as follows:
  - Metronidazole 2 g orally in a single dose, *plus*
  - Erythromycin base 500 mg orally four times a day for 7 days, *or*
  - Erythromycin ethylsuccinate 800 mg orally four times a day for 7 days
- Recommended regimens for the treatment of chlamydial infection in adolescents and adults are as follows:
  - Azithromycin 1 g orally in a single dose, *or*
  - Doxycycline 100 mg orally twice a day for 7 days
    - Alternative regimens include the following:
      - Erythromycin base 500 mg orally four times a day for 7 days, *or*
      - Erythromycin ethylsuccinate 800 mg orally four times a day for 7 days, *or*
      - Ofloxacin 300 mg orally twice a day for 7 days, *or*
      - Levofloxacin 500 mg orally for 7 days
- Recommended regimens for the treatment of chlamydial infection in children are as follows:
  - Children under 45 kg: erythromycin base 50 mg/kg/day orally divided four times daily for 10 to 14 days
  - Children who weigh more than 45 kg but who are younger than 8 years of age: azithromycin 1 g orally in a single dose
  - Children older than 8 years of age: azithromycin 1 g orally in a single dose, *or* doxycycline 100 mg orally twice a day for 7 days

REFERRAL

- Adolescent medicine specialist, especially in complicated cases
- Child protective services (social services) evaluation for possibility of sexual abuse in young children found to be infected with *N. gonorrhoeae* or *C. trachomatis*

PEARLS & CONSIDERATIONS

COMMENTS

- Most individuals with NGU are asymptomatic.
- Potential complications arising from urethritis may include epididymitis and Reiter's syndrome in males and pelvic inflammatory disease and infertility in females.

PATIENT/FAMILY EDUCATION

- Counsel patients that sexual activity is the most common mode of transmission.
- Each and every sexual contact of an infected individual needs to be evaluated and treated.
- Preventive measures that are most successful include abstinence, use of condoms, and good hygiene.

SUGGESTED READINGS

American Academy of Pediatrics: Chlamydia. *In* Pickering LK (ed): *Red Book 2003: Report of the Committee on Infectious Diseases,* 26th ed. Elk Grove Village, IL, American Academy of Pediatrics, 2003, pp 237–243.

Centers for Disease Control and Prevention: *2002 guidelines for treatment of sexually transmitted diseases.* MMWR Recommendations & Reports 51 (No. RR06): 1–80, May 10, 2002.

Centers for Disease Control and Prevention: Sexually Transmitted Diseases. Available at http://www.cdc.gov/od/owh/whstd.htm

Gaydos CA et al: Molecular amplification assays to detect chlamydial infections in urine specimens from high school female students and to monitor the persistence of chlamydial DNA after therapy. *J Infect Dis* 177:417, 1998.

Journal of the American Medical Association: Sexually Transmitted Disease Information Center. Available at www.ama-assn.org/special/std/treatmnt/guide/stdg3443.htm

Oh MK et al: High prevalence of *Chlamydia trachomatis* infections in adolescent females not having pelvic examinations: utility of PCR-based urine screening in an urban adolescent clinic setting. *J Adolesc Health* 21:80, 1997.

AUTHOR: **CYNTHIA CHRISTY, MD**

BASIC INFORMATION

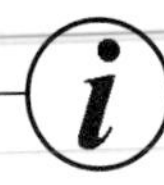

DEFINITION

Infection of the bladder or lower urinary tract is called *cystitis;* infection of the kidney or upper urinary tract is termed *acute pyelonephritis.*

SYNONYMS

Bladder infection
Cystitis
Kidney infection
Pyelonephritis

ICD-9-CM CODES
590.10 Acute pyelonephritis
595.0 Acute cystitis
599.0 Urinary tract infection, site not specific

EPIDEMIOLOGY & DEMOGRAPHICS

- Urinary tract infection (UTI) is the most common serious bacterial infection in febrile infants.
- Overall, prevalence is 5% in febrile infants.
- Prevalence is higher in young children when no apparent source of fever (no respiratory or gastrointestinal symptoms) is identified.
- High prevalence (17%) is seen in white girls less than 2 years of age with temperatures greater than 39°C.
- Uncircumcised boys have a fourfold higher risk than circumcised boys.
- Male infants younger than 2 months of age are more likely to develop a UTI than girls of the same age.
- In children 2 months to 2 years, girls have a fourfold higher risk than boys.

CLINICAL PRESENTATION

History

- Infants with UTI most likely to present with fever.
- Older children with UTI may report frequency, urgency, dysuria, or enuresis.
- Less common symptoms of UTI include:
  - Flank pain
  - Poor feeding
  - Vomiting
  - Failure to thrive
  - Abdominal pain
  - Jaundice

Physical Examination

- General appearance varies from normal to toxic appearance.
- Other signs of UTI include:
  - Fever
  - Shock
  - Irritability
  - Jaundice (neonate)
  - Costovertebral angle tenderness
  - Suprapubic tenderness

ETIOLOGY

- Organisms
  - *Escherichia coli* is responsible for 85%
  - Other gram-negative bacteria include *Klebsiella pneumoniae, Proteus* species, *Pseudomonas aeruginosa,* and *Enterobacter* species.
  - Gram-positive organisms (less common) include enterococci, staphylococci, and group B streptococci.
- Mechanisms: ascending infection
- Predisposing risk factors include:
  - Congenital anomalies (e.g., hydronephrosis, posterior urethral valves, vesicoureteral reflux)
  - Neurologic abnormalities (e.g., neurogenic bladder)
  - Dysfunctional elimination (which includes constipation and voiding dysfunction)
  - Indwelling catheters
  - Sexual activity

DIAGNOSIS

Dx

DIFFERENTIAL DIAGNOSIS

- Occult bacteremia
- Sepsis
- Other abdominal, pelvic, and retroperitoneal disease (e.g., acute gastroenteritis, appendicitis, pelvic inflammatory disease, vaginitis, cervicitis, urethritis)

WORKUP

Indications

- The presence of two or more of the following five variables should prompt a diagnostic evaluation:
  - Age under 1 year
  - White race
  - Temperature of 39°C or higher
  - Fever for more than 2 days
  - Absence of another source of fever on history or examination (i.e., absence of upper respiratory infection, acute otitis media, gastroenteritis)

Urine Collection Methods

- Infants and children with no bladder control: catheterized urine or suprapubic aspiration
- Older children: midstream, clean-catch specimen

LABORATORY TESTS

Urinalysis (UA)

- "Enhanced" UA
  - Preferred method: uses uncentrifuged urine and a hemocytometer, more sensitive and specific for UTI
  - Combination of pyuria and bacteriuria very suggestive of a UTI
  - Pyuria: more than 10 white blood cells (WBCs)/mm^3 (uncentrifuged urine)
  - Bacteriuria: any bacteria in any of 10 oil immersion fields (gram-stained smear)
- Standard UA
  - Pyuria: more than 5 WBCs/high-power field (centrifuged urine)
  - Bacteriuria: any bacteria/high-power field (unstained)
  - Urine dipstick for leukocyte esterase and nitrite: poor sensitivity for detecting UTI
- Urine culture: urine culture is considered positive if the following criteria are met:
  - Suprapubic specimen: any bacterial growth
  - Catheterized specimen: more than 50,000 colony-forming units (CFU)/mL of a single pathogen
  - Midstream specimen: more than 100,000 CFU/mL of a single pathogen

IMAGING STUDIES

- Although not entirely evidence-based, routine imaging is currently recommended for:
  - Children under 5 years of age with a febrile UTI
  - Girls under 3 years of age with a first UTI
  - Males of any age with a first UTI
  - Children with recurrent UTI
  - Children with UTI who do not respond promptly to therapy
- Renal ultrasound (US) is used to identify gross anatomic abnormalities. Because of the widespread use of prenatal US, it may be redundant if known to have a normal, late prenatal US. Obtain US in patients with poor clinical response within 48 hours of antimicrobial therapy.
- Voiding cystourethrogram (VCUG) is used to identify vesicoureteral reflux (VUR). Perform immediately after therapy, thus eliminating the need for prophylaxis. If unable to schedule immediately after therapy, keep patient on antimicrobial prophylaxis until VCUG can be done.
- ^{99m}Technetium 99m-dimercaptosuccinic acid (^{99m}Tc-DMSA) or ^{99m}Tc-glucoheptonate is used to identify acute pyelonephritis and renal scars. It is of limited value during acute pyelonephritis. It is useful to detect renal scars if performed at least 5 months after infection.
- Intravenous pyelography is no longer routinely used. It has been replaced by renal US because of its noninvasiveness and comparable accuracy.

TREATMENT

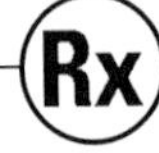

NONPHARMACOLOGIC THERAPY

- Frequent voiding

ACUTE GENERAL Rx

Oral Therapy

- Cefixime (double dose on day 1) is the only oral antimicrobial evaluated in a randomized, controlled trial for UTI in young children with fever and was shown to be equivalent to intravenous antibiotics in children beyond the neonatal period.
- Other possible antimicrobials include second and third generation cephalosporins or amoxicillin-clavulanate potassium.

- Resistance rates of *E. coli* to amoxicillin and trimethoprim-sulfamethoxazole (TMP-SMX) are 50% and 18%, respectively.
- Duration of treatment is 10 to 14 days.

Parenteral Therapy

- If toxic-appearing or unable to tolerate an oral antimicrobial.
- Second-generation (cefuroxime) or third-generation (cefotaxime, ceftriaxone) cephalosporin, ampicillin-sulbactam, or gentamicin may be used.
- Switch to oral medications when patient becomes afebrile. Continue oral treatment to complete 10- to 14-day course.

CHRONIC Rx

- Treat dysfunctional elimination if present
- Treat constipation
- Recommend timed voiding
- Consider urology referral
- If VUR is detected, need prophylaxis with nitrofurantoin (1 to 2 mg/kg/day) or TMP-SMX (2 mg/kg/day) for 1 year. Perform a radionuclide cystogram at 1 year to determine the need for continued prophylaxis.

COMPLEMENTARY & ALTERNATIVE MEDICINE

- Cranberry juice

DISPOSITION

Repeat urine culture within 48 to 72 hours if the clinical response is poor. Routine "test of cure" is not necessary.

REFERRAL

Consider referral to urologist for ureteral reimplantation in moderate or severe VUR or for management of dysfunctional elimination.

PEARLS & CONSIDERATIONS

COMMENTS

Sibling screening of patients with VUR is controversial.

PREVENTION

Treatment of voiding dysfunction and chronic constipation along with prompt evaluation and treatment of febrile episodes can reduce the risk of future renal scarring.

PATIENT/FAMILY EDUCATION

Instruct parents of preverbal children to bring child for evaluation early in the course of febrile episodes.

SUGGESTED READINGS

American Academy of Pediatrics: Practice guideline: the diagnosis, treatment, and evaluation of the initial urinary tract infection in febrile infants and young children. *Pediatrics* 103:843, 1999.

Hoberman A et al: Imaging studies after a first febrile urinary tract infection in young children [comment]. *N Engl J Med* 348:195, 2003.

Hoberman A et al: Oral versus initial intravenous therapy for urinary tract infections in young febrile children [comment]. *Pediatrics* 104:79, 1999.

Hoberman A et al: Enhanced urinalysis as a screening test for urinary tract infection. *Pediatrics* 91:1196, 1993.

AUTHORS: **NADER SHAIKH, MD, MPH** and **ALEJANDRO HOBERMAN, MD**

BASIC INFORMATION

DEFINITION

Urolithiasis is an abnormal development of calculi, or stones, in the urinary tract.

SYNONYMS

Kidney stones
Nephrolithiasis
Renal lithiasis
Renal stone (disease)
Urinary calculi

ICD-9-CM CODES
592 Calculus of kidney and ureter [excludes nephrocalcinosis (275.4)]
592.0 Nephrolithiasis NOS
592.1 Calculus of ureter
592.9 Urinary calculus, unspecified

EPIDEMIOLOGY & DEMOGRAPHICS

- The incidence is 1 in 1000 to 1 in 7600 pediatric hospital admissions in the U.S.
- Boys and girls are affected equally.
- Greater risk is seen in southern California and southeastern states.
- Caucasians > A.A. children.
- In developed countries, most stones are in the upper urinary tract.
- Bladder stones are endemic in Africa and Asia.
- Metabolic conditions are the most common cause in children.
- Urinary tract anomalies and infections increase risk of stone formation.

CLINICAL PRESENTATION

- Children do *not* usually present with the classic symptoms of renal colic.
- Pain can be abdominal, flank, or pelvic.
- Gross or microscopic hematuria common.
- UTI symptoms are noted in 50% fever, dysuria, urgency, frequency.
- Obstructive symptoms are less common: urinary retention, anuria, nausea, vomiting.
- Colicky or persistent abdominal pain may be described along the entire length of the ureter from the flank and abdominal wall to the lower abdomen, pelvis, and groin.
- Family, medication, and dietary history to assess risk.
- Blood pressure, height, and weight to assess systemic or chronic renal disease.
- Assess for congenital or anatomic abnormalities of the genital-urinary system.
- Abdominal, flank, or costovertebral angle tenderness may be present.

ETIOLOGY

- Concentration of precipitating substances in the urine forms stones.
- Calcium stones are the most common and include both calcium oxalate and phosphate.
  - Hypercalciuria can occur with or without hypercalcemia.
  - Diet-dependent hypercalciuria is more common in adults.
  - Hyperoxaluria; primary or secondary.
  - Hypocitraturia; decreased levels of stone inhibitor.
- Struvite stones are associated with UTIs.
  - Occur with urease-producing bacteria (*Proteus, Providencia, Klebsiella, Pseudomonas, Serratia, Streptococcus,* and *Mycoplasma*).
  - Composed of magnesium ammonium phosphate; precipitate at pH > 6.8
- Uric acid stones may occur in children receiving chemotherapy.
  - Hyperuricosuria with or without hyperuricemia
  - Precipitate at pH less than 5.8
- Cystine stones are usually associated with cystinuria, an autosomal recessive disorder and precipitate at pH less than 7.0.
- Rarely, stones are composed of xanthine, orotic acid, and dihydroxyadenine.

DIAGNOSIS

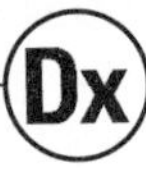

DIFFERENTIAL DIAGNOSIS

- Kidney disorder: pyelonephritis, obstruction (e.g., ureteropelvic or vesicoureteral stenosis)
- Gastrointestinal disease: appendicitis, volvulus, intussusception, gastroenterocolitis
- Genital tract disease: ovarian or testicular torsion, pelvic inflammatory disease, ectopic pregnancy

LABORATORY TESTS

- Perform stone analysis if possible.
- Urinalysis to assess pH, pyuria, bacteriuria, and crystals
- Urine culture when UTI is suspected
- 24-hour urine sample to analyze calcium, uric acid, phosphorus, citrate, sodium, cystine, and creatinine concentrations.
- Normal 24-hour urine calcium excretion is less than 4 mg/kg/day.
  - Spot urinary calcium:creatinine ratio is easier to obtain but less reliable.
- Normal infant calcium:creatinine ratio is less than 0.42.
- Normal child calcium:creatinine ratio is less than 0.21.
- Blood work to include complete blood count, blood urea nitrogen, creatinine, calcium, phosphorus, uric acid, and electrolytes.
- Consider parathyroid hormone level if serum or urine calcium is high.

IMAGING STUDIES

- Noncontrast helical computed tomography (CT) scan is highly sensitive.
- Intravenous urography is more invasive and less sensitive in children.
- Reliable initial tests include ultrasound and plain films. Most calcium stones can be seen on plain abdominal radiographs.
  - Cystine stones are weakly radiopaque.
  - Uric acid stones are radiolucent.

TREATMENT

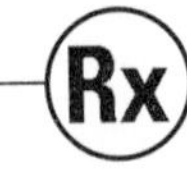

NONPHARMACOLOGIC THERAPY

- Indications for surgical stone removal include intractable pain, persistent obstruction, and persistent UTI.
- Shock-wave lithotripsy, percutaneous techniques, and endourologic procedures are replacing open stone surgery.
- Congenital anomalies in young children may necessitate open surgical repair.

ACUTE GENERAL Rx

- Pain management
- Oral or parenteral hydration, 1.5 to 2 times maintenance fluids
- Treatment of concomitant UTI

CHRONIC Rx

- High-fluid intake to keep urine volume high and specific gravity low
- For hypercalciuria: low-sodium diet; low-oxalate diet; hydrochlorothiazide (1 to 2 mg/kg/day); potassium citrate (1 to 4 mg/kg/day) in cases of hypocitraturia or renal acidosis contributing to calcium stone formation.
- For cystinuria: low-sodium diet; potassium citrate; chelating agents: considered with recurrent stones.
- For hyperuricosuria: potassium citrate; allopurinol (10 mg/kg/day).

COMPLEMENTARY & ALTERNATIVE MEDICINE

Cranberries and lemons have anti-lithogenic properties, especially against calcium oxalate stones.

DISPOSITION

Hospitalization for IV pain management, rehydration, or antibiotics may be necessary.

REFERRAL

- Pediatric urologist for congenital anomalies and surgical management
- Pediatric nephrologist for medical management of metabolic conditions

PEARLS & CONSIDERATIONS

COMMENTS

- Many systemic diseases and medications may increase the risk of stone formation.
- Provide parents with instructions and filters to strain urine for stones.

PREVENTION

Maintain adequate fluid intake and urine output at all times to prevent concentration.

PATIENT/FAMILY EDUCATION

National Institute of Diabetes & Digestive & Kidney Diseases: What I Need to Know about Kidney Stones. Available at www.niddk.nih.gov/kudiseases/pups/stones

SUGGESTED READING

Stapleton FB: Childhood stones. *Endocrinol Metab Clin North Am* 31(4):1001, 2002.

AUTHOR: **EDGARD A. SEGURA, MD**

BASIC INFORMATION

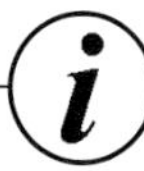

DEFINITION

West Nile virus is transmitted by the bite of infected mosquitoes. Most people who become infected have mild or no symptoms, but a few develop encephalitis, meningitis, or polio-like paralysis.

SYNONYMS

West Nile encephalitis
West Nile fever
West Nile meningoencephalitis

ICD-9-CM CODE
066.4 West Nile fever

EPIDEMIOLOGY & DEMOGRAPHICS

- Most infections are asymptomatic; 1 in 5 patients develop fever, and 1 in 150 patients develop central nervous system disease.
- Severe encephalitis and death occur most commonly in the elderly.
- Transmission occurs between birds and mosquitoes, with humans and horses as incidental hosts.
- The virus is spread by several genera of mosquitoes, most importantly *Culex* spp.
- The incubation period ranges from 2 days to 2 weeks.
- West Nile virus is found in Africa, Europe, the Middle East, Asia, Australia, and since 1999, in the Americas.
- In 2003 in the United States, 2707 cases of West Nile meningitis or encephalitis were reported, with 223 deaths.

CLINICAL PRESENTATION

- Febrile illness: fever, fatigue, myalgias, headache, back pain, pharyngitis, nausea, vomiting, diarrhea, abdominal pain, and maculopapular rash
- Central nervous system (CNS) disease (i.e., encephalitis, meningitis, or meningoencephalitis): fever, acute flaccid paralysis, meningismus, stupor, coma, seizures, nausea, vomiting, headache, myoclonus, and cranial nerve abnormalities
- Rare features: myocarditis, pancreatitis, and hepatitis

ETIOLOGY

- West Nile virus is an arthropod-borne flavivirus.
- Infection is caused by the bite of infected mosquitoes.

DIAGNOSIS Dx

DIFFERENTIAL DIAGNOSIS

- Nonspecific febrile viral illness
- Dengue fever
- St. Louis encephalitis
- Other arthropod-borne encephalitis viruses
- Lymphocytic meningitis

LABORATORY TESTS

- White blood cell count may be normal or mildly elevated.
- Cerebrospinal fluid (CSF) examination may show lymphocytic pleocytosis and mild protein elevation.
- Immunoglobulin M (IgM) antibodies are detected in serum or CSF by IgM antibody capture enzyme-linked immunosorbent assay (MAC-ELISA).
- Plaque reduction neutralization test may help in determining false-positive IgM results and in differentiating West Nile virus from other flavivirus infections.
- Polymerase chain reaction is used to detect viral RNA, but the method has a low sensitivity.
- Viral isolation is possible but not generally used for diagnosis.
- Electroencephalogram may show generalized slowing, especially in frontotemporal area.

IMAGING STUDIES

- Results of computed tomography of the brain are generally normal, even with CNS involvement.
- Magnetic resonance imaging is used to look for leptomeningeal and periventricular enhancement and the hyperintensity of basal ganglia and thalami on T2-weighted imaging.

TREATMENT Rx

NONPHARMACOLOGIC THERAPY

- Supportive care is the mainstay of therapy.
- No antiviral medications are licensed for the treatment of disease caused by the West Nile virus.
- Trials of intravenous immune globulin (with high titers of antibodies to West Nile virus) and interferon-alfa are ongoing.

DISPOSITION

- Mortality is most strongly associated with advanced age.
- The case-fatality rate is 2% to 12% for infections involving the CNS.
- Neurologic sequelae are common among survivors of CNS disease.

REFERRAL

- Suspected cases of West Nile virus infection should be referred to an infectious diseases specialist.
- Testing assistance is available through state health departments and the Centers for Disease Control and Prevention.
- West Nile virus infection is a reportable disease in most states. Contact the state health department for information on reporting.

PEARLS & CONSIDERATIONS

COMMENTS

- Flaccid paralysis with encephalitis suggests West Nile virus infection.
- Assay for IgM may be positive for persons vaccinated against yellow fever or Japanese encephalitis viruses and for those with closely related flavivirus infections.

PREVENTION

- Avoid the mosquito vector with personal protective measures, including clothing, DEET-containing repellents, screens, and not participating in outdoor activities during times when mosquitoes are most active.
- An equine vaccine is available, and research continues on a human vaccine.
- Eliminate mosquito breeding areas around homes and in communities.
- Community-level mosquito control programs are protective.

PATIENT/FAMILY EDUCATION

- Educate families about the spread of arboviral diseases.
- Educate patients and families about personal protective measures for mosquito avoidance.

SUGGESTED READINGS

American Academy of Pediatrics: Arboviruses. *In* Pickering LK (eds): *Red Book: 2003 Report of the Committee on Infectious Diseases,* 26th ed. Elk Grove Village, IL, American Academy of Pediatrics, 2003, pp 199–205.

Kim R et al: Spectrum of clinical manifestations of West Nile virus infection in children. *Pediatrics* 114:1673, 2004.

Peterson LR et al: West Nile virus: a primer for the clinician. *Ann Intern Med* 137:173, 2002.

Tsai TF et al: Flaviviruses (yellow fever, Dengue, Dengue hemorrhagic fever, Japanese encephalitis, West Nile encephalitis, St. Louis encephalitis, tick-borne encephalitis). *In* Mandel GL et al (eds): *Mandell, Douglas, and Bennett's Principles and Practices of Infectious Diseases,* 6th ed. Philadelphia, Elsevier, 2005, pp 1926–1950.

AUTHOR: **LORNA M. SEYBOLT, MD, MPH**

BASIC INFORMATION

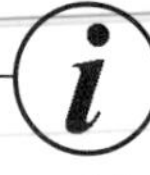

DEFINITION

Wilms' tumor is a malignant neoplasm of the kidney, derived from primitive metanephric blastema.

SYNONYM

Nephroblastoma

ICD-9-CM CODE
189.0 Malignant neoplasm of kidney, except pelvis

EPIDEMIOLOGY & DEMOGRAPHICS

- Wilms' tumor accounts for approximately 6% of pediatric cancers.
- The annual incidence is approximately 8 cases per 1 million children younger than 15 years.
- Total incidence is approximately 500 cases per year in the United States.
- The incidence among girls is slightly higher than among boys, especially for bilateral disease.
- The highest incidence in the United States is among blacks, followed by whites and then Asians.
- More than 75% of patients are diagnosed before 5 years of age; 90% are diagnosed before 7 years of age.
- The mean age of presentation is earlier for boys than girls.

CLINICAL PRESENTATION

History

- The patient may have asymptomatic abdominal fullness or mass, abdominal pain, hematuria, or fever.
- The patient may present with rapid abdominal enlargement and anemia, which may be related to hemorrhage in the tumor.
- Tumors may be detected during routine well-child visits.

Physical Examination

- The abdominal mass is usually palpable; it may be difficult to differentiate from hepatomegaly, splenomegaly, or other tumor by physical examination.
- The patient may have hypertension.
- Examination should include assessment for any associated physical anomalies, including aniridia, hemihypertrophy, or genitourinary abnormalities.

ETIOLOGY

- There are no identified environmental risk factors.
- Approximately 1% to 2% of patients have relatives with Wilms' tumor.
- An estimated 15% to 20% of patients have Wilms' tumor that is hereditary in nature but penetrance is incomplete.
- Between 10% and 13% of patients with Wilms' tumor have other anomalies and syndromes associated with the development of Wilms' tumor, and screening may be recommended for these patients.
    - Aniridia, genitourinary malformations, or a syndrome with those abnormalities and mental retardation (i.e., WAGR [**W**ilms' tumor, **a**niridia, **g**enital and/or urinary tract abnormalities, mental **r**etardation] syndrome)
    - Hemihypertrophy as an isolated finding or with overgrowth syndromes, including Beckwith-Wiedemann syndrome
    - Degenerative renal disease (i.e., Denys-Drash syndrome)
    - Trisomy 18
- Wilms' tumor suppressor genes are located at 11p13 (*WT1*) and 11p15 (*WT2*), but they account for only a minority of Wilms' tumors. Children with WAGR syndrome have a deletion at 11p13, which is also present in 5% to 10% of sporadic cases. The genetic locus of Beckwith-Wiedemann syndrome is 11p15.
- Loss of heterozygosity at chromosomes 16q and 1p is associated with a worse prognosis.

DIAGNOSIS

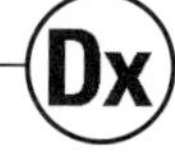

DIFFERENTIAL DIAGNOSIS

- Other malignant kidney tumors, including clear cell sarcoma and rhabdoid tumor of the kidney
- Mesoblastic nephroma (especially in children younger than 1 year) and cystic, partially differentiated nephroblastoma (i.e., low-risk or benign tumors)
- Other abdominal tumors, including neuroblastoma, lymphoma, hepatoblastoma, rhabdomyosarcoma

WORKUP

Pathology

- Favorable histology (FH) is indicated by an absence of anaplasia.
- Unfavorable histology (UH) is indicated by the presence of anaplasia, defined by gigantic polypoid nuclei within the tumor sample.
- Anaplasia may be focal or diffuse.

Staging

- Stage I: Tumor is limited to the kidney and completely resected; no tumor rupture and vessels of the renal sinus are not involved.
- Stage II: Tumor extends beyond the kidney but is completely resected. Tumor biopsy may have been done, or local tumor spillage may have occurred, but it is confined to the flank.
- Stage III: Residual nonhematogenous tumor, including any unresectable tumor, is present but confined to the abdomen.
- Stage IV: Hematogenous metastases (i.e., lung, liver, bone) or lymph node involvement outside the abdomen.
    - The lung is the most common site and the only site in approximately 80% of patients with metastatic disease.
    - Liver involvement, with or without lung metastases, occurs in 15% of patients.
- Stage V: Bilateral renal involvement is seen at diagnosis. Each side is then staged separately.

LABORATORY TESTS

There are no diagnostic laboratory tests, but a complete blood cell count, chemistries (including renal and liver function tests), and urinalysis are important components of a complete baseline evaluation.

IMAGING STUDIES

- Abdominal ultrasound, including Doppler, to evaluate inferior vena cava involvement
- Computed tomography (CT) of the abdomen and pelvis
- Chest radiograph
- CT of the chest

TREATMENT

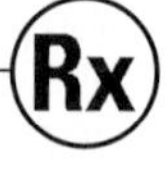

NONPHARMACOLOGIC THERAPY

- Radical nephrectomy is performed with examination of the contralateral kidney if the tumor is deemed resectable; biopsy only is done if the tumor is unresectable. Surgical recommendations evolve with efforts to perform more renal parenchyma-sparing surgeries.
- Surgery for bilateral tumors is individualized with the goal of sparing adequate renal parenchyma for normal renal function.
- Radiation therapy is indicated for stages II, III, and IV UH and for stages III and IV FH.
- Radiation therapy may be considered for pulmonary metastases visible on the chest radiograph or for pulmonary nodules visible on CT only that are unresponsive to chemotherapy.

ACUTE GENERAL Rx

Chemotherapy

- Chemotherapy regimens include vincristine and dactinomycin for stage I and II FH and stage I UH.
- Doxorubicin is added for stage II, III, and IV focal anaplasia and for stage III and IV FH.
- Stage II, III, and IV diffuse anaplasia is treated with vincristine, doxorubicin, cyclophosphamide, and etoposide.
- Chemotherapy usually is administered in the outpatient setting.

Prognosis

- Studies demonstrate an approximately 90% to 95% 5-year survival for Wilms' tumor patients as a group.
- Relapses beyond 5 years are rare.
- Patients with diffuse anaplasia are rare, but they have a poor prognosis.
- Prognosis after relapse is worse for patients who received doxorubicin or radiation therapy as part of their initial therapy.

DISPOSITION

- Obtain serial abdominal ultrasound or CT scans and chest radiographs or chest CT every 3 months for eight times and then every 6 months for four times.
- Late effects of chemotherapy are limited but may include cardiomyopathy in patients receiving doxorubicin and renal tubular dysfunction in patients receiving cyclophosphamide.
- Late effects of irradiation may include hypoplasia and potential reproductive difficulties in female patients, including pregnancy loss and premature delivery. There is a smaller risk of ovarian failure, pulmonary fibrosis, and second malignancies.
- Some restrictions may be recommended to single-kidney status, and renal function should be monitored. Renal failure is uncommon except in patients with identified syndromes, including Denys-Drash and WAGR.

REFERRAL

- All patients should be referred to pediatric oncologists and treated on National Wilms' Tumor Study protocols, as appropriate.
- A pediatric surgeon or pediatric urologist with experience in oncologic surgery should perform nephrectomy.

PEARLS & CONSIDERATIONS

COMMENTS

- Many patients with Wilms' tumor have the mass detected by a family member.
- Although only a small number of patients are diagnosed after hypertension is detected on routine examination, it is another reason to measure blood pressure during well-child visits.

PATIENT/FAMILY EDUCATION

- Most cases are sporadic, but bilateral, multicentric disease or disease diagnosed at younger ages is more likely to be heritable.
- A multimodal approach to therapy, including surgery, chemotherapy, and radiation therapy if necessary, has resulted in excellent cure rates for all stages of disease, including metastatic disease.
- Pediatric oncologists can refer patients and parents to local or national support organizations for children with cancer and their families. National organizations include the American Cancer Society and CureSearch, a component of the Children's Oncology Group (www.curesearch.org; www.cancer.org).

SUGGESTED READINGS

Grundy PE et al: Renal tumors. *In* Pizzo PA, Poplack DG (eds): *Principles and Practice of Pediatric Oncology,* 4th ed. Philadelphia, Lippincott Williams & Wilkins, 2002, pp 865–893.

Halperin EC: Wilms' tumor. *In* Halperin EC et al (eds): *Pediatric Radiation Oncology,* 4th ed. Philadelphia, Lippincott Williams & Wilkins, 2005, pp 379–421.

Kalapurakal JA et al: Management of Wilms' tumor: current practice and future goals. *Lancet Oncol* 5:37, 2004.

AUTHOR: **ANDREA S. HINKLE, MD**

BASIC INFORMATION

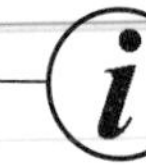

DEFINITION

Wilson disease is an autosomal recessive disorder of copper metabolism characterized by degenerative changes in the brain, liver disease, Kayser-Fleischer rings in the cornea, and sometimes, hemolysis.

SYNONYM

Hepatolenticular degeneration

ICD-9-CM CODE
275.1 Disorders of copper metabolism

EPIDEMIOLOGY & DEMOGRAPHICS

- Wilson disease affects 1 in 30,000 people.
- It occurs in all races and nationalities.
- It is an autosomal recessive disease with no sex predilection.
- Most cases are transmitted generation to generation, but some are caused by spontaneous mutations.
- Because it is autosomal recessive, most patients have no family history of the disease.
- Symptoms rarely manifest before age 5.
- Patients younger than 20 years tend to present with hepatic manifestations, sometimes with a brisk hemolytic anemia.
- Older individuals tend to have more neurologic and psychiatric manifestations.

CLINICAL PRESENTATION

History

- Abdominal mass or distention from asymptomatic hepatomegaly
- Jaundice, nausea, vomiting, and right upper quadrant pain associated with acute hepatitis
- Jaundice, edema, malaise, and pallor associated with hepatic failure and hemolytic anemia
- Esophageal bleeding and ascites from portal hypertension
- Neurologic manifestations, particularly those of a movement disorder, such as resting and intention tremors, spasticity, rigidity, chorea, dysphagia, and dysarthria
- Psychiatric disturbances, including syndromes indistinguishable from schizophrenia, manic-depressive disorder, and classic neuroses, as well as more bizarre behavioral disturbances
- Deterioration in school performance and marked behavioral changes

Physical Examination

- Hepatomegaly or hepatosplenomegaly
- Right upper quadrant tenderness
- Ascites
- Progressive renal failure, manifestations of Fanconi's syndrome detected on urinalysis
- Kayser-Fleischer rings in the cornea (i.e., slit-lamp examination is most often required, although detection is occasionally possible on routine examination)
- Rare: arthritis, endocrinopathies

ETIOLOGY

- Mutations occur in the *ATP7B* gene located at chromosome 13 at q14.3-q21.1.
- More than 200 different mutations have been identified.
- Gene encodes a P-type ATPase that plays a role in copper transport.
- Defective mobilization of copper from lysosomes in liver cells for excretion into bile leads to accumulation of copper in the liver.
- Copper is a potent inhibitor of enzymatic processes.
- When the liver's capacity for storing copper is exceeded, copper escapes the liver and causes damage to other organs, including the brain, kidneys, and eyes.

DIAGNOSIS

DIFFERENTIAL DIAGNOSIS

- Acute viral hepatitis, chronic hepatitis, α_1-Antitrypsin deficiency, porphyria, hepatic copper overload syndrome, indian childhood cirrhosis, copper poisoning

WORKUP

The diagnosis is fairly straightforward, as long as it is suspected.

LABORATORY TESTS

- The best screening test is to measure the serum level of ceruloplasmin. Most patients have a serum ceruloplasmin level that is decreased, less than 20 mg/dL.
- An ophthalmologic slit-lamp examination should be done to look for Kayser-Fleischer rings.
- Consider measuring urinary copper excretion.
- Liver biopsy should be considered. Hepatic copper concentration is the gold standard in diagnosing Wilson disease.
- There is no simple genetic test for Wilson disease. Markers close to the Wilson disease gene allow presymptomatic diagnosis in siblings.

TREATMENT

NONPHARMACOLOGIC THERAPY

- Restrict copper intake by avoiding shellfish, nuts, chocolate, liver, and other foods high in copper.
- If the copper content of local water is high, it may be necessary to demineralize.
- Liver transplantation may be undertaken for patients with fulminant hepatic disease or cirrhosis.

CHRONIC Rx

- Treatment consists of anticopper agents to remove excess copper from the body and to prevent it from accumulating again.
- The newest U.S. Food and Drug Administration (FDA)-approved drug is zinc acetate (Galzin), and it is considered the treatment of choice. Zinc acetate blocks absorption of copper, increases copper excretion in stool, and causes no serious side effects.
- Other drugs approved to treat Wilson disease include penicillamine and trientine. Both increase urinary excretion of copper, but can cause serious side effects.
- Tetrathiomolybdate, an experimental drug, also shows promise in treating Wilson disease.

DISPOSITION

- Wilson disease is fatal if untreated.
- The prognosis for patients receiving medical therapy depends on the progression of disease at the initiation of treatment and individual variation.
- Once initiated, therapy must be maintained for life.
- If treatment is begun early enough, symptomatic recovery is usually complete, and a life of normal length and quality can be possible.

REFERRAL

- Children with Wilson disease should be referred to a pediatric gastroenterologist specializing in this disorder.
- Consultations with a pediatric neurologist and hematologist may be warranted.

PEARLS & CONSIDERATIONS

COMMENTS

- Wilson disease should be considered in any child with an unexplained neurologic or psychiatric problem and evidence of elevated liver transaminases, hepatitis, or hepatomegaly.
- All patients with neurologic or psychiatric disturbance have Kayser-Fleischer rings; Kayser-Fleischer rings may be absent in the young patient with only liver disease.
- Unexplained hemolysis should always be regarded as a possible sign of Wilson disease.

PATIENT/FAMILY EDUCATION

- Most people with Wilson disease do not have a family history of the disease.
- The chance of a sibling of a child with Wilson disease being affected is 25%.
- Early treatment is important to prevent progression of the disease, and after treatment is initiated, it must continue for life.
- The Wilson's Disease Association has a support group (www.wilsonsdisease.org).

SUGGESTED READINGS

National Institute of Neurologic Diseases and Stroke Wilson's Disease. Available at www.ninds.nih.gov/disorders/wilsons/wilsons.htm

Wilson's Disease Association International. Available at www.wilsonsdisease.org

AUTHOR: **JEFFREY M. KACZOROWSKI, MD**

BASIC INFORMATION

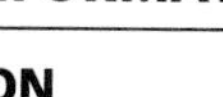

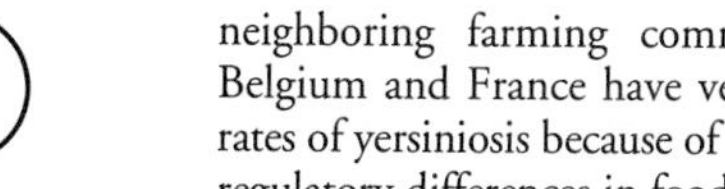

DEFINITION

Infection caused by *Yersinia enterocolitica* and, less commonly, by the closely related species *Yersinia pseudotuberculosis* is an increasingly recognized zoonosis causing food poisoning and mesenteric lymphadenitis. A separate species, *Yersinia pestis,* is responsible for the distinctly different disease, plague.

SYNONYMS

Bacterial enterocolitis
Nonplague yersiniosis

ICD-9-CM CODE
027.8 *Yersinia enterocolitica,* other specified zoonotic bacterial diseases

EPIDEMIOLOGY & DEMOGRAPHICS

- Disease reservoirs
  - *Y. enterocolitica* is widespread in nature.
  - The most common reservoir is the pig; sheep, cattle, horses, rodents, and household pets can also serve as reservoirs.
- Modes of transmission
  - Contaminated food or milk is a source; the organisms can persist and grow in refrigerated products. The most common foods associated with transmission are pork and cow's milk.
  - Transfusions of contaminated packed red blood cells or platelet concentrates; organisms can persist and grow despite refrigeration. This route of infection is rare but well described, occurring even with stored autologous transfusions.
  - The person-to-person (fecal-oral) route is rarely a mode of transmission.
- Incidence and prevalence
  - *Y. enterocolitica* is the fifth most common enteric bacterial cause of foodborne illness in the United States, after *Salmonella, Campylobacter, Shigella,* and *Escherichia coli* O157:H7.
  - Several hundred cases of *Y. enterocolitica* disease are reported yearly. Because it is not a nationally notifiable disease, exact figures are lacking.
  - The annual incidence in the United States has decreased in recent years (presumably because of stricter food-handling practices). The average annual incidence is about 0.4 per 100,000 children older than 5 years; however, the rate is 2.7 cases per 100,000 children between the ages of 1 and 4 years and as high as 25 cases per 100,000 infants younger than 1 year. The highest annual incidence is among U.S. black infants (142 cases per 100,000).
- Risk factors and affected groups
  - Infection is more common in general in temperate areas (e.g., Northern Europe, Canada, United States) than in tropical areas. However, variability in incidence rates exists; for example, geographically neighboring farming communities of Belgium and France have very different rates of yersiniosis because of cultural and regulatory differences in food handling.
  - Infants and young children are infected more often than older children and adults.
  - Black infants are infected more often than white or Hispanic infants, probably because of dietary customs, such as exposure to raw pork used to make chitterlings (i.e., intestines) at holiday gatherings.
  - Patients with iron overload states (e.g., hemochromatosis, thalassemia, renal failure with transfusion therapy) and those receiving iron chelation therapy with deferoxamine are more susceptible.

CLINICAL PRESENTATION

History

- Risk factors discussed earlier
- Ingestion of food associated with transmission in preceding 2 weeks
- Contact with preparers of high-risk food, such as pork chitterlings
- Findings on examination depend on the clinical syndrome.

Physical Examination

- Gastroenteritis
  - Enterocolitic diarrhea occurs with fever, abdominal pain, and mucus- and blood-containing stools, and sometimes with vomiting.
  - Incubation period is 3 to 7 days.
  - Symptoms persist for 1 to 3 weeks.
  - Gastroenteritis predominantly occurs in children younger than 5 years.
- Mesenteric lymphadenitis or pseudoappendicitis
  - Mimics acute appendicitis with fever, right lower quadrant pain, leukocytosis, but not diarrhea
  - Predominantly seen in children older than 6 to 10 years
  - Often misdiagnosed, resulting in laparotomy
- Extraintestinal infection
  - Bacteremia may occur with or without diarrhea and may lead to metastatic lesions, such as lymphadenitis, pharyngitis, osteomyelitis, septic arthritis, meningitis, peritonitis, and hepatic or splenic abscesses.
  - Invasive disease is more common after transfusions and in patients receiving iron overload or chelation therapy.
  - The mortality rate can approach 50%.
- Immunologic sequelae
  - Reactive arthritis, erythema nodosum, and Reiter's syndrome may occur after yersiniosis.
  - Adults with the HLA-B27 genotype are especially at risk for immunologic disorders.

ETIOLOGY

- *Y. enterocolitica* is a gram-negative, rod-shaped, aerobic bacterium.
- Serotypes 0:3, 0:8, and 0:9 predominate in human disease.
- Iron overload states and iron chelation therapy with deferoxamine enhance the virulence of *Y. enterocolitica.*

DIAGNOSIS

DIFFERENTIAL DIAGNOSIS

- Colitis
  - *Shigella*
  - *Salmonella*
  - *Campylobacter*
- Mesenteric adenitis
  - Appendicitis
  - Crohn's disease
  - Terminal ileitis
- Bacteremia with extraintestinal manifestations
  - Lymphadenitis
  - Peritonitis
  - Hepatic and splenic abscesses
  - Septic arthritis

LABORATORY TESTS

- Obtain bacterial cultures of blood.
- Obtain bacterial cultures of stool. Special media and selection techniques may be required, and the laboratory should be alerted to look for *Yersinia.*

IMAGING STUDIES

Abdominal computed tomography may help differentiate appendicitis from mesenteric lymphadenitis.

TREATMENT

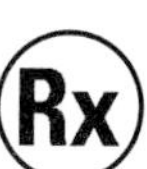

NONPHARMACOLOGIC THERAPY

Supportive therapy is provided for diarrhea, fever, and pain.

ACUTE GENERAL Rx

- Antibiotic therapy is indicated for bacteremia, systemic focal infections, infections in immunocompromised hosts, and severe cases of mesenteric adenitis.
- Uncomplicated cases of enterocolitis and mesenteric adenitis in older children may not require antibiotic therapy.
- Most *Y. enterocolitica* isolates are susceptible to trimethoprim-sulfamethoxazole, third-generation cephalosporins, and fluoroquinolones.

PEARLS & CONSIDERATIONS

COMMENTS

- Recent outbreaks of *Y. enterocolitica* febrile gastroenteritis have occurred in urban black children after Thanksgiving, Christmas, and New Year's holiday gatherings.
- Pork chitterlings, which are often prepared at such times, have been implicated as the

vehicle of spread of infection. Most children did not have direct contact with raw chitterlings. However, preparation of chitterlings is labor intensive and time consuming, and food-handling adults presumably infect the children.

PREVENTION

- Do not let children handle raw pork products (e.g., chitterlings).
- Thoroughly cook all pork products, and keep uncooked pork products separate from other foods.
- Wash hands, knives, and cutting boards after handling uncooked pork products.
- Avoid raw or unpasteurized milk.

PATIENT/FAMILY EDUCATION

- Centers for Disease Control and Prevention (disease information topic "A to Z" list): www.cdc.gov/az.do

SUGGESTED READINGS

Ackers ML et al: An outbreak of *Yersinia enterocolitica* O:8 infections associated with pasteurized milk. *J Infect Dis* 181:1834, 2000.

Butler T, Dennis DT: *Yersinia* species, including plague. *In* Mandell GL et al (eds): *Mandell, Douglas, and Bennett's Principles and Practice of Infectious Diseases,* 6th ed. Philadelphia, Elsevier, 2005.

Ray SM et al: Population-based surveillance for *Yersinia enterocolitica* infections in FoodNet sites, 1996–1999: higher risk of disease in infants and minority populations. *Clin Infect Dis* 38: S182, 2004.

Smego RA et al: Yersiniosis. I: Microbiological and clinicoepidemiological aspects of plague and non-plague *Yersinia* infections. *Eur J Clin Microbiol Infect Dis* 18:1, 1999.

Woods CR: Other *Yersinia* species. *In* Feigin RD et al (eds): *Textbook of Pediatric Infectious Diseases,* 5th ed. Philadelphia, WB Saunders, 2004.

AUTHOR: **GEOFFREY A. WEINBERG, MD**

Section II

Differential Diagnosis

ABDOMINAL MASS

The clinical classification of abdominal masses in children can be divided according to neonatal and postneonatal causes. Approximately one half of abdominal masses in newborns involve the urinary tract. Constipation is the most common cause of an abdominal mass in the older child.

NEONATAL

Urinary tract

Hydronephrosis (obstructive uropathy)
- Posterior urethral valves
- Ureterocele
- Prune belly syndrome

Renal cystic dysplasia
Polycystic kidney disease
Glomerulocystic kidney disease
Medullary cystic disease or juvenile nephronophthisis
Simple renal cysts
Wilms' tumor
Renal vein thrombosis
Renal hamartoma (mesoblastic nephroma)
Ectopic kidney
Other congenital abnormalities of kidneys
Renal or perinephric abscess
Distended bladder

Gastrointestinal system

Pyloric stenosis
Ileus (meconium)
Bowel duplication
Choledochal cyst
Hydrops of gallbladder

Hepatomegaly

Congestive heart failure
Sepsis
Congenital infections
- Cytomegalovirus
- Toxoplasmosis
- Enterovirus
- Herpes simplex virus
- Syphilis
- Rubella

Biliary atresia
Hemolytic anemia
Neonatal hepatitis
Peripheral hyperalimentation
Hepatic cysts
Hemangioma

Splenomegaly

Sepsis
Congenital infections (see "Hepatomegaly" earlier)
Hemolytic anemia
Portal vein thrombosis
- Omphalitis
- Umbilical vein catheterization

Neoplasms

Neuroblastoma
Teratoma
Renal tumors (mentioned earlier)

POSTNEONATAL

Urinary tract causes described earlier

Gastrointestinal system

Constipation
Intussusception
Pancreatic pseudocyst
Intestinal or appendiceal abscess
Ileus
Choledochal cyst
Hydrops of the gallbladder
Mesenteric cyst

Hepatomegaly (see Hepatomegaly and Hepatosplenomegaly in Section II)

Splenomegaly (see Splenomegaly, Isolated in Section II)

Genital tract

Pregnancy
Ovarian cyst
Ovarian torsion
Ovarian tumor
Pelvic abscess
Hematocolpos (imperforate hymen or vaginal atresia)

Neoplasms

Neuroblastoma
Teratoma
Lymphoma
Sarcoma
Adrenal tumor
Renal and ovarian tumors (mentioned earlier)

ABDOMINAL PAIN

Abdominal pain is any abdominal discomfort that may be acute or chronic, constant or intermittent, sudden or insidious. It may or may not be associated with other gastrointestinal (e.g., diarrhea, vomiting), genitourinary (e.g., dysuria, discharge, menorrhagia), infectious (e.g., fever, sore throat, headache, malaise), or systemic (e.g., lethargy, irritability, rash) findings.

CHRONIC

Common, general

Abdominal tumors or masses
Chronic pyelonephritis
Constipation
Dysmenorrhea
Endometriosis
Functional abdominal pain (i.e., chronic nonspecific abdominal pain of childhood and chronic recurrent abdominal pain)
Gastritis
Inflammatory bowel disease
Irritable colon
Lactose intolerance
Medications
- Antibiotics
- Bronchodilators
- Nonsteroidal anti-inflammatory drugs
- Ritalin

Peptic ulcer disease (*Helicobacter pylori* infection)
Psychogenic, anxiety related
Reflux esophagitis

Less common

Abdominal epilepsy
Abdominal migraine
Addison disease
Collagen vascular disease
Cystic fibrosis
- Hypoxia
- Medications
- Pneumonia
- With or without meconium plug or obstruction

Diskitis
Duplications along the gastrointestinal tract (usual presentation is obstruction)
Dysrhythmias (palpitations and nausea)
Heavy metal poisoning (lead, arsenic, mercury)
Hematocolpos
Mesenteric cysts
Other spinal cord or spinal diseases
- With or without constipation
- With or without urinary findings
- With or without gait abnormality

Porphyria
Superior mesenteric artery syndrome (especially with recent significant weight loss, usually with vomiting)

ACUTE

Many chronic causes of abdominal pain can manifest acutely. Other acute forms are listed here.

Infectious causes

Abdominal, pelvic, or abdominal wall abscess
Acute rheumatic fever
Appendicitis
Cholecystitis
Food poisoning
Hepatitis
Infectious gastroenteritis, gastroenterocolitis, enterocolitis
Pancreatitis (may be recurrent) or pancreatic cyst or pseudocyst
Pelvic inflammatory disease (PID), Fitz-Hugh-Curtis syndrome (perihepatitis)
Pericarditis
Peritonitis
- Acute bacterial
- Subacute bacterial

Pharyngitis or tonsillitis
Pneumonia
Pyelonephritis, cystitis (urinary tract infection)
Zoster

Obstruction

Acute hydrops
Adhesions
Choledochal or choledochal duct cyst
Cholelithiasis (may be recurrent)
Ectopic pregnancy
Inguinal or femoral hernia with bowel strangulation or torsion
Intussusception
Meckel's diverticulum
Ovary or ovarian cyst, torsion
Renal stones (may be recurrent)
Testicular torsion
Volvulus

Causes not specifically categorized

Abdominal muscle wall injury
Acute abdomen due to vaso-occlusive crisis in sickle cell disease
Diabetic ketoacidosis (DKA)

Duodenal hematoma
Electrolyte abnormalities (ileus with hypokalemia, cramping with hypocalcemia, acute abdomen with acidosis)
Familial dysautonomia
Hemolytic crises
Hemolytic uremic syndrome (HUS)
Hyperlipoproteinemia
Liver laceration or hematoma
Mesenteric artery occlusion
Mittelschmerz (recurrent)
Ovarian cyst rupture
Perforated viscus or abdominal blood vessel
Peritonitis due to bleeding
Spider bite (especially black widow)
Splenic rupture
Inflammatory causes
Hereditary angioneurotic edema (recurrent)
Peritoneal inflammation (rheumatologic, vascular, familial Mediterranean fever)
Vasculitis

ALOPECIA/HAIR LOSS

Alopecia refers to hair loss from the scalp. The differential diagnosis deals with acute causes of alopecia.

Tinea capitis (fungal infection)
Trauma
Traction alopecia
Trichotillomania
Chemical burn
Thermal burn
Radiation
Chemotherapy (anagen effluvium)
Alopecia areata (autoimmune)
Alopecia totalis (loss of all hair on the scalp)
Alopecia universalis (loss of all hair on the body)
Telogen effluvium
Significant stress (hospitalization, childbirth, surgery, malnutrition, psychosocial stress)
Drugs
- Valproic acid
- Coumadin
- Heparin
- Propranolol

Male-pattern baldness
Polycystic ovary syndrome (PCOS)
Systemic diseases
Systemic lupus erythematosus
Scleroderma (morphea)
Acrodermatitis enteropathica
Hypoparathyroidism

ALTERED MENTAL STATUS

Altered mental status includes several different states of consciousness. *Delirium* is confusion and irrational behavior that is sometimes accompanied by excitability. *Lethargy* refers to sleepiness and disinterest in the environment. *Stupor* or *obtundation* refers to a state of unconsciousness from which a child can momentarily be aroused. *Coma* is a prolonged state of unconsciousness.

Head trauma
Subdural hematoma
Epidural hematoma
Intracerebral hemorrhage
Intraventricular hemorrhage
Subarachnoid hemorrhage
Concussion
Contusion
Cerebral edema
Infectious causes
Sepsis
Meningitis
Encephalitis
Postinfectious encephalomyelitis
Brain abscess
Subdural empyema
Shigella infections
Drug intoxication, overdose, or reaction
Alcohol
Carbon monoxide
Sedatives
Benzodiazepines
Narcotics
Anticonvulsants
Anticholinergics
Neuroleptics
Psychedelics
Lead
Aspirin
Iron
Cocaine
Amphetamines
Organophosphates
Many others
Seizures
Status epilepticus
Postictal seizures
Neoplasms or brain tumors
Hydrocephalus or shunt malfunction
Hypertensive encephalopathy
Cerebrovascular disorders
Arteriovenous malformation
Venous thrombosis
Aneurysm
Stroke
Metabolic causes
Hypoglycemia
Diabetic ketoacidosis
Uremia
Hepatic encephalopathy
Reye's syndrome
Adrenal insufficiency
Hyponatremia and hypernatremia
Hypocalcemia and hypercalcemia
Hypomagnesemia
Inborn errors of metabolism
- Amino acid disorders
  - Urea cycle defects
  - Tyrosinemia
  - Nonketotic hyperglycinemia
- Organic acid disorders
  - Methylmalonic acidemia
  - Propionic acidemia
  - Maple syrup urine disease
  - Others
- Carbohydrate disorders
  - Galactosemia
  - Pyruvate dehydrogenase deficiency
  - Others
- Fatty acid disorders
  - Carnitine deficiencies
  - Acyl CoA dehydrogenase deficiency

Hypoxia or shock
Hypothermia or hyperthermia
Psychological causes
Psychosis
Conversion reaction
Other causes
Intussusception
Hemolytic uremic syndrome
Narcolepsy

AMENORRHEA

Amenorrhea is the absence of menses. *Primary amenorrhea* is defined as the absence of menarche by age 16 years in the presence of normal pubertal development *or* the absence of menarche by age 14 years in the absence of normal pubertal development *or* the absence of menarche 2 years after completion of sexual maturation. *Secondary amenorrhea* is defined as the absence of menstruation for at least three cycles or at least 6 months in females who have already established menstruation. It is helpful to divide the evaluation of amenorrhea into three categories: amenorrhea with normal pubertal development, amenorrhea with delayed pubertal development, and amenorrhea with abnormal genital examination findings.

Pregnancy
Hormonal contraception
Hypothalamic causes
Chronic or systemic illness
Eating disorder
Hypothalamic-pituitary axis immaturity
Infiltration (hemochromatosis)
Isolated gonadotropin-releasing hormone (GnRH) deficiency
Kallmann's syndrome (defect in olfaction)
Obesity
Strenuous exercise
Stress
Substance abuse
Tumor (craniopharyngioma)
Pituitary
Hypopituitarism
Infiltration (hemochromatosis)
Infarction
- Sheehan's syndrome
- Sickle cell disease

Tumor (prolactinoma)
Adrenal causes
Congenital adrenal hyperplasia
- Classic
- Nonclassic

Ovarian causes
Agenesis (46,XX)
Dysgenesis (Turner syndrome, 45,XO or variant)

Hyperandrogenic chronic anovulation (polycystic ovary syndrome)
Premature ovarian failure
Autoimmune disorders
Chemotherapy
Radiation
Tumor
Uterus, cervical, and vaginal abnormalities
Agenesis (Mayer-Rokitansky-Küster-Hauser syndrome)
Androgen insensitivity syndrome (testicular feminization)
Imperforate hymen
Synechiae (Asherman's syndrome)
Transverse vaginal septum
Other causes
Endocrinopathies
Thyroid disease
Cushing syndrome
Prader-Willi syndrome
Laurence-Moon-Biedl syndrome

ANEMIA

Anemia is a reduction in the number of red blood cells (RBC) or a low hemoglobin concentration. Anemia can be microcytic (small RBCs, low MCV), normocytic, or macrocytic (large RBCs, high MCV).
Microcytic anemia
Low reticulocyte count
Iron deficiency (nutritional, blood loss, hemorrhagic, gastrointestinal loss)
Lead poisoning
Celiac disease
Chronic disease
Protein malnutrition
Aluminum toxicity
Copper deficiency
Normal reticulocyte count
Thalassemia trait
Sideroblastic anemia
High reticulocyte count
Thalassemia syndromes
Hemoglobin C disorders
Normocytic anemia
Low reticulocyte count
Chronic disease
Red blood cell aplasia (transient erythroblastopenia of childhood, infection, drug induced)
Malignancy
Juvenile rheumatoid arthritis
Endocrinopathies
Renal failure
Normal reticulocyte count
Acute bleeding
Hypersplenism
Dyserythropoietic anemia II
High reticulocyte count
Antibody-mediated hemolysis
Hemoglobinopathies (sickle cell disease)
Membranopathies (spherocytosis, elliptocytosis)
Enzyme disorders
Glucose-6-phosphate dehydrogenase (G6PD) deficiency
Pyruvate kinase deficiency
Hypersplenism
Microangiopathic hemolytic anemias
Hemolytic uremic syndrome (HUS)
Thrombotic thrombocytopenic purpura (TTP)
Disseminated intravascular coagulation (DIC)
Kasabach-Merritt syndrome
Macrocytic anemia
Low reticulocyte count
Folate deficiency
Vitamin B_{12} deficiency
Aplastic anemia
Congenital bone marrow dysfunction (Diamond-Blackfan syndrome, Fanconi's syndrome)
Drug induced
Trisomy 21
Hypothyroidism
High reticulocyte count
Dyserythropoietic anemia I, III
Active hemolysis

ARTHRITIS

Arthritis is defined as swelling of a joint that is accompanied by limitation of motion, heat, pain, or tenderness. Arthralgia refers to pain or tenderness of a joint alone.
Trauma or mechanical causes
Hematoma or contusion
Fracture
Stress fracture
Osteochondritis dissecans
Dislocation
Ligament injuries (sprains)
Cartilage injuries
Chondromalacia patella
Muscle injuries (strains)
Tendon injuries
Hemarthrosis
Bursitis
Foreign body
Overuse syndromes
Osgood-Schlatter disease
Little league elbow
Infectious or postinfectious causes
Septic arthritis (bacterial)
Staphylococcus aureus
Group A streptococcus
Streptococcus pneumoniae
Group B streptococcus
Haemophilus influenzae type B
Neisseria gonorrhoeae
Neisseria meningitidis
Pseudomonas aeruginosa (puncture wounds)
Salmonella species (sickle cell disease)
Mycobacterium tuberculosis
Postinfectious bacterial causes
Group A streptococci (acute rheumatic fever)
Neisseria gonorrhoeae
Neisseria meningitidis
Chlamydia
Shigella
Salmonella
Yersinia
Campylobacter
Lyme disease
Rat bite fever
Mycoplasma
Viral or postviral causes
Rubella
Hepatitis B
Epstein-Barr virus
Cytomegalovirus
Parvovirus
Herpesvirus-6
Mumps
Enteroviruses
Adenovirus
Varicella zoster virus
Influenza viruses
Fungal causes
Bacterial endocarditis
Hemarthrosis or hematoma with infection
Rheumatic or collagen vascular disease
Juvenile rheumatoid arthritis
Systemic lupus erythematosus
Inflammatory bowel disease-associated arthritis
Behçet's syndrome
Henoch-Schönlein purpura
Kawasaki syndrome
Erythema nodosum-associated arthritis
Erythema multiforme (Stevens-Johnson syndrome)
Reiter's syndrome
Scleroderma
Dermatomyositis
Mixed connective tissue disorder
Ankylosing spondylitis
Polyarteritis nodosa
Sjögren's syndrome
Psoriatic arthritis
Pigmented villonodular synovitis
Hypermobility syndrome
Drugs
Serum sickness
Neoplasms
Leukemia
Neuroblastoma
Ewing's sarcoma
Osteogenic sarcoma
Other causes
Hemophilia (hemarthrosis)
Sickle cell disease
Ehlers-Danlos syndrome (dislocations)
Sarcoidosis
Familial Mediterranean fever

ATAXIA

Ataxia refers to impairment in coordination of movement without loss of muscle strength.
Drugs or toxins
Anticonvulsants
Barbiturates
Phenytoin
Carbamazepine
Valproate
Benzodiazepines
Heavy metal poisoning
Lead
Mercury
Arsenic
Substance abuse
Alcohol

Glue sniffing
Gasoline sniffing
Sedatives
Hypnotics
Drug withdrawal
Other agents
Infectious causes
Meningitis
Encephalitis
Herpesviruses
Enteroviruses
Arboviruses
Postinfectious encephalomyelitis
Labyrinthitis
Cerebellar abscess
Acute cerebellar ataxia
Central nervous system
Head trauma
Cerebellar hemorrhage
Posterior fossa subdural hematoma
Concussion
Tumor
Posterior fossa
Von Hippel-Lindau syndrome (cerebellar hemangioblastoma)
Hydrocephalus
Congenital anomalies of the cerebellum
Cerebellar dysgenesis
Dandy-Walker malformation
Chiari's malformation
Vascular malformation of cerebellum or cerebellar hemorrhage
Basilar artery migraine
Cerebral palsy
Metabolic disorders
Hypoglycemia
Vitamin B_{12} deficiency
Vitamin D deficiency
Amino acid disorders
Urea cycle defects
Hartnup disease
Organic acid disorders
Maple syrup urine disease
Isovaleric acidemia
Multiple carboxylase deficiency
Pyruvate metabolism disorders
Leigh disease (subacute necrotizing encephalomyelopathy)
Pyruvate dehydrogenase complex deficiency
Pyruvate decarboxylase deficiency
Systemic disorders
Friedreich's ataxia
Ataxia telangiectasia
Refsum's disease
Multiple sclerosis
Cockayne's syndrome
Angelman's syndrome
Abetalipoproteinemia
Lipidoses (Tay-Sachs disease)
Leukodystrophies
Conversion disorder or psychogenic causes

BACK PAIN

Back pain is less common in children than in adults. In general, the younger the child, the more likely back pain signifies serious pathology.

Traumatic, posttraumatic, and recurrent stress
Musculoskeletal strain
Contusion
Compression fracture
Spondylolysis
Spondylolisthesis
Herniated disk
Spinal epidural hematoma
Infectious causes
Spinal
Diskitis
Vertebral osteomyelitis
Epidural abscess
Tuberculosis
Extraspinal
Pyelonephritis
Pneumonia
Meningitis
Iliac osteomyelitis
Sacroiliac pyoarthrosis
Paraspinal abscess
Postinfectious (transverse myelitis)
Collagen vascular disease
Juvenile rheumatoid arthritis
Ankylosing spondylitis
Other spondylitis (inflammatory bowel disease, Reiter's syndrome, psoriasis)
Neoplasms
Vertebral tumors
Ewing's sarcoma
Osteogenic sarcoma
Eosinophilic granuloma
Osteoid osteoma
Osteoblastoma
Bone cysts
Spinal cord tumors
Neurofibromas
Gliomas
Lipomas
Teratomas
Extraspinal tumors
Neuroblastoma
Wilms' tumor
Leukemia
Lymphoma
Congenital and developmental spine disorders
Congenital anomalies of the spine
Scheuermann's disease (juvenile kyphosis)
Disk space calcification
Arteriovenous malformations
Systemic disorders
Sickle cell disease
Muscular dystrophies
Aortic aneurysm or dissection (hypertension, Marfan syndrome)
Referred pain
Gallbladder disease
Pancreatitis
Appendicitis
Renal colic
Gastrointestinal cramping
Psychogenic causes

BREAST MASS OR ENLARGEMENT

The differential diagnosis of a breast mass or enlargement is based on the age and sex of the child. Most breast masses in children and adolescents are benign. Obese children may sometimes appear to have breast enlargement without any breast tissue being present.

ANY AGE

Infection
Cellulitis
Abscess
Drugs
Estrogen-containing medicines
Spironolactone
Cimetidine
Imipramine
Phenothiazines
Isoniazid
Trauma
Hematoma
Fat necrosis
Contusion
Chronic liver disease
Tumors (rare)

INFANT

Physiologic hypertrophy
Primary tumor
Hemangioma

PREPUBERTY: MALE

Precocious puberty or prepubertal gynecomastia
Primary tumor
Lipoma
Neurofibroma

PREPUBERTY: FEMALE

Premature thelarche
Precocious puberty
Primary tumor
Lipoma
Neurofibroma

PUBERTY: MALE

Physiologic gynecomastia (can be asymmetric)
Klinefelter syndrome (47, XXY karyotype)
Tumor
Primary
Lipoma
Neurofibroma
Secondary (hormone-producing)
Adrenal
Testicular

PUBERTY: FEMALE

Physiologic (can be asymmetric)
Pregnancy
Lactational changes
Fibrocystic changes
Tumor
Fibroadenoma
Giant fibroadenoma

Cystosarcoma phyllodes
Intraductal papilloma
Lipoma
Breast carcinoma (rare)
Breast sarcoma (rare)
Intramammary lymph node

CHEST PAIN

Chest pain originates from inside or outside the chest. It may be referred from the abdomen.

Most common causes

Musculoskeletal (trauma, strain)
Psychogenic
Costochondritis
Esophagitis
Asthma
Cough
Pneumonia
Sickle cell disease

Trauma or mechanical causes

Chest wall strain
Costochondritis (Tietze's syndrome)
Direct trauma or muscle strain
Slipping rib syndrome
Precordial catch (Texidor's Twinge, benign pleuralgia)

Infectious causes

Devil's grip (epidemic pleurodynia, Bornholm disease)
Varicella zoster virus
Pleural effusion
Pneumonia
Pericarditis, myocarditis

Cardiac disease

Dysrhythmias (supraventricular tachycardia, premature ventricular contractions)
Structural abnormalities (hypertrophic congestive cardiomyopathy, aortic stenosis, pulmonary stenosis, mitral valve prolapse)
Coronary artery abnormalities
Coronary arteritis (Kawasaki disease)
Myocardial infarction, ischemia
Empyema, abscess
Myocarditis or pericarditis
Pneumopericardium
Rheumatic fever
Pulmonary hypertension
Dissecting aortic aneurysm
Marfan's syndrome
Ehlers-Danlos syndrome
Takayasu arteritis
Pheochromocytoma

Respiratory problems

Cough
Pneumonia
Asthma
Pleural effusion
Pneumothorax
Pneumomediastinum
Cystic fibrosis
Pulmonary embolism
Familial Mediterranean fever
Familial angioneurotic edema
Systemic lupus erythematosus

Gastrointestinal disorders

Esophagitis
Esophageal foreign bodies
Caustic ingestion
Esophageal ulceration, stricture
Achalasia
Peptic ulcer disease
Pancreatitis, pancreatic pseudocyst
Hiatal hernia
Pylorospasm

Idiopathic causes

Miscellaneous disorders

Thoracic tumor
Breast mass
Sickle cell crisis
Cigarette smoking
Anxiety, psychogenic causes (hyperventilation, depression, conversion reaction)

COMMON SKIN LESIONS

SKIN LESIONS ASSOCIATED WITH VESICLES AND BULLAE

A vesicle is a raised skin or mucous membrane lesion filled with clear fluid; a bulla is a lesion larger than 1 cm filled with clear fluid. Some may also involve pustules.

Bullous impetigo
Bullous pemphigoid
Burns
Carpet beetle bites (flaccid bullae)
Chronic bullous dermatosis of childhood
Coxsackievirus (hand-foot-mouth disease, many other coxsackievirus infections)
Dermatitis herpetiformis
Epidermolysis bullosa
  Dystrophic
  Generalized
  Localized
  Simplex
Friction blisters
Herpes gestationalis
Herpes simplex
IgA dermatosis
Incontinentia pigmenti (linear rows of blisters on extremities in first few months of life)
Miliaria crystallina
Papular urticaria (may look vesicular)
Pemphigus
  Benign familial
  Foliaceus
  Vulgaris
Polymorphous light eruption
Recurrent bullous eruption (Weber-Cockayne disease)
Staphylococcal scalded skin syndrome
Stevens-Johnson syndrome
Sucking blisters
Tinea pedis (occasionally manifests with pustules or vesicles on dorsum, not interdigital)
Toxic epidermal necrolysis
Varicella zoster virus (herpesvirus)
  Chickenpox
  Shingles

SKIN CONDITIONS ASSOCIATED WITH PUSTULES

A pustule is a raised lesion filled with white or yellow exudate. Many vesicular lesions may also involve pustules.

Abscess
Acne
Acropustulosis of infancy
Congenital candidiasis
Dyshidrotic eczema (pompholyx)
Erythema toxicum (newborn only)
Folliculitis
Hand-foot-mouth disease
Herpes simplex (HSVI and HSVII) virus infections
Kerion (often has pustules within boggy, red nodules)
Miliaria pustulosis
Palmoplantar pustulosis
Pustular melanosis (neonatal pustular melanosis)
Pustular psoriasis
Subcorneal pustulosis (Sneddon-Wilkinson disease)
Varicella Zoster

PAPULOSQUAMOUS SKIN LESIONS

A papular lesion is a solid, raised area, usually less than 1 cm in diameter, with distinct borders. The papule may be pink, red, violaceous, flesh colored, and hyperpigmented or hypopigmented. Papulosquamous disorders describe skin lesions with papules that have an accompanying scale.

Candida dermatitis (can manifest with collarette of scale on pink macule or papule)
Contact dermatitis
Dermatomyositis
Eczema or nummular eczema
Histiocytosis syndromes
Ichthyosis
Keratosis pilaris
Lichen planus
Lupus
Parapsoriasis
Pityriasis alba
Pityriasis rosea
Pityriasis rubra pilaris
PLEVA (pityriasis lichenoides et varioliformis acuta, Mucha-Haberman disease)
Psoriasis
Scabies
Seborrheic dermatitis
Secondary syphilis
Tinea corporis
Tinea versicolor

RED, RAISED LESIONS

Not including lesions listed previously, these papulosquamous lesions include erythema with and without scale.

Abscess
Acne
Angioedema
Angiofibroma
Atopic dermatitis (usually with scale)
Cellulitis and erysipelas
Diaper dermatitides (*Candida*, contact, psoriatic, seborrheic)
Erythema chronicum migrans (early rash of Lyme disease)
Erythema annulare

Erythema marginatum (rash associated with rheumatic fever)
Erythema multiforme
Erythema toxicum (neonatal)
Hemangioma (strawberry hemangioma)
Insect bites
Juvenile arthritis
Kawasaki disease
Lupus panniculitis
Miliaria rubra
Papular urticaria
Pyogenic granuloma
Rickettsial illnesses
- Rocky Mountain spotted fever
- Q fever
- Typhus
- Rickettsialpox

Scarlet fever and scarlatiniform exanthems (look like scarlet fever, but the cause is viral, often adenovirus or enteroviruses, especially coxsackievirus)
Secondary syphilis
Sunburn
Trauma
Urticaria
Viral exanthems
- They may be red or pink and can include any variety of macular (not raised, by definition), petechial (not raised, non-blanching), urticarial, morbilliform (measles-like), pustular, papular, ulcerative, and vesicular lesions.
- Viruses include adenoviruses, cytomegalovirus, Ebstein-Barr virus, enterovirus (especially coxsackievirus), echoviruses, human herpesvirus-6 (HHV-6), HHV-7, herpes simplex virus, rubeola, roseola (exanthem subitum), parvovirus B19 (fifth disease, erythema infectiosum), reoviruses, and varicella-zoster.

MACULAR LESIONS

Macular lesions are flat. They can be hyperpigmented or hypopigmented, and they may be red or pink.
Café au lait spots
Capillary hemangioma
Nevus flammeus (salmon patch)
Drug reaction or drug rash
Freckles
Nevi
Pityriasis alba (macule usually with slight scale)
Port wine stain
Postinflammatory hypopigmentation or hyperpigmentation
Tinea versicolor
Tuberous sclerosis (may have fine scale) and neurofibromatosis lesions
Viral exanthems
Vitiligo

COUGH

A reflexive action of deep inspiration followed by forced, rapid expiration, usually to protect and clear the airway of secretions, foreign material, or irritants.

Congenial anomalies: compression or abnormality of airway
Connection of airway to esophagus (tracheoesophageal fistula [TEF])
Tracheobronchomalacia
Interstitial lung disease
Aberrant mediastinal vessels
Pulmonary sequestration
Bronchopulmonary-foregut malformations
Bronchogenic cysts
Adductor vocal cord paralysis
Congenital mediastinal tumors
Other congenital sources
Cardiac malformations that lead to congestive heart failure
Aspiration because of neurogenic abnormality
Allergies
Rhinitis (allergic or vasomotor with postnasal drip)
Asthma or reactive airway (may begin with infectious upper airway disease)
Cough variant asthma (up to 40% of cases of chronic cough)
Allergic sinusitis
Infectious causes
Viral upper airway illnesses (upper respiratory infection)
- Respiratory syncytial virus (RSV)
- Human metapneumovirus (HMPV)
- Adenovirus
- Parainfluenza virus
- Influenza virus
- Rhinovirus
- Coronavirus

Sinusitis
- Streptococci
- *Moraxella*
- Nontypeable *Haemophilus influenzae*

Pneumonia and lower respiratory tract infections
- *Chlamydia* in young infant
- *Mycoplasma pneumoniae*
- *M. trachomatis* (infant)
- Viral pneumonia, bronchiolitis
- Bacterial pneumonias
  - *Streptococcus pneumoniae*
  - *Staphylococcus aureus*
  - *Haemophilus influenzae*
  - Gram-negative bacteria
  - Anaerobes
- Fungal infections

Whooping cough syndrome
- Pertussis
- Parapertussis
- RSV
- Adenovirus
- Influenza
- *Chlamydia*
- *Mycoplasma*
- Cystic fibrosis

Suppurative lung disease with bronchiectasis or abscess secondary to:
- Cystic fibrosis (CF)
- Dyskinetic cilia (immobile cilia, Kartagener syndrome)
- Foreign body

Granulomatous lung disease
- Tuberculosis
- Fungi (histoplasmosis, coccidiomycosis)

Paranasal sinus infection
Other causes usually associated with infections
Immunodeficiency syndromes
- Acquired immunodeficiency syndrome (AIDS)
- Immunoglobulin deficiencies
- T-cell abnormalities
- Combined B- and T-cell abnormalities
- Phagocyte defects

Abnormal mechanical clearance
- CF
- Immotile cilia
- Bronchiectasis

Foreign body aspiration or ingestion
Esophagus or tracheobronchial tree (most common in toddlers)
Tracheoesophageal (H-type) fistula
Tumors
Irritants
Chemical or physical
- Tobacco
- Firewood
- Dry or dusty air
- Volatile chemicals

Aspiration associated with gastroesophageal reflux disease (GERD)
Aspiration from swallowing abnormality or TEF
Psychogenic or habitual sources
Usually disappears during sleep
Brassy tone remarkable

DIARRHEA

Diarrhea is an abnormally high stool volume and water content, usually associated with increased frequency of stool, although normal amounts vary dramatically among children. Typical stool volumes for infants are 5 to 10 g/kg body weight per 24 hours and 100 to 200 g per day for adults. An amount that is greater than 10 g/kg/day for an infant or greater than 200 g/day for an older child usually means diarrhea. The most common causes of altered motility and absorption are colonization or invasion by bacteria, parasites, or viruses; inflammatory processes; or drugs.

HISTORY

Specific causes may be more likely with specific history.
Fever, crampy pain, tenesmus
- Inflammatory bowel diseases (Crohn's disease, ulcerative colitis)

Bloody stool
- *Shigella*
- *Escherichia coli*
- Amebiasis
- *Salmonella*
- *Yersinia*
- *Campylobacter*

Pain and fever (appendicitis-like)
- *Yersinia*

Multiple cases or outbreak
- In less than 6 hours: Staphylococcus, Bacillus
- In more than 6 hours: *Clostridium perfringens*

Seafood
Vibrio cholera (or similar)
Immunosuppression (malnutrition, acquired immunodeficiency syndrome [AIDS])
Salmonella
Rotavirus
Isoporosis
Cryptosporidium
Persistent diarrhea
Malnutrition
Diet changes
Milk ingestion
Antibiotic treatment
Poor appetite
Poor diet management

ACUTE DIARRHEA

Viral (acute gastroenteritis)
Rotavirus
Norwalk-like virus
Other viral causes
Bacterial
Salmonella spp. (antibiotics prolong carrier state; treat if dysentery, age < 6 months, immunosuppressed)
Shigella spp (trimethoprim-sulfamethoxazole [TMP-SMX], cephalosporin, amoxicillin or fluoroquinolone for severe disease or to prevent spread)
Yersinia (consider TMP-SMX, intravenous gentamicin, chloramphenicol)
Campylobacter (consider erythromycin ethylsuccinate, chloramphenicol, intravenous gentamicin)
C. difficile (50% newborns colonized, may be incidental; major treatment if infant discontinue antibiotic; may consider vancomycin or metronidazole)
E. coli 0157:H70 (antibiotics may increase risk of hemolytic uremic syndrome; treat only if toxic or septic or neonate with intravenous gentamicin or TMP-SMX)
Aeromonas (consider TMP-SMX)
Food poisoning, toxin mediated
Staphylococcus aureus
Bacillus cereus
C. perfringens
Other causes of acute diarrhea
Vibrio cholera
Giardia lamblia (furazolidone or metronidazole or use quinacrine)
Cryptosporidium
Entamoeba histolytica (metronidazole)
Inflammatory bowel disease
Consider if white blood cells or blood in stool but cultures are negative
Drug induced

CHRONIC DIARRHEA

Assess growth and development.
Onset in infancy, after infancy, school-age child or adolescent
Infancy
Congenital monosaccharidase or disaccharidase deficiencies
Pancreatic insufficiency (cystic fibrosis)
Na/H transport deficiencies
Chloride deficiency
Short gut
Microvillus abnormality
Chronic intractable diarrhea of the newborn (CIDN)
Malrotation or intermittent volvulus
After infancy
Overfeeding
Excessive juice intake
Specific food intolerance
Laxative abuse, Munchausen by proxy
Starvation stool, postinfectious enteropathy
Constipation with overflow encopresis
Irritable bowel syndrome
With growth insufficiency, workup may include the following:
Laboratory tests
Urinalysis, urine culture, blood urea nitrogen, creatinine (chronic renal insufficiency)
Calcium, phosphorus, alkaline phosphatase (rickets)
Electrolytes (acidosis, electrolyte abnormality)
Magnesium, zinc (fat malabsorption)
Carotene, cholesterol, human immunodeficiency virus (HIV), immunoglobulins, trypsinogen, sweat chloride, *C. difficile* toxin, small bowel aspirate and culture, IgA and transglutaminase (TTG) antibody, urine catecholamines, D-xylose
Stool ova and parasites
May also consider endoscopy or radiographic testing
Differential options include the following:
Cystic fibrosis
Immunodeficiency
AIDS/HIV
Celiac disease
Starvation stool
Giardia
Fat malabsorption
Celiac disease
Cystic fibrosis
Shwachman syndrome
Intestinal lymphangiectasia
Abetalipoproteinemia
Trypsinogen deficiency
Enterokinase deficiency
Acrodermatitis enteropathica (zinc deficiency)
Colitis or obstruction
Hirschsprung's disease
Inflammatory bowel disease
Milk protein allergy
Pseudo-obstruction
Secretory disorders (assess vasoactive polypeptide, prostaglandin, thyroid function testing, computed tomography of the abdomen)
Adrenal insufficiency
Thyroid disease
Tumor
Ganglioneuroma
Neuroblastoma
Carcinoid
Later childhood and adolescence
Laxative abuse (anorexia nervosa)
Irritable bowel (colon) syndrome
Inflammatory bowel disease
Other systemic disease
Giardia
Carbohydrate intolerance
Celiac disease
Eosinophilic gastroenteritis
Bacterial overgrowth
Food allergy

DYSURIA

Dysuria is pain with urination.
Infection
Urinary tract infection or cystitis
Viral
Bacterial
Enterobacteriaceae
Gram-positive organisms
Urethritis or vaginitis
Fungi *(Candida albicans)*
Bacterial
Gardnerella vaginalis
Neisseria gonorrhoeae
Chlamydia trachomatis
Syphilis (endourethral chancre)
Protozoa
Trichomonas vaginalis
Genital infection
Herpes simplex virus
Condyloma acuminata (genital warts)
Infection of paraurethral glands
Chemical irritation
Detergent
Fabric softener
Perfumed soaps
Bubble bath
Douches
Contraceptive jellies
Certain foods
Trauma or physical injury
Local injury
Masturbation
Meatal stenosis
Labial adhesion
Foreign body
Systemic disease
Reiter's syndrome
Crohn's disease
Hypercalciuria
Urinary stones

EAR PAIN

Ear pain, or otalgia, is common in children. Treatment of ear pain depends on the cause, which may be direct or indirect.
Direct causes
Acute otitis media
Serous otitis media
Otitis externa
Cellulitis of the ear
Mastoiditis
Herpes zoster infection of the ear or facial nerve
Barotrauma
Upper respiratory infection or nasal stuffiness
Airplane travel

Scuba diving
Foreign body
Object lodged in the ear canal
Cockroach or other insect
Impacted cerumen
Infected cyst
Neoplasms
Trauma
Indirect causes
Referred pain
Sore throat
Tooth pain
Temporomandibular joint dysfunction
Sinusitis
Parotitis
Lymphadenitis
Psychogenic causes

EDEMA, GENERALIZED

Edema is abnormal swelling from excessive accumulation of fluid in the interstitial space. Fluid usually appears in the dependent portions of extremities, especially the ankles or lower legs, or in distensible tissues, such as the eyelids, scrotum, labia, and abdomen.

Cardiac disease
Congestive heart failure
Pericardial effusion
Myocarditis
Renal disease
Nephrotic syndrome
Glomerulonephritis
Henoch-Schönlein purpura
End-stage renal failure
Renal vein thrombosis
Obstructive uropathy
Hepatic disease
Liver failure
Hepatitis
Biliary atresia
Gastrointestinal disease
Protein-losing enteropathy
Chronic protein malnutrition
Cystic fibrosis
Celiac disease
Enteritis of numerous types
Vascular disease
Vasculitis
Thrombosis
Lymphatic abnormalities
Turner syndrome
Noonan syndrome
Lymphedema
Primary or inherited form
Secondary forms caused by injury (infection, fibrosis, surgery, irradiation)
Allergic reaction
Hematologic disease
Hemolytic disease of the newborn
Pregnancy related
Normal pregnancy
Toxemia of pregnancy
Hereditary angioedema
Endocrine disease
Syndrome of inappropriate antidiuretic hormone (SIADH)
Hypothyroidism
Iatrogenic sources
Excess salt and water intake
Drugs
Steroids
Lithium
Contraceptives
Other causes
Vitamin E deficiency
Congenital albumin deficiency

GASTROINTESTINAL BLEEDING

Many food substances, such as red dyes, fruit juices, and beets, may mimic blood and confirmation of the presence of blood by Gastroccult (vomit) or guaiac (stool) tests is essential. Upper gastrointestinal tract bleeding occurs proximal to the ligament of Treitz (between the third and fourth segments of the duodenum); lower gastrointestinal bleeding occurs distal to this ligament. *Hematemesis* refers to bright red or brown blood in the vomit; it is usually seen with upper gastrointestinal tract bleeding. *Hematochezia* is bright red, brown, or dark red blood from the rectum; it is usually caused by bleeding in the lower gastrointestinal tract, but it can be seen with brisk upper gastrointestinal bleeding. *Melena* is the passage of black tarry material (product of degradation of blood in the small intestine) from the rectum; it is seen in cases of upper gastrointestinal tract bleeding.

BLEEDING FROM THE UPPER GASTROINTESTINAL TRACT

Oral or pharyngeal sources
Swallowed blood from the nose or oropharynx
Esophagus
Esophagitis
Esophageal varices
Stomach and duodenum
Gastritis
Ulcer
Mallory-Weiss tears (junction of esophagus and stomach)
Hemobilia (bleeding into the biliary tract)

BLEEDING FROM THE LOWER GASTROINTESTINAL TRACT

Small intestine
Cow's milk protein allergy
Necrotizing enterocolitis
Volvulus with malrotation
Meckel's diverticulum
Intussusception
Crohn's disease
Henoch-Schönlein purpura
Mesenteric thrombosis or embolism
Large intestine and rectum
Infectious colitis
Escherichia coli types
Salmonella species
Shigella species
Campylobacter jejuni
Clostridium difficile
Entamoeba
Parasites
Intussusception
Inflammatory bowel disease
Intestinal polyps
Juvenile polyps
Familial multiple adenomatous polyposis
Gardner's syndrome
Peutz-Jeghers syndrome
Benign lymphoid polyposis
Henoch-Schönlein purpura
Diverticulosis
Hemolytic uremic syndrome
Anus
Hemorrhoids
Fissure
Trauma or abuse

BLEEDING FROM THE UPPER OR LOWER GASTROINTESTINAL TRACT

Swallowed maternal blood
Vascular malformation
Arteriovenous malformations
Hemangiomas
Angiodysplasia
Rendu-Osler-Weber syndrome (hereditary hemorrhagic telangiectasia)
Duplication
Toxic ingestion or drugs
Aspirin or salicylates
Anticoagulants
Rat poison (superwarfarins)
Foreign body
Bleeding disorders
Hemorrhagic disease of the newborn
Disseminated intravascular coagulation
Hemophilia
Neoplasms

GENITAL SORES

Genital sores refers to lesions on female or male genitalia caused by infectious agents.

Herpes genitalis
Primary
Recurrent
Syphilis
Chancroid
Caused by *Haemophilus ducreyi*
Granuloma inguinale
Caused by *Calymmatobacterium granulomatis*
Genital warts or condyloma acuminatum
Frequently caused by human papillomavirus (HPV)
Lymphogranuloma venereum
Caused by *Chlamydia trachomatis*

HEADACHE

Most headaches in children do not indicate serious pathology. The differential diagnosis should initially focus on distinguishing serious causes from the more common causes. Table 2-1 reviews some characteristics that may be helpful in differentiating the common causes of headache.

TABLE 2-1 **Causes of Headache**

Characteristic	TYPE OF HEADACHE Migraine	Tension	Psychogenic
Location	Typically unilateral	Bilateral, often occipital	Bilateral, anywhere
Character	Throbbing	Pressure	Pressure or no particular
Severity	Moderate to severe	Mild to moderate	Usually mild
Aura	Sometimes	No	No
Associated symptoms	Vomiting, photophobia	Stress, muscle strain	Other somatic complaints, depression, anxiety

Vascular headache
Migraine
Common
Classic
Complicated
Hypertension
Vasculitis
Cerebral aneurysm
Embolus or infarction
Cluster headache
Intracranial infections
Meningitis
Encephalitis
Intracranial abscess
Altered intracranial pressure
Increased pressure
Tumor
Intracranial hemorrhage or hematoma
Intracranial abscess
Cerebral edema
Hydrocephalus
Pseudotumor cerebri
Venous sinus thrombosis
Decreased pressure
After lumbar puncture
Disorders of the head and neck
Eyestrain (rare)
Glaucoma
Sinus infections
Streptococcal pharyngitis
Dental caries
Malocclusion
Temporomandibular joint dysfunction
Cranial neuralgias (rare in pediatrics)
Muscular headache
Tension
Muscle strain
Activity
Posture
Prolonged position
Trauma
Intracranial hemorrhage or hematoma
Posttraumatic, concussion
Muscle strain (whiplash)
Psychogenic causes
Anxiety
Depression
Other causes
Systemic illness
Drugs
Poisoning
Hyperventilation
Hypoxia
Seizure, after seizure
Medical procedures (spinal tap)

HEMATURIA

Hematuria is the presence of red blood cells in the urine. Urine dipstick detects red blood cells, hemoglobin, and myoglobin; microscopy can reveal only red blood cells. Persistent hematuria, which is the presence of more than 2 to 5 red blood cells per high-power field on at least two of three consecutive spun urine specimens obtained over a 2-month period.

DIAGNOSTIC CONSIDERATIONS

Bleeding from glomeruli
Smoky (tea- or cola-colored), reddish brown urine
Red blood cell casts in urine
Proteinuria
Originates from red blood cells
May or may not coexist with hematuria
Combined with microscopic hematuria
Glomerulonephritis (most likely)
Acute tubular necrosis
Systemic diseases
Hemoglobinuria
Results from disorders causing hemolysis
Red cell membrane defects
Hemoglobinopathies
Immune hemolytic disorders
Mismatched blood transfusions
Disseminated intravascular coagulation
Sepsis
Malaria
Mechanical erythrocyte damage
Indicated by pink color of serum
Myoglobinuria
Caused by damage to muscles
Crush injury
Electrical burns
Prolonged seizures
Malignant hyperthermia
Myositis
Rhabdomyolysis
Extreme exercise
Presence determined by urine tests, normal-colored serum
Laboratory data to identify the source of urinary pigment indirectly
Low ratio of blood urea nitrogen to creatinine
High creatine phosphokinase level (damaged muscles release creatinine)
Causes of Hematuria
Infection
Cystitis
Pyelonephritis
Urethritis
Balanitis
Tuberculosis
Trauma
Kidney
Bladder
Urethra
Drugs or toxins
Nonsteroidal anti-inflammatory agents
Cyclophosphamide
Penicillins
Cephalosporins
Sulfa drugs
Furosemide
Aminoglycosides
Cyclosporin
Heavy metals
Vigorous exercise
Hypercalciuria
Calculi
Congenital
Infectious
Metabolic disorders
Hypercalciuria
Hyperuricosuria
Cystinuria
Hyperoxaluria
Idiopathic causes
Foreign body or instrumentation in the urethra or bladder
Urinary catheterization
Suprapubic aspiration
Tumor
Wilms' tumor
Leukemia
Hemangioma
Bladder cancer
Structural abnormality
Polycystic kidney disease
Cystic kidneys
Hydronephrosis
Ureteropelvic junction obstruction
Posterior urethral valves
Hemoglobinopathies
Sickle cell hemoglobinopathies
Others
Bleeding disorders

Hemophilias
Thrombocytopenias
Renal vessel thrombosis or infarction
Acute tubular necrosis
Drugs or toxins (see earlier)
Hypoxia
Hypoperfusion
Glomerulonephritis
Acute post-streptococcal inflammation
IgA nephropathy
Membranoproliferative disease
Henoch-Schönlein purpura
Alport's hereditary nephritis
Systemic diseases
Hemolytic uremic syndrome
Systemic lupus erythematosus
Polyarteritis nodosa
Wegener's granulomatosis
Goodpasture's syndrome
Benign familial hematuria
Benign nonfamilial hematuria

HEPATOMEGALY & HEPATOSPLENOMEGALY

Hepatomegaly is enlargement of the liver beyond its normal size. Hepatosplenomegaly is enlargement of the liver and the spleen. Causes of hepatomegaly without splenomegaly are indicated by (H). For splenomegaly without hepatomegaly, see Splenomegaly, Isolated in Section II.

Infectious causes
Viral infections
Epstein-Barr virus
Cytomegalovirus
Herpes simplex virus
Enterovirus
Varicella virus
Human immunodeficiency virus (HIV)
Congenital rubella
Hepatitis (H)
Bacterial infections
Sepsis
Endocarditis
Tuberculosis
Brucellosis
Congenital syphilis
Leptospirosis
Liver abscess (H)
Fitz-Hugh-Curtis syndrome (perihepatitis associated with gonorrhea or chlamydial infection)
Parasites
Toxoplasmosis
Visceral larva migrans
Chaga's disease
Amebiasis (H)
Malaria
Ascariasis (H)
Others
Fungal infection
Histoplasmosis
Rickettsial infection
Rocky Mountain spotted fever
Trauma or liver injury (H)
Hemolytic anemia
Neoplasms
Leukemia
Lymphoma
Neuroblastoma
Hemangioma (H)
Hepatic tumor (H)
Collagen vascular disease
Systemic lupus erythematosus
Juvenile rheumatoid arthritis
Cardiac causes
Congestive heart failure (H)
Pericardial tamponade (H)
Idiopathic neonatal hepatitis (H)
Chronic hepatitis (H)
Chronic active hepatitis
Chronic persistent hepatitis
Cirrhosis
Congenital hepatic fibrosis (h)
Hepatic cysts (H)
Drugs or toxins (H)
Acetaminophen
Ethanol
Carbon tetrachloride
Phenytoin
Valproate
Tetracycline
Isoniazid
Androgenic steroids
Antineoplastic or chemotherapeutic agents
Mushroom poisoning
Biliary tract obstruction (H)
Extrahepatic obstruction
Biliary atresia
Biliary hypoplasia
Gallstones
Intrahepatic obstruction
Intrahepatic biliary atresia
Alagille's syndrome
Byler's syndrome
Metabolic disorders
Amino acid disorders
Tyrosinemia
Carbohydrate disorders
Galactosemia (H)
Hereditary fructose intolerance (H)
Fructose-1,6-diphosphatase deficiency (H)
Glycogen storage diseases (H)
Others
Lipidoses
Niemann-Pick disease
Gaucher's disease
Farber's disease
Mucopolysaccharidoses
Mucolipidoses
Glycoproteinoses
Fucosidosis
Mannosidosis
Sialidosis
Acid lipase deficiency
Wolman's disease
Cholesterol ester storage disease (H)
Peroxisomal disorders
Zellweger syndrome (H)
Lipoprotein disorders
Type I hyperlipoproteinemia
Other causes
Peripheral hyperalimentation (H)
Malnutrition (H)
Cystic fibrosis (H)
Histiocytosis
Hemochromatosis (H)
Wilson disease (H)
α_1-Antitrypsin deficiency (H)
Reye's syndrome (H)
Sarcoidosis (H)

HOARSENESS

Hoarseness is a harsh-sounding voice, often with a decreased volume or whisper.

Infections
Laryngitis
Croup (laryngotracheitis)
Infectious mononucleosis
Epiglottitis
Bacterial tracheitis
Diphtheria
Voice strain or overuse
Excessive crying
Allergic reaction
Trauma
After intubation
Nasogastric or orogastric tube
Caustic substances or burns
Vocal cord paralysis (postoperative trauma)
Blunt neck trauma
Irritants
Tobacco smoke
Foreign body
Tumors
Benign
Laryngeal papilloma
Hemangioma
Vocal cord polyps
Others
Malignant (rare)
Congenital abnormalities
Laryngomalacia
Laryngeal web
Laryngeal cyst
Laryngocele
Laryngeal cleft
Congenital vocal cord paralysis
Neurologic abnormalities
Recurrent laryngeal nerve impingement
Aberrant great vessels
Cardiomegaly
Hemorrhage
Hilar adenopathy
Neoplasm
Recurrent laryngeal nerve dysfunction
Central nervous system disease
Arnold-Chiari malformation
Multiple sclerosis
Stroke
Tumor
Others
Motor nerve dysfunction
Botulism
Myasthenia gravis
Werdnig-Hoffmann disease
Muscular dystrophy
Toxins
Hypocalcemia
Angioneurotic edema
Genetic syndromes

Achondroplasia
Cri du chat syndrome
Others
Storage diseases
Lysosomal disorders
Sarcoidosis
Amyloidosis

HYPOGLYCEMIA

Hypoglycemia is defined as a serum or plasma glucose level less than 40 mg/dL or a whole blood glucose level below 35 mg/dL.

Hyperinsulinemia
Infant of a diabetic mother
Pancreatic or islet cell dysphasia or hyperplasia (formerly called nesidioblastosis)
Islet cell adenoma or adenomatosis
Beckwith-Weidemann syndrome
Exogenous administration of insulin
- Unintentional overdose
- Suicide attempt
- Munchausen syndrome by proxy

Poor intake or diminished glycogen stores
Low birth weight or small for gestational age
Hepatitis
Hepatic failure
- Congenital, infectious, or inborn error of metabolism (IEM)
- Cirrhosis
- Reye's syndrome
- α_1-Antitrypsin deficiency

Malnutrition
Malabsorption, chronic diarrhea
Insufficient glucose administration postoperatively
Ketotic hypoglycemia
Counter-regulatory hormone abnormalities
Hypothalamic defect or hypopituitarism
Growth hormone deficiency
Growth hormone receptor unresponsiveness (Laron dwarfism)
Cortisol deficiency
- Addison disease
- Adrenal failure
- Congenital adrenal insufficiency

Adrenocorticotropic hormone (corticotropin) deficiency or unresponsiveness
Thyroid hormone deficiency
Glucagon or catecholamine deficiency (both rare)
Inborn errors of metabolism
Glycogen storage diseases (GSD)
- GSD 6ype Ia, Ib (glucose-6-phosphatase deficiency)
- GSD type 0 (glycogen synthetase deficiency)
- Liver phosphorylase enzyme defects

Gluconeogenesis enzyme abnormalities
- Fructose-1,6-diphosphatase
- Phosphoenolpyruvate carboxykinase
- Pyruvate carboxylase

Galactosemia (galactose-1-phosphate uridyltransferase defect)
Hereditary fructose intolerance (fructose-1-phospate aldolase defect)
Amino acid and organic acid abnormalities
- Maple syrup urine disease (MSUD)
- Propionic acidemia
- Methylmalonic aciduria
- Tyrosinosis
- 3-Hydroxy-3-methlyglutaric aciduria
- Glutaric aciduria

Enzymatic defects in fat metabolism
- Carnitine deficiency
- Transferase deficiency
- Long-chain and medium-chain acyl CoA dehydrogenase deficiencies

Drugs or poisons
Salicylates
Alcohol (EtOH)
Propranolol
Hypoglycemic agents (sulfonylureas)
Pentamidine
Hypoglycin (Jamaican vomiting sickness from unripe ackees)
Other causes
Tumors
- Hepatoma
- Adrenocortical carcinoma
- Wilms' tumor
- Neuroblastoma
- Others

Cyanotic congenital heart disease

HYPOTONIA

Hypotonia is decreased resistance to passive movement. It is usually associated with joint hypermobility and decreased reflexes. It may or may not be associated with weakness (i.e., diminished muscle power).

Generalized brain insults
Hypoxic-ischemic encephalopathy
After seizures (post-ictal)
Sepsis
Meningitis
Hypotonic cerebral palsy
Spinal cord disorders
Trauma
Spinal dysraphism
- Meningomyelocele

Abscess
Neoplasm
Transverse myelitis
Anterior horn cell disorders
- Spinal muscular atrophy (Werdnig-Hoffman disease)
- Polio and other enteroviral infections

Peripheral nervous system disorders
Acute disorders
- Guillain-Barré syndrome

Chronic disorders
- Hereditary motor sensory neuropathy
  - Charcot-Marie-Tooth disease
  - Refsum's disease
- Leukodystrophies

Neuromuscular junction disorders
Botulism
Myasthenia gravis
Tick paralysis
Muscle disorders
Myopathies
- Congenital
- Mitochondrial
- Metabolic
- Glycogen storage diseases
- Carnitine deficiency

Periodic paralysis
- Hypokalemic
- Hyperkalemic
- Normokalemic

Muscular dystrophies
- Congenital
- Duchenne's
- Becker
- Limb-girdle
- Fascioscapulohumeral

Myotonic dystrophy
- Congenital
- Later-onset

Dermatomyositis
Polymyositis
Metabolic disorders
Amino acid disorders
Organic acid disorders
- Methylmalonic acidemia
- Propionic acidemia

Lipidoses
- Tay-Sachs disease
- Niemann-Pick disease

Leukodystrophies (Krabbe's disease)
Mucopolysaccharidoses
Mucolipidoses
Peroxisomal disorders
Endocrine disorders
Hypothyroidism
Hypopituitarism
Chromosomal disorders and syndromes
Down syndrome
Achondroplasia
Ehlers-Danlos syndrome
Marfan's syndrome
Opitz syndrome
Prader-Willi syndrome
Velocardiofacial (Shprintzen's syndrome)
Sotos syndrome
Others
Benign essential hypotonia

JAUNDICE & HYPERBILIRUBINEMIA

Jaundice refers to the yellow color of the skin and sclera caused by hyperbilirubinemia. Bilirubin is a breakdown product of heme, derived from red blood cells. Bilirubin is carried to the liver by albumin, where it is conjugated by glucuronyl transferase to a water-soluble form. Bilirubin is then excreted into the small intestine as bile and eliminated in the stool. Hyperbilirubinemia is classified as unconjugated (indirect) hyperbilirubinemia or conjugated (direct [directly measured]) hyperbilirubinemia.

NEONATAL UNCONJUGATED HYPERBILIRUBINEMIA

Physiologic jaundice
Increased bilirubin production
Cephalohematoma or other bleed with resorption of heme
Polycythemia

Delayed umbilical cord clamping
Twin-to-twin transfusion
Maternal-fetal transfusion
Maternal diabetes
Isoimmunization
Rh
ABO
Other reactions
Red blood cell enzyme defects
Glucose-6-phosphate dehydrogenase (G6PD) deficiency
Pyruvate kinase deficiency
Other defects
Red blood cell membrane defects
Hereditary spherocytosis
Hereditary elliptocytosis
Other defects
Decreased bilirubin conjugation
Glucuronyl transferase deficiency (Crigler-Najjar syndrome)
Type I
Type II
Transient familial hyperbilirubinemia (Lucy-Driscoll syndrome)
Decreased intestinal elimination
Intestinal obstruction
Pyloric stenosis
Duodenal atresia
Ileal atresia
Other obstructions
Lack of feeding
Delayed passage of meconium
Hirschsprung's disease
Meconium ileus
Other causes
Breast milk-associated jaundice
Hypothyroidism
Hypoalbuminemia
Drugs
Sulfa drugs
Cephalosporins
Sepsis
Hypoxia or acidosis

POSTNEONATAL UNCONJUGATED HYPERBILIRUBINEMIA

Increased bilirubin production
Hemolytic anemia (see Anemia in Differential Diagonsis [Section II])
Sepsis
Decreased bilirubin conjugation
Gilbert disease
Glucuronyl transferase deficiency (Crigler-Najjar syndrome)

NEONATAL CONJUGATED HYPERBILIRUBINEMIA

Infectious causes
Toxoplasmosis
Rubella
Cytomegalovirus
Herpesvirus
Syphilis
Varicella virus
Enterovirus
Hepatitis B virus
Sepsis or bacterial agents
Urinary tract infection
Biliary obstruction
Intrahepatic obstruction
Congenital biliary atresia–hypoplasia of intrahepatic biliary ducts
Alagille's syndrome
Byler's disease
Extrahepatic obstruction
Biliary atresia
Congenital malformations of the biliary tree
Total parenteral nutrition
Metabolic disorders
α_1-Antitrypsin deficiency
Cystic fibrosis
Zellweger syndrome
Galactosemia
Glycogen storage disease
Hereditary fructose intolerance
Tyrosinemia
Lipidoses
Niemann-Pick disease
Gaucher's disease
Neonatal hemosiderosis
Other causes
Idiopathic neonatal hepatitis
Inspissated bile syndrome (persistent direct hyperbilirubinemia associated with isoimmune hemolytic disease)
After asphyxia

POSTNEONATAL CONJUGATED HYPERBILIRUBINEMIA

Infectious causes
Hepatitis A, B, C, D, E
Epstein-Barr virus
Cytomegalovirus
Varicella virus
Peritonitis
Parasitic infections
Liver abscess
Chronic hepatitis
Chronic persistent hepatitis
Chronic active hepatitis
Drugs and chemicals
Acetaminophen
Phenytoin
Isoniazid
Carbon tetrachloride
Mushroom poisoning
Chemotherapy agents
Alcohol
Other chemicals
Biliary tract disease
Cholelithiasis
Cholecystitis
Choledochal cyst
Cholangitis
Pancreatic malformations or disease
Familial hepatic disorders
Dubin-Johnson syndrome
Rotor syndrome
Total parenteral nutrition
Cirrhosis
Neoplasms
Primary hepatic tumors
Metastatic disease
Metabolic disorders
Wilson disease
Hemochromatosis
Neonatal causes (see earlier)
Other causes
Reye's syndrome
Ischemic liver injury
Porphyria

KNEE PAIN

Knee pain is acute or chronic pain in or around the knee caused by one of multiple bone, tendon, ligament, muscle, or cartilage abnormalities (see Knee Maneuvers in Charts, Formulas, Laboratory Test and Values [Section IV]). The knee is a hinge joint with bony, ligamentous, muscle, and menisci involvement. Abnormal function, acute injury, or chronic inflammation of any element may cause knee pain, which also may be referred from disorders of the hip or back.

ASSOCIATED RISK FACTORS

Approximately 10% to 12% of patients presenting with musculoskeletal pain have knee pain.
Knee injuries account for 30% to 40% of sports medicine injuries in the pediatric and adolescent populations.
Hypermobility or hypermobile joint increases the risk of injury.
Injury, anomaly, or infection of bones, ligaments, tendons, and muscles may lead to knee pain.

ANATOMIC FACTORS

Bones involved in the knee
Femur: physis (growth plate) close to the knee joint
The distal femoral physis is the most active growth plate in body.
Medial and lateral condyles articulate with the tibial plateau.
Condyles are connected by the trochlear groove.
The anterior portion of the condyles and trochlear groove articulates with the patella.
Fusion occurs at approximately age 15 years in girls (range, 12 to 17 years) and age 17 years in boys (range, 15 to 20 years).
Tibia: proximal growth plate close to the knee joint
The physis is responsible for significant growth.
Flattened tibial plateau articulates with the femoral condyles.
Patella: initially cartilaginous, with ossification beginning as early as age 2 to 3 years
The patella, a sesamoid bone, is attached within the distal quadriceps.
It normally tracks parallel to the long axis of the lower extremity, moving caudad with flexion and cephalad with extension.
It articulates with the intertrochlear groove and femoral condyles.
Ligaments (static restraints that stabilize joints)

ICD-9-CM # 789.3 (0-9)

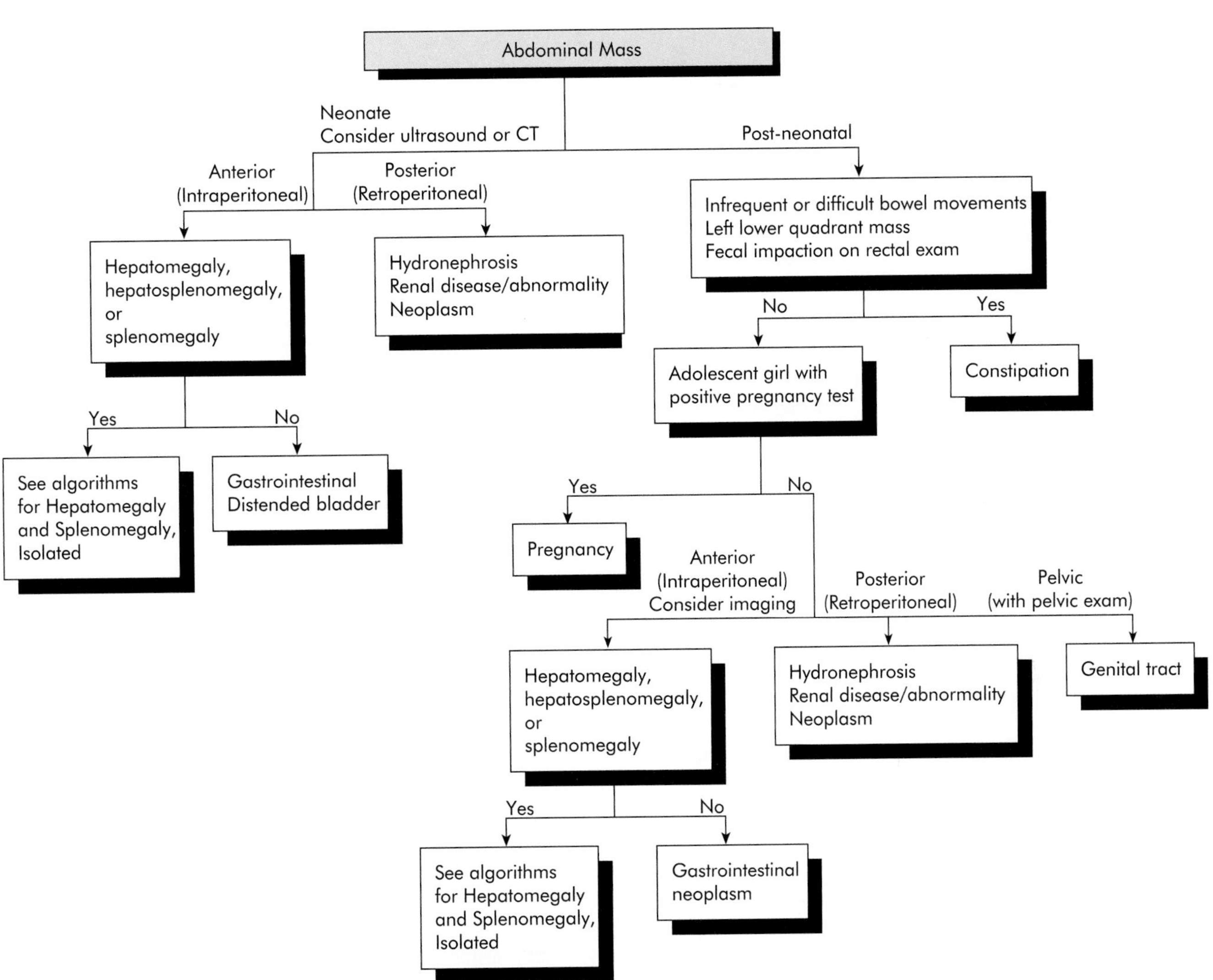

FIGURE 3-1 Abdominal Mass (see Abdominal Mass in Differential Diagnosis [Section II])

ICD-9-CM # 789.0 (0-9)

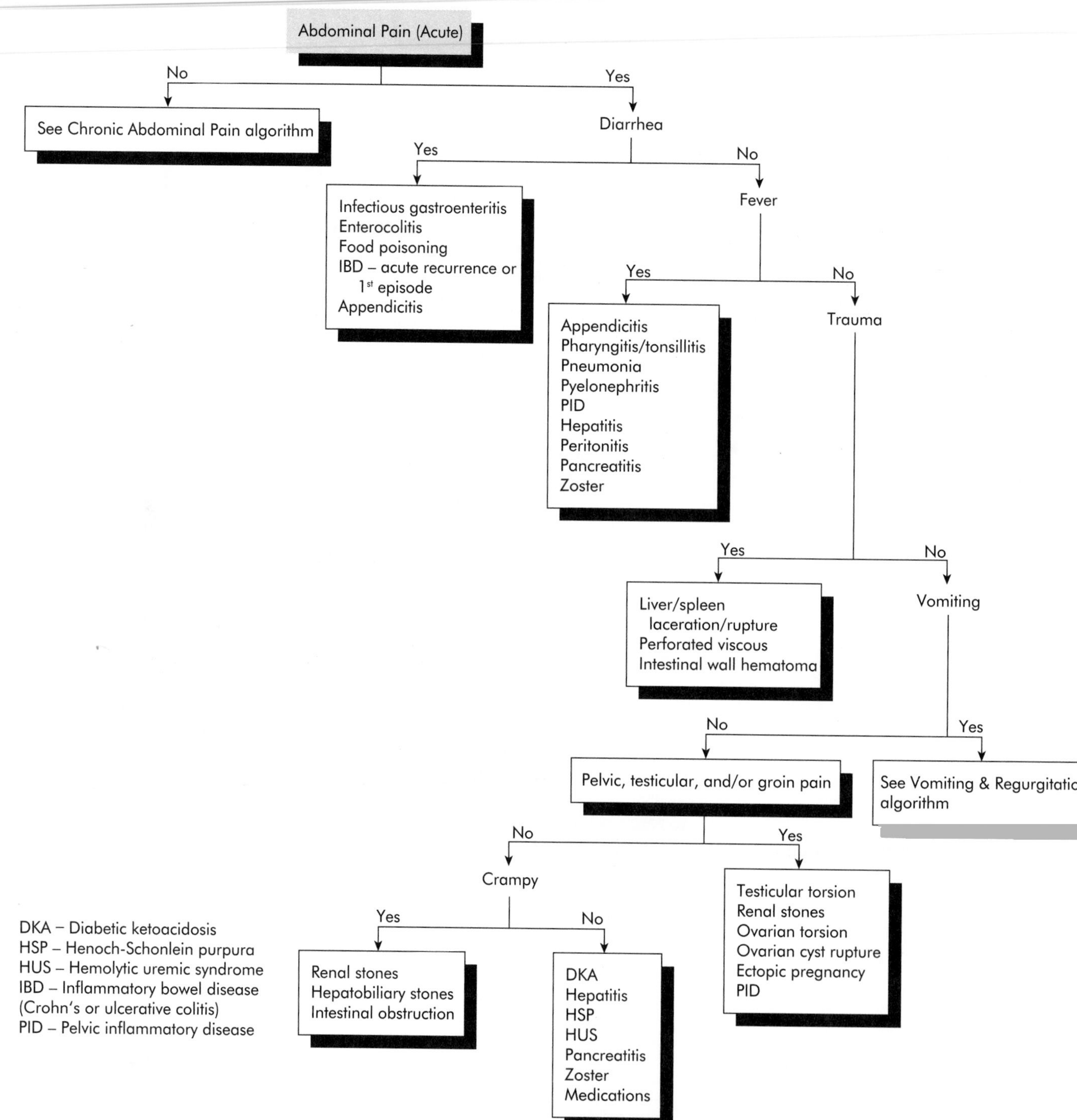

FIGURE 3-2 Abdominal Pain, Acute (see Abdominal Pain in Differential Diagnosis [Section II])

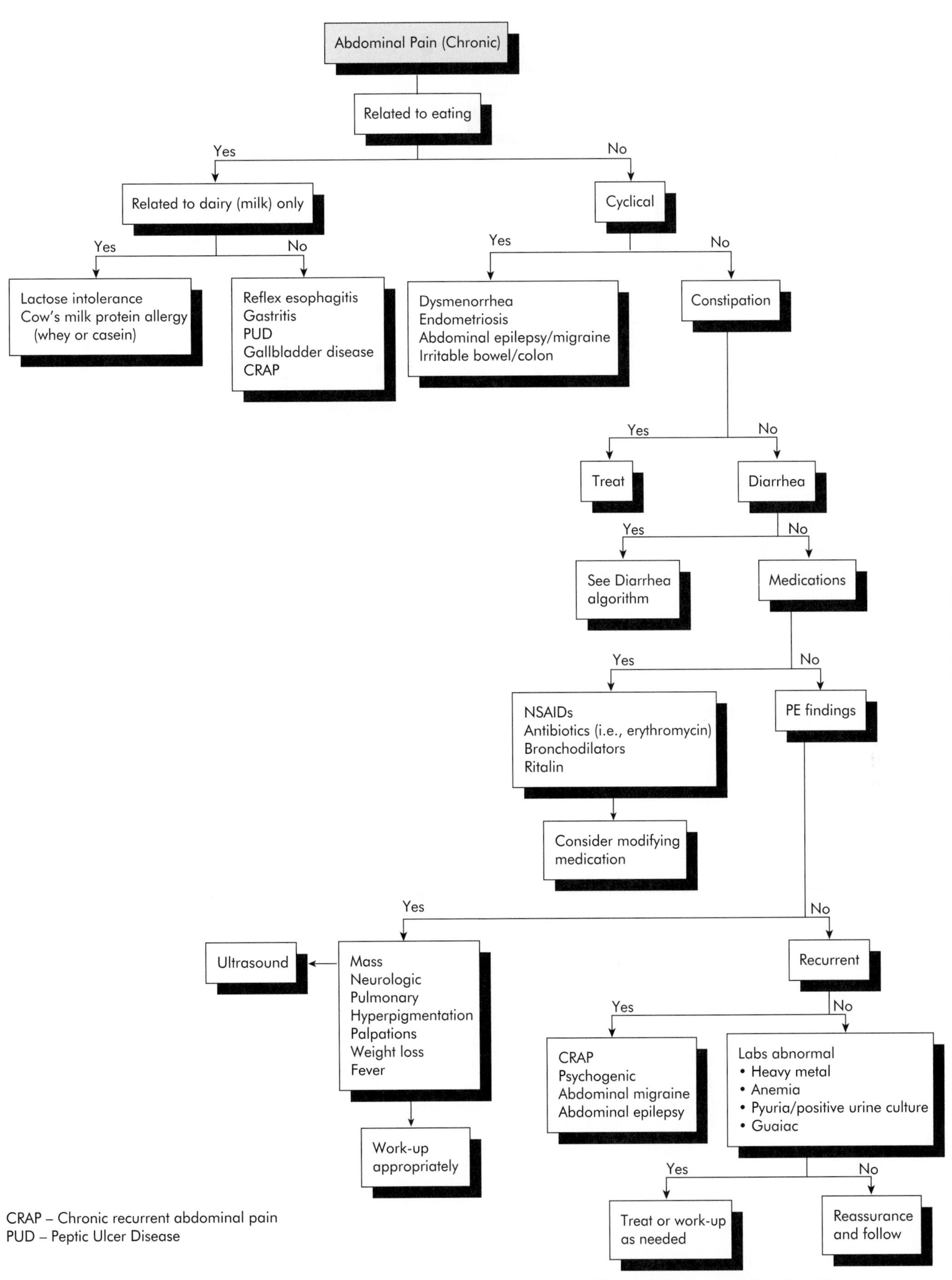

FIGURE 3-3 Abdominal Pain, Chronic (see Abdominal Pain in Differential Diagnosis [Section II])

ICD-9-CM # 704

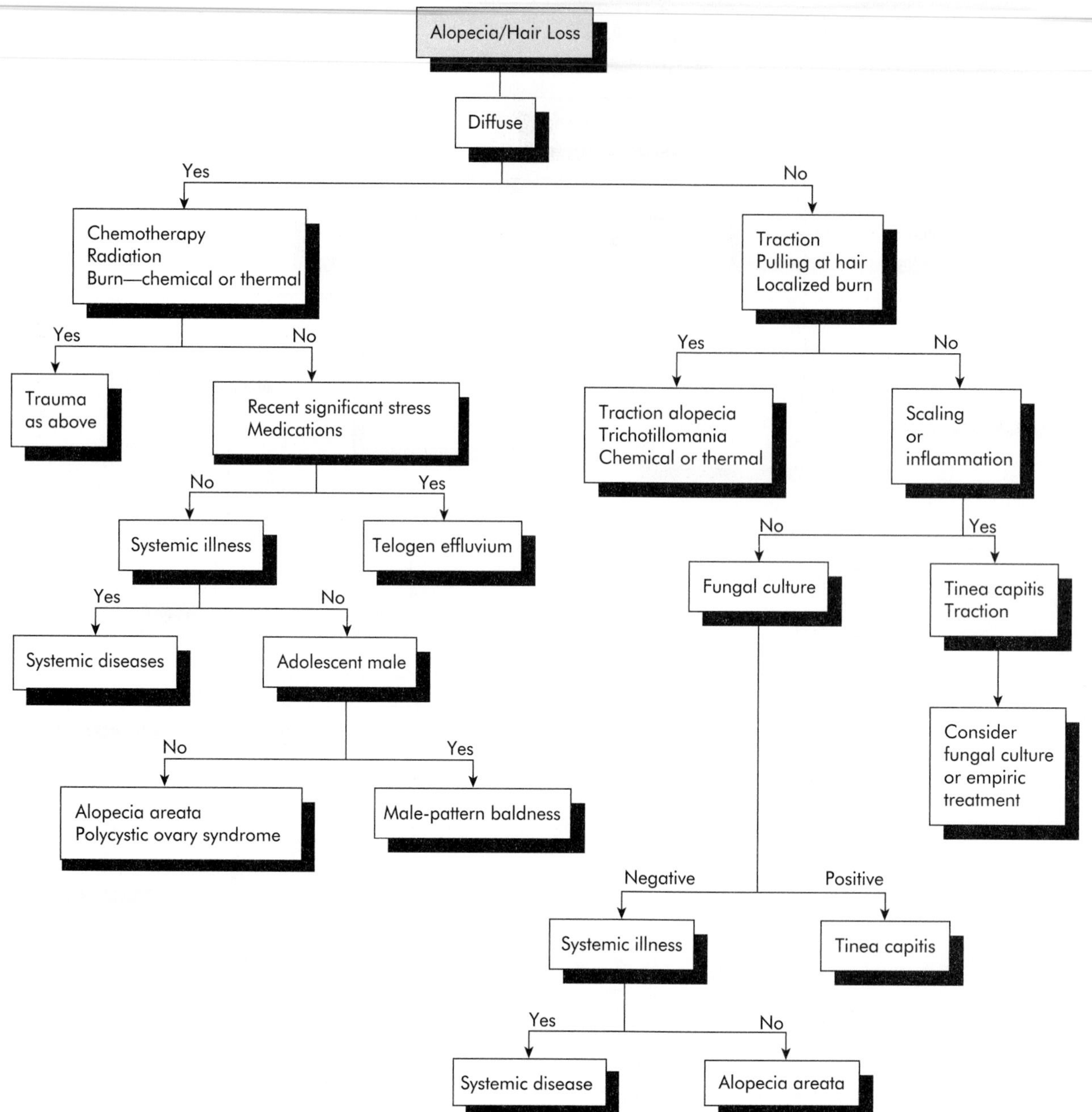

FIGURE 3-4 Alopecia/Hair Loss (see Alopecia/Hair Loss in Differential Diagnosis [Section II])

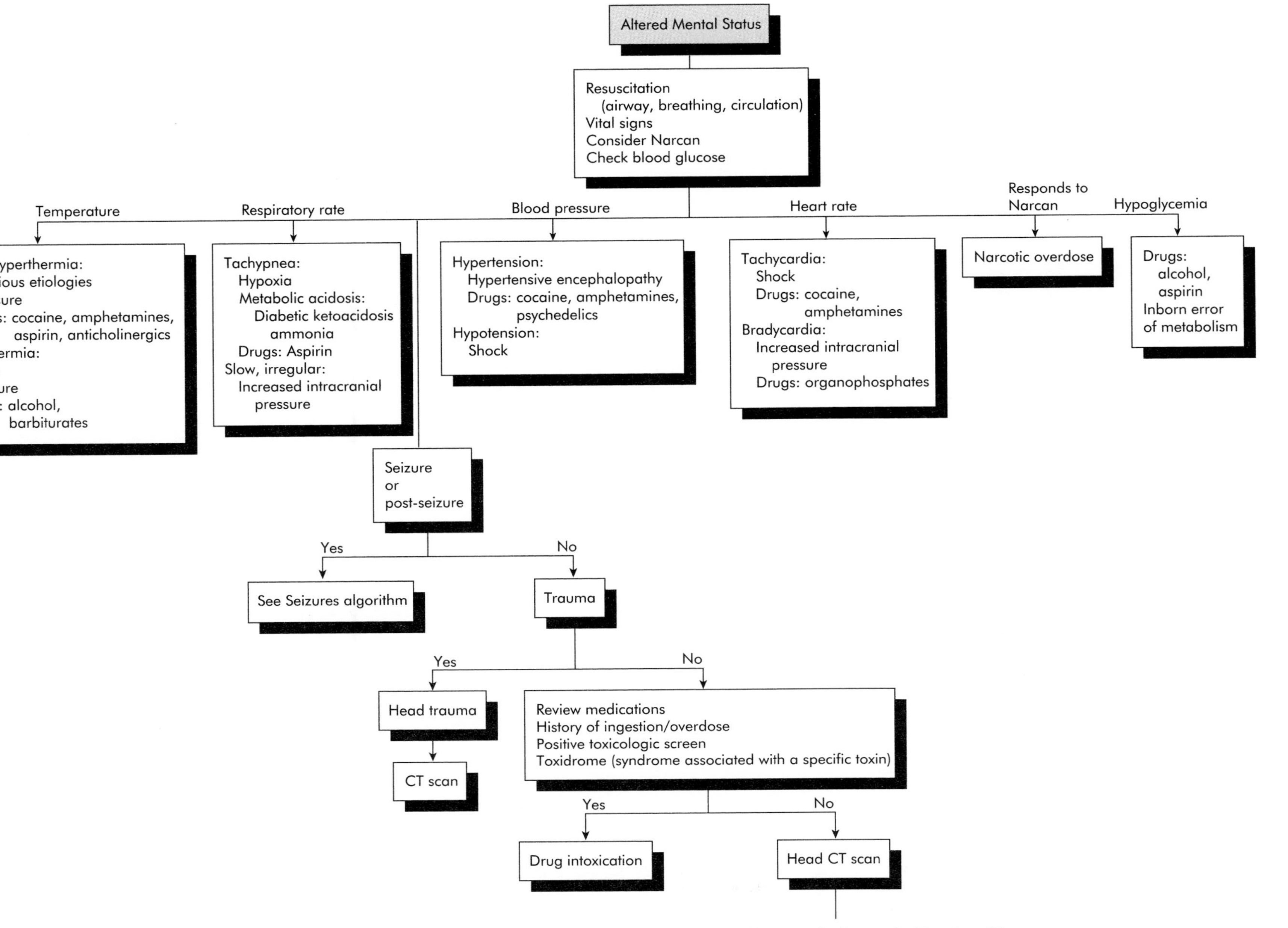

FIGURE 3-5 Altered Mental Status (see Altered Mental Status in Differential Diagnosis [Section II])

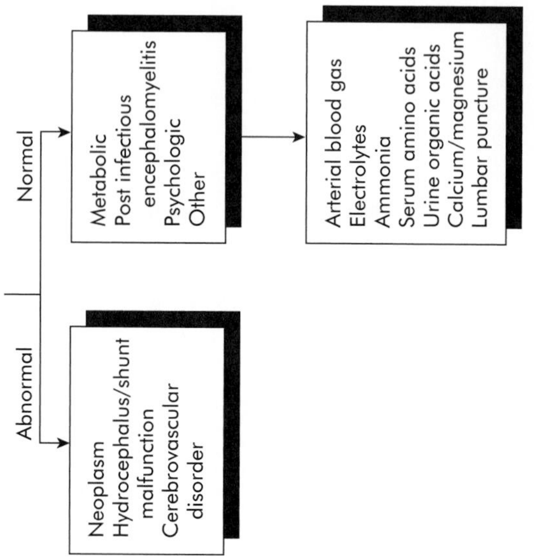

FIGURE 3-5 (Continued)

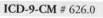

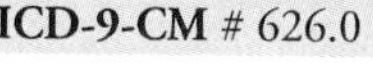

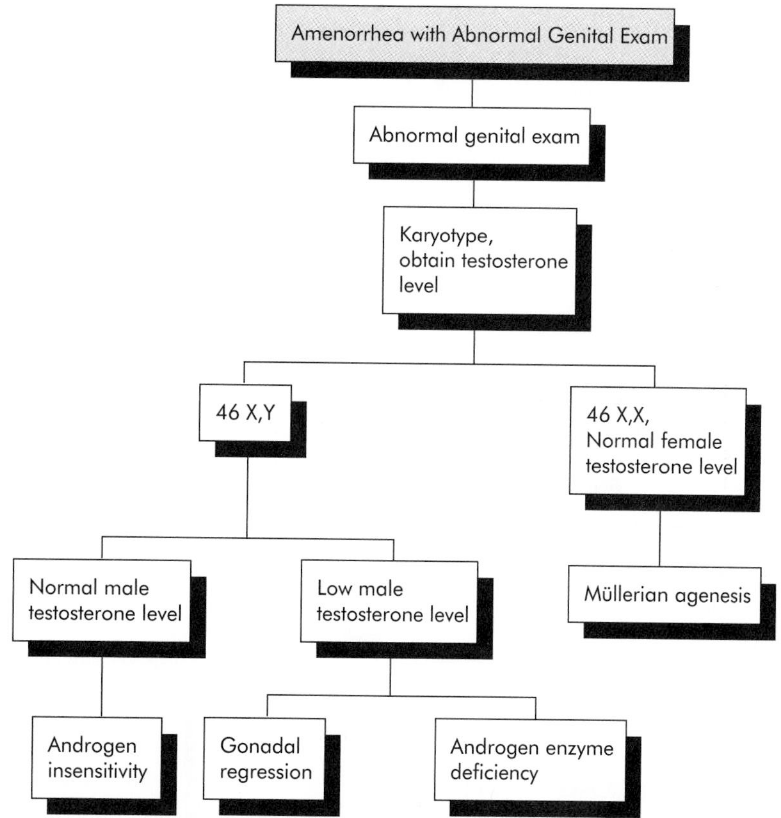

FIGURE 3-6 Amenorrhea with Abnormal Genital Exam (see Amenorrhea in Differential Diagnosis [Section II])

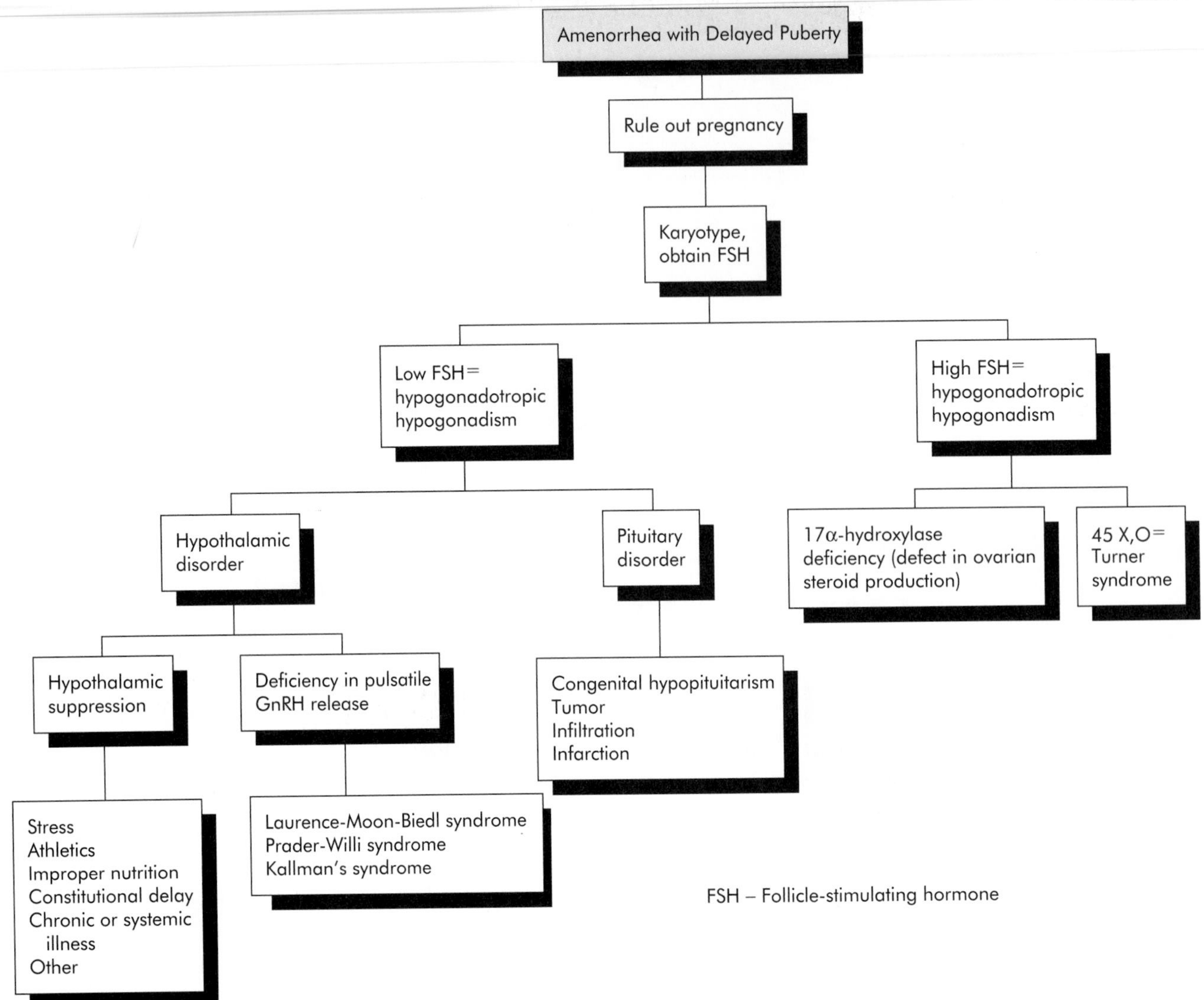

FIGURE 3-7 Amenorrhea with Delayed Puberty (see Amenorrhea in Differential Diagnosis [Section II])

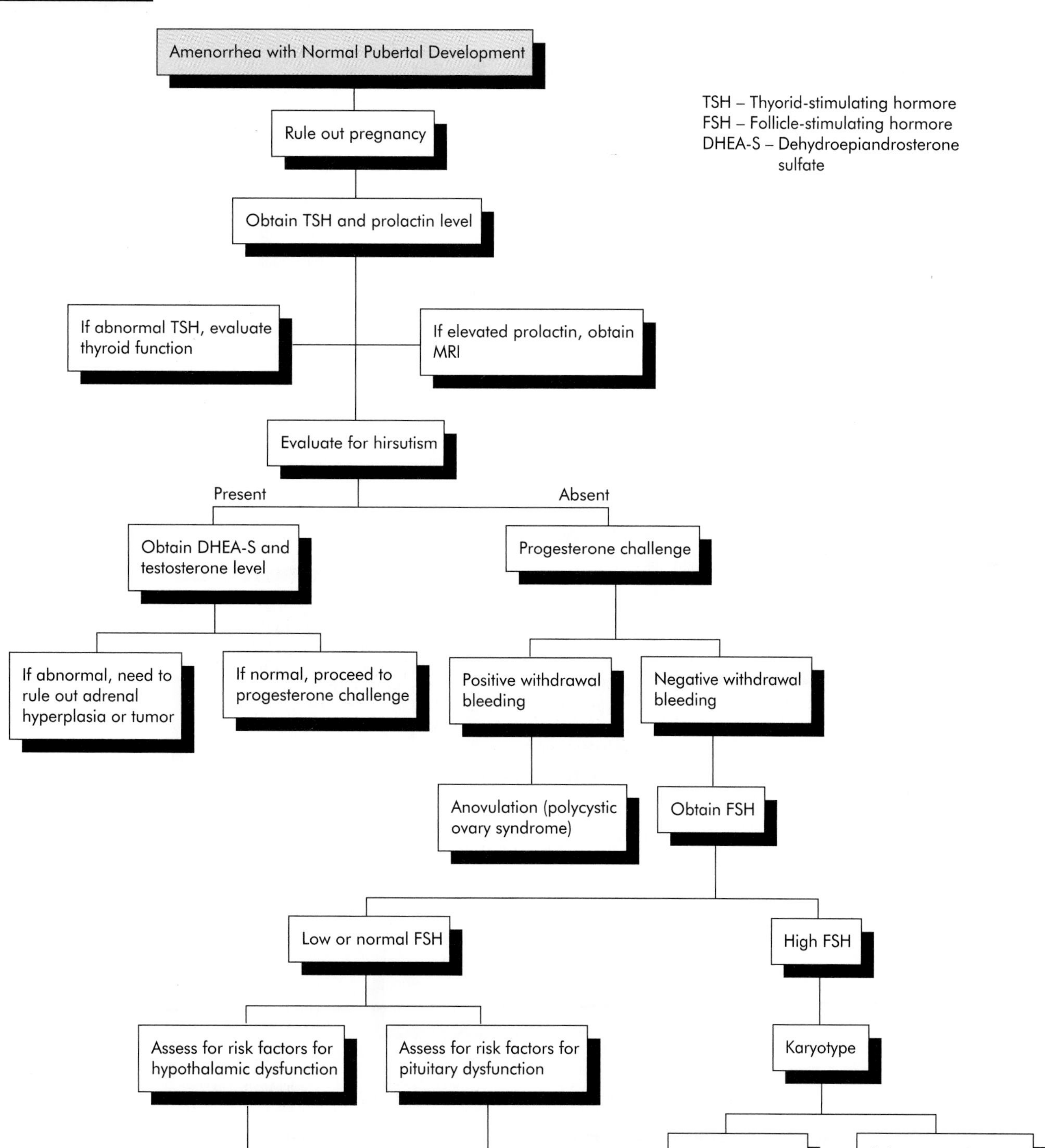

FIGURE 3-8 Amenorrhea with Normal Pubertal Development (see Amenorrhea in Differential Diagnosis [Section II])

ICD-9-CM # 716.9
716.1 Traumatic

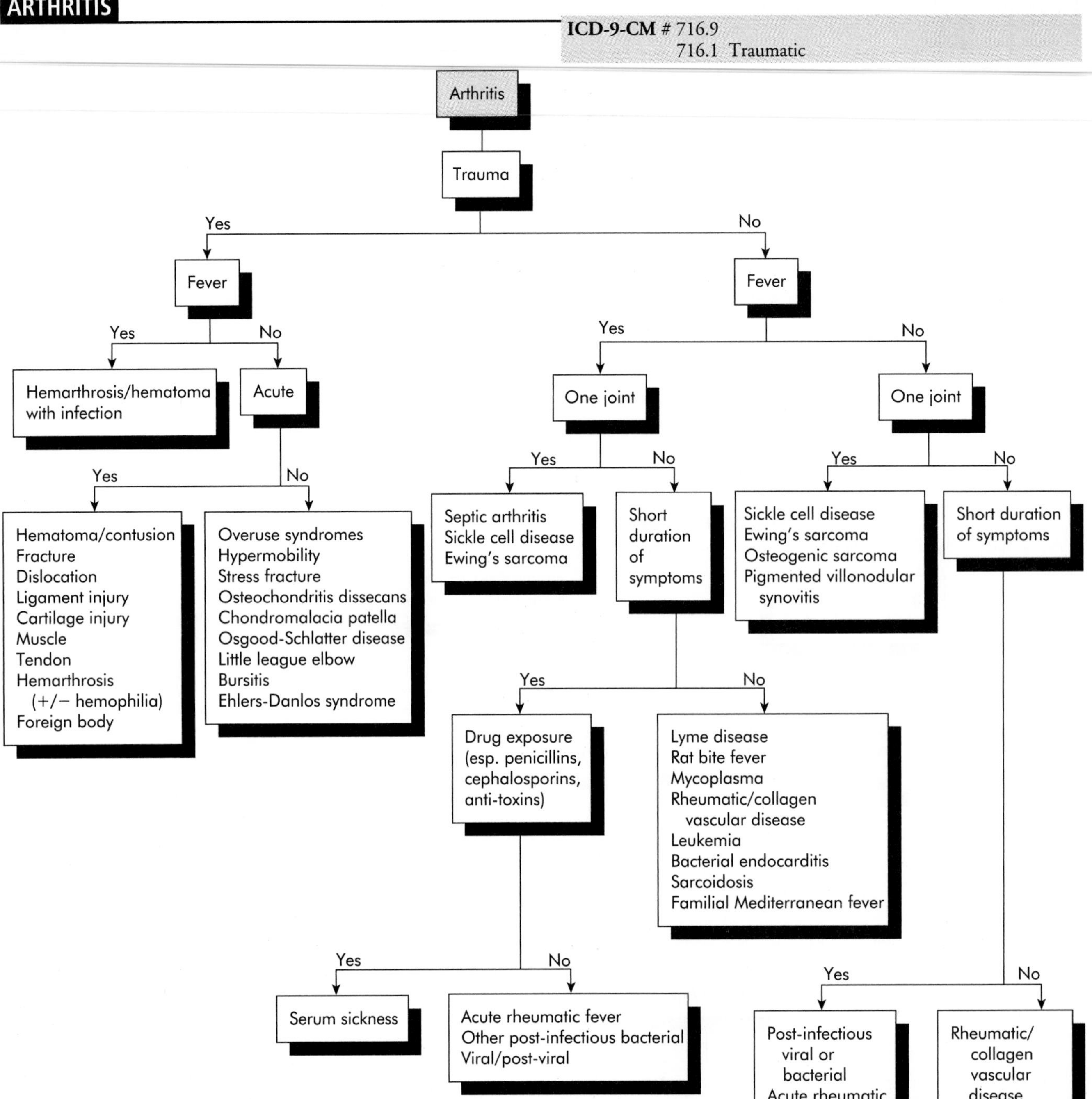

FIGURE 3-9 Arthritis (see Arthritis in Differential Diagnosis [Section II])

ICD-9-CM # 781.3

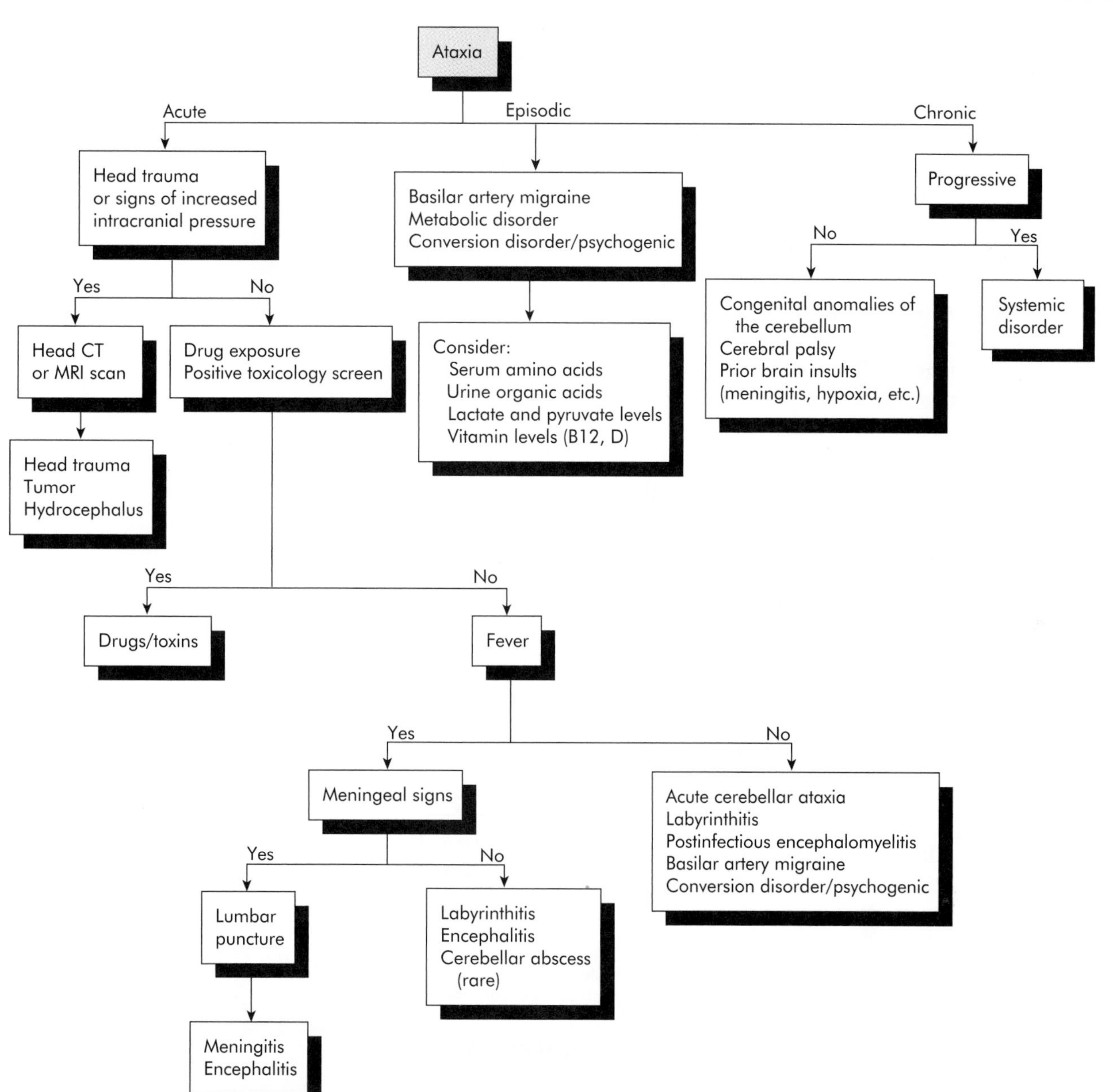

FIGURE 3-10 Ataxia (see Ataxia in Differential Diagnosis [Section II])

ICD-9-CM # 724.5

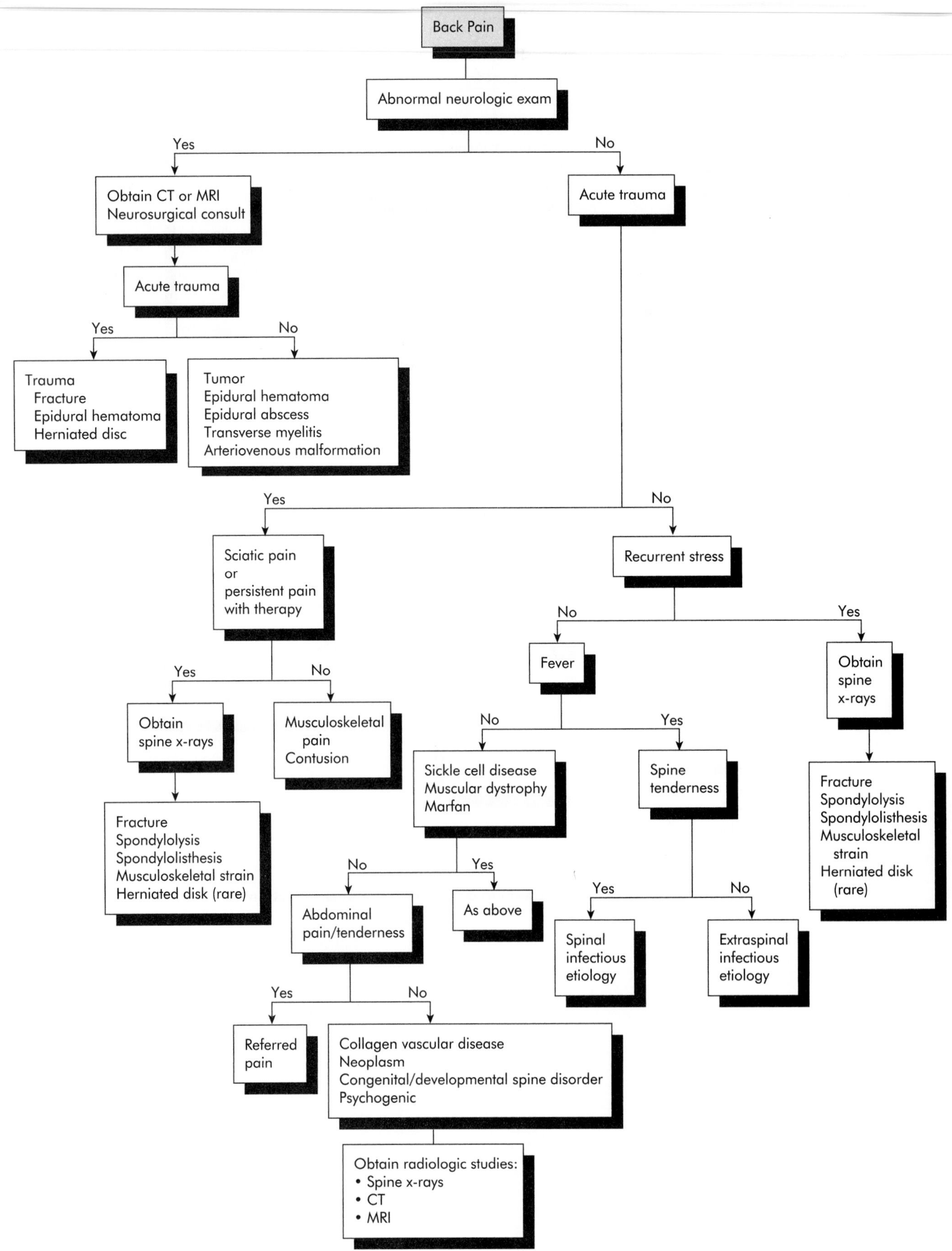

FIGURE 3-11 Back Pain (see Back Pain in Differential Diagnosis [Section II])

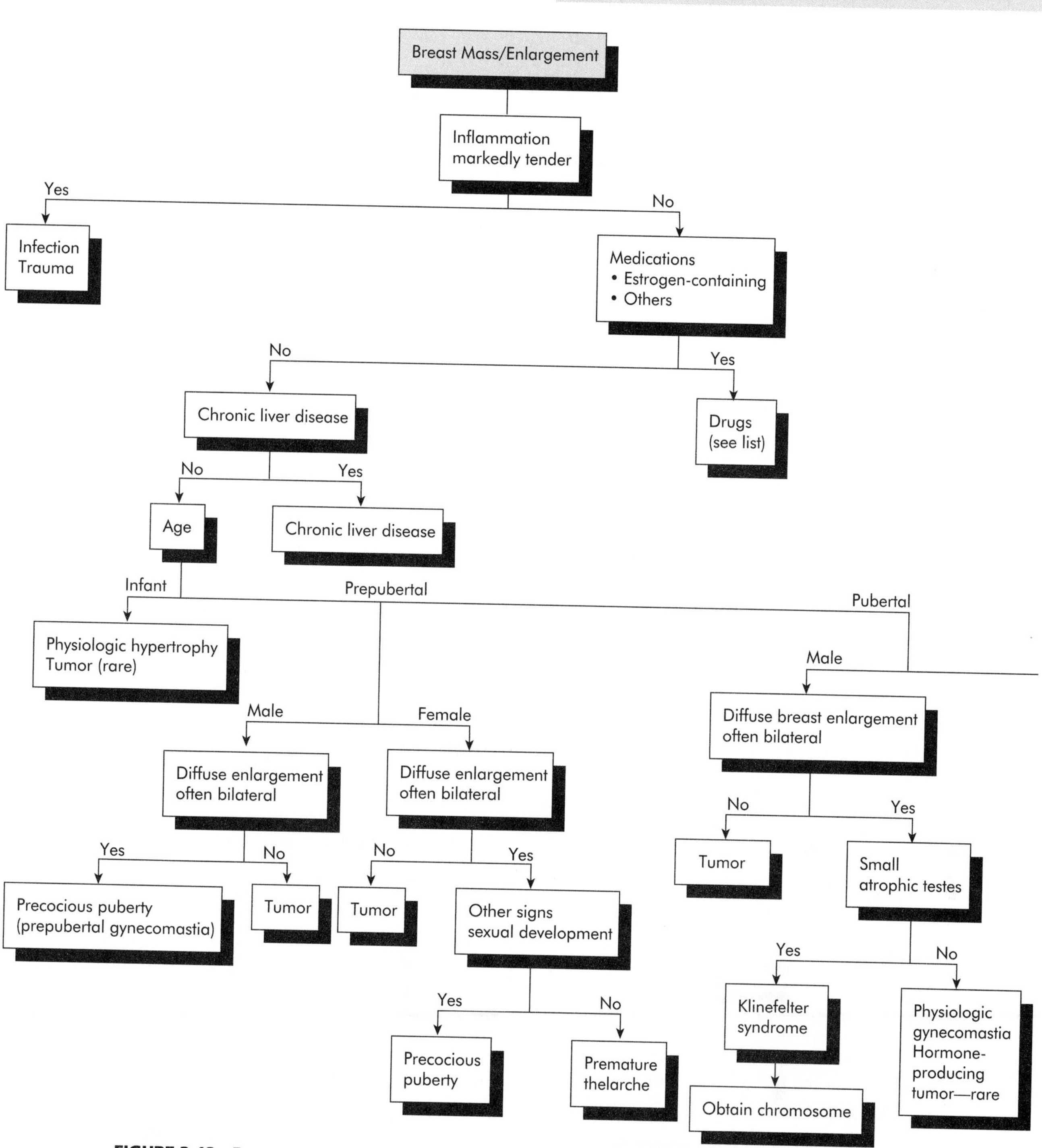

FIGURE 3-12 Breast Mass/Enlargement (see Breast Mass/Enlargement in Differential Diagnosis [Section II])

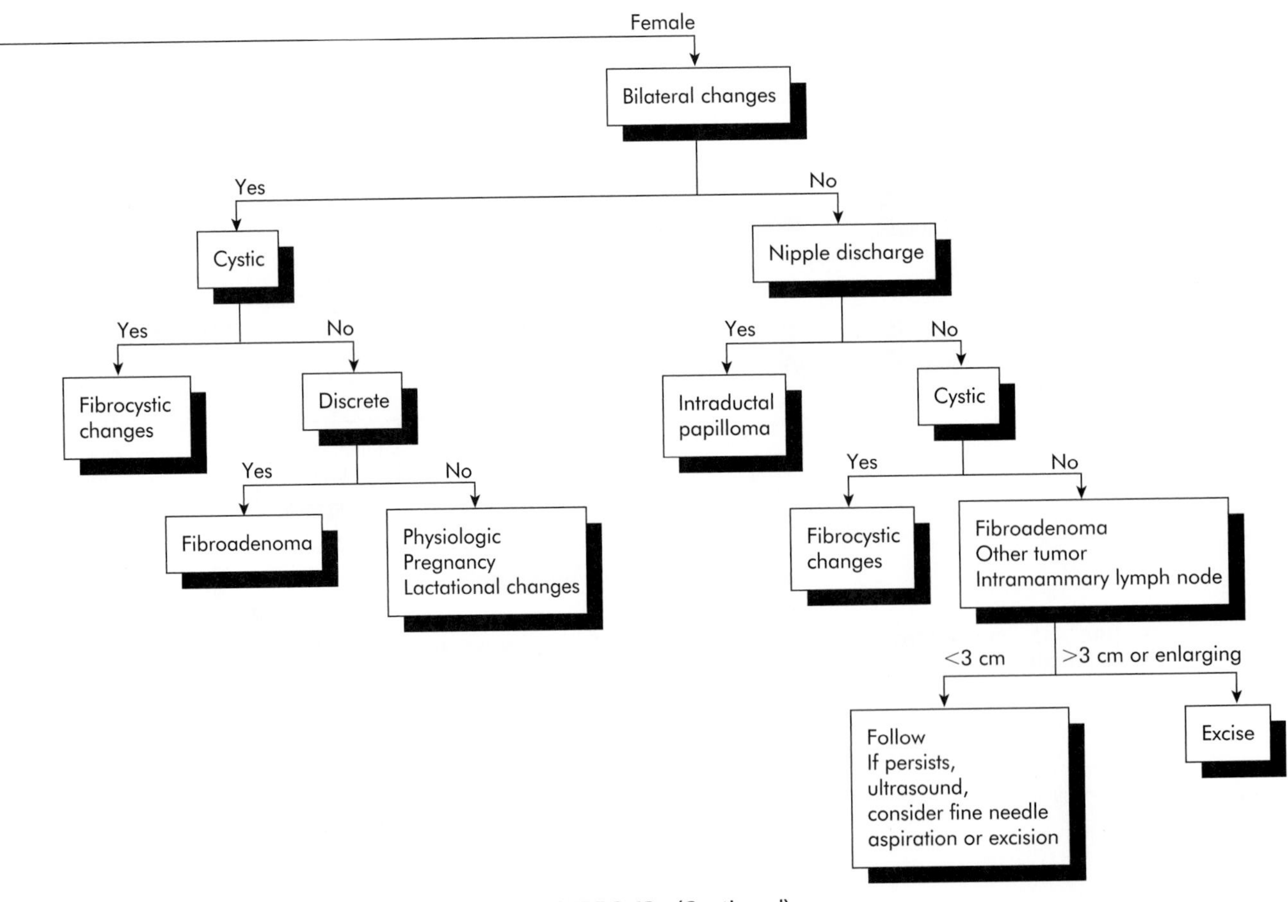

FIGURE 3-12 (Continued)

ICD-9-CM # 786.50

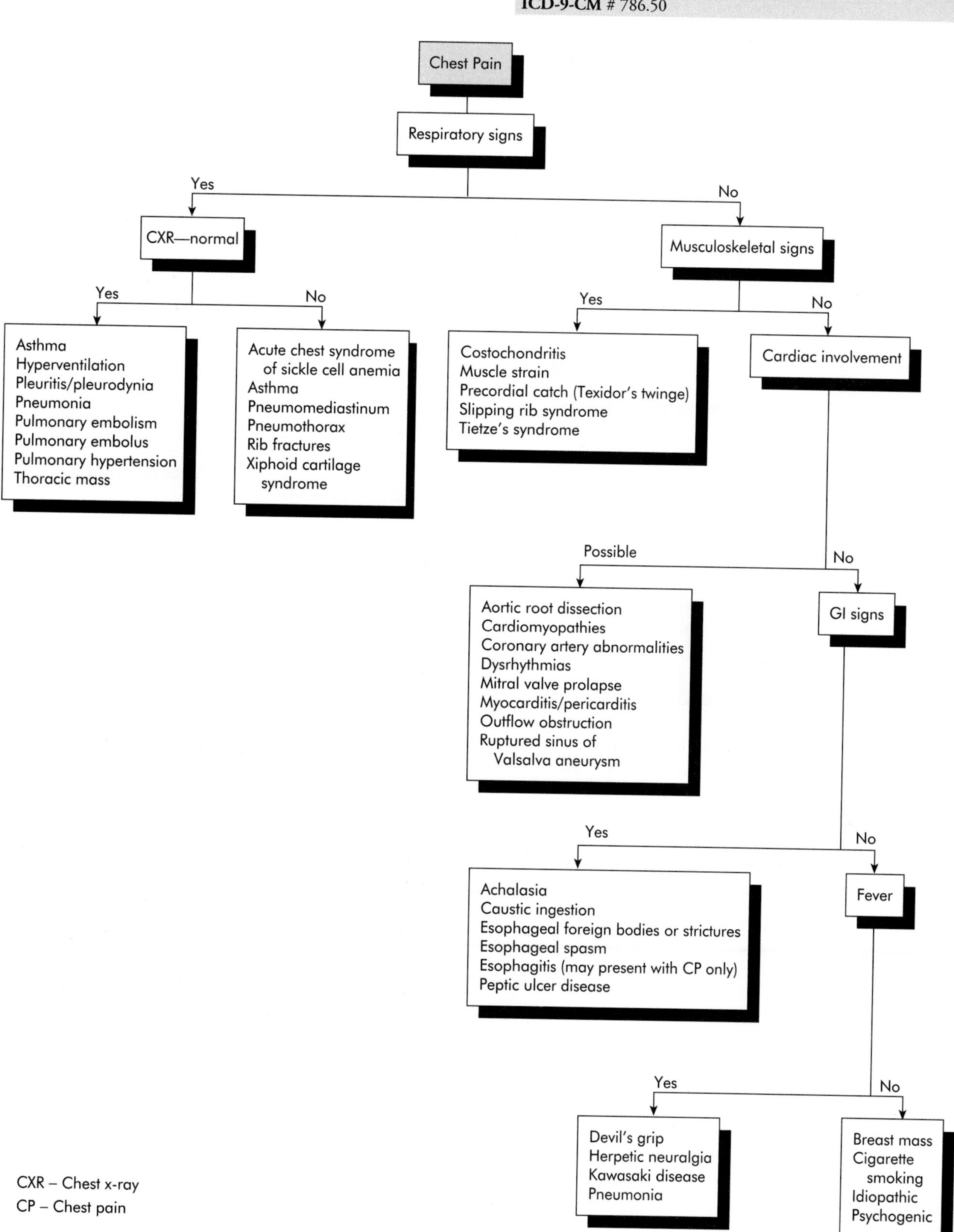

FIGURE 3-13 Chest Pain (see Chest Pain in Differential Diagnosis [Section II])

ICD-9-CM # 786.2

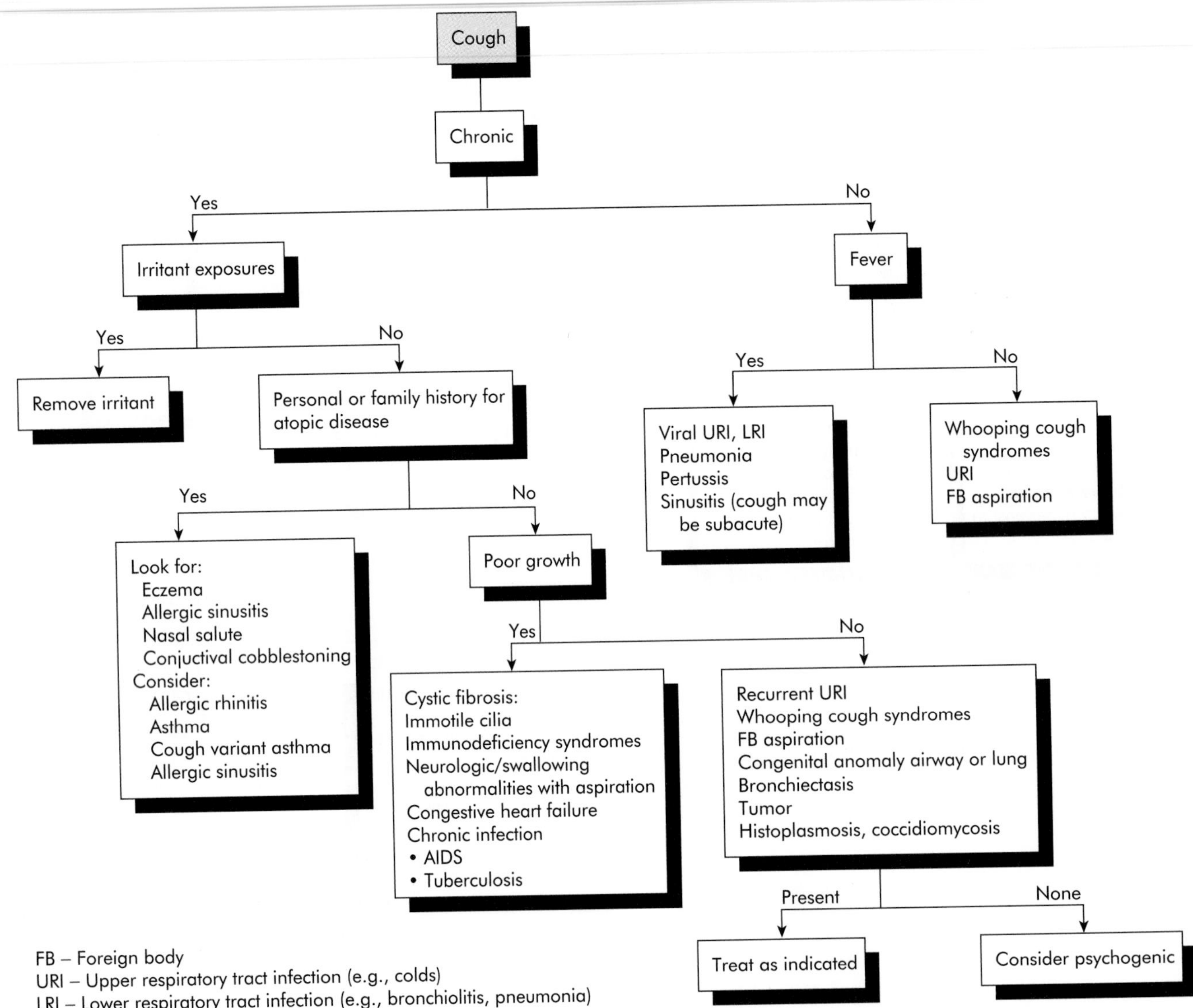

FIGURE 3-14 Cough (see Cough in Differential Diagnosis [Section II])

ICD-9-CM # 787.91

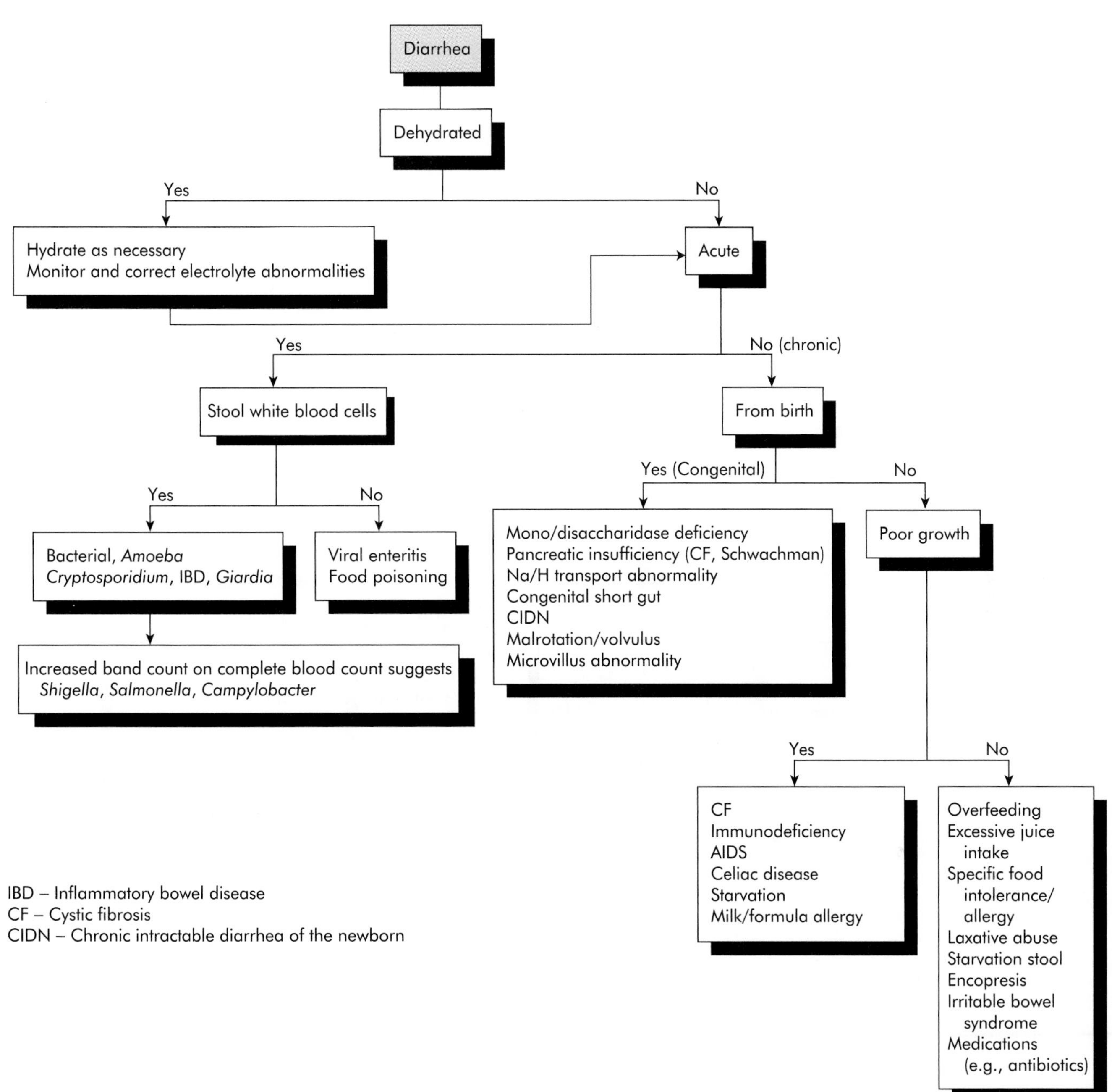

FIGURE 3-15 Diarrhea (see Diarrhea in Differential Diagnosis [Section II])

ICD-9-CM # 788.1

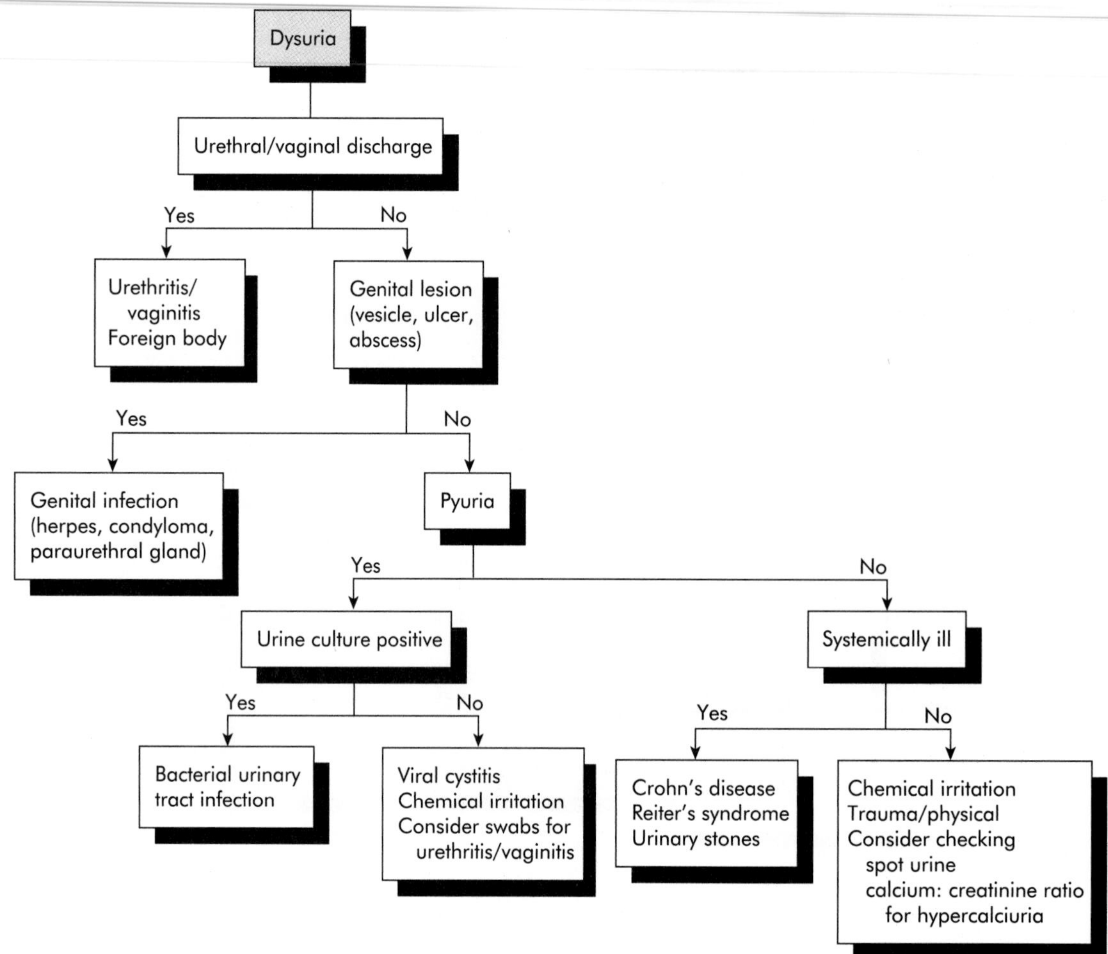

FIGURE 3-16 Dysuria (see Dysuria in Differential Diagnosis [Section II])

ICD-9-CM # 388.70

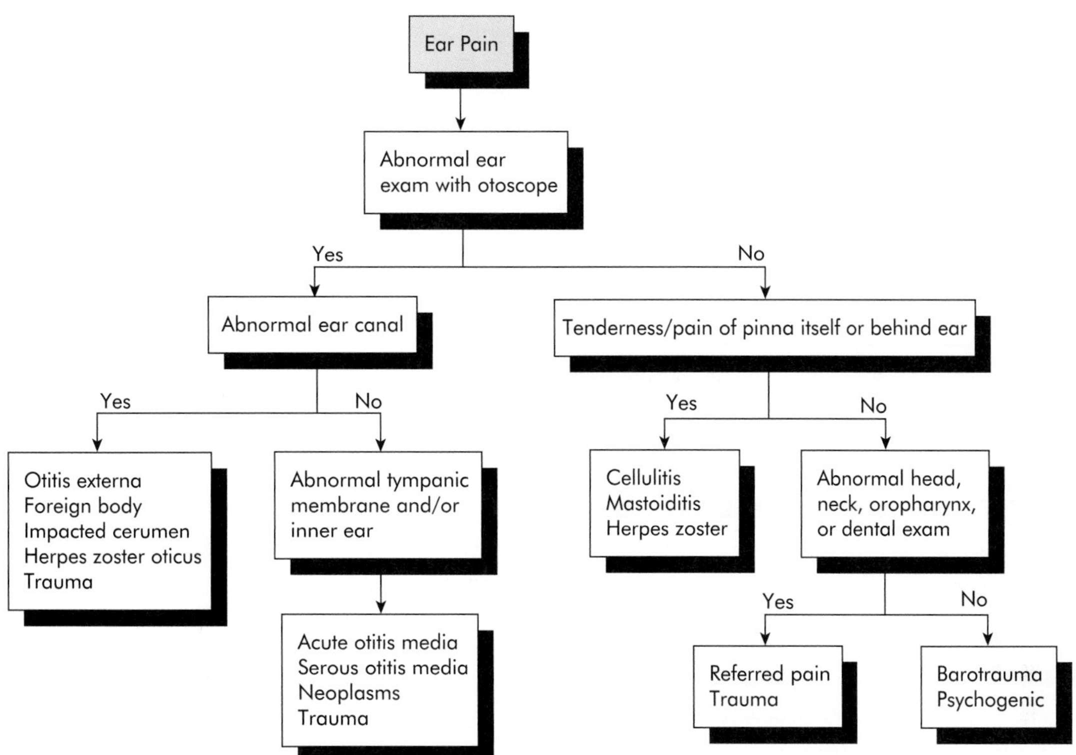

FIGURE 3-17 Ear Pain (see Ear Pain in Differential Diagnosis [Section II])

ICD-9-CM # 782.3
995.1 Allergic
428.0 Cardiac

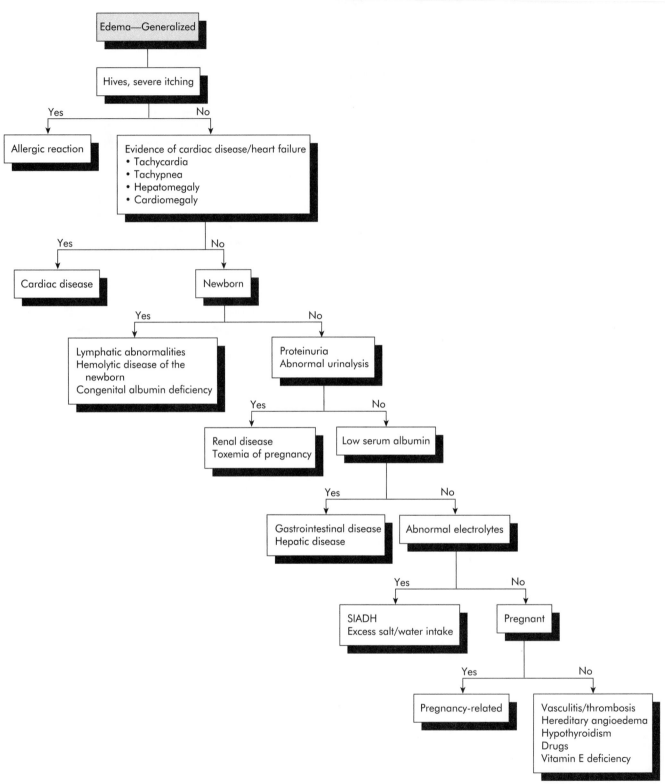

FIGURE 3-18 Edema—Generalized (see Edema—Generalized in Differential Diagnosis [Section II])

ICD-9-CM # 780.6 Fever
036.0 Petechiae

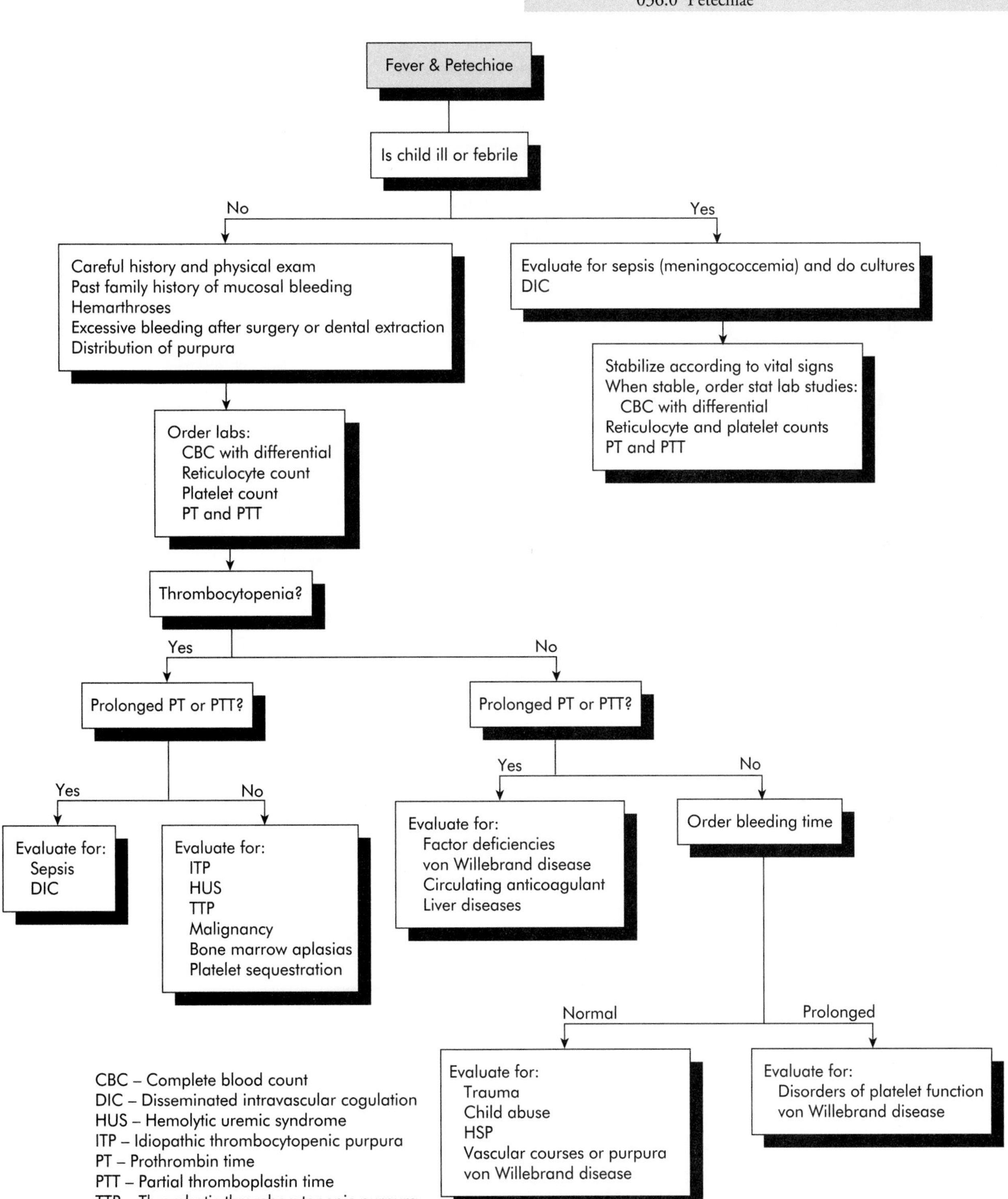

FIGURE 3-19 Fever & Petechiae (see Fever & Petechiae in Differential Diagnosis [Section II])

ICD-9-CM # 578.9

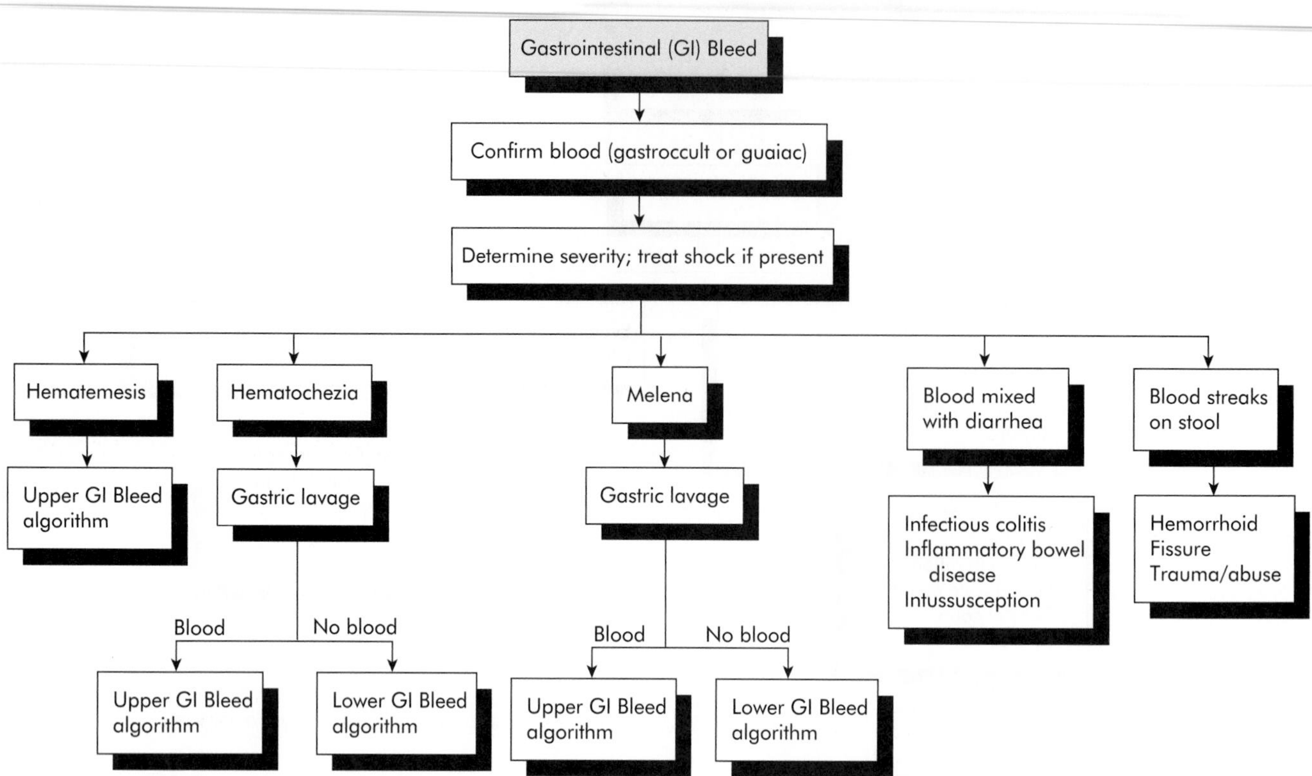

FIGURE 3-20 Gastrointestinal Bleed (see Gastrointestinal Bleeding in Differential Diagnosis [Section II])

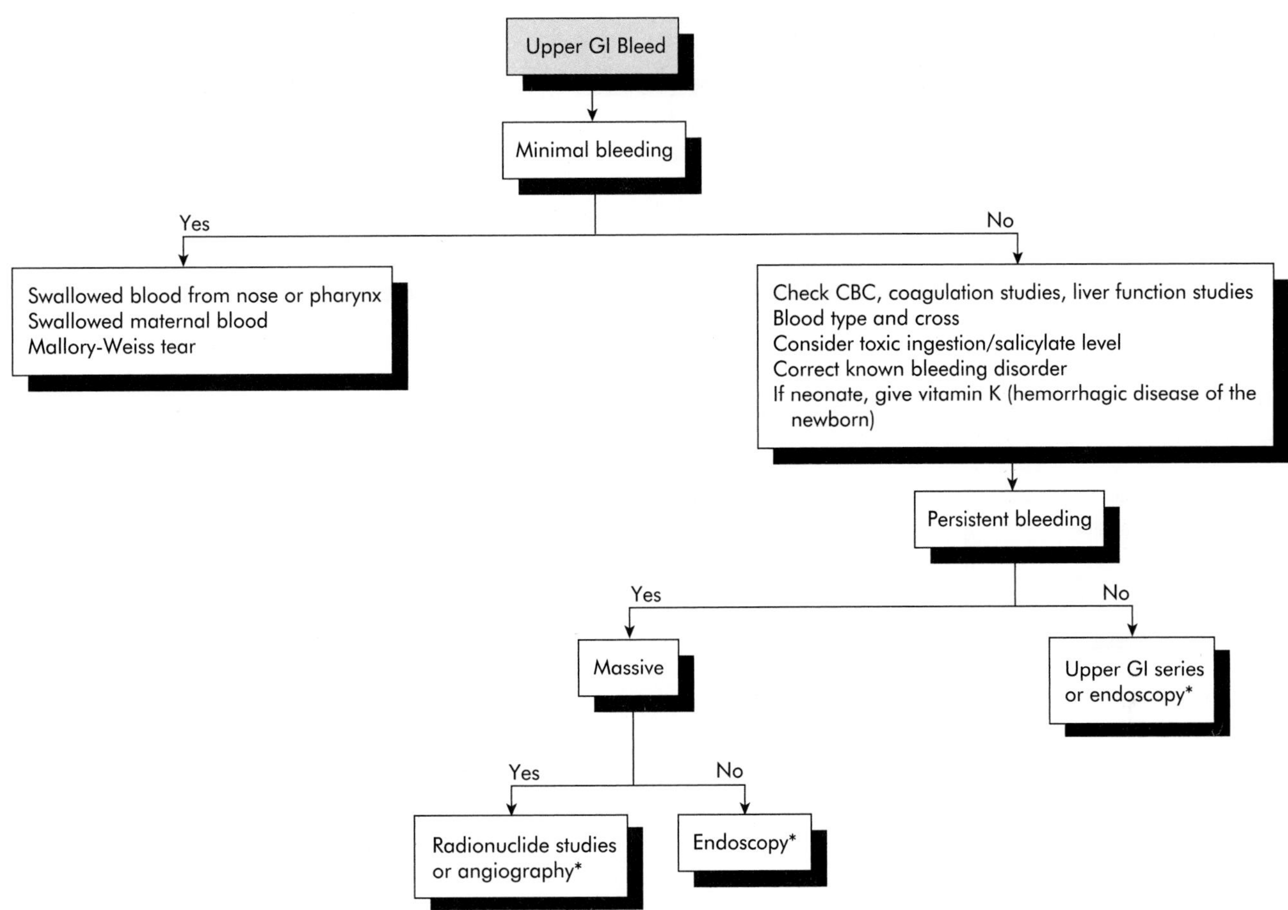

*To identify precise cause of bleeding: Esophagitis, Esophageal Varices, Gastritis, Ulcer, Hemobilia, Vascular Malformation, Duplication, Foreign Body, Neoplasm

FIGURE 3-20 (Continued)

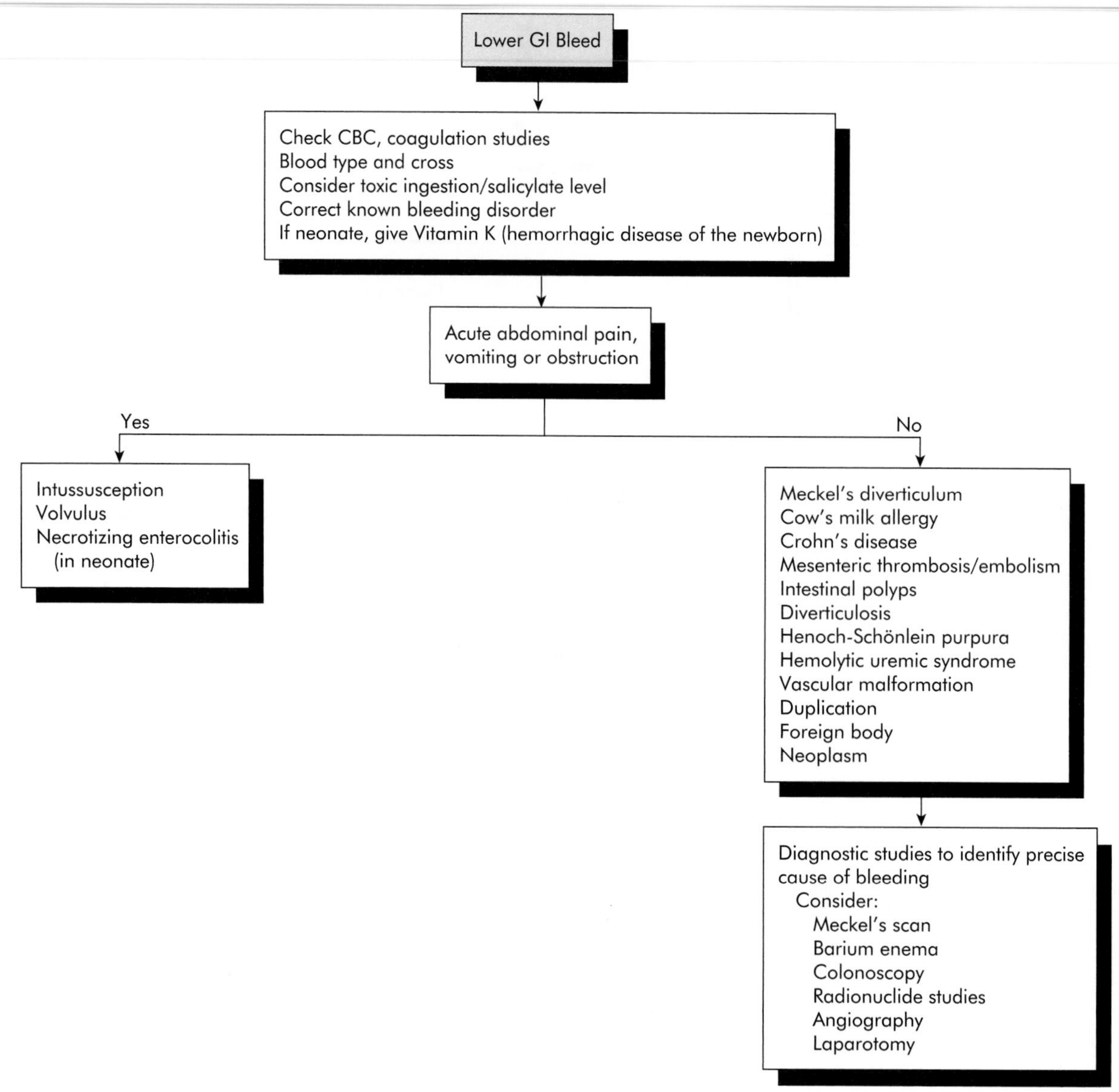

FIGURE 3-20 (Continued)

ICD-9-CM # 054.1 *Herpes genitalis*
078.19 Genital warts

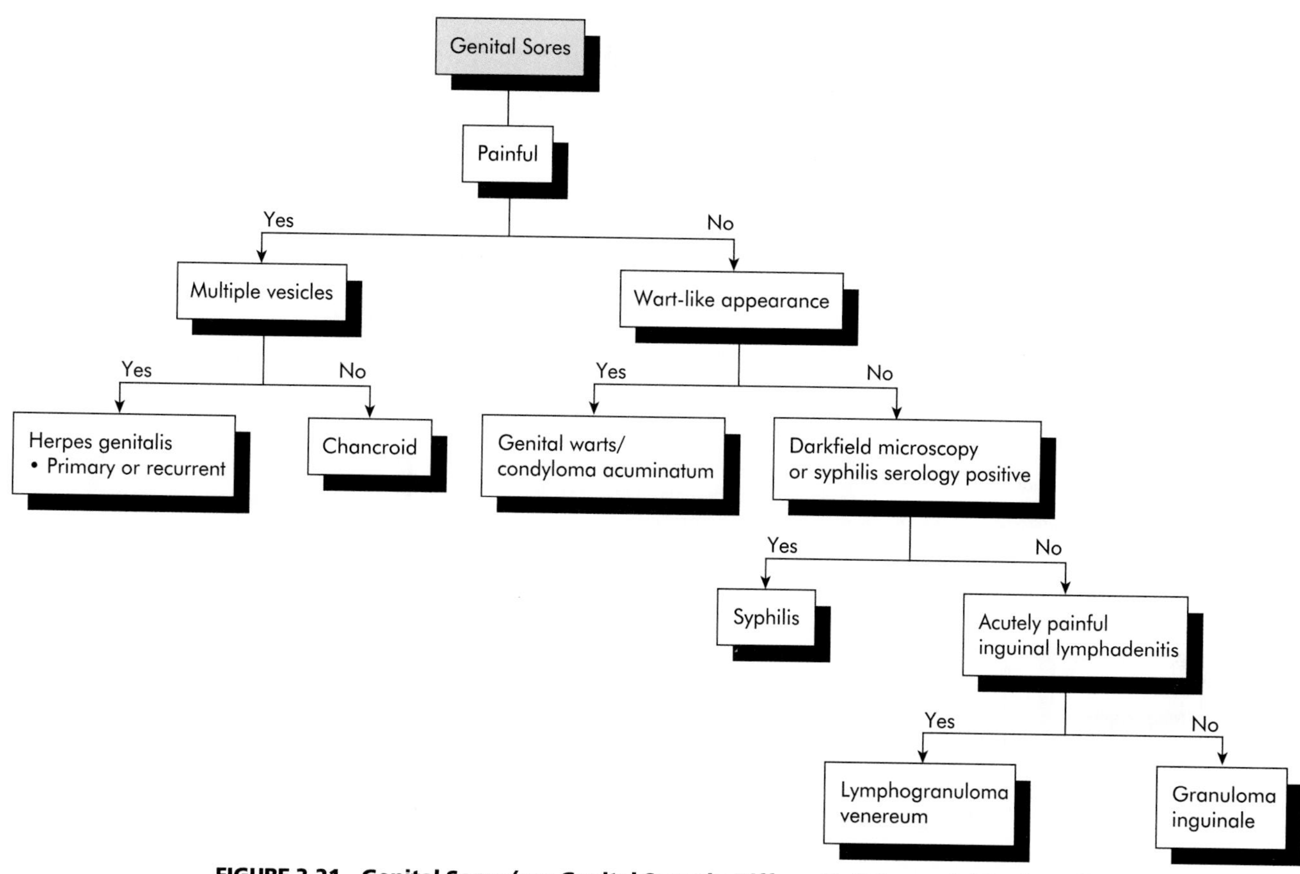

FIGURE 3-21 Genital Sores (see Genital Sores in Differential Diagnosis [Section II])

ICD-9-CM # 599.7

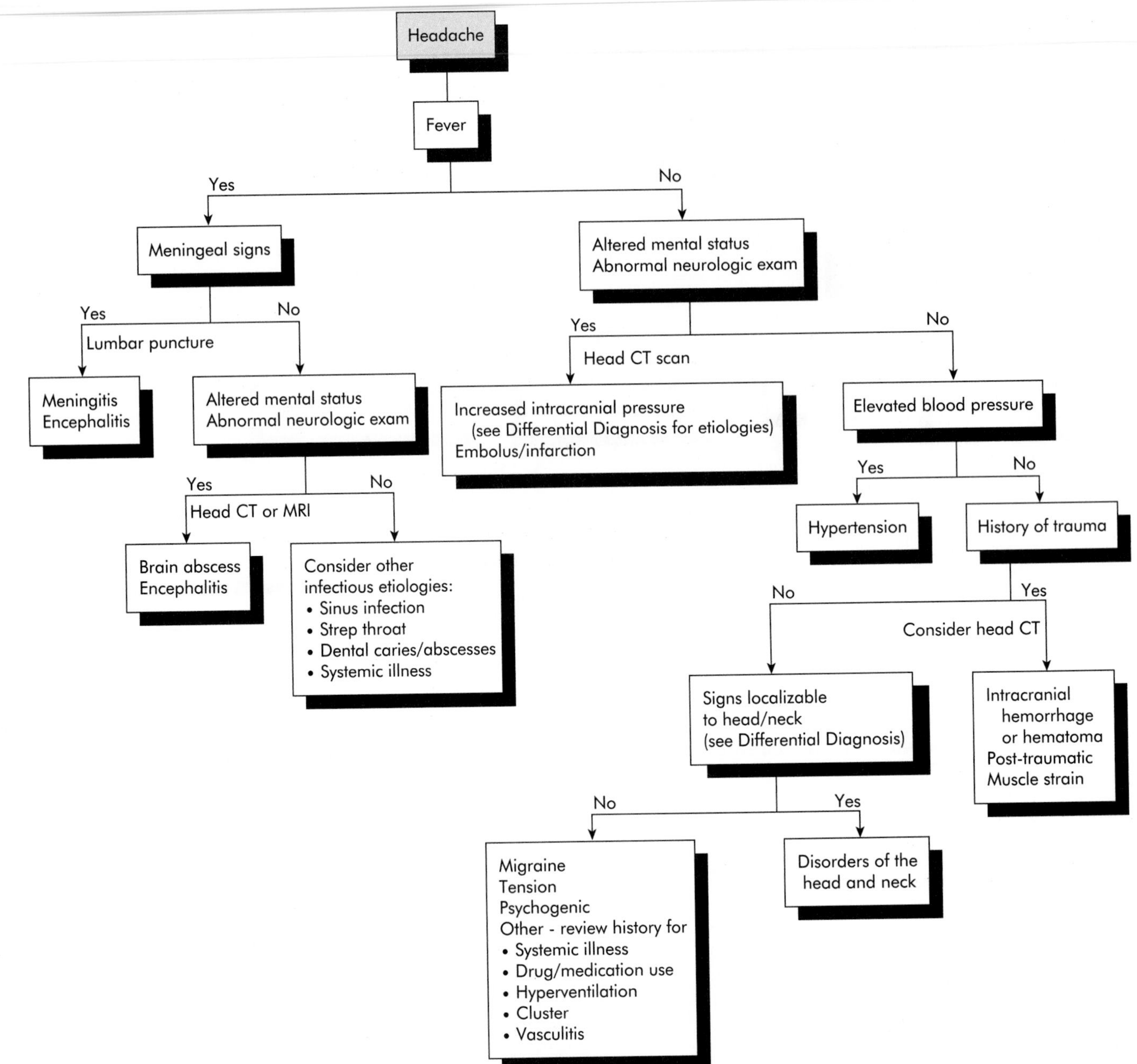

FIGURE 3-22 Headache (see Headache in Differential Diagnosis [Section II])

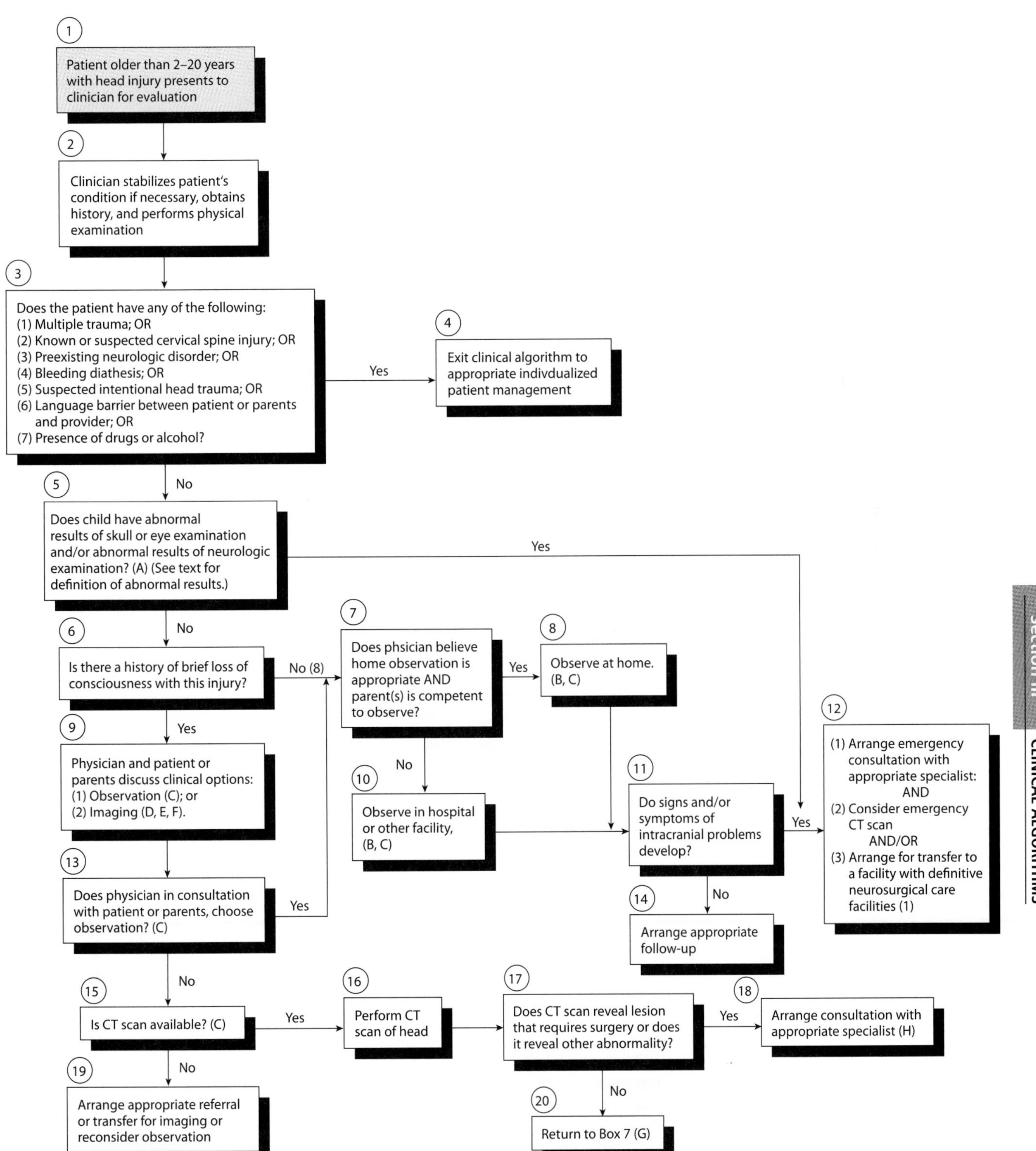
1
Patient older than 2–20 years with head injury presents to clinician for evaluation
2
Clinician stabilizes patient's condition if necessary, obtains history, and performs physical examination
3
Does the patient have any of the following:
(1) Multiple trauma; OR
(2) Known or suspected cervical spine injury; OR
(3) Preexisting neurologic disorder; OR
(4) Bleeding diathesis; OR
(5) Suspected intentional head trauma; OR
(6) Language barrier between patient or parents and provider; OR
(7) Presence of drugs or alcohol?
Yes
4
Exit clinical algorithm to appropriate indivdualized patient management
No
5
Does child have abnormal results of skull or eye examination and/or abnormal results of neurologic examination? (A) (See text for definition of abnormal results.)
Yes
No
6
Is there a history of brief loss of consciousness with this injury?
No (8)
7
Does phsician believe home observation is appropriate AND parent(s) is competent to observe?
Yes
8
Observe at home. (B, C)
Yes
9
Physician and patient or parents discuss clinical options: (1) Observation (C); or (2) Imaging (D, E, F).
No
10
Observe in hospital or other facility, (B, C)
11
Do signs and/or symptoms of intracranial problems develop?
Yes
12
(1) Arrange emergency consultation with appropriate specialist: AND
(2) Consider emergency CT scan AND/OR
(3) Arrange for transfer to a facility with definitive neurosurgical care facilities (1)
13
Does physician in consultation with patient or parents, choose observation? (C)
Yes
No
14
Arrange appropriate follow-up
No
15
Is CT scan available? (C)
Yes
16
Perform CT scan of head
17
Does CT scan reveal lesion that requires surgery or does it reveal other abnormality?
Yes
18
Arrange consultation with appropriate specialist (H)
No
19
Arrange appropriate referral or transfer for imaging or reconsider observation
No
20
Return to Box 7 (G)

FIGURE 3-22A Head Trauma

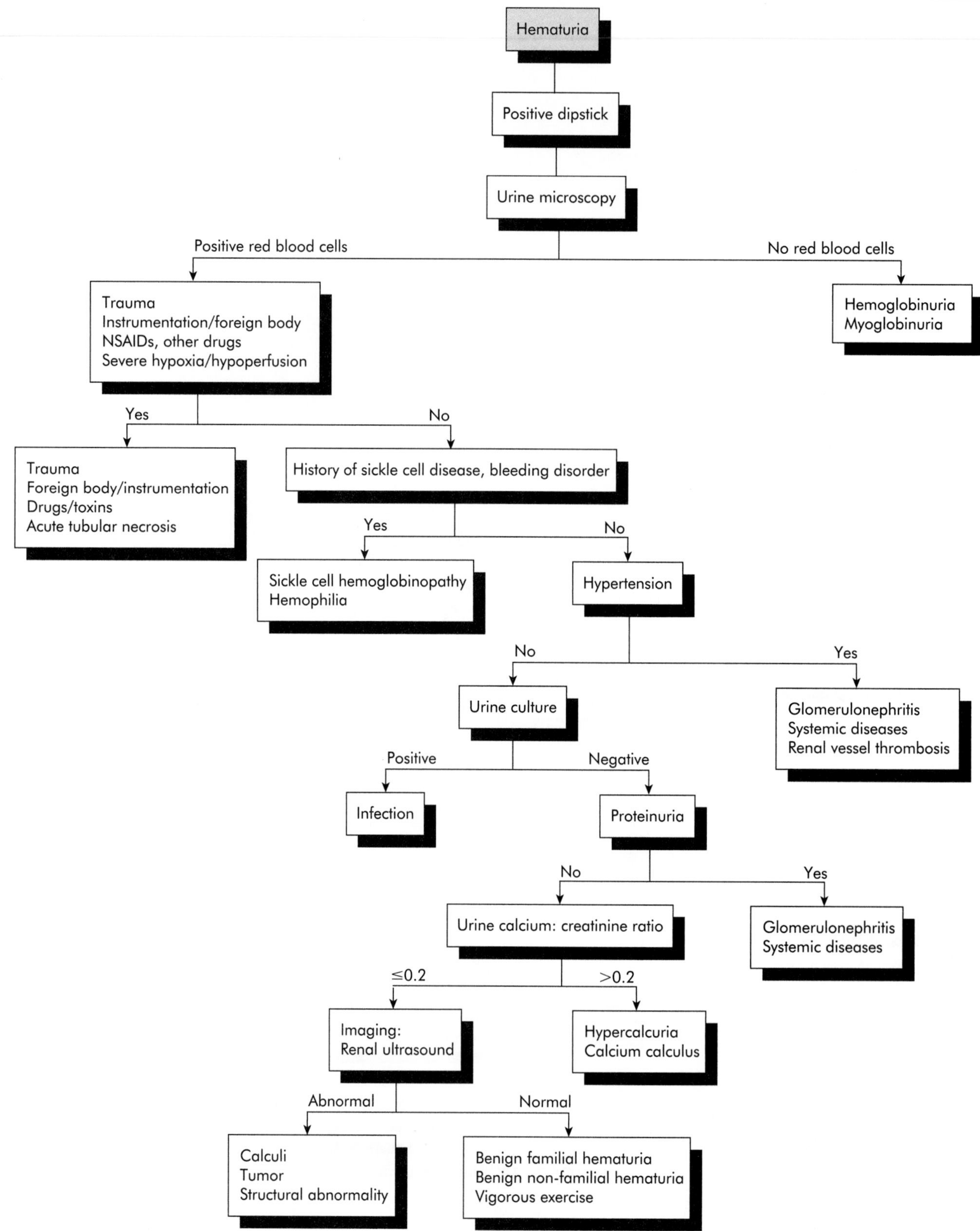

FIGURE 3-23 Hematuria (see Hematuria in Differential Diagnosis [Section II])

ICD-9-CM # 789.1
571.8 Hepatosplenomegaly

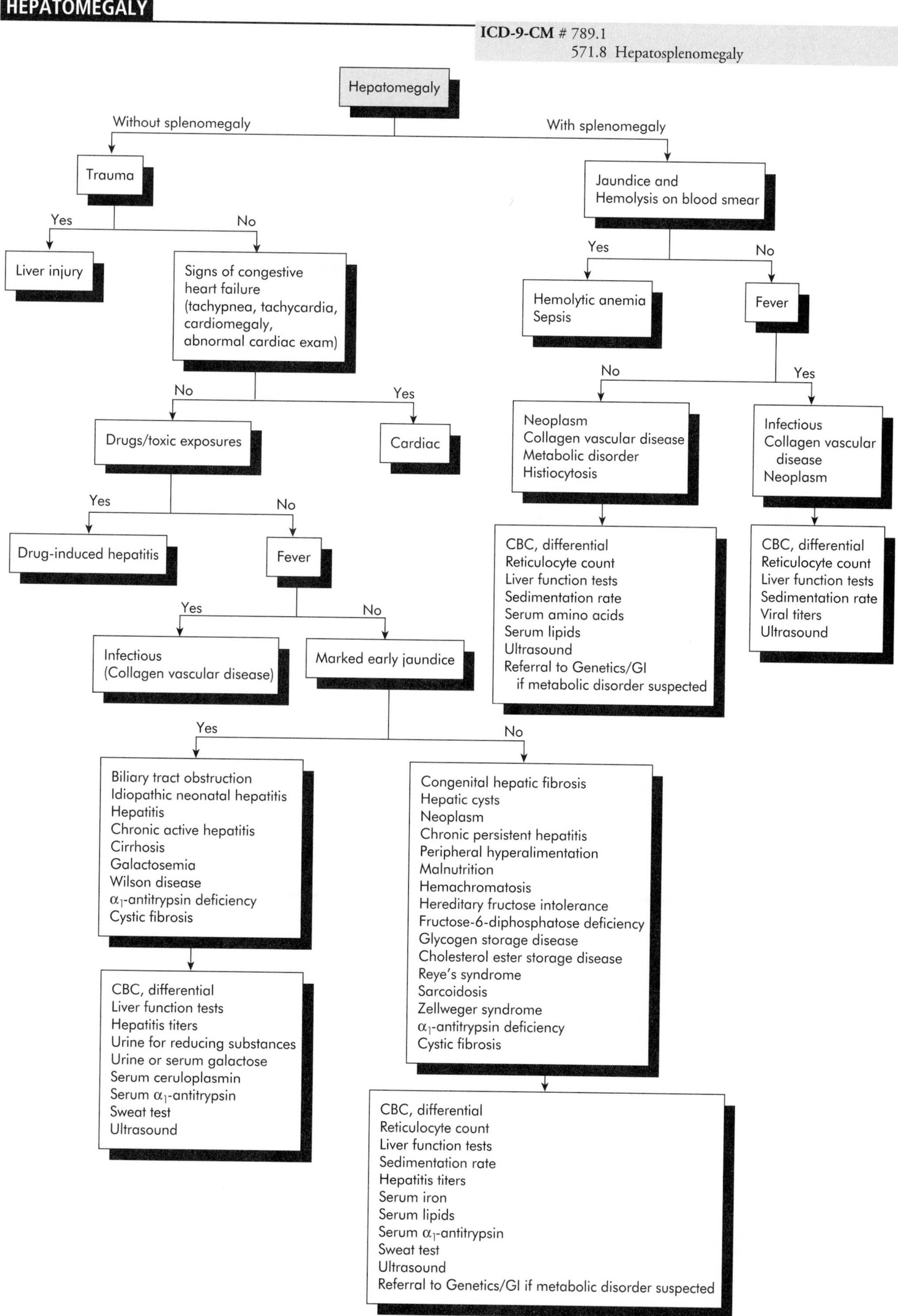

FIGURE 3-24 Hepatomegaly (see Hepatomegaly & Hepatosplenomegaly in Differential Diagnosis [Section II])

ICD-9-CM # 774.6 Neonatal
782.4 Jaundice

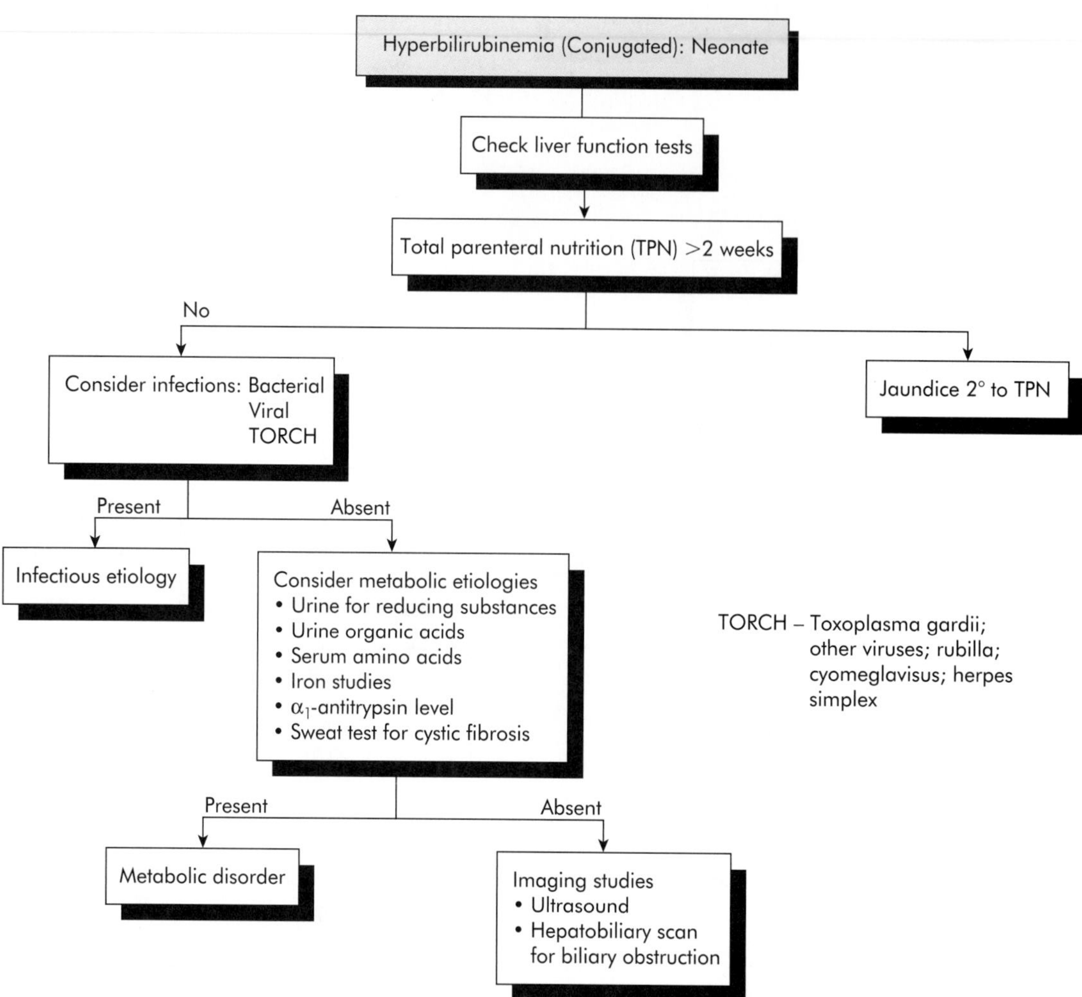

FIGURE 3-25 Hyperbilirubinemia (Conjugated): Neonate (see Jaundice/Hyperbilirubinemia in Differential Diagnosis [Section II])

HYPERBILIRUBINEMIA (CONJUGATED): POST-NEONATE

ICD-9-CM # 774.6 Neonatal
782.4 Jaundice

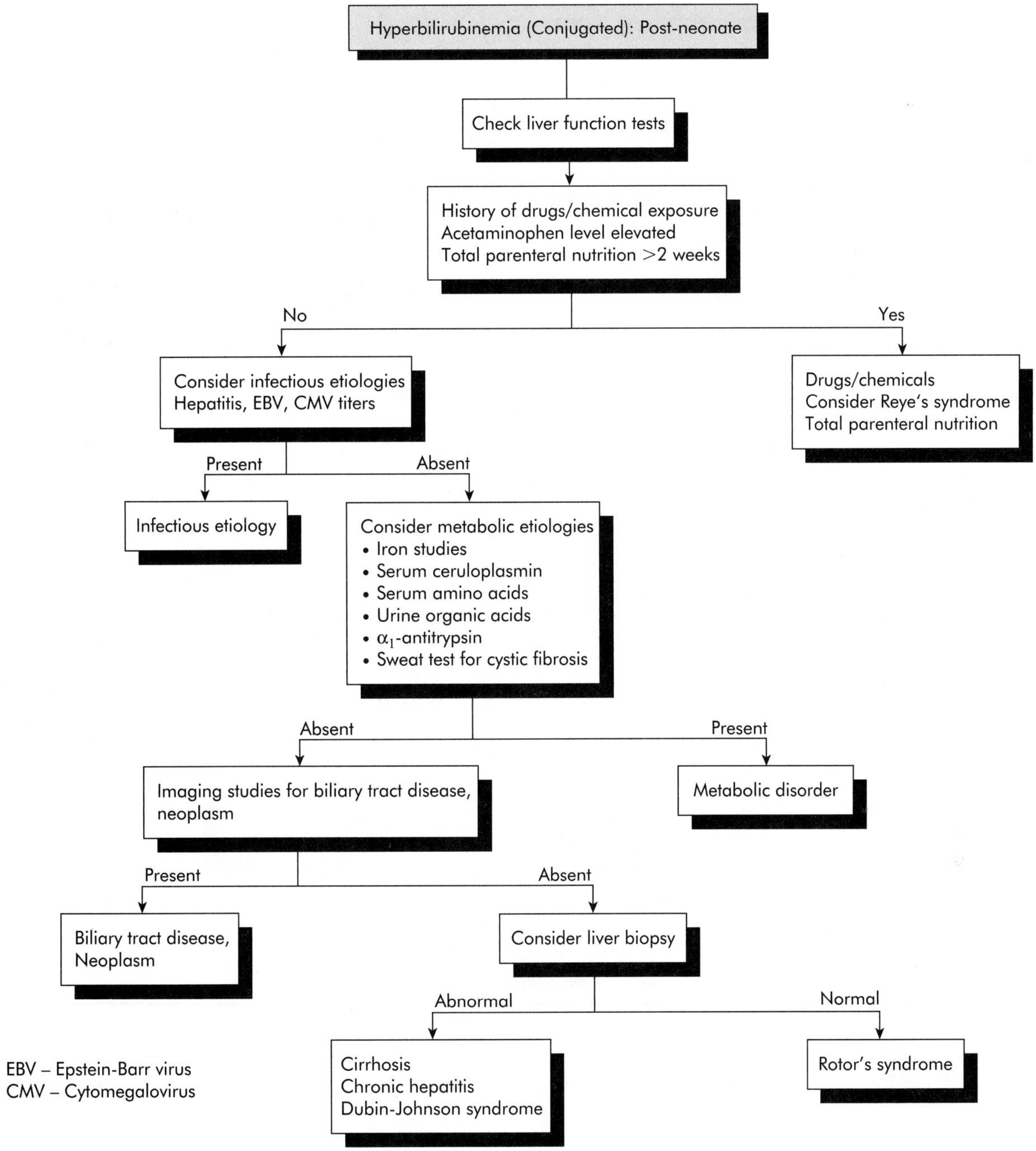

Hyperbilirubinemia (Conjugated): Post-neonate

Check liver function tests

History of drugs/chemical exposure
Acetaminophen level elevated
Total parenteral nutrition >2 weeks

- No → Consider infectious etiologies
  Hepatitis, EBV, CMV titers
  - Present → Infectious etiology
  - Absent → Consider metabolic etiologies
    - Iron studies
    - Serum ceruloplasmin
    - Serum amino acids
    - Urine organic acids
    - α_1-antitrypsin
    - Sweat test for cystic fibrosis
    - Absent → Imaging studies for biliary tract disease, neoplasm
      - Present → Biliary tract disease, Neoplasm
      - Absent → Consider liver biopsy
        - Abnormal → Cirrhosis
          Chronic hepatitis
          Dubin-Johnson syndrome
        - Normal → Rotor's syndrome
    - Present → Metabolic disorder
- Yes → Drugs/chemicals
  Consider Reye's syndrome
  Total parenteral nutrition

EBV – Epstein-Barr virus
CMV – Cytomegalovirus

FIGURE 3-26 Hyperbilirubinemia (Conjugated): Post-neonate (see Jaundice/Hyperbilirubinemia in Differential Diagnosis [Section II])

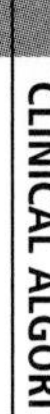

ICD-9-CM # 774.6 Neonatal
782.4 Jaundice

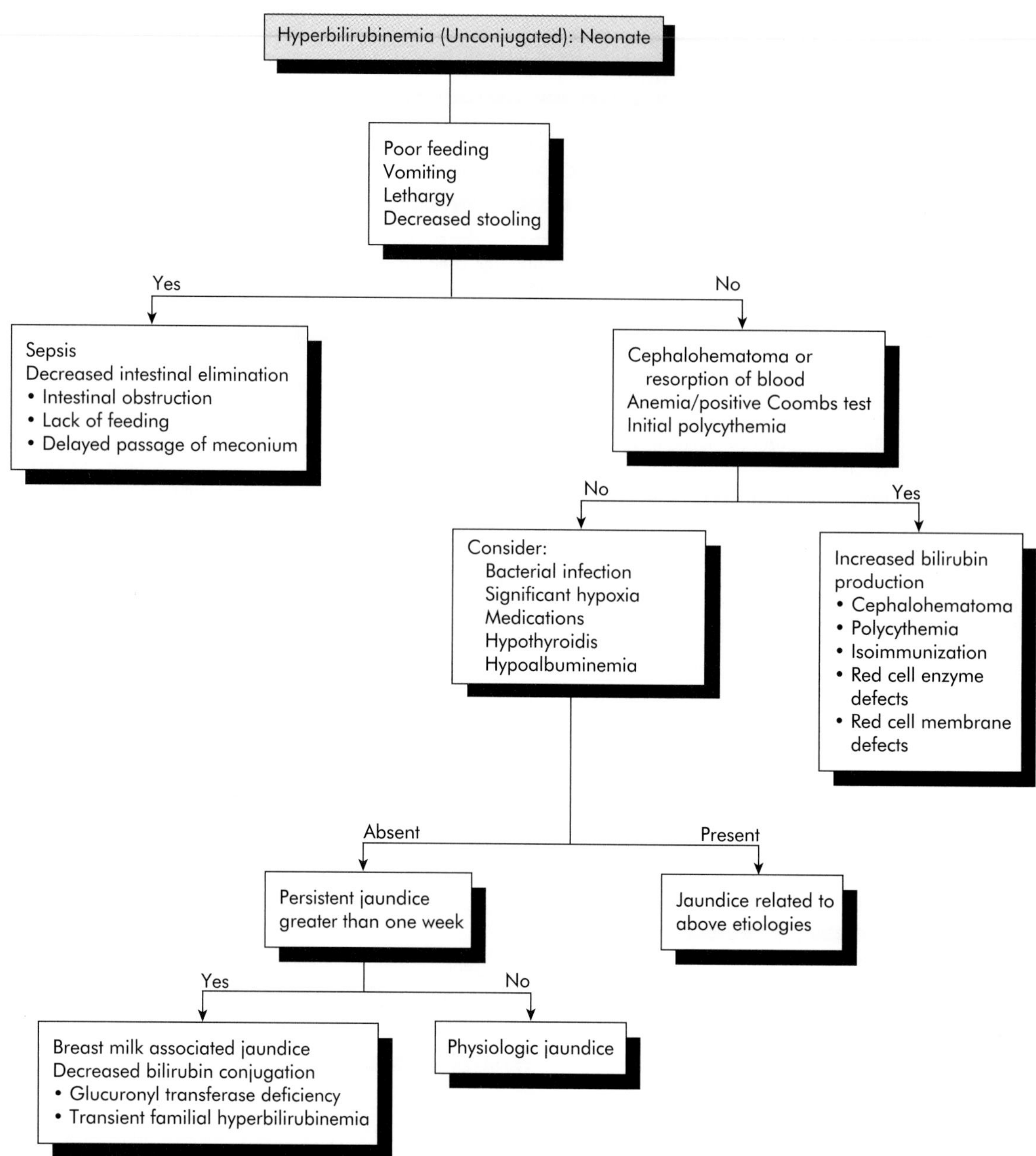

FIGURE 3-27 Hyperbilirubinemia (Unconjugated): Neonate (see Jaundice/Hyperbilirubinemia in Differential Diagnosis [Section II])

HYPERBILIRUBINEMIA (UNCONJUGATED): POST-NEONATE

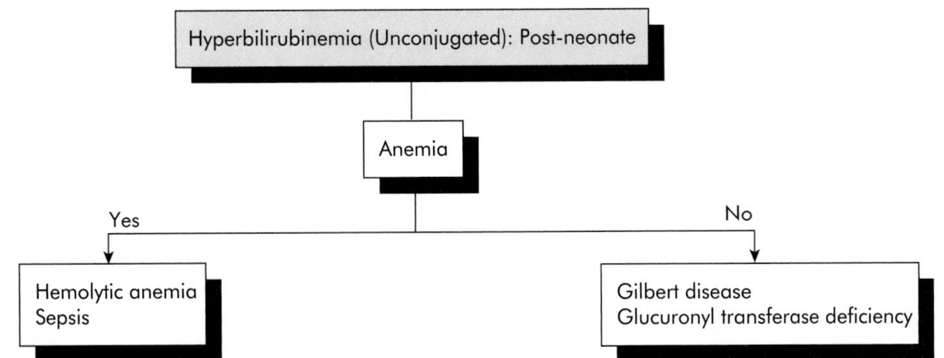

FIGURE 3-28 Hyperbilirubinemia (Unconjugated): Post-neonate (see Jaundice/Hyperbilirubinemia in Differential Diagnosis [Section II])

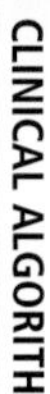

ICD-9-CM # 251.2

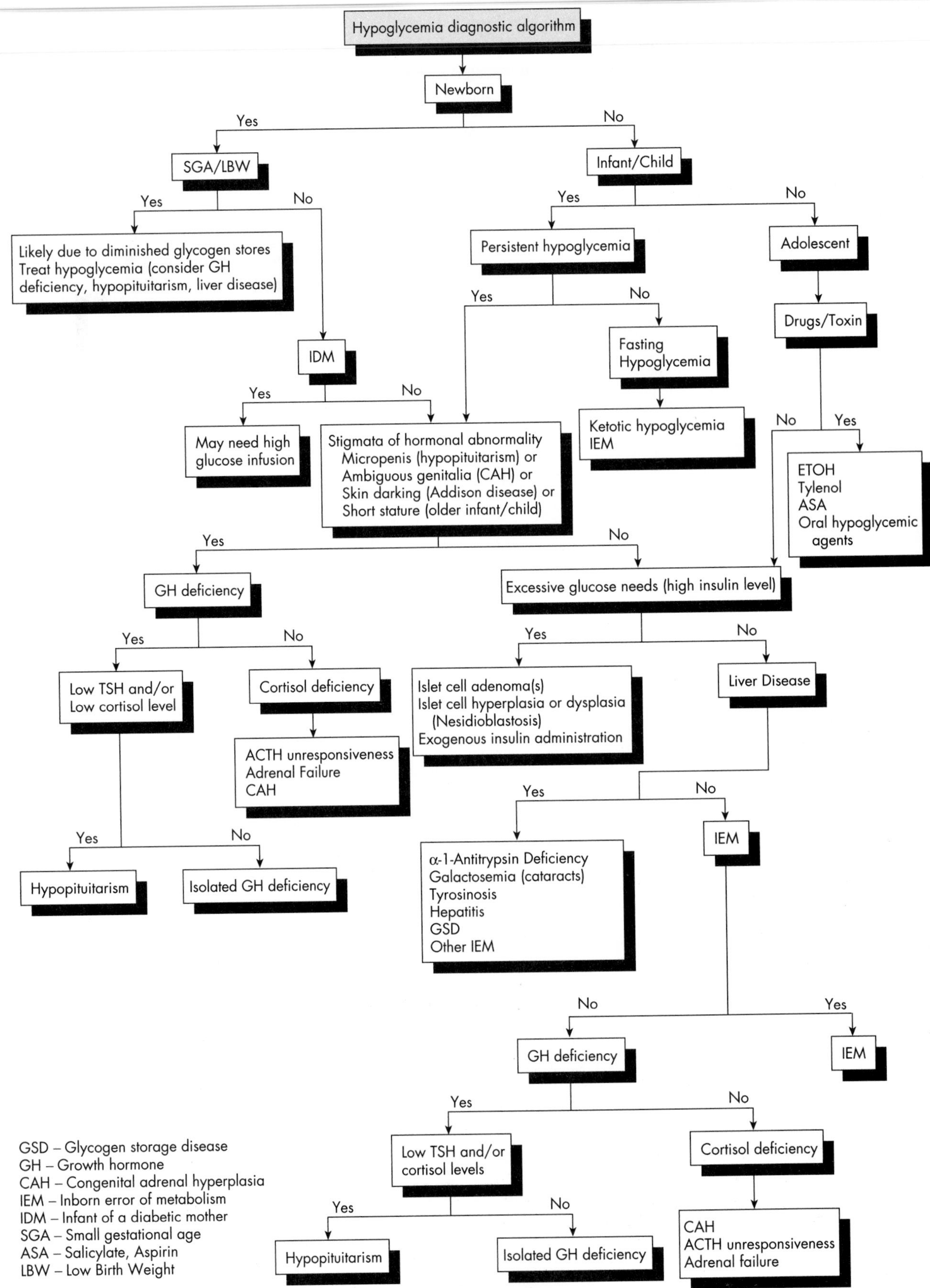

FIGURE 3-29 Hypoglycemia (see Hypoglycemia in Differential Diagnosis [Section II])

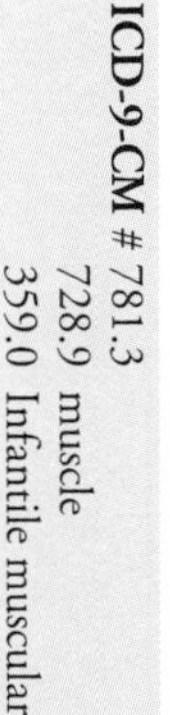
ICD-9-CM # 781.3
728.9 muscle
359.0 Infantile muscular

- Hypotonia
  - Weakness
    - Yes → Infant
      - Yes → Meningomyelocele, Spinal muscular atrophy, Botulism, Myasthenia gravis, Congenital myopathy, Congenital muscular dystrophy, Congenital myotonic dystrophy
        - → Consider/obtain: Creatine kinase, Spinal cord imaging, EMG, Nerve conduction studies, Muscle biopsy
      - No → Serum creatine kinase
        - Normal → Spinal cord disorder, Peripheral nerve disorder, Neuromuscular Junction disorder, Metabolic myopathy, Periodic paralysis, Myotonic dystrophy
          - → Consider/obtain: Spinal cord imaging, Serum potassium, EMG, Nerve conduction studies, Muscle biopsy
        - Abnormal → Muscular dystrophy, Mitochondrial myopathy, Polymyositis, Dermatomyositis
          - → Consider/obtain: EMG, Lactate/pyruvate levels, Muscle biopsy
    - No → Acute severe illness
      - No → Obtain: Thyroid function tests, serum amino acids, urine organic acids, chromosomes
        - Abnormal → Hypothyroidism/hypopituitarism, amino acid disorder, organic acid disorder, chromosome disorder
        - Normal → Progressive
          - Yes → Lipidoses, Leukodystrophies, Mucopolysaccharidoses, Mucolipidoses, Peroxisomal disorders
            - → Obtain: Head MRI
          - No → Syndrome, Hypotonic cerebral palsy, Benign essential hypotonia
      - Yes → Generalized brain insult

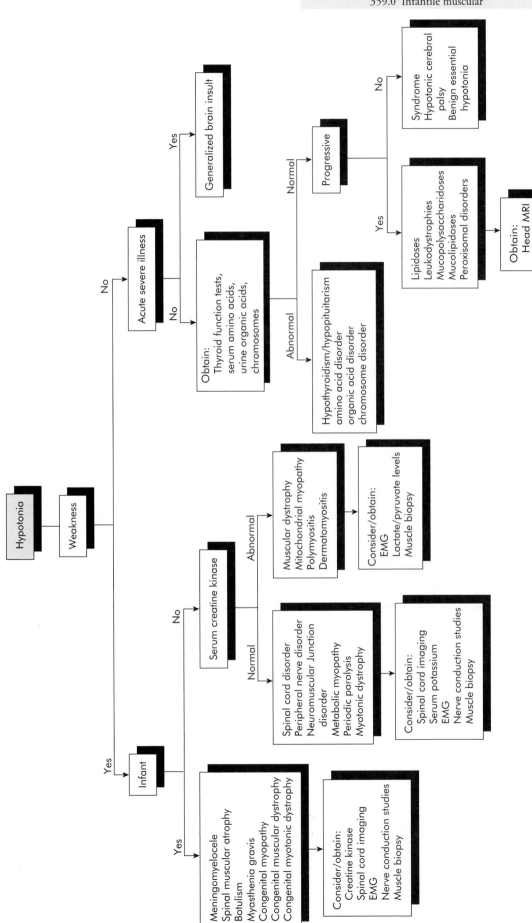

FIGURE 3-30 **Hypotonia (see Hypotonia in Differential Diagnosis [Section II])**

ICD-9-CM # 719.70

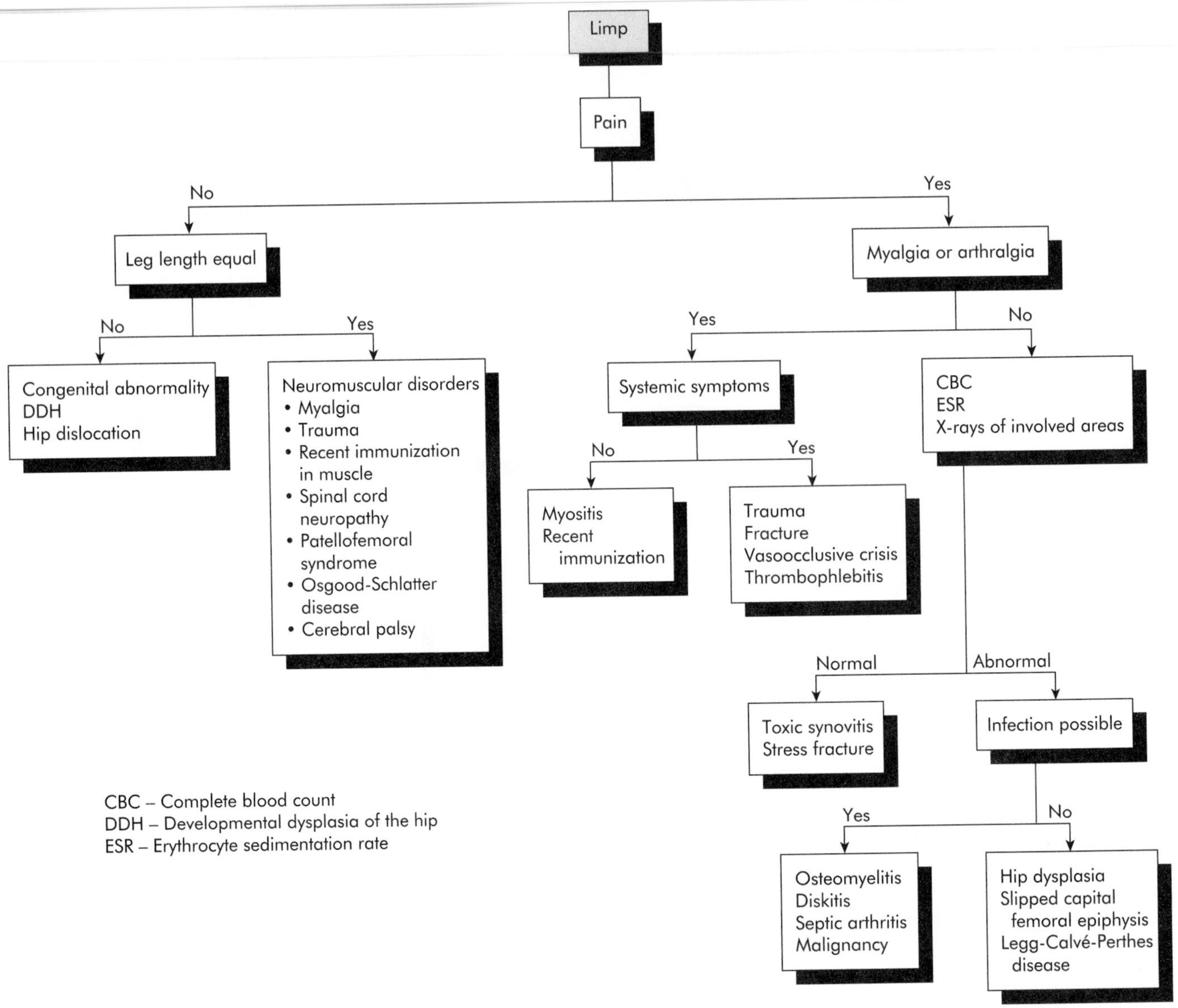

Limp

Pain

No → Leg length equal

- No → Congenital abnormality; DDH; Hip dislocation
- Yes → Neuromuscular disorders
  - Myalgia
  - Trauma
  - Recent immunization in muscle
  - Spinal cord neuropathy
  - Patellofemoral syndrome
  - Osgood-Schlatter disease
  - Cerebral palsy

Yes → Myalgia or arthralgia

- Yes → Systemic symptoms
  - No → Myositis; Recent immunization
  - Yes → Trauma; Fracture; Vasoocclusive crisis; Thrombophlebitis
- No → CBC; ESR; X-rays of involved areas
  - Normal → Toxic synovitis; Stress fracture
  - Abnormal → Infection possible
    - Yes → Osteomyelitis; Diskitis; Septic arthritis; Malignancy
    - No → Hip dysplasia; Slipped capital femoral epiphysis; Legg-Calvé-Perthes disease

CBC – Complete blood count
DDH – Developmental dysplasia of the hip
ESR – Erythrocyte sedimentation rate

FIGURE 3-31 Limp (see Limp in Differential Diagnosis [Section II])

ICD-9-CM # 756.0

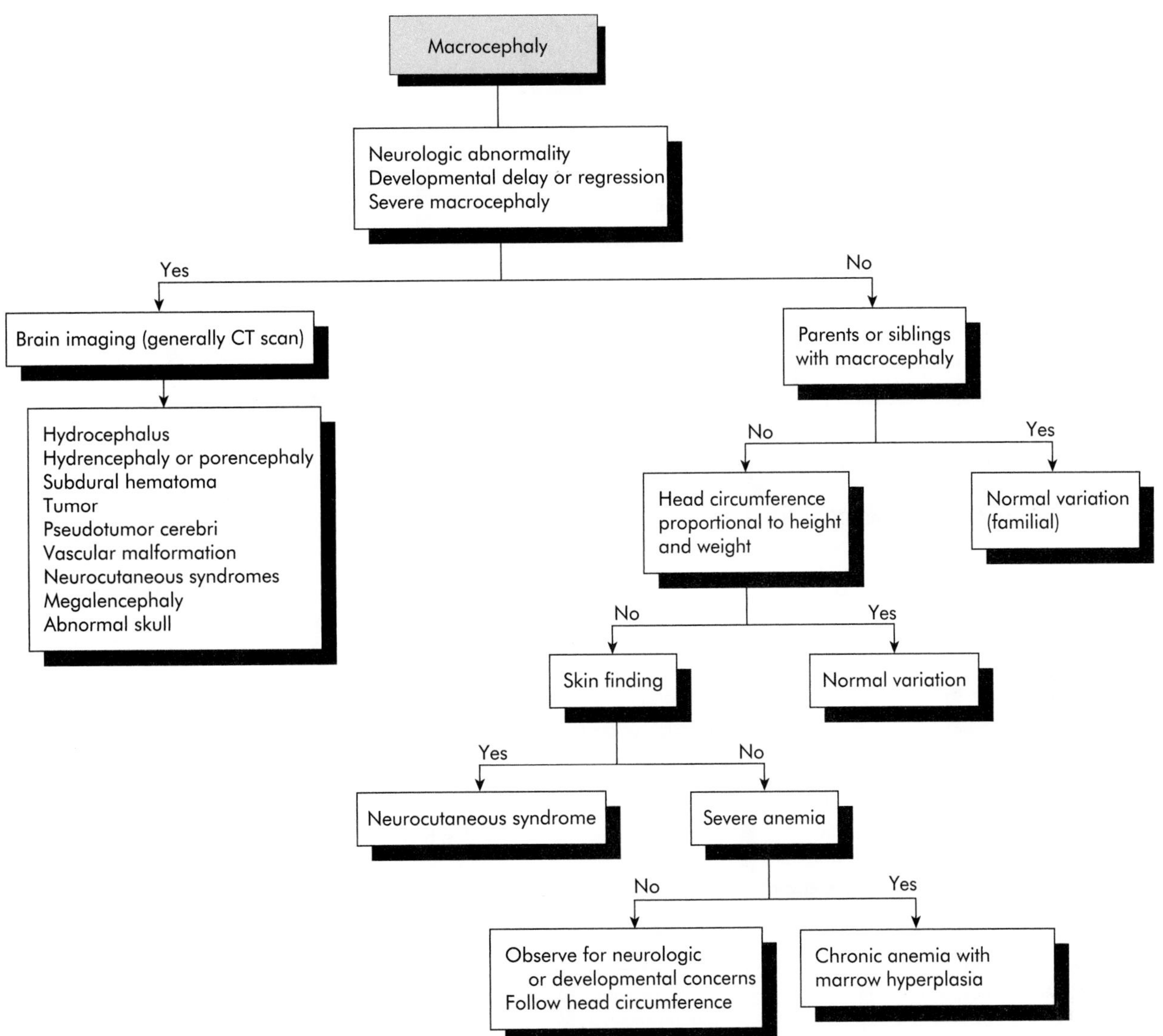

FIGURE 3-32 Macrocephaly (see Macrocephaly in Differential Diagnosis [Section II])

ICD-9-CM # 742.1

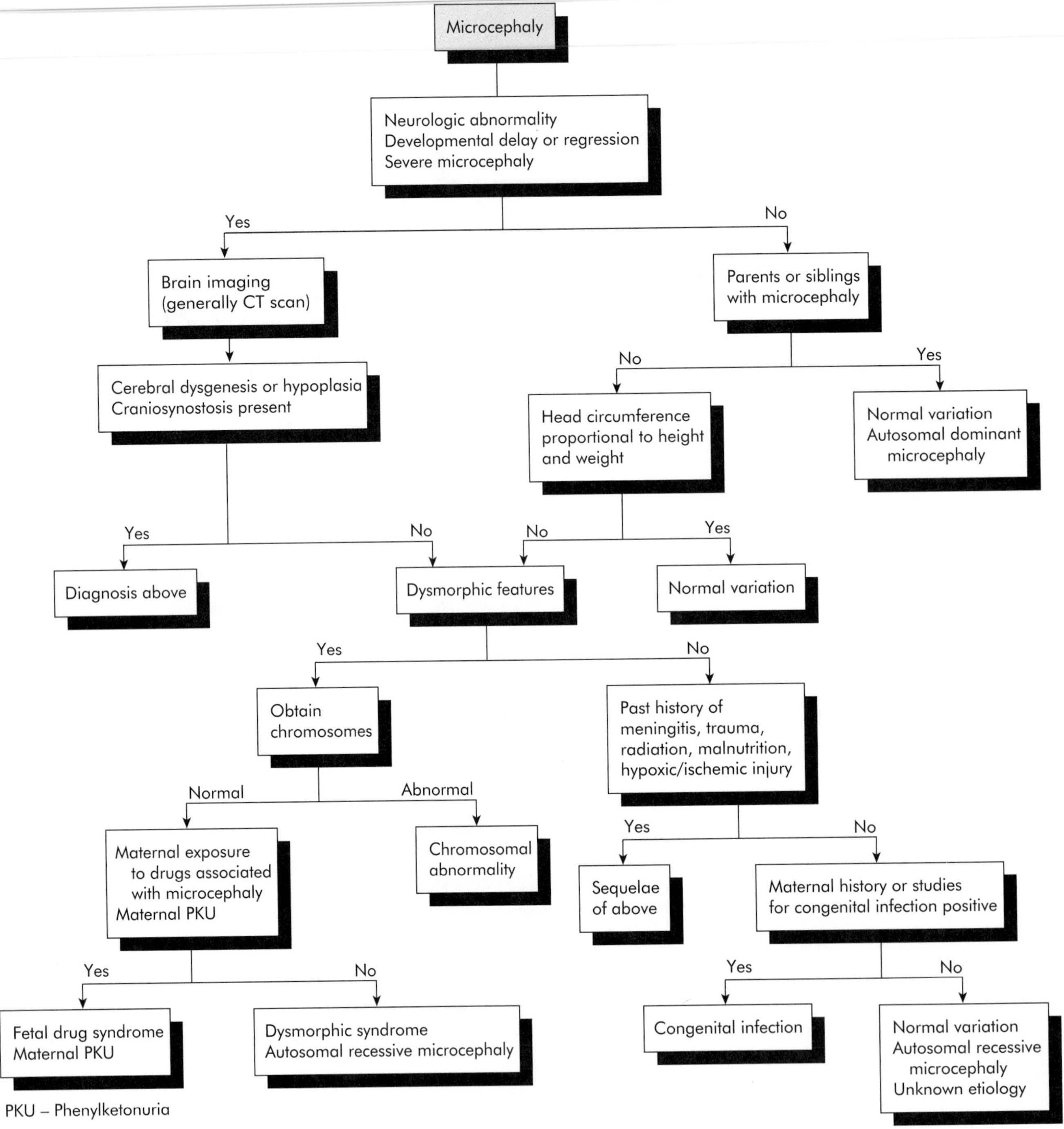

FIGURE 3-33 Microcephaly (see Microcephaly in Differential Diagnosis [Section II])

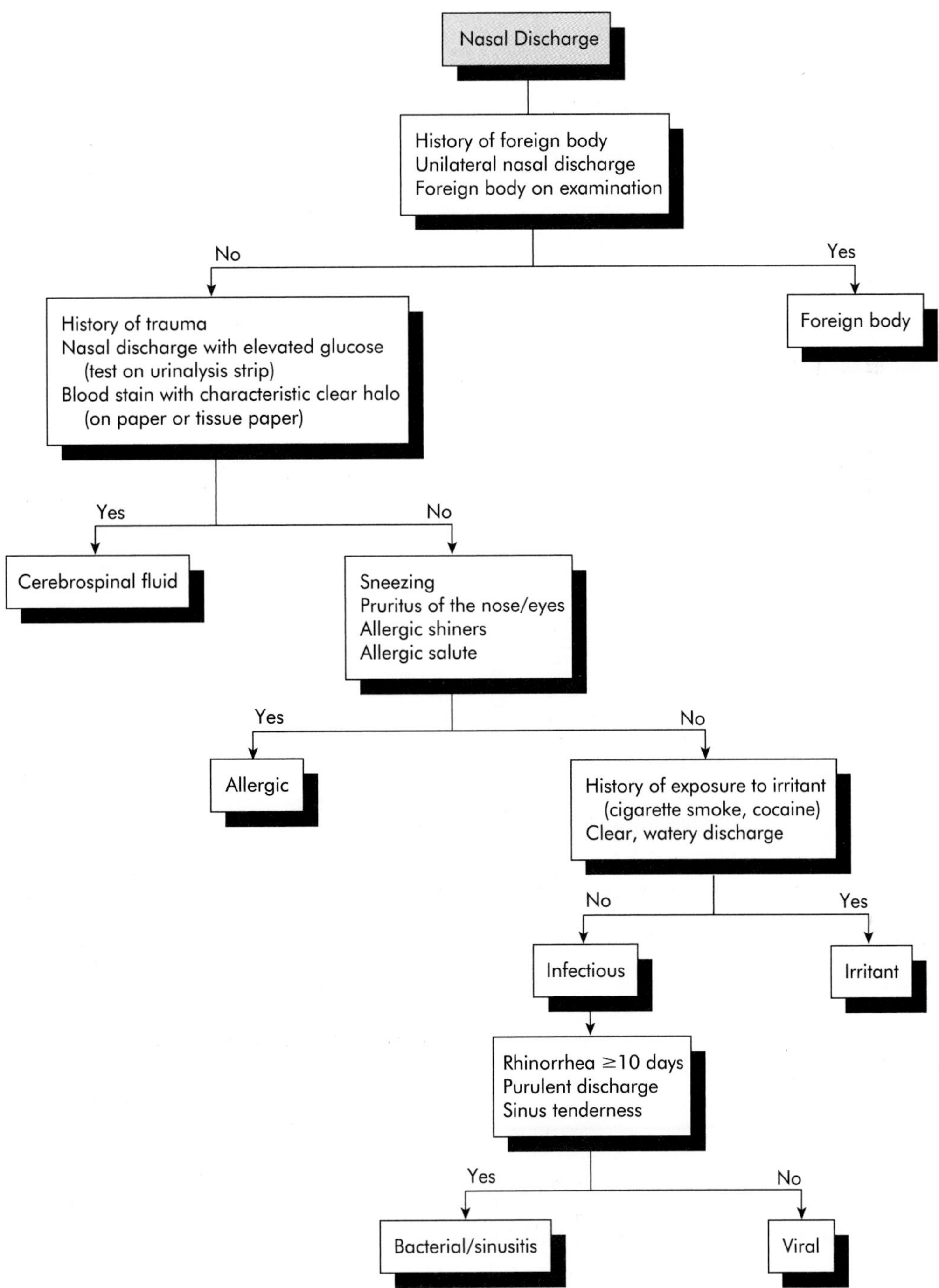

FIGURE 3-34 Nasal Discharge (see Nasal Discharge/Rhinorrhea in Differential Diagnosis [Section II])

ICD-9-CM # 784.2

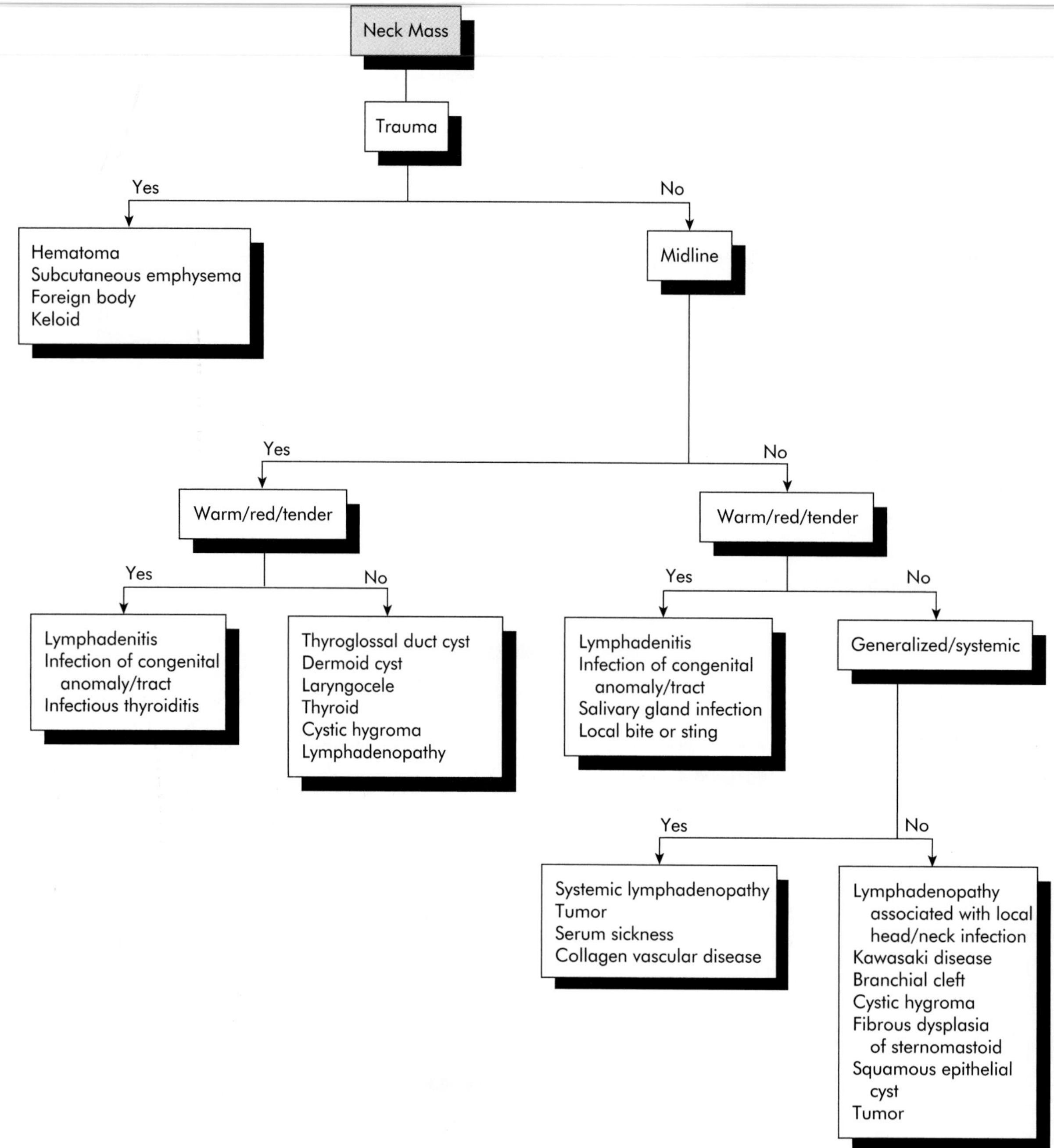

FIGURE 3-35 Neck Mass (see Neck Mass in Differential Diagnosis [Section II])

ICD-9-CM # 372.03

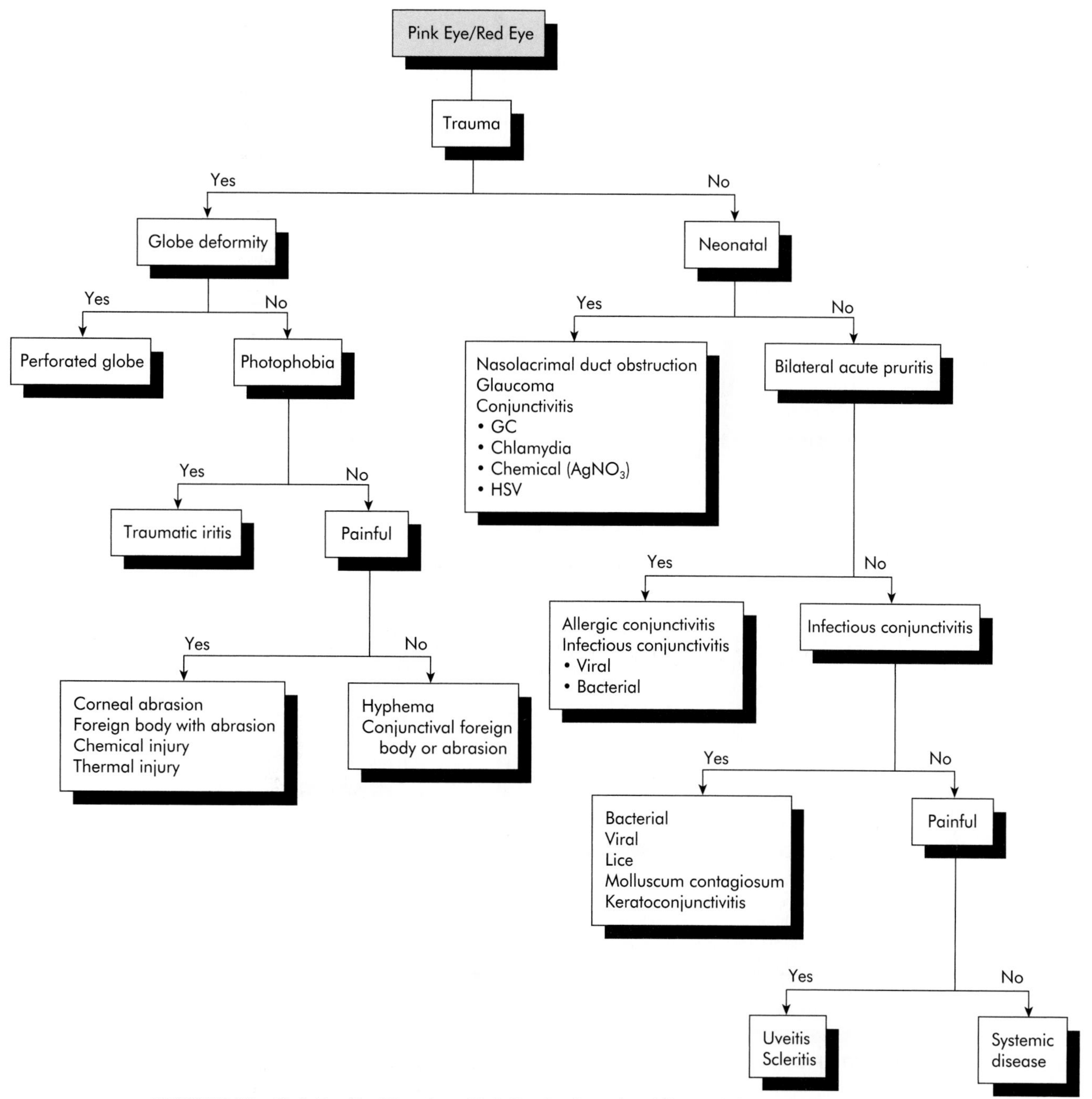

FIGURE 3-36 Pink Eye/Red Eye (see Pink Eye/Red Eye in Differential Diagnosis [Section II])

ICD-9-CM # 791.0

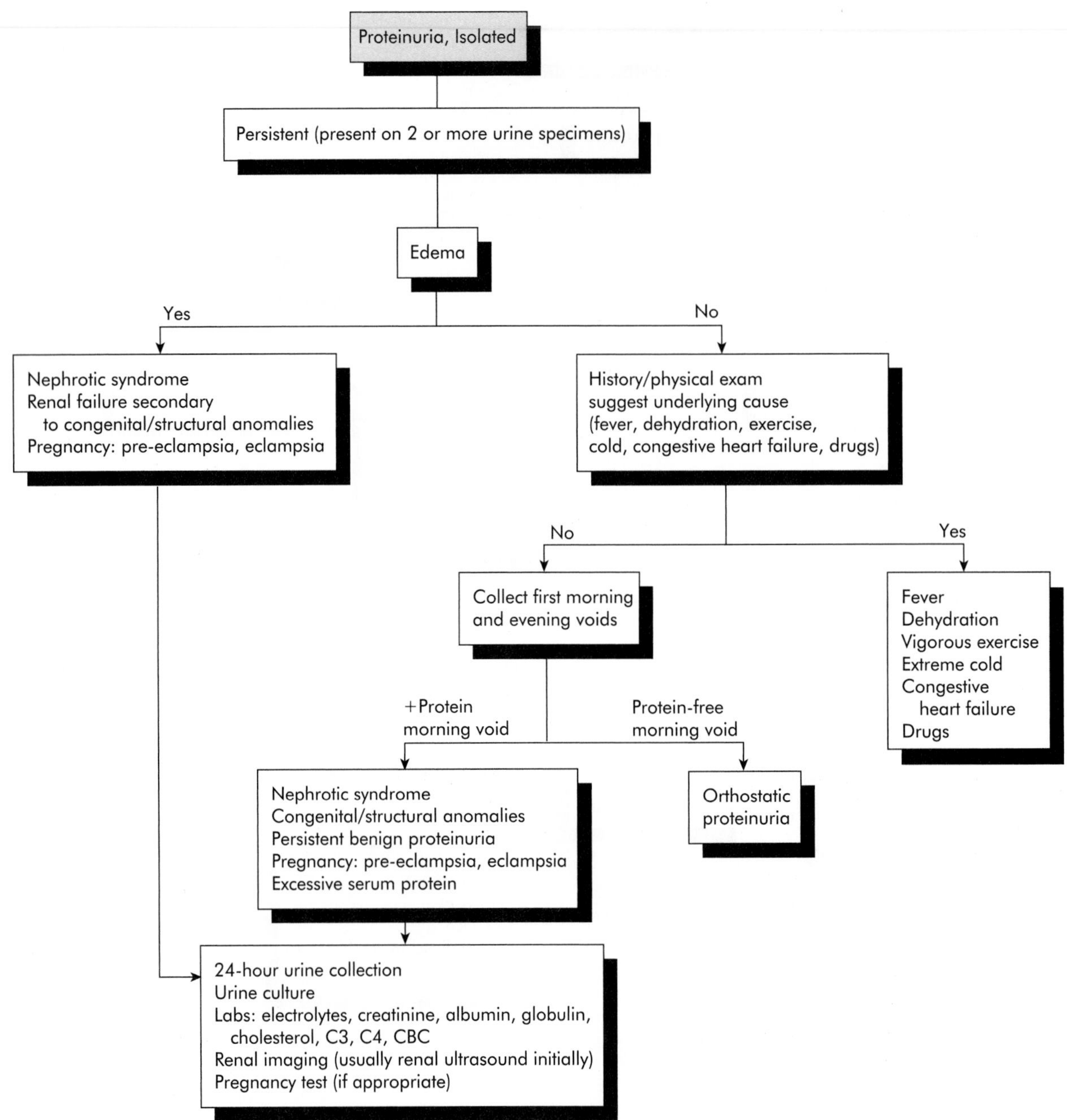

FIGURE 3-37 Proteinuria, Isolated (see Proteinuria, Isolated in Differential Diagnosis [Section II])

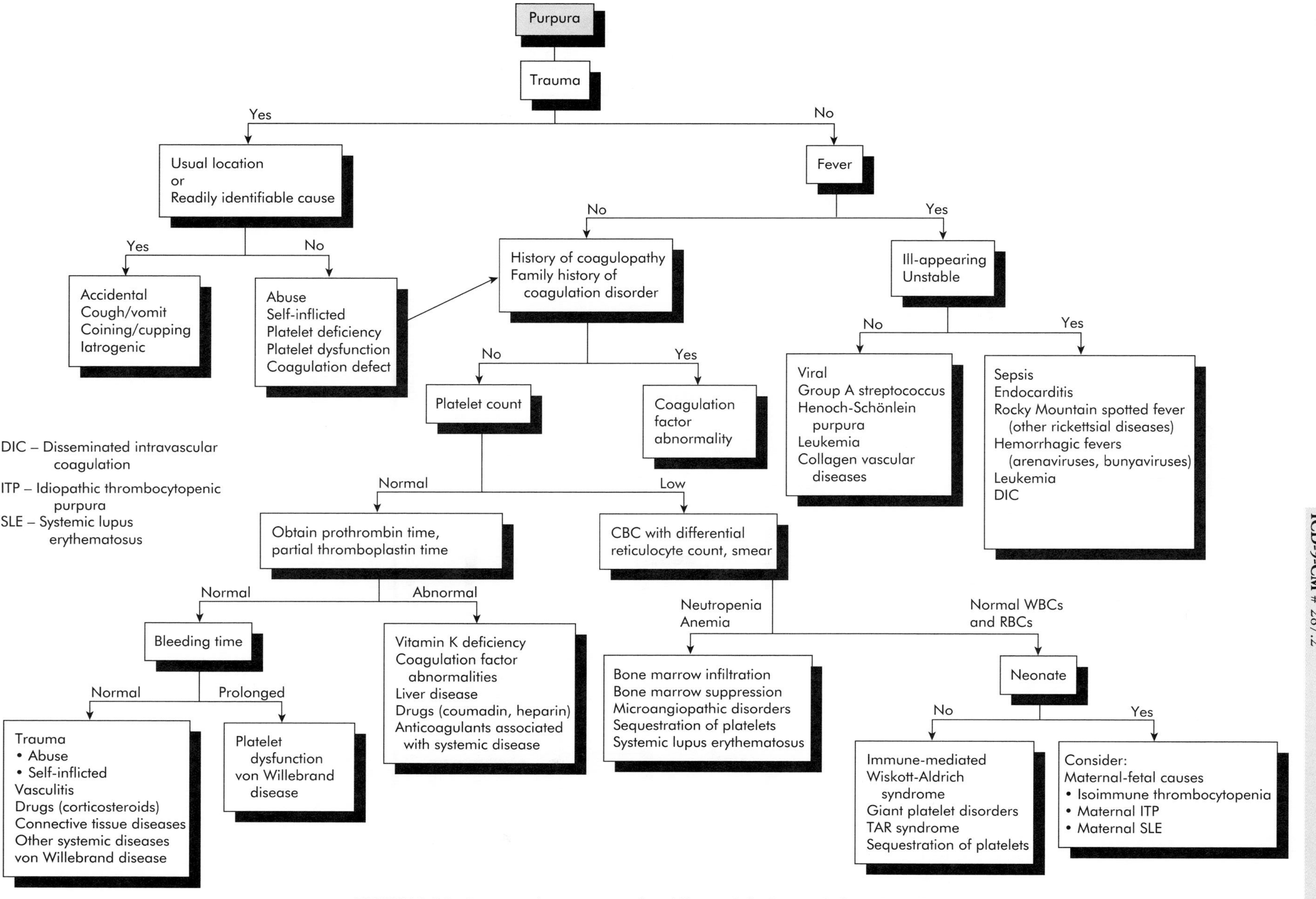

FIGURE 3-38 Purpura (see Purpura in Differential Diagnosis [Section II])

ICD-9-CM # 608.86

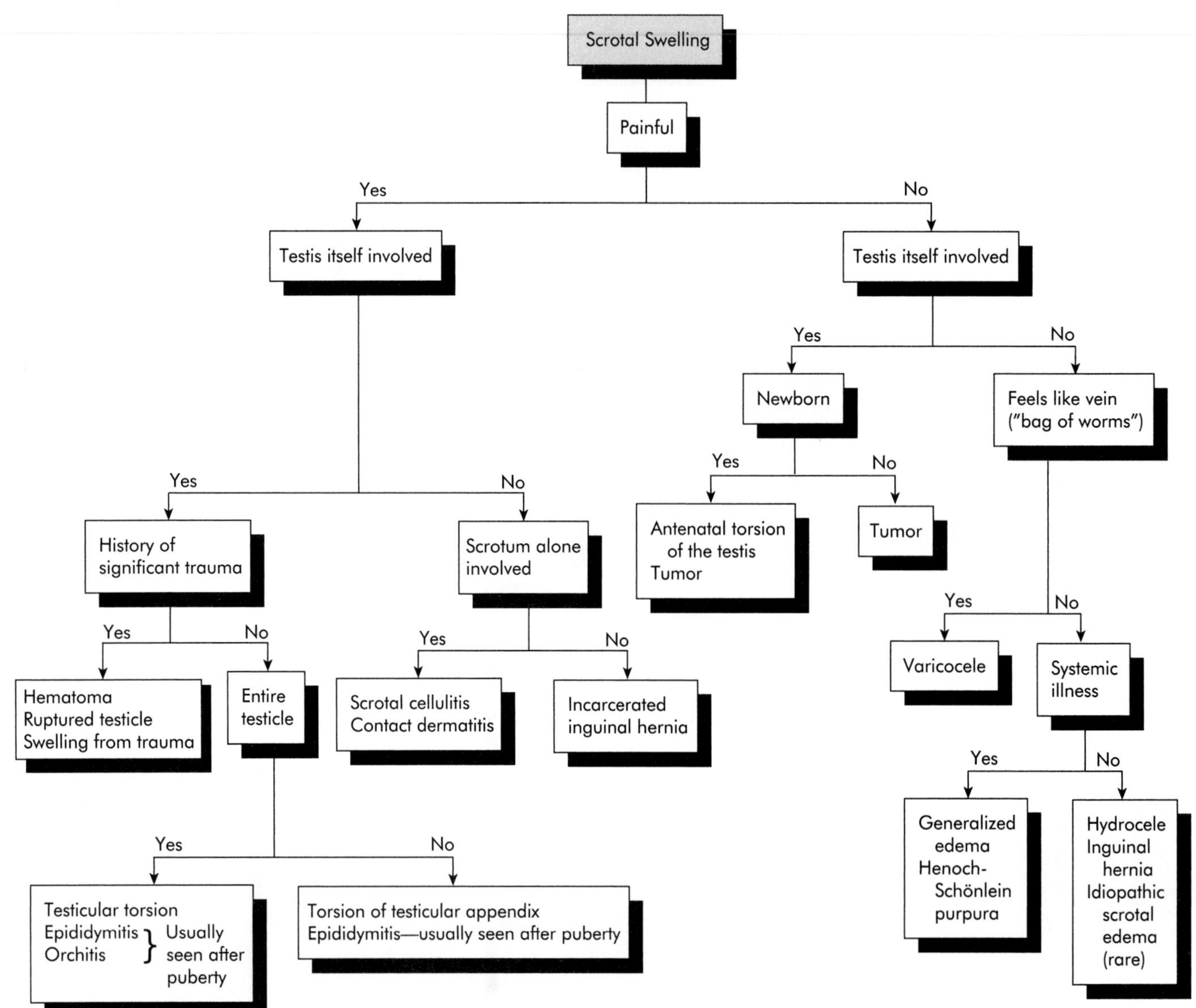

FIGURE 3-39 Scrotal Swelling (see Scrotal Swelling in Differential Diagnosis [Section II])

ICD-9-CM # 780.39

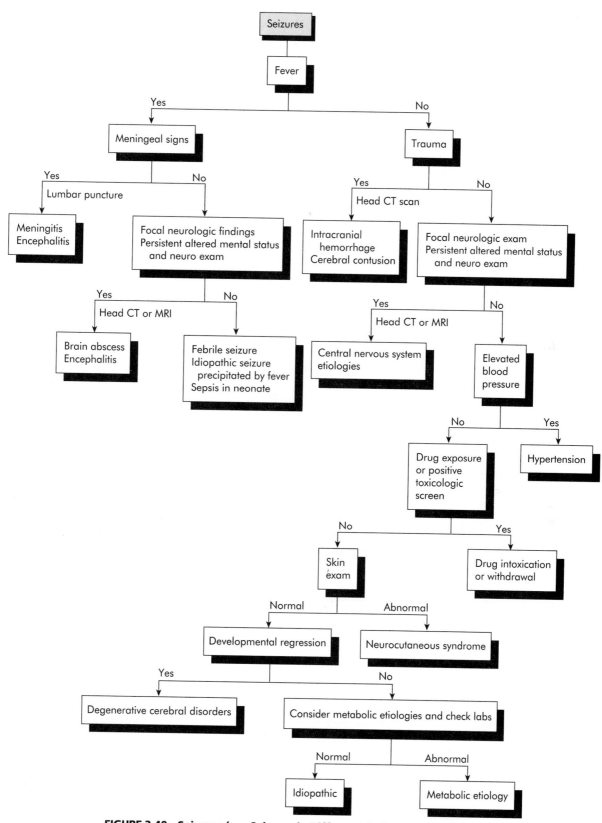

FIGURE 3-40 Seizures (see Seizures in Differential Diagnosis [Section II])

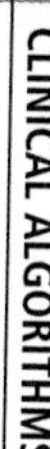

ICD-9-CM # 462

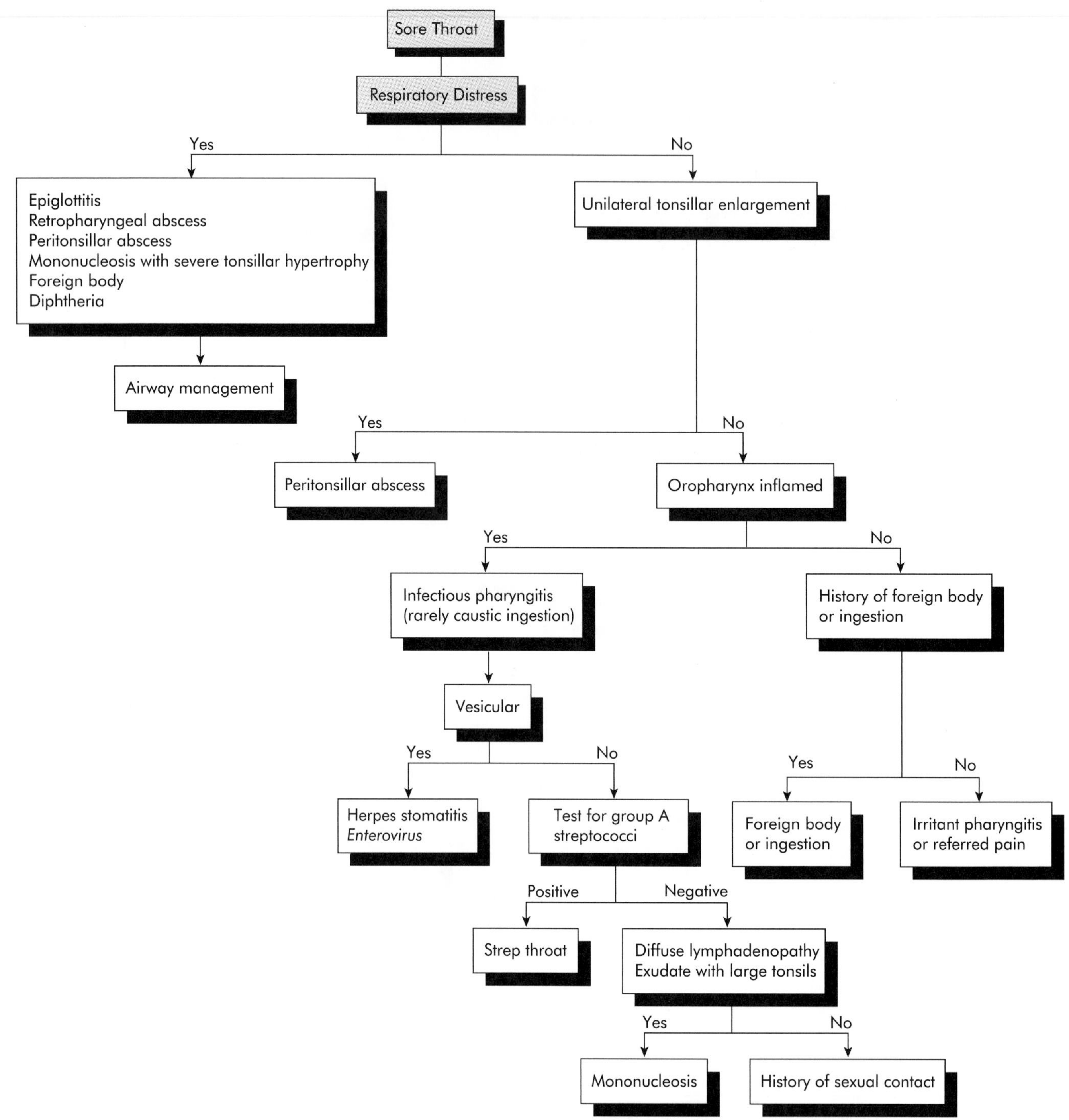

FIGURE 3-41 Sore Throat (see Sore Throat in Differential Diagnosis [Section II])

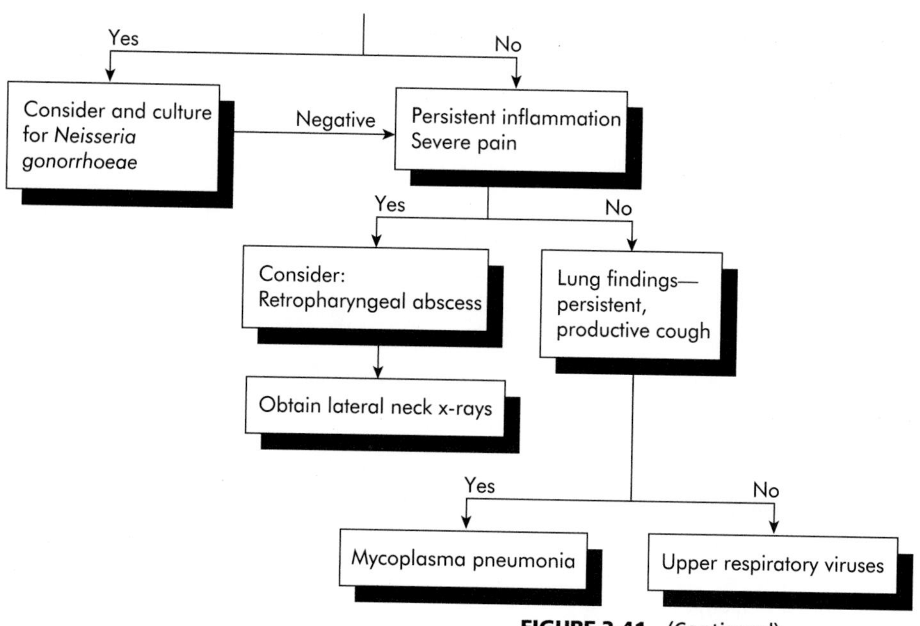

FIGURE 3-41 (Continued)

ICD-9-CM # 789.2

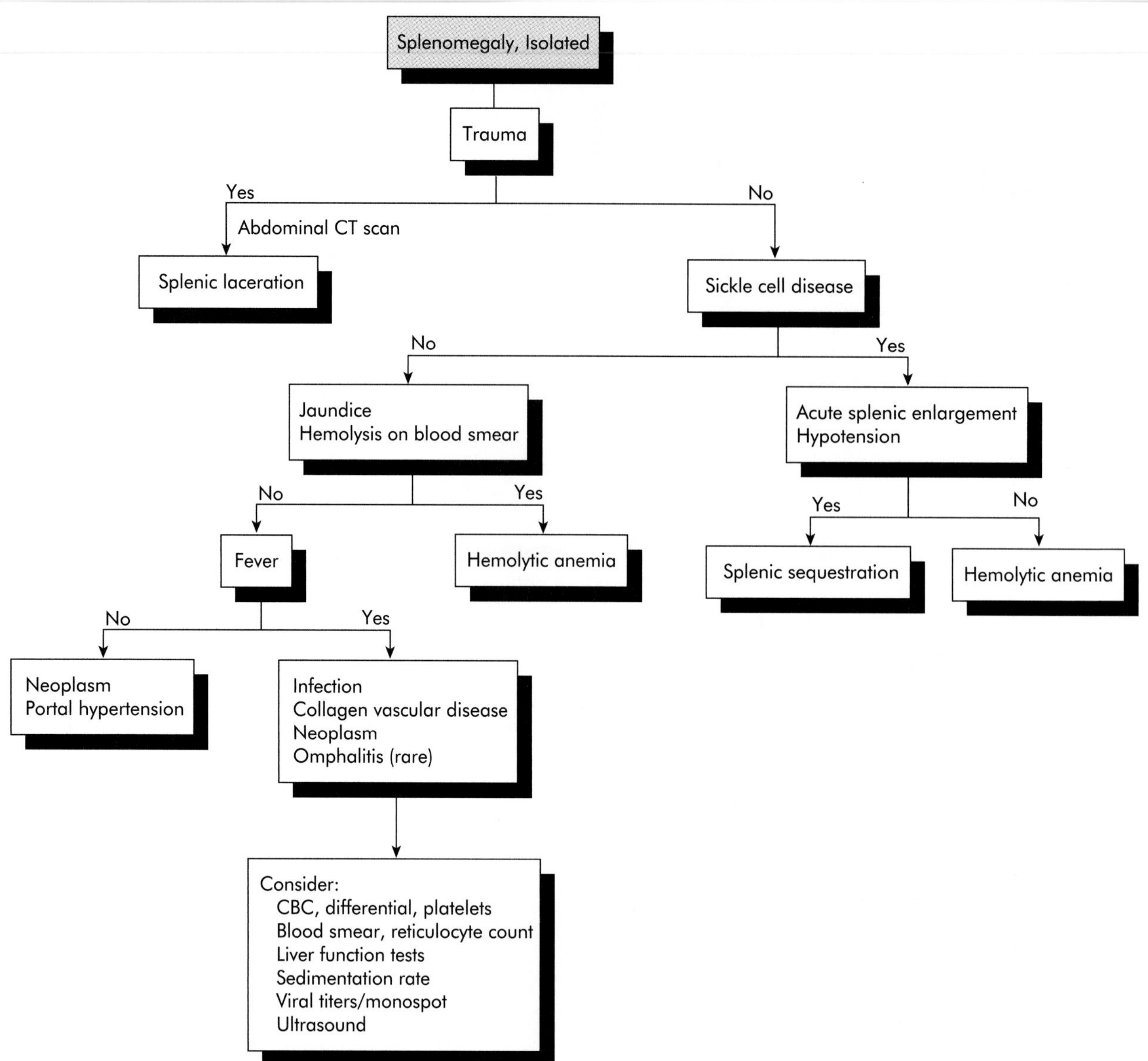

FIGURE 3-42 Splenomegaly, Isolated (see Splenomegaly, Isolated in Differential Diagnosis [Section II])

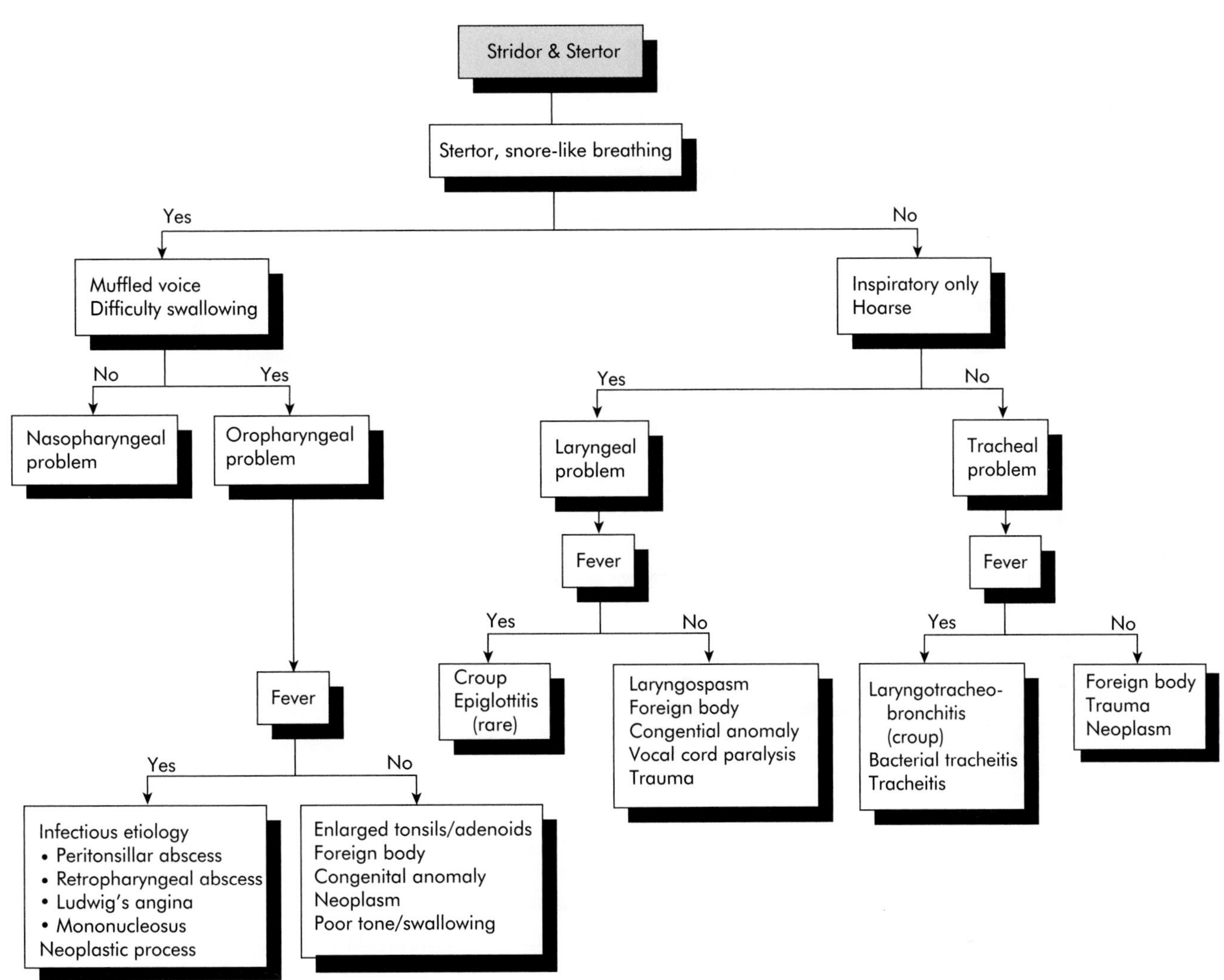

FIGURE 3-43 Stridor & Stertor (see Stridor & Stertor in Differential Diagnosis [Section II])

ICD-9-CM # 780.2

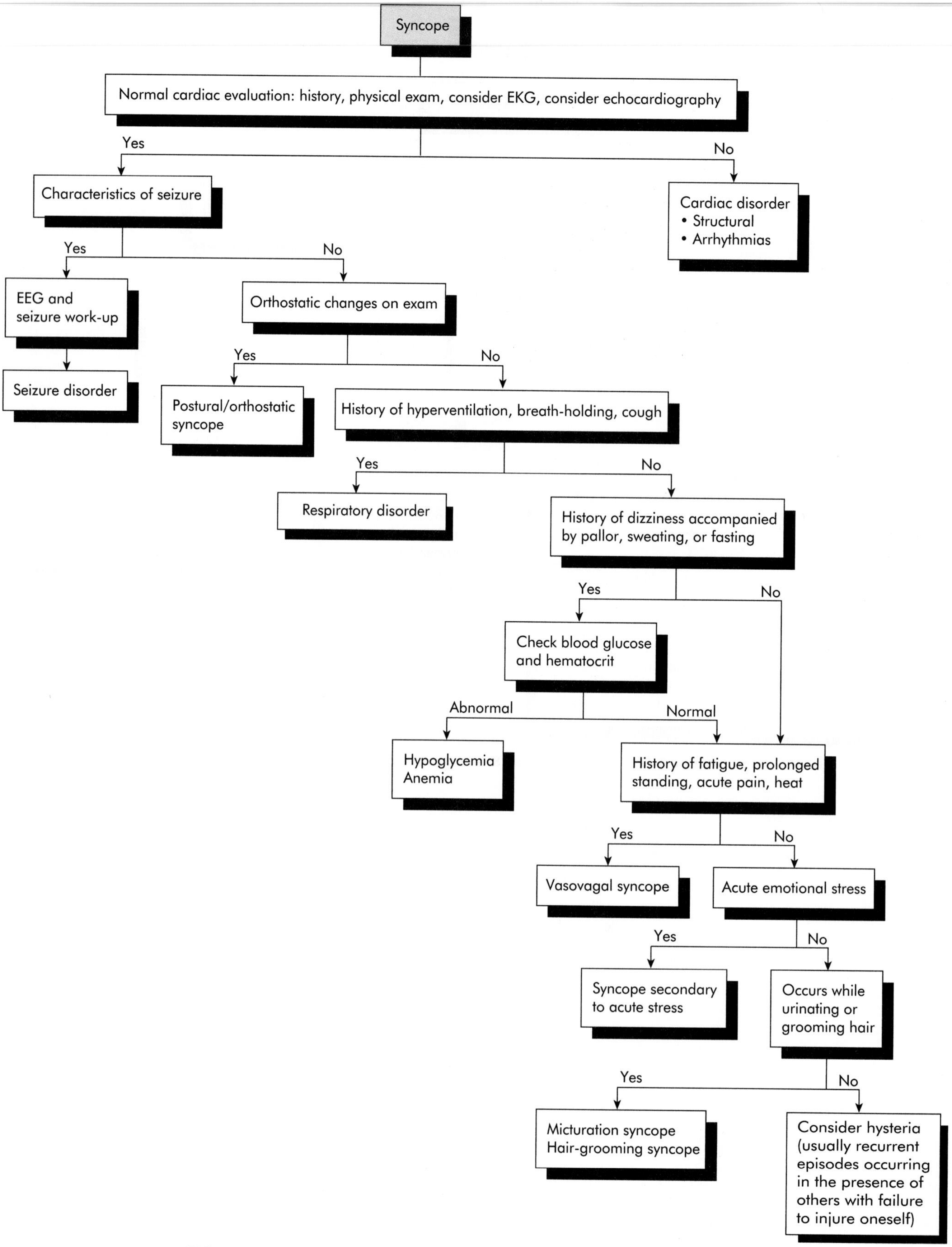

Syncope

Normal cardiac evaluation: history, physical exam, consider EKG, consider echocardiography

- Yes → Characteristics of seizure
  - Yes → EEG and seizure work-up → Seizure disorder
  - No → Orthostatic changes on exam
    - Yes → Postural/orthostatic syncope
    - No → History of hyperventilation, breath-holding, cough
      - Yes → Respiratory disorder
      - No → History of dizziness accompanied by pallor, sweating, or fasting
        - Yes → Check blood glucose and hematocrit
          - Abnormal → Hypoglycemia, Anemia
          - Normal → History of fatigue, prolonged standing, acute pain, heat
        - No → History of fatigue, prolonged standing, acute pain, heat
          - Yes → Vasovagal syncope
          - No → Acute emotional stress
            - Yes → Syncope secondary to acute stress
            - No → Occurs while urinating or grooming hair
              - Yes → Micturation syncope, Hair-grooming syncope
              - No → Consider hysteria (usually recurrent episodes occurring in the presence of others with failure to injure oneself)
- No → Cardiac disorder
  - Structural
  - Arrhythmias

FIGURE 3-44 Syncope (see S0yncope in Differential Diagnosis [Section II])

ICD-9-CM # 785.0

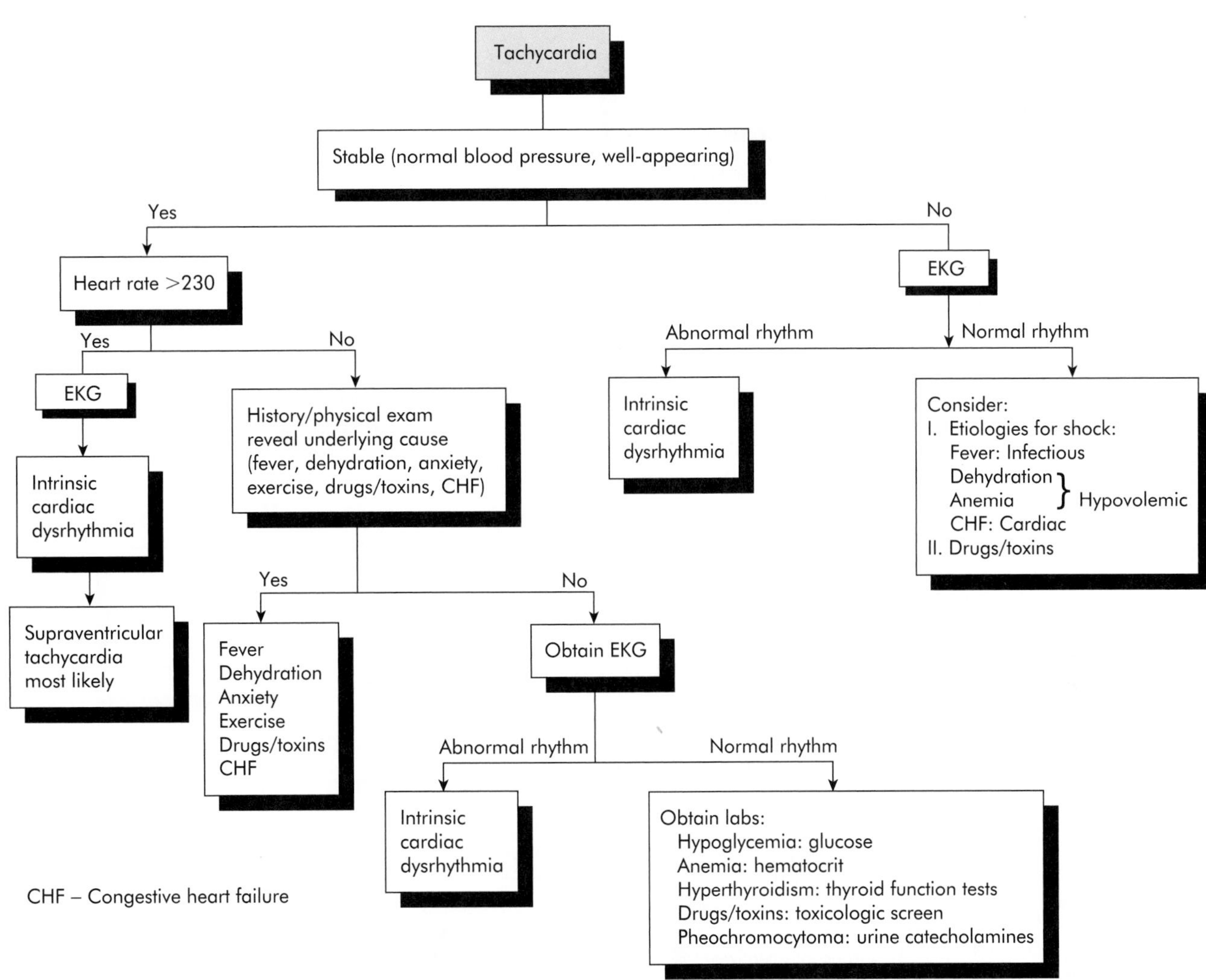

FIGURE 3-45 Tachycardia (see Tachycardia in Differential Diagnosis [Section II])

ICD-9-CM # 623.8 Vaginal bleeding
626.9 Uterine bleeding

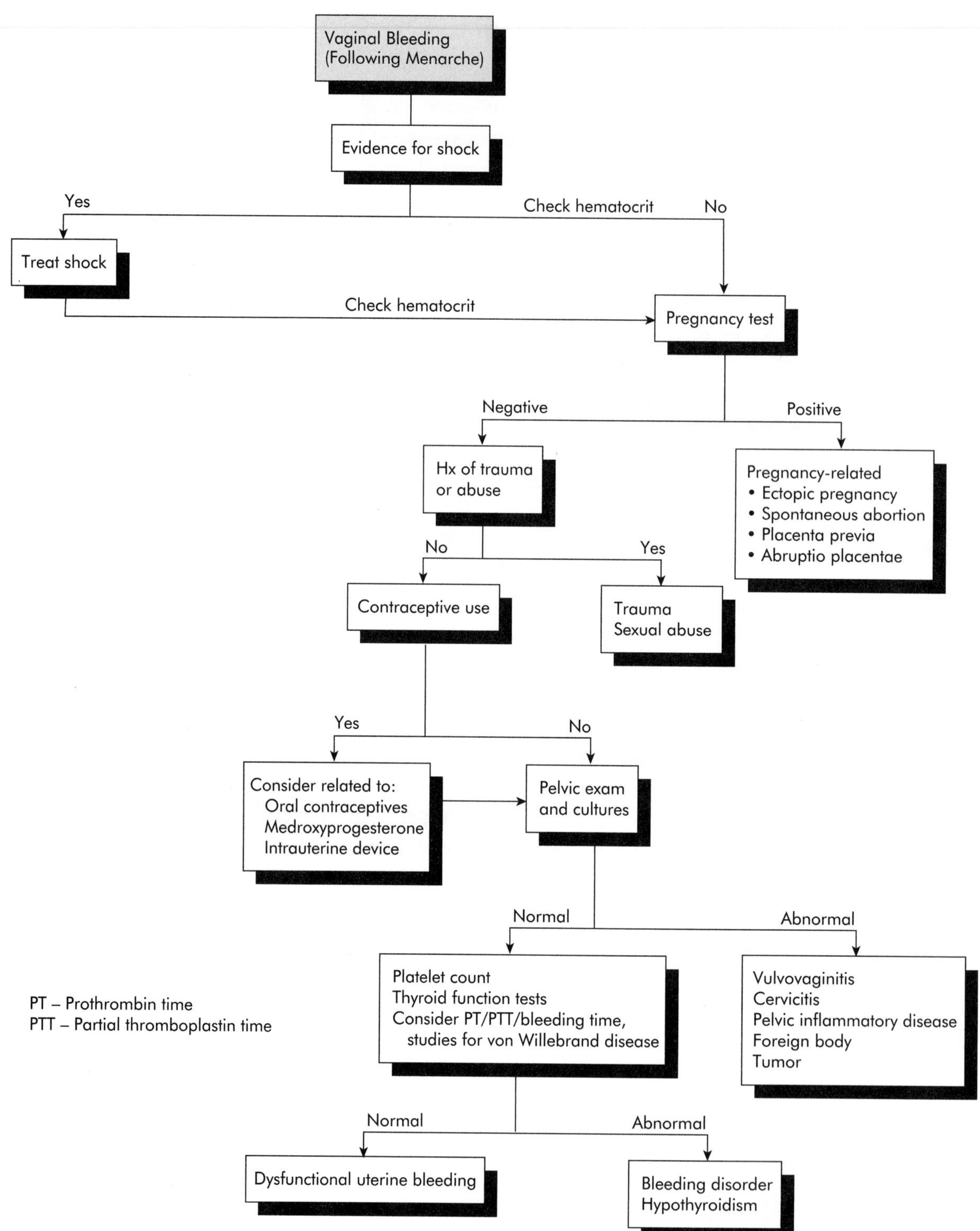

FIGURE 3-46 Vaginal Bleeding (Following Menarche) (see Vaginal Bleeding in Differential Diagnosis [Section II])

VAGINAL BLEEDING (PRIOR TO MENARCHE)

ICD-9-CM # 626.6 Unrelated to menstrual cycle

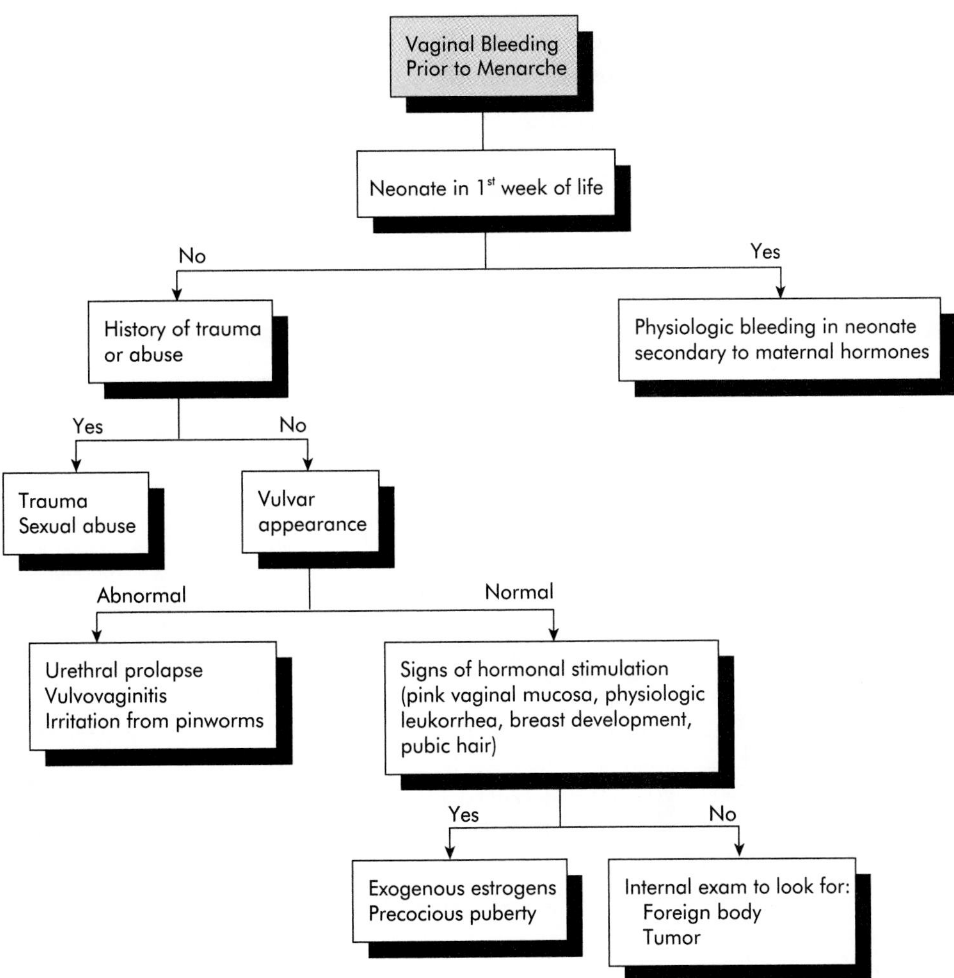

FIGURE 3-47 Vaginal Bleeding (Prior to Menarche) (see Vaginal Bleeding in Differential Diagnosis [Section II])

ICD-9-CM # 623.5

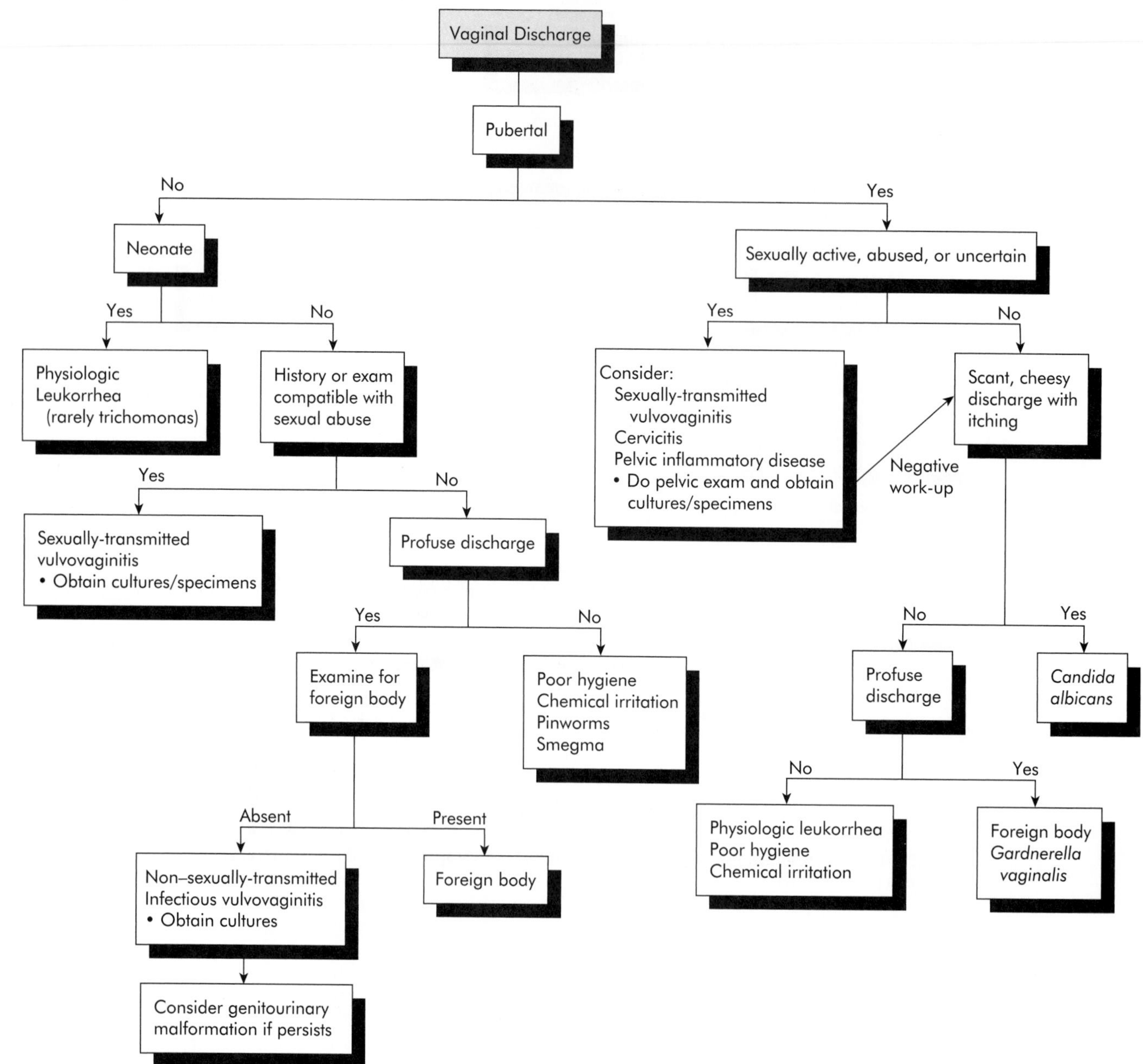

FIGURE 3-48 Vaginal Discharge (see Vaginal Discharge in Differential Diagnosis [Section II])

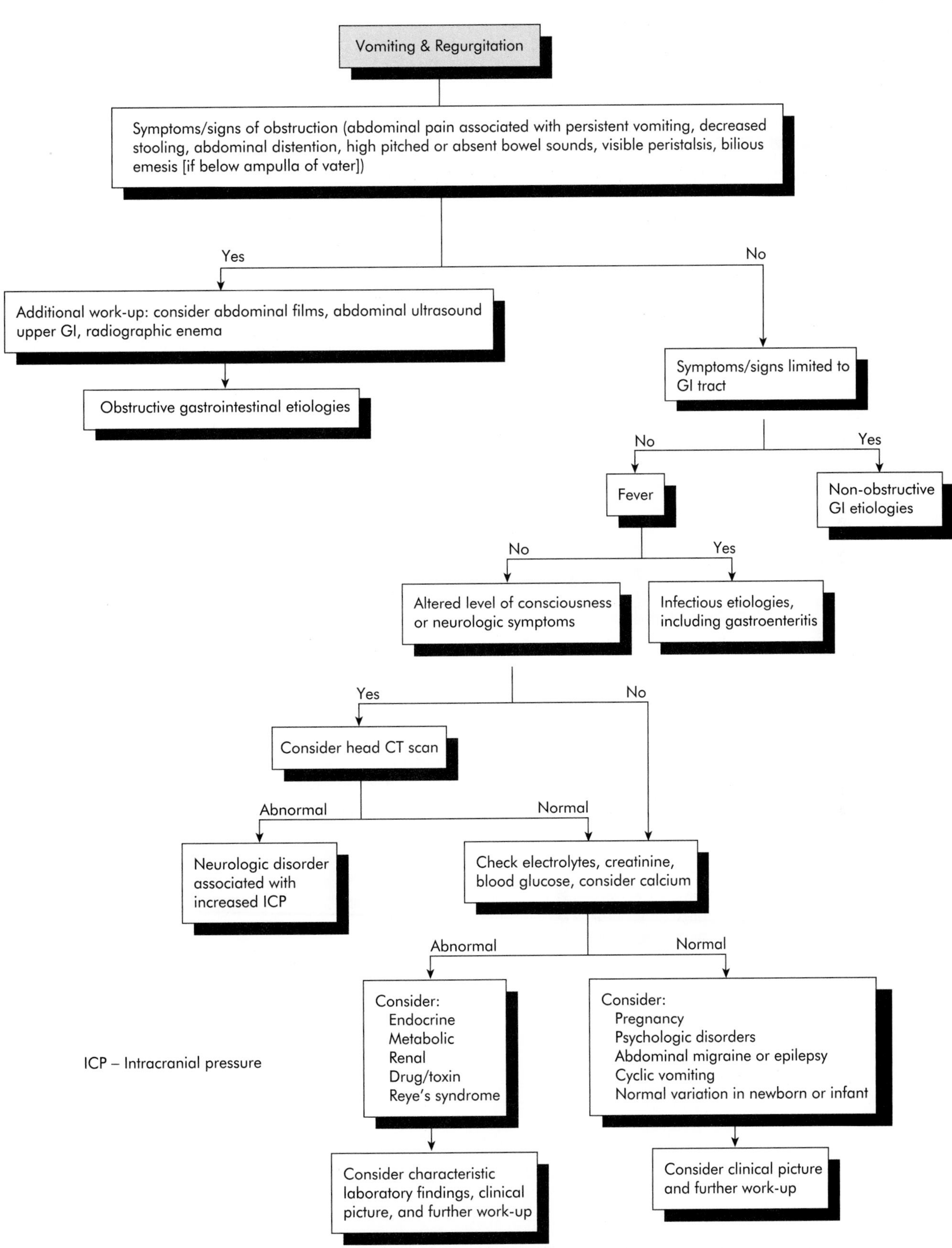

FIGURE 3-49 Vomiting & Regurgitation (see Vomiting & Regurgitation in Differential Diagnosis [Section II])

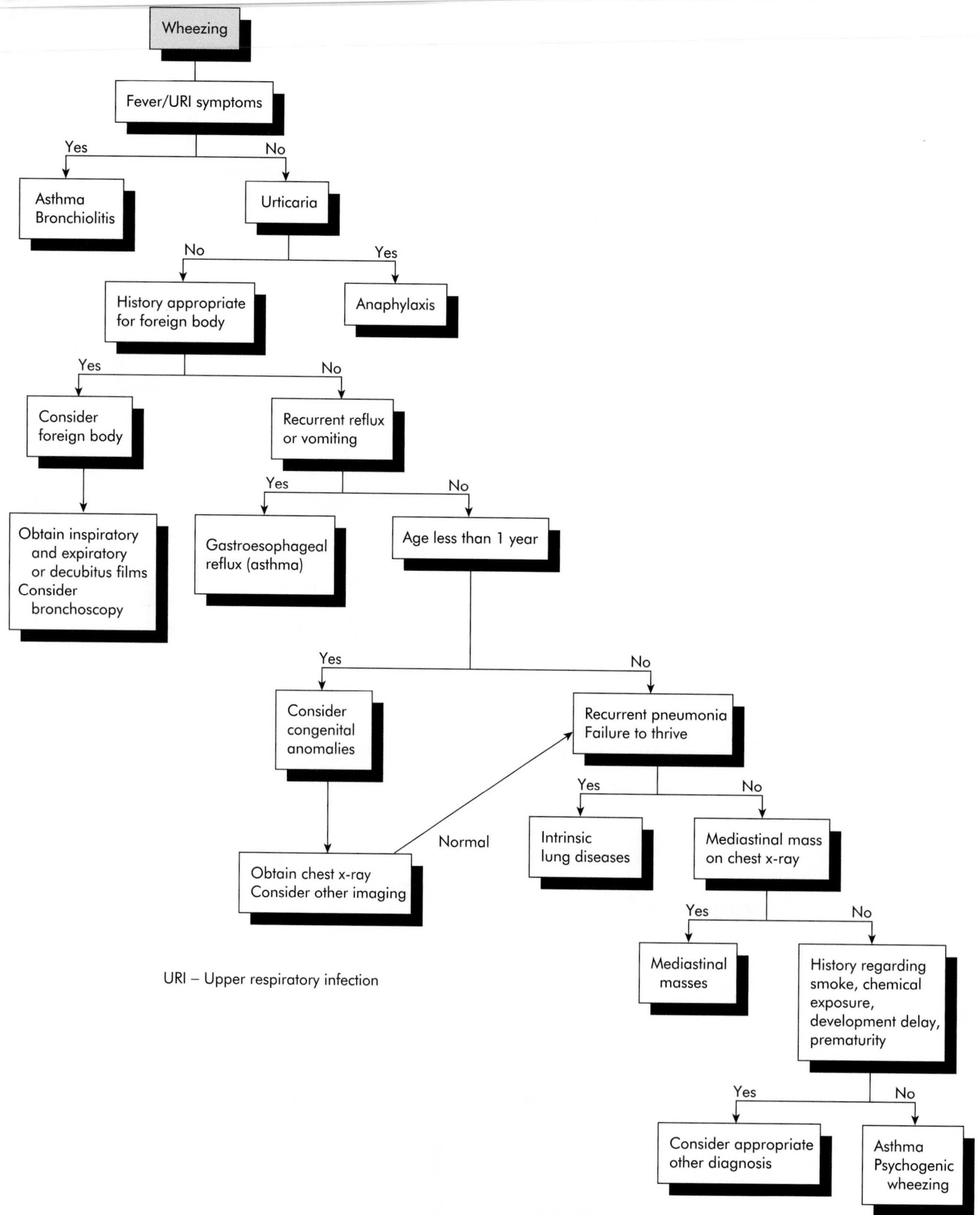

FIGURE 3-50 Wheezing (see Wheezing in Differential Diagnosis [Section II])

Section IV

Charts, Formulas, Tables and Tests

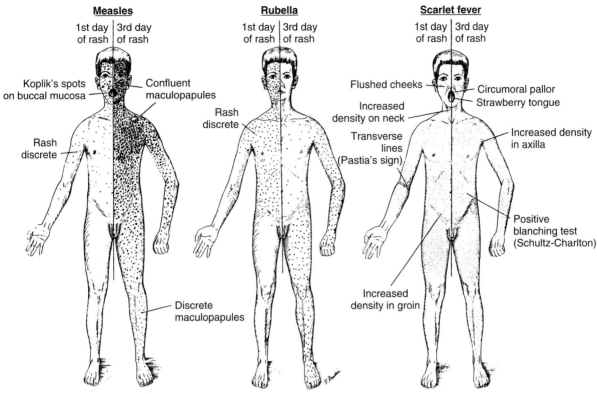

FIGURE 4-1 Location of rash on days 1 and 3 of measles, rubella, and scarlet fever. (From McMillan JA et al [eds]: *The whole pediatrician catalog: a compendium of clues to diagnosis and management.* Philadelphia, WB Saunders, 1979.)

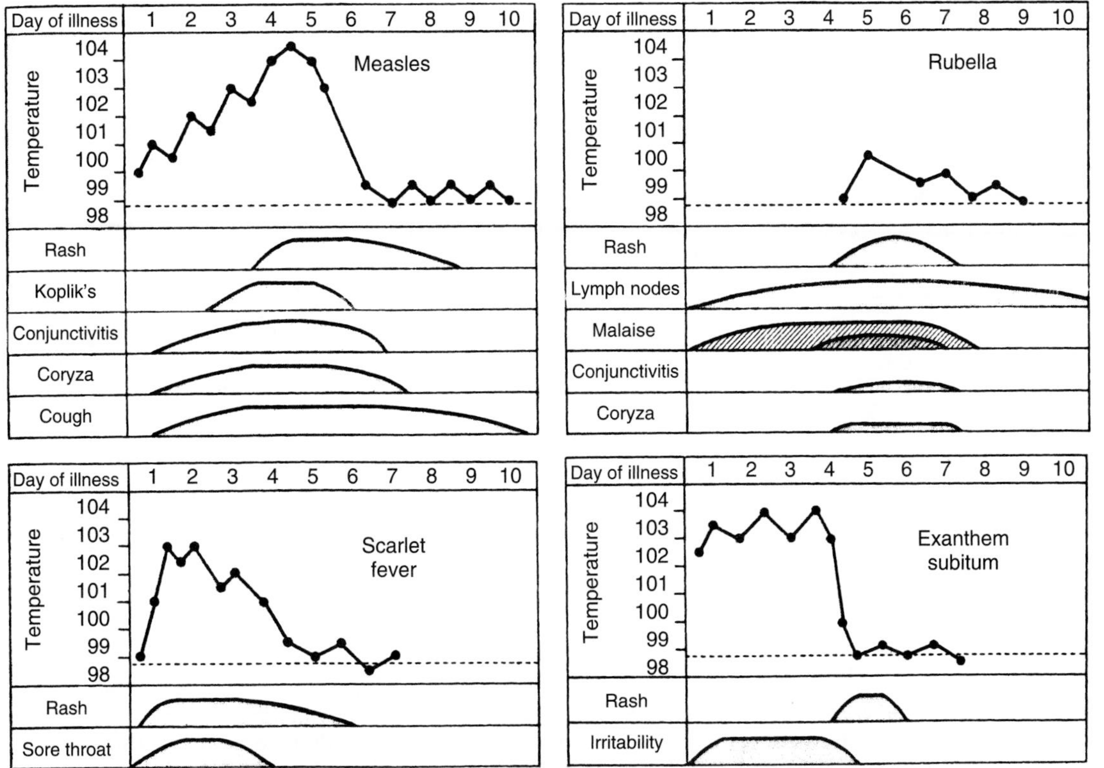

FIGURE 4-2 Prevalence of signs and symptoms in measles, rubella, scarlet fever, and exanthem subitum. (From McMillan JA et al [eds]: *The whole pediatrician catalog: a compendium of clues to diagnosis and management.* Philadelphia, WB Saunders, 1979.)

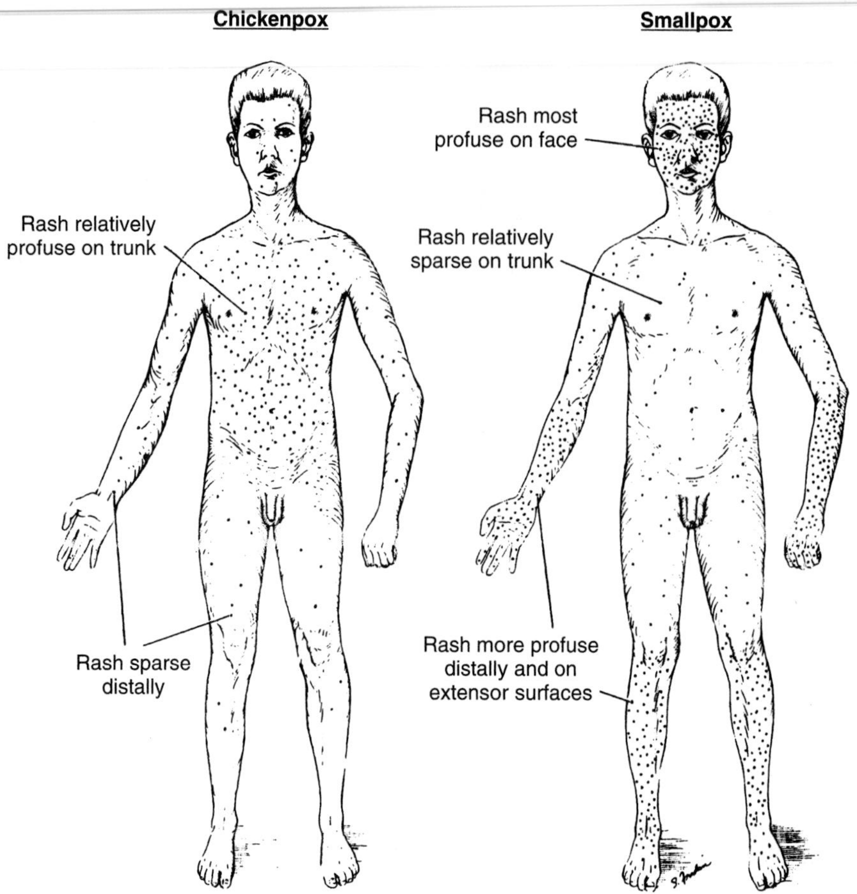

FIGURE 4-3 Location and intensity of rash in chickenpox and smallpox. (From McMillan JA et al [eds]: *The whole pediatrician catalog: a compendium of clues to diagnosis and management.* Philadelphia, WB Saunders, 1979.)

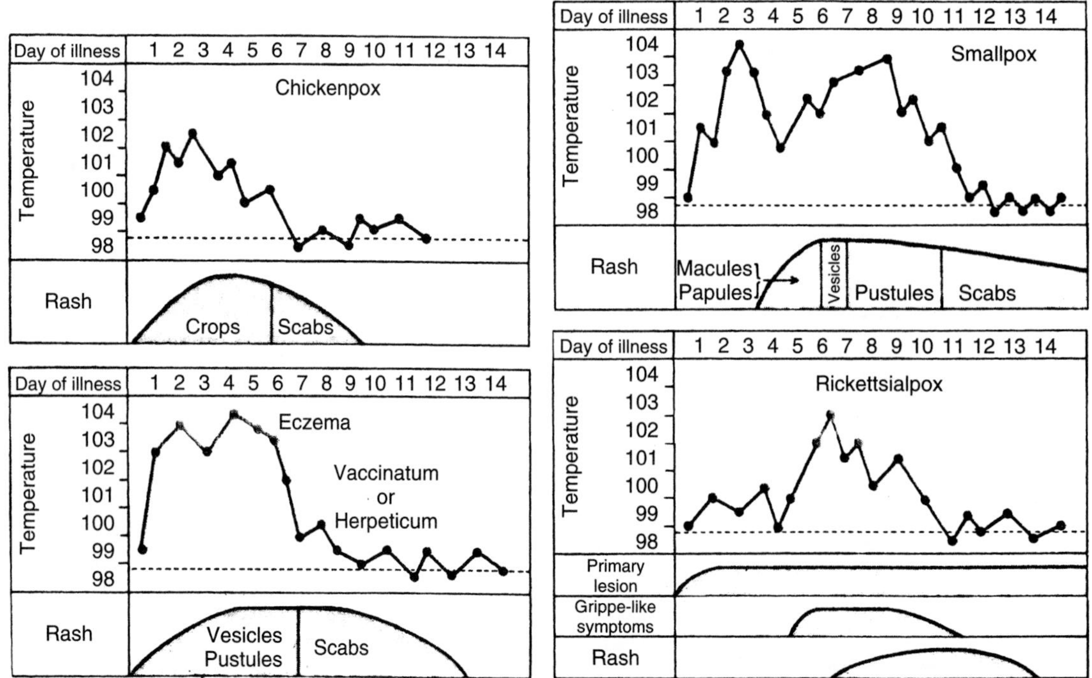

FIGURE 4-4 Prevalence of signs and symptoms in chickenpox, smallpox, eczema vaccinatum or herpeticum, and rickettsialpox. (From McMillan JA et al [eds]: *The whole pediatrician catalog: a compendium of clues to diagnosis and management.* Philadelphia, WB Saunders, 1979.)

TABLE 4-1 **Topical Glucocorticosteroid Potency**

Potency Group	Generic or Chemical Name	Concentration %	Formulation	Brand Name
I. HIGHEST	Betamethasone dipropionate augmented topical	0.05	G,O	Diprolene 0.05% G,O
	Clobetasol propionate topical	0.05	C,G,O	Clobex 0.05% L,SHMP
				Cormax 0.05% C,S
				Embeline 0.05% C,G,O,S
				Olux 0.05% F
				Temovate 0.05% C,G,O,S
	Diflorasone diacetate			Psorcon 0.05% O
	Fluocinonide			Vanos 0.1% C
	Halobetasol			Ultravate 0.05% C,O
II. HIGH	Amcinonide topical	0.1	O	Cyclocort 0.1% O
	Betamethasone dipropionate augmented topical	0.05	C	Diprolene 0.05% L
				Diprolene AF 0.05% C
	Betamethasone dipropionate topical	0.05	O	Diprosone 0.05% O
				Diprosone 0.1% A
				Maxivate 0.05% C*,O
	Betamethasone dipropionate calcipotriene topical			Taclonex 0.064%; 0.005% O
	Desoximetasone topical	0.25	C,O	Topicort 0.25% C,O
		0.05	G	Topicort 0.05% G
	Diflorasone topical	0.05	O	ApexiCon 0.05% O
				ApexiCon-E 0.05% C
				Florone 0.05% O
				Maxiflor 0.05% O
				Psorcon-E 0.05% C,O
				Psorcon 0.05% C
	Fluocinonide topical	0.05	C,G,L,O	Lidex 0.05% C,G,L,O
	Halcinonide topical	0.1	C,O	Halog 0.1% C,O
				Halog-E 0.1% C
	Mometasone topical	0.1	O	Elocon 0.1% O
	Triamcinolone acetonide topical			Aristocort-A 0.1% O; 0.5% C
III. HIGH/MED	Amcinonide topical	0.1	C,L	Cyclocort 0.1% C,O
	Betamethasone dipropionate topical	0.05	C	Diprosone 0.05% C
				Maxivate 0.05% C*,L
	Betamethasone valerate topical	0.1	O	Betatex, Valisone 0.1% O
	Desoximetasone topical	0.05	C	Topicort 0.05% C
	Diflorasone diacetate topical	0.05	C	Maxiflor 0.05% C
	Fluocinonide topical			Lidex E 0.05% C
	Flurandrenolide topical			Cordran 0.05% O[§]
	Fluticasone topical	0.005	O	Cutivate 0.005% O
	Halcinonide topical	0.1	S	Halog 0.1% S
	Mometasone topical	0.1	C,L	Elocon 0.1% C,L
	Triamcinolone acetonide topical	0.5	C	Kenalog 0.5% A,C
		0.1	O	Aristocort-A 0.1% O; 0.5% C
IV. MEDIUM	Betamethasone Benzoate			Uticort 0.025% G
	Betamethasone dipropionate topical	0.05	L	Diprosone 0.05% L
	Betamethasone valerate topical			Luxiq 0.12% F
	Clocortolone topical	0.1	C	Cloderm 0.1% C
	Desoximetasone			Topicort LP 0.05% C
	Fluocinolone topical	0.025	O,L	Synalar 0.025% O
	Flurandrenolide topical			Cordran 0.05% O[§]
	Hydrocortisone valerate topical	0.2	O	Westcort 0.2% O
	Mometasone furoate topical	0.1	O	Elocon 0.1% C,L
	Prednicarbate topical			Dermatop 0.1% O
	Triamcinolone acetonide topical	0.1	C	Aristocort A 0.1% C
				Kenalog 0.1% C,O

Continued

TABLE 4-1 **Topical Glucocorticosteroid Potency** *(Continued)*

Potency Group	Generic or Chemical Name	Concentration %	Formulation	Brand Name
V. MED/LOW	Alclometasone topical[#]	0.05	C,O	
	Betamethasone Benzoate			Uticort 0.025% C,L
	Betamethasone dipropionate topical	0.05	L	Diprosone 0.05% L
				Maxivate 0.05% L
	Betamethasone valerate topical	0.1	C	Betatrex 0.1% C,L
				Valisone 0.1% C,L
	Desonide topical	0.05	O	DesOwen 0.05% O
				Tridesilon 0.05% O
	Fluocinolone acetonide topical	0.025	C	Synalar 0.025% C
				Capex 0.01% SHMP
	Flurandrenolide topical			Cordran 0.05% C,L
	Fluticasone propionate topical	0.05	C	Cutivate 0.05% C
	Hydrocortisone butyrate topical	0.1	C,O,S	Locoid 0.1% C,O,S
				Locoid Lipocream 0.1% C
	Hydrocortisone probutate			Pandel cream 0.1% C
	Hydrocortisone valerate topical	0.2	C	Westcort 0.2% C
	Prednicarbate topical			Dermatop 0.1% C
	Triamcinolone acetonide topical	0.025	O	Aristocort 0.1% L
		0.1	L	Kenalog 0.1% L
VI. LOW	Alclometasone dipropionate topical[#]			Aclovate 0.05% C,O
	Betamethasone valerate topical	0.1	L	Valisone Lotion 0.1% L
	Desonide topical	0.05	C,L	DesOwen 0.05% C,L
				Tridesilon 0.05% C
				LoKara 0.05% L
	Fluocinolone topical	0.01	L	Synalar 0.01% C,S
	Triamcinolone topical	0.025	C,L	Aristocort A 0.025% C
				Kenalog 0.025% L
VII. LOWEST	Hydrocortisone topical OTC	0.5	C,L,O	Hycort 1% C,O
		1		Hytone 1%, 2.5% C,L,O
		2.5		Tucks anti-itch (OTC) 1% O
				Many, many brands
	Hydrocortisone/pramoxine topical			Analpram-HC 1% C
				Analpram-HC 2.5% C,L
				Pramosone 1%; 2.5% C,L,O
	Hydrocortisone/urea topical			Carmol HC 1% C

[*]Maxivate 0.05% C - listed as II in some sources and III in other sources.
[§]Cordan 0.05% O - listed as III in some sources and IV in other sources.
[#]Alclometasone topical 0.05% C,O - listed as V in some sources and VI in other sources.
A = AEROSOL
C = CREAM
F = FOAM
L = LOTION
O = OINTMENT
S = SOLUTION
SHMP = SHAMPOO

REFERENCES

1. Epocrates Inc. San Mateo, CA. Available at www.epocrates.com
2. Drug references. *In* Green SM (ed): *Pharmacopoeia Delux.* Lompoc, CA, Tarascon Publishing, 2002, pp 112–113.
3. Topical steroids. *In* Garfunkel LC et al (eds): *Pediatric Clinical Advisor.* St. Louis, Mosby, 2001, p 891.
4. Psoriasis. Available at www.psoriasis.org/treatment/psoriasis/steroids/potency.php

TABLE 4-2 **Developmental Milestones**

Age	Gross Motor	Visual-Motor/Problem-solving	Language	Social/Adaptive	Specific Guidance Issues
1 mo	Raises head slightly from prone, makes crawling movements	Birth: visually fixes 1 mo, has tight grasp, follows to midline	Alert to sound	Regards face	Car seats, fever control, thermometers, talking to baby, sleeping, stimulating mobiles
2 mo	Holds head in midline, lifts chest off table	No longer clenches fist tightly, follows object past midline	Smiles socially (after being stroked or talked to)	Recognizes parent	
3 mo	Supports on forearms in prone, holds head up steadily	Holds hands open at rest, follows in circular fashion, responds to visual threat	Coos (produces long vowel sounds in musical fashion)	Reaches for familiar people or objects, anticipates feeding	Car seats, diet, stimulating safe toys, babysitters
4 mo	Rolls front to back, supports on wrists and shifts weight	Reaches with arms in unison, brings hands to midline	Laughs, orients to voice	Enjoys looking around environment	
5 mo	Rolls back to front, sits supported	Transfers objects	Says "ah-goo," razzes, orients to bell (localizes laterally)	—	
6 mo	Sits unsupported, puts feet in mouth in supine position	Unilateral reach, uses raking grasp	Babbles	Recognizes strangers	Car seats, stair gates, electric cord and outlet covers, crawling, stranger anxiety, peek-a-boo, banging toys
7 mo	Creeps	—	Orients to bell (localized indirectly)	—	
8 mo	Comes to sit, crawls	Inspects objects	"Dada" indiscriminately	Fingerfeeds	
9 mo	Pivots when sitting, pulls to stand, cruises	Uses pincer grasp, probes with forefinger, holds bottle, throws objects	"Mama" indiscriminately, gestures, waves bye-bye, understands "no"	Starts to explore environment; plays gesture games (e.g., pat-a-cake)	Car seats, water bath safety, finger-foods, cup weaning, teeth care, first book, appropriate discipline, ipecac
10 mo	Walks when led with both hands held	—	"Dada"/"mama" discriminately; orients to bell (directly)	—	
11 mo	Walks when led with one hand held	—	One word other than "dada"/"mama," follows 1-step command with gesture	—	
12 mo	Walks alone	Uses mature pincer grasp, releases voluntarily, marks paper with pencil	Uses two words other than "dada"/"mama," immature jargoning (runs several unintelligible words together)	Imitates actions, comes when called, cooperates with dressing	Car seats, books, water safety, burns, scalds, decreased appetite, riding toys, pull toys, temper tantrums, nightmares
13 mo	—	—	Uses three words	—	
14 mo	—	—	Follows 1-step command without gesture	—	
15 mo	Creeps up stairs, walks backwards	Scribbles in imitation, builds tower of 2 blocks in imitation	Uses 4-6 words	15-18 mo: uses spoon, uses cup independently	
17 mo	—	—	Uses 7-20 words, points to 5 body parts, uses mature jargoning (includes intelligible words in jargoning)	—	

Continued

TABLE 4-2 **Developmental Milestones** *(Continued)*

Age	Gross Motor	Visual-Motor/Problem-solving	Language	Social/Adaptive	Specific Guidance Issues
18 mo	Runs, throws objects from standing without falling	Scribbles spontaneously, builds tower of 3 blocks, turns 2-3 pages at a time	Uses 2-word combinations	Copies parent in tasks (sweeping, dusting), plays in company of other children	
19 mo	—	—	Knows 8 body parts	—	
21 mo	Squats in play, goes up steps	Builds tower of 5 blocks	Uses 50 words, 2-word sentences	Asks to have food and to go to toilet	
24 mo	Walks up and down steps without help	Imitates stroke with pencil, builds tower of 7 blocks, turns pages one at a time, removes shoes, pants, etc.	Uses pronouns (I, you, me) inappropriately, follows 2-step commands	Parallel play	Car seats, books, playground safety, babysitter, giving up blanket, etc., appropriate discipline, learning to play with others
30 mo	Jumps with both feet off floor, throws ball overhand	Holds pencil in adult fashion, performs horizontal and vertical strokes, unbuttons	Uses pronouns appropriately, understands concept of "1," repeats 2 digits forward	Tells first and last names when asked; gets self drink without help	
3 yr	Can alternate feet when going up steps, pedals tricycle	Copies a circle, undresses completely, dresses partially, dries hands if reminded	Uses minimum 250 words, 3-word sentences; uses plurals, past tense; knows all pronouns; understands concept of "2"	Group play, shares toys, takes turns, plays well with others, knows full name, age, sex	
4 yr	Hops, skips, alternates feet going down steps	Copies a square, buttons clothing, dresses self completely, catches ball	Knows colors, says song or poem from memory, asks questions	Tells "tall tales," plays cooperatively with a group of children	Consideration should be given to discussing "private" areas and setting limits for those areas
5 yr	Skips alternating feet, jumps over low obstacles	Copies triangle, ties shoes, spreads with knife	Prints first name, asks what a word means	Plays competitive games, abides by rules, likes to help in household tasks	

From Bravo AM: Development. *In* Siberry GK, Iannone R (eds): *The Harriet Lane Handbook: A Manual for Pediatric House Officers,* 15th ed. St Louis, Mosby, 2000. Rounded norms from Capute AJ et al: *Dev Med Child Neurol* 28:762, 1986.

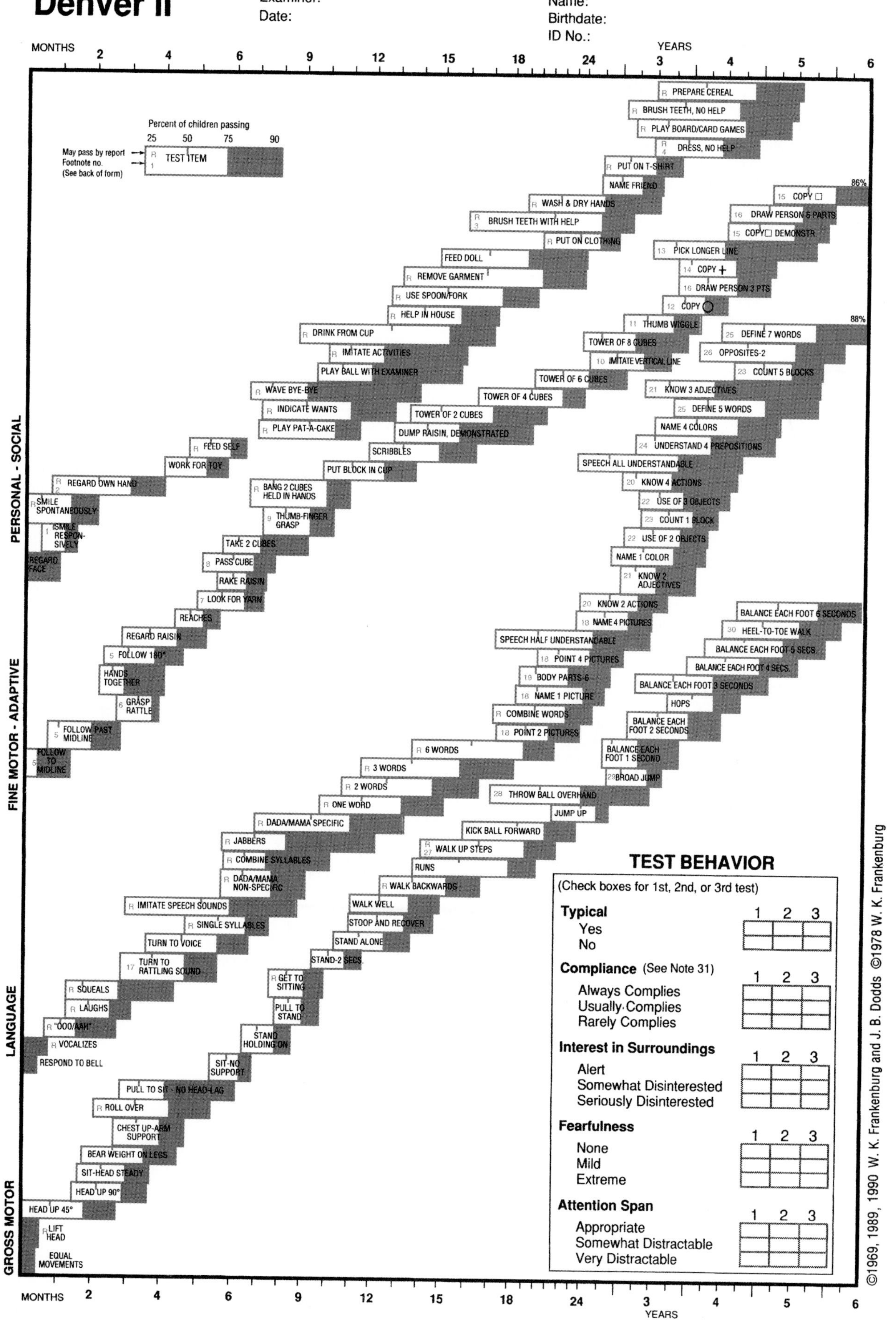

FIGURE 4-5A Denver II. Testing kits, test forms, and reference manuals (which must be used to ensure accuracy in administration of the test) for the DDST may be ordered from Denver Developmental Material, Inc., P.O. Box 6919, Denver, CO 80206-0919. (Copyright by William K. Frankenburg and J.B. Dodds.)

DIRECTIONS FOR ADMINISTRATION

1. Try to get child to smile by smiling, talking, or waving. Do not touch him/her.
2. Child must stare at hand several seconds.
3. Parent may help guide toothbrush and put toothpaste on brush.
4. Child does not have to be able to tie shoes or button/zip in the back.
5. Move yarn slowly in an arc from one side to the other, about 8" above child's face.
6. Pass if child grasps rattle when it is touched to the backs or tips of fingers.
7. Pass if child tries to see where yarn went. Yarn should be dropped quickly from sight from tester's hand without arm movement.
8. Child must transfer cube from hand to hand without help of body, mouth, or table.
9. Pass if child picks up raisin with any part of thumb and finger.
10. Line can vary only 30 degrees or less from tester's line.
11. Make a fist with thumb pointing upward and wiggle only the thumb. Pass if child imitates and does not move any fingers other than the thumb.

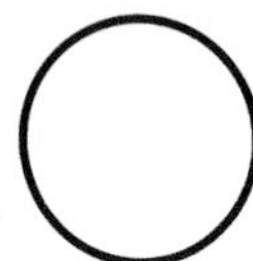

12. Pass any enclosed form. Fail continuous round motions.

13. Which line is longer? (Not bigger.) Turn paper upside down and repeat. (pass 3 of 3 or 5 of 6)

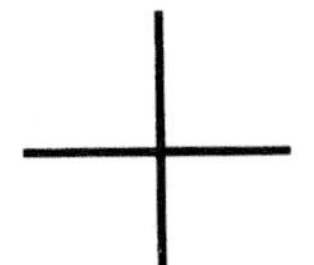

14. Pass any lines crossing near midpoint.

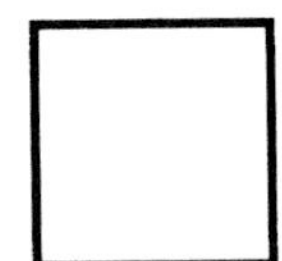

15. Have child copy first. If failed, demonstrate.

When giving items 12, 14, and 15, do not name the forms. Do not demonstrate 12 and 14.

16. When scoring, each pair (2 arms, 2 legs, etc.) counts as one part.
17. Place one cube in cup and shake gently near child's ear, but out of sight. Repeat for other ear.
18. Point to picture and have child name it. (No credit is given for sounds only.) If less than 4 pictures are named correctly, have child point to picture as each is named by tester.

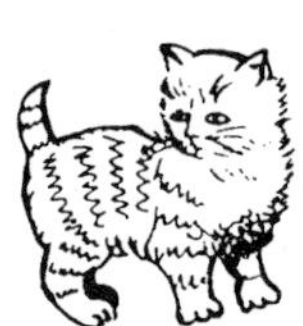
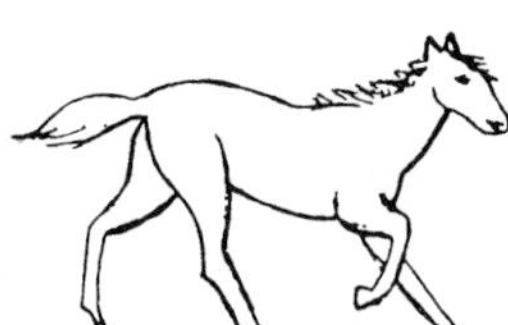
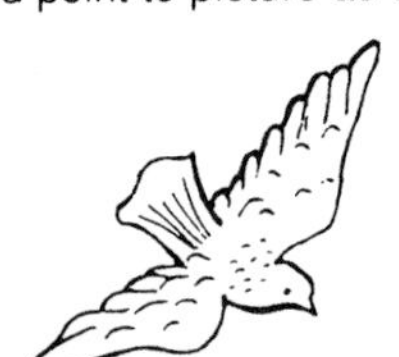
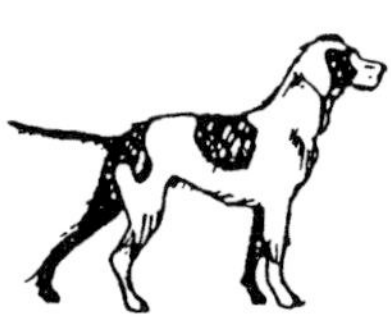
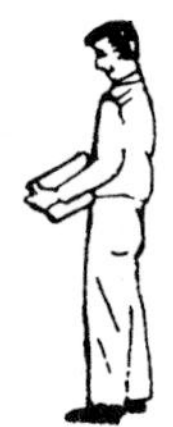

19. Using doll, tell child: Show me the nose, eyes, ears, mouth, hands, feet, tummy, hair. Pass 6 of 8.
20. Using pictures, ask child: Which one flies?... says meow?... talks?... barks?... gallops? Pass 2 of 5, 4 of 5.
21. Ask child: What do you do when you are cold?... tired?... hungry? Pass 2 of 3, 3 of 3.
22. Ask child: What do you do with a cup? What is a chair used for? What is a pencil used for? Action words must be included in answers.
23. Pass if child correctly places <u>and</u> says how many blocks are on paper. (1, 5).
24. Tell child: Put block **on** table; **under** table; **in front of** me, **behind** me. Pass 4 of 4. (Do not help child by pointing, moving head or eyes.)
25. Ask child: What is a ball?... lake?... desk?... house?... banana?... curtain?... fence?... ceiling? Pass if defined in terms of use, shape, what it is made of, or general category (such as banana is fruit, not just yellow). Pass 5 of 8, 7 of 8.
26. Ask child: If a horse is big, a mouse is __? If fire is hot, ice is __? If the sun shines during the day, the moon shines during the __? Pass 2 of 3.
27. Child may use wall or rail only, not person. May not crawl.
28. Child must throw ball overhand 3 feet to within arm's reach of tester.
29. Child must perform standing broad jump over width of test sheet (8 1/2 inches).
30. Tell child to walk forward, ∞∞∞∞→ heel within 1 inch of toe. Tester may demonstrate. Child must walk 4 consecutive steps.
31. In the second year, half of normal children are noncompliant.

OBSERVATIONS:

FIGURE 4-5B Instructions for administering the DDST. (Copyright by William K. Frankenburg and J.B. Dodds.)

LANGUAGE DEVELOPMENT: CLAMS/CAT*

CLAMS/CAT (Capute Scales) (Table 4-3): The Capute Scales are an assessment tool that gives quantitative developmental quotients for visual-motor/problem-solving and language abilities. The CLAMS (**C**linical **L**inguistic and **A**uditory **M**ilestone **S**cale) was developed, standardized, and validated for assessment of language development from birth to 36 months of age. The CAT (**C**linical **A**daptive **T**est) consists of problem-solving items, for ages from birth to 36 months, adapted from standardized infant psychologic tests.

- **Supplies:** The kit includes the following items: red ring, cup, 10 cubes, pegboard with six holes and two pegs, metal bell, crayon and paper, tissues, card with four pictures, card with six pictures, bottle and pellets, round stick, glass (made of Plexiglas), formboard with three shapes.
- **Responses:** Responses to the test item are recorded as "yes" for pass and "no" for fail. A basal age is determined when all items for 2 consecutive months are scored as "yes." Items for tests at the next higher age group are administered until two consecutive levels of all "no" responses are obtained. Items marked with an asterisk must be answered or demonstrated by the child and not per report of the parent/caregiver.
- **Scoring:** Scoring is done by calculating the basal age as the highest age group where a child accomplishes all of the test tasks correctly. The age equivalent is then determined by adding the decimal number (recorded in parentheses) next to each correctly scored item passed at age groups beyond the basal age to the basal age itself. This is done to calculate the language age equivalent and the problem-solving age equivalent. Each of these age equivalents is then divided by the child's chronologic age and multiplied by 100 to determine a developmental quotient (DQ). Again, a DQ less than 70% constitutes delay and warrants referral for evaluation to rule out MR or auditory/visual impairment. For example, a 6-month-old child who *can* orient to voice, laugh out loud, and orient toward bell laterally, but who *cannot* ah-goo or razz has a basal age (age where child accomplishes all tasks correctly) of 4 months. An additional 0.3 is added for the ability to orient toward bell laterally, as per the decimal number recorded in parentheses. Together, this gives an age-equivalent of 4.3. The DQ of this patient's linguistic and auditory skills is 4.3 (age equivalent) ÷ 6.0 (chronologic age) × 100 = 71.7.

*From Bravo AM: Development. *In* Siberry GK, Iannone R (eds): *The Harriet Lane Handbook: A Manual for Pediatric House Officers,* 15th ed. St Louis, Mosby, 2000.

TABLE 4-3 Clinical Linguistic and Auditory Milestone Scale (CLAMS)/Clinical Adaptive Test (CAT)

Age (mo)	CLAMS	Yes	No	CAT	Yes	No
1	1. Alert to sound (0.5)*	—	—	1. Visually fixates momentarily upon red ring (0.5)	—	—
	2. Soothes when picked up (0.5)	—	—	2. Chin off table in prone (0.5)	—	—
2	1. Social smile (1.0)*	—	—	1. Visually follows ring horizontally and vertically (0.5)	—	—
				2. Chest off table prone (0.5)	—	—
3	1. Cooing (1.0)	—	—	1. Visually follows ring in circle (0.3)	—	—
				2. Supports on forearms in prone (0.3)	—	—
				3. Visual threat (0.3)	—	—
4	1. Orients to voice (0.5)*	—	—	1. Unfisted (0.3)	—	—
	2. Laughs aloud (0.5)	—	—	2. Manipulates fingers (0.3)	—	—
				3. Supports on wrists in prone (0.3)	—	—
5	1. Orients toward bell laterally (0.3)*	—	—	1. Pulls down rings (0.3)	—	—
	2. Ah-goo (0.3)	—	—	2. Transfers (0.3)	—	—
	3. Razzing (0.3)	—	—	3. Regards pellet (0.3)	—	—
6	1. Babbling (1.0)	—	—	1. Obtains cube (0.3)	—	—
				2. Lifts cup (0.3)	—	—
				3. Radial rake (0.3)	—	—
7	1. Orients toward bell (1.0)* (upwardly/indirectly 90°)	—	—	1. Attempts pellet (0.3)	—	—
				2. Pulls out peg (0.3)	—	—
				3. Inspects ring (0.3)	—	—
8	1. "Dada" inappropriately (0.5)	—	—	1. Pulls out ring by string (0.3)	—	—
	2. "Mama" inappropriately (0.5)	—	—	2. Secures pellet (0.3)	—	—
				3. Inspects bell (0.3)	—	—
9	1. Orients toward bell (upward directly 180°) (0.5)*	—	—	1. Three finger scissor grasp (0.3)	—	—
	2. Gesture language (0.5)	—	—	2. Rings bell (0.3)	—	—
				3. Over the edge for toy (0.3)	—	—
10	1. Understands "no" (0.3)	—	—	1. Combine cube-cup (0.3)	—	—
	2. Uses "dada" appropriately (0.3)	—	—	2. Uncovers bell (0.3)	—	—
	3. Uses "mama" appropriately (0.3)	—	—	3. Fingers pegboard (0.3)	—	—
11	1. One word (other than "mama" and "dada") (1.0)	—	—	1. Mature overhand pincer movement (0.5)	—	—
				2. Solves cube under cup (0.5)	—	—
12	1. One-step command with gesture (0.5)	—	—	1. Releases one cube in cup (0.5)	—	—
	2. Two-word vocabulary (0.5)	—	—	2. Crayon mark (0.5)	—	—

Continued

TABLE 4-3 **Clinical Linguistic and Auditory Milestone Scale (CLAMS)/Clinical Adaptive Test (CAT)** *(Continued)*

Age (mo)	CLAMS	Yes	No	CAT	Yes	No
14	1. Three-word vocabulary (1.0)	—	—	1. Solves glass frustration (0.6)	—	—
	2. Immature jargoning (1.0)	—	—	2. Out-in with peg (0.6)	—	—
				3. Solves pellet-bottle with demonstration (0.6)	—	—
16	1. Four- to six-word vocabulary (1.0)	—	—	1. Solves pellet-bottle spontaneously (0.6)	—	—
	2. One-step command without gesture (1.0)	—	—	2. Round block on form board (0.6)	—	—
				3. Scribbles in imitation (0.6)	—	—
18	1. Mature jargoning (0.5)	—	—	1. Ten cubes in cup (0.5)	—	—
	2. Seven- to ten-word vocabulary (0.5)	—	—	2. Solves round hole in form board reversed (0.5)	—	—
	3. Points to one picture (0.5)*	—	—	3. Spontaneous scribbling with crayon (0.5)	—	—
	4. Body parts (0.5)	—	—	4. Pegboard completed spontaneously (0.5)	—	—
21	1. Twenty-word vocabulary (1.0)	—	—	1. Obtains object with stick (1.0)	—	—
	2. Two-word phrases (1.0)	—	—	2. Solves square in form board (1.0)	—	—
	3. Points to two pictures (1.0)*	—	—	3. Tower of three cubes (1.0)	—	—
24	1. Fifty-word vocabulary (1.0)	—	—	1. Attempts to fold paper (0.7)	—	—
	2. Two-step command (1.0)	—	—	2. Horizontal four cube train (0.7)	—	—
	3. Two word sentences (1.0)	—	—	3. Imitates stroke with pencil (0.7)	—	—
				4. Completes form board (0.7)	—	—
30	1. Uses pronouns appropriately (1.5)	—	—	1. Horizontal-vertical stroke with pencil (1.5)	—	—
	2. Concept of one (1.5)*	—	—	2. Form board reversed (1.5)	—	—
	3. Points to seven pictures (1.5)*	—	—	3. Folds paper with definite crease (1.5)	—	—
	4. Two digits forward (1.5)*	—	—	4. Train with chimney (1.5)	—	—
36	1. 250-word vocabulary (1.5)	—	—	1. Three cube bridge (1.5)	—	—
	2. Three-word sentence (1.5)	—	—	2. Draws circle (1.5)	—	—
	3. Three digits forward (1.5)*	—	—	3. Names one color (1.5)	—	—
	4. Follows two prepositional commands (1.5)*	—	—	4. Draw-a-person with head plus one other part of body (1.5)	—	—

From Bravo AM: Development. *In* Siberry GK, Iannone R (eds): *The Harriet Lane Handbook: A Manual for Pediatric House Officers,* 15th ed. St Louis, Mosby, 2000.

BLOCK SKILLS*

The structures should be demonstrated for the child. Figure 4-6 includes the developmental age at which each structure can usually be accomplished.

*From Siberry GK, Iannone R (eds): *The Harriet Lane Handbook: A Manual for Pediatric House Officers,* 15th ed. St Louis, Mosby, 2000.

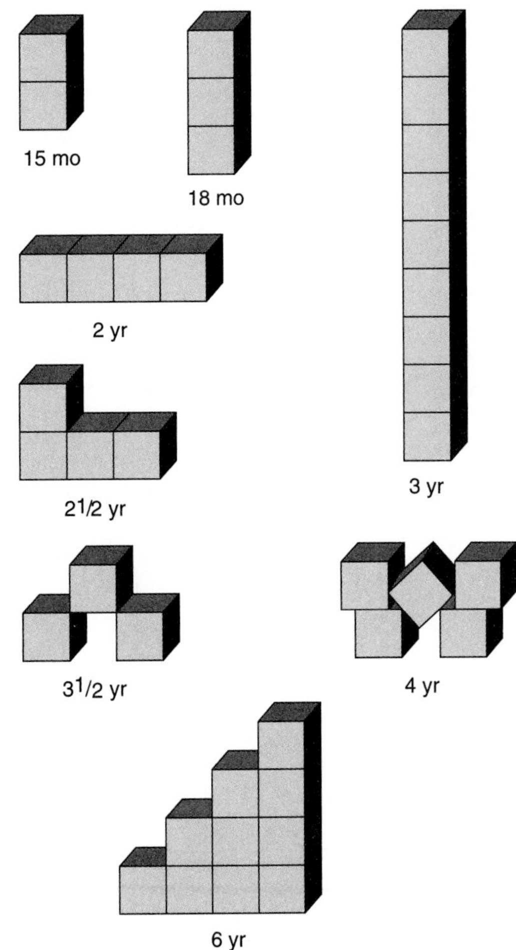

FIGURE 4-6 Block skills. (From Capute AJ, Accardo PJ: *The Pediatrician and the Developmentally Disabled Child: A Clinical Textbook on Mental Retardation.* Baltimore, University Press, 1979.)

GESELL FIGURES*

One should note that the examiner is not supposed to demonstrate the drawing of the figures (Fig. 4-7) for the patient; however, most developmentalists do demonstrate and do not feel that it makes a difference.

*From Siberry GK, Iannone R (eds): *The Harriet Lane Handbook: A Manual for Pediatric House Officers,* 15th ed. St Louis, Mosby, 2000.

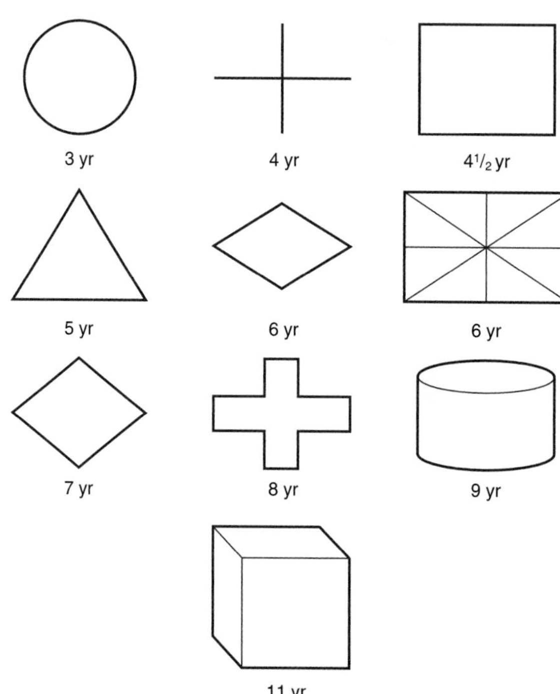

FIGURE 4-7 Gesell figures. (From Illingsworth RS: *The Development of the Infant and Young Child, Normal and Abnormal,* 5th ed. Baltimore, Williams & Wilkins, 1972; and Cattel P: *The Measurement of Intelligence of Infants and Young Children.* New York, The Psychological Corporation, 1960.)

GOODENOUGH-HARRIS DRAW-A-PERSON TEST*

- **Procedure:** Give the child a pencil (preferably a no. 2 with eraser) and a sheet of blank paper. Instruct the child to "Draw a person; draw the best person you can." Supply encouragement if needed (i.e., "Draw a whole person."); however, do not suggest specific supplementation or changes.
- **Scoring:** Ask the child to describe or explain the drawing to you. Give the child one point for each detail present using the guide in Table 4-4. (Maximum score = 51.)
- Age norms; see Table 4-5.

*From Straub DM: Adolescent medicine. *In* Siberry GK, Iannone R (eds): *The Harriet Lane Handbook: A Manual for Pediatric House Officers,* 15th ed. St Louis, Mosby, 2000.

TABLE 4-4 Goodenough-Harris Scoring

General:	☐ Head present	**Joints:**	☐ Elbow, shoulder, or both
	☐ Legs present		☐ Knee, hip, or both
	☐ Arms present	**Proportion:**	☐ Head: 10% to 50% of trunk area
Trunk:	☐ Present		☐ Arms: Approx. same length as trunk
	☐ Length greater than breadth		☐ Legs: 1-2 times trunk length; width less than trunk width
	☐ Shoulders		☐ Feet: 10% to 30% of leg length
Arms/legs:	☐ Attached to trunk		☐ Arms and legs in two dimensions
	☐ At correct point		☐ Heel
Neck:	☐ Present	**Motor coordination:**	☐ Lines firm and well connected
	☐ Outline of neck continuous with head, trunk, or both		☐ Firmly drawn with correct joining
Face:	☐ Eyes		☐ Head outline
	☐ Nose		☐ Trunk outline
	☐ Mouth		☐ Outline of arms and legs
	☐ Nose and mouth in two dimensions	**Ears:**	☐ Features
	☐ Nostrils		☐ Present
Hair:	☐ Present	**Eye detail:**	☐ Correct position and proportion
	☐ On more than circumference; nontransparent		☐ Brow or lashes
Clothing:	☐ Present		☐ Pupil
	☐ Two articles; nontransparent		☐ Proportion
	☐ Entire drawing nontransparent (sleeves and trousers)	**Chin:**	☐ Glance directed front in profile drawing
			☐ Present; forehead
	☐ Four articles	**Profile:**	☐ Projection
	☐ Costume complete		☐ Not more than one error
Fingers:	☐ Present		☐ Correct
	☐ Correct number		
	☐ Two dimension; length, breadth		
	☐ Thumb opposition		
	☐ Hand distinct from fingers and arm		

From Bravo AM: Development. *In* Siberry GK, Iannone R (eds): *The Harriet Lane Handbook: A Manual for Pediatric House Officers,* 15th ed. St Louis, Mosby, 2000.

TABLE 4-5 Goodenough Age Norms

Age (yr)	3	4	5	6	7	8	9	10	11	12	13
Points	2	6	10	14	18	22	26	30	34	38	42

From Taylor E: *Psychological Appraisal of Children with Cerebral Defects.* Boston, Harvard University, 1961. Adapted from Goodenough FL: *Measurement of Intelligence by Drawings.* Chicago, World Book Co, 1926.

EARLY ADOLESCENCE THROUGH YOUNG ADULTS

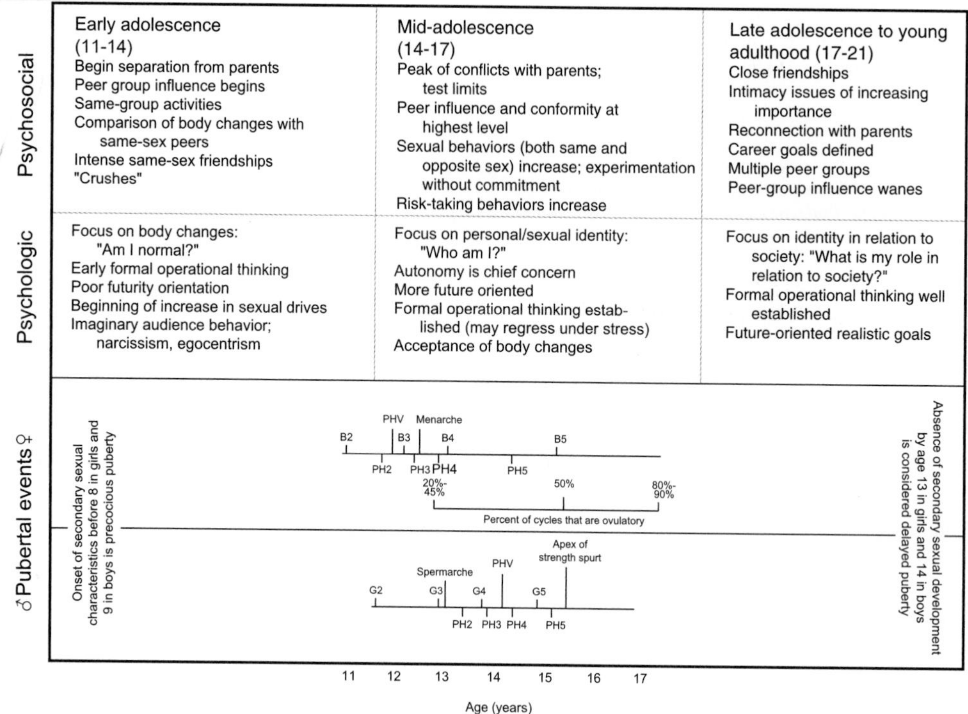

FIGURE 4-8 Pubertal events and Tanner stages. *B,* Breast (stage); *G,* genital (stage); *PH,* pubic hair (stage); *PHV,* peak height velocity. (Modified from Joffe A: Adolescent medicine. *In* Oski FA et al [eds]: *Principles and Practice of Pediatrics.* Philadelphia, JB Lippincott, 1994.)

BREAST DEVELOPMENT IN FEMALES

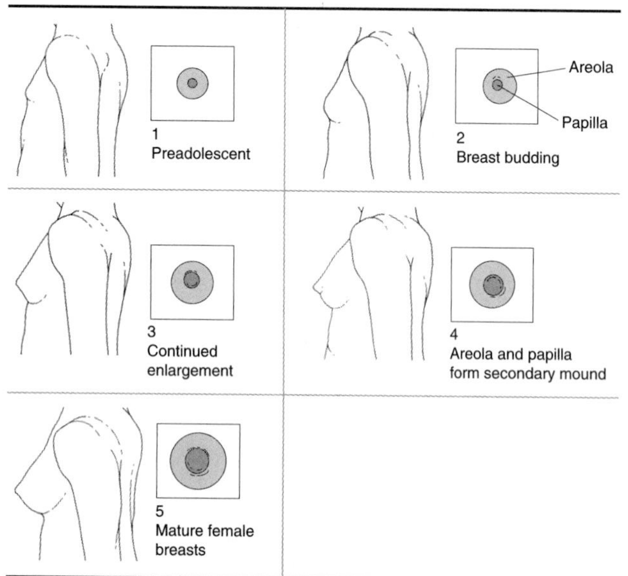

FIGURE 4-9 Tanner stages of breast development in females. (Modified from Johnson TR et al: *Children Are Different: Development Physiology,* 2nd ed. Columbus, Ohio, Ross Laboratories, Division of Abbott Laboratories, 1979. *In* Straub DM: Adolescent medicine. *In* Siberry GK, Iannone R [eds]: *The Harriet Lane Handbook: A Manual for Pediatric House Officers,* 15th ed. St Louis, Mosby, 2000.)

TABLE 4-6 Breast Development

Stage	Comment (mean age ± standard deviation)
I	Preadolescent; elevation of papilla only
II	Breast bud; elevation of breast and papilla as small mound; enlargement of areola diameter (11.15 ± 1.10)
III	Further enlargement and elevation of breast and areola; no separation of their contours (12.15 ± 1.09)
IV	Projection of areola and papilla to form secondary mound above level of breast (13.11 ± 1.15)
V	Mature stage; projection of papilla only as a result of recession of areola to general contour of breast (15.3 ± 1.74)

Modified from Marshall WA, Tanner JM: *Arch Dis Child* 44:291, 1969; and Marshall WA, Tanner JM: *Arch Dis Child* 45:13, 1970. *In* Oski FA (ed): *Principles and Practice of Pediatrics.* Philadelphia, JB Lippincott, 1994.

TABLE 4-7 Pubic Hair (Male and Female)

Stage	Comment (mean age ± standard deviation)
I	Preadolescent; vellus over pubes no further developed than that over abdominal wall (i.e., no pubic hair)
II	Sparse growth of long, slightly pigmented downy hair, straight or only slightly curled, chiefly at base of penis or along labia (male: 13.44 ± 1.09; female: 11.69 ± 1.21)
III	Considerably darker, coarser, and more curled; hair spreads sparsely over junction of pubes (male: 13.9 ± 1.04; female: 12.36 ± 1.10)
IV	Hair resembles adult in type; distribution still considerably less than in adult; no spread to medial surface of thighs (male: 14.36 ± 1.08; female: 12.95 ± 1.06)
V	Adult in quantity and type with distribution of the horizontal pattern (male: 15.18 ± 1.07; female: 14.41 ± 1.12)
VI	Spread up linea alba: "male escutcheon"

Modified from Marshall WA, Tanner JM: *Arch Dis Child* 44:291, 1969; and Marshall WA, Tanner JM: *Arch Dis Child* 45:13, 1970. *In* Oski FA (ed): *Principles and Practice of Pediatrics*. Philadelphia, JB Lippincott, 1994.

PUBIC HAIR DEVELOPMENT IN FEMALES

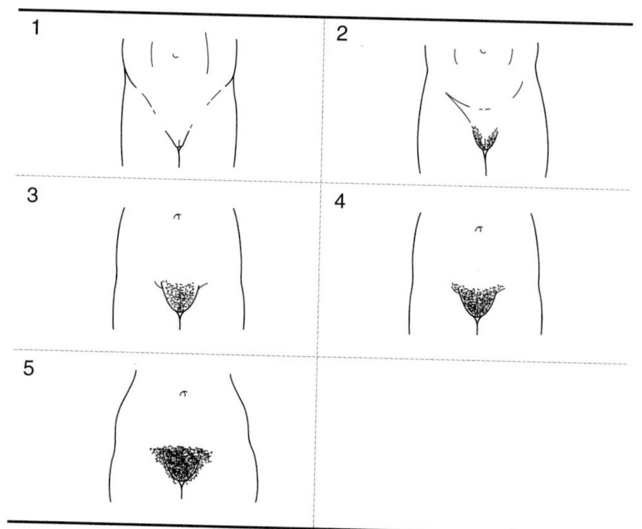

FIGURE 4-10 Tanner stages of pubic hair development in females. (Modified from Neinstein LS: *Adolescent Health Care: A Practical Guide*, 2nd ed. Baltimore, Urban & Schwarzenberg, 1991. *In* Straub DM: Adolescent medicine. *In* Siberry GK, Iannone R [eds]: *The Harriet Lane Handbook: A Manual for Pediatric House Officers*, 15th ed. St Louis, Mosby, 2000.)

PUBLIC HAIR & GENITAL DEVELOPMENT IN MALES

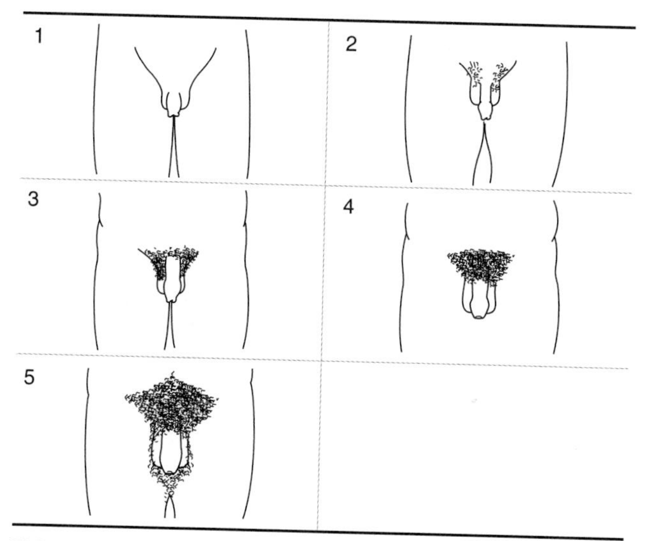

FIGURE 4-11 Pubic hair and genital development in males. (Modified from Neinstein LS: *Adolescent Health Care: A Practical Guide*, 2nd ed. Baltimore, Urban & Schwarzenberg, 1991. *In* Straub DM: Adolescent medicine. *In* Siberry GK, Iannone R [eds]: *The Harriet Lane Handbook: A Manual for Pediatric House Officers*, 15th ed. St Louis, Mosby, 2000.)

TABLE 4-8 Genital Development (Male)

Stage	Comment (mean age ± standard deviation)
I	Preadolescent; testes, scrotum, and penis about same size and proportion as in early childhood
II	Enlargement of scrotum and testes; skin of scrotum reddens and changes in texture; little or no enlargement of penis (11.64 ± 1.07)
III	Enlargement of penis, first mainly in length; further growth of testes and scrotum (12.85 ± 1.04)
IV	Increased size of penis with growth in breadth and development of glans; further enlargement of testes and scrotum and increased darkening of scrotal skin (13.77 ± 1.02)
V	Genitalia adult in size and shape (14.92 ± 1.10)

Modified from Marshall WA, Tanner JM: *Arch Dis Child* 44:291, 1969; and Marshall WA, Tanner JM: *Arch Dis Child* 45:13, 1970. *In* Oski FA (ed): *Principles and Practice of Pediatrics*. Philadelphia, JB Lippincott, 1994.

TABLE 4-9 Chronology of Human Dentition of Primary or Deciduous and Secondary or Permanent Teeth

	AGE AT ERUPTION		AGE AT SHEDDING	
	Maxillary	Mandibular	Maxillary	Mandibular
Primary Teeth				
Central incisors	6–8 mo	5–7 mo	7–8 yr	6–7 yr
Lateral incisors	8–11 mo	7–10 mo	8–9 yr	7–8 yr
Cuspids (canines)	16–20 mo	16–20 mo	11–12 yr	9–11 yr
First molars	10–16 mo	10–16 mo	10–11 yr	10–12 yr
Second molars	20–30 mo	20–30 mo	10–12 yr	11–13 yr
Secondary Teeth				
Central incisors	7–8 yr	6–7 yr		
Lateral incisors	8–9 yr	7–8 yr		
Cuspids (canines)	11–12 yr	9–11 yr		
First premolars (bicuspids)	10–11 yr	10–12 yr		
Second premolars (bicuspids)	10–12 yr	11–13 yr		
First molars	6–7 yr	6–7 yr		
Second molars	12–13 yr	12–13 yr		
Third molars	17–22 yr	17–22 yr		

From Behrman RE et al: *Nelson Textbook of Pediatrics*, 15th ed. Philadelphia, WB Saunders, 1996.

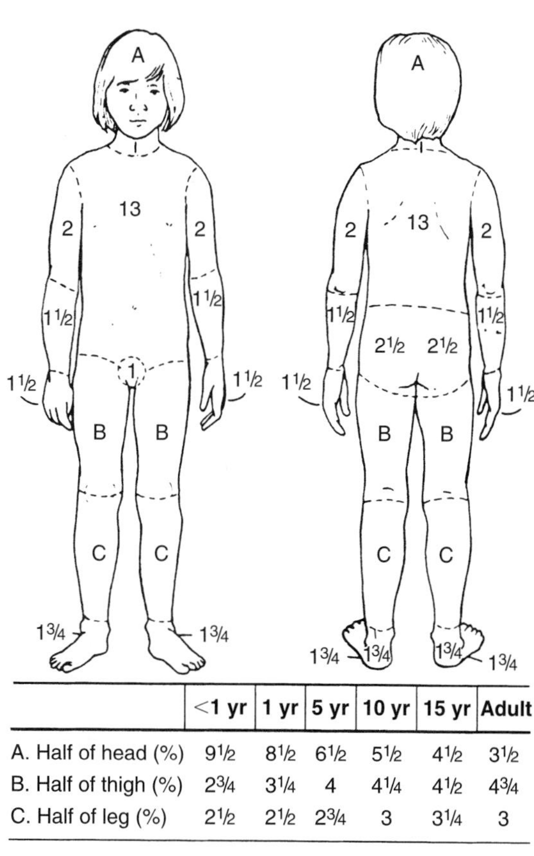

	<1 yr	1 yr	5 yr	10 yr	15 yr	Adult
A. Half of head (%)	9½	8½	6½	5½	4½	3½
B. Half of thigh (%)	2¾	3¼	4	4¼	4½	4¾
C. Half of leg (%)	2½	2½	2¾	3	3¼	3

FIGURE 4-12 Burn assessment chart. (From Barkin RM, Rosen P: *Emergency Pediatrics,* 5th ed. St Louis, Mosby, 1999.)

TABLE 4-10 **Glasgow Coma Scale**

	Adults and Children	Toddlers and Infants
Eyes opening score		
4	spontaneously	spontaneously
3	to verbal command	to shout
2	to pain	to pain
1	no response	no response
Motor response score		
6	obeys	spontaneous movement
5	localizes pain	localizes pain
4	flexion withdrawal	flexion withdrawal
3	decorticate	decorticate
2	decerebrate	decerebrate
1	no response	no response
Verbal response score		
5	oriented/appropriate words	smiles/coos appropriately
4	disoriented/inappropriate words	cries and consolable
3	inappropriate words/persistent cries	cries and inconsolable
2	incomprehensible sounds/grunts	grunts/moans
1	no response	no response

BOX 4-1 Commonly Used Formulas

- Alveolar-arterial oxygen gradient (Aa gradient)

$$\text{Aa gradient} = \left[(713)(FIO_2) - \left(\frac{PaCO_2}{0.8}\right)\right] - PaO_2$$

Normal Aa gradient = 5-15 mm
FIO_2 = Fraction of inspired oxygen (normal = 0.21-1.0)
$PaCO_2$ = Arterial carbon dioxide tension (normal = 35-45 mm Hg)
PaO_2 = Arterial partial pressure oxygen (normal = 70-100 mm Hg)
Differential diagnosis of Aa gradient:

ABNORMALITY	15% O_2	100% O_2
Diffusion defect	Increased gradient	Correction of gradient
Ventilation/perfusion mismatch	Increased gradient	Partial or complete correction of gradient
Right-to-left shunt (intracardiac or pulmonary)	Increased gradient	Increased gradient (no correction)

- Anion gap (AG)

$$AG = Na^+ - (Cl^- + HCO_3^-)$$

- Creatinine clearance (CCr)

$$CCr = \frac{UV}{P} \times \frac{1.73}{S.A} = \text{ml/min/1.73 m}^2$$

U (mg/dl) = Urine creatinine concentration
V (ml/min) = Total urine volume ÷ length of collection time
P (mg/dl) = Serum creatinine
S.A. (m^2) = Surface area

- Serum osmolality

$$Osm = 2(Na^+ + K^+) + \frac{\text{Glucose}}{18} + \frac{\text{BUN}}{2.8}$$

- Sodium correction in hyperglycemic patients

$$\text{Corrected } Na^+ = \text{Measured } Na^+ + 1.6 \times \frac{\text{Glucose} - 140}{100}$$

- Fractional excretion of sodium

$$FE_{Na} = \frac{U_{Na}/P_{Na}}{U_{Cr}/P_{Cr}} \times 100$$

- Water deficit in hypernatremic patients

$$\text{Water deficit (in liters)} = 0.6 \times \text{Body weight (kg)} \times \left(\frac{\text{Measured serum sodium}}{\text{Normal serum sodium}} - 1\right)$$

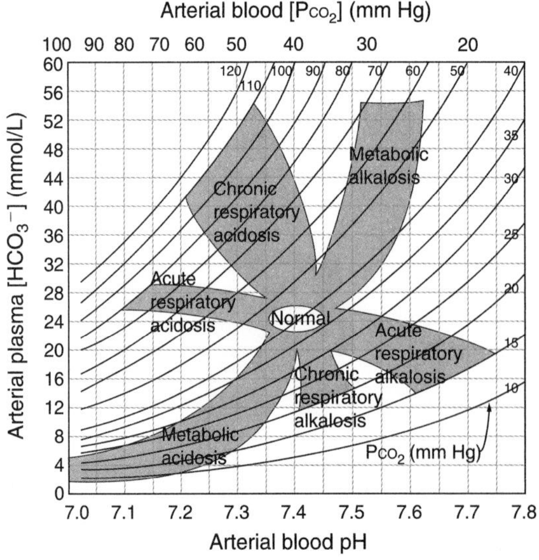

FIGURE 4-13 Acid-base nomogram. (Modified from Brenner BN, Floyd CR Jr [eds]: *The kidney,* vol 1. Philadelphia, WB Saunders, 1991. *In* Siberry GK, Iannone R [eds]: *The Harriet Lane Handbook: A Manual for Pediatric House Officers,* 15th ed. St Louis, Mosby, 2000.)

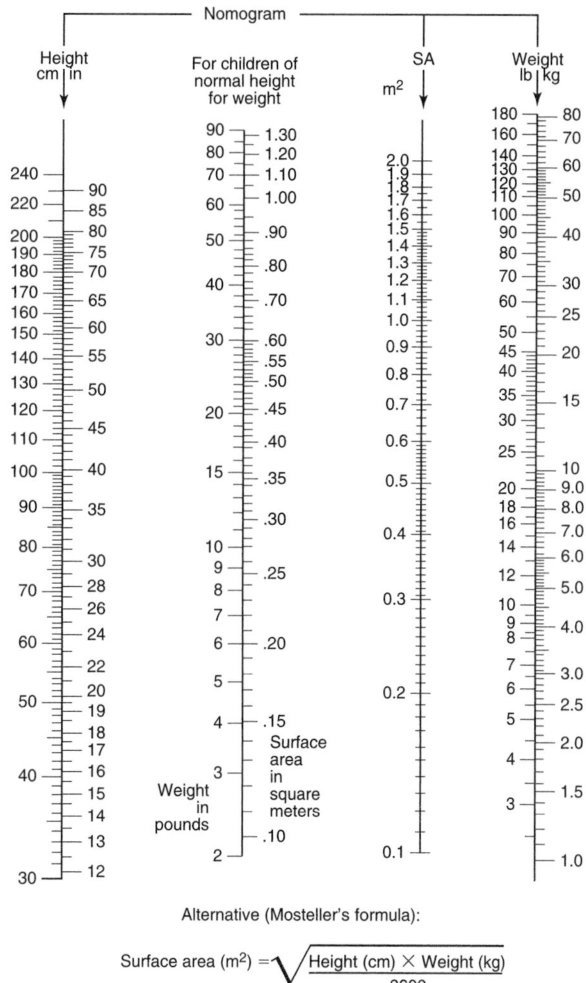

$$\text{Surface area } (m^2) = \sqrt{\frac{\text{Height (cm)} \times \text{Weight (kg)}}{3600}}$$

FIGURE 4-14 Body surface area nomogram and equation. (Data from Briars GL, Bailey BJ: *Arch Dis Child* 70:246, 1994; *In* Siberry GK, Iannone R [eds]: *The Harriet Lane Handbook: A Manual for Pediatric House Officers,* 15th ed. St Louis, Mosby, 2000.)

TABLE 4-11 Glomerular Filtration Rates (GFR) by Age

NORMAL VALUES OF GFR		
Age	**GFR (Mean) (mL/min/1.73m^2)**	**Range (mL/min/1.73m^2)**
Neonates <34 wk gestational age		
2-8 days	11	11-15
4-28 days	20	15-28
30-90 days	50	40-65
Neonates >34 wk gestational age		
2-8 days	39	17-60
4-28 days	47	26-68
30-90 days	58	30-86
1-6 mo	7	39-114
6-12 mo	103	49-157
12-19 mo	127	62-191
2 yr-adult	127	89-165

From Holliday MA et al: Pediatric nephrology. Baltimore: Williams & Wilkins; 1994.
From Renal function tests. *In* Gunn VL, Nechyba C (eds): *The Harriet Lane Handbook: A Manual for Pediatric House Officers,* 16th ed. Philadelphia, Mosby, 2002.

TABLE 4-12 Average Peak Expiratory Flow Rates for Normal Children

Height (in)	PEFR (L/min)
43	147
44	160
45	173
46	187
47	200
48	214
49	227
50	240
51	254
52	267
53	280
54	293
55	307
56	320
57	334
58	347
59	360
60	373
61	387
62	400
63	413
64	427
65	440
66	454
67	467

From Voter KZ: *Pediatr Rev* 17(2):53–63, 1996; and Renal Function Tests. *In* Gunn VL, Nechyba C (eds): *The Harriet Lane Handbook: A Manual for Pediatric House Officers,* 16th ed. Philadelphia, Mosby, 2002.

WEIGHT-FOR-AGE PERCENTILES

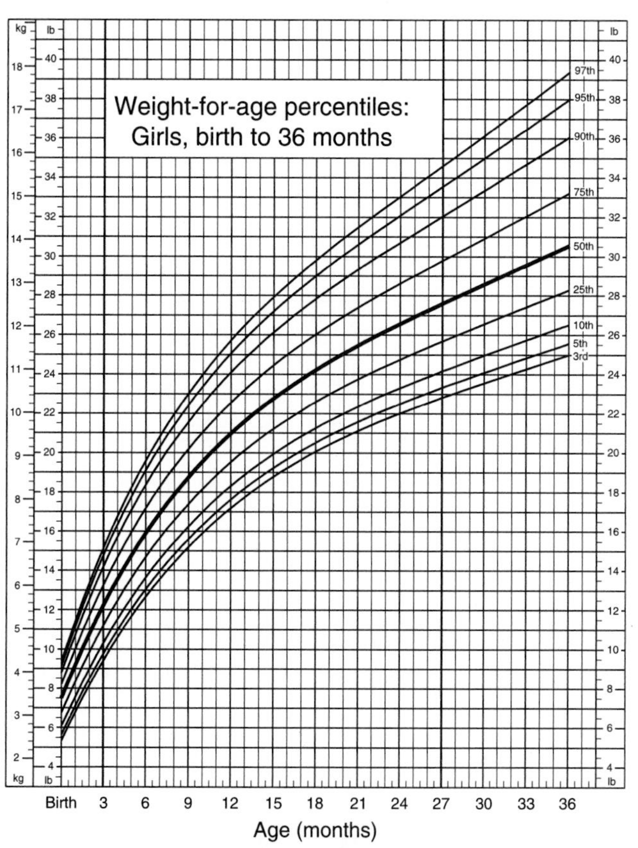

FIGURE 4-15 Weight-for-age percentiles, girls, birth to 36 months, CDC growth charts: United States. (Developed by the National Center for Health Statistics in collaboration with the National Center for Chronic Disease Prevention and Health Promotion, 2000.)

LENGTH-FOR-AGE PERCENTILES

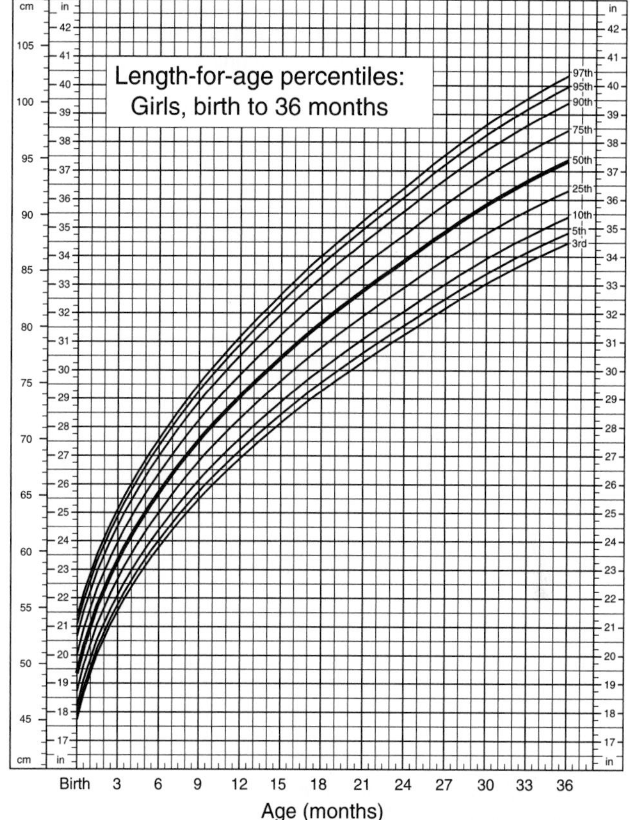

FIGURE 4-16 Length-for-age percentiles, girls, birth to 36 months, CDC growth charts: United States. (Developed by the National Center for Health Statistics in collaboration with the National Center for Chronic Disease Prevention and Health Promotion, 2000.)

HEAD CIRCUMFERENCE-FOR-AGE PERCENTILES

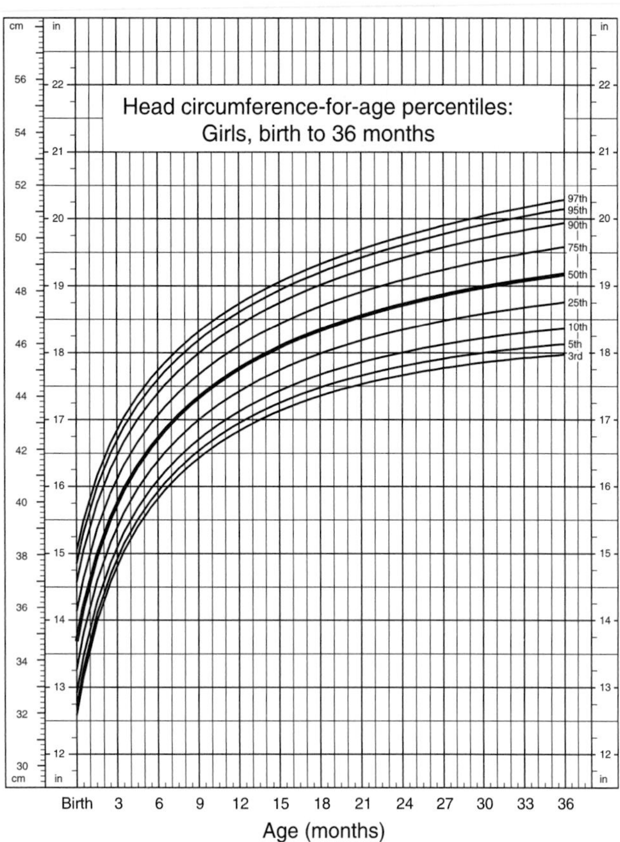

FIGURE 4-17 Head circumference-for-age percentiles, girls, birth to 36 months, CDC growth charts: United States. (Developed by the National Center for Health Statistics in collaboration with the National Center for Chronic Disease Prevention and Health Promotion, 2000.)

WEIGHT-FOR-LENGTH PERCENTILES

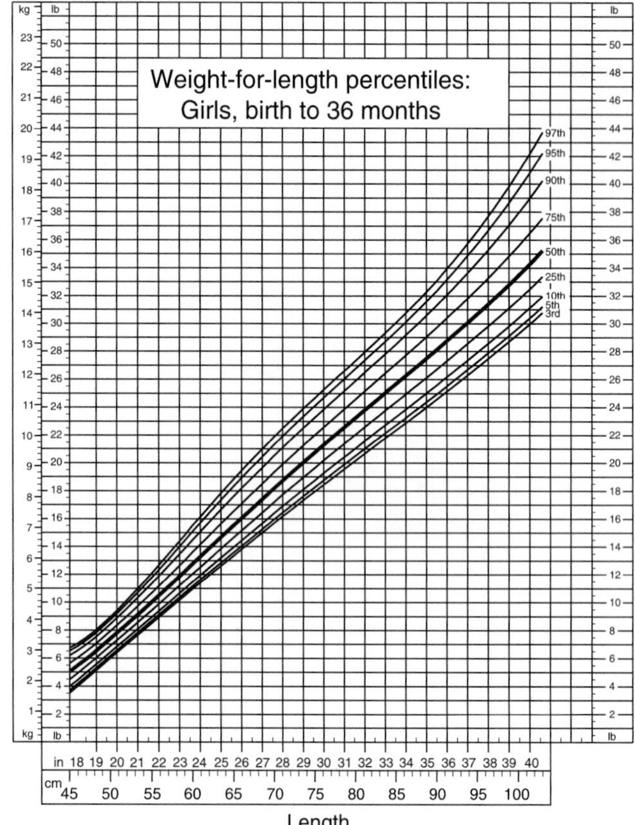

FIGURE 4-18 Weight-for-length percentiles, girls, birth to 36 months, CDC growth charts: United States. (Developed by the National Center for Health Statistics in collaboration with the National Center for Chronic Disease Prevention and Health Promotion, 2000.)

WEIGHT-FOR-AGE PERCENTILES

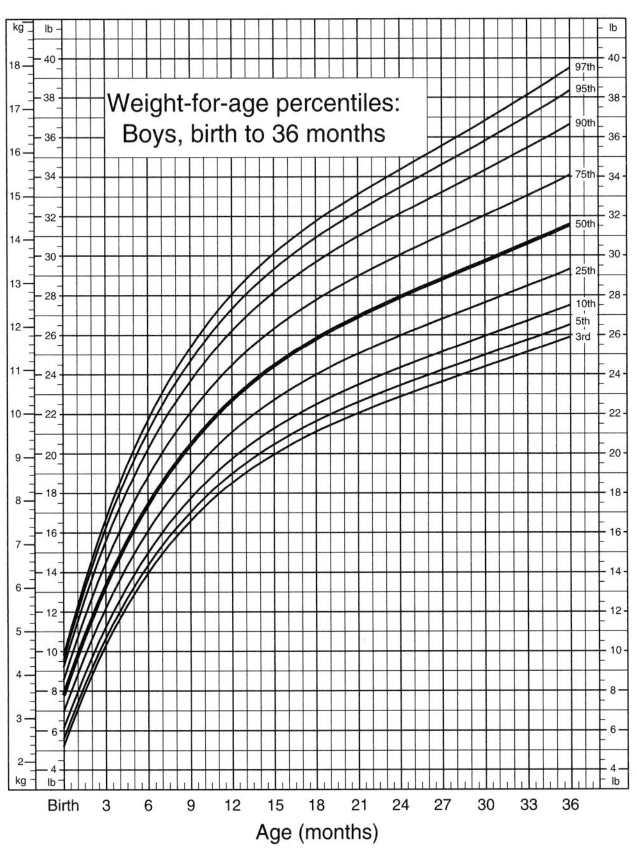

FIGURE 4-19 Weight-for-age percentiles, boys, birth to 36 months, CDC growth charts: United States. (Developed by the National Center for Health Statistics in collaboration with the National Center for Chronic Disease Prevention and Health Promotion, 2000.)

LENGTH-FOR-AGE PERCENTILES

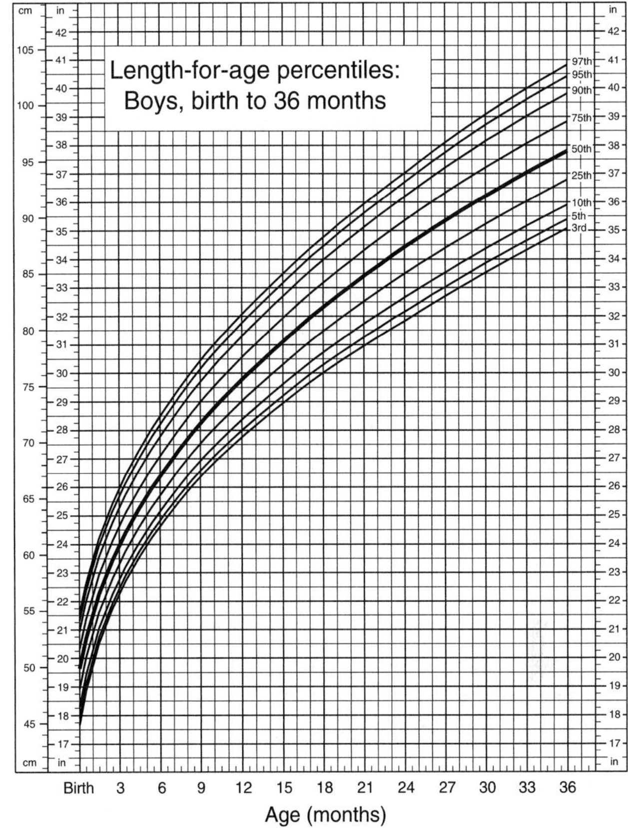

FIGURE 4-20 Length-for-age percentiles, boys, birth to 36 months, CDC growth charts: United States. (Developed by the National Center for Health Statistics in collaboration with the National Center for Chronic Disease Prevention and Health Promotion, 2000.)

HEAD CIRCUMFERENCE-FOR-AGE PERCENTILES

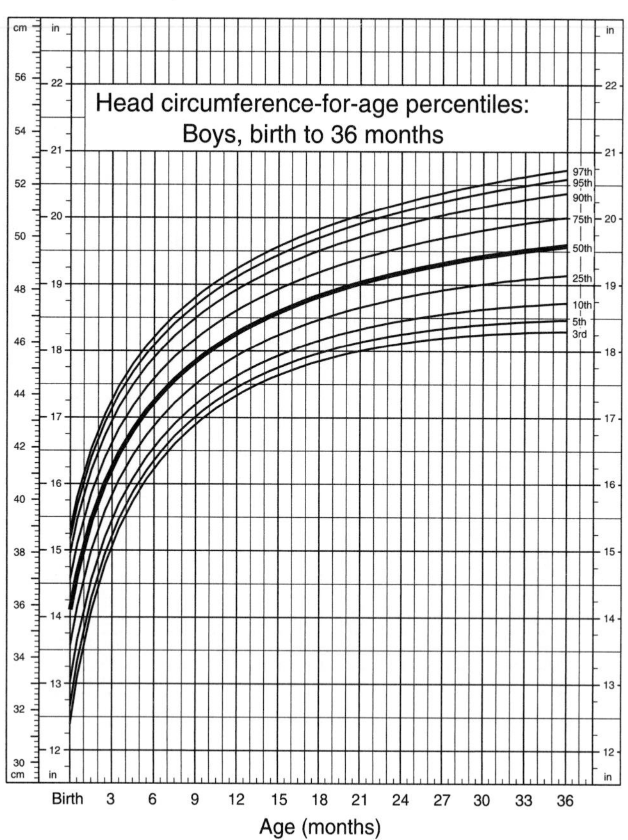

FIGURE 4-21 Head circumference-for-age percentiles, boys, birth to 36 months, CDC growth charts: United States. (Developed by the National Center for Health Statistics in collaboration with the National Center for Chronic Disease Prevention and Health Promotion, 2000.)

WEIGHT-FOR-LENGTH PERCENTILES

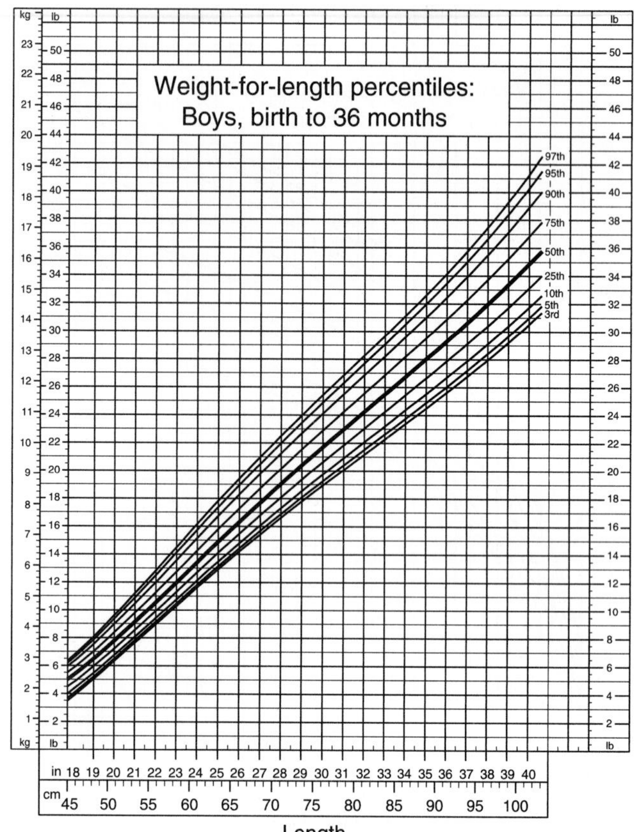

FIGURE 4-22 Weight-for-length percentiles, boys, birth to 36 months, CDC growth charts: United States. (Developed by the National Center for Health Statistics in collaboration with the National Center for Chronic Disease Prevention and Health Promotion, 2000.)

WEIGHT-FOR-AGE PERCENTILES

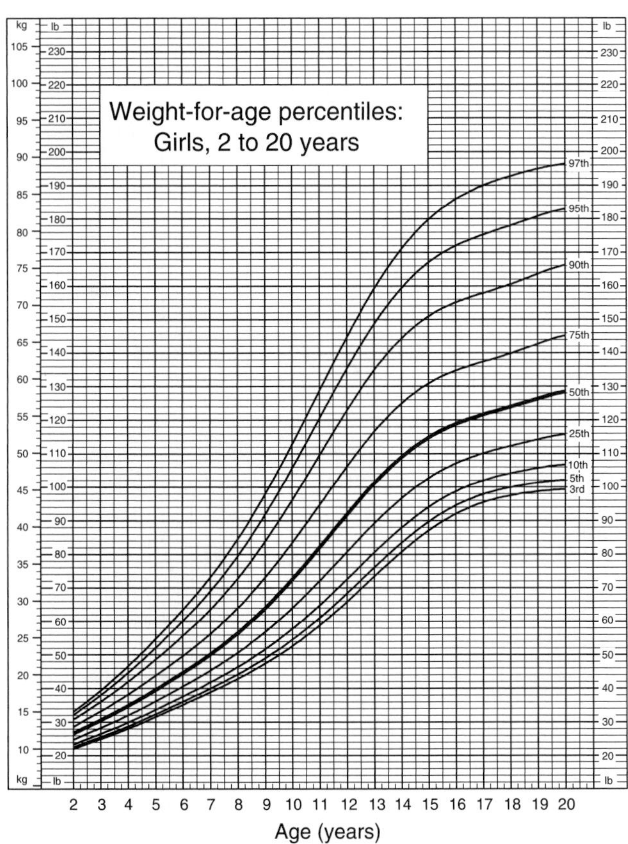

FIGURE 4-23 Weight-for-age percentiles, girls, 2 to 20 years, CDC growth charts: United States. (Developed by the National Center for Health Statistics in collaboration with the National Center for Chronic Disease Prevention and Health Promotion, 2000.)

STATURE-FOR-AGE PERCENTILES

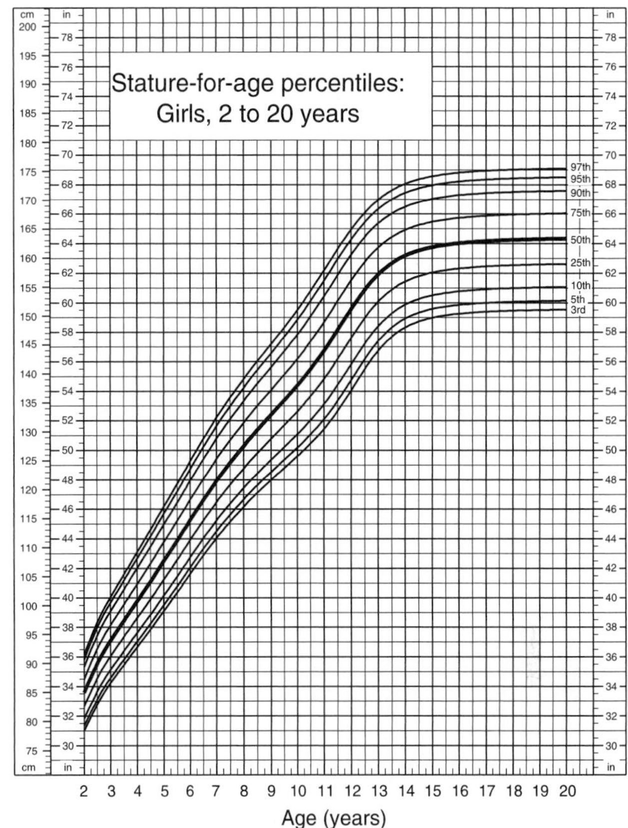

FIGURE 4-24 Stature-for-age percentiles, girls, 2 to 20 years, CDC growth charts: United States. (Developed by the National Center for Health Statistics in collaboration with the National Center for Chronic Disease Prevention and Health Promotion, 2000.)

WEIGHT-FOR-STATURE PERCENTILES

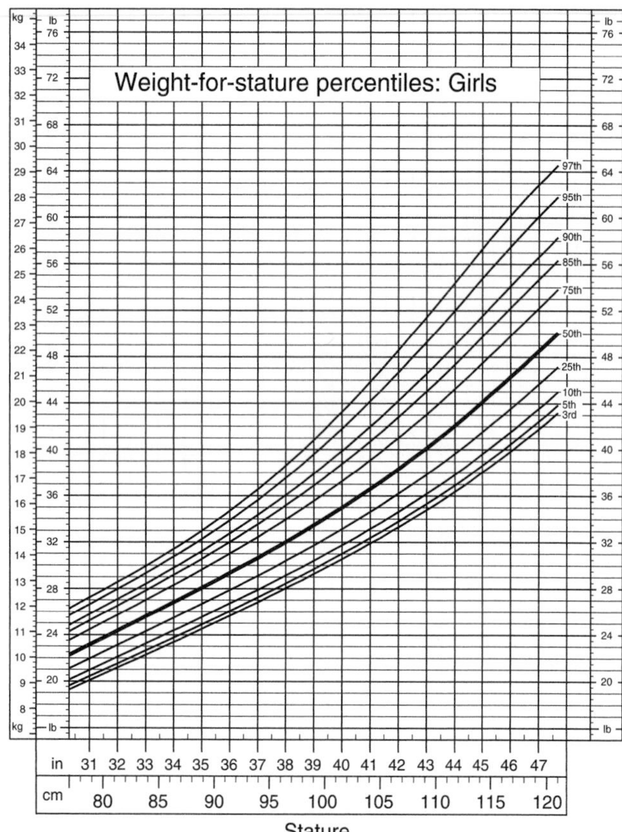

FIGURE 4-25 Weight-for-stature percentiles, girls, CDC growth charts: United States. (Developed by the National Center for Health Statistics in collaboration with the National Center for Chronic Disease Prevention and Health Promotion, 2000.)

BODY MASS INDEX-FOR-AGE PERCENTILES

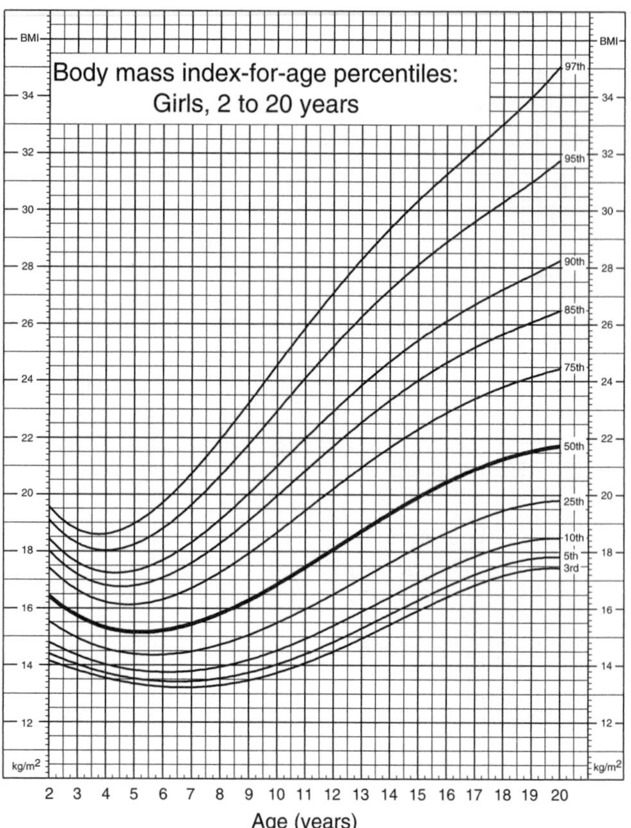

FIGURE 4-26 Body mass index-for-age percentiles, girls, 2 to 20 years, CDC growth charts: United States. (Developed by the National Center for Health Statistics in collaboration with the National Center for Chronic Disease Prevention and Health Promotion, 2000.)

WEIGHT-FOR-AGE PERCENTILES

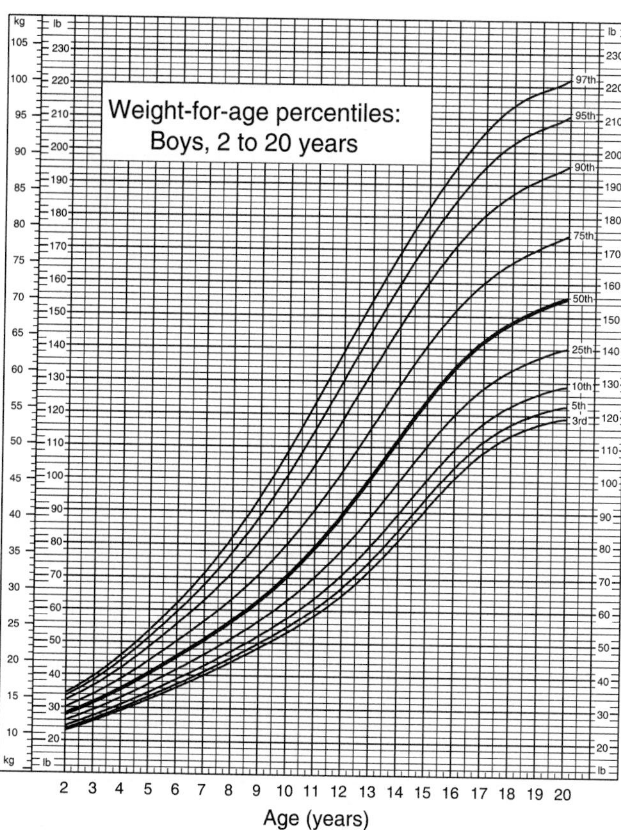

FIGURE 4-27 Weight-for-age percentiles, boys, 2 to 20 years, CDC growth charts: United States. (Developed by the National Center for Health Statistics in collaboration with the National Center for Chronic Disease Prevention and Health Promotion, 2000.)

STATURE-FOR-AGE PERCENTILES

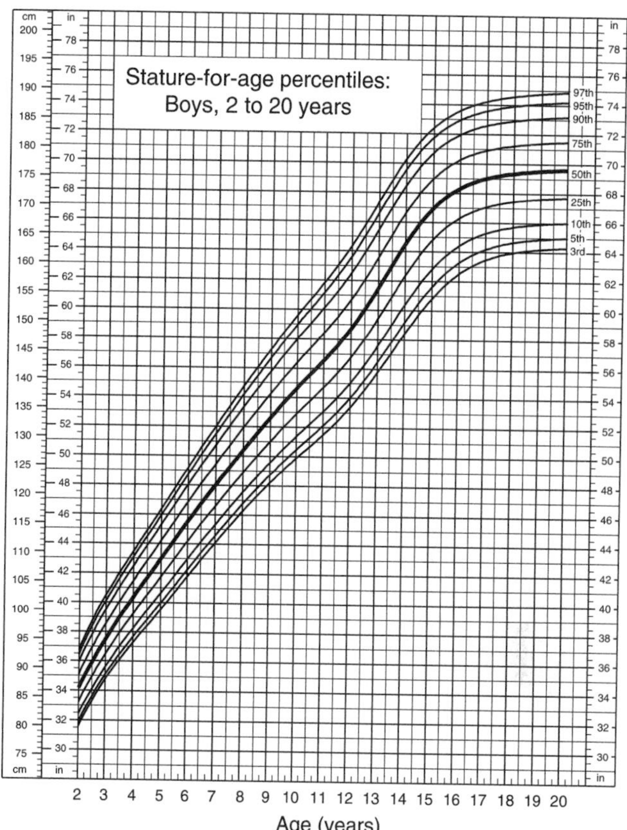

FIGURE 4-28 Stature-for-age percentiles, boys, 2 to 20 years, CDC growth charts: United States. (Developed by the National Center for Health Statistics in collaboration with the National Center for Chronic Disease Prevention and Health Promotion, 2000.)

WEIGHT-FOR-STATURE PERCENTILES

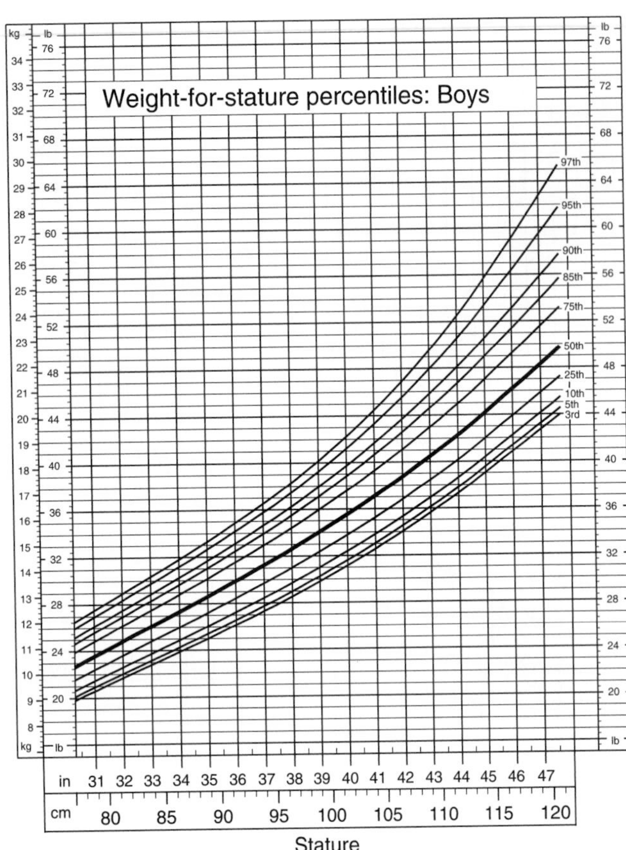

FIGURE 4-29 Weight-for-stature percentiles, boys, CDC growth charts: United States. (Developed by the National Center for Health Statistics in collaboration with the National Center for Chronic Disease Prevention and Health Promotion, 2000.)

BODY MASS INDEX-FOR-AGE PERCENTILES

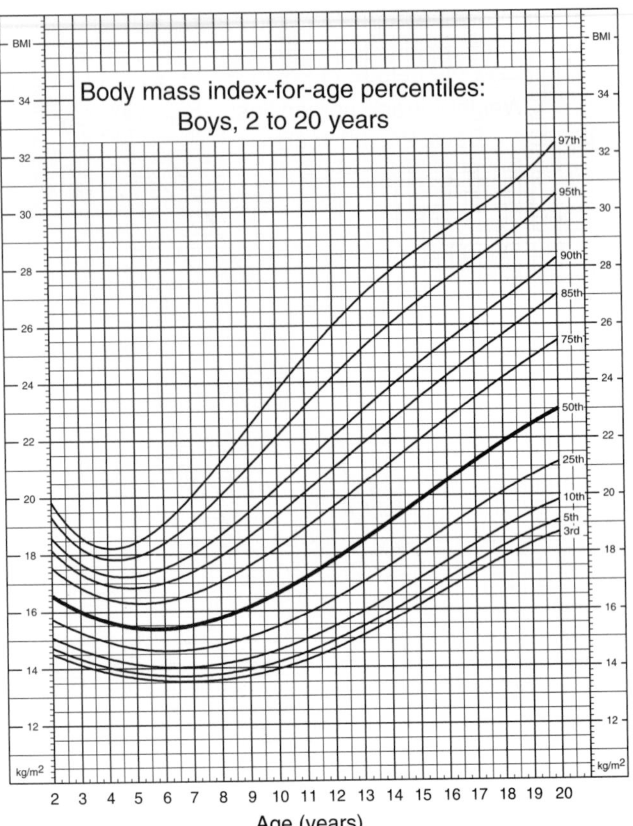

FIGURE 4-30 Body mass index-for-age percentiles, boys, 2 to 20 years, CDC growth charts: United States. (Developed by the National Center for Health Statistics in collaboration with the National Center for Chronic Disease Prevention and Health Promotion, 2000.)

HEAD CIRCUMFERENCE

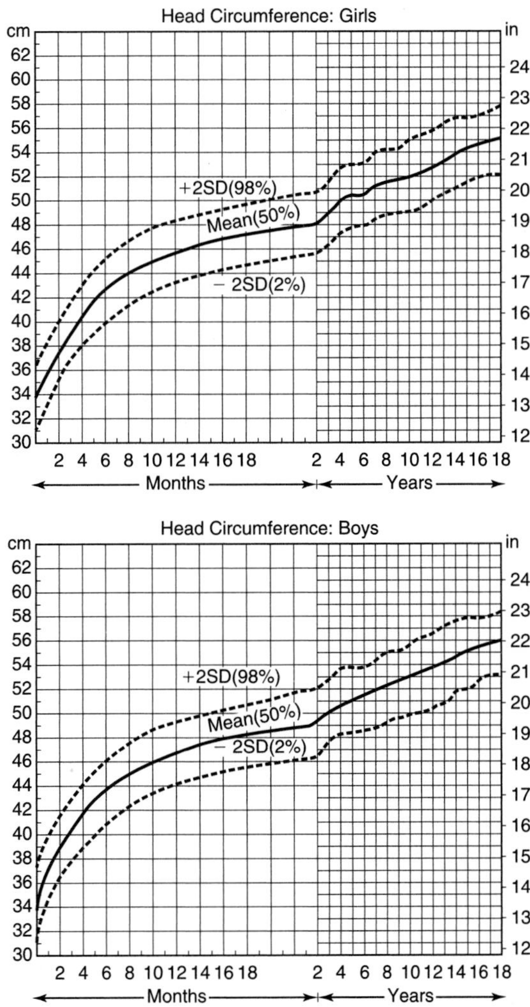

FIGURE 4-31 Head circumference for boys and girls, 2 to 18 years. (Modified from Niehaus G: *J Pediatr* 41:106, 1968. *In* Siberry GK, Iannone R [eds]: *The Harriet Lane Handbook: A Manual for Pediatric House Officers,* 15th ed. St Louis, Mosby, 2000.)

Height Velocity Curves

GIRLS 2 TO 18 YEARS

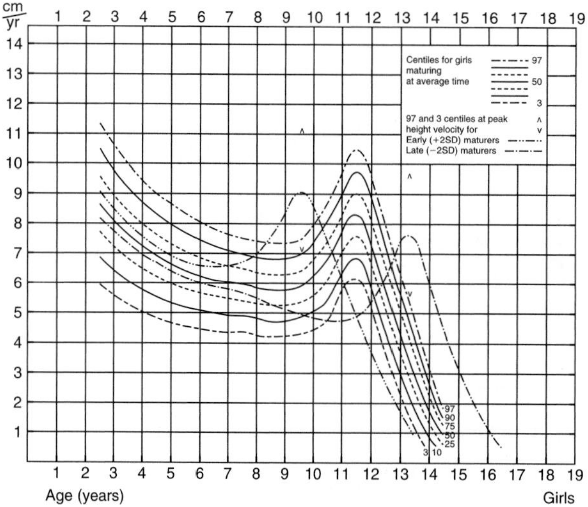

FIGURE 4-32 Height velocity for girls 2 to 18 years. (Modified from Tanner JM, Davis PS: *J Pediatr* 107:317, 1985. Courtesy Castlemead Publications, 1985. Distributed by Sereno Laboratories. *In* Siberry GK, Iannone R [eds]: *The Harriet Lane Handbook: A Manual for Pediatric House Officers,* 15th ed. St Louis, Mosby, 2000.)

BOYS 2 TO 18 YEARS

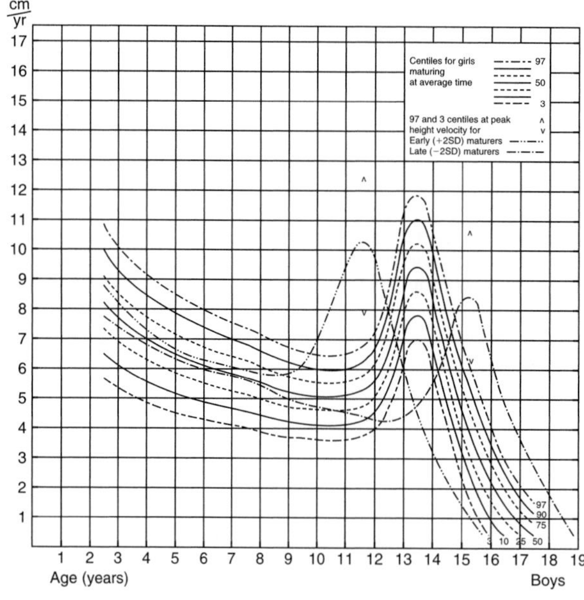

FIGURE 4-33 Height velocity for boys 2 to 18 years. (Modified from Tanner JM, Davis PS: *J Pediatr* 107:317, 1985. Courtesy Castlemead Publications, 1985. Distributed by Sereno Laboratories. *In* Siberry GK, Iannone R [eds]: *The Harriet Lane Handbook: A Manual for Pediatric House Officers,* 15th ed. St Louis, Mosby, 2000.)

LENGTH, WEIGHT, & HEAD CIRCUMFERENCE—PRETERM INFANTS

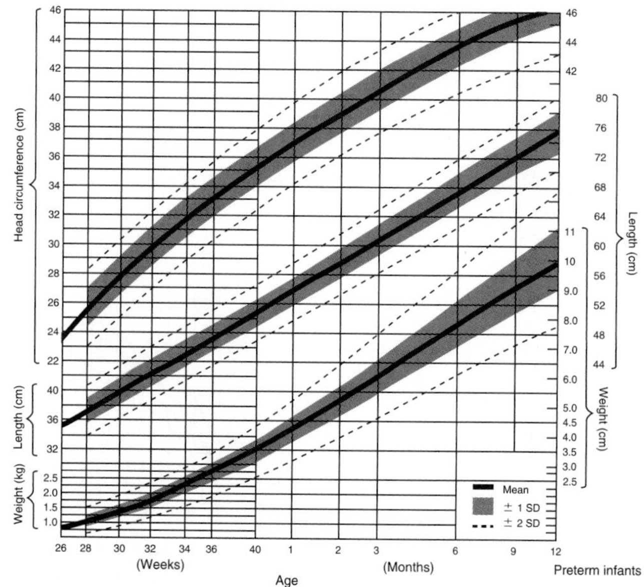

FIGURE 4-34 Length, weight, and head circumference for preterm infants. (Modified from Babson SG, Benda GI: *J Pediatr* 89:815, 1976. *In* Siberry GK, Iannone R [eds]: *The Harriet Lane Handbook: A Manual for Pediatric House Officers,* 15th ed. St Louis, Mosby, 2000.)

Achondroplasia Growth Charts

HEIGHT FOR GIRLS BIRTH TO 18 YEARS

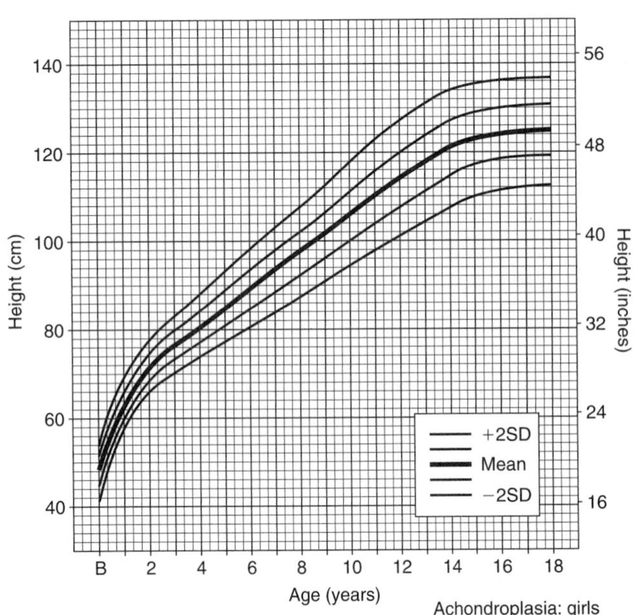

FIGURE 4-35 Height for girls with achondroplasia, from birth to 18 years. (From Horton WA et al: *J Pediatr* 93:435, 1978. *In* Siberry GK, Iannone R [eds]: *The Harriet Lane Handbook: A Manual for Pediatric House Officers,* 15th ed. St Louis, Mosby, 2000.)

HEIGHT FOR BOYS BIRTH TO 18 YEARS

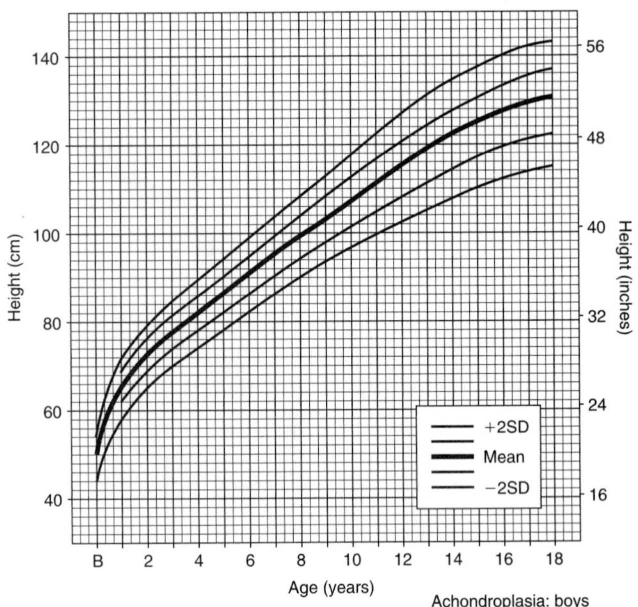

FIGURE 4-37 Height for boys with achondroplasia, from birth to 18 years. (From Horton WA et al: *J Pediatr* 93:435, 1978. *In* Siberry GK, Iannone R [eds]: *The Harriet Lane Handbook: A Manual for Pediatric House Officers,* 15th ed. St Louis, Mosby, 2000.)

HEAD CIRCUMFERENCE FOR GIRLS BIRTH TO 18 YEARS

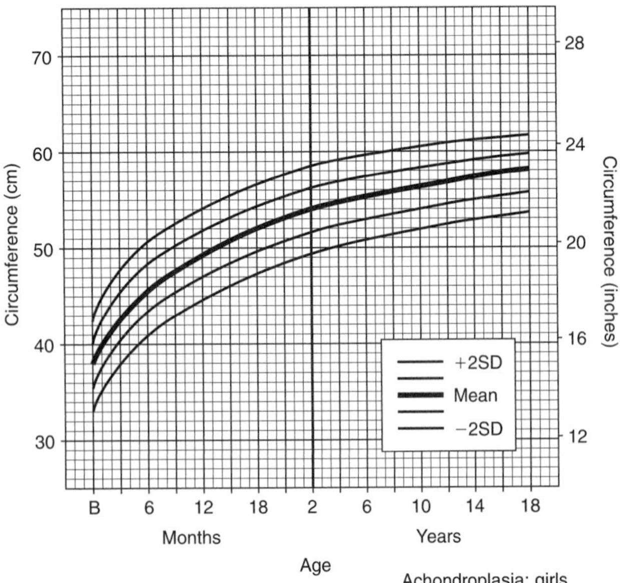

FIGURE 4-36 Head circumference for girls with achondroplasia, from birth to 18 years. (From Horton WA et al: *J Pediatr* 93:435, 1978. *In* Siberry GK, Iannone R [eds]: *The Harriet Lane Handbook: A Manual for Pediatric House Officers,* 15th ed. St Louis, Mosby, 2000.)

HEAD CIRCUMFERENCE FOR BOYS BIRTH TO 18 YEARS

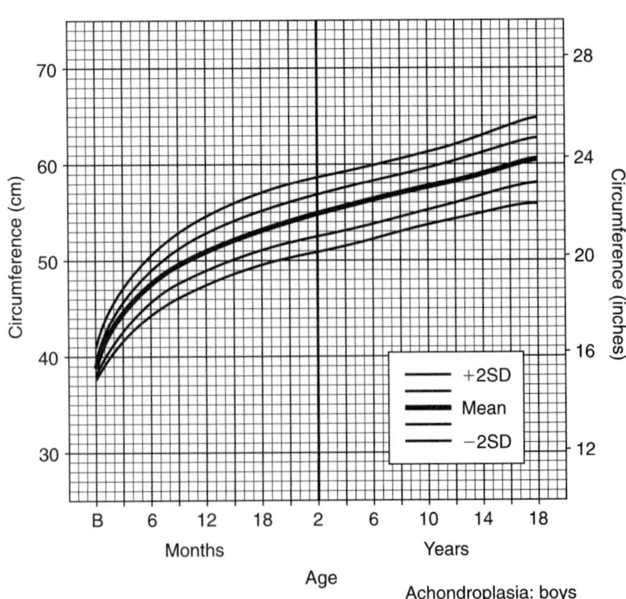

FIGURE 4-38 Head circumference for boys with achondroplasia, from birth to 18 years. (From Horton WA et al: *J Pediatr* 93:435, 1978. *In* Siberry GK, Iannone R [eds]: *The Harriet Lane Handbook: A Manual for Pediatric House Officers,* 15th ed. St Louis, Mosby, 2000.)

Down Syndrome Growth Charts

LENGTH & WEIGHT FOR GIRLS 0 TO 36 MONTHS

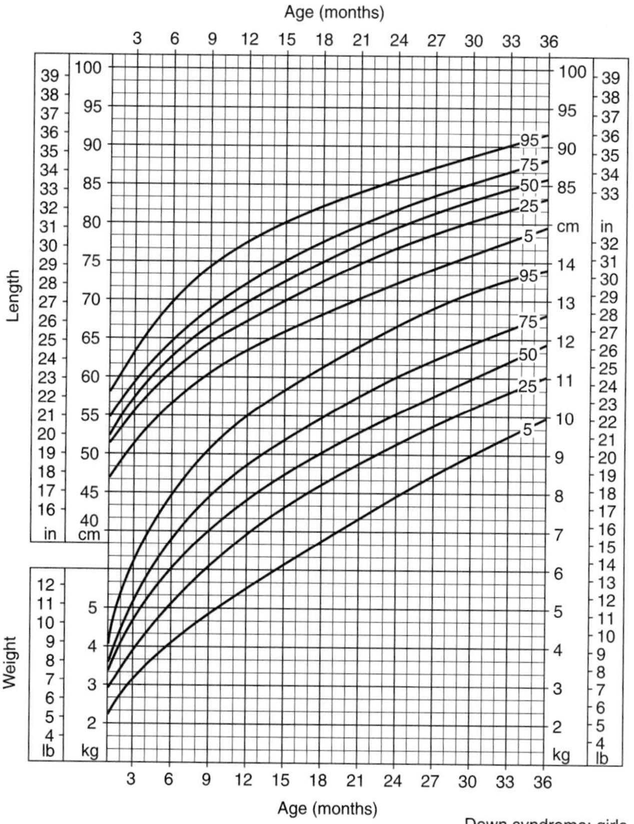

FIGURE 4-39 Length and weight for girls with Down syndrome, from birth to 36 months. (Modified from Cronk C et al: *Pediatrics* 81:102, 1988. *In* Siberry GK, Iannone R [eds]: *The Harriet Lane Handbook: A Manual for Pediatric House Officers,* 15th ed. St Louis, Mosby, 2000.)

HEAD CIRCUMFERENCE FOR GIRLS 0 TO 36 MONTHS

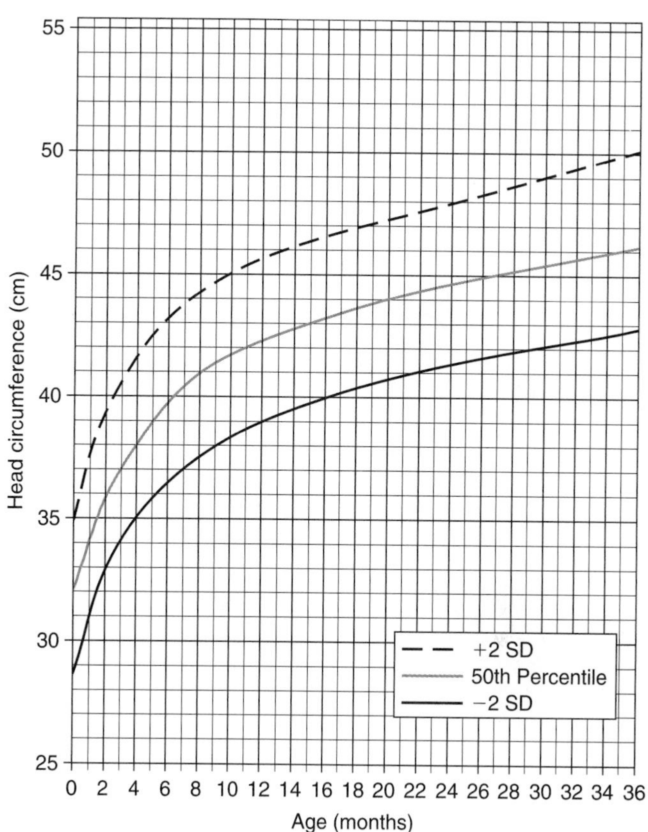

FIGURE 4-40 Head circumference for girls with Down syndrome, from birth to 36 months.

Down Syndrome Growth Charts

LENGTH & WEIGHT FOR BOYS 0 TO 36 MONTHS

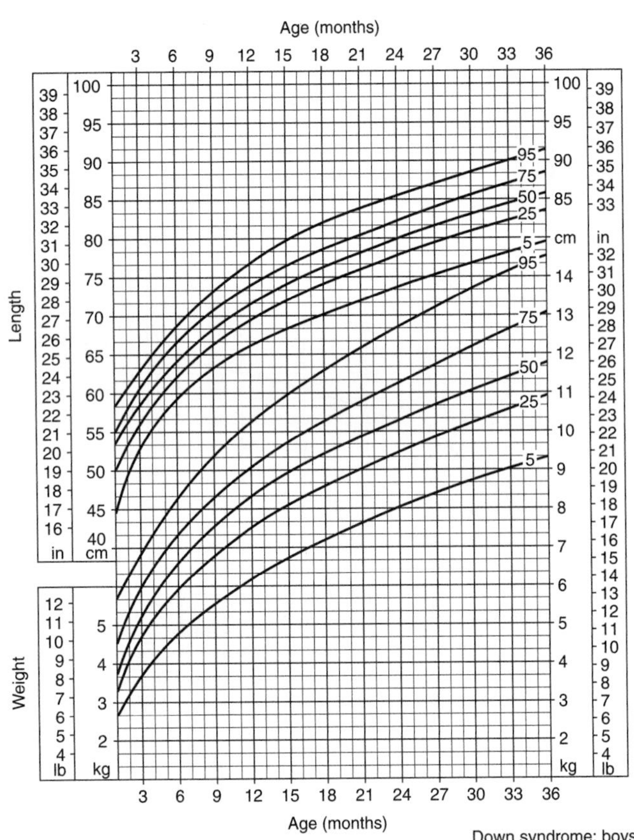

FIGURE 4-41 Length and weight for boys with Down syndrome, from birth to 36 months. (Modified from Cronk C et al: *Pediatrics* 81:102, 1988. *In* Siberry GK, Iannone R [eds]: *The Harriet Lane Handbook: A Manual for Pediatric House Officers,* 15th ed. St Louis, Mosby, 2000.)

HEAD CIRCUMFERENCE FOR BOYS 0 TO 36 MONTHS

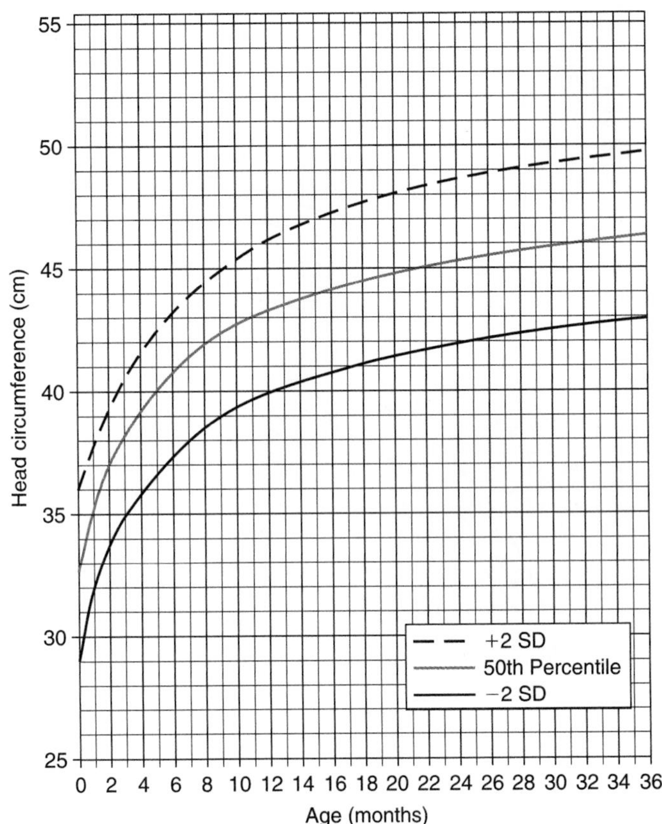

FIGURE 4-42 Head circumference for boys with Down syndrome, from birth to 36 months.

Down Syndrome Growth Charts

STATURE & WEIGHT FOR GIRLS 2 TO 18 YEARS

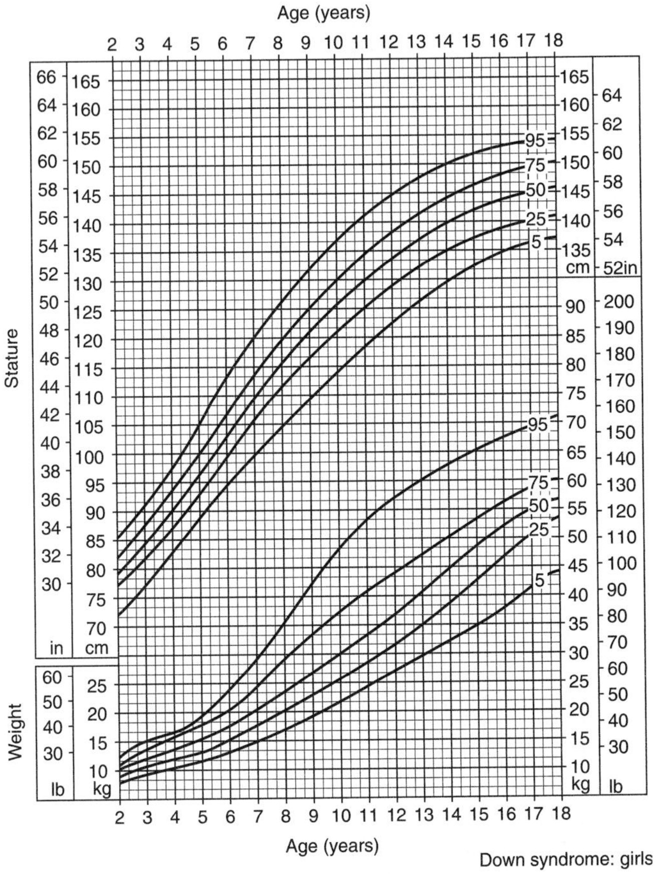

FIGURE 4-43 Stature and weight for girls with Down syndrome, from 2 to 18 years. (Modified from Cronk C et al: *Pediatrics* 81:102, 1988. *In* Siberry GK, Iannone R [eds]: *The Harriet Lane Handbook: A Manual for Pediatric House Officers,* 15th ed. St Louis, Mosby, 2000.)

STATURE & WEIGHT FOR BOYS 2 TO 18 YEARS

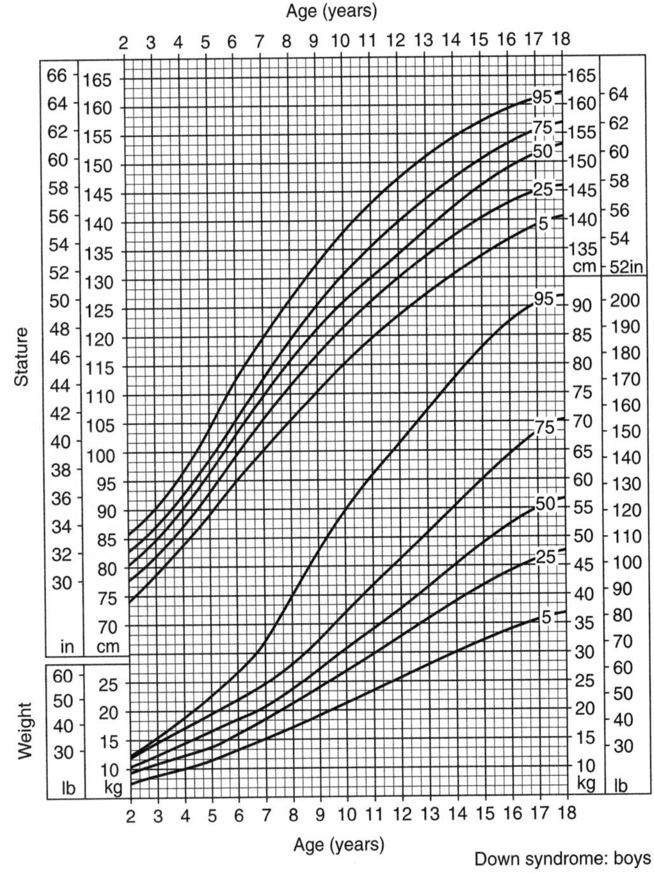

FIGURE 4-44 Stature and weight for boys with Down syndrome, from 2 to 18 years. (Modified from Cronk C et al: *Pediatrics* 81:102, 1988. *In* Siberry GK, Iannone R [eds]: *The Harriet Lane Handbook: A Manual for Pediatric House Officers,* 15th ed. St Louis, Mosby, 2000.)

PHYSICAL GROWTH (HEIGHT) FOR GIRLS WITH TURNER SYNDROME 2 TO 18 YEARS

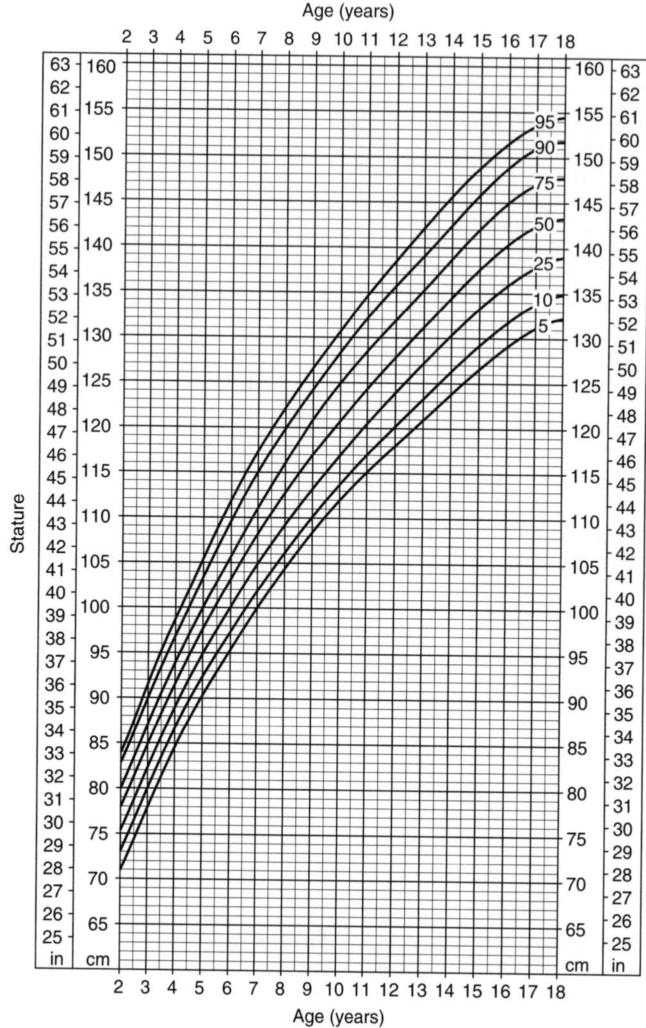

FIGURE 4-45 Stature for girls with Turner syndrome, from 2 to 18 years. (From Lyon AJ, Preece MA, Grant DB: *Arch Dis Child* 60:932, 1985. Courtesy Greentech, Inc., 1987. *In* Siberry GK, Iannone R [eds]: *The Harriet Lane Handbook: A Manual for Pediatric House Officers,* 15th ed. St Louis, Mosby, 2000.)

NOMOGRAM FOR BODY MASS INDEX

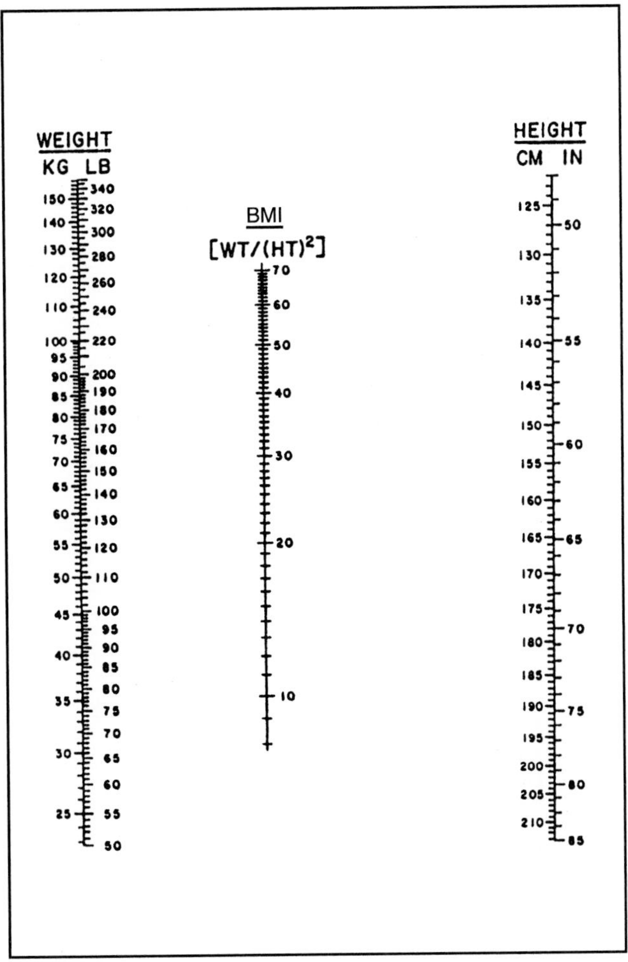

FIGURE 4-46 Nomogram for body mass index (BMI). (From Bray GA: *Obesity in America.* NIH Publication No. 79-359, Nov 1979.)

BMI FORMULA

$$BMI = \frac{Weight(kg)}{[(m)]^2}$$

TABLE 4-13 **Body Mass Index (BMI, in kg/m²) for Selected Statures and Weights**

Weight kg (lb)	HEIGHT m (in)																											
	1.24 (49)	1.27 (50)	1.30 (51)	1.32 (52)	1.35 (53)	1.37 (54)	1.40 (55)	1.42 (56)	1.45 (57)	1.47 (58)	1.50 (59)	1.52 (60)	1.55 (61)	1.57 (62)	1.60 (63)	1.63 (64)	1.65 (65)	1.68 (66)	1.70 (67)	1.73 (68)	1.75 (69)	1.78 (70)	1.80 (71)	1.83 (72)	1.85 (73)	1.88 (74)	1.90 (75)	1.93 (76)
20 (45)	13	13	12	12	11	11	10	10	10	9	9	9	8															
23 (50)	15	14	13	13	12	12	12	11	11	10	10	10	9	9	9	9	8											
25 (55)	16	15	15	14	14	13	13	12	12	12	11	11	10	10	10	9	9	9										
27 (60)	18	17	16	16	15	15	14	13	13	13	12	12	11	11	11	10	10	10	9	9								
29 (65)	19	18	17	17	16	16	15	15	14	14	13	13	12	12	12	11	11	10	10	10	10							
32 (70)	21	20	19	18	17	17	16	16	15	15	14	14	13	13	12	12	12	11	11	11	10	10						
34 (75)	22	21	20	20	19	18	17	17	16	16	15	15	14	14	13	13	12	12	12	11	11	11	10					
36 (80)	24	22	21	21	20	19	19	18	17	17	16	16	15	15	14	14	13	13	13	12	12	11	11	11				
39 (85)	25	24	23	22	21	21	20	19	18	18	17	17	16	16	15	15	14	14	13	13	13	12	12	12	11			
41 (90)	27	25	24	23	22	22	21	20	19	19	18	18	17	17	16	15	15	14	14	14	13	13	13	12	12	12		
43 (95)	28	27	25	25	24	23	22	21	20	20	19	19	18	17	17	16	16	15	15	14	14	14	13	13	13	12	12	
45 (100)	29	28	27	26	25	24	23	22	22	21	20	20	19	18	18	17	17	16	16	15	15	14	14	14	13	13	13	12
48 (105)	31	30	28	27	26	25	24	24	23	22	21	21	20	19	19	18	17	17	16	16	16	15	15	14	14	13	13	13
50 (110)	32	31	30	29	27	27	25	25	24	23	22	22	21	20	19	19	18	18	17	17	16	16	15	15	15	14	14	13
52 (115)	34	32	31	30	29	28	27	26	25	24	23	23	22	21	20	20	19	18	18	17	17	16	16	16	15	15	14	14
54 (120)	35	34	32	31	30	29	28	27	26	25	24	24	23	22	21	20	20	19	19	18	18	17	17	16	16	15	15	15
57 (125)	37	35	34	33	31	30	29	28	27	26	25	25	24	23	22	21	21	20	20	19	19	18	17	17	17	16	16	15
59 (130)	38	37	35	34	32	31	30	29	28	27	26	26	25	24	23	22	22	21	20	20	19	19	18	18	17	17	16	16
61 (135)	40	38	36	35	34	33	31	30	29	28	27	27	25	25	24	23	22	22	21	20	20	19	19	18	18	17	17	16
64 (140)	41	39	38	36	35	34	32	31	30	29	28	27	26	26	25	24	23	22	22	21	21	20	20	19	19	18	18	17
66 (145)	43	41	39	38	36	35	34	33	31	30	29	28	27	27	26	25	24	23	23	22	21	21	20	20	19	19	18	18
68 (150)	44	42	40	39	37	36	35	34	32	31	30	29	28	28	27	26	25	24	24	23	22	21	21	20	20	19	19	18
70 (155)	46	44	42	40	39	37	36	35	33	33	31	30	29	29	27	26	26	25	24	23	23	22	22	21	21	20	19	19
73 (160)	47	45	43	42	40	39	37	36	35	34	32	31	30	29	28	27	27	26	25	24	24	23	22	22	21	21	20	19
77 (170)	50	48	46	44	42	41	39	38	37	36	34	33	32	31	30	29	28	27	27	26	25	24	24	23	23	22	21	21
79 (175)		49	47	46	44	42	40	39	38	37	35	34	33	32	31	30	29	28	27	27	26	25	24	24	23	22	22	21
82 (180)		51	48	47	45	44	42	40	39	38	36	35	34	33	32	31	30	29	28	27	27	26	25	24	24	23	23	22

TABLE 4-13 **Body Mass Index (BMI, in kg/m²) for Selected Statures and Weights** *(Continued)*

Weight kg (lb)	HEIGHT m (in)																											
	1.24 (49)	1.27 (50)	1.30 (51)	1.32 (52)	1.35 (53)	1.37 (54)	1.40 (55)	1.42 (56)	1.45 (57)	1.47 (58)	1.50 (59)	1.52 (60)	1.55 (61)	1.57 (62)	1.60 (63)	1.63 (64)	1.65 (65)	1.68 (66)	1.70 (67)	1.73 (68)	1.75 (69)	1.78 (70)	1.80 (71)	1.83 (72)	1.85 (73)	1.88 (74)	1.90 (75)	1.93 (76)
84 (185)			50	48	46	45	43	42	40	39	37	36	35	34	33	32	31	30	29	28	27	26	26	25	25	24	23	23
86 (190)				49	47	46	44	43	41	40	38	37	36	35	34	32	32	31	30	29	28	27	27	26	25	24	24	23
88 (195)				51	49	47	45	44	42	41	39	38	37	36	35	33	32	31	31	30	29	28	27	26	26	25	25	24
91 (200)					50	48	46	45	43	42	40	39	38	37	35	34	33	32	31	30	30	29	28	27	27	26	25	24
93 (205)						50	47	46	44	43	41	40	39	38	36	35	34	33	32	31	30	29	29	28	27	26	26	25
95 (210)							49	47	45	44	42	41	40	39	37	36	35	34	33	32	31	30	29	28	28	27	26	26
98 (215)							50	48	46	45	43	42	41	40	38	37	36	35	34	33	32	31	30	29	28	28	27	26
100 (220)								49	47	46	44	43	42	40	39	38	37	35	35	33	33	31	31	30	29	28	28	27
102 (225)								51	49	47	45	44	42	41	40	38	37	36	35	34	33	32	31	30	30	29	28	27
104 (230)									50	48	46	45	43	42	41	39	38	37	36	35	34	33	32	31	30	30	29	28
107 (235)										49	47	46	44	43	42	40	39	38	37	36	35	34	33	32	31	30	30	29
109 (240)										50	48	47	45	44	43	41	40	39	38	36	36	34	34	33	32	31	30	29
111 (245)											49	48	46	45	43	42	41	39	38	37	36	35	34	33	32	31	31	30
113 (250)											50	49	47	46	44	43	42	40	39	38	37	36	35	34	33	32	31	30
116 (255)												50	48	47	45	44	42	41	40	39	38	37	36	35	34	33	32	31
118 (260)													49	48	46	44	43	42	41	39	39	37	36	35	34	33	33	32
120 (265)													50	49	47	45	44	43	42	40	39	38	37	36	35	34	33	32
122 (270)														50	48	46	45	43	42	41	40	39	38	37	36	35	34	33
125 (275)															49	47	46	44	43	42	41	39	38	37	36	35	35	33
127 (280)															50	48	47	45	44	42	41	40	39	38	37	36	35	34
129 (285)															50	49	47	46	45	43	42	41	40	39	38	37	36	35
132 (290)																50	48	47	46	44	43	42	41	39	38	37	36	35
134 (295)																50	49	47	46	45	44	42	41	40	39	38	37	36
136 (300)																	50	48	47	45	44	43	42	41	40	39	38	37

From Green M (ed): *Bright Futures: Guidelines For Health Supervision of Infants, Children, and Adolescents,* 1994. National Center for Education in Maternal and Child Health.

TABLE 4-14 Hearing Evaluation in Office

Test	Method	Interpretation
Weber's test	512-Hz tuning fork placed on top of the head; patient is asked which ear tone is heard	*Normal:* sound heard in midline *Conductive loss:* sound heard on affected side *Neurosensory loss:* sound heard on unaffected side
Rinne's test	512-Hz tuning fork held against mastoid; when sound is no longer heard, duration of bone conduction is noted; fork transferred to ½ inch from ear; air conduction should be twice as long as bone and louder	*Air > bone:* normal (+) test *Bone > air:* conductive hearing loss (−) test
Whispered voice	Occlude opposite ear; whisper softly, from 2 feet away; do not use a question that is answered by "yes" or "no"	Usually indicates 20-dB hearing loss if not perceived
Watch tick	Hold watch 2 inches from ear	Indicates high-frequency loss if not perceived; if heard, 98% chance of hearing all lower frequencies normally
Schwabach's test	512-Hz tuning fork is pressed alternately to examiner's mastoid, then to patient's mastoid	When hearing is normal, both patient and examiner cease to hear the tuning fork at the same time; if patient hears the tuning fork longer than an examiner with normal hearing, this indicates middle ear (conductive) loss; if examiner with normal hearing hears the tuning fork longer, the patient has sensorineural loss

From Driscoll CE et al: *The Fmily Practice Desk Reference,* 3rd ed. St Louis, Mosby, 1996.

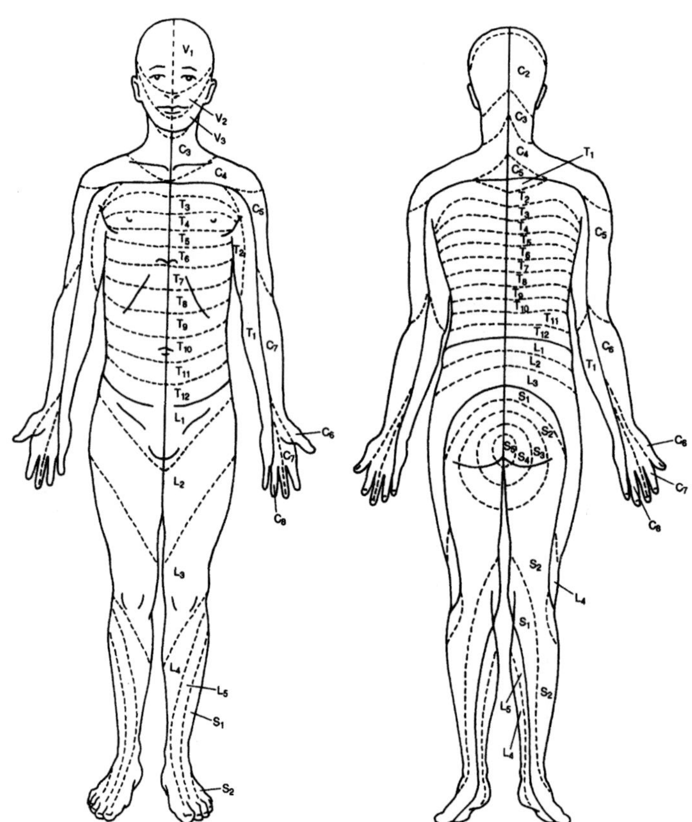

FIGURE 4-47 Spinal dermatomes. (From Siberry GK, Iannone R [eds]: *The Harriet Lane Handbook: A Manual for Pediatric House Officers,* 15th ed. St Louis, Mosby, 2000.)

TABLE 4-15 Movement Abnormalities

Movement	Speed	Location	Direction	Stereotype	Rhythmicity	Interval
Athetosis	Slow	Most prominent in distal limbs	Axial rotations (writhing) and hyperextension	Common; continuous movement in extremity	Not rhythmic	Continuous, amplitude increased by excitement
Ballismus	Rapid	Proximal, especially at shoulder; also at hip; sometimes trunk, face, and muscles of respiration	Hurling, flinging, throwing, kicking, circumducting	Constant location; movements vary	Not rhythmic	0.5-120 seconds
Chorea	Rapid	Generalized; may be unilateral	Primarily at right angles to axis; also facial grimacing; flexion and extension	None; movements generally dance from joint to joint; when proximal and severe may appear semipurposeful	Not rhythmic	0.5-5 seconds
Dystonia	Rapid, slow; very slow relaxation	Trunk, head, extremities	Any, often twisting	Common; because of location of movements, relative strength of contracting muscles	Irregular	Irregular
Myoclonus	Very rapid	Localized or generalized	Any	Stereotyped	Irregular	0.5-5 seconds
Tic	Rapid	Usually in area supplied by motor cranial nerve (face, shoulder, neck)	Rotational; away	Stereotyped	Irregular	1 second to minutes
Tremor	Variable	Usually localized, often in hand	Complex or simple	Extreme stereotype	Very rhythmic; may be irregular	0.1-1 second

From McMillan JA et al (eds): *The Whole Pediatrician Catalog: A Compendium of Clues to Diagnosis and Management.* Philadelphia, WB Saunders, 1979.

TABLE 4-16 Postural Reactions

Postural reaction	Age of appearance	Description	Importance
Head righting	6 wk–3 mo	Lifts chin from tabletop in prone position	Necessary for adequate head control and sitting
Landau response	2–3 mo	Extension of head, then trunk and legs when held prone	Early measure of developing trunk control
Derotational righting	4–5 mo	Following passive or active head turning, the body rotates to follow the direction of the head	Prerequisite to independent rolling
Anterior propping	4–5 mo	Arm extension anteriorly in supported sitting	Necessary for tripod sitting
Parachute	5–6 mo	Arm extension when falling	Facial protection when falling
Lateral propping	6–7 mo	Arm extension laterally in protective response	Allows independent sitting
Posterior propping	8–10 mo	Arm extension posteriorly	Allows pivoting in sitting

From Bravo AM: Development. *In* Siberry GK, Iannone R (eds): *The Harriet Lane Handbook: A Manual for Pediatric House Officers,* 15th ed. St Louis, Mosby, 2000.

TABLE 4-17 Primitive Reflexes

Primitive reflexes	Elicitation	Response	Timing
Moro reflex (MR, "embrace" response) of fingers, wrists, and elbows	Supine: sudden neck extension; allow head to fall back about 3 cm	Extension, adduction, and then abduction of UEs, with semiflexion	Present at birth; disappears by 3–6 mo
Galant reflex (GR)	Prone suspension: stroking paravertebral area from thoracic to sacral region	Produces truncal incurvature with concavity towards stimulated side	Present at birth; disappears by 2–6 mo
Asymmetric tonic neck reflex (ATNR, "fencer" response)	Supine: rotate head laterally about 45°–90°	Relative extension of limbs on chin side and flexion on occiput side	Present at birth; disappears by 4–9 mo
Symmetric tonic neck reflex (STNR, "cat" reflex)	Sitting: head extension/flexion	Extension of UEs and flexion of LEs/ flexion of UEs and LE extension	Appears at 5 mo; not present in most normal children; disappears by 8–9 mo
Tonic labyrinthine supine (TLS)	Supine: extension of the neck (alters relation of labyrinths)	Tonic extension of trunk and LEs, shoulder retraction and adduction, usually with elbow flexion	Present at birth; disappears by 6–9 mo
Tonic labyrinthine prone (TLP)	Prone: flexion of the neck	Active flexion of trunk with protraction of shoulders	Present at birth; disappears by 6–9 mo
Positive support reflex (PSR)	Vertical suspension; bouncing hallucal areas on firm surface	Neonatal: momentary LE extension followed by flexion	Present at birth; disappears by 2–4 mo
		Mature: extension of LEs and support of body weight	Appears by 6 mo
Stepping reflex (SR, walking reflex)	Vertical suspension; hallucal stimulation	Stepping gait	Disappears by 2–3 mo
Crossed extension reflex (CER)	Prone; hallucal stimulation of a LE in full extension	Initial flexion, adduction, then extension of contralateral limb	Present at birth; disappears by 2–3 mo
Plantar grasp (PG)	Stimulation of hallucal area	Plantar flexion grasp	Present at birth; disappears by 9 mo
Palmar grasp	Stimulation of palm	Palmar grasp	Present at birth; disappears by 4 mo
Lower extremity placing (LEP)	Vertical suspension; rubbing tibia or dorsum of foot against edge of tabletop	Initial flexion, then extension, the placing of LE on tabletop	Appears at 1 day
Upper extremity placing (UEP)	Rubbing lateral surface of forearm along edge of tabletop from elbow to wrist to dorsum	Flexion, extension, then placing of hand on tabletop	Appears at 3 mo
Downward thrust (DT)	Vertical suspension; thrust LEs downward	Full extension of LEs	Appears at 3 mo

From Bravo AM: Development. *In* Siberry GK, Iannone R (eds): *The Harriet Lane Handbook: A Manual for Pediatric House Officers,* 15th ed. St Louis, Mosby, 2000.
LE, Lower extremity; UE, upper extremity.

TABLE 4-18 Medical Conditions and Sports Participation

This table is designed to be understood by medical and nonmedical personnel. In the *Explanation* sections below, "needs evaluation" means that a physician with appropriate knowledge and experience should assess the safety of a given sport for an athlete with the listed medical condition. Unless otherwise noted, this is because of the variability of the severity of the disease or of the risk of injury among the specific sports in Box 4-2, or both.

Condition	May participate?
Atlantoaxial instability (instability of the joint between cervical vertebrae 1 and 2)	Qualified yes
Explanation: Athlete needs evaluation to assess risk of spinal cord injury during sports participation.	
Bleeding disorder	Qualified yes
Explanation: Athlete needs evaluation.	
Cardiovascular diseases	
Carditis (inflammation of the heart)	No
Explanation: Carditis may result in sudden death with exertion.	
Hypertension (high blood pressure)	Qualified yes
Explanation: Those with significant essential (unexplained) hypertension should avoid weight and power lifting, body building, and strength training. Those with secondary hypertension (hypertension caused by a previously identified disease) or severe essential hypertension need evaluation.	
Congenital heart disease (structural heart defects present at birth)	Qualified yes
Explanation: Those with mild forms may participate fully; those with moderate or severe forms, or who have undergone surgery, need evaluation. The 26th Bethesda Conference defined mild, moderate, and severe disease for common cardiac lesions.	
Arrhythmia (irregular heart rhythm)	Qualified yes
Explanation: Those with symptoms (chest pain, syncope, dizziness, shortness of breath, or other symptoms of possible dysrhythmia) or evidence of mitral regurgitation (leaking) on physical examination need evaluation. All others may participate fully.	
Heart murmur	Qualified yes
Explanation: If the murmur is innocent (does not indicate heart disease), full participation is permitted. Otherwise, the athlete needs evaluation (see "Congenital Heart Disease" and "Mitral Valve Prolapse" above).	
Cerebral palsy	Qualified yes
Explanation: Athlete needs evaluation.	
Diabetes mellitus	Yes
Explanation: All sports can be played with proper attention to diet, blood glucose concentration, hydration, and insulin therapy. Blood glucose concentration should be monitored every 30 min during continuous exercise and 15 min after completion of exercise.	
Diarrhea	Qualified no
Explanation: Unless disease is mild, no participation is permitted, because diarrhea may increase the risk of dehydration and heat illness (see "Fever" below).	
Eating disorders	Qualified yes
Anorexia nervosa	
Bulimia nervosa	
Explanation: These patients need both medical and psychiatric assessment before participation.	
Eyes	Qualified yes
Functionally one-eyed athlete	
Loss of an eye	
Detached retina	
Previous eye surgery or serious eye injury	
Explanation: A functionally one-eyed athlete has a best corrected visual acuity of <20/40 in the worse eye. These athletes would suffer significant disability if the better eye was seriously injured as would those with loss of an eye. Some athletes who have previously undergone eye surgery or had a serious eye injury may have an increased risk of injury because of weakened eye tissue. Availability of eye guards approved by the American Society for Testing Materials (ASTM) and other protective equipment may allow participation in most sports, but this must be judged on an individual basis.	
Fever	No
Explanation: Fever can increase cardiopulmonary effort, reduce maximum exercise capacity, make heat illness more likely, and increase orthostatic hypotension during exercise. Fever may rarely accompany myocarditis or other infections that may make exercise dangerous.	
Heat illness, history of	Qualified yes
Explanation: Because of the increased likelihood of recurrence, the athlete needs individual assessment to determine the presence of predisposing conditions and to arrange a prevention strategy.	
Hepatitis	Yes
Explanation: Because of the apparent minimal risk to others, all sports may be played that the athlete's state of health allows. In all athletes, skin lesions should be covered properly and athletic personnel should use universal precautions when handling blood or body fluids with visible blood.	

Continued

TABLE 4-18 **Medical Conditions and Sports Participation** *(Continued)*

Condition	May Participate?
HIV infection	Yes
Explanation: Because of the apparent minimal risk to others, all sports may be played that the state of health allows. In all athletes, skin lesions should be properly covered and athletic personnel should use universal precautions when handling blood or body fluids with visible blood.	
Kidney: absence of one	Qualified yes
Explanation: Athlete needs individual assessment for contact/collision and limited contact sports.	
Liver: enlarged	Qualified yes
Explanation: If the liver is acutely enlarged, participation should be avoided because of risk of rupture. If the liver is chronically enlarged, individual assessment is needed before collision/contact or limited contact sports are played.	
Malignant neoplasm	Qualified yes
Explanation: Athlete needs individual assessment.	
Musculoskeletal disorders	Qualified yes
Explanation: Athlete needs individual assessment.	
Neurologic disorders	
History of serious head or spine trauma, severe or repeated concussions, or craniotomy.	Qualified yes
Explanation: Athlete needs individual assessment for collision/contact or limited contact sports, and also for noncontact sports if there are deficits in judgment or cognition. Recent research supports a conservative approach to management of concussion.	
Seizure disorder, well controlled	Yes
Explanation: Risk of convulsion during participation is minimal.	
Seizure disorder, poorly controlled	Qualified yes
Explanation: Athlete needs individual assessment for collision/contact or limited contact sports. Avoid the following noncontact sports: archery, riflery, swimming, weight or power lifting, strength training, or sports involving heights. In these sports, occurrences of a convulsion may be a risk to self or others.	
Obesity	Qualified yes
Explanation: Because of the risk of heat illness, obese persons need careful acclimatization and hydration.	
Organ transplant recipient	Qualified yes
Explanation: Athlete needs individual assessment.	
Ovary: absence of one	Yes
Explanation: Risk of severe injury to the remaining ovary is minimal.	
Respiratory	
Pulmonary compromise including cystic fibrosis	Qualified yes
Explanation: Athlete needs individual assessment, but generally all sports may be played if oxygenation remains satisfactory during a graded exercise test. Patients with cystic fibrosis need acclimatization and good hydration to reduce the risk of illness.	
Asthma	Yes
Explanation: With proper medication and education, only athletes with the most severe asthma will have to modify their participation.	
Acute upper respiratory infection	Qualified yes
Explanation: Upper respiratory obstruction may affect pulmonary function. Athlete needs individual assessment for all but mild disease (see "Fever" earlier).	
Sickle cell disease	Qualified yes
Explanation: Athlete needs individual assessment. In general, if status of the illness permits, all but high exertion, collision/contact sports may be played. Overheating, dehydration, and chilling must be avoided.	
Sickle cell trait	Yes
Explanation: It is unlikely that individuals with sickle cell trait (AS) have an increased risk of sudden death or other medical problems during athletic participation except under the most extreme conditions of heat, humidity, and possibly increased altitude. These individuals, like all athletes, should be carefully conditioned, acclimatized, and hydrated to reduce any possible risk.	
Skin: boils, herpes simplex, impetigo, scabies, molluscum contagiosum	Qualified yes
Explanation: While the patient is contagious, participation in gymnastics with mats, martial arts, wrestling, or other collision/contact or limited contact sports is not allowed.	
Spleen, enlarged	Qualified yes
Explanation: Patients with acutely enlarged spleens should avoid all sports because of risk of rupture. Those with chronically enlarged spleens need individual assessment before playing collision/contact or limited contact sports.	
Testicle: absent or undescended	Yes
Explanation: Certain sports may require a protective cup.	

From American Academy of Pediatrics, Committee on Sports Medicine and Fitness: *Pediatrics* 107:1205, 2001.

BOX 4-2 Classification of Sports by Contact

Contact/Collision	Limited Contact		Noncontact	
Basketball	Baseball	Racquetball	Archery	Race walking
Boxing*	Bicycling	Skateboarding	Badminton	Riflery
Diving	Canoeing/kayaking (white water)	Skating	Body building	Rope jumping
Field hockey	Cheerleading	Ice	Bowling	Running
Football	Fencing	Inline	Canoeing/kayaking (flat water)	Sailing
Tackle	Field events	Roller	Crew/rowing	Scuba diving
Ice hockey†	High jump	Skiing	Curling	Swimming
Lacrosse	Pole vault	Cross-country	Dancing	Table tennis
Martial arts	Floor hockey	Downhill	Field events	Tennis
Rodeo	Football	Water	Discus	Track
Rugby	Flag	Snowboarding	Javelin	Weight lifting
Ski jumping	Gymnastics	Softball	Shot put	
Soccer	Handball	Squash	Golf	
Team handball	Horseback riding	Ultimate Frisbee	Orienteering	
Water polo		Volleyball	Power lifting	
Wrestling		Windsurfing/surfing		

From American Academy of Pediatrics, Committee on Sports Medicine and Fitness: *Pediatrics* 107:1205, 2001.

*Participation not recommended.

†The AAP recommends limiting the amount of body checking allowed for hockey players 15 years and younger to reduce injuries.

BOX 4-3 Concussion and Return to Play

Little evidence is available to support any specific guideline for return to play (RTP) after traumatic brain injury (concussion). What is accepted is the need to allay risk of further injury. Grading signs and systems for severity of concussion are variable making direct comparisons between different guidelines problematic. Most use amnesia, confusion, and loss of consciousness (LOC) to grade severity. Evaluation includes orientation, concentration, immediate memory, and delayed recall. A thorough neurologic exam and exertional testing are also part of the evaluation for concussion. A summary of three commonly quoted and referenced guidelines are displayed here.

	Source/Definition	1st Concussion	2nd Concussion	3rd Concussion
Grade 1 "Mild" Concussion	American Academy of Neurology (AAN), 1997[1] • Transient confusion • No LOC • Symptoms resolve within 15 minutes	Removed and examined at 5 minute intervals. Return to sports that day if symptoms resolve within 15 minutes and assessment remains normal at rest and exertion.	Removed from sports until asymptomatic for 1 week.	Within same season disqualify for season. Question remains on RTP if athlete plays more than one sport: should RTP be after 3–4 months or after one year.
	Colorado Guidelines[2] • Confusion • No amnesia • No LOC	Return to play only if no symptoms or amnesia appear within 20 minutes. May return if asymptomatic for 1 week. End season if abnormal CT or MRI.	May return after 1 symptom-free week.	Disqualify from contact sports for at least 3 months and only RTP if asymptomatic at both rest and exertion.
	Cantu Update, 2001[3] • No LOC • Symptoms (including post traumatic amnesia, concussion signs, or concussion symptoms) lasting <30 minutes		Return to play in 2 weeks if no symptoms for 1 week. Consider terminating season.	Terminate season. If asymptomatic may RTP following season.
Grade 2 "Moderate" Concussion	**Source/Definition** AAN • Transient confusion • No LOC • Duration of mental status abnormalities or symptoms >15 minutes	**1st Concussion** Return only after asymptomatic for 1 full week.	**2nd Concussion** Removed until asymptomatic for 2 weeks.	**3rd Concussion**
	Colorado • Confusion and post-traumatic amnesia • No LOC	Return to play after 1 week if asymptomatic within 1 day.	Consider ending season. Possible return after 1 month if symptom-free and no evidence of intracranial pathology if imaging was done.	End season.
	Cantu • LOC less than 1 minute • Post-traumatic amnesia or concussion symptoms or signs >30 minutes, <24 hours.	Return to play after asymptomatic at rest and with exertion for 1 week.	Return to play in 1 month minimum if asymptomatic for 1 week, but consider ending season.	End season.

BOX 4-3 **Concussion and Return to Play** *(Continued)*

	Source/Definition	1st Concussion	2nd Concussion	3rd Concussion
Grade 3 "Severe" Concussion	AAN • LOC either brief (seconds) or prolonged (minutes or more).	Removed until asymptomatic 1 full week for brief and 2 full weeks for prolonged loss of consciousness. If any intracranial pathology on CT or MRI, removed for season and discouraged from future return to any contact sport.	Removed until asymptomatic for 1 month. If any intracranial pathology on CT or MRI, removed for season and discouraged from future return to any contact sport.	
	Colorado • Any LOC	Removed for 1 month if asymptomatic for 2 weeks and cleared by neurosurgeon or neurologist.	End season. Possible return next season if asymptomatic, but may discourage any return to contact sports.	
	Cantu • LOC for ≥1 minute or amnesia for >24 hours. • Post concussion signs or symptoms lasting longer than 7 days.	Removed for one month. If symptoms at rest and exertion resolved for at least 2 weeks may return to play then.	End season. Possible return to play if asymptomatic next season but discourage from contact sports.	Possibly permanently disqualified from contact sports.

REFERENCES

1. Quality Standards Subcommittee: Practice Parameter: The management of concussion in sports (summary statement). *Am Acad Neuro* 48:581–585, 1997.
2. The School Health and Sports Medicine Committee, Colorado Medical Society. *Guidelines for the Management of Concussion in Sports.* 1990.
3. Cantu RC: Posttraumatic retrograde and anterograde amnesia: pathophysiology and implications in grading and safe return to play. *J Athletic Training* 36:244–248, 2001.
4. Guskiewicz KM et al: Recommendations on management of sport-related concussion: summary of the National Athletic Trainers' Association position statement. *Neurosurgery* 55:891–896, 2004.
5. Harmon KG: Assessment and management of concussion in sports. *Am Family Physician* 60:887–892, 894, 1999.
6. Guskiewicz KM et al: National Athletic Trainers' Association position statement: management of sport-related concussion. *J Athletic Training* 39:280–297, 2004.

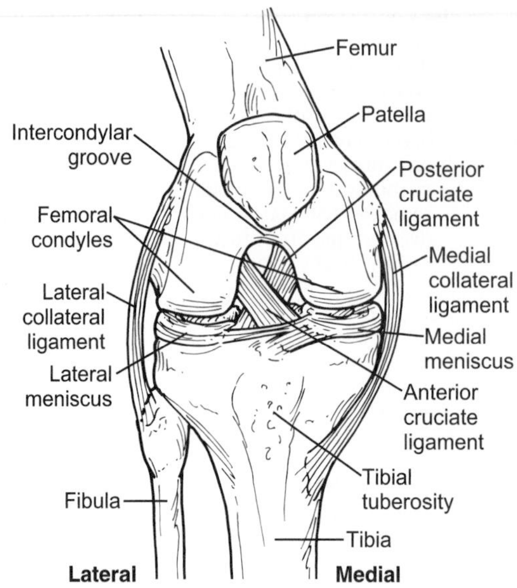

FIGURE 4-48 Knee joint, open and partially flexed.

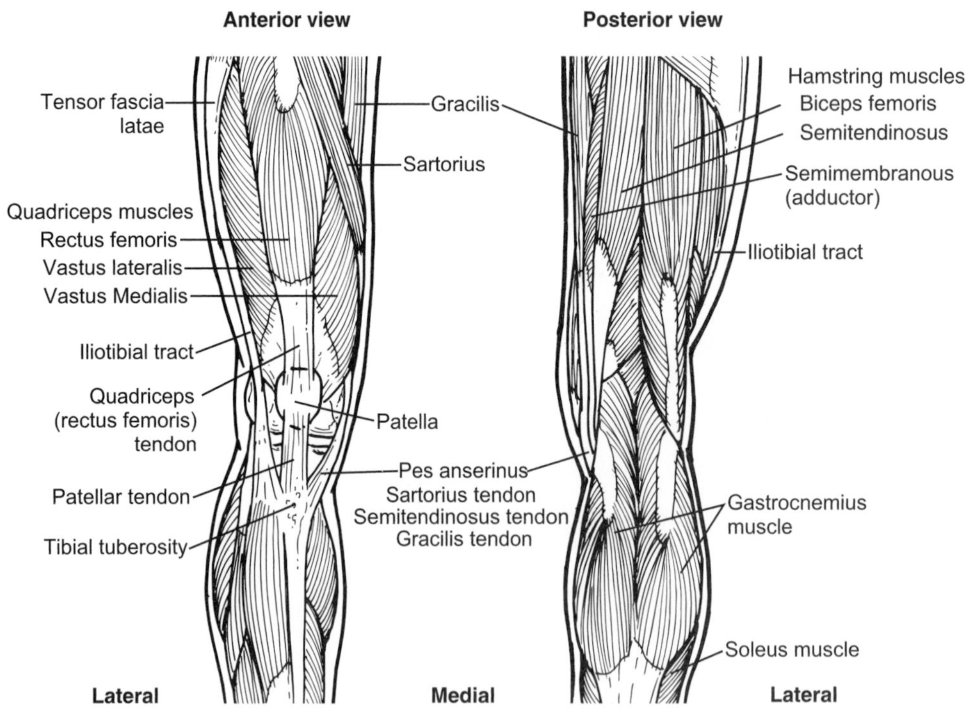

FIGURE 4-49 Muscles of the knee.

BOX 4-4 **Knee Maneuvers**

Knee Valgus Stress Test	To test medial collateral ligament
Patient:	Supine, leg extended and supported by examiner
Examiner:	Beside extremity tested, with one hand on distal lateral femur and other on medial tibia below the joint line
Technique:	Apply medial pressure on femur while distracting tibia laterally. Note amount of opening of medial knee. It should be minimal. Compare with other leg.
Knee Varus Stress Test	To test lateral collateral ligament
Patient:	Supine, leg extended and supported by examiner
Examiner:	Beside extremity tested, with one hand on distal medial femur and other on the lateral tibia below the joint line
Technique:	Apply lateral pressure on the femur while distracting the tibia medially. Note amount of opening of lateral knee. It should be minimal. Compare with other leg.
McMurray Sign	To test for tears in medial and lateral menisci
Patient:	Supine and relaxed with knee completely bent
Examiner:	Standing at the side of the injured limb
Technique:	Grasp the heel and rotate the foot externally while abducting the leg and extending the knee. A click or pain is significant for lateral tear. Opposite maneuver can be positive for medial tear and is done by rotating the foot internally and abducting the leg while extending the knee.
Apprehension Test	To test for patella subluxation
Patient:	Seated
Examiner:	Hand on affected patella
Technique:	Gently push the patella laterally. A start of apprehension is positive. If negative, examiner can extend the knee and then passively flex the knee while gently pushing the patella laterally.
Anterior Drawer Sign	To test the anterior cruciate
Patient:	Supine, hip flexed 45 degrees, knee flexed 90 degrees
Examiner:	Sitting on patient's ipsilateral foot
Technique:	Place hands around the tibia just below the joint line. Apply anterior force and note the amount of anterior motion. Always compare with other knee.
Lachman's Test	When the knee cannot be flexed
Patient:	Supine, hip and knee extended
Examiner:	Standing beside patient
Technique:	Grasp the femur with one hand and the tibia below the joint line. Apply a distracting force to the tibia and note the excursion.
Posterior Drawer Sign	To test the posterior cruciate
Patient:	Supine, hip flexed 45 degrees, knee flexed 90 degrees
Examiner:	Sitting on patient's ipsilateral foot
Technique:	Same as anterior drawer sign, except apply posterior force on tibia.

From Driscoll CE et al: *The Family Practice Desk Reference,* 3rd ed. St Louis, Mosby, 1996.

ANKLE INJURY ASSESSMENT

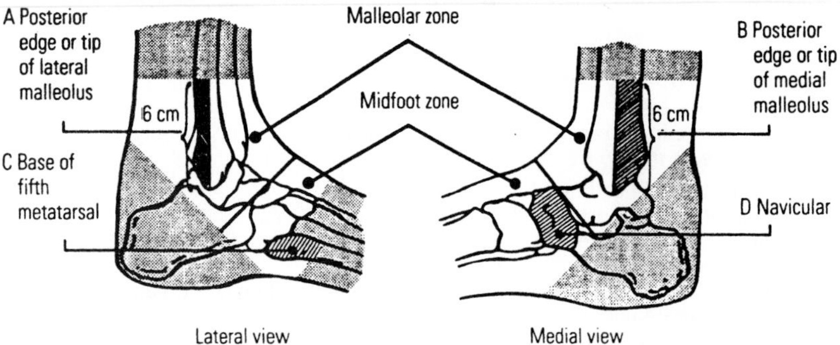

An ankle radiographic series is only required if there is any pain in the malleolar zone and any of these findings is present:

(1) bone tenderness at A
(2) bone tenderness at B
(3) inability to bear weight both immediately and in the ED

A foot radiographic series is only required if there is any pain in midfoot zone and any of these findings is present:

(1) bone tenderness at C
(2) bone tenderness at D
(3) inability to bear weight both immediately and in the ED

FIGURE 4-50 Ottawa ankle rules. (Courtesy Stiell IG, Greenberg GH, McKnight RD, Wells GA, Ottowa Civic Hospital, Ottowa, Ontario, Canada.)

SCOLIOSIS ASSESSMENT

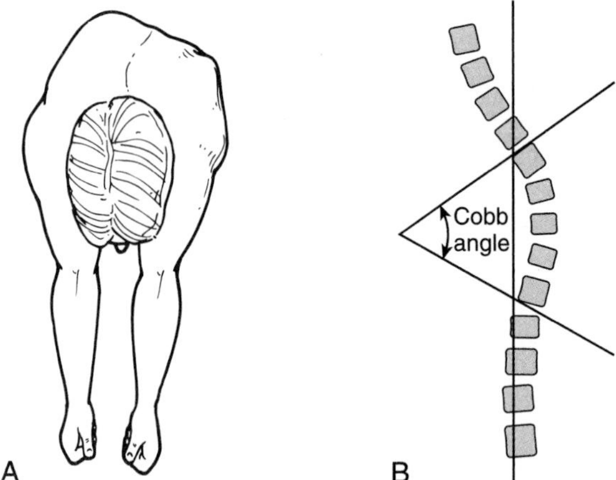

FIGURE 4-51 A. Forward bending test. This emphasizes any asymmetry of the paraspinous muscles and rib cage. **B. Cobb angle.** This is measured using the superior and inferior endplates of the most tilted vertebrae at the end of each curve. (A: Modified from American Academy of Family Physicians: Preparticipation Physical Exam, 2nd ed. Kansas City, MO, American Academy of Family Physicians, 1997.)

TABLE 4-19 **Common Causes of Microcytic Anemia**

	Iron deficiency	ß-Thalassemia Trait	Chronic Inflammation
Reticulocyte count	Low	Normal to ↑	Normal
RDW	↑	↓	Normal
Ferritin	↓	Normal to ↑	Normal to ↑
FEP	↑	Normal	↑
Iron	↓	Normal	↓
TIBC	↑	Normal	↓
Electrophoresis	Normal	↑ HbA_2	Normal
ESR	Normal	Normal	↑
Smear	Hypochromic, target cells, microcytic, fine basophilic stippling	Normochromic, microcytic, coarse basophilic stippling	Variable

From Ebel BE, Raffini L: Hematology. *In* Siberry GK, Iannone R (eds): *The Harriet Lane Handbook: A Manual for Pediatric House Officers,* 15th ed. St Louis, Mosby, 2000.
ESR, Erythrocyte sedimentation rate; FEP, free erythrocyte protoporphrin; Hb, hemoglobin; RDW, red cell distribution width; TIBC, total iron-binding capacity.

TABLE 4-20 **Neonatal Hemoglobin (Hb) Electrophoresis Patterns***

FA	Fetal Hb and adult normal Hb; the normal newborn pattern.
FAV	Indicates the presence of both HbF and HbA. However, an anomalous band (V) is present, which does not appear to be any of the common Hb variants.
FAS	Indicates fetal Hb, adult normal HbA and HbS, consistent with benign sickle cell trait.
FS	Fetal and sickle HbS without detectable adult normal HbA. Consistent with homozygous sickle Hb genotype (S/S) or sickle ß-thalassemia, with manifestations of sickle cell anemia during childhood.
FC[†]	Designates the presence of HbC without adult normal HbA. Consistent with clinically significant homozygous HbC genotype (C/C), resulting in a mild hematologic disorder presenting during childhood.
FSC	HbS and HbC present. This heterozygous condition could lead to the manifestations of sickle cell disease during childhood.
FAC	HbC and adult normal HbA present, consistent with benign HbC trait.
$FSAA_2$	Heterozygous HbS/ß-thalassemia, a clinically significant sickling disorder.
FAA_2	Heterozygous HbA/ß-thalassemia, a clinically benign hematologic condition.
F[†]	Fetal HbF is present without adult normal HbA. Although this may indicate a delayed appearance of HbA, it is also consistent with homozygous ß-thalassemia major, or homozygous hereditary persistence of fetal HbF.
FV[†]	Fetal HbF and an anomalous Hb variant (V) are present.
AF	May indicate prior blood transfusion. Submit another filter paper blood specimen when the infant is 4 mo of age, at which time the transfused blood cells should have been cleared.

From Ebel BE, Raffini L: Hematology. *In* Siberry GK, Iannone R (eds): *The Harriet Lane Handbook: A Manual for Pediatric House Officers,* 15th ed. St Louis, Mosby, 2000.
*Hemoglobin variants are reported in order of decreasing abundance; for example, FA indicates more fetal than adult hemoglobin.
†Repeat blood specimen should be submitted to confirm the original interpretation.

TABLE 4-21 **Evaluation of Liver Tests**

Enzyme	Source	Increased	Decreased	Comments
AST/ALT	Liver Heart Skeletal muscle Pancreas Red blood cells Kidney	Hepatocellular injury Rhabdomyolosis Muscular dystrophy Hemolysis Liver cancer	Vitamin B_6 deficiency Uremia	ALT more specific than AST for liver AST > ALT in hemolysis AST/ALT >2 in 90% of alcohol disorders in adults
Alkaline phosphatase	Liver Osteoblasts Small intestine Kidney Placenta	Hepatocellular injury Bone growth, disease, trauma Pregnancy Familial	Low phosphate Wilsons disease Zinc deficiency Hypothyroidism Pernicious anemia	Highest in cholestatic conditions Must be differentiated from bone source
GGT	Bile ducts Renal tubules Pancreas Small intestine Brain	Cholestasis Newborn period Induced by drugs	Estrogen therapy Artificially low in hyperbilirubinemia	Not found in bone Increased in 90% primary liver disease Biliary obstruction Intrahepatic cholestasis Induced by alcohol Specific for hepatobiliary disease in nonpregnant patient
5′-NT	Liver cell membrane Intestine Brain Heart Pancreas	Cholestasis		Specific for hepatobiliary disease in nonpregnant patient
NH_3	Bowel Bacteria Protein metabolism	Hepatic disease secondary to urea cycle dysfunction Hemodialysis Valproic acid treatment Urea cycle enzyme deficiency Organic acidemia and carnitine deficiency		Converted to urea in liver

From Gleason BK: Gastroenterology. *In* Siberry GK, Iannone R (eds): *The Harriet Lane Handbook: A Manual for Pediatric House Officers,* 15th ed. St Louis, Mosby, 2000.
Alk phos, Alkaline phosphatase; AST/ALT, aspartate aminotransferase/alanine aminotransferase; GGT, γ-glutamyl transpeptidase; 5′-NT, 5′-nucleotidase.

FETAL HEMOGLOBIN (APT TEST)*

- **Purpose:** To differentiate fetal blood from swallowed maternal blood.
- **Method:** Mix specimen with an equal quantity of tap water and centrifuge or filter. Add 1 part of 0.25 mMol/L (1%) NaOH to 5 parts of supernatant.
  Note: Specimen must be bloody, and supernatant must be pink for proper interpretation.
- **Interpretation:** A pink color persisting over 2 minutes indicates fetal hemoglobin. Transition from pink to yellow within 2 minutes indicates adult hemoglobin.

*From Gleason BK: Gastroenterology. *In* Siberry GK, Iannone R (eds): *The Harriet Lane Handbook: A Manual for Pediatric House Officers,* 15th ed. St Louis, Mosby, 2000.

BEDSIDE COLD AGGLUTININ TEST

- One milliliter of the patient's blood is drawn into a tube containing anticoagulant (the tube used for prothrombin determinations is best).
- Before cooling, examination of the tube shows a smooth coating of the tube by red cells.
- The blood is cooled to 4°C by placing it in a standard refrigerator.
- After 3 to 4 minutes, the tube is examined for evidence of macroscopic agglutination as the tube is rolled.
- The tube is then rewarmed to 37°C in an incubator or by exposure to body heat, and the agglutination disappears.
- A positive result correlates with a laboratory titer of 1:64 or greater.

OSMOTIC FRAGILITY

METHODOLOGY

The osmotic fragility test assesses the presence or absence of spherocytes and roughly gauges their quantity in the red cell population. Increasing proportions of red blood cells lyse upon exposure to increasingly hypo-osmotic saline solutions.

The test does not distinguish between spherocytes in hereditary spherocytosis and in acquired autoimmune hemolytic anemia; the test only indicates that a proportion of the red cells have decreased surface-to-volume ratios and are more susceptible to lysis in hypo-osmotic solutions. Cells with increased surface-to-volume ratios, such as occur in thalassemias and iron deficiency, may also show decreased osmotic fragility.

CLINICAL SIGNIFICANCE

Erythrocyte osmotic fragility is most often requested in the workup of possible cases of hereditary spherocytosis.

REFERENCES

1. Elghetany MT, Davey FR: Erythrocytic disorders. *In* Henry JB (ed): *Clinical Diagnosis and Management by Laboratory Methods,* 19th ed. Philadelphia, WB Saunders, 1996.
2. Kjeldsberg C et al: *Practical Diagnosis of Hematologic Disorders,* 3rd ed. Chicago, ASCP Press, 2000.

SCHILLING TEST

WHY THE SCHILLING TEST IS PERFORMED*

The Schilling test is performed to evaluate vitamin B_{12} absorption. Ingested vitamin B_{12} combines with intrinsic factor (produced in the stomach) and is absorbed in the distal ileum.

HOW THE SCHILLING TEST IS PERFORMED

- The patient may fast (except for water) for 8 hours before starting the test, then he or she may eat normally.
- An intramuscular injection of nonradioactive vitamin B_{12} is given to bind available vitamin B_{12} receptor sites. This facilitates rapid excretion of radioactive vitamin B_{12}, if it is absorbed, because there are no places in the body for it to adhere.
- Urinary B_{12} levels are measured after oral ingestion of a small amount of radioactive vitamin B_{12}.
  - Either the one-stage Schilling test (without intrinsic factor) or the two-stage Schilling test (with intrinsic factor) may be used.
  - A 24-hour urine sample is needed.

NORMAL VALUES

Excretion of 8% to 40% of the radioactive vitamin B_{12} within 24 hours is normal.

INTERFERING FACTORS

- Renal insufficiency (inadequate kidney function)
- Hypothyroidism
- Laxatives (may decrease the rate of absorption)

WHAT ABNORMAL RESULTS MEAN

Pernicious anemia results when absorption of vitamin B_{12} is inadequate. This may be caused by malabsorption, intestinal inflammation, a deficiency of vitamin B_{12} in the diet, or a deficiency of intrinsic factor.

Abnormal one- and two-stage Schilling tests may indicate the following:

- Biliary disease
- Celiac disease (sprue)
- Hypothyroidism
- Liver disease

Lower-than-normal amounts of vitamin B_{12} absorption may indicate the following:

- Biliary disease, resulting in malabsorption (inadequate absorption of nutrients from the intestinal tract)
- Intestinal malabsorption (e.g., related to sprue or celiac disease)
- Liver disease (causing malabsorption)
- Pernicious anemia

Additional conditions under which the test may be performed include the following:

- Anemia of B_{12} deficiency
- Blind loop syndrome
- Megaloblastic anemia

*From *Mosby's Medical Encyclopedia.* St Louis, Mosby, 1998.

TABLE 4-22 Respiratory Rates by Age and Gender

Age (yr)	Boys	Girls
0–1	31 ± 8	30 ± 6
1–2	26 ± 4	27 ± 4
2–3	25 ± 4	25 ± 3
3–4	24 ± 3	24 ± 3
4–5	23 ± 2	22 ± 2
5–6	22 ± 2	21 ± 2
6–7	21 ± 3	21 ± 3
7–8	20 ± 3	20 ± 2
8–9	20 ± 2	20 ± 2
9–10	19 ± 2	19 ± 2
10–11	19 ± 2	19 ± 2
11–12	19 ± 3	19 ± 3
12–13	19 ± 3	19 ± 2
13–14	19 ± 2	18 ± 2
14–15	18 ± 2	18 ± 3
15–16	17 ± 3	18 ± 3
16–17	17 ± 2	17 ± 3
17–18	16 ± 3	17 ± 3

From Iliff A, Lee V: *Child Dev* 23:240, 1952. *In* Siberry GK, Iannone R (eds): *The Harriet Lane Handbook: A Manual for Pediatric House Officers*, 15th ed. St Louis, Mosby, 2000.

TABLE 4-23 Heart Rates by Age

Age	2%	Mean	98%
<1 day	93	123	154
1–2 days	91	123	159
3–6 days	91	129	166
1–3 wks	107	148	182
1–2 mos	121	149	179
3–5 mos	106	141	186
6–11 mos	109	134	169
1–2 yrs	89	119	151
3–4 yrs	73	108	137
5–7 yrs	65	100	133
8–11 yrs	62	91	130
12–15 yrs	60	85	119

From Chiang LK, Dunn AE: Cardiology. *In* Siberry GK, Iannone R (eds): *The Harriet Lane Handbook: A Manual for Pediatric House Officers*, 15th ed. St Louis, Mosby, 2000.

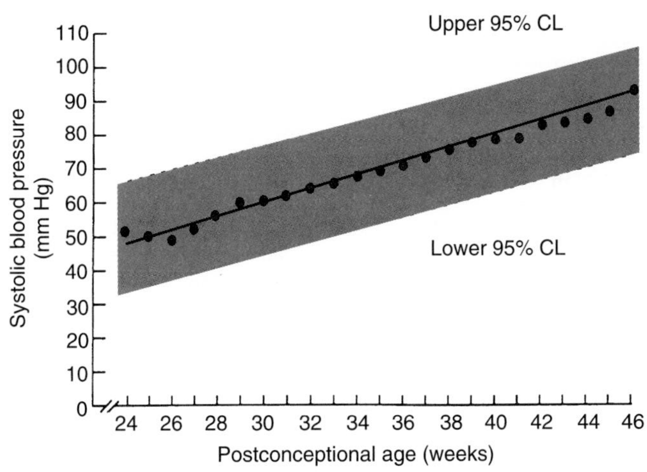

FIGURE 4-52 Linear regression of mean systolic blood pressure on postconceptual age (gestational age in weeks + weeks after delivery). (From Zubrow AB et al: *J Perinatol* 15:470, 1995.)

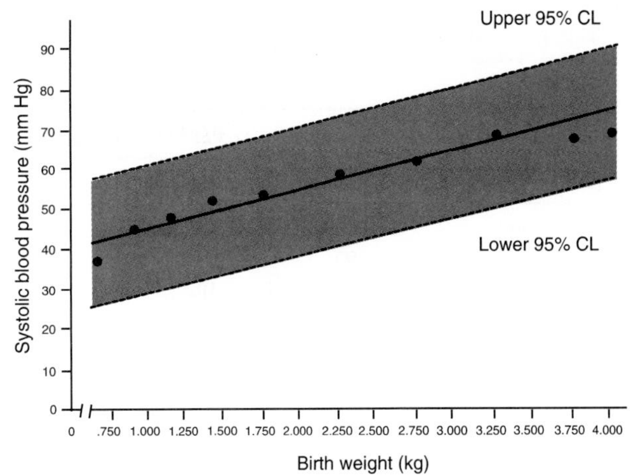

FIGURE 4-53 Linear regression of mean systolic blood pressure on birth weight on day 1 of life. (From Zubrow AB et al: *J Perinatol* 15:470, 1995.)

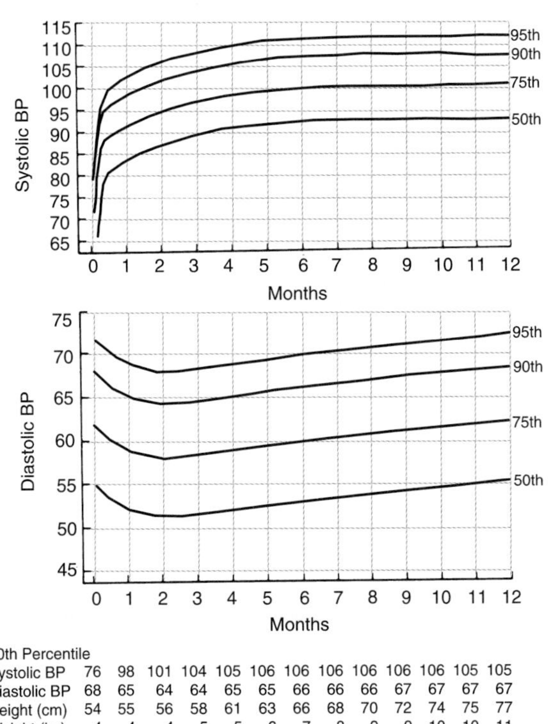

90th Percentile													
Systolic BP	76	98	101	104	105	106	106	106	106	106	106	105	105
Diastolic BP	68	65	64	64	65	65	66	66	66	67	67	67	67
Height (cm)	54	55	56	58	61	63	66	68	70	72	74	75	77
Weight (kg)	4	4	4	5	5	6	7	8	9	9	10	10	11

FIGURE 4-54 Age-specific percentiles of blood pressure (BP) measurements in girls from birth to 12 months of age; Korotkoff phase IV (K4) used for diastolic BP. (From Horan MJ: *Pediatrics* 79:1, 1987.)

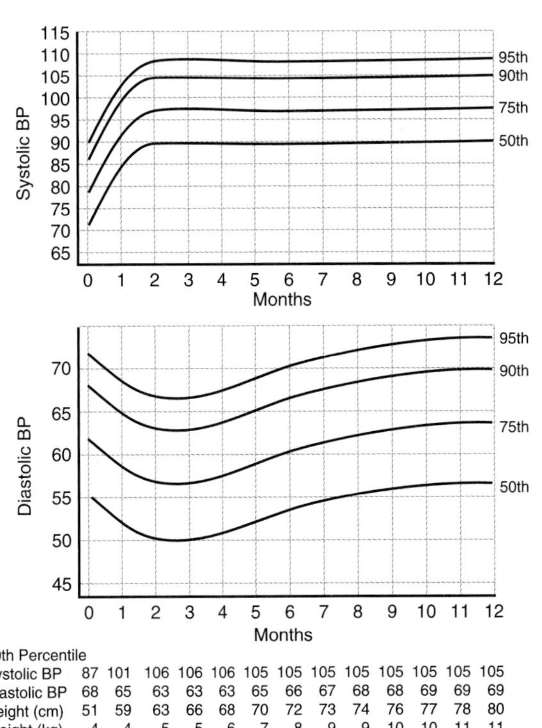

90th Percentile													
Systolic BP	87	101	106	106	106	105	105	105	105	105	105	105	105
Diastolic BP	68	65	63	63	63	65	66	67	68	68	69	69	69
Height (cm)	51	59	63	66	68	70	72	73	74	76	77	78	80
Weight (kg)	4	4	5	5	6	7	8	9	9	10	10	11	11

FIGURE 4-55 Age-specific percentiles of blood pressure (BP) measurements in boys from birth to 12 months of age; Korotkoff phase IV (K4) used for diastolic BP. (From Horan MJ: *Pediatrics* 79:1, 1987.)

TABLE 4-24 Blood Pressure Levels for Girls by Age and Height Percentile

		Systolic BP, mm Hg							Diastolic BP, mm Hg						
		PERCENTILE OF HEIGHT							PERCENTILE OF HEIGHT						
Age (yr)	BP Percentile	5th	10th	25th	50th	75th	90th	95th	5th	10th	25th	50th	75th	90th	95th
1	50th	83	84	85	86	88	89	90	38	39	39	40	41	41	42
	90th	97	97	98	100	101	102	103	52	53	53	54	55	55	56
	95th	100	101	102	104	105	106	107	56	57	57	58	59	59	60
	99th	108	108	109	111	112	113	114	64	64	65	66	66	67	67
2	50th	85	85	87	88	89	91	91	43	44	44	45	46	46	47
	90th	98	99	100	101	103	104	105	57	58	58	59	60	61	61
	95th	102	103	104	105	107	108	109	61	62	62	63	64	65	65
	99th	109	110	111	112	114	115	116	69	69	70	70	71	72	72
3	50th	86	87	88	89	91	92	93	47	48	48	49	50	50	51
	90th	100	100	102	103	104	106	106	61	62	62	63	64	64	65
	95th	104	104	105	107	108	109	110	65	66	66	67	68	68	69
	99th	111	111	113	114	115	116	117	73	73	74	74	75	76	76
4	50th	88	88	90	91	92	94	94	50	50	51	52	52	53	54
	90th	101	102	103	104	106	107	108	64	64	65	66	67	67	68
	95th	105	106	107	108	110	111	112	68	68	69	70	71	71	72
	99th	112	113	114	115	117	118	119	76	76	76	77	78	79	79
5	50th	89	90	91	93	94	95	96	52	53	53	54	55	55	56
	90th	103	103	105	106	107	109	109	66	67	67	68	69	69	70
	95th	107	107	108	110	111	112	113	70	71	71	72	73	73	74
	99th	114	114	116	117	118	120	120	78	78	79	79	80	81	81
6	50th	91	92	93	94	96	97	98	54	54	55	56	56	57	58
	90th	104	105	106	108	109	110	111	68	68	69	70	70	71	72
	95th	108	109	110	111	113	114	115	72	72	73	74	74	75	76
	99th	115	116	117	119	120	121	122	80	80	80	81	82	83	83
7	50th	93	93	95	96	97	99	99	55	56	56	57	58	58	59
	90th	106	107	108	109	111	112	113	69	70	70	71	72	72	73
	95th	110	111	112	113	115	116	116	73	74	74	75	76	76	77
	99th	117	118	119	120	122	123	124	81	81	82	82	83	84	84
8	50th	95	95	96	98	99	100	101	57	57	57	58	59	60	60
	90th	108	109	110	111	113	114	114	71	71	71	72	73	74	74
	95th	112	112	114	115	116	118	118	75	75	75	76	77	78	78
	99th	119	120	121	122	123	125	125	82	82	83	83	84	85	86
9	50th	96	97	98	100	101	102	103	58	58	58	59	60	61	61
	90th	110	110	112	113	114	116	116	72	72	72	73	74	75	75
	95th	114	114	115	117	118	119	120	76	76	76	77	78	79	79
	99th	121	121	123	124	125	127	127	83	83	84	84	85	86	87
10	50th	98	99	100	102	103	104	105	59	59	59	60	61	62	62
	90th	112	112	114	115	116	118	118	73	73	73	74	75	76	76
	95th	116	116	117	119	120	121	122	77	77	77	78	79	80	80
	99th	123	123	125	126	127	129	129	84	84	85	86	86	87	88
11	50th	100	101	102	103	105	106	107	60	60	60	61	62	63	63
	90th	114	114	116	117	118	119	120	74	74	74	75	76	77	77
	95th	118	118	119	121	122	123	124	78	78	78	79	80	81	81
	99th	125	125	126	128	129	130	131	85	85	86	87	87	88	89
12	50th	102	103	104	105	107	108	109	61	61	61	62	63	64	64
	90th	116	116	117	119	120	121	122	75	75	75	76	77	78	78
	95th	119	120	121	123	124	125	126	79	79	79	80	81	82	82
	99th	127	127	128	130	131	132	133	86	86	87	88	88	89	90

Continued

TABLE 4-24 **Blood Pressure Levels for Girls by Age and Height Percentile** *(Continued)*

		Systolic BP, mm Hg							Diastolic BP, mm Hg						
		PERCENTILE OF HEIGHT							PERCENTILE OF HEIGHT						
Age (yr)	**BP Percentile**	**5th**	**10th**	**25th**	**50th**	**75th**	**90th**	**95th**	**5th**	**10th**	**25th**	**50th**	**75th**	**90th**	**95th**
13	50th	104	105	106	107	109	110	110	62	62	62	63	64	65	65
	90th	117	118	119	121	122	123	124	76	76	76	77	78	79	79
	95th	121	122	123	124	126	127	128	80	80	80	81	82	83	83
	99th	128	129	130	132	133	134	135	87	87	88	89	89	90	91
14	50th	106	106	107	109	110	111	112	63	63	63	64	65	66	66
	90th	119	120	121	122	124	125	125	77	77	77	78	79	80	80
	95th	123	123	125	126	127	129	129	81	81	81	82	83	84	84
	99th	130	131	132	133	135	136	136	88	88	89	90	90	91	92
15	50th	107	108	109	110	111	113	113	64	64	64	65	66	67	67
	90th	120	121	122	123	125	126	127	78	78	78	79	80	81	81
	95th	124	125	126	127	129	130	131	82	82	82	83	84	85	85
	99th	131	132	133	134	136	137	138	89	89	90	91	91	92	93
16	50th	108	108	110	111	112	114	114	64	64	65	66	66	67	68
	90th	121	122	123	124	126	127	128	78	78	79	80	81	81	82
	95th	125	126	127	128	130	131	132	82	82	83	84	85	85	86
	99th	132	133	134	135	137	138	139	90	90	90	91	92	93	93
17	50th	108	109	110	111	113	114	115	64	65	65	66	67	67	68
	90th	122	122	123	125	126	127	128	78	79	79	80	81	81	82
	95th	125	126	127	129	130	131	132	82	83	83	84	85	85	86
	99th	133	133	134	136	137	138	139	90	90	91	91	92	93	93

The 90th percentile is 1.28 SD, the 95th percentile is 1.645 SD, and the 99th percentile is 2.326 SD over the mean.

For research purposes, the SDs in Table B1 allow one to compute BP Z scores and percentiles for girls with height percentiles given in Table 4 (ie, the 5th, 10th, 25th, 50th, 75th, 90th, and 95th percentiles). These height percentiles must be converted to height Z scores given by: 5% = −1.645; 10% = −1.28; 25% = −0.68; 50% = 0; 75% = 0.68; 90% = 1.28; and 95% = 1.645 and then computed according to the methodology in steps 2 through 4 described in Appendix B. For children with height percentiles other than these, follow steps 1 through 4 as described in Appendix B.

The 4th Report on the Diagnosis, Evaluation, and Treatment of High Blood Pressure in Children and Adolescents. National High Blood Pressure Education Program Working Group on High Blood Pressure in Children and Adolescents. *Pediatrics* 114:555–576, 2004.

TABLE 4-25 Blood Pressure Levels for Boys by Age and Height Percentile

		Systolic BP, mm Hg							Diastolic BP, mm Hg						
		PERCENTILE OF HEIGHT							PERCENTILE OF HEIGHT						
Age (yr)	**BP Percentile**	**50th**	**10th**	**25th**	**50th**	**75th**	**90th**	**95th**	**5th**	**10th**	**25th**	**50th**	**75th**	**90th**	**95th**
1	50th	80	81	83	85	87	88	89	34	35	36	37	38	39	39
	90th	94	95	97	99	100	102	103	49	50	51	52	53	53	54
	95th	98	99	101	103	104	106	106	54	54	55	56	57	58	58
	99th	105	106	108	110	112	113	114	61	62	63	64	65	66	66
2	50th	84	85	87	88	90	92	92	39	40	41	42	43	44	44
	90th	97	99	100	102	104	105	106	54	55	56	57	58	58	59
	95th	101	102	104	106	108	109	110	59	59	60	61	62	63	63
	99th	109	110	111	113	115	117	117	66	67	68	69	70	71	71
3	50th	86	87	89	91	93	94	95	44	44	45	46	47	48	48
	90th	100	101	103	105	107	108	109	59	59	60	61	62	63	63
	95th	104	105	107	109	110	112	113	63	63	64	65	66	67	67
	99th	111	112	114	116	118	119	120	71	71	72	73	74	75	75
4	50th	88	89	91	93	95	96	97	47	48	49	50	51	51	52
	90th	102	103	105	107	109	110	111	62	63	64	65	66	66	67
	95th	106	107	109	111	112	114	115	66	67	68	69	70	71	71
	99th	113	114	116	118	120	121	122	74	75	76	77	78	78	79
5	50th	90	91	93	95	96	98	98	50	51	52	53	54	55	55
	90th	104	105	106	108	110	111	112	65	66	67	68	69	69	70
	95th	108	109	110	112	114	115	116	69	70	71	72	73	74	74
	99th	115	116	118	120	121	123	123	77	78	79	80	81	81	82
6	50th	91	92	94	96	98	99	100	53	53	54	55	56	57	57
	90th	105	106	108	110	111	113	113	68	68	69	70	71	72	72
	95th	109	110	112	114	115	117	117	72	72	73	74	75	76	76
	99th	116	117	119	121	123	124	125	80	80	81	82	83	84	84
7	50th	92	94	95	97	99	100	101	55	55	56	57	58	59	59
	90th	106	107	109	111	113	114	115	70	70	71	72	73	74	74
	95th	110	111	113	115	117	118	119	74	74	75	76	77	78	78
	99th	117	118	120	122	124	125	126	82	82	83	84	85	86	86
8	50th	94	95	97	99	100	102	102	56	57	58	59	60	60	61
	90th	107	109	110	112	114	115	116	71	72	72	73	74	75	76
	95th	111	112	114	116	118	119	120	75	76	77	78	79	79	80
	99th	119	120	122	123	125	127	127	83	84	85	86	87	87	88
9	50th	95	96	98	100	102	103	104	57	58	59	60	61	61	62
	90th	109	110	112	114	115	117	118	72	73	74	75	76	76	77
	95th	113	114	116	118	119	121	121	76	77	78	79	80	81	81
	99th	120	121	123	125	127	128	129	84	85	86	87	88	88	89
10	50th	97	98	100	102	103	105	106	58	59	60	61	61	62	63
	90th	111	112	114	115	117	119	119	73	73	74	75	76	77	78
	95th	115	116	117	119	121	122	123	77	78	79	80	81	81	82
	99th	122	123	125	127	128	130	130	85	86	86	88	88	89	90
11	50th	99	100	102	104	105	107	107	59	59	60	61	62	63	63
	90th	113	114	115	117	119	120	121	74	74	75	76	77	78	78
	95th	117	118	119	121	123	124	125	78	78	79	80	81	82	82
	99th	124	125	127	129	130	132	132	86	86	87	88	89	90	90
12	50th	101	102	104	106	108	109	110	59	60	61	62	63	63	64
	90th	115	116	118	120	121	123	123	74	75	75	76	77	78	79
	95th	119	120	122	123	125	127	127	78	79	80	81	82	82	83
	99th	126	127	129	131	133	134	135	86	87	88	89	90	90	91

Continued

TABLE 4-25 **Blood Pressure Levels for Boys by Age and Height Percentile** *(Continued)*

		Systolic BP, mm Hg							Diastolic BP, mm Hg						
		PERCENTILE OF HEIGHT							PERCENTILE OF HEIGHT						
Age (yr)	**BP Percentile**	**50th**	**10th**	**25th**	**50th**	**75th**	**90th**	**95th**	**5th**	**10th**	**25th**	**50th**	**75th**	**90th**	**95th**
13	50th	104	105	106	108	110	111	112	60	60	61	62	63	64	64
	90th	117	118	120	122	124	125	126	75	75	76	77	78	79	79
	95th	121	122	124	126	128	129	130	79	79	80	81	82	83	83
	99th	128	130	131	133	135	136	137	87	87	88	89	90	91	91
14	50th	106	107	109	111	113	114	115	60	61	62	63	64	65	65
	90th	120	121	123	125	126	128	128	75	76	77	78	79	79	80
	95th	124	125	127	128	130	132	132	80	80	81	82	83	84	84
	99th	131	132	134	136	138	139	140	87	88	89	90	91	92	92
15	50th	109	110	112	113	115	117	117	61	62	63	64	65	66	66
	90th	122	124	125	127	129	130	131	76	77	78	79	80	80	81
	95th	126	127	129	131	133	134	135	81	81	82	83	84	85	85
	99th	134	135	136	138	140	142	142	88	89	90	91	92	93	93
16	50th	111	112	114	116	118	119	120	63	63	64	65	66	67	67
	90th	125	126	128	130	131	133	134	78	78	79	80	81	82	82
	95th	129	130	132	134	135	137	137	82	83	83	84	85	86	87
	99th	136	137	139	141	143	144	145	90	90	91	92	93	94	94
17	50th	114	115	116	118	120	121	122	65	66	66	67	68	69	70
	90th	127	128	130	132	134	135	136	80	80	81	82	83	84	84
	95th	131	132	134	136	138	139	140	84	85	86	87	87	88	89
	99th	139	140	141	143	145	146	147	92	93	93	94	95	96	97

The 90th percentile is 1.28 SD, the 95th percentile is 1.645 SD, and the 99th percentile is 2.326 SD over the mean.

For research purposes, the SDs in Table B1 allow one to compute BP Z scores and percentiles for boys with height percentiles given in Table 3 (ie, the 5th, 10th, 25th, 50th, 75th, 90th, and 95th percentiles). These height percentiles must be converted to height Z scores given by: 5% = −1.645; 10% = −1.28; 25% = −0.68; 50% = 0; 75% = 0.68; 90% = 1.28; and 95% = 1.645, and then computed according to the methodology in steps 2 through 4 described in Appendix B. For children with height percentiles other than these, follow steps 1 through 4 as described in Appendix B.

The 4th Report on the Diagnosis, Evaluation, and Treatment of High Blood Pressure in Children and Adolescents. National High Blood Pressure Education Program Working Group on High Blood Pressure in Children and Adolescents. *Pediatrics* 114:555–576, 2004.

Section V

Prevention

PART A • Adolescent

Routine Adolescent Health Visit

CONTENT FOR ROUTINE ADOLESCENT HEALTH VISIT*

- **MEDICAL HISTORY:** Immunizations, chronic illness, chronic medications (including hormonal contraception), recent dental care, hospitializations, surgeries
- **FAMILY HISTORY:** Psychiatric disorders, suicide, alcoholism/substance abuse
- REVIEW OF SYSTEMS
  - **Dietary habits:** Typical foods consumed, types and frequency of meals skipped, vomiting, use of laxatives or other weight-loss methods, dietary sources of calcium
  - **Recent weight gain or loss**
- PSYCHOSOCIAL/MEDICOSOCIAL HISTORY (HEADSS)
  - **H(ome)**
    - Household composition
    - Family dynamics and relationships with adolescent
    - Living/sleeping arrangements
    - Guns in the home
  - **E(ducation)**
    - School attendance/absences
    - Ever failed a grade(s)? Grades as compared to last year's
    - Attitude toward school
    - Favorite, most difficult, best subjects
    - Special educational needs
    - Goals: Vocational/technical school, college, career
  - **A(ctivities)**
    - Physical activity, exercise, hobbies
    - Sports participation
    - Job
    - Weapon carrying and fighting
  - **D(rugs)**
    - Cigarettes/smokeless tobacco: Age at first use, packs per day
    - Alcohol and/or other drugs: Use at school or parties; use by friends, self; kind (i.e., beer, wine coolers), frequency, and quantity used. If yes, CAGE: Have you ever felt the need to **C**ut down; have others **A**nnoyed you by commenting on your use; have you ever felt **G**uilty about your use; have you ever needed an **E**yeopener (alcohol first thing in the morning)?
  - **S(exuality)**
    - Sexual feelings: Opposite or same sex
    - Sexual intercourse: Age at first intercourse, number of lifetime and current partners, recent change in partners
    - Contraception/sexually transmitted disease (STD) prevention
    - History of STDs
    - Prior pregnancies, abortions; ever fathered a child?
    - History of/current nonconsensual intimate physical contact/sex
  - **S(uicide)/depression**
    - Feelings about self: Positive and negative
    - History of depression or other mental health problems, prior suicidal thoughts, prior suicide attempts
    - Sleep problems: Difficulty getting to sleep, early waking
- PHYSICAL EXAMINATION (MOST PERTINENT ASPECTS)
  - **Skin:** Acne (type and distribution of lesions)
  - **Thyroid**
  - **Spine:** Scoliosis (see p. 812 for assessment and treatment)
  - **Breasts:** Tanner stage, masses
  - **External genitalia**
    - Pubic hair distribution: Tanner stage
    - Testicular examination: Tanner stage, masses
  - **Pelvic examination:** Sexually active, gynecologic compliant
- LABORATORY TESTS
  - **Purified protein derivative (PPD):** If high risk
  - **Hemoglobin/hematocrit:** Once during puberty for boys, once after menarche for girls.
  - **Sexually active adolescents:** Serologic tests for syphilis annually; offer HIV testing, especially if syphilis or other ulcerative genital disease.
    - Males: First part voided urinalysis/leukocyte esterase screen with positive results confirmed by detection tests for gonorrhea and chlamydia (i.e., cultures, ligase/polymerase chain reaction)
    - Females: Detection tests for gonorrhea and chlamydia (i.e., cultures, LCR/PCR), wet preparation, potassium hydroxide (KOH), cervical Gram stain, Papanicolaou smear, midvaginal pH
- IMMUNIZATIONS
  - **Tetanus, diptheria, and acellular pertussis (Tdap):** Booster age 11-15 years
  - **Measles:** Two doses of live attenuated vaccine are required after first birthday. Use measles, mumps, rubella (MMR) vaccine if not previously immunized for mumps or rubella. Assess pregnancy status, and do not administer rubella vaccine to woman anticipating pregnancy within 90 days.
  - **Hepatitis B vaccine:** Recommended for all adolescents (three doses) if not previously vaccinated.
  - **Varicella vaccine:** Two doses at least 1 month apart are recommended for adolescents $\geq$13 years old with no history of disease.
  - **HPV:** Human papilloma virus vaccine is now recommended for all girls after 9 to 11 years
- ANTICIPATORY GUIDANCE
  - **Sexuality** (e.g., abstinence, STD/pregnancy prevention)
  - **Nutrition:** Excessive/inadequate calories, balanced diet, calcium
  - **Coping skills/violence prevention**
  - **Safety:** Driving/seat belts, guns, bicycle helmets
  - **Substance abuse prevention**

*From Straub DM: Adolescent medicine. *In* Siberry GK, Iannone R (eds): *The Harriet Lane Handbook: A Manual for Pediatric House Officers,* 15th ed. St Louis, Mosby, 2000.

Recommended Childhood and Adolescent Immunization Schedule

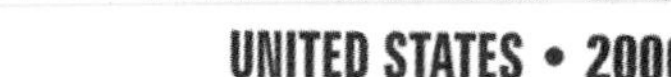

UNITED STATES • 2006

CDC

Vaccine ▼ / Age ▶	Birth	1 month	2 months	4 months	6 months	12 months	15 months	18 months	24 months	4–6 years	11–12 years	13–14 years	15 years	16–18 years
Hepatitis B[1]	HepB	HepB		*HepB[1]*		HepB					HepB Series			
Diphtheria, Tetanus, Pertussis[2]			DTaP	DTaP	DTaP		DTaP			DTaP	Tdap		Tdap	
Haemophilus influenzae type b[3]			Hib	Hib	*Hib[3]*	Hib								
Inactivated Poliovirus			IPV	IPV		IPV				IPV				
Measles, Mumps, Rubella[4]						MMR				MMR			MMR	
Varicella[5]							Varicella				Varicella			
Meningococcal[6]							Vaccines within broken line are for selected populations		MPSV4		MCV4		MCV4 / MCV4	
Pneumococcal[7]			PCV	PCV	PCV	PCV			PCV		PPV			
Influenza[8]						Influenza (Yearly)					Influenza (Yearly)			
Hepatitis A[9]										HepA Series				

This schedule indicates the recommended ages for routine administration of currently licensed childhood vaccines, as of December 1, 2005, for children through age 18 years. Any dose not administered at the recommended age should be administered at any subsequent visit when indicated and feasible. ▬ Indicates age groups that warrant special effort to administer those vaccines not previously administered. Additional vaccines may be licensed and recommended during the year. Licensed combination vaccines may be used whenever any components of the combination are indicated and other components of the vaccine are not contraindicated and if approved by the Food and Drug Administration for that dose of the series. Providers should consult the respective ACIP statement for detailed recommendations. Clinically significant adverse events that follow immunization should be reported to the Vaccine Adverse Event Reporting System (VAERS). Guidance about how to obtain and complete a VAERS form is available at www.vaers.hhs.gov or by telephone, 800-822-7967.

Range of recommended ages | Catch-up immunization | 11–12 year old assessment

1. **Hepatitis B vaccine (HepB).** ***AT BIRTH:*** **All newborns** should receive monovalent HepB soon after birth and before hospital discharge. **Infants born to mothers who are HBsAg-positive** should receive HepB and 0.5 mL of hepatitis B immune globulin (HBIG) within 12 hours of birth. **Infants born to mothers whose HBsAg status is unknown** should receive HepB within 12 hours of birth. The mother should have blood drawn as soon as possible to determine her HBsAg status; if HBsAg-positive, the infant should receive HBIG as soon as possible (no later than age 1 week). **For infants born to HBsAg-negative mothers**, the birth dose can be delayed in rare circumstances but only if a physician's order to withhold the vaccine and a copy of the mother's original HBsAg-negative laboratory report are documented in the infant's medical record. ***FOLLOWING THE BIRTHDOSE:*** The HepB series should be completed with either monovalent HepB or a combination vaccine containing HepB. The second dose should be administered at age 1–2 months. The final dose should be administered at age $\geq$24 weeks. It is permissible to administer 4 doses of HepB (e.g., when combination vaccines are given after the birth dose); however, if monovalent HepB is used, a dose at age 4 months is not needed. **Infants born to HBsAg-positive mothers** should be tested for HBsAg and antibody to HBsAg after completion of the HepB series, at age 9–18 months (generally at the next well-child visit after completion of the vaccine series).
2. **Diphtheria and tetanus toxoids and acellular pertussis vaccine (DTaP).** The fourth dose of DTaP may be administered as early as age 12 months, provided 6 months have elapsed since the third dose and the child is unlikely to return at age 15–18 months. The final dose in the series should be given at age $\geq$4 years.

   Tetanus and diphtheria toxoids and acellular pertussis vaccine (Tdap – adolescent preparation) is recommended at age 11–12 years for those who have completed the recommended childhood DTP/DTaP vaccination series and have not received a Td booster dose. Adolescents 13–18 years who missed the 11–12-year Td/Tdap booster dose should also receive a single dose of Tdap if they have completed the recommended childhood DTP/DTaP vaccination series. Subsequent **tetanus and diphtheria toxoids (Td)** are recommended every 10 years.
3. ***Haemophilus influenzae*** **type b conjugate vaccine (Hib).** Three Hib conjugate vaccines are licensed for infant use. If PRP-OMP (PedvaxHIB® or ComVax® [Merck]) is administered at ages 2 and 4 months, a dose at age 6 months is not required. DTaP/Hib combination products should not be used for primary immunization in infants at ages 2, 4 or 6 months but can be used as boosters after any Hib vaccine. The final dose in the series should be administered at age $\geq$12 months.
4. **Measles, mumps, and rubella vaccine (MMR).** The second dose of MMR is recommended routinely at age 4–6 years but may be administered during any visit, provided at least 4 weeks have elapsed since the first dose and both doses are administered beginning at or after age 12 months. Those who have not previously received the second dose should complete the schedule by age 11–12 years.
5. **Varicella vaccine.** Varicella vaccine is recommended at any visit at or after age 12 months for susceptible children (i.e., those who lack a reliable history of chickenpox). Susceptible persons aged $\geq$13 years should receive 2 doses administered at least 4 weeks apart.
6. **Meningococcal vaccine (MCV4).** Meningococcal conjugate vaccine (MCV4) should be given to all children at the 11–12 year old visit as well as to unvaccinated adolescents at high school entry (15 years of age). Other adolescents who wish to decrease their risk for meningococcal disease may also be vaccinated. All college freshmen living in dormitories should also be vaccinated, preferably with MCV4, although **meningococcal polysaccharide vaccine (MPSV4)** is an acceptable alternative. Vaccination against invasive meningococcal disease is recommended for children and adolescents aged $\geq$2 years with terminal complement deficiencies or anatomic or functional asplenia and certain other high risk groups (see *MMWR* 2005;54 [RR-7]:1-21); use MPSV4 for children aged 2–10 years and MCV4 for older children, although MPSV4 is an acceptable alternative.
7. **Pneumococcal vaccine.** The heptavalent **pneumococcal conjugate vaccine (PCV)** is recommended for all children aged 2–23 months and for certain children aged 24–59 months. The final dose in the series should be given at age $\geq$12 months. **Pneumococcal polysaccharide vaccine (PPV)** is recommended in addition to PCV for certain high-risk groups. See *MMWR* 2000; 49(RR-9):1-35.
8. **Influenza vaccine.** Influenza vaccine is recommended annually for children aged $\geq$6 months with certain risk factors (including, but not limited to, asthma, cardiac disease, sickle cell disease, human immunodeficiency virus [HIV], diabetes, and conditions that can compromise respiratory function or handling of respiratory secretions or that can increase the risk for aspiration), healthcare workers, and other persons (including household members) in close contact with persons in groups at high risk (see *MMWR* 2005;54[RR-8]:1-55). In addition, healthy children aged 6–23 months and close contacts of healthy children aged 0–5 months are recommended to receive influenza vaccine because children in this age group are at substantially increased risk for influenza-related hospitalizations. For healthy persons aged 5–49 years, the intranasally administered, live, attenuated influenza vaccine (LAIV) is an acceptable alternative to the intramuscular trivalent inactivated influenza vaccine (TIV). See *MMWR* 2005;54(RR-8):1-55. Children receiving TIV should be administered a dosage appropriate for their age (0.25 mL if aged 6–35 months or 0.5 mL if aged $\geq$3 years). Children aged $\leq$8 years who are receiving influenza vaccine for the first time should receive 2 doses (separated by at least 4 weeks for TIV and at least 6 weeks for LAIV).
9. **Hepatitis A vaccine (HepA).** HepA is recommended for all children at 1 year of age (i.e., 12–23 months). The 2 doses in the series should be administered at least 6 months apart. States, counties, and communities with existing HepA vaccination programs for children 2–18 years of age are encouraged to maintain these programs. In these areas, new efforts focused on routine vaccination of 1-year-old children should enhance, not replace, ongoing programs directed at a broader population of children. HepA is also recommended for certain high risk groups (see *MMWR* 1999; 48[RR-12]1-37).

The Childhood and Adolescent Immunization Schedule is approved by:
Advisory Committee on Immunization Practices www.cdc.gov/nip/acip • American Academy of Pediatrics www.aap.org • American Academy of Family Physicians www.aafp.org

FIGURE 5-1 Recommended childhood and adolescent immunization schedule, 2006.

Recommended Immunization Schedule for Children and Adolescents Who Start Late or Who Are More Than 1 Month Behind

UNITED STATES • 2006

The tables below give catch-up schedules and minimum intervals between doses for children who have delayed immunizations. There is no need to restart a vaccine series regardless of the time that has elapsed between doses. Use the chart appropriate for the child's age.

CATCH-UP SCHEDULE FOR CHILDREN AGED 4 MONTHS THROUGH 6 YEARS

Vaccine	Minimum Age for Dose 1	Minimum Interval Between Doses			
		Dose 1 to Dose 2	Dose 2 to Dose 3	Dose 3 to Dose 4	Dose 4 to Dose 5
Diphtheria, Tetanus, Pertussis	6 wks	4 weeks	4 weeks	6 months	6 months[1]
Inactivated Poliovirus	6 wks	4 weeks	4 weeks	4 weeks[2]	
Hepatitis B[3]	Birth	4 weeks	8 weeks (and 16 weeks after first dose)		
Measles, Mumps, Rubella	12 mo	4 weeks[4]			
Varicella	12 mo				
Haemophilus influenzae type b[5]	6 wks	**4 weeks** if first dose given at age <12 months **8 weeks (as final dose)** if first dose given at age 12-14 months **No further doses needed** if first dose given at age ≥15 months	**4 weeks[6]** if current age <12 months **8 weeks (as final dose)[6]** if current age ≥12 months and second dose given at age <15 months **No further doses needed** if previous dose given at age ≥15 mo	**8 weeks (as final dose)** This dose only necessary for children aged 12 months–5 years who received 3 doses before age 12 months	
Pneumococcal[7]	6 wks	**4 weeks** if first dose given at age <12 months and current age <24 months **8 weeks (as final dose)** if first dose given at age ≥12 months or current age 24–59 months **No further doses needed** for healthy children if first dose given at age ≥24 months	**4 weeks** if current age <12 months **8 weeks (as final dose)** if current age ≥12 months **No further doses needed** for healthy children if previous dose given at age ≥24 months	**8 weeks (as final dose)** This dose only necessary for children aged 12 months–5 years who received 3 doses before age 12 months	

CATCH-UP SCHEDULE FOR CHILDREN AGED 7 YEARS THROUGH 18 YEARS

Vaccine	Minimum Interval Between Doses		
	Dose 1 to Dose 2	Dose 2 to Dose 3	Dose 3 to Booster Dose
Tetanus, Diphtheria[8]	4 weeks	6 months	**6 months** if first dose given at age <12 months and current age <11 years; otherwise **5 years**
Inactivated Poliovirus[9]	4 weeks	4 weeks	IPV[2,9]
Hepatitis B	4 weeks	8 weeks (and 16 weeks after first dose)	
Measles, Mumps, Rubella	4 weeks		
Varicella[10]	4 weeks		

1. **DTaP.** The fifth dose is not necessary if the fourth dose was administered after the fourth birthday.
2. **IPV.** For children who received an all-IPV or all-oral poliovirus (OPV) series, a fourth dose is not necessary if third dose was administered at age ≥4 years. If both OPV and IPV were administered as part of a series, a total of 4 doses should be given, regardless of the child's current age.
3. **HepB.** Administer the 3-dose series to all children and adolescents <19 years of age if they were not previously vaccinated.
4. **MMR.** The second dose of MMR is recommended routinely at age 4–6 years but may be administered earlier if desired.
5. **Hib.** Vaccine is not generally recommended for children aged ≥5 years.
6. **Hib.** If current age <12 months and the first 2 doses were PRP-OMP (PedvaxHIB® or ComVax® [Merck]), the third (and final) dose should be administered at age 12–15 months and at least 8 weeks after the second dose.
7. **PCV.** Vaccine is not generally recommended for children aged ≥5 years.
8. **Td.** Adolescent tetanus, diphtheria, and pertussis vaccine (Tdap) may be substituted for any dose in a primary catch-up series or as a booster if age appropriate for Tdap. A five-year interval from the last Td dose is encouraged when Tdap is used as a booster dose. See ACIP recommendations for further information.
9. **IPV.** Vaccine is not generally recommended for persons aged ≥18 years.
10. **Varicella.** Administer the 2-dose series to all susceptible adolescents aged ≥13 years.

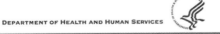

DEPARTMENT OF HEALTH AND HUMAN SERVICES

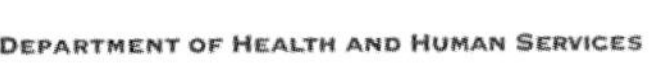

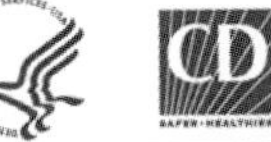

CENTERS FOR DISEASE CONTROL AND PREVENTION

Report adverse reactions to vaccines through the federal Vaccine Adverse Event Reporting System. For information on reporting reactions following immunization, please visit www.vaers.hhs.gov or call the 24-hour national toll-free information line 800-822-7967. Report suspected cases of vaccine-preventable diseases to your state or local health department.

For additional information about vaccines, including precautions and contraindications for immunization and vaccine shortages, please visit the National Immunization Program Website at www.cdc.gov/nip or contact 800-CDC-INFO (800-232-4636) (In English, En Español — 24/7)

FIGURE 5-2 Recommended immunization schedule for children/adolescents who start late or who are more than 1 month behind, 2006.

TABLE 5-1 Schedule for Catch-Up Administration of Pneumococcal Conjugate Vaccine (Prevnar) in Unvaccinated Infants and Children

Age at First Dose	Primary Series	Booster Dose
2-6 mo	Three doses, 2 mo apart*	One dose at 12-15 mo†
7-11 mo	Two doses, 2 mo apart*	One dose at 12-15 mo†
12-23 mo	Two doses, 2 mo apart	—
24-59 mo		
Healthy children	One dose	—
Children with sickle cell disease, asplenia, human immunodeficiency virus (HIV) infection, chronic illness, or immunocompromising condition‡	Two doses, 2 mo apart	—

*For the primary series in children vaccinated before they are 12 months old, the minimum interval between doses is 4 weeks.
†The booster dose should be administered at least 8 weeks after the primary series is completed.
‡Recommendations do not include children who have undergone bone marrow transplantation.
Adapted from Centers for Disease Control and Prevention (CDC): Preventing pneumococcal disease among infants and young children. *MMWR Morb Mortal Wkly Rep* 49(RR-9):24, 2000.

TABLE 5-2 Administration Schedule for Pneumococcal Conjugate Vaccine (Prevnar) When a Lapse in Immunization Has Occurred

Age at Presentation	Pneumococcal Conjugate Vaccine Immunization History	Recommended Regimen
7-11 mo	One dose	One dose at 7 to 11 mo, followed by a booster at 12 to 15 mo with a minimal interval of 2 mo
	Two doses	One dose at 7 to 11 mo, followed by a booster at 12 to 15 mo with a minimal interval of 2 mo
12-23 mo	One dose before 12 mo	Two doses at least 2 mo apart
	Two doses before 12 mo	One dose at least 2 mo after the most recent dose
24-59 mo	Any incomplete schedule	One dose*

*Children with certain chronic illnesses or immunosuppressing conditions should receive two doses at least 2 months apart.
Adapted from Centers for Disease Control and Prevention (CDC): Recommendations of the Advisory Committee on Immunization Practices (ACIP). *MMWR Morb Mortal Wkly Rep* 49(RR-9):24, 2000.

TABLE 5-3 Using Pneumococcal Polysaccharide Vaccine in High-Risk Children 2 Years and Older Who Have Been Immunized with Pneumococcal Conjugate Vaccine (Prevnar)

Health Status	PPV Schedule	Revaccinate with PPV
Healthy	None	No
Sickle cell disease, anatomic or functional asplenia, HIV infection, immunocompromising conditions	One dose of PPV given at least 2 mo after PCV	Yes*
Chronic illness	One dose of PPV given at least 2 mo after PCV	No

HIV, human immunodeficiency virus; PCV, pneumococcal conjugate vaccine; PPV, pneumococcal polysaccharide vaccine.
*If patient is older than 10 years, a single revaccination should be given at least 5 years after the previous dose; if patient is 10 years or younger, revaccinate 3 to 5 years after the previous dose. Regardless of when the vaccine is administered, a second dose of PPV should not be given less than 3 years after the previous PPV dose.
Adapted from Centers for Disease Control and Prevention (CDC). *MMWR Morb Mortal Wkly Rep* 49(RR-9):24, 2000.

TABLE 5-4 **Guide to Contraindications and Precautions for Commonly Used Vaccines**

Vaccine	True Contraindications and Precautions*	Vaccines Can Be Administered
For all vaccines	Contraindications[†] Serious allergic reaction (e.g., anaphylaxis) after a previous vaccine dose Serious allergic reaction (e.g., anaphylaxis) to a vaccine component Precautions[‡] Moderate or severe acute illness with or without fever	Mild acute illness with or without fever Mild to moderate local reaction (i.e., swelling, redness, soreness); low-grade or moderate fever after previous dose Lack of previous physical examination for well-appearing person Current antimicrobial therapy Convalescent phase of illness Premature birth (hepatitis B vaccine is an exception in certain circumstances)[§] Recent exposure to an infectious disease History of penicillin allergy, other nonvaccine allergies, relative with allergies, receiving allergen extract immunotherapy
Diphtheria, tetanus toxoids, and acellular pertussis vaccine (DTaP)	Contraindications Severe allergic reaction after a previous dose or to a vaccine component Encephalopathy (e.g., coma, decreased level of consciousness, prolonged seizures) within 7 days of administration of previous dose of DTP or DTaP Progressive neurologic disorder, including infantile spasms, uncontrolled epilepsy, progressive encephalopathy; defer DTaP until neurologic status clarified and stabilized Precautions Fever of >40.5°C ≤48 hours after vaccination with a previous dose of DTP or DTaP Collapse or shocklike state (i.e., hypotonic hyporesponsive episode) Duration ≤48 hours after receiving a previous dose of DTP or DTaP Seizure ≤3 days of receiving a previous dose of DTP/DTaP[‖] Persistent, inconsolable crying lasting ≤48 hours after receiving a previous dose of DTP or DTaP Moderate or severe acute illness with or without fever	Temperature <40.5° C, fussiness or mild drowsiness after a previous dose of diphtheria toxoid–tetanus toxoid–pertussis vaccine (DTP) or DTaP Family history of seizures[‖] Family history of sudden infant death syndrome Family history of an adverse event after DTP or DTaP administration Stable neurologic conditions (e.g., cerebral palsy, well-controlled convulsions, developmental delay)
Pediatric diphtheria-tetanus toxoid (DT); adult tetanus-diphtheria toxoid (Td)	Contraindications Severe allergic reaction after a previous dose or to a vaccine component Precautions Guillain-Barré syndrome ≤6 weeks after previous dose of tetanus toxoid–containing vaccine Moderate or severe acute illness with or without fever	
Inactivated poliovirus vaccine (IPV)	Contraindications Severe allergic reaction to previous dose or vaccine component Precautions Pregnancy Moderate or severe acute illness with or without fever	
Measles-mumps-rubella vaccine (MMR[#])	Contraindications Severe allergic reaction to previous dose or vaccine component Pregnancy Known severe immunodeficiency (e.g., hematologic and solid tumors, congenital immunodeficiency, long-term immunosuppressive therapy** or severely symptomatic human immunodeficiency virus [HIV] infection) Precautions Recent (≤11 months) receipt of antibody-containing blood product (specific interval depends on product) History of thrombocytopenia or thrombocytopenic purpura Moderate or severe acute illness with or without fever	Positive tuberculin skin test Simultaneous TB skin testing[††] Breastfeeding Pregnancy of recipient's mother or other close or household contact Recipient is child-bearing-age female Immunodeficient family member or household contact Asymptomatic or mildly symptomatic HIV infection Allergy to eggs

Continued on following page

TABLE 5-4 **Guide to Contraindications and Precautions for Commonly Used Vaccines** *(Continued)*

Vaccine	True Contraindications and Precautions*	Vaccines Can Be Administered
Haemophilus influenzae type b vaccine (Hib)	Contraindications Severe allergic reaction to previous dose or vaccine component Age <6 weeks Precautions Moderate or severe acute illness with or without fever	
Hepatitis B	Contraindications Severe allergic reaction to previous dose or vaccine component Precautions Infant weighing <2000 g Moderate or severe acute illness with or without fever	Pregnancy Autoimmune disease (e.g., systemic lupus erythematosus, rheumatoid arthritis)
Hepatitis A	Contraindications Severe allergic reaction to previous dose or vaccine component Precautions Pregnancy Moderate or severe acute illness with or without fever	
Varicella[@]	Contraindications Severe allergic reaction to previous dose or vaccine component Substantial suppression of cellular immunity Pregnancy Precautions Recent (≤11 months) receipt of antibody-containing blood product (specific interval depends on product) Moderate or severe acute illness with or without fever	Pregnancy of recipient's mother or other close or household contact Immunodeficient family member or household contact[‡‡] Asymptomatic or mildly symptomatic HIV infection Humoral immunodeficiency (e.g., agammaglobulinemia)
Pneumococcal conjugate vaccine (PCV)	Contraindications Severe allergic reaction to previous dose or vaccine component Precautions Moderate or severe acute illness with or without fever	
Influenza	Contraindications Severe allergic reaction to previous dose or vaccine component, including egg protein Precautions Moderate or severe acute illness with or without fever	Nonsevere (e.g., contact) allergy to latex or thimerosal Concurrent administration of Coumadin or aminophylline
Pneumococcal polysaccharide vaccine (PPV)	Contraindications Severe allergic reaction to previous dose or vaccine component Precautions Moderate or severe acute illness with or without fever	

*Events or conditions listed as precautions should be reviewed carefully. Benefits and risks of administering a specific vaccine to a person under these circumstances should be considered. If the risk from the vaccine is believed to outweigh the benefit, the vaccine should not be administered. If the benefit of vaccination is believed to outweigh the risk, the vaccine should be administered. Whether and when to administer DTaP to children with proven or suspected underlying neurologic disorders should be decided on a case-by-case basis.

†A contraindication is a condition in a recipient that increases the risk for a serious adverse reaction. A vaccine is not administered when a contraindication exists. For a full definition and examples, consult the Centers for Disease Control and Prevention (CDC): Vaccine side effects, adverse reactions, contraindications, and precautions: recommendations of the advisory committee on immunization practices (ACIP). *MMWR Morb Wkly Rep* 45 (RR12):1–42, 1996.

‡A precaution is a condition in a recipient that may increase the risk for a serious adverse reaction or that may compromise the ability of the vaccine to produce immunity. Injury may result, or a person may experience a more severe reaction to the vaccine than otherwise expected; however, the risk for this happening is less than expected with a contraindication. Under normal circumstances, vaccinations should be deferred when a precaution is identified. However, vaccination may be indicated in the presence of a precaution because the benefit of protection from the vaccine outweighs the risk for an adverse reaction. For a full definition and examples, consult the Centers for Disease Control and Prevention (CDC): Vaccine side effects, adverse reactions, contraindications, and precautions: recommendations of the advisory committee on immunization practices (ACIP). *MMWR Morb Wkly Rep* 45 (RR12):1–42, 1996.

§Hepatitis B vaccination should be deferred for infants weighing less than 2000 g if the mother is documented to be negative for hepatitis B surface antigen (HBsAg) at the time of the infant's birth. Vaccination can commence at the chronologic age of 1 month. For infants born to HBsAg-positive women, hepatitis B immunoglobulin and hepatitis B vaccine should be administered at or soon after birth, regardless of weight. Consult the Centers for Disease Control and Prevention (CDC): Vaccine side effects, adverse reactions, contraindications, and precautions: recommendations of the advisory committee on immunization practices (ACIP). *MMWR Morb Wkly Rep* 45 (RR12):1–42, 1996.

‖Acetominophen or another appropriate antipyretic can be administered to children with a personal or family history of seizures at the time of DTaP vaccination and every 4 to 6 hours for 24 hours thereafter to reduce the possibility of fever after vaccination. (Data from American Academy of Pediatrics: Active immunization. *In* Pickering LK (ed): *2000 Red Book: Report of the Committee on Infectious Diseases*, 25th ed. Elk Grove Village, IL, American Academy of Pediatrics, 2000).

#MMR and varicella vaccines can be administered on the same day. If not administered on the same day, these vaccines should be separated by ≥28 days.

**Substantially immunosuppressive steroid dose is considered to be more than 2 weeks of daily receipt of 20 mg or 2 mg/kg body weight of prednisone or an equivalent.

††Measles vaccination can suppress tuberculin reactivity temporarily. Measles-containing vaccine can be administered on the same day as tuberculin skin testing. If testing cannot be performed until after the day of the MMR vaccination, the test should be postponed for more than 4 weeks after the vaccination. If an urgent need exists to skin test, do so with the understanding that reactivity may be reduced by the vaccine.

‡‡If a vaccine recipient experiences a presumed vaccine-related rash 7 to 25 days after the vaccination, avoid direct contact with immunocompromised persons for the duration of the rash.

TABLE 5-5 Immunizations for Immunocompromised Infants and Children

Vaccine	Routine	HIV/AIDS	Severe Immunosuppression*	Asplenia	Renal Failure	Diabetes
Routine Infant Immunizations						
DTaP/DTP (DT/T/Td)	Recommended	Recommended	Recommended	Recommended	Recommended	Recommended
IPV	Recommended	Recommended	Recommended	Use as indicated	Use as indicated	Use as indicated
MMR/MR/M/R	Recommended	Recommended or considered	Contraindicated	Recommended	Recommended	Recommended
Hib	Recommended	Recommended	Recommended	Recommended	Recommended	Recommended
Hepatitis B	Recommended	Recommended	Recommended	Recommended	Recommended	Recommended
Varicella	Recommended	Contraindicated or considered†	Contraindicated	Contraindicated	Use if indicated	Use if indicated
Rotavirus	Recommended	Contraindicated	Contraindicated	Contraindicated	Use if indicated	Use if indicated
Other Childhood Immunizations						
Pneumococcus‡	Use if indicated	Recommended	Recommended	Recommended	Recommended	Recommended
Influenza§	Use if indicated	Recommended	Recommended	Recommended	Recommended	Recommended

AIDS, acquired immunodeficiency syndrome; DT, pediatric diphtheria-tetanus toxoid; DTaP, diphtheria, tetanus toxoids, and acellular pertussis vaccine; Hib, Haemophilus influenzae type b vaccine; HIV, human immunodeficiency virus; IPV, inactivated poliovirus vaccine; MMR, measles-mumps-rubella vaccine; Td, adult tetanus-diphtheria toxoid.

*Severe immunosuppression can result from congenital immunodeficiency, HIV infection, leukemia, lymphoma, aplastic anemia, generalized malignancy, alkylating agents, antimetabolites, irradiation, or large amounts of corticosteroids.

†Varicella vaccine should be considered for asymptomatic or mildly symptomatic HIV-infected children in CDC class N1 or A1 with age-specific $CD4^+$ T-lymphocyte percentages of ≥25%. Eligible children should receive two doses of varicella vaccine with a 3-month interval between doses.

‡Recommended for persons ≥2 years old.

§Not recommended for infants <6 months old.

Adapted from Centers for Disease Control and Prevention (CDC): Recommendations of the Advisory Committee on Immunization Practices (ACIP): Use of vaccines and immune globulins in persons with altered immunity. *MMWR Morb Mortal Wkly Rep* 42(RR-4):15, 1993.

TABLE 5-6 Suggested Intervals Between Immune Globulin Administration and Measles Immunization (MMR, MMRV, or Monovalent Measles Vaccine)

Indication for Immunoglobulin	Route	DOSE		Interval, mo*
		U or mL	mg IgG/kg	
Tetanus (as TIG)	IM	250 U	10	3
Hepatitis A prophylaxis (as IG)				
Contact prophylaxis	IM	0.02 mL/kg	3.3	3
International travel	IM	0.06 mL/kg	10	3
Hepatitis B prophylaxis (as HBIG)	IM	0.06 mL/kg	10	3
Rabies prophylaxis (as RIG)	IM	20 IU/kg	22	4
Varicella prophylaxis (as VariZIG)	IM	125 U/10 kg (maximum 625 U)	20–40	5
Measles prophylaxis (as IG)				
Standard	IM	0.25 mL/kg	40	5
Immunocompromised host	IM	0.50 mL/kg	80	6
RSV prophylaxis (palivizumab monoclonal antibody)	IM	—	15 mg/kg (monoclonal)	None
Cytomegalovirus immune globulin	IV	3 mL/kg	150	6
Blood transfusion				
Washed RBCs	IV	10 mL/kg	Negligible	0
RBCs, adenine-saline added	IV	10 mL/kg	10	3
Packed RBCs	IV	10 mL/kg	20–60	5
Whole blood	IV	10 mL/kg	80–100	6
Plasma or platelet products	IV	10 mL/kg	160	7
Replacement (or therapy) of immune deficiencies (as IGIV)	IV	—	300–400	8
ITP (as IGIV)	IV	—	400	8
ITP	IV	—	1000	10
ITP or Kawasaki disease	IV	—	1600–2000	11

HBIG, hepatitis B IG; IG, immune globulin; IgG, immunoglobulin G; IGIV, IG intravenous; IM, intramuscular; ITP, immune (formerly termed "idiopathic") thrombocytopenic purpura; IV, intravenous; MMR, measles-mumps-rubella; MMRV, measles-mumps-rubella-varicella; RBCs, red blood cells; RIG, rabies IG; RSV, respiratory syncytial virus; TIG, tetanus immune globulin.

*These intervals should provide sufficient time for decreases in passive antibodies in all children to allow for an adequate response to measles vaccine. Physicians should not assume that children are fully protected against measles during these intervals. Additional doses of IG or measles vaccine may be indicated after exposure to measles.

TABLE 5-7 **Recommendations for Measles Immunization**

Category	Recommendations
Unimmunized, no history of measles (12–15 mo of age)	A 2-dose schedule (with MMR) is recommended The first dose is recommended at 12–15 mo of age; the second is recommended at 4–6 y of age
Children 6–11 mo of age in epidemic situations or prior to international travel	Immunize (with monovalent measles vaccine or, if not available, MMR); reimmunization (with MMR) at 12–15 mo of age is necessary, and a third dose is indicated at 4–6 y of age
Children 4–12 y of age who have received 1 dose of measles vaccine at ≥12 mo of age	Reimmunize (1 dose)
Students in college and other post-high school institutions who have received 1 dose of measles vaccine at ≥12 mo of age	Reimmunize (1 dose)
History of immunization before the first birthday	Consider susceptible and immunize (2 doses)
History of receipt of inactivated measles vaccine or unknown type of vaccine, 1963–1967	Consider susceptible and immunize (2 doses)
Further attenuated or unknown vaccine given with IG	Consider susceptible and immunize (2 doses)
Allergy to eggs	Immunize; no reactions likely
Neomycin allergy, nonanaphylactic	Immunize; no reactions likely
Severe hypersensitivity (anaphylaxis) to neomycin or gelatin	Avoid immunization
Tuberculosis	Immunize; if patient has untreated tuberculosis disease, start anti-tuberculosis therapy before immunizing.
Measles exposure	Immunize and/or give IG, depending on circumstances
HIV-infected	Immunize (2 doses) unless severely immunocompromised
Personal or family history of seizures	Immunize; advise parents of slightly increased risk of seizures
Immunoglobulin or blood recipient	Immunize at the appropriate interval

HIV, human immunodeficiency virus; IG, immune globulin; MMR, measles-mumps-rubella vaccine.

TABLE 5-8 **Administration of Multiple Vaccines and Immune Globulins**

Vaccine Combination	Recommended Minimum Interval Between Doses
≥2 Inactivated vaccines	None; may be administered simultaneously or at any interval between doses. If possible, cholera, parenteral typhoid, and plague vaccines should be given on separate occasions to avoid accentuating their side effects.
Inactivated and live vaccines	None; may be administered simultaneously or at any interval between doses. Cholera vaccine with yellow fever vaccine is the exception. These vaccines should be given separately at least 3 weeks apart; otherwise the antibody response to each may be suboptimal.
≥2 Live vaccines parenteral	May be administered simultaneously. If given separately, there must be an interval at least 4 weeks between them.
Live vaccine and purified protein derivative (PPD)	May be administered simultaneously. If given separately, the PPD should be given 4 to 6 weeks after the live vaccine.
Antibody-containing products and killed vaccine	None; may be administered simultaneously or at any interval between doses.
Antibody-containing products and live vaccine	If simultaneous administration of measles-containing vaccine or varicella vaccines is unavoidable, administer at different sites and revaccinate or test for seroconversion after the recommended interval.

Adapted from Centers for Disease Control and Prevention (CDC): General Recommendations on Immunization: Recommendations of the Advisory Committee on Immunization Practices (ACIP) and the American Academy of Family Physicians (AAFP). *MMWR Morb Mortal Wkly Rep* 51(RR-2):1–35, 2002.

TABLE 5-9 Cardiac Conditions Associated with Endocarditis

ENDOCARDITIS PROPHYLAXIS		
Recommended		**Not recommended**
High Risk	**Moderate Risk**	**Negligible Risk***
Prosthetic cardiac valves, including bioprosthetic and homograft valves Previous bacterial endocarditis Complex cyanotic congenital heart disease (e.g., single ventricle states, transposition of the great arteries, tetralogy of Fallot) Surgically constructed systemic pulmonary shunts or conduits	Most other congenital cardiac malformations (other than those in the high-risk and negligible-risk categories) Acquired valvular dysfunction (e.g., rheumatic heart disease) Hypertrophic cardiomyopathy Mitral valve prolapse with valvular regurgitation and/or thickened leaflets†	Isolated secundum atrial septal defect Surgical repair of atrial septal defect, ventricular septal defect, or patent ductus arteriosus (without residua and beyond 6 mo of age) Previous coronary artery bypass graft surgery Mitral valve prolapse without valvular regurgitation† Physiologic, functional, or innocent heart murmurs† Previous Kawasaki disease without valvular dysfunction Previous rheumatic fever without valvular dysfunction Cardiac pacemakers (intravascular and epicardial) and implanted defibrillators

*No greater risk than the general population.
†For further details, see Dajani AS et al: Prevention of bacterial endocarditis. Recommendations by the American Heart Association. *JAMA* 277:1794–1801, 1997.
American Academy of Pediatrics: Cardiac conditions associated with endocarditis (Table 5.2). *In* Pickering LK et al (eds): *Red Book: 2006 Report of the Committee on Infectious Diseases*, 27th ed. Elk Grove Village, IL, American Academy of Pediatrics, 2006, p 831.

TABLE 5-10 Dental Procedures and Endocarditis Prophylaxis

ENDOCARDITIS PROPHYLAXIS	
Recommended*	**Not Recommended**
Dental extractions Periodontal procedures, including surgery, scaling and root planing, probing, and routine maintenance Dental implant placement and reimplantation of avulsed teeth Endodontic (root canal) instrumentation or surgery only beyond the apex Subgingival placement of antimicrobial fibers or strips Initial placement of orthodontic bands but not brackets Intraligamentary local anesthetic injections Prophylactic cleaning of teeth or implants during which bleeding is anticipated	Restorative dentistry† (operative and prosthodontic) with or without retraction cord‡ Local anesthetic injections (nonintraligamentary) Intracanal endodontic treatment; postplacement and buildup Placement of rubber dams Postoperative suture removal Placement of removable prosthodontic or orthodontic appliances Taking of oral impressions Fluoride treatments Taking of oral radiographs Orthodontic appliance adjustment Shedding of primary teeth

*Prophylaxis is recommended for patients with high- and moderate-risk cardiac conditions.
†This includes restoration of decayed teeth (filling cavities) and replacement of missing teeth.
‡Clinical judgment may indicate antimicrobial use in some circumstances that may create significant bleeding.
American Academy of Pediatrics: Dental procedures and endocarditis prophylaxis (Table 5.3). *In* Pickering LK et al (eds): *Red Book: 2006 Report of the Committee on Infectious Diseases*, 27th ed. Elk Grove Village, IL, American Academy of Pediatrics, 2006, p 832.

TABLE 5-11 **Other Procedures and Endocarditis Prophylaxis**

	ENDOCARDITIS PROPHYLAXIS	
	Recommended*	**Not Recommended**
Respiratory tract	Tonsillectomy, adenoidectomy, or both Surgical operations that involve respiratory mucosa Bronchoscopy with a rigid bronchoscope	Endotracheal intubation Bronchoscopy with a flexible bronchoscope, with or without biopsy[†] Tympanostomy tube insertion
Gastrointestinal tract[‡]	Sclerotherapy for esophageal varices Esophageal stricture dilation Endoscopic retrograde cholangiography with biliary obstruction Biliary tract surgery Surgical operations that involve intestinal mucosa	Transesophageal echocardiography[†] Endoscopy with or without gastrointestinal tract biopsy[†]
Genitourinary tract	Prostate surgery Cystoscopy Urethral dilation	Vaginal hysterectomy[†] Vaginal delivery[†] Cesarean delivery In uninfected tissue: Urethral catheterization Uterine dilatation and curettage Therapeutic abortion Sterilization procedures Insertion or removal of intrauterine devices
Other		Cardiac catheterization, including balloon angioplasty Implanted cardiac pacemakers, implanted defibrillators, and coronary stents Incision or biopsy of surgically scrubbed skin Circumcision

*Prophylaxis is recommended for high- and moderate-risk cardiac conditions.
†Prophylaxis is optional for high-risk patients.
‡Prophylaxis is recommended for high-risk patients; optional for medium-risk patients.
American Academy of Pediatrics: Other procedures and endocarditis prophylaxis (Table 5.4). *In* Pickering LK et al (eds): *Red Book: 2006 Report of the Committee on Infectious Diseases*, 27th ed. Elk Grove Village, IL, American Academy of Pediatrics, 2006, p 833.

TABLE 5-12 **Endocarditis Prophylactic Regimens for Dental, Oral Respiratory Tract, or Esophageal Procedures**

Situation	Agent	Regimen*
Standard general prophylaxis	Amoxicillin	Adults: 2.0 g; children: 50 mg/kg of body weight, orally, 1 h before procedure
Unable to take oral medications	Ampicillin	Adults: 2.0 g, intramuscularly (IM) or intravenously (IV); children: 50 mg/kg, IM or IV, within 30 min before procedure
Allergic to penicillin	Clindamycin	Adults: 600 mg; children: 20 mg/kg, orally, 1 h before procedure
	OR	
	Cephalexin[†] or cefadroxil[†]	Adults: 2.0 g; children: 50 mg/kg, orally, 1 h before procedure
	OR	
	Azithromycin or clarithromycin	Adults: 500 mg; children: 15 mg/kg, orally, 1 h before procedure
Allergic to penicillin and unable to take oral medications	Clindamycin	Adults: 600 mg; children: 20 mg/kg, IV, within 30 min before procedure
	OR	
	Cefazolin[†]	Adults: 1.0 g; children: 25 mg/kg, IM or IV, within 30 min before procedure

*Total dose for children should not exceed adult dose.
†Cephalosporins should not be used for people with immediate-type hypersensitivity reaction (urticaria, angioedema, or anaphylaxis) to penicillins.
American Academy of Pediatrics: Prophylactic regimens for dental, oral, respiratory tract, or esophageal procedures (Table 5.5). *In* Pickering LK et al (eds): *Red Book: 2006 Report of the Committee on Infectious Diseases*, 27th ed. Elk Grove Village, IL, American Academy of Pediatrics, 2006, p 834.

TABLE 5-13 Hepatitis B Vaccine Schedules for Infants, by Maternal Hepatitis B Surface Antigen (HBsAg) Status*

	SINGLE-ANTIGEN VACCINE		SINGLE-ANTIGEN + COMBINATION	
Maternal HBsAg Status	**Dose**	**Age**	**Dose**	**Age**
Positive	1[†]	Birth (≤12 h)	1[†]	Birth (≤12 h)
	HBIG[‡]	Birth (≤12 h)	HBIG	Birth (≤12 h)
	2	1–2 mo	2	2 mo
	3[§]	6 mo	3	4 mo
			4[§]	6 mo (Pediarix) or 12–15 mo (Comvax)
Unknown[‖]	1[†]	Birth (≤12 h)	1[†]	Birth (≤12 h)
	2	1–2 mo	2	2 mo
	3[§]	6 mo	3	4 mo
			4[§]	6 mo (Pediarix) or 12–15 mo (Comvax)
Negative	1[†,#]	Birth (before discharge)	1[†,#]	Birth (before discharge)
	2	1–2 mo	2	2 mo
	3[§]	6–18 mo	3	4 mo
			4[§]	6 mo (Pediarix) or 12–15 mo (Comvax)

HBIG, hepatitis B immune globulin.

*Centers for Disease Control and Prevention: A comprehensive immunization strategy to eliminate transmission of hepatitis B virus infection in the United States. Recommendations of the Advisory Committee on Immunization Practices (ACIP) part 1: immunization of infants, children, and adolescents. *MMWR Recomm Rep* 54(RR-16):1–23, 2005.

†Recombivax HB or Engerix-B should be used for the birth dose. Comvax and Pediarix cannot be administered at birth or before 6 weeks of age.

‡Hepatitis B Immune Globulin (0.5 mL) administered intramuscularly in a separate site from vaccine.

§The final dose in the vaccine series should not be administered before 24 weeks (164 days) of age.

‖Mothers should have blood drawn and tested for HBsAg as soon as possible after admission for delivery; if the mother is found to be HBsAg-positive, the infant should receive HBIG as soon as possible but no later than 7 days of age.

#On a case-by-case basis and only in rare circumstances, the first dose may be delayed until after hospital discharge for an infant who weighs ≥2000 g and whose mother is HBsAg negative, but only if a physician's order to withhold the birth dose and a copy of the mother's original HBsAg-negative laboratory report are documented in the infant's medical record.

American Academy of Pediatrics: Hepatitis B vaccine schedules for infants, by maternal hepatitis B surface antigen (HBsAg) status (Table 3.19). *In* Pickering LK et al (eds): *Red Book: 2006 Report of the Committee on Infectious Diseases*, 27th ed. Elk Grove Village, IL, American Academy of Pediatrics, 2006, p 348.

TABLE 5-14 Recommendations for Hepatitis B Prophylaxis after Percutaneous Exposure to Blood That Contains or Might Contain HBsAg*

	TREATMENT WHEN SOURCE IS		
Exposed Person	**HBsAg Positive**	**HBsAg Negative**	**Unknown or Not Tested**
Unimmunized	Administer HBIG[†] (1 dose), and initiate hepatitis B vaccine series	Initiate hepatitis B vaccine series	Initiate hepatitis B vaccine series
Previously immunized			
Known responder	No treatment	No treatment	No treatment
Known nonresponder	HBIG (1 dose) **and** initiate reimmunization[‡] or HBIG (2 doses)	No treatment	If known high-risk source, treat as if source were HBsAg positive
Response unknown	Test exposed person for anti-HBs[§] • If inadequate, HBIG[†] (1 dose) **and** vaccine booster dose[‖] • If adequate, no treatment	No treatment	Test exposed person for anti-HBs[§] • If inadequate, vaccine booster dose[‖] • If adequate, no treatment

Anti-HBs, antibody to HBsAg; HBIG, hepatitis B immune globulin; HBsAg, hepatitis B surface antigen.

*Centers for Disease Control and Prevention: Updated US Public Health Service guidelines for the management of occupational exposures to HBV, HCV, and HIV and recommendations for postexposure prophylaxis. *MMWR Recomm Rep* 50(RR-11):1–52, 2001.

†Dose of HBIG, 0.06 mL/kg, intramuscularly.

‡The option of giving 1 dose of HBIG (0.06 mL/kg) and reinitiating the vaccine series is preferred for nonresponder who has not completed a second 3-dose vaccine series. For people who previously completed a second vaccine series but failed to respond, 2 doses of HBIG (0.06 mL/kg) are preferred, 1 dose as soon as possible after exposure and the second 1 month later.

§Adequate anti-HBs is ≥10 mIU/mL.

‖The person should be evaluated for antibody response after the vaccine booster dose. For people who receive HBIG, anti-HBs testing should be performed when passively acquired antibody from HBIG no longer is detectable (e.g., 4–6 months); for people who did not receive HBIG, anti-HBs testing should be performed 1 to 2 months after the vaccine booster dose. If anti-HBs is inadequate (>10 mIU/mL) after the vaccine booster dose, 2 additional doses should be administered to complete a 3-dose reimmunization series.

TABLE 5-15 **Recommended HIV Postexposure Prophylaxis for Percutaneous Injuries**

	INFECTION STATUS OF SOURCE				
Exposure Type	**HIV-Positive Class 1***	**HIV-Positive Class 2***	**Source of Unknown HIV Status†**	**Unknown Source‡**	**HIV Negative**
Less severe§	Recommend basic 2-drug PEP	Recommend expanded 3-drug PEP	Generally, no PEP warranted; however, consider basic 2-drug PEP‖,# for source with HIV risk factors**	Generally, no PEP warranted; however, consider basic 2-drug PEP# in settings where exposure to HIV-infected persons is likely	No PEP warranted
More severe**	Recommend expanded 3-drug PEP	Recommend expanded 3-drug PEP	Generally, no PEP warranted; however, consider basic 2-drug PEP‖,# for source with HIV risk factors	Generally, no PEP warranted; however, consider basic 2-drug PEP# in settings where exposure to HIV-infected persons is likely	No PEP warranted

HIV, human immunodeficiency virus; PEP, postexposure prophylaxis (see Box 5-1).
*HIV-positive, class 1: asymptomatic HIV infection or known low viral load (e.g., <1500 RNA copies/mL). HIV-positive, class 2: symptomatic HIV infection, acquired immunodeficiency syndrome, acute seroconversion, or known high viral load. If drug resistance is a concern, obtain expert consultation. Initiation of PEP should not be delayed pending expert consultation, and because expert consultation alone cannot substitute for face-to-face counseling, resources should be available to provide immediate evaluation and follow-up care for all exposures.
†Source of unknown HIV status (e.g., deceased source person with no samples available for HIV testing).
‡Unknown source (e.g., a needle from a sharps disposal container).
§Less severe (e.g., solid needle and superficial injury).
‖If PEP is offered and taken and the source is later determined to be HIV-negative, PEP should be discontinued.
#The designation "consider PEP" indicates that PEP is optional and should be based on an individualized decision made by the exposed person and the treating clinician.
**More severe (e.g., large-bore hollow needle, deep puncture, visible blood on device, needle used in patient's artery or vein).

TABLE 5-16 **Recommended HIV Postexposure Prophylaxis for Mucous Membrane Exposures and Nonintact Skin Exposures***

	INFECTION STATUS OF SOURCE				
Exposure Type	**HIV-Positive Class 1†**	**HIV-Positive Class 2†**	**Source of Unknown HIV Status‡**	**Unknown Source§**	**HIV Negative**
Small volume‖	Consider basic 2-drug PEP#	Recommend basic 2-drug PEP	Generally, no PEP warranted; however, consider basic 2-drug PEP# for source with HIV risk factors**	Generally, no PEP warranted; however, consider basic 2-drug PEP# in settings where exposure to HIV-infected persons is likely	No PEP warranted
Large volume††	Recommend basic 2-drug PEP	Recommend expanded 3-drug PEP	Generally, no PEP warranted; however, consider basic 2-drug PEP# for source with HIV risk factors**	Generally, no PEP warranted; however, consider basic 2-drug PEP# in settings where exposure to HIV-infected persons is likely	No PEP warranted

HIV, human immunodeficiency virus; PEP, postexposure prophylaxis (see Box 5-1).
*For skin exposures, follow-up is indicated only if there is evidence of compromised skin integrity (e.g., dermatitis, abrasion, open wound).
†HIV-positive, class 1: asymptomatic HIV infection or known low viral load (e.g., <1500 RNA copies/mL). HIV-positive, class 2: symptomatic HIV infection, acquired immunodeficiency syndrome, acute seroconversion, or known high viral load. If drug resistance is a concern, obtain expert consultation. Initiation of PEP should not be delayed pending expert consultation, and because expert consultation alone cannot substitute for face-to-face counseling, resources should be available to provide immediate evaluation and follow-up care for all exposures.
‡Source of unknown HIV status (e.g., deceased source person with no samples available for HIV testing).
§Unknown source (e.g., splash from inappropriately disposed blood).
‖Small volume (i.e., a few drops).
#The designation "consider PEP" indicates that PEP is optional and should be based on an individualized decision made by the exposed person and the treating clinician.
**If PEP is offered and taken and the source is later determined to be HIV negative, PEP should be discontinued.
††Large volume (i.e., major blood splash).

BOX 5-1 Situations for Which Expert Consultation for Human Immunodeficiency Virus Postexposure Prophylaxis Is Advised*

- Delayed (i.e., later than 24 to 36 hours) exposure report
  - The interval after which there is no benefit from postexposure prophylaxis (PEP) is undefined.
- Unknown source (e.g., needle in sharps disposal container or laundry)
  - Decide about the use of PEP on a case-by-case basis.
  - Consider the severity of the exposure and the epidemiologic likelihood of human immunodeficiency virus (HIV) exposure.
  - Do not test needles or other sharp instruments for HIV.
- Known or suspected pregnancy in the exposed person
  - Does not preclude the use of optimal PEP regimens.
  - Do not deny PEP solely on the basis of pregnancy.
- Resistance of the source virus to antiretroviral agents
  - The influence of drug resistance on transmission risk is unknown.
  - Selection of drugs to which the source person's virus is unlikely to be resistant is recommended if it is known or suspected to be resistant to one or more of the drugs considered for the PEP regimen.
  - Resistance testing of the source person's virus at the time of the exposure is not recommended.
- Toxicity of the initial PEP regimen
  - Adverse symptoms, such as nausea and diarrhea, are common with PEP.
  - Symptoms often can be managed without changing the PEP regimen by prescribing antimotility and antiemetic agents.
  - In other situations, modification of dose intervals (i.e., administering a lower dose of drug more frequently throughout the day, as recommended by the manufacturer) may help alleviate symptoms.

*Seek local experts or call the National Clinicians' Postexposure Prophylaxis Hotline (PEPline): 1-888-448-4911.

TABLE 5-17 Recommended Daily Dosage of Influenza Antiviral Medications for Treatment and Chemoprophylaxis in the United States

	AGE GROUP (YEARS)				
Antiviral Agent	**1–6**	**7–9**	**10–12**	**13–64**	**≥65**
Zanamivir* treamtent, influenza A and B	N/A†	10 mg (two inhalations) twice daily	10 mg (two inhalations) twice daily	10 mg (two inhalations) twice daily	10 mg (two inhalations) twice daily
Chemoprophylaxis, influenza A and B	Ages 1-4: N/A†	Ages 5-9: 10 mg (two inhalations) once daily	10 mg (two inhalations) once daily	10 mg (two inhalations) once daily	10 mg (two inhalations) once daily
Oseltamivir*,‡ treatment, influenza A and B	Dose varies by child's weight§	Dose varies by child's weight§	Dose varies by child's weight§	75 mg twice daily	75 mg twice daily
Chemoprophylaxis, influenza A and B	Dose varies by child's weight‖	Dose varies by child's weight‖	Dose varies by child's weight‖	75 mg once daily	75 mg once daily

*Zanamivir (Relenza, inhaled powder) is manufactured by GlaxoSmithKline. Oseltamivir is manufactured by Roche Pharmaceuticals (Tamiflu, tablet). This information is based on data published by the U.S. Food and Drug Administration (http://www.fda.gov). Zanamivir is administered through oral inhalation by using a plastic device included in the medication package. Patients can benefit from instruction and demonstration of the correct use of the device. Zanamivir is not recommended for persons with underlying airway disease.
†Not applicable.
‡A reduction in the dose of oseltamivir is recommended for persons with creatinine clearance values less than 30 mL/min.
§The treatment dosing recommendations of oseltamivir for children weighing 15 kg or less is 30 mg twice daily; for children weighing more than 15 to 23 kg, the dose is 45 mg twice daily; for children weighing more than 23 to 40 kg, the dose is 60 mg once daily; and for children weighing more than 40 kg, the dose is 75 mg once daily.
‖The chemoprophylaxis dosing recommendations of oseltamivir for children weighing 15 kg or less is 30 mg once daily; for children weighing more than 15 to 23 kg, the dose is 45 mg once daily; for children weighing more than 23 to 40 kg, the dose is 60 mg once daily; and for children weighing more than 40 kg, the dose is 75 mg once daily.

TABLE 5-18 Duration of Prophylaxis for Persons Who Have Had Rheumatic Fever: Recommendations of the American Heart Association

Category	Duration
Rheumatic fever without carditis	5 or until age 21, whichever is longer
Rheumatic fever with carditis but without residual heart disease (no valvular disease*)	10 yr or well into adulthood, whichever is longer
Rheumatic fever with carditis and residual heart disease (persistent valvular disease*)	At least 10 yr since last episode and at least until age 40; sometimes lifelong prophylaxis

*Clinical or echocardiographic evidence.
Modified from Dajani A et al: *Pediatrics* 96:758, 1995.

TABLE 5-19 **Chemoprophylaxis for Recurrences of Rheumatic Fever**

Drug	Dose	Route
Benzathine penicillin G	1,200,000 U every 4 wk*	Intramuscular
OR		
Penicillin V	250 mg twice a day	Oral
OR		
Sulfadiazine or sulfisoxazole	0.5 g once a day for patients ≤27 kg (60 lb) 1.0 g once a day for patients >27 kg (60 lb)	Oral
For persons allergic to penicillin and sulfonamide drugs		
Erythromycin	250 mg twice a day	Oral

*In high-risk situations, administration every 3 weeks is recommended.
Modified from Dajani A et al: *Pediatrics* 96:758, 1995.

TABLE 5-20 **Vaccinations for International Travel**

Disease*	Areas Affected†	Prophylaxis Recommended	Ideal Time Between Last Vaccine Dose and Travel
Tetanus	All	All travelers; vaccine series/booster	Probably 30 days for series Anamnestic response to booster
Measles	All	Born after 1956; ensure immunity by antibody titer, diagnosed measles, or two doses of vaccine	As MMR, 7–14 days
Rubella	All	Born after 1956 and any female of child-bearing age; rubella titer or one dose of vaccine	As MMR, 7–14 days
Mumps	All	Born after 1956; ensure immunity by antibody titer, diagnosed mumps, or one dose of vaccine	As MMR, 7–14 days
Varicella	All	All travelers; antibody titer, reported illness, or vaccine series	7–14 days
Hepatitis B	5% to 20% of population are carriers in Africa, Middle East except Israel, all Southeast Asia, Amazon basin, Haiti, and Dominican Republic; 1% to 5% of population are carriers in south-central and southwest Asia, Israel, Japan, Americas, Russia, and eastern and southern Europe	Travelers for more than 6 mo in close contact with population or for less time but with high-risk activities (close household contact, seeking dental or medical care, sex); vaccine series	Probably 30 days
Hepatitis A	Developing countries	Travelers to rural areas; eating and drinking in settings of poor sanitation; vaccine or pooled immune globulin (IG)	Vaccine, 30 days Pooled IG, 2 days
Influenza	Tropics throughout the year; southern hemisphere from April to September	Travelers for whom vaccine is otherwise indicated; give current vaccine and revaccinate in fall as usual	7–14 days
Meningococcus*	Sub-Saharan African belt (Senegal to Ethiopia) from December to June; required for pilgrims to Saudi Arabia during Hajj; epidemics reported in other African nations, India, Nepal, and Mongolia	All travelers; vaccine	7–10 days
Rabies	Endemic dog rabies exists in Mexico, El Salvador, Guatemala, Peru, Colombia, Ecuador, India, Nepal, Philippines, Sri Lanka, Thailand, and Vietnam	Travelers staying for more than 30 days or at high risk for exposure to domestic or wild animals; vaccine series/booster	7–14 days
Poliomyelitis	Developing countries not in Western Hemisphere; at risk all year in tropics; in temperate zones, incidence increases in summer and fall	All travelers; vaccine series/booster	Parenteral vaccine series, 28 days Anamnestic response to booster

TABLE 5-20 Vaccinations for International Travel *(Continued)*

Disease*	Areas Affected†	Prophylaxis Recommended	Ideal Time Between Last Vaccine Dose and Travel
Typhoid fever	Many countries in Asia, Africa, Central America, and South America	Travelers with prolonged stay in rural areas with poor sanitation; vaccine series/booster	Oral vaccine, 7 days Parenteral vaccine, probably 14 days
Yellow fever*	North and central South America, forest-savannah zones of Africa; some countries in Africa, Asia, and Middle East require travelers from endemic areas to be vaccinated	All travelers; vaccine/booster at approved yellow fever vaccination centers; travelers with infants <9 months old should be strongly advised against travel to yellow-fever endemic zone	10 days
Japanese encephalitis	Seasonally in most areas of Asia, Indian subcontinent, and western Pacific islands; in temperate zones, incidence increases in summer and early fall; in tropics, year-round incidence	Travelers staying for more than 30 days in high-risk rural areas; staying outdoors during transmission season; vaccine series; no data on efficacy for infants <1 year old	10 days
Cholera*	Certain undeveloped countries	If required by local authorities, one dose usually suffices; primary series only for those living in high-risk areas under poor sanitary conditions or those with compromised gastric defense mechanisms (e.g., achlorhydria, antacid therapy, previous ulcer surgery); booster every 6 mo	Probably 30 days
Plague	Africa, Asia, and Americas in rural mountainous or upland areas	Travelers whose research or field activities bring them in contact with rodents; vaccine series/booster; consider taking tetracycline (500 mg four times daily) for chemoprophylaxis (inferred from clinical experience in treating plague)	Probably 30 days

MMR, measles-mumps-rubella vaccine.
*Only yellow fever vaccine is required for entry by any country, cholera vaccine may be required by some local authorities, and meningococcus vaccine is required for pilgrims to Mecca, Saudi Arabia, during Hajj. However, it is important to follow CDC recommendations for all vaccines to prevent disease. If a required vaccine is contraindicated or withheld for any reason, attempts should be made to obtain a waiver from the country's consulate or embassy.
†Because areas affected can change and for more specific details, consult the CDC's traveler's hotline (www.cdc.gov/travel/vaccinat/htm; 877-FYI-TRIP).
From Noble J: Primary Care Medicine, 3rd ed. St Louis, Mosby, 2001.

TABLE 5-21 Vaccines for Children Who Travel

Vaccine*	Description	Dosing	Comments and Contraindications	LENGTH OF TRAVEL: Brief (<2 wk)	Intermediate (2 wk-3 mo)	Long-term Residential (>3 mo)
Routine						
Polio†	OPV: live attenuated, oral IPV: inactivated, injection	IPV at 2, 4 mo; OPV at 12-18 mo, 4-6 yr; may accelerate to q 4-8 wk × 3 doses	IPV at 2 and 4 mo decreases risk of polio in undiagnosed immunocompromised infants; AAP recommendation may change to IPV only	+	+	+
Diphtheria-tetanus-pertussis†	DPT: D, T toxoid + whole cell P	DTaP recommended at 2, 4, 6, 15-18 mo and 4-6 yr; Td booster at age 12, then every 10 yr	May accelerate to dose every 4 wk × 3 doses if necessary; decreased incidence of vaccine-related reactions with DTaP	+	+	+
	DTaP: DT toxoid + acellular P					
	Td: booster					
Haemophilus influenzae b†	Hib polysaccharide: protein conjugate	0.5 mL IM at 2, 4, 6, 12-15 mo	Typically given as combination with DTaP	+	+	+

Continued on following page

TABLE 5-21 **Vaccines for Children Who Travel** *(Continued)*

Vaccine*	Description	Dosing	Comments and Contraindications	LENGTH OF TRAVEL Brief (<2 wk)	Intermediate (2 wk-3 mo)	Long-term Residential (>3 mo)
Hepatitis B	Recombivax HB: inactivated viral antigen	3 doses: 0, 1, 6 mo; if <11 yr old: 0.25 mL IM; if >11 yr old: 0.5 mL IM	Some protection after just 1 or 2 doses; may accelerate Engerix-B to 0, 1, 2, 12 mo	+	+	+
	Engerix-B: same	3 doses: 0, 1, 6 mo; if <11 yr old: 0.5 mL IM; if >11 yr old: 1.0 mL IM				
Measles-mumps-rubella[†]	Live attenuated viruses	0.25 mL IM at 12-15 mo old, then booster at 4-6 or 11-12 yr old	May accelerate to 6-12 mo, repeat 1 mo later, then per usual schedule; give at least 2-3 wk before IgG	+	+	+
Varicella	Live attenuated virus	12 mo-12 yr old: 0.5 mL SC as single dose	Give at least 2-3 wk before IgG; may be given with MMR using different sites; avoid if immunocompromised	+	+	+
		>12 yr old: 2 doses 4-8 wk apart				
Routine for Travel						
Hepatitis A	Havrix: inactive virus (720ELU)	>2 yr old: 2 × 0.5 mL doses 6-12 mo apart	Preferred for hepatitis A protection if over age 2 yr	+	+	+
	Vaqta (24U)		Protects in 4 wk after dose 1			
Immune globulin (IgG)	Antibodies	<2 yr old: 0.02 mL/kg for <3 mo of travel; 0.06 mL/kg every 5 mo and 3 days before travel	Hepatitis A protection for those <2 yr old; beware of timing with live virus vaccines			
Required or Geographically Indicated						
Yellow fever	Live virus	>9 mo old: 0.5 mL SC at least 10 days before departure; booster every 10 yr	Required for parts of sub-Saharan Africa, tropical South America; may give when 4-9 mo old if traveling to epidemic area; <9 mo old: risk of vaccine-related encephalitis	+	+	+
Typhoid	Heat inactivated	6 mo-2 yr old: 2 × 0.25 mL SC 4 wk apart, booster every 3 yr	Fever, pain with heat killed; significantly fewer side effects with ViCPS and Ty21a; important for Latin America, Asia, Africa; vaccine not a substitute for eating and drinking cleanly	±	+	+
	ViCPS: polysaccharide	2-6 yr old: 0.5 mL IM × 1 booster every 2 yr				
	Ty21a: oral live attenuated	>6 yr old: 1 capsule q 2 days × 4; booster every 5 yr				
Meningococcal	Serogroups A, C, Y, W-135: polysaccharide	>2 years old: 0.5 mL SC; booster in 1 yr if 1st dose after age 4 yr, otherwise in 5 yr	Use for central Africa, Saudi Arabia for the Hajj, Nepal, and epidemic areas; minimal efficacy in children <2 yr old	±	±	±

TABLE 5-21 **Vaccines for Children Who Travel** *(Continued)*

Vaccine*	Description	Dosing	Comments and Contraindications	LENGTH OF TRAVEL: Brief (<2 wk)	Intermediate (2 wk-3 mo)	Long-term Residential (>3 mo)
Japanese encephalitis	Inactivated virus	1-3 yr old: 0.5 mL SC at 0, 7, 14-30 days	Indicated for parts of India and rural Asia if stay <1 mo; no safety data for children <1 yr old; high rate of hypersensitivity	±	±	+
		>3 years old: 1.0 mL SC at 0, 7, 14-30 days				
		Last dose >10 days before travel				
Cholera	Inactivated bacteria	>6 mo old: 0.2 mL SC	Vaccine of questionable efficacy; not recommended by CDC or WHO; do not use in children <6 mo old			
Lyme disease	LYMErix: antigenic protein[†]	>15 yr old: 0.5 mL IM at 0, 1, 12 mo	Indicated for frequent, prolonged exposure to Lyme-endemic area, not brief exposures			
Extended Stay						
Rabies	HDCV: human diploid cell	1 mL IM in deltoid muscle at 0, 7, 21-28 days if >1-mo stay	If exposed and immunized: give vaccine, 1 mL IM at 0, 3 days	±	+	+
			If exposed and not immunized: give rabies Ig (RIG), 20 IU/kg: one half at site and one half IM; give vaccine, 1 mL IM at 0, 3, 7, 14, 28 days			

AAP, American Academy of Pediatrics; DTaP, diphtheria, tetanus toxoids, and acellular pertussis vaccine; HDCV, human diploid cell vaccine; Hib, *Haemophilus influenzae* type b vaccine; IM, intramuscularly; IPV, inactivated polio vaccine; MMR, measles-mumps-rubella vaccine; OPV, oral polio vaccine; SC, subcutaneously; +, recommended; ±, consider.

*Consult Centers for Disease Control and Prevention (CDC) for current and specific vaccine recommendations for destination country.

[†]Not readily available.

From Auerbach PS: Wilderness Medicine, 4th ed. St. Louis, Mosby, 2004.

TABLE 5-22 **Accelerated Schedule of Routine Childhood Immunizations If Necessary for Travel**

Vaccine	Routine Schedule	Accelerated Schedule
Diphtheria-tetanus-pertussis	DTaP: 2, 4, 6, 15-18 mo old	DTaP: 6 wk old, with 4 wk between 1st, 2nd, and 3rd doses; and 6 mo between 3rd and 4th doses
	DTaP: 4-6 yr old (booster)	DTaP: 4 yr old
	DT every 10 yr	DT every 5 yr if at high risk
Poliomyelitis	IPV: at 2 and 4 mo, 6-18 mo, and 4-6 yr old	IPV: 6 wk old, with 1 mo between 1st and 2nd doses and 6 mo between 2nd and 3rd doses
	No additional boosters unless traveling to an endemic area	A single IPV lifetime booster for adolescents and adults who have completed primary immunization
Measles-mumps-rubella	MMR: 12-15 mo old, with second dose at age 4-6 yr	Two doses at ≥12 mo old, 4 wk apart
	Not routinely recommended for children <12 mo old	May give first measles as early as age 6 mo, with additional two doses ≥12 mo old
Haemophilus influenzae type b	2, 4, 6 (if HbOC or PRP-T), and 12-15 mo old	HbOC and PRP-T: 6 wk old, with 1 mo between the 1st and 2nd and the 2nd and 3rd doses; booster at ≥12 mo old (≥2 mo from the 3rd dose)
		PRO-OMP: 6 wk old, with 1 mo between the 1st and 2nd doses; booster at ≥12 mo old (≥2 mo from the 3rd dose)
Hepatitis B	Birth, 1-2 mo, 6 mo old	0, 1, and 4 mo old
Varicella	12-18 mo old	12 mo old (two doses 1 mo apart for persons ≥13 yr old)
Rotavirus	2, 4, 6 mo old	6 wk old, with 2nd and 3rd doses each separated by 3 wk

DT, pediatric diphtheria-tetanus toxoid; DTaP, diphtheria, tetanus toxoids, and acellular pertussis vaccine; HbOC, *Haemophilus influenzae* type b oligosaccharide conjugate vaccine; Hib, *Haemophilus influenzae* type b vaccine; IPV, inactivated poliovirus vaccine; MMR, measles-mumps-rubella vaccine; PRO-OMP, hepatitis B vaccine in combination with Hib; PRP-T, Hib vaccine prepared by chemically conjugating the capsular polysaccharide of Hib to tetanus toxoid.

From Behrman RE: Nelson Textbook of Pediatrics, 16th ed. Philadelphia, WB Saunders, 2000.

TABLE 5-23 **Classification of Formulas by Carbohydrate**

	Lactose	Sucrose and Glucose Polymers	Glucose Polymers	Minimal Carbohydrates
Common ingredient names		See glucose polymers	Glucose polymers Maltodextrins Corn syrup solids Modified tapioca starch	
Comments	Requires lactase enzyme for digestion Contraindicated in galactosemia	Requires sucrase enzyme for digestion (see also glucose polymers)	Easily digested For individuals with lactose malabsorption	For severe carbohydrate intolerance
Infants	America's Store Brand formulas (generic) Enfamil Enfamil AR Enfamil Enfacare Enfamil Premature Evaporated milk formula Neorure* Nestlé Carnation Follow-Up Nestlé Carnation Good Start Similac Similac PM 60/40 Similac Special Care	Alimentum America's Store Brand Soy Isomil Isomil DF (Fiber) Nestlé Carnation Alsoy Nestlé Carnation Follow-Up Soy Portagen	Enfamil Lactofree Neocate Nutramigen Pregestimil ProSobee Similac Lactose Free	MJ3232A RCF
Toddlers and young children	Cow's milk Next Step* Similac 2	Compleat Pediatric† Isomil 2 Kindercal TF (Fiber) Neocate One Plus Next Step Soy Nutren Junior PediaSure (also w/Fiber) Pediatric EO_{28} Peptamen Junior‡ ProPeptide for Kids Resource Just for Kids	EleCare KetoCal Neocate Junior Pepdite One+ Vivonex Pediatric	
Older children and adolescents	Carnation Instant Breakfast Scandishake	Boost Boost Plus Boost High Protein Other formulas shown in Table 5-29	Criticare HN Crucial Deliver 2.0 L-Emental faa Glucerna Glytrol Isocal Jevity (fiber) Nestlé Carnation Modulen IBD Nutren (all) Osmolite Promote Peptamen ProPeptide Replete Tolerex Ultracal Vivonex Plus Vivonex TEN	

*Also contains glucose polymers.
†Also contains fruit and vegetable purees.
‡Unflavored contains glucose polymers only.

TABLE 5-24 **Classification of Formulas by Protein**

	Cow's Milk Protein	Soy Protein	Hydrolysate	Free Amino Acids
Common ingredient names	Cow's milk protein Nonfat milk Demineralized whey Reduced mineral whey Sodium, calcium, magnesium caseinate Casein	Soy protein Soy protein isolate	Casein hydrolysate, hydrolyzed whey, meat, or soy	
Comments	Requires normal protein digestion and absorption	Requires normal protein digestion and absorption Not recommended for premature infants, those with cystic fibrosis, or those on synthroid	For individuals with protein allergy and/or malabsorption	For individuals with severe protein allergy and/or severe protein malabsorption
Infants	America's Store Brand formulas (generic) Enfamil Enfamil AR Enfamil Enfacare Enfamil Lactofree Enfamil Premature Evaporated milk formula Nestlé Carnation Follow-Up Nestlé Carnation Good Start Portagen Similac Similac Lactose Free Similac Neosure Similac PM 60/40 Similac Special Care	America's Store Brand Soy Isomil Isomil DF Nestlé Carnation Alsoy Nestlé Carnation Follow-Up Soy ProSobee RCF	Alimentum MJ3232A Nutramigen Pregestimil	Neocate
Toddlers and young children	Compleat Pediatric* Cow's milk KetoCal Kindercal Next Step Nutren Junior PediaSure Resource Just for Kids Similac 2	Next Step Soy Isomil 2	Pepdite One+ Peptamen Junior Pro-Peptide for Kids	Vivonex Pediatric EleCare Neocate Junior Neocate One+ Pediatric EO_{28}
Older children and adolescents	See Table 5-29	Ensure† Ensure with Nutraflora FOS† Ensure Plus† Isocal† Osmolite† Promote†	Criticare HN Crucial Peptamen ProPeptide Vital HN	L-Emental faa Tolerex Vivonex TEN Vivonex Plus

*Blenderized protein diet of meat, vegetables, and fruit.
†Also contains cow's milk.

TABLE 5-25 **Classification of Formulas by Fat**

	Long-Chain Triglycerides	Medium-Chain and Long-Chain Triglycerides
Common ingredient names:	Butterfat Canola oil Coconut oil Corn oil Palm olein Safflower oil Soy oil Sunflower oil	Fractioned coconut oil Medium-chain triglycerides (MCT oil)
Comments:	Requires normal fat digestion and absorption	For individuals with fat malabsorption Bile digestion not required Absorbed directly into portal circulation
Infants:	America's Store Brand formulas (generic) America's Store Brand Soy Enfamil Enfamil AR Enfamil Lactofree Evaporated milk formula Isomil (all) Neocate Nestlé Carnation Alsoy Nestlé Carnation Follow-Up Nestlé Carnation Follow-Up Soy Nestlé Carnation Good Start Nutramigen ProSobee RCF Similac Similac Lactose Free Similac PM 60/40	Alimentum Enfamil Enfacare Enfamil Premature MJ3232A Neosure Portagen Pregestimil Similac Special Care
Toddlers and young children:	Compleat Pediatric Cow's milk Isomil 2 KetoCal Next Step Next Step Soy Similac 2	Elecare Kindercal Neocate Junior Neocate One+ powder Nutren Junior PediaSure Pediatric EO_{28} Peptamen Junior Pepdite One+ ProPeptide for Kids Resource Just For Kids Vivonex Pediatric
Older children and adolescents:	Carnation Instant Breakfast Criticare HN Ensure Ensure with Fiber Ensure Plus Glucerna L-Emental Tolerex Vivonex Plus Vivonex TEN Boost Boost High-Protein Boost Plus Nepro Scandishake Suplena	Crucial Deliver 2.0 faa Isocal Jevity Glytrol Nestlé Modulen FBD Nutren 2.0 Nutren 1.0 (with Fiber) Osmolite Peptamen Promote ProPeptide Replete Subdue Traumacal Ultracal Vital HN

TABLE 5-26 **Infant Formula Analysis (per Liter)**

Formula	kcal/mL (kcal/oz)	Protein g (% kcal)	Carbohydrates g (% kcal)	Fat g (% kcal)	Na (mEq)	K (mEq)	Ca (mg)	P (mg)	Fe (mg)	Osmolality (mOsm/kg water)	Suggested Uses
Alimentum (Ross)	0.67 (20)	19 (11) Casein hydrolysate l-Cystine, l-Tyr, l-Trp	69 (41) Sucrose 67% Modified tapioca starch	37 (48) MCT oil (33%) Saff oil (39%) Soy oil (28%)	13	20	708	506	12	370	Infants with food allergies, protein or fat malabsorption
America's Store Brand (Wyeth Nutritionals)	0.67 (20)	14.6 (9) Nonfat milk Whey protein concentrate	71 (42) Lactose	35 (47) Oleo oil Coconut oil HO saff+ Sun oil Soy oil	6.5	14	425	284	12	—	Infants with normal GI tract
America's Store Brand for Older Infants (Wyeth Nutritionals)	0.68 (20)	22 (13) Cow's milk protein	69 (40) Lactose Corn syrup solids	37 (48) Oleo Coconut oil HO soy	9.6	21.5	816	571	12	280	Infants 4-6 mo and older with normal GI tract
America's Store Brand Soy (Wyeth Nutritionals)	0.67 (20)	18 (11) Soy protein isolate l-Methionine	69 (41) Corn syrup solids Sucrose	35 (47) Palm olein HO saff or HO sun Coconut oil Soy oil	6.5	14	608	425	12		Infants with allergy to cow's milk, lactose malabsorption, galactosemia
Enfacare with iron (Mead Johnson)	0.74 (22)	21 (11) Nonfat milk Demineralized whey	79 (43) Maltodextrin Lactose Citrates	39 (46) HO sun oil Soy oil MCT oil Coconut oil	11	20	890	490	13	230	Infants with conditions such as prematurity
Enfamil AR (Mead Johnson)	0.67 (20)	16.8 (10) Nonfat milk	74 (44) Lactose (57%) Rice starch (30%) Maltodextrins (13%)	34 (46) Palm olein (45%) Soy oil (20%) Coconut oil (20%) HO sun oil (15%)	12	19	530	360	12	240	When a thickened feeding is desired (should not be concentrated >24 kcal/oz)
Enfamil with Iron [low iron] (Mead Johnson)	0.67 (20)	14 (9) Nonfat milk Demineralized whey	73 (44) Lactose	36 (48) Palm olein (45%) Soy oil (20%) Coconut oil (20%) HO sun oil (15%)	8	19	530	360	12 [5]	300	Infants with normal GI tract

Continued on following page

TABLE 5-26 Infant Formula Analysis (per Liter) *(Continued)*

Formula	kcal/mL (kcal/oz)	Protein g (% kcal)	Carbohydrates g (% kcal)	Fat g (% kcal)	Na (mEq)	K (mEq)	Ca (mg)	P (mg)	Fe (mg)	Osmolality (mOsm/kg water)	Suggested Uses
Enfamil with Iron 24 [low iron] (Mead Johnson)	0.8 (24)	17 (9) Nonfat milk whey	88 (43) Lactose	43 (48) Palm olein (45%) Soy oil (20%) HO sun oil (15%) Coconut oil (20%)	10	23	630	430	15 [6]	360	Infants with normal GI tract requiring additional calories
Enfamil Lactofree (Mead Johnson)	0.67 (20)	14 (9) Milk protein isolate	74 (43) Corn syrup solids	36 (48) Palm olein (45%) Soy oil (20%) Coconut oil (20%) HO sun oil (15%)	9	19	550	370	12	200	Infants with lactose malabsorption
Enfamil Premature Formula 20 [w/Fe] (Mead Johnson)	0.67 (20)	20 (12) Demineralized whey Nonfat milk	75 (44) Corn syrup solids Lactose	35 (44) MCT oil (40%) Soy oil Coconut oil	11	18	1120	560	1.7 [12]	260	Preterm infants
Enfamil Premature Formula 24 [w/Fe] (Mead Johnson)	0.8 (24)	24 (12) Demineralized whey Nonfat milk	9 (44) Corn syrup solids Lactose	41 (44) MCT oil (40%) Soy oil Coconut oil	14	21	1340	670	2 [15]	310	Preterm infants
Evaporated milk formula: 13 oz evaporated whole milk, 19 oz water, 2 tbsp corn syrup	0.67 (20)	27 (16) Cow's milk	72 (43) Lactose Corn syrup	31 (41) Butterfat	21	32	1066	832	0.8		Infants with normal GI tract; need vitamin C and iron supplement
Isomil (Ross)	0.67 (20)	17 (10) Soy protein isolate Methionine	70 (41) Corn syrup Sucrose	37 (49) Soy oil (30%) Coconut oil (30%) HO saff oil (40%)	13	19	709	507	12	200	Infants with allergy to cow's milk, lactose malabsorption, galactosemia
Isomil DF (Ross)	0.67 (20)	18 (11) Soy protein isolate Methionine	68 (40) Corn syrup Sucrose Soy fiber	37 (49) Soy oil (60%) Coconut oil (40%)	13	19	709	507	12	240	Short-term management of diarrhea; contains fiber

MJ3232A (Mead Johnson)	0.42 (12.7)	19 (18) Casein hydrolysate l-Cystine, l-Tyr, l-Trp	28 (27) Tapioca starch CHO selected by physician	28 (55) MCT oil (85%) Corn oil (15%)	13	19	640	430	13	250	Infants with severe CHO intolerance (CHO must be added)
Neocate (SHS North America)	0.69 (21)	20 (12) Free amino acids	78 (47) Corn syrup solids	30 (41) Saff oil Coconut oil Soy oil	11	26	837	628	12	375	Infants with severe food allergies
Nestlé Carnation Alsoy (Nestlé)	0.67 (20)	21 (11) l-Methionine Soy protein isolate	68 (44) Sucrose Maltodextrin	36 (45) Palm olein (47%) Soy oil (26%) Coconut oil (21%) HO saff oil (6%)	10	20	702	413	13	270	Infants with allergy to cow's milk, lactose malabsorption, galactosemia
Nestlé Carnation Follow-Up (Nestlé)	0.67 (20)	18 (10) Nonfat milk	89 (53) Corn syrup Lactose	28 (37) Palm olein (47%) Soy oil (26%) Coconut oil (21%) HO saff oil (6%)	11	23	811	603	13	326	Infants 4–12 months with normal GI tract
Nestlé Carnation Follow-Up Soy (Nestlé)	0.67(20)	21(12) Soy protein isolate Methionini	81(48) Maltodextrin Sucrose	29(40) Palm olein (47%) Soy oil (26%) Coconut oil (21%) HO saff oil (6%)	12	20	905	603	13	200	Infants 4–12 months with allergy to cow's milk, lactose malabsorption, galactosemia
Nestlé Carnation Good Start (Nestlé)	0.67 (20)	Partially hydrolyzed whey	74 (44) Lactose Maltodextrins	35 (46) Palm olein (47%) Soy oil (26%) Coconut oil (21%) HO saff oil (6%)	7	17	429	241	10	300	Infants with normal GI tract
Nutramigen (Mead Johnson)	0.67 (20)	19 (11) Casein hydrolysate l-Cystine, l-Tyr, l-Trp	75 (44) Corn syrup solids Modified cornstarch	34 (45) Palm olein (45%) Soy oil (20%) Coconut oil (20%) HO sun oil (15%)	14	19	640	430	12	320	Infants with food allergies

Continued on following page

TABLE 5-26 Infant Formula Analysis (per Liter) *(Continued)*

Formula	kcal/mL (kcal/oz)	Protein g (% kcal)	Carbohydrates g (% kcal)	Fat g (% kcal)	Na (mEq)	K (mEq)	Ca (mg)	P (mg)	Fe (mg)	Osmolality (mOsm/kg water)	Suggested Uses
Portagen (Mead Johnson)	0.67 (20)	24 (14) Na caseinate	78 (46) Corn syrup solids Sucrose	32 (40) MCT oil (86%) Corn oil (14%)	16	22	640	470	13	230	Infants with fat malabsorption, intestinal lymphatic obstruction, chylothorax
Pregestimil (Mead Johnson)	0.67 (20)	19 (11) Casein hydrolysate l-Cystine, l-Tyr, l-Trp	69 (41) Corn syrup solids (60%) Modified corn starch (20%) Dextrose (20%)	38 (48) MCT oil (55%) Corn oil (10%) Soy oil (25%) HO saff oil (10%)	11	19	766	500	12	320	Infants with food allergies, protein or fat malabsorption
ProSobee (Mead Johnson)	0.67 (20)	17 (10) l-Methionine soy protein isolate	73 (42) Corn syrup solids	37 (48) Palm olein (45%) Soy oil (20%) Coconut oil (20%) HO sun oil (15%)	10	21	710	560	12	200	Infants with allergy to cow's milk, lactose malabsorption, galactosemia
RCF* [w/Fe] (Ross)	0.4 (12)	20 (20) Soy isolate	Selected by physician	36 (80) Soy oil Coconut oil	13	19	709	507	12	*	Infants with severe CHO intolerance (CHO must be added); Modified for ketogenic diet
Similac with Iron [low iron] (Ross)	0.67 (20)	14 (8) Nonfat milk Whey protein	73 (43) Lactose	36 (49) Soy oil (30%) Coconut oil (30%) HO saff oil (40%)	7	18	527	284	12 [5]	300	Infants with normal GI tract

Similac with Iron 24 (Ross)	0.8 (24)	22 (11) Nonfat milk	85 (42) Lactose	42 (47) Soy oil (60%) Coconut oil (40%)	12	27	726	565	15	380	Infants with normal GI tract requiring additional calories
Similac Lactose Free (Ross)	0.67 (20)	14.5 (9) Milk protein isolate	72.3 (43) Corn syrup solids (55%) Sucrose (45%)	36.5 (49) Soy oil (60%) Coconut oil (40%)	9	18	568	378	12	200	Infants with lactose malabsorption
Similac Neosure (Ross)	0.73 (22)	19 (10) Nonfat mlk Whey protein concentrate	77 (41) Lactose (50%) Maltodextrins (50%)	41 (49) MCT oil (25%) Soy oil (45%) Coconut oil (30%)	11	27	784	463	13	25	Preterm infants, after hospital discharge, until goal catch-up growth
Similac PM 60/40 (Ross)	0.67 (20)	15 (9) Whey protein concentrate Na caseinate	69 (41) Lactose	38 (50) Soy oil (12%) Coconut oil (38%) Corn oil (50%)	7	15	378	189	5	280	Infants who require lowered calcium and phosphorus levels
Similac Special Care 20 [w/ Fe] (Ross)	0.67 (20)	18 (11) Nonfat milk Whey protein concentrate	72 (42) Corn syrup solids (50%) Lactose (50%)	37 (49) MCT oil (50%) Soy oil (30%) Coconut oil (20%)	13	22	1216	676	2.5 (12)	235	Preterm infants
Similac Special Care 24 [w/ Fe] (Ross)	0.8 (24)	22 (11) Nonfat milk Whey protein concentrate	86 (42) Corn syrup solids (50%) Lactose (50%)	44 (49) MCT oil (50%) Soy Oil (30%) Coconut oil (20%)	15	27	1452	806	3 (15)	280	Preterm infants

Ca, calcium; CHO, carbohydrate; Fe, iron; GI, gastrointestinal; MCT, medium chain triglycerides; Na, sodium; K, potassium; P, phosphorus; Saff, safflower; Soy oil, soybean oil; Sun, sunflower.
*Available as concentrated liquid. Nutrient values vary depending on amount of added carbohydrate (CHO) and water. A total of 12 fl oz of concentrated liquid with 15 g CHO and 12 fl oz water yields 20 kcal/fl oz formula with 68 g CHO/L. For most current information, refer to formula websites or labels.

TABLE 5-27 **Human Milk and Fortifiers Analysis (per Liter)**

Formula	kcal/mL (kcal/oz)	Protein g (% kcal)	Carbohydrate g (% kcal)	Fat g (% kcal)	Na (mEq)	K (mEq)	Ca (mg)	P (mg)	Fe (mg)	Osmolality (mOsm/kg water)	Suggested Uses
Human milk (mature)	0.69 (20)	10 (6) Human milk protein	72 (42) Lactose	39 (54) Human milk fat	7	13	280	147	0.4	286	Infants
Human milk* (preterm)	0.67(20)	14 (8) Human milk protein	66 (40) Lactose	39(52) Human milk fat	11	15	248	128	1.2	290	Preterm infants
Enfamil Human Milk Fortifier [per packet] (Mead Johnson)	3.5 (–)	0.3 (29) Whey protein isolate Na caseinate	0.26 (30) Corn syrup solids	0.16 (42) From caseinate	0.12	0.13	23	11	0.36	—	Fortifier for preterm human milk
Similac Natural Care Human Milk Fortifier (Ross)	0.8 (24)	22 (11) Nonfat milk Whey protein concentrate	86 (42) Corn syrup solids (50%) Lactose (50%)	44 (47) MCT oil (50%) Soy oil (30%) Coconut oil (20%)	15	26.6	1694	935	3	280	Fortifier for preterm human milk
Preterm Human Milk + Enfamil Human Milk Fortifier (1 pkt/25 mL)	0.79 (24)	27 (13) Human milk protein, Whey protein concentrate Na caseinate	82 (41) Lactose Corn syrup solids	41 (46) Human milk fat	165	18	1140	590	15	410	Preterm infants
Preterm Human Milk + Similac Human Milk Fortifier (1 packet/25 mL)	0.79 (24)	23 (12) Nonfat milk Whey protein concentrate Human milk protein	82 (41) Lactose Corn syrup solids	41 (47) MCT oil Human milk fat	17	30	1380	776	4.6	385	Preterm infants
Preterm Human Milk + Similac Natural Care 75:25 ratio	0.7 (21)	16 (9) Human milk protein Nonfat milk Whey protein concentrate	71 (40) Lactose Corn syrup solids	40 (51) Human milk fat MCT oil, Soy oil Coconut oil	12	18	610	330	1.65	288	Preterm infants
Preterm Human Milk + Similac Natural Care 50:50 ratio	0.74 (22)	18 (10) Human milk protein Nonfat milk Whey protein concentrate	71 (40) Lactose Corn syrup solids	41 (50) Human milk fat MCT oil Soy Oil Coconut oil	13	21	971	531	2.1	285	Preterm infants

Ca, calcium; Fe, iron; MCT, medium chain triglycerides; Na, sodium; K, potassium; P, phosphorus; Soy, soybean.
*Composition of human milk varies with maternal diet, state of lactation, within feedings, diurnally, and among mothers.
From Ross Products Division, Abbott Laboratories, Inc.

TABLE 5-28 **Toddler and Young Child Formula Analysis (per Liter)**

Formula	kcal/mL (kcal/oz)	Protein g (% kcal)	Carbohydrate g (% kcal)	Fat g (% kcal)	Na (mEq)	K (mEq)	Ca (mg)	P (mg)	Fe (mg)	Osmolality (mOsm/kg water)	Suggested Uses
Compleat Pediatric (Novartis)	1 (30)	38 (15) Beef Na caseinate Ca caseinate	130 (50) Vegetables Fruit Hydrolyzed cornstarch Apple juice	39 (35) HO sun oil Soy oil MCT oil	30	38	1000	1000	13	380	For those who desire a blenderized tube feeding
Cow's milk, whole	0.63 (19)	34 (22) Cow's milk	48 (31) Lactose	34 (49) Butterfat	22	40	1226	956	0.5	285	Children >1 year of age with normal GI tract
Elecare (Ross)	1 (30)	30 (15) Free l-amino acids	107 (43) Corn syrup solids	47.6 (42) HO saff oil (39%) MCT oil (33%) Soy oil (28%)	20	39	1082	808	18	596	Children with malabsorption, protein allergy
Isomil 2 (Ross)	0.67 (20)	17 (10) Soy protisolate Methionine	70 (41) Corn syrup (80%) Sucrose (20%)	37 (49) HO saff (40%) Coconut (30%) Soy oil (30%)	13	19	912	608	12	200	Milk sensitive 6–18 mo eating cereal and baby foods
KetoCal (SHS North America)	1.44 (43)	30 (8.4) Cow's milk protein	6 (1.6) Corn syrup solids	144 (90) Soybean oil	26	55	1600	1300	22	197	Children on ketogenic diet
Kindercal TF [contains fiber] (Mead Johnson)	1.06 (32)	30 (11) Milk protein concentrate	135 (52) Maltodextrins Sucrose	44 (37) Canola oil (40%) HO sun oil (28%) Corn oil (12%) MCT oil (20%)	16	34	1010	850	11	345 (institutional and retail) 440 (vanilla) 520 (chocolate)	Tube feeding and oral supplement for children with normal GI tract
Neocate Junior (SHS North America)	1 (30)	30 (12) Free amino acids	104 (42) Corn syrup solids	50 (46) Canola oil MCT oil (25%) Saff oil	18	35	1130	940	14	602	Children with malabsorption, protein allergy
Neocate One+ Powder (SHS North America)	1 (30)	25 (10) Free amino acids	146 (58) Corn syrup solids	35 (22) MCT oil (35%) Canola oil Saff oil	9	24	620	620	8	610	Children with malabsorption, protein allergy

Continued on following page

TABLE 5-28 **Toddler and Young Child Formula Analysis (per Liter)** *(Continued)*

Formula	kcal/mL (kcal/oz)	Protein g (% kcal)	Carbohydrate g (% kcal)	Fat g (% kcal)	Na (mEq)	K (mEq)	Ca (mg)	P (mg)	Fe (mg)	Osmolality (mOsm/kg water)	Suggested Uses
Next Step (Mead Johnson)	0.67 (20)	18 (10) Nonfat milk protein	75 (45) Lactose Corn syrup solids	34 (45) Palm olein (45%) Soy oil (20%) Coconut oil (20%) HO sun oil (15%)	12	23	810	570	12	270	Toddlers with normal GI tract
Next Step Soy (Mead Johnson)	0.67 (20)	22 (13) Soy protein isolate	80 (47) Corn syrup solids Sucrose	30 (40) Palm olein (45%) Soy oil (20%) Coconut oil (20%) HO sun oil (15%)	13	26	780	610	12	260	Toddlers with cow's milk allergy, galactosemia
Nutren Junior [also with fiber] (Nestlé)	1 (30)	30 (12) Casein (50%) Whey (50%)	128 (51) Maltodextrins Sucrose (soy polysaccharides)	42 (37) Soy oil MCT oil (25%) Canola oil Soy lecithin	20	34	1000	800	14	350	Tube feeding and oral supplement for children with normal GI tract
PediaSure [also with fiber] (Ross)	1 (30)	30 (12) Na caseinate Whey protein concentrate	110 (44) Maltodextrins Sucrose (soy fiber)	50 (44) HO saff oil (50%) Soy oil (30%) MCT oil (20%)	17	34	970	800	14	335 (institutional) 430 (retail/oral)	Tube feeding and oral supplement for children with normal GI tract
Pediatric EO_{28} (SHS North America)	1 (30)	25 (10) Free amino acids	146 (58) Maltodextrins Sucrose	35 (32) MCT oil Canola oil HO saff oil	9	24	620	620	8	820	Children with malabsorption, protein allergy

Pepdite One+ (SHS North America)	1 (30)	31 (12) Hydrolized meat and soy protein Free amino acids	106 (42) Corn syrup solids	50 (46) MCT oil Canola oil Saff oil	18	35	1130	940	14	432–440	Children with malabsorption
Peptamen Junior [also with fiber] (Nestlé)	1 (30)	30 (12) Enzymatically hydrolyzed whey protein	138 (55) Maltodextrin Sucrose (flavored) Cornstarch	38.5 (33) MCT oil (60%) Soy oil Canola oil Lecithin	20	33	1000	800	14	260 (unflavored) 360 (flavored)	Children with malabsorption
Propeptide for Kids (Hormel Health Labs)	1 (30)	30 (12) Enzymatically hydrolyzed whey protein	137.5 (55) Maltodextrin Sucrose Cornstarch	38.5 (33) MCT oil (18.5%) Soy oil (22%) Canola oil (60%) Lecithin	20	34	1000	800	14	360	Children with malabsorption
Resource Just for Kids (Novartis)	1 (30)	30 (12) Na caseinate Ca caseinate Whey protein concentrates	110 (44) Hydrolyzed cornstarch Sucrose	50 (44) HO sun oil Soy oil MCT oil	17	33	1140	800	14	390	Tube feeding and oral supplement for children with normal GI tract
Similac 2	0.67 (20)	14 (8) Nonfat milk Whey protein concentrate	72 (43) Lactose	37 (49) HO saff (40%) Coconut oil (30%) Soy oil (30%)	7	18	797	432	12	300	6–18 months eating cereal and baby foods
Vivonex Pediatric (Novartis)	0.8 (24)	24 (12) Free amino acids	130 (63) Maltodextrins Modified starch	24 (25) MCT oil (68%) Soy oil (32%)	17	31	970	800	10	360	Children with malabsorption, protein allergy

Ca, calcium; Fe, iron; GI, gastroinstinal; MCT, medium chain triglycerides; Na, sodium; K, potassium; P, phosphorus; Saff, safflower; Soy oil, soybean oil; Sun, sunflower.

TABLE 5-29 Older Child and Adult Formula Analysis (per Liter)

Formula	kcal/mL (kcal/oz)	Protein g (% kcal)	Carbohydrate g (% kcal)	Fat g (% kcal)	Na (mEq)	K (mEq)	Ca (mg)	P (mg)	Fe (mg)	Osmolality (mOsm/kg water)	Suggested Uses
Boost (Mead Johnson)	1 (30)	42 (17) Milk protein concentrate	171 (67) Corn syrup solids Sucrose	17 (16) Canola oil HO sun oil Corn oil	24	43	1248	1040	15	610	Oral supplement
Boost High Protein (Mead Johnson)	1 (30)	61 (24) Na caseinate Ca caseinate Milk protein concentrate	139 (55) Corn syrup solids Sucrose	23 (21) Canola oil HO sun oil Corn oil	31	41	1390	1310	19	540	Oral supplement or tube feeding for patients with increased protein needs
Boost Plus (Mead Johnson)	1.5 (45)	59 (16) Na caseinate Ca caseinate Milk protein concentrate	200 (50) Corn syrup solids Sucrose	58 (34) Canola oil HO sun oil Corn oil	31	41	1390	1310	19	720	Oral supplement or tube feeding for patients with high calorie needs, normal GI tract, volume fluid restriction
Carnation Instant Breakfast [w/whole milk] (Nestlé)	1.2 (36)	53 (18) Cow's milk	161 (54) Lactose Maltodextrin Sucrose	34 (26) Butterfat	42	67	1632	1400	17	590	High-calorie supplement for patients with normal GI tract
Criticare HN (Mead Johnson)	1.06 (32)	38 (14) Hydrolyzed casein Amino acids	220 (81.5) Maltodextrin Modified cornstarch	5 (4.5) Saff oil	27	34	530	530	9.7	650	Patients with malabsorption IBD, short bowel
Crucial (Nestlé)	1.5 (45)	94 (25) Enzymatically hydrolyzed casein arginine glutamine	135 (36) Maltodextrin Corn starch	68 (39) Marine oil MCT oil (50%) Soybean oil	51	48	1000	1000	18	490	Volume-restricted critically ill patients
Deliver 2.0 (Mead Johnson)	2 (60)	75 (15) Ca caseinate Na caseinate	200 (40) Corn syrup	101 (45) Soy oil (70%) MCT oil (30%)	35	43	1010	1010	18	640	Oral supplement or tube feeding for patients with fluid restriction or liver disease increased calorie needs
Ensure (Ross)	1.06 (32)	37 (14) Na caseinate Ca caseinate Soy protein isolate Whey protein concentrate	167 (64) Corn syrup Maltodextrin Sucrose	25 (22) HO saff oil (40%) Canola oil (40%) Corn oil (20%)	36	40	1250	1250	18.7	590	Oral supplement or tube feeding for patients with normal GI tract

Ensure Fiber [with FOS] (Ross)	1.06 (32)	37 (14) Na caseinate Ca caseinate Soy protein isolate	175 (64) Maltodextrin (65%) Sucrose (29%) Soy fiber (2%) Oat fiber (2%) Fructooligosaccharides (2%)	25 (22) Corn oil (20%) HO saff oil (40%) Canola oil (40%)	37	40	1458	1250	19	500	Oral supplement or tube feeding with fiber, normal GI tract
Ensure Plus (Ross)	1.5 (45)	54 (15) Na caseinate Ca caseinate Soy protein isolate	208 (56) Corn syrup Sucrose Maltodextrin	48 (29) Corn oil (25%) Canola oil (50%) HO saff (25%)	43	47	833	833	19	680	Oral supplement or tube feeding for patients with higher calorie needs, normal GI tract
faa (Nestlé)	1.0 (30)	50 (20) Free amino acids	176 (70) Maltodextrin	11(10) Soy oil MCT oil	24	38	800	700	18	700	Tube feeding or oral supplement for malabsorption, not for protein allergy
Glucerna (Ross)	1 (30)	42 (17) Na caseinate Ca caseinate	96 (34) Soy fiber Fructose Maltodextrin	54 (49) HO saff oil (85%) Canola oil (10%) Lecithin (5%)	40	40	705	705	13	355	Patients with impaired glucose tolerance, also contains fiber
Glytrol (Nestlé)	1.0 (30)	45 (18) Ca potassium caseinates	100 (40) Maltodextrin Modified corn starch Fructose Gum arabic Soy polysaccharide pectin	48 (42) Canola oil HO saff MCT oil Soy lecithin	32	36	720	720	13	380	Tube feeding or oral supplement for patients with impaired glucose tolerance
Isocal (Mead Johnson)	1.06 (32)	34 (13) Na caseinate Ca caseinate Soy protein	135 (50) Maltodextrin	44 (37) MCT oil (20%) Soy oil (80%)	23	34	630	530	10	270	Tube feeding for patients with normal GI tract
Jevity (Ross)	1.06 (32)	44 (17) Na caseinate Ca caseinate	155 (54) Corn syrup Maltodextrin Soy fiber	35 (29) HO saff oil (48%) Canola oil (29%) MCT oil (20%) Lecithin (3%)	40	40	910	760	14	300	Tube feeding with fiber, normal GI tract
I-Emental (Hormel Health Labs)	1 (30)	38 (15) Free amino acids	210 (82) Maltodextrins	2.85 (3) Saff oil	20	20	500	500	9	630	Patients with malabsorption, protein allergy
Nepro (Ross)	2 (60)	70 (14) Ca caseinate Mg caseinate Na caseinate Milk protein isolate	108 (44)	96 (43) HO saff oil (67%) Canola oil (29%) Lecithin (4%)	36	27	1370	685	19	665	Patients with renal failure undergoing dialysis

Continued on following page

TABLE 5-29 Older Child and Adult Formula Analysis (per Liter) *(Continued)*

Formula	kcal/mL (kcal/oz)	Protein g (% kcal)	Carbohydrate g (% kcal)	Fat g (% kcal)	Na (mEq)	K (mEq)	Ca (mg)	P (mg)	Fe (mg)	Osmolality (mOsm/kg water)	Suggested Uses
Nestlé Modulen IBD (Nestlé)	1 (30)	36 (14) Acid casein with TGF-β_2	108(44) Corn syrup Sucrose	46 (42) Milk fat MCT oil Corn oil Soy oil Lecithin	15	31	888	600	12	370	Patients with Crohn's disease
Nutren 1.0 [with fiber] (Nestlé)	1 (30)	40 (16) K caseinate Ca caseinate	127 (51) Maltodextrin Corn syrup solids (soy polysaccharide)	38 (33) Canola oil MCT oil (25%) Corn oil	38	32	668	668	12	315–370	Standard tube feeding with fiber
Nutren 2.0 (Nestlé)	2 (60)	80 (16) K caseinate Ca caseinate	196 (39) Corn syrup solids Maltodextrin Sucrose	106 (45) MCT oil (75%) Canola oil Corn oil Soy lecithin	57	49	1340	1340	24	745	Oral supplement or tube feedings for patients with fluid restriction or increased calorie needs
Osmolite (Ross)	1.06 (32)	37 (14) Na caseinate Ca caseinate Soy protein isolate	151 (57) Maltodextrin	35 (29) HO saff oil (48%) Canola oil (29%) MCT oil (20%) Lecithin (3%)	28	26	535	535	9.6	300	Tube feeding for patients with normal GI tract
Peptamen (Nestlé)	1 (30)	40 (16) Enzymatically hydrolyzed whey protein	127 (51) Maltodextrin Corn starch	39 (33) MCT oil (70%) Soybean oil (30%)	24	39	800	700	18	270–380	Patients with malabsorption
Promote (Ross)	1 (30)	63 (25) Na caseinate Ca caseinate Soy protein isolate	130 (52) Maltodextrin Sucrose	26 (23) HO saff oil (47%) Canola oil (28%) MCT oil (19%) Lecithin (6%)	43	50	1200	1200	18	340	Tube feeding or oral supplement for patients with increased protein needs
ProPeptide [unflavored] (Hormel Health Labs)	1 (30)	40 (16) Hydrolyzed whey	127 (51) Maltodextrins Starch	39 (33) Sun oil (30%) MCT oil (70%)	22	32	800	700	14	270	Patients with malabsorption
Replete [with fiber] (Nestlé)	1 (30)	62 (25) Ca Potassium Caseinate	113 (40) Maltodextrin Corn syrup solids	34 (30) Canola oil MCT oil Soy lecithin	38	39	1000	1000	18	300–398	Tube feeding or oral supplement for patients with increased protein needs

Scandishake [w/whole milk] (Scandipharm)	2.5 (75)	50 (8) Cow's milk	292 (47) Lactose Maltodextrin Soy oil	125 (45) Coconut oil Saff oil Palm oil	240	103	391	479	Trace	1094	High-calorie supplement and for fat malabsorption
Subdue (Mead Johnson)	1 (30)	50 (20) Hydrolyzed whey protein concentrate	127 (50) Maltodextrin Corn starch Sucrose	34 (30) Canola oil HO sun oil Corn oil MCT oil	48	41	1081	1040	15	330	Patients with malabsorption, IBD
Suplena (Ross)	2 (60)	30 (6) Na caseinate Ca caseinate	255 (51) Maltodextrin Sucrose (10%)	96 (43) HO saff oil (86%) Soy oil (10%) Lecithin (4%)	34	29	1430	730	19	600	Patients with renal failure not undergoing dialysis
Tolerex (Novartis)	1 (30)	21 (8) Free amino acids	230 (91) Maltodextrin	1.5 (1) Saff oil	20	30	560	560	10	550	Patients with chylothorax, malabsorption, or severe food allergy
Traumacal (Mead Johnson)	1.5 (45)	82 (22) Na caseinate Ca caseinate	144 (38) Corn syrup Sucrose	68 (40) Soy oil (70%) MCT oil (30%)	51	36	750	750	9	560	Patients with increased protein and calorie needs
Ultracal (Mead Johnson)	1.06 (32)	45 (17) Na caseinate Ca caseinate Milk protein concentrate	132 (50) Maltodextrin Soy fiber Microcrystalline cellulose Acacia	39 (33) MCT oil (30%) Canola oil (35%) HO sun oil (25%) Corn oil (10%)	59	47	1000	1000	18	360	Oral supplement or tube feeding with fiber, normal GI tract
Vital HN (Ross)	1 (30)	42 (17) Hydrolyzed whey, meat, and soy protein (87%) Free amino acids (13%)	185 (74) Maltodextrin, Sucrose, Lactose (<0.5%)	11 (9) Saff oil (55%) MCT oil (45%)	25	36	667	667	12	500	Patients with malabsorption, IBD
Vivonex Plus (Novartis)	1 (30)	45 (18) Free amino acids	190 (76) Maltodextrin modified cornstarch	6.7 (6) Soy oil	27	27	560	560	10	650	Patients with malabsorption or severe food allergy
Vivonex TEN (Novartis)	1 (30)	38 (15) Free amino acids	210 (82) Maltodextrin modified cornstarch	2.8 (3) Saff oil	26	24	500	500	9	630	Patients with malabsorption or severe food allergy

Ca, calcium; Fe, iron; GI, gastroinstinal; IBD, irritable bowel disease; K, potassium; MCT, medium chain triglycerides; Na, sodium; P, phosphorus; Saff, safflower; Soy oil, soybean oil; Sun, sunflower.

TABLE 5-30 **Oral Rehydration Solutions**

Solution	kcal/mL (kcal/oz)	Carbohydrate (g/L)	Na (mEq/L)	K (mEq/L)	Osmolality (mOsm/kg H_2O)
CeraLyte-70 (Cera)	0.16 (4.9)	Rice digest 40	70	20	232
CeraLyte-50 (Cera)	0.16 (4.9)	Rice digest, Glucose 40	50	20	200
Enfalyte (Mead Johnson)	0.12 (3.7)	Rice syrup solids 30	50	25	200
Oral Rehydration Salts (WHO) (Jianas)	0.06 (2)	Dextrose 20	90	20	330
Pedialyte Unflavored (Ross)	0.1 (3)	Dextrose 25	45	20	250
Rehydralyte (Ross)	0.1 (3)	Dextrose 25	75	20	305

K, potassium; Na, sodium.

BOX 5-2 **MyPyramid for Kids Guidelines Based on a 1,800-Calorie Diet**

Grains
- 6 ounces a day, half of which should be whole grain
- 1 ounce equivalent is about 1 slice of bread; 1 cup dry cereal; or ½ cup cooked rice, pasta, cereal
- Search ingredient lists to determine if bread is "whole" grain. Brown does not always mean whole grain.

Vegetables
- 2½ cups a day
- Colorizing plates with colorful vegetables such as dark green broccoli and spinach, and orange carrots and sweet potatoes

Fruits
- 1½ cups a day
- Juice should contain 100% fruit juice, no sweeteners.

Milk
- 3 cups a day; for children over 8 years old
- 2 cups for children ages 2 to 8 years old
- 1 cup yogurt or 1½ ounces cheese = 1 cup milk
- Use low-fat or fat-free milk, yogurt, or cheese.

Meat and Beans
- 5 ounces every day
- Eat lean or low-fat meat, chicken, turkey, and fish for protein and have it baked, broiled, or grilled—not fried.
- Nuts, seeds, peas, and beans are all sources of protein, too.

Other
- Obtain healthy oils from fish, nuts, corn oil, soybean oil, and canola oil.
- Read Nutrition Facts labels for fat and sugar content.
- Choose food and beverages that are low in added sugars and other caloric sweeteners
- Exercise at least 60 minutes a day: walking, running, rollerblading, or dancing.

For the full MyPyramid charts, go to http://www.myPyramid.gov

TABLE 5-31 Following the DASH Eating Plan

Food Group	Daily Servings	Serving Sizes	Examples and Notes	Significance in the DASH Eating Plan*
Grains and grain products	7–8	1 slice bread 1 ounce dry cereal[†] 0.5 cup cooked rice, pasta, or cereal	Whole wheat bread, English muffin, pita bread, bagel, cereals, grits, oatmeal, crackers, unsalted pretzels, popcorn	Major source of energy and fiber
Vegetables	4–5	1 cup raw leafy vegetable 0.5 cup cooked vegetable 6 ounces vegetable juice	Tomatoes, potatoes, carrots, green peas, squash, broccoli, turnip greens, collards, kale, spinach, artichokes, green beans, lima beans, sweet potatoes	Rich sources of potassium, magnesium, and fiber
Fruits	4–5	6 ounces fruit juice 1 medium fruit 0.25 cup dried fruit 0.5 cup fresh, frozen, or canned fruit	Apricots, bananas, dates, grapes, oranges, orange juice, grapefruit, grapefruit juice, mangos, melons, peaches, pineapples, prunes, raisins, strawberries, tangerines	Important sources of potassium, magnesium, and fiber
Low-fat or fat-free dairy foods	2–3	8 ounces milk 1 cup yogurt 1.5 ounces cheese	Fat-free (skim) or low-fat (1%) milk, fat-free or low-fat buttermilk, fat-free or low-fat regular or frozen yogurt, low-fat and fat-free cheese	Major sources of calcium and protein
Meats, poultry, and fish	2 or less	3 ounces cooked meats, poultry, or fish	Select only lean; trim away visible fats; broil, roast, or boil instead of frying; remove skin from poultry	Rich sources of protein and magnesium
Nuts, seeds, and dry beans	4–5 per week	0.33 cup or 1.5 ounces nuts 2 Tbsp or 0.5 ounce seeds 0.5 cup cooked dry beans, peas	Almonds, filberts, mixed nuts, peanuts, walnuts, sunflower seeds, kidney beans, lentils	Rich sources of energy, magnesium, potassium, protein, and fiber
Fats and oils[‡]	2–3	1 tsp soft margarine 1 Tbsp low-fat mayonnaise 2 Tbsp light salad dressing 1 tsp vegetable oil	Soft margarine, low-fat mayonnaise, light salad dressing, vegetable oil (e.g., olive, corn, canola, safflower)	DASH has 27% of calories as fat, including fat in or added to foods
Sweets	5 per week	1 Tbsp sugar 1 Tbsp jelly or jam 0.5 ounce jelly beans 8 ounces lemonade	Maple syrup, sugar, jelly, jam, fruit-flavored gelatin, jelly beans, hard candy, fruit punch, sorbet ices	Sweets should be low in fat content

*The Dietary Approaches to Stop Hypertension (DASH) eating plan is based on 2000 calories per day. The number of daily servings in a food group may vary from those listed, depending on an individual's caloric needs. This chart can help in planning menus and can be taken to the store when shopping.

[†]Equals 0.5 to 1.25 cups, depending on cereal type. Check the product's nutritional fact label.

[‡]Fat content changes serving counts for fats and oils. For example, 1 Tbsp of regular salad dressing equals 1 serving; 1 Tbsp of a low-fat dressing equals 0.5 serving; 1 Tbsp of a fat-free dressing equals 0 servings.

TABLE 5-32 DASH Eating Plan: Number of Servings for Other Calorie Levels

	SERVINGS PER DAY	
Food Group	**1600 Calories/Day**	**3100 Calories/Day**
Grains and grain products	6	12–13
Vegetables	3–4	6
Fruits	4	6
Low-fat or fat-free dairy foods	2–3	3–4
Meats, poultry, and fish	1–2	2–3
Nuts, seeds, and dry beans	3 per week	1
Fat and oils	2	4
Sweets	0	2

DASH, dietary approaches to stop hypertension.

TABLE 5-33 Where Is the Sodium?

Food Groups	Sodium (mg)*
Grains and Grain Products	
Cooked cereal, rice, pasta, unsalted, 0.5 cup	0–5
Ready-to-eat cereal, 1 cup	100–360
Bread, 1 slice	110–175
Vegetables	
Fresh or frozen, cooked without salt, 0.5 cup	1–70
Canned or frozen with sauce, 0.5 cup	140–460
Tomato juice, canned 0.75 cup	820
Fruit	
Fresh, frozen, canned, 0.5 cup	0–5
Low-Fat or Fat-Free Dairy Foods	
Milk, 1 cup	120
Yogurt, 8 ounces	160
Natural cheeses, 1.5 ounces	110–450
Processed cheeses, 1.5 ounces	600
Nuts, Seeds, and Dry Beans	
Peanuts, salted, 0.3 cup	120
Peanuts, unsalted, 0.3 cup	0–5
Beans, cooked from dried, or frozen, without salt, 0.5 cup	0–5
Beans, canned, 0.5 cup	400
Meats, Fish, and Poultry	
Fresh meat, fish, poultry, 3 ounces	30–90
Tuna canned, water pack, no salt added, 3 ounces	35–45
Tuna canned, water pack, 3 ounces	250–350
Ham, lean, roasted, 3 ounces	1020

*Only a small amount of sodium occurs naturally in foods. Most sodium is added during processing.

TABLE 5-34 Reducing Sodium When Eating Out

Ask how foods are prepared.

Ask that foods be prepared without adding salt, MSG, or salt-containing ingredients. Most restaurants are willing to accommodate requests.

Know the terms that indicate a high-sodium content: pickled, curried, soy sauce, broth.

Move the saltshaker away from the table.

Limit condiments with salt-containing ingredients, such as mustard, catsup, pickles, and sauces.

Choose fruits or vegetables instead of salty snack foods.

TABLE 5-35 **Label Language for Salt**

Phrase*	What It Means
Sodium	
Sodium free or salt free	Less than 5 mg per serving
Very low sodium	35 mg or less of sodium per serving
Low sodium	140 mg or less of sodium per serving
Low sodium meal	140 mg or less of sodium per 3½ oz (100 g)
Reduced or less sodium	At least 25% less sodium than the regular version
Light in sodium	50% less sodium than the regular version
Unsalted or no salt added	No salt added to the product during processing
Fat	
Fat free	Less than 0.5 g per serving
Low saturated fat	1 g or less per serving
Low fat	3 g or less per serving
Reduced fat	At least 25% less fat than the regular version
Light in fat	One half of the fat compared with the regular version

*Food labels can help you choose items lower in sodium and in saturated and total fat. Look for these labels on cans, boxes, bottles, bags, and other packaging.

TABLE 5-36 **Step 1 and Step 2 Diets**

Nutrient	Step 1 Diet	Step 2 Diet
Calories	Adequate to promote normal growth and development	Same
Total fat	≤30% of calories	Same
Saturated fat	<10% of calories	<7% of calories
Polyunsaturated fat	Up to 10% of calories	Same
Monounsaturated	Remaining fat calories	Same
Cholesterol	<300 mg/day	<200 mg/day
Carbohydrates	Approximately 55% of calories	Same
Protein	About 15%–20% of calories	Same

Adoption, Intercountry/International

DEFINITION

Adoption is the legal process by which a child, biologically related to one set of parents, becomes a member of another family. Intercountry adoption is the adoption of a child born in one country by a family living in another country.

EPIDEMIOLOGY & DEMOGRAPHICS

- Increasing numbers of children are being adopted internationally.
- More than 20,000 children per year are adopted: 20,099 in 2002; 21,616 in 2003; and 22,884 in 2004.
- Trends include the adoption of children from Russia, eastern European countries, China, South Korea, South America, and Central America.
- Guidelines for eligibility for intercountry adoption are determined by the country of the child's birth and by the country in which the adopting family lives (see "Suggested Readings").

ADOPTION ISSUES FOR THE PHYSICIAN

- There is a lack of understanding regarding need for comprehensive evaluation of adopted children. A full diagnostic evaluation should be undertaken on every child adopted internationally at the time of arrival, regardless of the child's apparent health.
- Many of the diagnoses made for internationally adopted children are silent infections, putting the child and family at risk for long-term sequelae if not recognized and treated.
- Supports are needed to assist families with mental health issues for which they may be ill prepared.
- Frequently, billing for initial evaluations and laboratory studies must be resubmitted for insurance review, along with a letter outlining the child's risk. To avoid resubmission, use ICD-9-CM codes for specific diagnoses; insurance companies may reject V codes.

CLINICAL PRESENTATION

History

- At the time of the initial evaluation, the health care provider should review all written, video, and photographic information available, even if the accuracy of this information is suspect.
- The physician should review medical information, birth history (if available), laboratory and other diagnostic test results, and treatments (e.g., for prenatal exposure to alcohol and drugs).
- The information available in the child's medical history varies according to the country of birth.
  - South Korea sends detailed and accurate information.
  - China provides little information. Birth and family histories are unavailable because children may have been abandoned before location in an orphanage and subsequent adoption.
  - For Russia and eastern Europe, information varies from detailed records with a video to limited data.
- Medical terms used are often unfamiliar to health care providers familiar with Western medicine.
  - Terms used may imply social or medical risk but not necessarily medical diagnoses.
  - In South or Central America, information may or may not be accurate.
- Specific risks depend on the child's history (e.g., nutrition, abuse and neglect, exposure to alcohol and drugs), not on country of birth.
- Plot all growth parameters (e.g., length or height, weight, head circumference) before adoption.
  - Use standard Centers for Disease Control (CDC) growth charts, not ethnic growth charts.
  - Institutionalized children often have growth delays. Estimate 1 month delay for each 3 to 4 months in an institution. Microcephaly may be a marker for developmental disability.
- Increased incidence of fetal alcohol syndrome (FAS) and fetal alcohol spectrum disorder (FASD) occurs among these children.
- Other possible in utero exposures or infections should be assessed.

Physical Examination

- A complete, unclothed physical examination should be done within a month after arrival in the adoptive home. Many physicians see children within 2 weeks of arrival.
- Measure height or length, weight, and head circumference, plotting the findings on CDC growth charts.
- Examine the child for visible signs of infectious diseases and infestations, such as scabies, lice, impetigo, and scalp furuncles.
- Examine the child for visible signs of abuse or neglect.
  - Document bruises visible at the time of arrival (to prevent potential allegations of abuse against the adoptive parents).
  - If there is evidence of previous abuse, consider a skeletal survey.
  - Document gray-green (blue-gray) spots in children of Asian, Hispanic, and African descent. Spots may be evident on the buttocks, back, arms, and legs.
  - If there is an unusual pattern of spots or bruises, document with photos.
- Perform a careful neurologic evaluation for weakness, asymmetry, and neurologic deficits.
- Evaluate vision.
- Evaluate hearing.
- Perform a dental evaluation for children with teeth.
  - Remind dental professionals that internationally adopted children may have lived in an area without fluoridation.
  - There is a particular risk for baby bottle tooth decay because of the use of propped bottles and poor dental hygiene in orphanages.
- Perform a developmental assessment.
  - For children up to age 3 years, consider referral to early intervention programs for assessment and intervention.
  - Children adopted internationally are at particular risk for sensory processing problems. Refer to occupational therapy for sensory integration evaluation if symptoms of tactile defensiveness or sensory overload persist.
  - Comprehensive developmental evaluations should be obtained for children who are considerably developmentally delayed.

LABORATORY & DIAGNOSTIC STUDIES

- A full assessment should be undertaken for all internationally adopted children, regardless of clinical appearance at the time of the initial office evaluation.
- The workup is based on the risks to the child, gleaned from the history, physical examination results, and the country of origin.
- Infectious disease risks should be assessed (also consult the current *Red Book*).
  - Rapid plasma reagent (RPR) or Venereal Disease Research Laboratory (VDRL), and the fluorescent treponemal antibody tests are used to evaluate for congenital syphilis.
  - Tests are performed for hepatitis B surface antigen, surface antibody, and core antibody (even if performed before adoption).
  - Assess for hepatitis C antibody, particularly in Asian children and children with any history of prenatal drug or alcohol exposure.
- Providers who see numerous adoptees usually check hepatitis C titers.
- Human immunodeficiency virus (HIV) status should be checked with an enzyme-linked immunosorbent assay (ELISA).
- The purified protein derivative (PPD) test is the most overlooked screening test. A blood test for tuberculosis is awaiting U.S. Food and Drug Administration approval.
  - PPD should be done regardless of whether the child has had the Bacille Calmette-Guérin (BCG) vaccine or known exposure.

  - Delay in PPD testing is permissible only for children with a freshly healing BCG scar.
  - A positive PPD result is 10 mm of induration.
  - If positive, a chest radiograph is needed to determine if there is active disease.
- If the chest radiograph is negative, the recommendation is to treat latent tuberculosis for 9 months with isoniazid (10 to 15 mg/kg/day).
  - Liquid form may cause diarrhea.
  - Obtain baseline liver function tests.
- Test stool for ova and parasites.
  - Three specimens are collected 48 to 72 hours apart.
  - Include *Giardia* and *Cryptosporidium* antigens.
  - Obtain samples for testing even in the absence of diarrhea.
  - Consider stool for bacterial culture, particularly if diarrhea is present.
- Assess nutritional, environmental, and genetic risks.
  - Obtain a complete blood cell count and hemoglobin electrophoresis for children of Asian or African descent.
  - Assess the lead level.
  - Consider calcium, phosphorus, and alkaline phosphatase testing for children who are malnourished or at risk for rickets.
  - Assess the thyroid-stimulating hormone (TSH) level for children previously living in areas of low iodine (e.g., China, Russia, eastern Europe).
  - A metabolic screen (with appropriate age-adjusted norms) is recommended for children younger than 1 year to detect inborn errors screened by standard newborn metabolic screening in the United States.

INTERVENTIONS & THERAPY

- Promote family attachment by minimizing visitors.
- Parents should feed, comfort, address toileting needs, and give affection until the child shows signs of attachment to the parents.
- Do not push the child to be independent.
  - The child should be encouraged to depend on the new parents for all of his or her needs.
  - Delay elective surgeries (e.g., circumcision) until the child has adjusted to the new family.
- Sleep problems are common.
  - Parents may need to consider flexible sleeping arrangements, and during the adjustment period, families should consider sharing bedrooms.
  - Parents should avoid allowing child to "cry it out." Parents should encourage adjustment of child to the new family and home but allow adequate sleep for other family members.
- Feeding may require adjustments.
  - Some children may not have been fed textured foods.
  - They may need slow introduction of solid foods.
  - Children may habitually hoard food as a reaction to prior deprivation. They may fill their cheeks or hide food in their rooms.
- Immunizations are usually needed.
  - Children immunized in other countries might have been given vaccines that were not stored properly, were not efficacious, or were not given at appropriate intervals.
  - Vaccine records are often invalid, with the possible exception of those for children who lived in foster care in South Korea.
  - There are two methods for approaching immunization status: re-immunize or obtain titers.
  - Re-immunize with all standard vaccines. For children who did receive three or four previous doses of diphtheria and tetanus toxoids and acellular pertussis (DTaP) vaccine, there may be an increase in local reaction to this vaccine.
  - Obtain titers to document immunity to diphtheria, tetanus, hepatitis B (surface antibody), polio (neutralizing antibody), hepatitis A, measles, mumps, rubella, and varicella.
  - Titers should be done at an age when testing can pick up the child's antibody levels, not those of the biologic mother.
  - Vaccine titers may not be covered by insurance companies.
  - Titers should only be performed if dates of immunizations are available to verify that the vaccines were actually given (with the exception of varicella and hepatitis A).
  - Children should be immunized according to Advisory Committee on Immunization Practices (ACIP) recommendations.
  - Follow the "catch-up" schedule (outlined in the *Red Book* of the American Academy of Pediatrics) for all children requiring immunization or re-immunization.
  - Longer-term follow-up may be required. If results for hepatitis B, hepatitis C, HIV, and tuberculosis exposure were negative at initial evaluation, retest 6 months later.
    - Evaluate the possibility for exposure just before adoption.
    - Malnourished children may be anergic.
    - Monitor closely during the first few months for tuberculosis.
  - Defer PPD testing if the previous PPD result was positive and child is on isoniazid.
- During the first few months after arrival, monitor the child closely for issues related to growth, development, and mental health adjustment.
  - If growth delays persist beyond 6 months, further workup is needed.
  - Refer the child and parents to speech, occupational, and physical therapy as needed.
- Children may need special services because they are at extremely high risk for mental health problems.
  - Posttraumatic stress disorder is common.
  - Attachment disorders occur frequently.
  - Many issues relate to the loss of the previous family, culture, and home.
- Clinicians should wait 1 year before deciding that the age reported (of an older child) is accurate. Consider changing the assigned age if the results of the bone age assessment and dental examination are in variance with the reported age by more than 1 year.

SUGGESTED READINGS

Adoptive Families. Available at www.adoptivefamilies.org

American Academy of Pediatrics Section on Adoption and Foster Care. Available at www.aap.org/sections/adoption/default.htm

American Academy of Pediatrics: Families and adoption: the pediatrician's role in supporting communication. *Pediatrics* 112:1437, 2003.

American Academy of Pediatrics: The medical evaluation of the adopted child: current recommendations. Available at www.aap.org

Bledsoe JM, Johnston BD: Preparing families for international adoption. *Pediatr Rev* 25:242, 2004.

Families with Children from China. Available at www.fwcc.org

Fetal Alcohol Syndrome. Available at http://depts.washington.edu/fasdpn/

Glennen S: Language development and delay in internationally adopted infants and toddlers: a review. *Am J Speech Lang Pathol* 11:333, 2002.

International Adoption Information US Department of State, Bureau of Consular Affairs. Available at http://travel.state.gov/family/adoption/info/info_458.html

Jenista JA: The immigrant, refugee, or internationally adopted child. *Pediatr Rev* 22:419, 2001.

Joint Council on International Children's Services (information about how to adopt, agencies involved in international adoption). Available at www.jcics.org

Kranowitz C: *The Out of Sync Child.* New York, Perigee, 1998.

Kranowitz C: *The Out of Sync Child Has Fun.* New York, Perigee, 2003.

Medical issues in international adoptions. *Pediatr Ann* 29: whole issue 2000.

Miller LC: *The Handbook of International Adoption Medicine.* New York, Oxford University Press, 2005.

National Adoption Information Clearinghouse. Available at http://naic.acf.hhs.gov/

Pickering LK et al (ed): *2003 Red Book: Report of the Committee on Infectious Diseases,* 26th ed. Elk Grove Village, IL, American Academy of Pediatrics, 2003. (The Red Book is updated every 3 years.)

Sensory Integration. Available at www.sensoryint.com

Travel information. Available at www.cdc.gov/travel

AUTHOR: **DEBORAH BORCHERS, MD**

Contraception

DEFINITION

Contraception is the voluntary prevention of conception or impregnation. There are both hormonal and barrier means to prevent pregnancy.

TYPES OF BIRTH CONTROL

- Condom
- Cervical cap
- Diaphragm
- Female condom
- Oral contraceptive pills (OCs, "the pill")
- Intrauterine device (IUD)
  - Levonorgestrel intrauterine system (LNG-IUS)
- Emergency contraception (i.e., emergency contraceptive pills [ECPs])
- Combined hormonal contraceptives
  - Combined oral contraceptive (COC) pill
  - Transdermal patch ("the patch")
  - Vaginal ring
- Progestin-only contraceptive methods
  - Progestin-only pill (POP, "minipill")
  - Depo-Provera (DMPA, Depo)
  - Implanon (similar to an older implanted contraceptive, Norplant)
- Abstinence

EPIDEMIOLOGY

- Contraceptive use among adolescents increased between 1995 and 2002.
- Adolescents were more likely to use a method for the first and most recent episodes of intercourse in 2002 (see Table 5-37).
- Use of condoms and very effective contraceptives, such as injectable methods, increased between 1995 and 2002.
- In 2002, approximately 74% of female adolescents and 82% of male adolescents between the ages of 15 and 19 years used contraception for their first episode of intercourse (Table 5-37).
- The younger the age at first intercourse, the higher the proportion of adolescents not using any method at first intercourse.
- Use of dual methods (i.e., a condom and a hormonal method) increased between 1995 and 2002.
- At last sexual intercourse, 83% of female adolescents and 91% of male adolescents between the ages of 15 and 19 who had been sexually active in previous 3 months used contraception (Table 5-38).
- Barriers to contraception include inadequate knowledge, poor access (e.g., cost, transportation, confidentiality), and adolescent development (e.g., peer pressure, denial of risk).

HORMONAL CONTRACEPTION

- Hormonal contraception inhibits ovulation, thickens cervical mucus, inhibits sperm capacitation, slows tubal motility (delaying sperm transport), disrupts transport of the fertilized ovum, and causes endometrial changes that hamper implantation.
- Failure rates are shown in Table 5-39 and discussed later.
- COC pills include estrogen and progestin. OCs contain 20 to 35 μg of ethinyl estradiol.
  - Monophasic, triphasic, 28- and 21-day packs, and extended-cycle packaging (91 days; 84 hormonal pills and 7 placebo pills) are available.
  - If estrogen side effects are problematic, use a lower dose (20 μg) of estrogen.
  - Extended-dosing regimen (e.g., Seasonale) uses a monophasic formulation in which 84 days of hormonal pills are taken before 7 days of placebo.
  - Newer progestins (e.g., norgestimate, desogestrel, drospirenone) have fewer androgen effects.
  - Drospirenone, a derivative of spironolactone, has anti-mineralocorticoid activity, which may be helpful with fluid retention experienced by some COC users.
- Contraceptive patch (e.g., Ortho Evra).
  - The outer protective layer of polyester has a medicated adhesive layer containing ethinyl estradiol and norelgestromin (i.e., metabolite of norgestimate).
  - A new patch is applied to the skin weekly for 3 weeks, followed by 1 week off for a withdrawal bleed.
- Vaginal ring (e.g., NuvaRing).
  - The flexible, soft ring is made of plastic (i.e., ethylene vinyl acetate); it is 54 × 4 mm.
  - It contains ethinyl estradiol and etonogestrel (i.e., metabolite of desogestrel).
  - The ring is inserted in the vagina for 3 weeks and then removed for 1 week for a withdrawal bleed.
- Hormonal doses in the patch and the ring are low, because hormones are more bioavailable and avoid first-pass liver affects by direct absorption from the skin or vaginal mucosa.

TABLE 5-37 Types of Contraception Relied on for the First Episode of Intercourse by Adolescents between 15 and 19 Years Old

Gender	Condom	Oral Contraceptives	Dual Methods	Withdrawal
Female	66%	17%	13%	8%
Male	71%	15%	10%	10%

Adapted from Abma JC et al: Teenagers in the United States: sexual activity, contraceptive use, and childbearing, 2002. National Center for Health Statistics. *Vital Health Stat* 23:24, 2004.

TABLE 5-38 Types of Contraception Relied on during the Most Recent Episode of Intercourse by Adolescents between 15 and 19 Years Old

Gender	Condom	Oral Contraceptives	Other Hormonal Methods*	Dual Methods	Other Methods†
Female	54%	34%	9%*	20%	2%
Male	71%	31%	6%*	24%	2%

*Other hormonal methods include Depo-Provera, Lunelle, Norplant, emergency contraception, and the contraceptive patch.
†Other methods exclude use of male condom or hormonal methods: e.g., includes sterilization, spermicide, periodic abstinence, diaphragm, cervical cap, IUD, female condom.
Adapted from Abma JC et al: Teenagers in the United States: sexual activity, contraceptive use, and childbearing, 2002. National Center for Health Statistics. *Vital Health Stat* 23:24, 2004.

TABLE 5-39 **Contraceptive Failure Rates**

Method	Lowest Expected (%)	Usual (%)
OCs: COC and POP	0.3	8
Ortho Evra patch	0.3	8
NuvaRing	0.3	8
Depo-Provera	0.3	3
Implanon*		
Male condom	2	15
Female condom	5	21
IUD (copper)	0.6	0.8
IUD (progesterone, Mirena)	0.1	0.1
Diaphragm	6	16
Cap		
Parous	26	32
Nulliparous	9	16
Sponge		
Parous	20	32
Nulliparous	9	16
Spermicides	18	29
Withdrawal	4	27
Periodic abstinence		25
None	85	85

COC, combined oral contraceptive pill; IUD, intrauterine device; OC, oral contraceptive pill; POP, progestin-only pill.
*No pregnancies in the first 70,000 cycles studied.
Adapted from Hatcher RA et al: *Contraceptive Technology*, 18th ed. New York, Ardent Media, 2004.

- POPs (i.e., minipill)
  - Less efficacious than combined OCs.
  - More breakthrough bleeding than combined OCs.
- Depo-Provera can provide contraception.
  - Medroxyprogesterone acetate (150 mg) is administered intramuscularly every 12 weeks.
- Implanon (i.e., implantable rod) became available in 2005.
  - Etonogestrel (a progestin) in a single 4-cm rod is implanted subdermally in the arm.
  - It is effective for 3 years.

COMMON CONCERNS

- Regimens to make up missed pills can be complicated, depending on the number of pills missed and the week of the pill cycle. A simplified regimen is outlined in the 18th edition of *Contraceptive Technology*, edited by Hatcher.
  - If no intercourse in 5 days
    - Missed 1 to 4 pills: Take 2 hormonal pills together and then finish the pack taking 1 pill per day; use a back-up method for 7 days.
    - Missed more than 4 pills: Take 2 hormonal pills together and then finish the pack taking 1 pill per day. Then skip the placebo pills in the old pack and start new pack; use a back-up method for 7 days.
  - For intercourse in the past 5 days, use emergency contraception immediately and then follow the previous instructions starting the next day.
- Breast cancer and contraception
  - COCs, patch, ring
    - Little or no effect on breast cancer
    - No increased risk in 35- to 64-year-old current or former users
    - Small apparent increased risk in current users likely due to detection bias; tumors in OC users more likely localized to the breast
    - No relationship to family history of breast cancer or age of initiation of use
  - Depo
    - There was no increased overall relative risk in the World Health Organization (WHO) collaborative study.
    - One other study showed an increased risk in those younger than 35 years, with the greatest risk among those using Depo for 6 or more years.
    - Apparent increase may represent acceleration of breast cancer presentation by promotion of growth in existing tumors.
- Cardiovascular, thromboembolic, or metabolic disorders
  - OCs, patch, ring
    - Healthy, nonsmoking women are not at increased risk for myocardial infarction or stroke; smokers older than 35 years are at highest risk for myocardial infarction.
    - All contraceptives with ethinyl estradiol increase the risk of blood clots.
    - Inherited thrombogenic disorders significantly increase this risk.
    - Any patient with a history of thrombophlebitis or thromboembolism should not use estrogen-containing contraceptives (patch, pill, or ring).
    - Those with a family history of deep venous thrombosis (DVT) or pulmonary embolism (PE) in a first-degree relative should be evaluated for an inherited clotting disorder before use.
    - Less than 5% develop hypertension.
    - Low-dose pills produce minimal changes in lipids.
    - Low-dose OCs do not adversely affect carbohydrate metabolism.
    - OCs are metabolized in the liver and may produce adverse outcomes when liver function is compromised.
    - Improvement in bone density can be seen, but there are mixed results, and concerns have been raised about the prevention of osteoporosis, particularly at the lowest doses of ethinyl estradiol.
  - Depo
    - It may decrease high-density lipoprotein (HDL) and increase low-density lipoprotein (LDL) cholesterol levels.
    - It can cause individuals to be hypoestrogenic.
    - Because of the lipid changes and hypoestrogenic effects of Depo, there is concern about possible increased risks of adverse effects

in individuals with a history of cerebrovascular accident, those with current or past ischemic heart disease, and diabetics with nephropathy, retinopathy, or neuropathy and other vascular disease. There is limited evidence for a small increased risk of cardiovascular events in those with significant hypertension.
    - Some progestins may increase the risk of venous thrombosis, but this risk is much lower than with combined hormonal contraception.
    - There is a slightly exaggerated insulin response to the glucose tolerance test.
    - Progestins are metabolized in the liver and may produce adverse outcomes when liver function is compromised.
- Decrease in bone density
  - Depo
    - The affect on long-term bone density accrual in adolescents unclear.
    - A black box warning has been issued by the U.S. Food and Drug Administration (FDA) about the bone density issue.
    - All Depo users should take in adequate calcium and exercise.
    - WHO guidelines place Depo in a category of benefits that outweigh risks for adolescents.
- Menstrual pattern
  - OCs
    - Initial breakthrough bleeding usually resolves after the first few months, and OCs are used to regulate menses.
    - Patch users may have more breakthrough bleeding than COC users in first two cycles.
    - Minipill users have more breakthrough bleeding than COC users.
    - Ring users have better cycle control than OC users.
    - No specific OC is best at eliminating spotting or breakthrough bleeding.
    - In evaluating spotting and breakthrough bleeding, rule out vaginitis, cervicitis, missed pills, and other medications or conditions blocking hormone absorption.
    - Menses become shorter and lighter over time.
  - Depo
    - Approximately 70% of patients have irregular menses (i.e., amenorrhea or spotting).
    - Between 30% and 50% have amenorrhea during year 1 and 70% by the end of year 2.
    - Bleeding can be treated with nonsteroidal anti-inflammatory drugs (NSAIDs), Premarin, or OCs.
- Infertility
  - No hormonal methods cause infertility.
  - Delay in return of regular ovulatory cycles is more common with Depo compared with OCs or Implanon.
- Weight gain
  - Low-dose OCs do not cause significant weight gain; some individuals experience mild fluid retention, which may be helped by using an OC containing drospirenone.
  - Depo may cause significant weight gain as a result of increased appetite.
- Headaches
  - Combined hormonal contraceptives
    - Migraine with aura is associated with an increased risk of ischemic stroke and is a contraindication for all combined hormonal contraceptives (Table 5-40).
    - Estrogen withdrawal may be associated with migraine. Mircette has fewer nonhormonal days (ethinyl estradiol present in last week of 28-day cycle), which may be helpful.
  - Depo
    - Migraine with aura is in a category of advantages that outweigh risks for Depo initiation but in the category of risks that usually outweigh advantages for method continuation.
      - Progestins may be associated with an increased frequency of severe headaches.
- Depression
  - OCPs: no evidence that there is significant increase
  - Depo

TABLE 5-40 World Health Organization Contraindications to Hormonal Contraception

Condition	Combined	Depo	POP
Breast cancer (current)	4	4	4
Active viral hepatitis	4	3	3
Viral hepatitis carrier	1	1	1
Current DVT or PE	4	3	3
History of DVT or PE	4	2	2
Known thrombogenic mutation	4	2	2
Surgery with prolonged immobilization	4	2	2
CVA, ischemic heart disease	4	3	2/3 I/C
Migraine with aura	4/4 I/C	2/3 I/C	2/3 I/C
Diabetes with vascular disease*	3/4	3	2
Diabetes without vascular disease	2	2	2
Hypertension (160/100+ mm Hg)	4	3	2
Hypertension (140-159/90-99 mm Hg)	3	2	1
Current gallbladder disease, symptomatic	3	2	2
Current gallbladder disease, asymptomatic	2	2	2
Unexplained vaginal bleeding	2	3	2
Cervical intraepithelial neoplasia	2	2	1
Depressive disorders	1	1	1

C, continuation; CVA, cerebrovascular accident; Depo, Depo-Provera; DVT, deep venous thrombosis; I, initiation; PE, pulmonary embolism; POP, progestin-only pill.

*Assess by severity of disease: 1, no restriction; 2, advantages generally outweigh theoretical or proven risks; 3, theoretical or proven risks usually outweigh advantages; 4, unacceptable health risk.

Adapted from World Health Organization, Reproductive Health and Research: *Medical Eligibility Criteria for Contraceptive Use*, 3rd ed. Geneva, World Health Organization, 2004.

- Overall rates are not increased, but some individuals may have increased depression with Depo.
- Depo is more of a problem because it cannot be discontinued immediately; consider a trial of oral progesterone if this is a concern before injection.

- Drug interactions
  - OC, patch, ring
    - Hepatic enzyme-inducing drugs may decrease efficacy.
    - Drugs associated with decreased efficacy include anti-tuberculosis medications (e.g., rifampin), antifungals (e.g., griseofulvin), anticonvulsants, anti-HIV protease inhibitors, and St. John's Wort.
    - Efficacy is not reduced with short-term or long-term use of broad-spectrum antibiotics in the absence of vomiting or diarrhea.
    - Combined hormonal contraceptives may alter hepatic clearance of other medications, resulting in lower or higher serum levels of other medications (e.g., fluoroquinolones, anticonvulsants, theophylline, antipsychotic drugs).
  - Depo: no significant interactions

Method-Specific Concerns

- Patch
  - Local skin hypersensitivity
  - The patch can detach, and an extra patch is needed for replacement to ensure efficacy.
  - It is less effective for women who weigh more than 198 pounds.
- Ring
  - The patient must be comfortable with vaginal insertion.
  - It can be removed for a maximum of 3 hours during sexual intercourse.
  - Complaints include leukorrhea (4.6%), vaginitis (5.8%), and vaginal discomfort (4%).
- Minipill
  - Compliance, including taking the pill at the same time every day, is important for efficacy.

Method-Specific Benefits

- Combined hormonal contraceptives may lead to improvement in benign breast disease, endometriosis, dysmenorrhea, dysfunctional bleeding, anemia, bone density, ovarian cysts, pelvic inflammatory disease, acne, hirsutism, and uterine and ovarian cancer.
- The patch and the ring may provide easier compliance than OCs, because the patch is changed only weekly and the ring is in place for 3 weeks.
- Depo-Provera leads to improvement in dysmenorrhea, endometrial cancer, anemia, breast tenderness, pelvic inflammatory disease (PID), seizures, and sickle cell disease (i.e., decreases sickling and increases red blood cell survival).
  - Compliance is easier than with OCPs.
  - Confidentiality is better because the method is not visible.

EMERGENCY CONTRACEPTION

Methods

- ECPs
  - Standard COC pills that contain norgestrel or levonorgestrel (Table 5-41).
  - Progestin only methods include levonorgestrel OC and Plan B.
- Copper IUD

Proposed Mechanisms of Action

- ECPs
  - Inhibit or delay ovulation
  - Cause changes in endometrium preventing implantation (conflicting studies)
  - Cause luteolysis
  - Prevent fertilization, including impaired sperm migration and function
  - Do not disrupt existing pregnancy
- Copper IUDs
  - Prevent fertilization
  - Interfere with implantation

Efficacy of Contraception

- Reduces risk of pregnancy as follows
  - At least 75%: combined OC
  - Approximately 89%: Plan B
  - Approximately 99%: copper IUD

Prescribing Information

- Ideally, take pills within 72 hours of unprotected sex. Studies have shown effectiveness for up to 120 hours (5 days).
  - COC (see Table 5-41), two doses 12 hours apart, may need to use antiemetic 30 to 60 minutes before the ECP dose
  - Plan B: 1 pill every 12 hours for total of 2 pills
    - Studies have shown good efficacy for giving both pills together at one time.
    - Plan B has significantly less nausea and vomiting than COC.
    - The only contraindication is known pregnancy because ECP will be ineffective.
- Advantages generally outweigh risks even for women with contraindications to combined hormonal contraceptives such as migraine with aura and severe liver disease.
- Progestin-only ECP may be preferable in an adolescent with history of thromboembolic disease.
- Insert a copper IUD within 5 to 7 days of unprotected intercourse.
- The Emergency Contraceptive Hotline is 800-NOT2-LATE.
- Consider a prophylactic prescription of ECP.

TABLE 5-41 **Emergency Contraception Using Standard Oral Contraceptive Pills**

Trade Name	Formulation	Pills per Dose
Ovral, Ogestrel	0.05 mg ethinyl estradiol, 0.50 mg norgestrel	2 white pills
Lo/Ovral, Low-Ogestrel, Cryselle	0.03 mg ethinyl estradiol, 0.30 mg norgestrel	4 white pills
Nordette, Levelen	0.03 mg ethinyl estradiol, 0.15 mg levonorgestrel	4 light orange pills
Levora	0.03 mg ethinyl estradiol, 0.15 mg levonorgestrel	4 white pills
Portia, Seasonale	0.03 mg ethinyl estradiol, 0.15 mg levonorgestrel	4 pink pills
Trivora	0.03 mg ethinyl estradiol, 0.125 mg levonorgestrel	4 pink pills
Trilevlen, Triphasil	0.03 mg ethinyl estradiol, 0.125 mg levonorgestrel	4 yellow pills
Enpresse	0.03 mg ethinyl estradiol, 0.125 mg levonorgestrel	4 orange pills
Alesse, Levlite, Lessina	0.02 mg ethinyl estradiol, 0.10 mg levonorgestrel	5 pink pills
Aviane	0.02 mg ethinyl estradiol, 0.10 mg levonorgestrel	5 orange pills
Ovrette	0.075 mg norgestrel	20 yellow pills

NONHORMONAL CONTRACEPTION

Methods

- Condoms
  - Male: latex, polyurethane, natural skin
  - Female: polyurethane
- Spermicides
  - Nonoxynol-9
  - Suppository, film, foam, jelly
  - No advantage for spermicidal condoms; some individuals sensitive to ingredients
- Diaphragm
  - Dome-shaped latex cup used with spermicide
  - Fit by clinician; sizes 50 to 95 mm in diameter
  - Arching, coil, and flat spring, wide-seal rim versions
- Cervical cap
  - Dome-shaped latex cap used with spermicide
  - Fit by trained clinician; four sizes available
  - About 6% to 10% of women cannot be fit.
  - Effective for 48 hours without additional spermicide
- IUD
  - Copper: copper T, effective for 10 years
  - Progesterone: levonorgestrel (Mirena), effective for 5 years
- Sponge
  - Polyurethane sponge containing nonoxynol-9
  - Effective for 24 hours after insertion
  - To be reintroduced into the market in the near future

Mechanisms of Action

- Barrier: condom, diaphragm, cap
- Spermicidal: spermicide, IUD, diaphragm, sponge, cap
- Thicken cervical mucus and prevention of ovulation through systemic absorption of progesterone: progesterone IUD (Mirena)
- Inhibit fertilization: IUD

Method-Specific Issues

- Male condom
  - The physician needs to discuss and demonstrate proper use.
  - When used with full dose of spermicide, it is 98% to 99% effective against pregnancy.
  - Polyurethane is available if a person is allergic to latex.
  - Condoms cannot be used with oil-based lubricants, except the polyurethane brand.
  - Spermicidal condoms may increase the risk of human immunodeficiency virus (HIV) transmission if inflammation occurs in an individual sensitive to spermicide.
- Female condom
  - The physician needs to explain and demonstrate proper use.
  - Correct use is more difficult than with the male condom.
  - It can be noisy and may need extra lubricant.
  - The patient needs to be comfortable touching the genitalia to insert the condom.
  - Inserted before sex.
  - It can be used with oil-based lubricants.
- Spermicide
  - Foam or jelly immediately active
  - Film or suppository active in 10 to 15 minutes
  - For individuals sensitive or allergic, may have increased HIV transmission risk due to vulvovaginal epithelial disruption
  - Increased HIV transmission associated with use two or more times per day in studies
- Diaphragm
  - Refitting required postpartum or with 10-pound weight change
  - Cannot use with oil-based lubricant
  - Must use with spermicide for optimal efficacy; can add additional spermicide for each sexual act
  - Can be inserted up to 6 hours before sex
  - Must be left in place 6 hours after sex
  - Increased risk of toxic shock syndrome
  - Increased risk of urinary tract infection (UTI), bacterial vaginosis, and yeast infection
- Cap
  - More difficult to insert than diaphragm
  - Must use with spermicide for optimal efficacy
  - Cannot use with oil-based lubricants
  - Must be inserted before sex; need at least 30 minutes between insertion and sexual intercourse
  - Must be left in place 6 hours after sex
  - Increased risk of toxic shock syndrome
- Sponge
  - Must be left in place 6 hours after intercourse
  - Risk of toxic shock
  - Can be difficult to remove
  - Can cause vaginal dryness
  - Increased risk of UTI, yeast, and bacterial vaginosis
- IUD
  - Popularity returning
  - Easy compliance
  - Risks: perforation, pain, bleeding, expulsion
    - More expulsions occur if the patient is nulliparous or has excessive menstrual flow.
    - LNG-IUS can decrease menstrual flow and result in amenorrhea.
    - The risk of PID is greatest at time of insertion.
  - Absolute contraindications: malignant disease of the uterus or cervix, abnormal uterine anatomy, vaginal bleeding of unclear origin, pregnancy, active PID or sexually transmitted infections (STIs), or cervicitis within previous 3 months
  - Relative contraindications: multiple sexual partners
  - Most appropriate: parous woman, mutually monogamous relationship

PRESCRIPTION & USE OF COMBINED ORAL CONTRACEPTIVES, THE PATCH, & THE VAGINAL RING

Indications & Contraindications

- Refrain from providing COC (all contraception containing estrogen) for unacceptable health risk (WHO category 4).
  - History of or current thrombophlebitis or thromboembolic disease; known thrombogenic mutation
  - Current or history of stroke or ischemic heart disease; structural heart disease with complications
  - Current breast or liver cancer
  - Acute liver disease, benign hepatic adenoma, or severe cirrhosis
  - Diabetes with complications (e.g., nephropathy, retinopathy, neuropathy)
  - Migraine with aura
  - Major surgery with prolonged immobilization
  - Hypertension with pressures of 160+/100+ mm Hg
  - Breastfeeding less than 6 weeks postpartum
- Theoretical or proven risks outweigh the advantages of the method (WHO category 3).
  - History of hypertension when blood pressure cannot be evaluated or even when adequately controlled and can be evaluated (pressures 149-159/90-99 mm Hg)
  - Hyperlipidemia (assessed by type, severity, and presence of other cardiovascular risk factors)
  - Migraine without aura in persons younger than 35 years while taking combined hormonal contraceptives
  - History of breast cancer without evidence of disease in past 5 years
  - Symptomatic gallbladder disease, history of cholestasis related to combined hormonal contraceptive, or mild cirrhosis
  - Concurrent use of drugs that affect liver enzymes
  - Breastfeeding 6 weeks to 6 months postpartum

- Advantages generally outweigh the theoretical or proven risks (WHO category 2).
  - Diabetes without complications
  - Major surgery without prolonged immobilization
  - Sickle cell disease
  - Hyperlipidemia (see earlier)
  - Undiagnosed breast mass
  - Breastfeeding longer than 6 months postpartum
  - Smoking in patient younger than 35 years
  - Obesity
  - Family history of DVT or PE in first-degree relative (and negative result for personal coagulopathy workup); superficial thrombophlebitis
  - Uncomplicated structural heart disease
  - Migraine without aura in patient younger than 35 years at initiation of method
  - Unexplained vaginal bleeding; cervical intraepithelial neoplasia
  - Asymptomatic gallbladder disease
  - History of pregnancy-related cholestasis
  - Antiretroviral or griseofulvin therapy

Instructions for Use of Combined Oral Contraceptives

- Starting on Sunday is the most common method; the patient can also begin on the first day of menses.
- Start with low-dose estrogen pill (25 to 35 μg).
- The usual formulation is 21 days of hormonal pills plus 7 days of inactive pills.
- Advise the patient about need for back-up methods during first week of use and the need for STI prevention with consistent condom use.
- Good medical history, blood pressure, and weight are crucial elements at baseline.
- A pelvic examination is not needed before prescribing hormonal contraception.
- An examination (at least annually) is important for detecting STIs.
- Urine-based STI testing may be sufficient for gonorrhea and *Chlamydia,* along with a vaginal smear for wet mount analysis to evaluate for *Trichomonas* and other causes of vaginitis.
- Perform a Pap smear within 3 years of the onset of sexual activity.
- Two or three visits a year are needed to monitor for compliance, blood pressure, weight, and side effects.

Instructions for Use of the Patch

- Use of the patch may begin on Sunday or the first day of menses.
- If switching from COC, apply 4 to 5 days after taking the last active pill.
- If switching from Depo, apply when due for the next shot.
- Apply the patch to a clean area of skin (e.g., lower abdomen, upper back, upper arm, upper buttock).
  - Do not apply to the chest near the breast. Place a new patch in a rotating location for 3 weeks in a row, followed by a patch-free week for initiating a withdrawal bleed.
  - If the patch is off for less than 24 hours, replace with a new patch, no back-up needed, and keep same patch change day.
  - If the patch is off for more than 24 hours, replace with a new patch and start a new 4-week cycle. Use back-up for 7 days, and record the new patch change day; consider ECP use if sexually active.
  - If late starting a new patch cycle, apply a patch immediately, use back-up for 7 days, and consider ECP use.
  - If less than 48 hours late, change the patch on week 2 or 3 of the cycle, put on a new patch, keep same patch change day, and back-up is not needed.
  - If more than 48 hours late, change the patch on week 2 or 3 of cycle, put on a new patch, and start new 4-week cycle. Consider ECP if sexually active, use back-up contraception for 7 days, and record the new patch change day.
  - If late removing the patch for the fourth week of the cycle, remove the patch and reapply a new patch on the usual change day. No back-up contraception or ECP is needed.

Instructions for Use of the Vaginal Ring

- Insert during first 5 days of menstrual cycle.
- If switching from COC, insert on the day scheduled to start a new pack; if switching from POP, insert on the day of the last pill in the pack.
- If switching from Depo, insert on the day due for the next shot.
- Keep the ring in place for 3 weeks, and then remove it for 7 days to initiate menses.
- The ring may be removed for up to 3 hours for sexual activity. If it is out for more than 3 hours, reinsert it, and use 7 days of a back-up method. Rinse with cool or lukewarm (not hot) water before inserting.

Side Effects of Hormonal Contraceptives: Aches

- **A**bdominal pain (e.g., mesenteric or pelvic vein thrombosis, benign liver tumor, gallbladder disease)
- **C**hest pain (e.g., pulmonary embolism, myocardial infarction, angina, breast mass)
- **H**eadaches (e.g., stroke, migraine headaches with aura, hypertension, retinal vein thrombosis)
- **E**ye symptoms (e.g., stroke, retinal vein or artery thrombosis, migraine with aura, poor-fitting contacts)
- **S**evere leg pain (e.g., thrombophlebitis of the lower extremity, venous thrombosis)

Clinical Pearls & Pitfalls

- All low-dose combined hormonal contraceptives are safe and effective in healthy adolescents.
- Counsel patients about dual methods using condoms and hormonal contraception to protect from STIs, HIV infection, and pregnancy.
- A pelvic examination is not necessary before prescribing hormonal contraception.
- ECP should be discussed with patients.
- Potential problems with bone mineral density should be discussed with patients using Depo.
- The IUD (particularly Mirena) is not absolutely contraindicated in adolescents.

Instructions for Emergency Contraception Use

- Recommend an antiemetic dose 30 to 60 minutes before the first dose of emergency contraception containing estrogen.
- The first dose should be taken as soon as possible after unprotected sex, ideally within the first 72 hours, but it may be taken up to 120 hours.
- The second dose should be taken 12 hours after the first dose.
- Do not take any extra pills.
- Both doses of progestin-only ECP can be taken simultaneously.
- Use only one type of pill.
- Recommend the use of condoms, spermicides, or a diaphragm during sex after taking ECP until the next menstrual period.
- Ensure a regular birth control method for the future.
- The patient may resume use of OCs, the patch, or the ring the next day if ECP was used while on one of those methods.
- Perform a pregnancy test if there is no menstrual period within 3 weeks of ECP treatment.

SUGGESTED READINGS

Abma JC et al: Teenagers in the United States: sexual activity, contraceptive use, and childbearing, 2002. National Center for Health Statistics. *Vital Health Stat* 23:24, 2004.

Hatcher RA et al: *Contraceptive Technology,* 18th ed. New York, Ardent Media, 2004.

World Health Organization, Reproductive Health and Research: *Medical Eligibility Criteria for Contraceptive Use,* 3rd ed. Geneva, World Health Organization, 2004.

AUTHOR: **PAULA K. BRAVERMAN, MD**

Divorce

DEFINITION

Divorce is a major stressor in separating adults and their children. It is second only to death in terms of the severity of the stress and the amount of time required to adjust.

RISKS ASSOCIATED WITH DIVORCE & CHILDREN'S ADJUSTMENT

- A meta-analysis of 95 studies involving more than 13,000 children shows that divorce poses specific risks for children socially, emotionally, and academically (Table 5-42).
  - Compared with children whose parents remain married, children of divorced parents have significantly lower academic achievement, psychological adjustment, self-concept, conduct, and social competencies.
  - Children of divorced parents have a two to three times greater rate of needing mental health services than children from nondivorced families.
- Risks for children are also related to parental conflict, economic hardship, parental mental health problems, and difficulties in parent-child relationships.
  - Children exposed to high levels of parental conflict have elevated cortisol levels.
  - A child's likelihood of illness the week after exposure to parents' verbal conflict is triple the usual rate.
  - A high level of parental conflict is a risk factor for children, whether parents are married, separated, or divorced.
  - If conflict is reduced after a divorce, these risks for children decrease.
  - Children of divorced parents have higher rates of school dropout and out-of-wedlock pregnancies.
  - Risks may continue into adulthood, with the quality of parent-child relationships affected.
    - There is a 39% increase in the risk of mental health problems at age 23.
    - There is an 85% increase in the risk of mental health problems at age 33.
  - Children from divorced families have a shorter life span by more than 4 years.
  - Variability in child outcome is shaped by risk factors and protective factors.

EPIDEMIOLOGY & DEMOGRAPHICS

- Every year, 1.5 million, or approximately 2%, of children in the United States experience parental divorce.
- By age 16, 38% of white children and 75% of African American children face the end of their parents' marriage.
- Fifty percent of children spend a portion of their childhood in single-parent families because of the high rate of divorce and the high rate of single parents at birth.
- Between 20% and 25% of children demonstrate an increased risk for adjustment problems after the break-up of their parents' marriage. Difficulties can endure with
  - Higher risk for lower socioeconomic status (SES)
  - Poorer subjective well-being
  - Increased number of marital problems
  - Greater likelihood of divorce in their own marriages

POTENTIAL OUTCOMES

- In the short term, children experience considerable distress. Common reactions include the following:
  - Sadness
  - Anger
  - Anxiety about what will happen to them
  - Confusion
  - Guilt
  - Loyalty conflicts
  - Somatic symptoms (headaches and stomachaches)
- Common reactions among preschool youngsters include the following:
  - Regression
  - Misconceptions about the divorce
  - Fears of abandonment
- School adjustment and academic difficulties often occur among school-aged children.
- Long-term outcomes vary considerably and are based on a number of risk and protective factors.
  - How the parents handle family changes
  - How well the parents contain their conflict
  - How well parents keep their children's needs a top priority and nurture healthy relationships with their children through warm, authoritative parenting
  - Economic stability

INTERVENTIONS

- Pediatric health care professionals may be the first resource a family seeks. Pediatricians are often seen by parents as trusted child advocates and personal confidantes.
- Reinforce parenting practices that help children develop healthy adjustment after the break-up.

TABLE 5-42 Three Categories of Protective and Risk Factors Identified in Divorce Research with Children

Individual Factors	Family Factors	Extrafamilial Support Factors
Protective Factors		
Active coping style	Encapsulated or minimal conflict	Contact with positive adult caretakers
Effective coping skills	Psychological well-being of residential parent	Support network: family, schools, and community
Accurate attributions, realistic perceptions of control	Solid, supportive parent-child relationships	Preventive interventions combining group support and skills training
Hopes for the future, "good natured" temperament	Effective parenting; household structure or stability	Proactive social and legal policies
Risk Factors		
Pre-divorce adjustment problems	Interparental conflict: overt and covert	Lack of caring adults to whom child feels connected
Attitudes and coping style	Diminished capacity to parent	Violent, unsafe neighborhoods
Age—each age has own risk factors	Impaired parent-child relationships	Lack of supportive friends or family
Difficult temperament	Economic decline, domestic violence	No access to supportive services

- Encourage parents to foster children's resilience by protecting the child from conflict, from taking sides, from being used as an informant, and for delivering support payments.
- Ongoing conflict impedes child's healthy development.
  - Avoid criticizing the child's other parent. Children interpret this as disapproval of a part of themselves.
  - Remind parents that divorce can be beneficial when it results in an end to on-going conflict by creating more harmonious home environments for child.
  - Act respectfully and develop a businesslike relationship with their child's other parent.
- Communicate in a way that keeps the child from being in the middle of disagreements.
- Remind parents to care for themselves physically and emotionally, so they can best care for their children.
  - Practice healthy stress management.
  - Avoid the use of drugs or alcohol.
  - Encourage the parents to seek support and professional help for getting through an intensely emotional and stressful time.
- Nurture positive parent-child relationships by talking with children about their feelings and family changes.
  - Assist the child in focusing on his or her strengths.
  - Encourage parents to spend time with each child engaged in an enjoyable activity of the child's choice and to practice effective parenting with warmth, nurturance, and effective limit setting.
  - Parents should set clear and consistent limits and expectations of appropriate behavior.
  - Parents should monitor and communicate with adolescents regularly.
  - Parents should listen to children and show understanding and empathy.
- Parents should maintain household structure and routines.
  - Eat meals together
  - Maintain regular bedtimes
  - Limit TV and other screen time
- Allow children time to adjust to the separation before introducing them to new partners.
  - Children may feel displaced by a parent's new partner.
  - Ideally, parents should make their children the top priority when they are with them.
- Understand warning signs of significant adjustment difficulties, when additional or specialized professional help is needed.
  - Refer to a psychologist or other licensed mental health professional specializing in issues of children and divorce.
  - Encourage parents to seek help preventively, before problems become severe.
  - Emphasize that seeking help when needed is a sign of strength, not weakness.
- Warning signs for adults include the following:
  - Severe or chronic anger, depression, or suicide intent (seek help emergently)
  - Problem behaviors or negative mood becomes chronic instead of periodic
  - Decreased ability to care for children or to be effective at work
  - No symptom improvement
  - Feelings of hopelessness, helplessness, or inability to cope
- Warning signs for children include the following:
  - Desire to hurt self (seek help emergently)
  - Negative changes in the child's mood or behavior that persist for more than 3 months
  - Increase in somatic complaints, such as headaches or stomachaches
  - Prolonged sadness, anger, or resentment
  - Prolonged difficulty sleeping or frequent nightmares
  - Expression of strong negative feelings ("I hate my life.")
  - Sudden drop in school performance or motivation
  - Severe regression in young children
  - Increasingly or very withdrawn, anxious, or aggressive
  - Lack of desire to engage in social, athletic, school, or family activities
  - Refusal to spend time with a parent
- Parents should reassure children in words and behaviors that they are loved and will continue to be cared for, despite family changes.
- Inform parents of local resources for assisting families through transition, such as parent education programs for divorcing parents, support groups for separating couples, and children's support groups that many communities and schools provide.
- Develop a specific parenting plan that allows both parents to be actively involved in their children's lives, if it is safe to do so.
- Situations of abuse, domestic violence, or a parent with major mental illness require special consideration.
- If violence or abuse is not a factor, alternatives to litigation can be helpful, such as mediation and collaborative law.

RESOURCES

- The American Psychological Association has a web site with relevant articles on marriage, divorce, and parenting (www.apa.org/topics/topicdivorce.html).
- The Association of Family and Conciliation Courts (AFCC) has a web site that includes resources for parents and children, including Uptoparents.org, an interactive site that provides parenting information, and Fameleschange.ca, an educational web site for children, teens, and adults. The AFCC web site is http://www.afccnet.org/resources/resources_parents.asp
- Joint Custody Association, 10606 Wilkins Avenue, Los Angeles, CA 90024; 310-475-5352; http://www.jointcustody.org
- Parents Without Partners, 1650 South Dixie Highway, Suite 510, Boca Raton, FL 33432; 561-391-8833; http://www.parentswithoutpartners.org
- Stepfamily Association of America, 650 J Street, Suite 205, Lincoln, NE 68508; 1-800-735-0329; http://www.saafamilies.org
- Support groups for children: Encourage parents to check with their schools or mental health association to see what is available in their community.
- www.collaborativepractice.com

SUGGESTED READINGS

Amato PR, Keith B: Consequences of parental divorce for children's well-being: a meta-analysis. *Psychol Bull* 110:26, 1991.

Bumpass L: Children and marital disruption. A replication and update. *Demography* 21:71, 1984.

Chase-Lansdale PL et al: Effects of divorce on mental health throughout the life course. *Am Sociol Rev* 63:239, 1995.

Flinn MV, England BG: Childhood stress: endocrine and immune system responses to psychosocial events. *In* Wilce JM (ed): *Social & Cultural Lives of Immune Systems.* London, Routledge Press, 2003, pp 107–147.

Pedro-Carroll JL: The promotion of wellness in children and families: challenges and opportunities. *Am Psychologist* 56:993, 2001.

Schwartz JE et al: Sociodemographic and psychosocial factors in childhood as predictors of adult mortality. *Am J Public Health* 85:1237, 1995.

AUTHOR: **JOANNE PEDRO-CARROLL, PhD**

Domestic Violence

DEFINITION

Domestic violence (DV) occurs when an intimate partner commits a physical, sexual, emotional, economic, or psychological assault on the other partner through the use of a pattern of controlling behaviors, including force, coercion, threats, or intimidation. DV may be referred to as spousal abuse, intimate partner violence, or family violence. Children who live in homes where violence is occurring are acutely aware of the abuse and may suffer significant physical and mental effects.

EPIDEMIOLOGY & DEMOGRAPHICS

- DV is a pediatric issue. An estimated 3.3 to 10 million children annually witness violence in their homes.
- Teen dating violence is common. Between 20% and 25% of female high school students report being physically or sexually abused by a dating partner.
- Most victims of DV are women. More than one half of female victims are living in households with children younger than 12 years old.
- DV affects all races, all social classes, all age groups, the disabled and well-bodied, and heterosexual and homosexual partners.
- In the United States, one fourth to one third of all women have been sexually or physically abused by an intimate partner at some point in their lives.
- DV is the leading cause of injury for women between the ages of 15 and 44, resulting in 2 million injuries and almost 1300 deaths annually. Women are 10 times more likely to be killed by an intimate partner. Three women are murdered by their (ex) husband or (ex) boyfriends each day.
- There are many misconceptions and biases about DV victims and their ability or inability to leave violent relationships. The following are facts:
  - Women who leave their abusers are at a 75% greater risk of being killed by the batterer than those who stay.
  - Many women lack the economic means to survive, especially those with dependent children.
  - Fifty percent of all homeless women and children are on the streets because of violence in the home.

POTENTIAL OUTCOMES

- Children in violent homes may suffer from a wide range of lifelong effects, including poor academic achievement and behavioral, emotional, social, and psychological dysfunction.
- The child's reactions to this exposure are affected by the severity and chronicity of the abuse, as well as the age, sex, and developmental stage of the child.
- Several signs and symptoms that may occur include:
  - Sleep difficulties
  - Somatic complains (i.e., headache and stomachache)
  - Distractibility, inability to focus, "daydreaming"
  - Depression
  - Anxiety or aggression
  - Poor peer relationships
- Domestic violence and child abuse are intricately connected, with a significant number of children becoming victims of abuse at a rate 6 to 10 times greater than in the general population. Studies indicate that in homes with DV, there is a 30% to 60% co-occurrence of child abuse.
  - Children may be injured, physically disciplined, or hurt in attempts to intervene.
  - The U.S. Advisory Board on Child Abuse suggests that domestic violence may be the single major precursor to child abuse and neglect fatalities in this country.
- Pregnancy is a high-risk time for women in violent relationships. More than 325,000 pregnant women are physically abused annually. This violence can lead to intrauterine complications, including second- and third-trimester bleeding, miscarriage, preterm labor, and low birth weight.
- Abused women are among the unhealthiest women in the United States. They experience more physical health problems and have a higher occurrence of mental health issues, such as depression, suicide attempts, and drug and alcohol abuse, than women who are not abused.
- DV can adversely affect parenting.
  - Decreased recognition of stressors in a child's life
  - Attachment or bonding difficulties
  - Increased likelihood of physical punishment
  - Reversal of parent-child roles

INTERVENTIONS & POTENTIAL SOLUTIONS

- In 1998, the American Academy of Pediatrics (AAP) recommended that all pediatricians routinely screen for DV as part of their anticipatory guidance.
- By screening, identifying, and intervening, children can be spared significant lifetime complications of their exposure.

Barriers to Screening & Solutions to These Barriers

- Fear of offending: Because DV occurs in all ages, races, ethnicities, and socioeconomic groups, DV screening should be a routine part of a complete history for all families. Studies have shown that physicians are poor predictors of which families are at risk for DV and that stereotypes cannot be used to determine who to screen.
- Lack of time: Development of routine screening questions and office protocols for screening, follow-up, and referral to services is necessary.
- Lack of education about DV: Pediatricians do not need to be experts on DV, but they should know effective screening methods and understand some of the dynamics and biases associated with DV.
  - Women may not disclose violence, but by screening, they are made aware that this is an important issue they can discuss with health care providers when ready.
  - Many women do not leave violent relationships for a variety of reasons, but health care providers can still help them to keep their children and themselves safer.
- Mothers should be screened at every well child check, when signs or symptoms raise concerns (i.e., bruising on child or mother), and when a new intimate partner is identified.
- Adolescents should be screened at every well-child check, if a new intimate partner is identified, or during any visits while pregnant and when signs or symptoms raise concerns.
- Attempt assessment with children out of the room. If this is not practical, more general questions need to be asked. If the mother gives cues she is uncomfortable, alternative methods of screening or discussion should be approached.
- There are several methods of screening.
  - Most importantly, ask the question in an effective and efficient manner that becomes routine for all patients.
  - Be direct in your questioning.
  - Understand your state's domestic and child abuse laws; in some states, health care workers are mandated to report domestic abuse and children's exposure to DV.
  - Be aware of local and national resources.
- Examples of office-based screening questions with anticipatory guidance
  - "I ask all my patients this question because I want you to know this is a safe place where help is available. Your health and well-being are important to me and may affect your children's safety and health."
  - "Because violence is so common, we have started to ask all patients about violence in the home."

- "Are you in a relationship in which you are being hurt physically or emotionally?"
- "Have you ever been emotionally or physically abused by your partner? By this I mean have you ever been hit, kicked, slapped, punched, or isolated from your family or someone important to you by your partner?"

- Several screening tools have been effectively implemented at primary care pediatric offices.
- Adaptations from the American Medical Association's recommended DV screening questions have successfully revealed DV among women who were screened in the pediatric office setting (Parkinson et al, 2001; Siegel et al, 1999).
- The Child Safety Questionnaire uses four similar questions (Wahl et al, 2004).
  - Have you ever been in a relationship with someone who has hit you, kicked you, slapped you, punched you, or threatened to hurt you?
  - Are you currently in such a relationship?
  - When you were pregnant, did anyone ever physically hurt you?
  - Are you in a relationship with someone who yells at you, calls you names, or puts you down?
- What to do with abnormal screening results
  - The pediatrician's job is not to fix the problem but to be available.
  - Validate and support the victim.
  - Listen nonjudgmentally.
  - Encourage communication.
  - Begin to help victims understand their situation, to educate them, and address the impact of DV on children.
  - Assess for safety.
  - Report the case if mandated; inform the mother, assess for a possible increase in violence, and arrange for safety.
  - Refer the patient to the appropriate resource.
    - Social work
    - Local DV support groups or shelter
    - Mental health counseling
    - Legal services
  - Document so that other providers will be aware of any disclosure, but develop a protocol for confidentiality because the batterer may have access to the child's records.

PRIMARY RESOURCES FOR PHYSICIANS' OFFICES

- Identifying and responding to domestic violence: Consensus Recommendations for Child and Adolescent Health (http://endabuse.org/programs/healthcare/files/Pediatric.pdf)
- Developed by the Family Violence Prevention Fund's National Health Resource Center on Domestic Violence, these recommendations are the first of their kind to address how to assess children and youth for domestic violence, and they specifically offer recommendations on assessing adults for victimization with children present.
- Toolkit to End Violence Against Women (http://toolkit.ncjrs.org/) is a web-based toolkit with 16 chapters that provide recommendations for strengthening prevention efforts and improving services for victims. Readers can quickly pinpoint topics of interest and download the related discussions and action items.
- Electronic Palm DV Assessment Tool (http://endabuse.org/programs/printable/display.php3?DocID=349)
- Intimate partner violence: An Assessment Tool for Providers, PALM version (www.endabuse.org/health/ipv/ipv-doc.doc)

VICTIM RESOURCES

- National Domestic Violence Hotline: http://www.ndvh.org/; 1-800-799-SAFE (1-800-799-7233); TTY: 1-800-787-3224. Staff provides callers with crisis intervention, information about domestic violence, and referrals to local programs 24 hours each day, 7 days each week. Telephone assistance is available in many languages, including Spanish.

SUGGESTED READINGS

American Academy of Pediatrics, Committee on Child Abuse and Neglect: The role of the pediatrician in recognizing and intervening on behalf of abused women. *Pediatrics* 101:1091, 1998.

American Medical Association: *Diagnostic and Treatment Guidelines on Domestic Violence.* Chicago, American Medical Association, 1992, pp 4–19.

Augustyn M, Groves BM: If we don't ask, they aren't going to tell: screening for domestic violence. *Contemp Pediatr* 23:43, 2005.

Erikson MJ et al: Barriers to DV screening in the pediatric setting. *Pediatrics* 108:98, 2001.

Groves B et al: *Identifying and Responding to Domestic Violence: Consensus Recommendations for Child and Adolescent Health.* San Francisco, CA, Family Violence Prevention Fund, 2002.

Parkinson GW et al: Maternal domestic violence screening in an office-based pediatric practice. *Pediatrics* 108:e43, 2001. Available at http://pediatrics.aappublications.org/cgi/content/full/108/3/e43

Rennison C: *Intimate partner violence, 1993–2001.* Publication No. NCJ197838. Washington, DC, Bureau of Justice Statistics, Department of Justice (US), 2003.

Siegel RM et al: Screening for DV in the community pediatric setting. *Pediatrics* 104:874, 1999.

Silverman JG et al: Dating violence against adolescent girls and associated substance use, unhealthy weight control, sexual risk behavior, pregnancy, and suicidality. *JAMA* 286:527–529, 2001.

Tjaden P, Thoennes N: Extent, nature, and consequences of intimate partner violence: findings from the National Violence Against Women Survey, research report. *Report for grant 93-IJ-CX-0012, funded by the U.S. Department of Justice, National Institute of Justice, and the Centers for Disease Control and Prevention.* Publication No. NCJ 181867. Washington, DC, U.S. Department of Justice, 2000a. Available at http://www.ojp.usdoj.gov/nij/pubs-sum/181867.htm

U.S. Advisory Board on Child Abuse and Neglect, U.S. Department of Health and Human Services: *A Nation's Shame: Fatal Child Abuse and Neglect in the United States: Fifth Report, 1995.* Washington, DC, U.S. Department of Health and Human Services, 2004.

U.S. Department of Health and Human Services. Office of Disease Prevention and Health Promotion. Available at http://www.healthypeople.gov

Wahl RA et al: Clinic-based screening for domestic violence: use of a child safety questionnaire. *BMC Med* 2:25, 2004.

AUTHOR: **DANIELLE THOMAS-TAYLOR, MD**

Foster Care

DEFINITION

Foster care is government-subsidized and -regulated temporary care for children who have been removed from their families for reasons of abuse and neglect. The goals of foster care are the health, safety, and permanency of children. Permanency is achieved by reunification with the birth family or through adoption. Reunification can be achieved by informal or formal placement with a relative (i.e., kinship care) or through independent living. The three main types of foster care that exist are family foster care, kinship care, and residential group care, and the term *foster care* is used for all three. There are about four times as many children in kinship care as are in family foster care. Kinship care includes care by relatives, neighbors, and friends. Kinship care may be informal placement with a relative or formal placement through legal guardianship or foster care placement. Informal arrangements or guardianship are not subsidized in this context in most states.

EPIDEMIOLOGY & DEMOGRAPHICS

- Serious neglect and abuse are the most common reasons why children are removed from their parents' care.
- The main risk factor for placement into foster care include family and social stressors.
- Typical stressors include the following:
  - Serious family dysfunction
  - Domestic violence
  - Parental mental health disorders
  - Parental addiction to licit and illicit substances
  - Parental criminal activity
- Efforts to prevent foster care placement have resulted in increased numbers of children being placed in kinship care in the past decade.
- Daily in the United States, more than 500,000 children are living in foster home care. Yearly, more than 800,000 children experience placement in a foster home.
- The average length of stay in foster care is 33 months, and it ranges from a few days to many years.
- Fifty-two percent of those in foster care are male, and they range in age from birth to 21 years; most states discharge youths at age 18.
- Most children in foster care reside in large urban settings.
- In 2000, 1% of the U.S. child population was in foster care.
  - Utah had the overall lowest rate (0.25%).
  - Wisconsin and the District of Columbia had the highest rates (2.7%).
- Children in foster care have high rates of physical health problems (35% to 60%), mental health problems (60% to 80%), developmental problems (60%), all of which are accompanied by poor long-term outcomes.
- Prevalence rates of mental health disorders particularly posttraumatic stress disorder (PTSD), are significantly higher among those who were formerly in foster care than in the general population.
  - Among youths previously in foster care, 54% have one or more mental health disorders, compared with 22% in the general population.
  - Twenty-five percent have PTSD, compared with 7% in the general population.
  - A comparable rate of major depression (20%) has been found among those who were formerly in foster care and in the general population.
- Poor outcomes are attributable to adversities before placement and within foster care.
- All children in foster care experience separation and loss. All deal with uncertainty.

BARRIERS

- Consent and confidentiality
- Transience of the foster care population, caseworkers, and foster families
- Lack of funding: Medicaid often not sufficient to cover health care needs, including physical, emotional, and dental care
- Lack of care coordination and poor communication among providers
  - Health care providers
  - Child protective service (CPS)
  - Legal services
  - Schools, teachers, early intervention services or programs
  - Legal authority
  - Child care providers and facilities
  - Court Appointed Special Advocate (CASA) program

POTENTIAL ADVERSE OUTCOMES

- Data indicate that overall health and well-being does not improve in foster care.
- Many psychosocial, medical, and educational problems are not addressed.
- Mental health issues include the following:
  - Adolescents: common problems include conduct disorder, attention deficit/hyperactivity disorder (AD/HD), depression, anxiety, and PTSD.
  - Younger children: common problems include adjustment disorder not otherwise specified, AD/HD, and oppositional defiant disorder.
- Physical health problems include the following:
  - Higher rates exist for all chronic conditions; prevalence rates of chronic conditions range from 30% to 80% of the foster care population.
  - Fifteen percent of children are 5% under average height and weight on entry to foster care.
  - Rates of hearing and vision problems, seizures disorders, and neurologic disorders are higher than in general population.
- Educational problems include the following:
  - Although some children in foster care do have improved school attendance and improved school functioning, most are at risk for significant behavior difficulties, leading to and including suspension.
  - Youths who have previously been in foster care are at risk for poor educational outcomes in part because of multiple school and placement changes.
  - Although most (85%) youths in foster care complete high school, 28.5% complete high school by passing the General Educational Development Credential (GED) tests, compared with 5% in general population.
  - Completion of post-secondary education is low, with 1.8% obtaining at least a Bachelor's degree compared with 27.5% of 25- to 34-year-old adults in the general population.
- Problems with health coverage and homelessness include the following:
  - Youths who "age out" of foster care are at risk for lacking health insurance. One third of young adults who had previously been in foster care had no health insurance, compared with 18% of 18 to 44 year olds in general population.
  - More than 20% of young adults experienced homelessness after leaving foster care.

INTERVENTIONS & SOLUTIONS

- Because mental health problems are prevalent among children and youth in foster care, all children should have comprehensive developmental and mental health assessments. Screen frequently, and refer children for timely intervention of mental disorders.
- Screen for educational failure and challenges.
  - School changes may be frequent, leading to significant disruptions in learning.
  - Primary care physicians (PCPs) can help facilitate educational success by encouraging families to keep children in school.

- The McKinney-Vento Homeless Assistance Act seeks to overcome educational challenges that homeless youths face.
- Children in foster care can opt to stay in their school of origin until the end of the academic year, even if the school district must provide transportation to do so.
- Emphasize self-efficacy of children and youths by encouraging participation in extracurricular activities.
- Refer to the health care guidelines promoted by the American Academy of Pediatrics (AAP) to care for children in foster care (Healthy Foster Care America: www.aap.org/advocacy/HFCA/).
  - Maintain open communication between PCPs and caseworkers by sharing developmental, mental health, and physical health information.
  - Provide anticipatory guidance around foster care-specific issues, such as consent and confidentiality, visitation with parents, and mental health needs.
  - Emphasize the importance of maintaining schedules across environments (i.e., between foster family and birth family schedules).
- PCPs can help to prepare children and families for known transitions, including the following:
  - Visitation with parents or siblings
  - Changes in foster care placement
  - Discharge from foster care to birth families, adoptive families, or relatives
  - Teens aging out of foster care
  - Court dates

SUGGESTED READINGS

American Academy of Pediatrics, Committee on Early Childhood, Adoption and Dependent Care: Developmental issues for young children in foster care. *Pediatrics* 106:1145, 2000.

American Academy of Pediatrics, District II, New York State. Task Force on Health Care for Children in Foster Care: *Fostering Health: Health Care for Children and Adolescents in Foster Care.* Chicago, American Academy of Pediatrics, 2005.

Child Welfare League of America: *CWLA Standards for Health Care Services for Children in Out-of-Home Care.* Washington, DC, Child Welfare League of America, June 1998.

Dicker S et al: Improving the Odds for the Healthy Development of Young Children in Foster Care. *Promoting the Emotional Well-Being of Children and Families, Policy Paper No. 2. National Center for Children in Poverty: Columbia University Mailman School of Public Health.* New York, Columbia University, January 2002, pp 1–28.

Healthy Foster Care America. Available at www.aap.org/advocacy/HFCA/

Huber J, Grimm B: Children and family services reviews, part V: Most states fail to meet the mental health needs for foster children. *Youth Law News* xx:1–36, 2004.

Pecora PJ et al: Improving Family Foster Care: Findings from the Northwest Foster Care Alumni Study. Seattle, WA, Casey Family Programs, xxxx. Available at http://www.casey.org

Simms M et al: Health care needs of children in the foster care system. *Pediatrics* 106:909, 2000.

Smithgall C et al: *Educational Experiences of Children in Out-of-Home Care.* Chicago, Chapin Hall Center for Children at the University of Chicago, 2004, pp 1–77. Available at www.chapinhall.org

AUTHORS: **SANDRA H. JEE, MD, MPH** and **MOIRA A. SZILAGYI, MD, PhD**

Incarcerated Parents

DEFINITION

It is projected that the proportion of children with incarcerated parents will continue to grow, because women prisoners are the fastest growing incarcerated population. The number of female prisoners is growing at a faster rate than that of male prisoners (106% versus 75%). Between 1991 and 1999, the number of children with a mother in jail doubled.

EPIDEMIOLOGY & DEMOGRAPHICS

- One million children had a parent in a state or federal prison in 1999. This was 2.1% of an estimated 72 million children in the United States.
- Fifty-five percent of state prisoners and 63% of federal prisoners are parents.
- Of women who are incarcerated, 75% are mothers.
- Most parents in state prisons were previously incarcerated. This suggests that children experience the unexpected, often traumatic loss of a parent several times.
- Contacts of incarcerated parents with their children are limited.
  - Fifty-four percent of mothers and 57% of fathers in state prison have never had a visit with their children.
  - Sixty percent of parents are imprisoned more than 100 miles from their last home.
  - Forty percent of mothers and 60% of fathers did not have weekly contact (i.e., phone, mail, or visit) with their children.
- Demographic profiles of women in prison have characteristic patterns.
  - The typical incarcerated woman is 25 to 29 years old, is a single parent with one to three children, and comes from a single-parent household herself.
  - More than one half have been physically abused, and 42% have been sexually abused.
  - Most of the mothers regularly use or abuse alcohol or drugs, and they have done so since their early teen years. Drug offenders are responsible for 55% of the increase seen in incarcerated women.
- For children with an incarcerated father, 77% live with the mother and 15% live with a grandparent or other relative.
- For children with an incarcerated mother, 17% live with the father, 6% live in foster care, 53% live with a grandparent, and 26% live with other relatives.

POTENTIAL OUTCOMES

- Trauma is associated with parental incarceration. There is sudden, sometimes violent separation from the caregiver.
- Children often are present at the time of arrest.
  - Unstable care may be provided after the arrest. The child often is moved from home to home.
  - Research suggests that the mother's arrest is more disruptive than the father's arrest.
  - Seventy-five percent of children report symptoms of depression, difficulty sleeping and concentrating, flashbacks, and poor school performance.
- Children experiencing parental incarceration are at increased risk for several problems.
  - School failure
  - Gang involvement
  - Drug use or abuse
  - Teen pregnancy
  - Entering into the juvenile criminal justice system
- These children are five times more likely than their peers to end up in prison.
- One in 10 children will be incarcerated before reaching adulthood.
- Little is known about the other effects on children of incarcerated parents, including:
  - Access to health care
  - Immunization rates
  - Mental health and mental illness
  - Behavioral disabilities
  - Emotional damage
- Most law enforcement agencies do not gather family information from a prisoner.
  - Officers are rarely required to ask about children at the time of an arrest.
  - Officers are responsible for "reasonably ensuring the safety of children left unattended following a caretaker's arrest" according to a 1979 ruling.
- Parental rights can be terminated while the parent is in prison. The Federal Adoption and Safe Families Act of 1997 states that the rights can be terminated when a child is in foster care 15 of the previous 22 months.

INTERVENTIONS FOR CHILDREN

- Children should understand that the parent's incarceration is not their fault.
- Inform the child about the incarcerated parent.
- The child should visit and maintain contact with the incarcerated parent when permitted, wanted, and appropriate. Understand when and how the child will have contact with the parent.
- The child should be told what will stay the same and what will change while the parent is incarcerated.
- Children need to know where and with whom they will be living and where they will be going to school.
- The child needs verbal reassurance that it is okay to love the parent and to be angry. Encourage the child to express his or her feelings about the parent's incarceration.
- Help to find representation for the rights of the child.
- Further study is needed to consider the impact on children of incarcerated parents and to evaluate the effectiveness of programs.
  - Visitation programs
  - Mentoring programs
  - Counseling interventions
  - Child-parent reunification programs
- Children of Incarcerated Parents Bill of Rights is a document describing the issues facing children of incarcerated parents from the child's perspective, with suggestions for steps to be taken to protect these children. A copy of the Bill of Rights can be found at www.cwla.org/programs/incarcerated/cop_billofrights.htm

INTERVENTIONS FOR INCARCERATED PARENTS

- Educate, counsel, and lend emotional, monetary, and legal support to start a new life.
- Provide intensive drug treatment and community-based alternatives to incarceration.
- Provide parenting classes because most incarcerated parents were not well parented and have few role models.
- From Spiritus Christi Prison Outreach: Women of Conviction Project—What Women Say They Need: "Ask me if I have ever been parented? Have I ever been a child in the parent-child relationship? Ask a woman what does love mean to you? As most of us just don't know what love is, because the people who have said they have loved us have not cared for us" (from an anonymous incarcerated mother).

RESOURCES

How to Explain Jails and Prisons to Children: A Caregiver's Guide. Oregon Department of Corrections, Children of Incarcerated Parents Project: http://egov.oregon.gov/DOC/TRANS/PROGMS/oam_children.shtml

SUGGESTED READINGS

Center for Children of Incarcerated Parents. Available at www.e-ccip.org
Child Welfare League of America. Available at www.cwla.org
Family and Corrections Network. Available at www.fcnetwork.org
Mumola CJ: Bureau of Justice Special Report: Incarcerated Parents and Their Children. *National Criminal Justice (NCJ 182335).* Washington, DC, US Department of Justice, August 2000, pp 1–12.
Sazie E et al: *How to Explain Jails and Prisons to Children. A Caregiver's Guide.* Oregon Department of Corrections Children of Incarcerated Parents Project, 2003, pp 1–15. Available at http://egov.oregon.gov/DOC/TRANS/PROGMS/oam_children.shtml
Simmons CW: Children of Incarcerated Parents. CRB note vol 7. Sacramento, California Research Bureau, March 2000, pp 1–11.
Spiritus Christi Prison Outreach: *Women of Conviction Project: Reducing the Rate of Incarceration and Recidivism of Women Offenders—What Women Say They Need.* Rochester, NY, Center for Government Research, 2000, pp 1–81.
Status Report on Female Offenders. Available at www.dc.state.fl.us/pub/females/status102001
Women's Prison Association & Home, Inc., Family to Family: *Partnerships between Corrections and Child Welfare,* part 2. Baltimore, MD, Annie E. Casey Foundation. Available at www.aecf.org/initiatives/familytofamily/tools/16937.pdf.

AUTHOR: **HEATHER MICHALAK, MD**

Maternal Depression

DEFINITION

The spectrum of depressive disorders in mothers includes postpartum blues, perinatal depression (prenatal and postpartum), postpartum psychosis, and maternal depression.

RISK PROFILES

- Postpartum blues
  - Develops in 70% of women
  - Can last up to 4 weeks (usually 1 to 2 weeks)
  - Typically does not interfere with the mother's ability to function
- Perinatal depression in the prenatal period
  - Affects 20% to 25% of women
  - Peaks during the third trimester
  - Associated with poor prenatal care, substance abuse, and preterm delivery
- Perinatal depression in the postpartum period
  - Occurs in 12% to 15% of women
  - Usually develops insidiously, but may appear acutely within the first 3 postpartum months
  - Lasts, on average, 7 months if untreated
  - More persistent and debilitating than postpartum blues
  - Signs and symptoms indistinguishable from major depression: feeling worthless, sad, "low," "down"; loss of interest or pleasure in usual activities; excessive or inappropriate guilt; general fatigue, loss of energy; thoughts of dying
  - Anxiety, including worries or obsessions about the infant; ambivalent or negative feelings about infant; intrusive or unpleasant fears or thoughts about harming infant
  - Can interfere with the mother's ability to care for herself or her child
- Postpartum psychosis
  - Incidence: 1 or 2 cases per 1000 births
  - Manifests within 2 weeks of delivery
  - Acute onset of major disturbances in thinking and behavior, hallucinations, and delusions
  - As a psychiatric emergency, requires immediate action to prevent suicide and infanticide
- Maternal depression
  - Chronic or acute depression in women with dependent children
  - Many negative consequences for children of depressed mothers across all ages and includes difficulty with bonding and emotional development, behavior problems, and mental illness
- General features of depressive disorders
  - Consider genetic and parenting factors.
  - More chronic or severe problems have longer lasting and more serious effects.
  - Protective factors for the child include the presence of a non-ill caregiver, a strong sense of self, and activities such as school or work.
  - Exacerbating factors for the child include interpartner violence, substance abuse, and divorce.

EPIDEMIOLOGY

- Depression, a leading cause of disease burden for women 15 to 44 years of age, occurs in 10% to 15%.
- Between 8% and 12% of women may experience postpartum depression, with increases in depressive symptoms occurring in up to 24% of mothers.
- The cause is unclear, but it may involve a complex interaction of biochemical, interpersonal, and social factors.
- Women at the highest risk are those with a personal or family history of depression, previous episode of postpartum depression, low socioeconomic status, lower educational level, poor maternal health status, and other stressful life events.

INTERVENTIONS

- At every well-child visit
  - Ask the mother directly if she is feeling overwhelmed, stressed, anxious or depressed.
  - Observe maternal-child interactions.
  - Ask specific questions about coping and feeling. Do not just ask, "How are you doing?"
  - Listen. Mothers will talk about concerns, especially if they feel the provider is not judgmental.
  - Ask the mother about her resources: family members, child care, and financial.
  - Assess for other stressors: marital difficulties, substance abuse, and interpartner violence.
  - Ask specifically about a history of depression.
  - Ask about suicide ideation.
  - Assure mothers that they are not alone and that there is support if they need it.
  - Help mothers meet other mothers and learn about other community resources (e.g., support groups).
  - Encourage mothers to get help they may need to be the best mother they can be.
  - Consider using a standardized screening tool to assess the mother's symptoms.
- Screening tools include the Edinburgh Postpartum Depression Scale (EPDS).
  - Easy to use 10-item questionnaire
  - High scores predict depression
  - Good sensitivity (93% to 100%) and specificity (83% to 90%) for major depression
- Another screening tool is the U.S. Preventive Task Force Questions.
  - During the past 2 weeks, have you ever felt down, depressed, or hopeless?
  - During the past 2 weeks, have you felt little interest or pleasure in doing things.
- Other depression screening tools may be helpful (e.g., CES-D, Beck). Remember that screening tools detect symptoms but do not make a diagnosis.
- If the mother screens positive or you are in any way concerned
  - Ask the mother if she has a primary care provider of her own and obtain permission to communicate with that provider.
  - Initiate a referral to a mental health professional, support group, or other therapeutic agency with the mother's consent.
  - Obtain approval to speak with other family members who may be supportive.
  - Provide print and online resources that may be useful.
  - Let the mother know that depression is treatable.
  - Refer immediately if the mother shows severe impairment, psychosis, or suicidal or homicidal ideation.
  - Schedule frequent follow-up office visits with the mother and her child or children.

RESOURCES FOR MOTHERS

- Postpartum Support International: Organization offers support and information to those dealing with postpartum depression (http://www.postpartum.net/).
- National Women's Health Information Center. Available at http://www.4woman.gov/faq/postpartum.htm; for frequently asked questions on postpartum depression, phone: 1-800-994-9662.
- Center for Postpartum Health: Addresses the physical, mental, and emotional needs of pregnant and postpartum women and their families, facilitating the transition from pregnancy to parenthood (http://www.postpartumhealth.com/).
- Online PPD Support Group: Offers information, support, and assistance to those dealing with postpartum mood disorders,

their families, friends, physicians, and counselors (http://www.ppdsupportpage.com/).

- Postpartum Education for Parents: This organization is run by parent volunteers, and it offers services and advice for new parents (http://www.sbpep.org; phone: 1-805-564-3888).
- Henry AD et al (eds): *Parenting Well When You're Depressed: A Complete Resource for Maintaining a Healthy Family.* xxx, xxx, xxxx.

SUGGESTED READINGS

Beck Depression Inventory (BDI). Available at http://www.mindmendtherapy.com/page12_beck.html (most recent version is copyrighted).

Center for Epidemiological Studies Depression Scale (CES-D). Available at http://www.hepfi.org/nnac/pdf/sample_cesd.pdf (link to a PDF sample of the CES-D).

Chaudron L: Postpartum depression: what pediatricians need to know. *Pediatr Rev* 24:154, 2003.

GHI: Providers: Recognizing Postpartum Depression. Available at http://www.ghi.com/providers/diagnosis/ppo/pr_dia_ppo_postpart.html (link to information about postpartum depression and the Edinburgh Postpartum Depression Scale).

Goodman S, Gotlib I: *Children of Depressed Parents: Mechanisms of Risk and Implications for Treatment.* Washington, DC, American Psychological Association, 2002, p 351.

Heneghan A et al: Do pediatricians recognize mothers with depressive symptoms? *Pediatrics* 106:1367, 2000.

McLennan J, Offord D: Should postpartum depression be targeted to improve child mental health? *J Am Acad Child Adolesc Psychiatry* 41:28, 2002.

U.S. Preventive Task Force: *Screening for Depression Recommendations and Rationale.* Rockville, MD, Agency for Healthcare Research and Quality, May 2002. Available at http://ahrq.gov/clinic/3rduspstf/depressrr.htm

Weissman M et al: Remissions in maternal depression and child psychopathology (A ATAR*D-Child Report). *JAMA* 295:1389, 2006.

Wisner K et al: Postpartum depression. *N Engl J Med* 347:194, 2002.

AUTHOR: **AMY HENEGHAN, MD**

Refugee Health

DEFINITION

A *refugee* is a person, who because of "a well-founded fear of being persecuted for reasons of race, religion, nationality, membership of a particular social group, or political opinion, is outside the country of his nationality and is unable to or, owing to such fear, is unwilling to avail himself of the protection of that country. . ." (1951 Convention Relating to the Status of Refugees). Refugees come to the United States seeking protection from persecution and in search of freedom, peace, and better opportunities for their families. Although the terms *refugee* and *immigrant* are often used interchangeably, the two are fundamentally different and are treated differently under international law. When referring to refugee populations, a few terms are important. An *asylee* is similar to a refugee; it describes a foreign-born resident who cannot return to his or her country for the same reasons as a refugee. However, an asylee is not granted this status until after arriving in the United States (a refugee receives the status before entering the United States). A *parolee* is a person born outside the United States who is allowed to enter under emergency or humanitarian conditions or when entry is thought to be in the public's best interest. *Immigrants* are those who choose to move to improve their future prospects. *Refugees* must move to save their lives or protect their freedom. Refugees fleeing war or persecution are in the utmost of vulnerable situations. They have no protection from their own country, and it is often their homeland that is threatening to persecute them.

EPIDEMIOLOGY & DEMOGRAPHICS

- The United Nations High Commissioner for Refugees (UNHCR) estimates that there were 9.2 million refugees globally at the beginning of 2005.
- The number of people "of concern" to UNHCR was 19.2 million, which is approximately 1 of every 350 persons on Earth. In addition to the 9.2 million refugees (48%), this includes 839,200 asylum seekers (4%), 1.5 million recently returned refugees (8%), 5.6 million internally displaced persons (29%), and 2 million others of concern (11%).
- More than one half of the world's refugees are children.
- The United States was the fifth leading refugee hosting country in 2004, home to an estimated 421,000 refugees.
- In 2004, there were 56,000 new asylum applications submitted in the United States.

POTENTIAL CHALLENGES

- Refugee children often face difficulty in accessing health care services because of language and cultural barriers, fear of investigation regarding legal status, and economic issues.
- Refugee children often arrive with infectious diseases, and U.S.-trained pediatricians often lack sufficient knowledge for diagnosis and treatment.
- Many children from less developed countries do not have up-to-date immunizations according to U.S. standards.
- Children of refugee families have often been uprooted from their homes because of war or violence, and in the aftermath of emergencies, refugee children are left with significant psychological trauma and have critical mental health issues that need to be addressed.

INTERVENTIONS

- Before entry into the United States, all refugees undergo a mandatory overseas health screening conducted by a physician with the Intergovernmental Organization for Migration (IOM). This examination is valid for 6 months before a refugee's departure.
- The protocol for this Overseas Visa Medical Examination (OVME) includes the following:
  - Review of immunizations, although refugees are not required to comply with vaccine requirements at the time of the OVME
  - Medical history
  - Screening for mental disorders
  - Physical examination, including an examination for Hansen's disease (i.e., leprosy)
  - Chest radiograph for those older than 15 years and for those older than 2 years if a Southeast Asian refugee
  - Sputum smears for acid-fast bacilli if the chest radiograph suggests active tuberculosis (TB)
  - Test for syphilis for those older than 15 years
  - Human immunodeficiency virus (HIV) testing for those older than 15 years
- Asylum seekers are not required to have the OVME because they are already in the United States at the time of their application.
- The U.S. Public Health Service, through the Centers of Disease Control and Prevention (CDC), has 18 official ports of entry for refugees coming to the United States, and they are located at major international airports and border crossings.
- As refugees pass through one of the ports of entry, copies of the OVME are forwarded onto the Refugee Health Coordinator in the state where the refugee is destined.
- After a refugee has arrived in the United States, he or she is entitled to a comprehensive health assessment, which is done as soon as possible after arrival, but always within 90 days.
  - Although the examination is not mandatory, it is strongly encouraged.
  - The importance of the domestic examination is underscored by the fact that several months might have passed since the OVME, and the refugee might have contracted other communicable diseases in the interim period.
  - The domestic examination allows provision of health care to improve the refugee's health and provides protection of the U.S. population from imported infections.
- Each state has guidelines for screening refugees and for reimbursement of providers who perform screenings. Some states direct that screenings be performed at county health departments. For state-specific information, contact the State Refugee Health Coordinator (http://www.acf.dhhs.gov/programs/orr/partners/).
- General guidelines for screening a newly arrived refugee child include the following:
  - Medical and family history
  - Physical examination, including
    - Vision screen
    - Hearing test
    - Dental assessment
    - Assessment of developmental stage and milestones
    - Mental health assessment
  - Immunization assessment and update (see Part B Immunization and Infections Diseases and Prevention in Primary & Secondary Prevention Topics [Section V])
    - Existing immunization records should be reviewed.
    - Documented immunizations given outside of the United States are considered valid as long as the vaccine was given at the correct age and interval.
    - With no documentation, the child is considered *unvaccinated*, even if a parent claims child was vaccinated or had a vaccine-preventable illness.
    - Patients who received any live vaccines (MMR, varicella) in the preceding 4 weeks should not have a TB skin test (TBST), because tuberculin reactivity may be suppressed, leading to a false-negative result. If the TBST was done first, it is unnecessary to wait before administering live vaccines. A TBST can be administered at the same time as any vaccine, without causing reactivity suppression.
  - TB screening (see Tuberculosis in Diseases and Disorders [Section I])
    - Refugee children are at considerable risk for tuberculosis compared with American children.

- All refugee children older than 6 months of age should receive a TBST and have the result read by a trained provider within 48 to 72 hours.
- Many children from developing countries receive the Bacille Calmette-Guérin (BCG) vaccine; this is not a contraindication to a TBST.
- The vaccine is most effective at preventing serious sequelae from disseminated TB, but it does not prevent latent TB infection, which can later reactivate.
- Although the BCG vaccine may cross-react with the purified protein derivative of a TBST, reactions of more than 10 mm are more likely to be caused by latent TB infection.
- The recommendations for further evaluation and treatment of children with a positive TBST result are the same for all children, regardless of BCG vaccination status.
- Children are much more likely to have extrapulmonary TB and atypical presentations than adults.

- Hepatitis B screening
  - Hepatitis B virus (HBV) is highly endemic in many of the countries of origin from which refugees come to the United States. In highly endemic areas, most infections occur in infants and children before the fifth birthday.
  - All refugee children should be tested for HBV by obtaining serologic tests for HBsAg, anti-HBs, and anti-HBc.
  - Results may include the following: positive HBsAg: child is currently infected with HBV virus; positive anti-HBs: child is immune (has had natural disease or has been vaccinated); or positive anti-HBc: child has had natural disease. If only anti-HBc is positive, the child should be considered unprotected and should receive the vaccine series because of the possibility of isolated falsely positive anti-HBc tests.
  - The hepatitis B vaccination series may be initiated at the first visit if not already done. If serologic tests subsequently document previous immunity, HBV immunization may be discontinued. This is the most cost-effective approach.
- Screening for sexually transmitted diseases
  - Data on the need for universal HIV testing of refugees and adoptees are conflicting. All adolescents older than 15 years are tested for syphilis and HIV in the mandatory OVME before departure. However, younger children are not uniformly tested, and for individuals of all ages, some in-country HIV test results have been found to be incorrect or falsified.
  - Consider risk factors for HIV infection among children, especially those who may have acquired the disease vertically or through breastfeeding.
  - When testing for HIV, specify screening for both HIV-1 and HIV-2. This is especially important for refugees from sub-Saharan Africa, where HIV-2 is most likely to occur.
  - Use clinical judgment about retesting and about screening for other sexually transmitted diseases (STDs) after the child is in the United States. Decisions should be made on a case-by-case basis.
- Parasite screening
  - The most commonly found parasites among refugee children are *Ascaris, Trichuris, Giardia, Entamoeba,* schistosomiasis, and hookworm.
  - Ectoparasites (lice and scabies) are also common among refugee populations.
  - Have all newly arrived refugee children submit at least two (if not three) stool samples at least 24 hours apart for ova and parasite (O&P) detection (even if asymptomatic).
  - Obtain a complete blood cell count with a differential count at the first visit to evaluate for eosinophilia.
  - Children with negative stool samples but who have peripheral blood eosinophilia need to undergo further evaluation to determine the cause, because tissue-invasive and many other parasites are not excluded by negative stool O&P results.
- Lead screening: The CDC has recommended the following interim practice for screening until federal standards for testing and risk assessment among refugees is implemented:
  - A blood lead level (BLL) should be obtained for all refugee children 6 months to 16 years of age on arrival to the United States.
  - For children younger than 6 years, a BLL should be repeated 90 days after arrival, and a follow-up BLL should be done 3 to 6 months after placement into a permanent home.
  - Refugee children between the ages of 6 months and 5 years should be started on a pediatric multivitamin with iron immediately after arrival.
- Malaria screening in symptomatic children
  - Approximately 90% of all malaria cases occur in tropical Africa.
  - Worldwide, malaria is one of the top five killers for children younger than 5 years.
  - Refugee children are best screened for malaria on a case-by-case basis, taking into consideration a suspicious history, fever of unknown origin, and travel from a highly endemic region.
  - For symptomatic patients, obtain several thin blood smears for identifying malarial parasites. A single blood film may be falsely negative for malaria.

SOURCES FOR PATIENTS & PARENTS

- United Nations High Commissioner for Refugees: www.unhcr.org
- Centers for Disease Control and Prevention (CDC) has multiple sites
  - Division of Global Migration and Quarantine: www.cdc.gov/ncidod/dq/ includes specific health care recommendations for certain refugees, including Somali Bantu, Hmong, and the lost boys and girls of Sudan.
  - Division of Parasitic Diseases: www.cdc.gov/ncidod/dpd/
  - National Center for HIV, STD, and TB Prevention: www.cdc.gov/nchstp/od/
- U.S. Committee for Refugees and Immigrants: www.refugees.org
- International Organization for Migration: www.iom.int/
- The U.S. Public Health Service Advisory Committee on Immunization Practices: www.immunize.org
- The Center for Victims of Torture: www.cvt.org

SUGGESTED READINGS

Barnett ED: Infectious disease screening for refugees resettled in the United States. *Clin Infect Dis* 39:833, 2004.

Centers for Disease Control and Prevention: Lead: Fact Sheets. *Lead Exposure among Refugee Children.* Atlanta, CDC, 2005. Available at www.cdc.gov/lead/factsheets/refugeechildrenfactsheet.htm

Garg PK et al: Risk of intestinal helminth and protozoan infection in a refugee population. *Am J Trop Med Hyg* 73:386, 2005.

Minnesota Department of Health, Refugee Health Program: Minnesota Refugee Health Provider Guide. St. Paul, MN, minnesota Department of Health Refugee Health Program, 2004. Phone: 612-676-5414.

United Nations High Commissioner for Refugees, 2004 Global Refugee Trends: *Overview of Refugee Populations, New Arrivals, Durable Solutions, Asylum-Seekers, Stateless and Other Persons of Concern to UNHCR.* Geneva, Population and Geographical Data Section, Division of Operational Support, United Nations High Commissioner for Refugees, June 2005.

United Nations High Commissioner for Refugees: *Refugee Children: Guidelines on Protection and Care.* Geneva, Population and Geographical Data Section, Division of Operational Support, United Nations High Commissioner for Refugees, January 1, 1994.

AUTHOR: **ANN BUCHANAN, MD**

Smoking Cessation

RISKS & HEALTH BURDEN

- Tobacco is the leading cause of death and disease in the United States (430,00 deaths annually).
- Roughly 25% of Americans smoke.
- In 2002, 3.6 million adolescents smoked, and 28% of high school students used some form of tobacco.
- Each day, 2300 teens start smoking, and one third of these become addicted.
- Almost 90% of all adult smokers started during their teens, and 60% started before age 14.
- Most preschoolers recognize cigarettes; more than 55% think they will smoke as adults.
- Second-hand smoke (SHS) facts
  - A tobacco industry executive's (1996) response to a question about how infants could avoid SHS was, "At some point, they begin to crawl."
  - SHS contains more than 4000 compounds, 11 of which are known carcinogens.
  - SHS was classified as a group A carcinogen in 1992.
  - Between 8000 and 26,000 new cases of asthma are attributed to SHS each year.
  - Three thousand nonsmoking adults die of lung cancer each year from SHS.
  - Children exposed to SHS have higher rates of sudden infant death syndrome (SIDS), acute otitis media, asthma, respiratory infections, and caries.
  - In 82% of the cases in which a young person lives with a smoker, the smoker is a parent.

ROLE OF PEDIATRICIANS

- Pediatricians see two patients each day who will eventually die of a tobacco-related illness.
  - Pediatricians see almost 25% of all smokers through child visits; many of the parents see their child's pediatrician more than their own physicians.
  - An estimated 43% of children live in homes with a smoking parent or family member.
  - Only one third of pediatric residents counseled cessation to their patients or their families. Of these, less than one half assessed the motivation to quit, and only 16% asked parents to set a quit date.
- Only 4% of visits for well-child care and asthma and a mere 0.3% of visits for otitis media included tobacco counseling.
  - About 80% of adult and 54% of high school smokers want to quit.
  - About 46% of smokers try to quit each year, many "cold turkey," but only 5% succeed.
  - A smoker attempts to quit five to seven times before ultimately becoming successful.
  - A physician's advice to quit can increase cessation rates by up to 30%.
  - Roughly 25% of smokers who receive advice from a physician to quit will make an attempt to do so.

INTERVENTIONS

- Cessation interventions
  - The five As for brief intervention: ask, advise, assess, assist, arrange
  - The five Rs for resistance: relevance, risks, rewards, roadblocks, repetition
  - The five Ds to fight the urge: delay, drink water, do something else, deep breathe, discuss
- The five As
  - Ask (identify tobacco status at each visit)
    - 0 to 5 year olds: Ascertain potential smoke exposures (from parents or other adults).
    - 5 to 12 year olds: Ask children if they know any smokers, what their thoughts are on harms of smoking, and whether they will smoke as adults or have they already tried smoking.
    - Adolescents: Question teens on any patterns of use (e.g., weekends, sports) or smokeless tobacco use.
  - Advise (finding your own strong statement)
    - 0 to 5 year olds: Encourage maintenance of a smoke-free environment; focus on role models and the benefits of not smoking for parent and child health.
    - 5 to 12 year olds: Focus on short-term smoking side effects (e.g., smell, teeth, fingers); discuss smoking effect on sport performance; warn of the likelihood of addiction; and praise nonsmokers and parents who teach nonsmoking.
    - Adolescents: Question teens on any patterns of use (e.g., weekends, sports) or smokeless tobacco use.
  - Assess (are they willing to quit at this time)
    - All: Do parents think the child is at risk for smoking?
    - Older than 12 years: Assess the stages of change: pre-contemplation, contemplation, preparing to act, action, maintenance (helpful in establishing intermediate goals, and work in the 5 Rs if resistant to cessation).
  - Assist (where the bulk of the action is)
    - Encourage setting a quit date within 2 weeks.
    - Promote total abstinence. Tapering to 10 to 15 cigarettes per day often is harder than going cold turkey.
    - Remove cigarettes from common smoking zones (e.g., jackets, car, workplace, porch, bathroom).
    - Use pharmaceutical and counseling aides (phone, internet, support groups).
    - Provide self-help pamphlets and referrals to parents' own physicians.
    - Assisting prevention for the non-smoker—how to counter peer pressure and "just say no."
  - Arrange
    - Follow-up during the week of the quit date and again during the first month.
    - Relapse is common. It takes an average of seven attempts to successfully quit.
    - Assess why relapse occurred and what can be learned from experience to avoid relapse the next time.
    - Refer to community agencies, and use other adjuncts (e.g., over-the-counter medications, phone help lines, web sources).
- The five Rs
  - Relevance: why quitting is personally relevant
  - Risks: negative consequences of use (as identified by patient)
  - Rewards: patient-identified benefits of quitting
  - Roadblocks: barriers or impediments to quitting
  - Repetition: Repeat the five Rs at every visit and remind that many attempts often are needed before success is achieved.
- The five Ds and anticipating difficulties with cessation
  - Help prospective quitters anticipate withdrawal symptoms: irritability, headache, insomnia, drowsiness, constipation, diarrhea, and increased appetite.
    - Symptoms tend to be worse in smokers who have first cigarette within 30 minutes of waking.
    - Symptom severity usually fades over 10 minutes but can persist up to 4 weeks.
    - Tapering to 10 to 15 cigarettes per day is often harder than going cold turkey.
  - The five Ds to curb the urge
    - Delay: The urge usually passes in the first few minutes.
    - Drink water: Encourage sips of water or other low-caloric drinks to ward off the urge.

- Do something else: Have patients find an alternative activity to distract themselves from the need to light up.
- Deep breathe: Use relaxation techniques to gain control over the urges.
- Discuss: Have smokers enlist a friend with whom they can share their feelings and thoughts.

PREVENTING THE EFFECTS OF SECOND-HAND SMOKE

- Encourage smoke-free homes and smoke-free cars.
  - Although 70% of all U.S. households completely ban smoking in their homes, among households in which a smoker lives, only 46% have rules against smoking in the home.
  - Focus on all smoke exposures for children, rather than asking only if the parent smokes.
  - Ask the child if anyone smokes around her or him.
- Seek counseling.
  - There is a strong dose-response relationship between the effectiveness and intensity of tobacco-dependence counseling (i.e., minutes of contact).
  - Use problem solving and skills training (e.g., coping skills, lifestyle changes) to reduce smoking stress and identify situations likely to cause relapse.
  - Employ individual, group, telephone, or web-based counseling and social support as part of and outside treatment.
- Advocate pharmacotherapy.
  - Tobacco (not nicotine) is responsible for most adverse health effects.
  - Both nicotine and bupropion taken over long periods are safer than cigarette smoking.
  - All forms of nicotine replacement therapy (NRT) have been more effective than placebo in aiding abstinence, on average by more than 50%.
  - First-line, Food and Drug Administration (FDA)-approved options are listed in Table 5-43.

TABLE 5-43 Pharmacologic Approaches to Smoking Cessation Approved by the U.S. Food and Drug Administration

Pharmacotherapy	Pros	Side Effects	Dosage	Duration	Availability	Cost
Bupropion SR (Zyban)	Can be used with NRT Smaller degree of weight gain Easy to use	Insomnia, dry mouth, headache Contraindicated if history of seizure or eating disorder	150 mg each morning × 3 days, then 150 mg bid Start 1–2 wk before quit date	7–12 wk Maintenance up to 6 mo	Rx only Covered by Medicaid	\$3.50/day
Nicotine gum	Aids oral stimulation Can control own dose Mint, orange flavors	Dyspepsia Mouth soreness Needs to be used correctly	2-mg gum: for 1–24 cigs/day 4-mg gum: for 25+ cigs/day (max 24 pieces/day for either dose)	Up to 12 wk	OTC Covered by Medicaid	Name brand: Nicorette \$48 to \$52 for 110 pieces Store brand: \$58 for 168 pieces
Nicotine lozenge	Aids oral stimulation Can control own dose	Dyspepsia	2 mg: if first cig later than 30 min of waking 4 mg: if first cig within 30 min of waking	1 lozenge/1–2 hr (wk 1–6) 1 lozenge/2–4 hr (wk 7–8) 1 lozenge/4–8 hr (wk 10–12) Use up to 12 wk	OTC Not covered by Medicaid	Store brand or name brand (Commit): \$40 for 72 lozenges
Nicotine patch	Easy to use 1 patch/day Automatically gives right dose Helps with morning cravings	24-Hour patch may cause insomnia Skin irritation common No oral gratification	21 mg: pack+/day 14 mg: 10–15 cigs/day 7 mg: <10 cigs/day Use 1 patch/16–24 hr	8 wk	OTC Covered by Medicaid	\$30 to \$48 per 2-week supply
Nicotine inhaler	Simulates behavioral and sensory aspect of smoking Can control own dose	Contraindicated if history of severe reactive airway disease (inhaled nicotine can cause bronchospasm) May not be enough for heavy smokers Slow absorption of nicotine by mouth	10 mg/cartridge 6–16 cartridges/day for first 6–12 wk (max: 16/day) Taper dose over next 12 wk	3–6 mo	Rx only Covered by Medicaid	Name brand: Nicotrol Inhaler Menthol flavored \$125 per inhaler (168 cartridges)
Nicotine nasal spray	Fast relief (rapid rise in plasma nicotine is similar to smoking) Can control own dose	Initial nasal irritation Increased potential for prolonging nicotine dependence (compared with other NRT)	10 mg/mL 1–2 doses/hr Max 5 doses/hr or 40 doses/day	3–6 mo	Rx only Covered by Medicaid	Name brand: Nicotrol NS 10 mg/mL \$33 per bottle (200 sprays)

cigs, cigarettes; NRT, nicotine replacement therapy; OTC, over the counter; Rx, prescription.

 - Nicotine gum
 - Nicotine lozenge
 - Nicotine patch
 - Nicotine inhaler
 - Nicotine nasal spray
 - Bupropion SR (Zyban®)
- Second-line (not FDA approved) options are available.
 - Clonidine
 - Nortriptyline
- Chantix (Varenicline)
 - Newly Approved, oral tablet
 - Selective nicotinic-receptor modulator

SOURCES FOR PATIENTS & PARENTS

- Comprehensive site offers links to an extensive array of smoking-cessation sites, including quit lines, cessation guides, government and public fact sites. PowerPoint and other presentations are available for public use. The site is geared for professionals, patients, and consumers: www.kidslivesmokefree.org
- Valuable site allows teens to learn about smoking facts and watch entertaining but informative anti-smoking visuals: www.thetruth.com
- Youth-oriented site focuses on second-hand smoke issues: www.dontpassgas.org
- Site created from tobacco settlement funds is dedicated to preventing youth smoking and aiding smoking cessation: www.americanlegacy.org
- Government web sites: www.surgeongeneral.gov/tobacco and www.smokefree.gov

SUGGESTED READINGS

Centers for Disease Control and Prevention (CDC): Tobacco use, access, and exposure to tobacco in media among middle and high school students—United States, 2004. *MMWR Morb Mortal Wkly Rep* 54:297, 2005.

Fiore et al: *Clinical Practice Guideline: Treating Tobacco Use and Dependence.* Washington, DC, U.S., Department of Health and Human Services, June 2000.

Klein J: Tobacco prevention and cessation in pediatric patients. *Pediatr Rev* 25:16, 2004.

Rennard S: Overview of smoking cessation. UpToDate.

Sackey J: Behavioral approach to smoking cessation. UpToDate.

Verardo et al: *Health Care Provider's Tool Kit for Delivering Smoking Cessation Services.* Sacrament, CA, Next Generation California Tobacco Control Alliance, 2003.

AUTHOR: **ROBERT HUMPHREYS, MD** and **SUSANNE TANSKI, MD**

Index

Note: Page numbers followed by the letter f refer to figures and those followed by t refer to tables.

B

D

E

F

G

H

I

J

K

L

M

N

Q

R

S

W

X

Y

Z